The Royal Marsden Hospital Manual of Clinical Nursing Procedures

Fifth Edition

Edited by

Jane Mallett
PhD, MSc, BSc, RN
Nursing and Rehabilitation
Research and Development Manager
The Royal Marsden Hospital

and

Lisa Dougherty
MSc, RN, RM, Onc Cert
Clinical Nurse Specialist
Intravenous Services
The Royal Marsden Hospital

b
**Blackwell
Science**

© 1992, 1996, 2000 The Royal Marsden Hospital
Blackwell Science Ltd
Editorial Offices:
Osney Mead, Oxford OX2 0EL
25 John Street, London WC1N 2BS
23 Ainslie Place, Edinburgh EH3 6AJ
350 Main Street, Malden
  MA 02148 5018, USA
54 University Street, Carlton
  Victoria 3053, Australia
10, rue Casimir Delavigne
  75006 Paris, France

Other Editorial Offices:

Blackwell Wissenschafts-Verlag GmbH
Kurfürstendamm 57
10707 Berlin, Germany

Blackwell Science KK
MG Kodenmacho Building
7–10 Kodenmacho Nihombashi
Chuo-ku, Tokyo 104, Japan

Iowa State University Press
A Blackwell Science Company
2121 S. State Avenue
Ames, Iowa 50014-8300, USA

The right of the Author to be identified as the
Author of this Work has been asserted in
accordance with the Copyright, Designs and
Patents Act 1988.

First Edition published by Harper and Row Ltd 1984
Second Edition published 1988
Reprinted by HarperCollins 1990
Third Edition published by Blackwell Scientific Publications 1992
Fourth Edition published by Blackwell Science 1996
Fifth Edition published 2000
Reprinted 2001

Set in 9/10pt Goudy Old Style
by Best-Set Typesetter Ltd, Hong Kong
Printed and bound in Great Britain by
Redwood Books, Trowbridge, Wilts.

DISTRIBUTORS

Marston Book Services Ltd
PO Box 269
Abingdon
Oxon OX14 4YN
(Orders: Tel: 01235 465500
           Fax: 01235 465555)

USA
  Blackwell Science, Inc.
  Commerce Place
  350 Main Street
  Malden, MA 02148 5018
  (Orders: Tel: 800 759 6102
                   781 388 8250
             Fax: 781 388 8255)

Canada
  Login Brothers Book Company
  324 Saulteaux Crescent
  Winnipeg, Manitoba R3J 3T2
  (Orders: Tel: 204 837-2987
             Fax: 204 837-3116)

Australia
  Blackwell Science Pty Ltd
  54 University Street
  Carlton, Victoria 3053
  (Orders: Tel: 03 9347 0300
             Fax: 03 9347 5001)

A catalogue record for this title is available
from the British Library

ISBN 0-632-05235-X (pb)
ISBN 0-632-05236-8 (ringbinder)

Library of Congress
Cataloging-in-Publication Data
The Royal Marsden hospital manual of clinical nursing
procedures. – 5th ed. / edited by Jane Mallett and Lisa Dougherty.
     p. ; cm.
  Includes Bibliographical references and index.
  ISBN 0-632-05235-X (pbk: alk. paper)
  ISBN 0-632-05236-8 (ringbinder)
  Nursing – Technique – Handbooks, manuals, etc.
I. Mallett, Jane, RGN.   II. Bailey, Christopher.   III. Royal
Marsden NHS Trust.   IV. Royal Marsden NHS Trust manual
of clinical nursing procedures.
[DNLM: 1. Nursing Care – methods.   2. Nursing Process.
3. Nursing Theory.   4. Patient Care Planning.
WY 100 R986 2000]
RT42. R68 2000-06-19
610.73 – dc21

                                              00-023642

For further information on
Blackwell Science, visit our website:
www.blackwell-science.com

Contents

Quick Reference to the Guidelines

Contributors to Fifth Edition

Edited by

Jane Mallett, *PhD, MSc, BSc, RN*
Nursing and Rehabilitation Research and Development
Manager, The Royal Marsden Hospital

Lisa Dougherty, *MSc, RN, RM, Onc Cert*
Clinical Nurse Specialist Intravenous Services, The Royal
Marsden Hospital

Contributors

Amanda Baxter, *BSc, RN, RMN, Onc Cert*
Clinical Nurse Specialist Pelvic Care
                    (CHAPTERS 5, 6, 9, 27, 28, 39, 43)

Peter Blake, *MD, MBBS, BSc, FRCR*
Head of Radiotherapy Services   (CHAPTER 33)

Susan Broom, *RN*
Sister Day Surgery Unit   (CHAPTER 30)

Siobhan Carroll, *RN, BSc, Onc Cert*
formerly CNS Breast Care Services   (CHAPTERS 1, 38)

Anne Chandler, *BSc, RN, Onc Cert*
Pain Management Research Nurse   (CHAPTER 29)

Jill Cooper, *DipCOT, SROT*
Head Occupational Therapist   (CHAPTERS 11, 47)

Shelley Dolan, *MSc, BA, RN, ENB 100, ENB ITU, Onc
Cert*
Nurse Consultant, Critical Care
                    (CHAPTERS 8, 15, 28, 31, 35, 44)

Lisa Dougherty, *MSc, RN, RM, Onc Cert*
Clinical Nurse Specialist Intravenous Services
                    (CHAPTERS 10, 12, 20, 36, 44, 45)

Elizabeth Doyle, *BSc, RN, DN, Onc Cert*
Clinical Nurse Specialist Community Liaison
                    (CHAPTERS 11, 15)

Nicola Gale, *BSc, RN, Onc Cert*
Ward Sister, Pinkham Day Unit   (CHAPTER 28)

Jag Grewal, *BA, RN, ENB 188, A 13*
Teaching Sister, Operating Theatres   (CHAPTER 30)

Douglas Guerrero, *MSc, BSc, RN, DN, Onc Cert, COD
Cert, Counselling Cert*
Clinical Nurse Specialist Neuro-Oncology
                    (CHAPTERS 23, 26, 38, 42)

Sarah Hart, *MSc, BSc, RN, FETC, Onc Cert, Infect Cont
Cert*
Clinical Nurse Specialist Infection Control and Radiation
Protection   (CHAPTERS 3, 4, 18, 27, 33, 34, 37)

Sonja Hoy, *BSc, RN, Onc Cert, PGC Man Health Services,
HIV/AIDS Cert*
formerly Ward Sister, Miles Ward   (CHAPTER 41)

Margaret James, *RN, Paed Onc Cert, ENB N10*
Sister Nuclear Medicine   (CHAPTER 34)

Fiona Kinnaird, *BSc, RN, Onc Cert*
formerly Sister Nuclear Medicine   (CHAPTER 34)

Diana Laverty, *BSc, RN, Onc Cert*
Clinical Nurse Specialist Palliative Care
                    (CHAPTERS 15, 20, 29, 32, 42, 47)

Nicholas Lodge, *MSc, BSc, RN, EN(G), Onc Cert*
Clinical Group Research Nurse Gynaecology
                    (CHAPTER 33)

Jane Machin, *BA, Dip CCS, Reg MCSLT, DALF*
Senior Oncology Speech and Language Therapist
                    (CHAPTER 40)

Elizabeth MacKenzie, *BSc, RN, Onc Cert, ENB 100*
Ward Sister High Dependency Unit (CHAPTERS 21, 35)

Jane Mallett, *PhD, MSc, BSc, RN*
Research and Practice Development Manager
                    (CHAPTER 12)

Rachel Mead, *BSc, RN, Dip Onc*
Acting Clinical Nurse Specialist, Breast Care Services
                    (CHAPTER 38)

Amene Mir, *PhD, BA*
Chaplain   (CHAPTER 22)

Wayne Naylor, *RN, BSc, Dip Nurs, Onc Cert*
Wound Management Research Nurse   (CHAPTER 17)

Sinead Parry, *BSc, RN, DN*
Clinical Nurse Specialist Community Liaison
                    (CHAPTER 11)

Emma Pennery, *MSc, RN, ENB A11, ENB 931,
Counselling Cert*
Lecturer Practitioner Cancer Care   (CHAPTERS 1, 7)

Helen Jayne Porter, *MSc, RN, Onc Cert*
formerly Clinical Nurse Specialist High Dose
Chemotherapy   (CHAPTERS 19, 24)

Jane Power, *BSc, SRD*
formerly Senior Dietitian (CHAPTER 27)

Joanne Preece, *DMS, BSc, MIOSH, RSP*
Health and Safety Adviser (CHAPTER 18)

Frances Rhys-Evans, *MSc, RN, Onc Cert, ENB 100*
formerly Clinical Nurse Specialist/Ward Manager Head &
Neck and Thyroid Cancer (CHAPTERS 17, 24)

Tim Root, *BSc, MRPharmS*
Chief Pharmacist (CHAPTER 12)

Mave Salter, *MSc, BSc, RN, DN Cert, Cert Ed, Onc Cert,
ENB 216, Dip Counselling*
Clinical Nurse Specialist Community Liaison
(CHAPTERS 11, 39)

Kate Scott, *BSc, RN, RMN, Onc Cert, Counselling Cert*
Clinical Nurse Specialist Psychological Care
(CHAPTER 46)

Katie Sharma, *BA, RN, OHNC, MIOSH*
formerly Back Care Adviser (CHAPTER 25)

Clare Shaw, *BSc, SRD*
Chief Dietitian (CHAPTER 27)

Ramani Sitamvaram, *BSc, RN, Onc Cert*
Clinical Nurse Specialist Gastro-Intestinal Cancer
(CHAPTER 2)

Jane Skelley, *RN, Onc Cert*
Staff Nurse, Wiltshaw Ward (CHAPTER 10)

Caroline Soady, *BSc, RN*
Clinical Nurse Specialist Head, Neck and Thyroid
(CHAPTERS 13, 27, 40, 47)

Val Speechley, *MA, RN, RCNT, Onc Cert*
Patient Information Officer (CHAPTER 1)

Moira Stephens, *DPSN, RN, Onc Cert, ENB 934*
Clinical Nurse Specialist High Dose Chemotherapy
(CHAPTER 23)

Mavis Stork, *BSc, RN, RM*
formerly Theatre Services Manager (CHAPTER 30)

Karen Summerville, *RN, DN, Onc Cert, Gynae Cert,
Stoma Care Cert*
formerly Clinical Nurse Specialist, Pelvic Cancer
(CHAPTER 2)

Sara Travis, *BSc, RN, Onc Cert, Counselling Cert*
Clinical Nurse Specialist Palliative Care
(CHAPTERS 11, 14, 15, 22)

Christine Viner, *MSc, RN, FETC, Onc Cert*
Clinical Nurse Specialist Ambulatory Chemotherapy
(CHAPTER 20)

Mary Woods, *BSc, RN, Onc Cert*
Senior Clinical Nurse Specialist Lymphoedema Services
(CHAPTER 16)

Contributors to Previous Editions

First Edition edited by
A. Phylip Pritchard
Research Assistant, Department of Nursing Research

Valerie-Anne Walker
Research Assistant, Department of Nursing Research

Second Edition edited by
A. Phylip Pritchard
Assistant to the Director of In-Patient Services/Chief
Nursing Officer

Jill A. David
Director of Nursing Research

Third Edition edited by
A. Phylip Pritchard
Formerly Co-ordinator of European Educational
Initiatives, The Royal Marsden Hospital
and
Executive Secretary, European Oncology Nursing Society

Jane Mallett
Research and Practice Development Co-ordinator

Fourth Edition edited by

Jane Mallett
Research and Practice Development Manager

Christopher Bailey
Macmillan Research Practitioner, Macmillan Practice
Development Unit, Centre for Cancer and Palliative Care
Studies, Institute of Cancer Research

Contributors
Caroline Badger, formerly Senior Nurse (Lymphoedema)

Christopher Bailey, Macmillan Research Practitioner,
Institute of Cancer Research

Sophie Baty, Sister (Recovery Theatre)

Amanda Baxter, Clinical Nurse Specialist (Pelvic Cancer)

Chris Berry, formerly Back Care Advisor

Peter Blake, Consultant Clinical Oncologist

Judith Bibbings, formerly Sister (Gastro-intestinal/Genito-
urinary)

Yannette Booth, formerly Lecturer in Cancer Nursing

Derryn Borley, formerly Assistant Director of Nursing
Services

Monica Burchall, formerly Sister (High Dependency)

Nancy Burnett, Senior Nurse Manager

Antoinette Byrne, formerly Dietitian

Jill Carter, formerly Clinical Nurse Specialist (Palliative
Care)

Patrick Casey, formerly Clinical Nurse Specialist/Unit
Manager (Gastro-intestinal/Genito-urinary)

Gay Curling, Clinical Nurse Specialist (Breast Diagnostic
Unit)

Lisa Curtis, formerly Macmillan Lecturer, Institute of
Cancer Research

Tonia Dawson, Clinical Nurse Specialist (Pelvic Cancer)

Barbara Dicks, Director of Patient Services/Chief Nursing
Officer

Emma Dilnutt, formerly Clinical Nurse Specialist
(Palliative Care)

Anne Doherty, formerly Staff Nurse (Operating Theatres)

Shelly Dolan, Clinical Nurse Specialist (High
Dependency and Critical Care)

Lisa Dougherty, Clinical Nurse Specialist/Manager
(Intravenous Services)

Nuala Durkin, formerly Clinical Nurse Specialist/Unit
Manager (High Dependency)

Jean Edwards, Senior Nurse Manager/Private Patient Co-
ordinator

Sarah Faithfull, CRC Nursing Fellow, Institute of Cancer
Research

Deborah Fenlon, formerly Group Clinical Nurse Specialist
(Breast Care Services)

Jacqueline Green, Senior Dietitian

Douglas Guerrero, Clinical Nurse Specialist/Ward
Manager (Rehabilitation and Neuro-oncology)

Rachel Hair, formerly Senior Nurse (Neuro-oncology)

Sarah Hart, Clinical Nurse Specialist (Infection
Control/Radiation Protection)

Cathryn Havard, formerly Senior Nurse (Gastro-
intestinal/Genito-urinary)

Pauline Hill, Clinical Nurse Specialist (Community Liaison)

Sian Horn, formerly Sister (High Dependency)

Elizabeth Houlton, formerly Senior Nurse (Community Liaison/Self-Care Unit)

Nest Howells, formerly Information Officer, CancerLink

Jennifer Hunt, Director, Nursing Research Initiative for Scotland

Maureen Hunter, Rehabilitation Services Manager

Lorraine Hyde, Sister (Intravenous Services)

Elizabeth Janes, formerly Dietitian

Penelope A. Jones, formerly Clinical Nurse Specialist (Community Liaison/Palliative Care)

Margareta Johnstone, formerly Clinical Nurse Specialist (High Dependency Unit)

Danny Kelly, formerly Lecturer in Cancer Nursing, Institute of Cancer Research

Diane Laverty, Clinical Nurse Specialist (Palliative Care)

Annie Leggett, formerly Clinical Nurse Specialist (Intravenous Therapy)

Anne Lister, formerly Clinical Nurse Specialist/Unit Manager (Palliative Care)

Nicholas Lodge, Clinical Group Research Nurse (Gynaecology)

E. Lopez-Verdugo, Senior Technician/Theatre Manager

Jane Mallett, Research and Practice Development Manager

Jane Machin, Senior Oncology Speech and Language Therapist

Glynis Markham, formerly Director of Nursing Services

Elizabeth MacKenzie, Manager (High Dependency Unit)

Catherine Miller, formerly Senior Nurse (Continuing Care)

Marion Morgan, formerly Research Sister (Gynaecology)

Katrina Neal, formerly Clinical Nurse Specialist/Unit Manager (Palliative Care)

Helen Jayne Porter, formerly Clinical Nurse Specialist (High Dose Chemotherapy)

Judith Pretty, formerly Clinical Nurse Specialist (Head and Neck)

Frances Rhys-Evans, formerly Clinical Nurse Specialist/Ward Manager (Head & Neck and Thyroid Cancer)

Helen Roberts, formerly Senior Nurse (Head and Neck)

Tim Root, Chief Pharmacist

Ray Rowden, formerly Director of Nursing Services

Miriam Rushton, formerly Senior Nurse (Gynaecology)

Lena Salter, formerly Patient Services Manager

Mave Salter, Clinical Nurse Specialist (Community Liaison)

Kate Scott, Clinical Nurse Specialist/Lecturer/Practitioner (Psychological Care)

Clare Shaw, Chief Dietitian

Val Speechley, Patient Information Officer

James Smith, formerly Chaplain

Mavis Stork, formerly Theatre Services Manager

June Toovey, formerly Sister (Intravenous Therapy Team)

Anne Topping, formerly Senior Nurse (Gastro-intestinal/Genito-urinary)

Jennie Treleaven, Consultant Haematologist

Robert Tunmore, formerly Clinical Nurse Specialist (Psychological Support)

Beverley van der Molen, formerly Clinical Nurse Specialist/Unit Manager (General Oncology)

Richard Wells, formerly Rehabilitation Services Manager

Isabel White, Head of Undergraduate Cancer Care Studies

Jane Wilson, formerly Group Theatre Manager

Mary Woods, Clinical Nurse Specialist (Lymphoedema Services)

Miriam Wood, formerly Ward Manager (Breast Care Services)

Karen Wright, formerly Research Assistant, Nursing Research Unit

Karen Young, formerly Physiological Measurement Technician

Foreword to Fifth Edition

The essence of nursing at The Royal Marsden Hospital is the relationship between the nurse, the patient and their loved ones, and the way in which they form a true partnership to negotiate care. However, it is against this, perhaps philosophical, backdrop that there is an emerging interest throughout the UK in ensuring that the fundamentals of nursing practice, such as expertise in carrying out clinical procedures, are given high priority.

This, the Fifth Edition, of *The Royal Marsden Hospital Manual of Clinical Nursing Procedures* has been published at an ideal time. Health care providers and government health bodies in the UK, Europe and beyond are focussing their energies on evidence-based practice and there is a pressing need for nurses to have quick and easy access to the most up-to-date information on clinical procedures. In the UK, evidence-based practice is a key component of Clinical Governance, which is our consistent and methodical approach to ensuring that patient care is of the highest possible quality. Indeed, evidence-based practice is also at the core of many of the other aspects of Clinical Governance including risk management, continuing professional development and clinical effectiveness.

In 1999, The Royal Marsden Hospital Strategy for Nursing was published. In that document we made a commitment to sharing good practice locally, nationally and internationally. The publication of *The Royal Marsden Hospital Manual of Clinical Nursing Procedures* is not only a practical demonstration of that commitment, but also clearly highlights our quest to constantly improve our own clinical practice.

This edition is the product of an enormous amount of effort by nurses throughout The Royal Marsden Hospital, especially Jane Mallett and Lisa Dougherty. As always, it is with great pride, that I am able to support their work.

Dickon Weir-Hughes
Chief Nurse / Director of Quality Assurance
The Royal Marsden Hospital (London & Surrey)

Foreword to Third Edition

Once again it is my great pleasure to write the foreword to *The Royal Marsden Hospital Manual of Clinical Nursing Procedures*.

This, the third edition, represents a continuation of a successful tradition which dates back to its first publication in 1984. Since that time the nursing profession has developed its scientific and professional base, and the third edition of the manual has sought to reflect this development. A number of new chapters have been added including the Management of Chronic Oedema and Arterial Lines. Other chapters have been thoroughly revised to incorporate up-to-date information and research findings on which a firm base for clinical practice can be founded. As we have emphasized previously, the comments and suggestions of those who use the manual are invaluable in guiding us towards ever improved future editions. We will endeavour to incorporate them into the fourth edition as it begins to take shape.

Robert Tiffany, OBE
Director of Patient Services/Chief Nursing Officer

Foreword to Fourth Edition

It is with great pleasure that I write the foreword to this, the fourth edition of *The Royal Marsden NHS Trust Manual of Clinical Nursing Procedures*.

Since the first publication in 1984 not only have we seen the advent of the 'health market', but also significant changes have occurred in the form of nursing's contribution to the organization of health care. Possibly one of the most notable changes is the growth of nurse-led care where nurses in community, and hospital inpatient and outpatient settings have shown beyond a doubt that skilled nursing practice does not merely make economic sense, but can make a unique contribution to the way patients experience disease.

Proofs of the manual's success has to lie in its widespread use, and every effort has been made to ensure that this fourth edition is an improvement on its forerunners. New and revised chapters will, we trust, guarantee its continued popularity as nursing rises to the challenges which the new millennium will inevitably bring.

Barbara Dicks
Director of Patient Services/Chief Nursing Officer

Acknowledgements

The Royal Marsden Hospital Manual of Clinical Nursing Procedures is the outcome of constant review and refinement to produce Guidelines for the best evidence-based practice. Therefore, production of the Manual involved much more than simply writing chapters but a complete appraisal of research literature, national and local guidelines and audit results, etc., as well as utilizing a wealth of experience with regard to patient care. This is only possible through the expertise and commitment of many professionals at The Royal Marsden Hospital, some of whom are contributing for the first time, while others have been involved since the first edition in 1984. The text reflects contributors' beliefs concerning the continuing development of excellence in patient care. In this was each chapters represents not only the theory underpinning practice, but also quality in care, and the perceptions and ideals of professionals who are specialists in their fields. We extend our many thanks to our contributors for providing evidence-based text and procedures that guide best practice and further develop and expand on work on previous editions.

Thanks must also go to Phylip Pritchard, (formerly Co-ordinator of European Educational Initiatives, The Royal Marsden Hospital) editor of the first, second and third editions, to whose very special talents this work is a continuing tribute. Others that have also led the development of the Manual from its initial conception to the work it is today. Therefore thanks must go to Jennifer Hunt (formerly Director of Nursing Studies, The Royal Marsden Hospital), who collected and collated the hospital's procedures, to Valerie-Anne Walker (formerly Research Assistant, The Royal Marsden Hospital) and Jill David (formerly Director of Nursing Research, The Royal Marsden Hospital) who were joint editors of, and contributors to, the second and third editions, and to the many health care professionals who have contributed over the years. However, without the vision to support this project from its conception to realization *The Royal Marsden Hospital Manual of Clinical Nursing Procedures* would not be at the leading edge of practice today and for this our gratitude must go to Mr Robert Tiffany who was the Director of Patient Services and Chief Nursing Officer during its early development.

In an effort to strive for excellence this book is reviewed by external referees who are expert in the relevant areas and we are greatly indebted to these reviewers who have remained anonymous, for their constructive, critical and helpful comments.

Finally, our thanks go to Griselda Campbell, Julie Musk and Gill Mullin at Blackwell Science for their advice and support in all aspects of the publishing process.

Jane Mallett
Lisa Dougherty

The Royal Marsden Hospital Strategy for Nursing: Principles of Person-Focussed Care

As nurses we believe that:

1 People affected by cancer, that is patients, families and friends, should be cared for with respect and as individuals, with nursing care being negotiated, planned and implemented in response to their physical, emotional, psychosocial, cultural and spiritual needs.
2 The wellness and quality of life of the person affected by cancer is of paramount concern when planning and delivering nursing care.
3 The affects of cultural and societal influences on the needs of a person affected by cancer should be recognized and accommodated.

Nurses at The Royal Marsden Hospital will pursue clinical excellence in cancer care through:

1 Collaborative, evidence-based care and the dissemination of nursing knowledge and good practice.

2 Promotion of a safe environment via clinical governance strategies.
3 Evaluation of clinical effectiveness through review of nursing interventions and organization of care.
4 Utilization of specialist nursing knowledge, skills and understanding.
5 Commitment of life-long learning and nursing education, professional development and clinical supervision.
6 Promotion of leadership skills.
7 Development of enhanced communication networks and nursing information systems.
8 Provision of support for nurses.

Introduction

The concept of clinical governance is to improve the quality of patient care. In nursing this is underpinned by evidence-based knowledge and practice, and through research. *The Royal Marsden Hospital Manual of Clinical Nursing Procedures* utilizes this approach as a foundation for procedures in both the hospital and community setting. The Manual is also a resource for nurses starting out on their training as well as a comprehensive reference work for those with more extensive experience.

The Fifth Edition of this text builds upon previous work. New chapters have been included and others have been expanded to encompass current aspects and recent developments in patient care. In addition, to improve clarity and accessibility there has been some reorganization of chapters. New chapters include Spinal Cord Compression Management (Chapter 38) and Gene Therapy for the Management of Cancer (Chapter 18). The latter is a rapidly growing modality of treatment, which has particular implications for patient care due to the hazards of handling, and administration of, this innovative therapy. Pain Assessment and Management (Chapter 29) has been expanded to incorporate the management of both acute and chronic pain using pharmacological and complementary therapies, thus maintain, the procedures within a holistic framework. Haematological Procedures: Specialist, Diagnostic and Therapeutic (Chapter 19) now encompasses bone marrow and peripheral stem cell diagnostic and harvesting procedures and replaces the chapter on bone marrow. Infusion Devices (Chapter 20) highlights not only the range of devises utilized in infusion therapies but also the MDA classification and requirements for training and maintenance. Finally, three former chapters (Arterial Lines, IV Management and Central Venous Catheterization) have been collated more logically to create one chapter entitled Vascular Access Devices: Insertion and Management (Chapter 44). This also includes procedures for cannulation and midline and PICC insertion which are now commonly performed by nurses and illustrate one aspect of nurses' roles in advancing practice. All other procedures have been reviewed, chapters updated and many have been extensively revised.

This edition aims to continue the high standards that were provided by the work of the previous four editions, and to contribute to the continuing development of a conceptual framework for nursing care. The format remains substantially unchanged. Every procedure has two sections: (1) reference material and (2) guidelines. Some procedures also have a third section devoted to nursing care plans.

Reference material

The reference material section consists of a review of the literature and other relevant material. Whenever possible, research findings have been utilized. A list of references and further reading is included at the end to indicate the source of the information and to assist the reader to follow up the topic if more detail is required Where no research evidence has been available the procedures have been based on extensive experience and systematic review.

Guidelines

The guidelines section provides a list of the equipment needed, followed by a detailed step-by-step account of the procedure and the rationale for the proposed action.

Nursing care plan

The nursing care plan section gives a list of the problems that may occur, their possible causes and suggestions for their resolution and prevention. Items from this sheet can be used on the patient's own nursing care plan.

Procedures have been arranged in alphabetical order although some have been group together, for example the procedures on blood pressure, respiration, temperature, urinalysis, ECGs and now glucose monitoring will be found under the general heading of Observations (Chapter 28).

All relevant procedures begin with the action 'Explain and discuss the procedure with the patient', the rationale for this being 'to ensure that the patient understands the procedure and gives his/her valid consent'. This is intended to reflect a patient-focussed approach to obtaining appropriate consent and is addressed in more depth in Chapter 1.

This book is intended as a reference and guide to quality care and not as a replacement for education. None of the procedures in this book, from the most basic to the most technical, should be undertaken without appropriate instruction and supervision.

We hope that *The Royal Marsden Hospital Manual of Clinical Nursing Procedures* will continue to stimulate further debate. To this end the editors welcome the opportunity to respond to specific points from readers.

Lisa Dougherty
Jane Mallett

Care in Context: Assessment, Communication and Consent

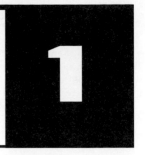

Introduction

Nursing practice encompasses a process of judgement which facilitates identification and assessment of patients' potential needs and expectations in order that they may be adequately and appropriately addressed before, during and after any episode of nursing care. Crucial to the delivery of high quality nursing intervention is the notion of assessment; thus the first section of this chapter explores the knowledge and skills required to assess the needs of individuals with particular reference to cancer nursing practice.

The second section of this chapter highlights communication skills, which may be useful in allowing patients to express their needs during the experience of illness and the importance of regarding patients as individuals with unique expectations and problems.

The third section focuses on issues surrounding valid consent in the context of consent to examination and treatment. The overall aims of this chapter are to foster an awareness of an individualized approach to nursing care of the person with cancer and their families and friends. The procedures outlined in this book, therefore, should be seen as part of a larger picture, which encompasses an appreciation of the unique experience of illness.

Assessment

Approaching patient assessment

A conceptual nursing model is designed as a set of concepts and statements that integrate them into a meaningful configuration (Fawcett 1995). Different conceptual models have emerged over time, implying that there is a perceived value in the coexistence of a variety of perspectives.

Assessment strategies and terminology are adopted from the model in question. For example, Peplau (1992) defines 'Orientation' as the phase where the patient and/or family has a perceived need, which is directly affected by the patient's and nurse's attitudes about giving or receiving aid. The expression of needs, in this model, is dependent on the therapeutic relationship developed between patient and nurse.

Nursing models may be adapted to a suitable area of care. For example, the concept of self-care, espoused by Orem (1991) may be particularly suited to the area of cancer rehabilitation, but not for areas where patients are most dependent, such as critical care. Nursing models

provide a framework to the process of assessment, enabling appropriate interventions and achievement of outcomes. In summary they guide the overall process of care.

It is vital that nurses are aware of the rationale for choosing to implement a particular nursing model for their area of practice, because this choice will largely determine the nature of patient assessment in their day-to-day work. If the model is inappropriate, it may well follow that the assessment data collected are less effective than they could be (Tierney 1998).

Many studies emphasize the importance of effective, two-way communication in cancer nursing (Wilkinson 1992; Jarrett & Payne 1995; Larsson et al. 1998), and that staff should be trained in the field of therapeutic communication, to ask patients and their families specific questions about their perceptions (Wilkinson 1995). Collecting information and offering explanations was seen in one study of nursing care as one of the most frequent forms of nurse behaviour in contact with patients expressing their worries. However, clarification and reflection of the feelings of the patient, which deepen the understanding of the problem and help in the expression of hidden emotions and the integration of them with other aspects of their experience occurred rarely (Motyka et al. 1997). Larsson et al. (1998, p. 863) summarize the approach to assessment in cancer care succinctly by stating that: 'Even though various tools facilitate the communication with the patient, the use of assessment tools alone is not sufficient to capture the whole spectrum of patient perceptions concerning their care'.

The planned assessment interview, which often takes place when a patient is admitted, is an opportunity to collect detailed, specific information, in order that the most effective interventions can be offered. Patients and their families often see this planned interaction as a time to obtain clear answers to questions about their illness and treatment. The assessment interview allows the nurse–patient relationship to be established on the basis of mutual concern for the patient's well-being. However, there must be structure to the interview. It has a beginning and ending, and should progress logically, ensuring meaning to the participants. There is a difference between being document/form focused and patient focused, while both are essential prerequisites to an assessment. The venue for this meeting, if possible, must be chosen with care with the criteria of privacy and preservation of dignity paramount. In an attempt to emphasize the importance of good communication in the nurse's repertoire of assessment skills (which will be discussed in more detail in the next section) it is all too easy to forget the need to be equally effective in observation (Kemp & Richardson 1994). Clinical observation means using all the senses to gain information which may not be available in any other way and which, if not considered, may result in some serious omission in the achievement of an accurate picture of the patient's condition.

It may also be the case that the information gathered is incomplete, either because the patient was not well enough to continue the interview or because it was inappropriate to examine certain physical and psychological aspects of the patient's problems at the time. The nurse has a responsibility to ensure that this fact does not go unrecognized and a mechanism is in place to ensure that the document is duly completed. The patient also needs to be assured of the use to which the data will be put (Kemp & Richardson 1994).

There may be times when it is not possible to obtain vital information from the patient directly; they may be unconscious or unable to speak clearly, if at all. In such situations, the appropriate details will have to be obtained from relatives or friends. Note should be made in the record of the name and relationship of the person who gave the information, as conflicting information may be given by different individuals.

The first interview enables the nurse to obtain a baseline of information against which new and changing information can be compared. It facilitates thinking and planning ahead, and consideration of the patient's likely outcome of care, for example problems on discharge. Some problems may not be disclosed by the patient and may only be identified when the nurse and patient relationship develops and the patient trusts the nurse.

Functions of assessment

The functions of nursing assessment can be summarized as follows:

1 To ascertain patient, family and friends' needs and potential needs
2 To provide information on which to plan interventions and thus to achieve appropriate outcomes
3 To document and record the relevant areas assessed, to act as a baseline for reassessment and evaluation of care given
4 To act as an instrument for the safety, continuity and quality of patient care
5 To facilitate the structuring of knowledge for nursing practice, as well as for teaching and research
6 To fulfil legal and professional obligation.

(Heartfield 1996; Allen 1998.)

Assessment and nursing diagnosis

Assessment can appropriately be regarded as part of diagnosis. All nurses go through a process of problem identification; gathering information during their assessment of a patient and then looking for suitable terminology to describe that information (Heath 1998). Nursing diagnoses

are a way of communicating such information and many nursing establishments in Britain are considering incorporating this concept into nursing care (Hardwick 1998). The North American Nursing Diagnosis Association (NANDA) defines nursing diagnosis as a clinical judgement about patients' responses to actual or potential health problems. A nursing diagnosis provides the basis for selection of nursing interventions to achieve outcomes for which the nurse is accountable (Carpenito 1993). A standardized language such as the nursing diagnosis classification system provides nurses with a common language for communicating the nursing needs of patients. The North American definition of nursing diagnosis refers to clinical judgement, which Katoaka-Yahirom & Saylor (1995) suggest is related to problem solving in nursing and is composed of critical thinking, a specific knowledge base, experience, competencies, attitudes and standards. Through using thorough assessment skills to identify patient problems, nurses are more likely to conclude a nursing diagnosis with which to drive planned nursing interventions (Katoaka-Yahirom & Saylor 1995). It appears that the formulation of nursing interventions is dependent on adequate information collection and clinical judgement in patient assessment in order that specific patient outcomes may be derived and appropriate nursing interventions are undertaken to assist the patient to achieve those outcomes (Hardwick 1998).

Nursing in Great Britain, based on the nursing process and models of nursing care, endeavours to include all these components within nursing care. As yet, in Great Britain the term nursing diagnosis is not highly visible to nurses as part of the nursing process, as no definitive classification (or taxonomy) of nursing diagnosis is in general use. There is a profusion of literature concerning nursing diagnosis from a North American perspective, but very little published literature originating in the UK (Hardwick 1998).

Confusion exists in the UK due to the interchangeable use of the terms 'nursing diagnosis' and 'nursing problems' and cultural and logistic differences between North America and the UK (Hogston 1997). The use of 'patient problems or needs', Hogston (1997) asserts, is also a common language used within nursing to facilitate communication within nursing and nursing care. As patient problems/needs may involve solutions or treatments from disciplines other than nursing, the concept of 'patient problem' is similar to but broader than nursing diagnosis. Nursing diagnosis is purely concerned with problems that may be dealt with by nursing expertise (Leih & Salentijn 1994; Table 1.1).

Table 1.1 Characteristics of conditions labelled as nursing diagnoses (Gordon 1994)

---

1 Nurses can identify the condition through a process of diagnostic reasoning (assessment, problem identification).
2 The condition can be resolved primarily by nursing interventions.
3 Nurses assume accountability for patient/outcomes.
4 Nurses assume responsibility for research on the condition and its treatment.

Nursing diagnoses or problems/needs identification are made after sufficient data become available. Nursing assessment includes gathering, validating and organizing data, identifying patterns and reporting and recording relevant data (Alfaro-Lefevre 1994). Careful judgement is required about a cluster of signs and symptoms before diagnosis or problem/need identification. Assessment that gets at the deeper meaning of superficial cues and includes the meanings attributed to events by the patient/client is associated with greater diagnostic accuracy and thus more effective intervention (Gordon 1994).

The endeavour in assessment should be to focus on the patients' perception of their functioning in the activities of daily life and on the relevance for patient care (Ehrenberg et al. 1996). This view is supported by Lauri et al. (1997), who investigated nurses' and patients' views of patients' needs in hospital. They found that the most significant differences between nurses' and patients' views occurred in the area of reactions to functional health status, with regard to feelings of despair and powerlessness, changes in outer appearance and non-involvement in decision-making.

However, in order to obtain a good understanding of the patient's situation, it is necessary to analyse each problem (for nursing relevance) and need in context, where possible, together with the patient and/or significant other persons (Ehrenberg et al. 1996).

Whether nursing diagnosis and/or problem/need identification is used in practice, the assessment document/computer program available should reflect the language in use for clarification and communication. Furthermore, it is essential that assessment documentation is sensitive to the facets of a particular client group, in this case people affected by cancer, their families and friends. The assessor should possess knowledge and some understanding of the particular client group and the treatments that they are undergoing, so that diagnostic reasoning and critical thinking skills are enhanced (O'Neill & Dluhy 1997). It is incumbent on nurse managers to provide education about the assessment process/documentation in use, to endorse overall standards of care. The nurse also has a responsibility to be aware of any new developments in the assessment process/documentation tool in use.

Assessment in cancer nursing practice

Assessing the needs and potential needs of people affected by cancer (that is patient, family and friends), is a dynamic activity based on a professional model of practice in which a qualified professional is responsible and accountable for a caseload of patients for the duration of their care (Hunter 1998). This is an ongoing and a central component of everyday care which nurses achieve by using skills of observation and communication, and by applying relevant theoretical knowledge (O'Neill & Dluhy 1997).

Assessment in cancer care has a number of attributes as follows:

1 It should be concerned with quality and quantity of life; it is a dimension of care and potential survival.

2 Assessment is governed by the notion of patients' needs and potential needs and those of the family and friends and should adopt a holistic approach.
3 It should be concerned with optimal functioning and the promotion of independence.
4 It should be a dynamic process, characterized by individualized care, which is relevant at any stage in the disease and should start ideally at diagnosis or before.
5 It should be a process in which the patient ideally plays an active role.
6 It must be patient focused and multidisciplinary.
7 Cancer is a family issue and this is reflected in the assessment strategy.
8 Assessment techniques and documentation vary according to setting; day care, outpatient, inpatient; short or long stay; critical care or rehabilitative. Shortened inpatient stays and admission guidelines have markedly increased the number of outpatient and day care patients (Smith & Richardson 1996). However, underlying principles and patient focused techniques remain the same.

In the acute phase of cancer care, it has been demonstrated that certain changes in function are common, whether physical, psychosocial or spiritual. In this acute phase, accurate assessment enables appropriate and therapeutic interventions to achieve outcomes (Smith & Richardson 1996; Burton & Watson 1998; Larsson et al. 1998).

Cancer is a chronic illness for many people, more patients are living with cancer for longer. The assessment process and interventions here aim ideally to move patients out of the sick role and into effective day-to-day self-management of their illness (Davies et al. 1997; Hunter 1998).

With the goal of optimal functioning, any health care professional involved in patient care will play a part in assessment. Although, in practice, any or all of the health-care professionals involved could carry out an initial assessment, in most cases this responsibility lies with the nurse (Hunter 1998). The assessment is a time-consuming process, but it must be remembered that a comprehensive and effective initial assessment will mean that patient needs are identified at the earliest possible opportunity and that appropriate intervention is timely. Referral can then be made to specialist nurses, therapists or other professionals as appropriate, in order to continue the assessment process in more depth (Hunter 1998).

Assessment is often described as having physical, psychological, emotional, spiritual, social and cultural dimensions. In reality, however, it may not be possible to make clear distinctions between dimensions, when caring for an individual patient (Jenner 1998). Problems or needs identified in one domain may have direct effects on other domains. For example, a patient with breast cancer, having chemotherapy, reports to the nurse that they are experiencing nausea and vomiting, with each course of chemotherapy. Anxiety, fatigue and consequential anorexia and poor nutritional intake are also complications of this side-effect. The patient is concerned about not being able to care for her young daughter adequately due to the physical effects of treatment. She may consider not having any more treatment. Careful assessment of the patient's needs requires a holistic approach to identify the interrelated components of these complications/side-effects, to maximize any appropriate interventions and to minimize the risks of psychological morbidity. In this way, the acceptability of the treatment plan and the patient's quality of life are improved. It may therefore be more useful to view assessment as a holistic process with particular aspects demanding more focus on specific occasions. Assessing people with cancer requires skills which allow the nurse to enable the patient to 'tell their story' and their concerns so that the most appropriate interventions can be planned.

Documentation and assessment

Formal checklists and documents are available to guide nursing assessment. They can be useful for gathering baseline data, and as ongoing measures of patients' needs. Ongoing assessment of patient need is particularly important when disease processes are unpredictable and characterized by repeated admissions to hospital. During these times the patient and family may experience disruption in every aspect of their life, including work and relationships. Whilst assessment schedules may allow these issues to be addressed, they must be used in a way that allows ongoing changes to be noted and regular evaluations to be taken into account (Bowling 1997; Frank-Stromborg & Olsen 1997).

The Multidisciplinary Care Plan and Patient Assessment Form now in use at the Royal Marsden Hospital is shown in Fig. 1.1. This includes sections to assess physical health, such as nutritional needs or sleep patterns; social assessment pertaining to financial concerns and childcare; religious, spiritual and cultural issues; and psychological status including body image and sexual concerns. This document has been improved from the previous format and it is now in booklet form. This minimizes confusion, achieves uniformity and provides more space for documentation of specific needs and for greater detail when appropriate. Specific sections on risk/safety assessment and on discharge needs have been developed following recognition that these areas need to be highlighted as having an impact on the planning of care.

The document also includes a separate readmission assessment to identify new and ongoing areas of care. A short-stay admission assessment document, a day care assessment document and outpatient assessment document are also incorporated. It is important to point out that, although assessment in each of these individual areas will differ because of the context and time limitations imposed, the documents (which are contained in the patient's records) should be viewed as part of an ongoing strategic assessment between, for example, outpatient visits and inpatient stays.

Detailed guidelines and flowcharts have been developed to ensure appropriate use and assimilation of the assessment document. These are shown in Fig. 1.2. The use of such guidelines illustrates the importance of education with regards to the use of specific documentation tools. In addition, the importance of electronic patient records to facilitate accurate and swift document of diagnosis, interventions and outcomes has been recognized and is under development.

The adequacy and effectiveness of patient records are obviously a multidisciplinary responsibility. Information from other members of the health care team is valuable, and may help to avoid repeating assessments. However, nurses have a personal and professional responsibility for the accuracy of nursing care records (UKCC 1993). If nursing records, including assessments, are inaccurate or inadequate, patient safety will be compromised. There would also be greater difficulty in demonstrating any effect of nursing care delivery. Furthermore, poor records can create major problems when complaints about care are being investigated or in instances of litigation (Hocking & Shamash 1998).

Other approaches to assessment have recently been described. One of these utilizes patient held records, which facilitate the transfer of information when a patient is discharged from hospital either to their own home or to another health care setting (Williams *et al.* 1994; Hayward 1998). These are in use in the Paediatric Unit at the Royal Marsden Hospital and are being developed in other areas.

Another approach is the use of multidisciplinary critical care pathways. These are defined as the identification and documentation of the sequence of standardized interdisciplinary processes or events that must occur for a particular case type or cohort of patients to move along a continuum towards a desired outcome in a defined period of time (Roebuck 1998).

A key requirement is an approach that staff find useful and appropriate in their particular area of practice (Smith & Richardson 1996; Allen 1998). It must be sensitive enough to discriminate between different clinical needs and flexible enough to be updated on a regular basis. In this regard, specialist wards or specialist nurses may use specific assessment documentation and/or tools to decipher pertinent information relevant to their skills and practice. For example, specialist practitioners, working in the field of lung cancer, who manage the symptom of breathlessness, use a detailed assessment approach designed to elicit the impact and meaning of the symptom for the patient and to ameliorate associated symptoms (Scullion & Henry 1998).

As information technology has developed into a multimedia approach it has opened up new opportunities for health care applications. The electronic patient record provides the caring professions with the potential to record sounds, provide frequently updated graphic displays of physiological data and sequential visual records such as still and moving images (Barnett 1997). Data can be sent to the general practitioner or district nurse. The data in a clinical nursing database can also be used for other purposes, such as care by other disciplines, quality assurance, management, policy-making and research. In addition, the electronic patient record will allow collation of data across patient groups to facilitate changes in clients' needs and evaluation of interventions for patients. However, the nurse must be able to validate the data about the care process before they can be used for other purposes. For the organizational aspects, there is agreement that multidisciplinary care plans are preferred, not only the single care plan for the nurse (Goossen *et al.* 1997). Although this era of information technology represents an exciting opportunity for nurses, there are some contentious issues surrounding the implementation of such systems. Examples of these include the potential negative influence of computer use on care delivery, lack of nursing terminology, poor involvement of nurses in decisions about systems and lack of evidence of the benefits of nursing information systems (Goossen *et al.* 1997).

Sources of assessment data

The information that is used in the assessment of patients is derived from a wide range of diverse sources. Nurse researchers and clinicians have developed a broad spectrum of tools to assess the problems frequently encountered by people with cancer. Examples of such assessment tools are given in Table 1.2. While it is unrealistic to assume that the use of tools like these is always feasible in everyday practice, it should be acknowledged that the use of an appropriate tool may be necessary to assess a particular patient's needs.

Tools link assessment of clinical variables with measurement of clinical interventions (Frank-Stromborg & Olsen 1997). For example, a nurse caring for a leukaemic patient who has had high dose chemotherapy may use the assessment tool described by Eilers *et al.* (1988), which provides a baseline assessment of the patient's normal oral status and allows regular and ongoing evaluation. Daily changes can be observed, medication prescribed and referrals made quickly and efficiently where appropriate.

The choice of assessment tool should be based on the variable to be measured in a particular patient group, the tool's purpose, measurement framework, conceptual base, reliability, validity and sensitivity (Frank-Stromborg & Olsen 1997). The use of assessment instruments can also assist health care professionals in practice development and research, by developing a body of knowledge concerning outcomes of intervention.

Table 1.2 Examples of assessment tools in cancer care

Topic	Reference
Revised grief experience inventory, for use in palliative care	Lev *et al.* (1993)
Piper fatigue scale, measuring subjective fatigue in cancer patients	Piper (1997)
Morrow assessment of nausea and emesis follow-up (anticipatory)	Chin *et al.* (1992)
Sexual behaviours questionnaire, used to assess effects of cancer therapy on women with breast cancer	Wilmoth (1994)
Oral assessment guide	Eilers *et al.* (1988)
Pain assessment chart	Walker *et al.* (1987)

Asking patients to describe their needs and difficulties may be particularly helpful when dealing with complex problems such as anxiety and stress. Information of this kind can also be collected in a health diary, which patients can use to record their needs and experiences since their last appointment (Richardson & Wilson-Barnett 1995; Burton & Watson 1998). Effective assessment strategies, therefore, mean gathering appropriate data from patients (George 1995). Whatever method is adopted to guide formal assessment, it remains a crucial part of effective nursing practice.

Summary

Nurses have a central role to play in helping patients to manage the demands of the procedures described in this book. The key to success in this role is accurate assessment of patients' needs and a commitment to meeting them with sensitivity. Taking time to explore individual needs is one way of demonstrating caring in everyday practice. The diverse range of technical procedures that patients may be subjected to should act as a reminder not to lose sight of the unique person undergoing such procedures. Caring for a person involves respect for their rights using communication that is open, honest and facilitative. This notion will now be explored in more depth.

Communication

Communication is recognized as an important aspect of heath care with far reaching effects (Jarman 1995). It has been frequently suggested that the use of communication skills by nurses is an integral and essential part of the care they provide, fundamental to all nursing practice and the concern of all nurses working in all specialties (Macleod Clark & Sims 1988; Brereton 1995; Naish 1996; Wilkinson 1999).

Communicating involves both verbal and non-verbal messages that convey feelings and information. The purpose of successful communication is to ensure appropriate social contact and professional interaction to meet the needs of patients and their families (Macleod Clark *et al.* 1991; Wilkinson *et al.* 1998). This section will explore the needs for, and effect of, communication in a cancer setting. It also considers the importance of therapeutic communication skills in differing circumstances and reasons as to why communication may break down between health care professionals and patients.

The need for clear communication

The topic of communication in health care has been widely researched and evaluated and the beneficial effects of good communication have been clearly demonstrated (Naish 1996). It is suggested that effective communication makes a positive contribution to an individual's recovery by acting as a buffer against fear and confusion (Nichols 1993). The provision of clear information and explanation on admission to hospital and prior to medical procedures may result

The Royal Marsden Hospital - Multidisciplinary Care Plan Information Sheet

Attach Patient Label

Name:

GP Name:

Address:

DOB:

Marital Status:

Address:

Religion:

Tel No.:

Tel. No.:

Communication: (sight/hearing/speech/language)

Age:

Consultant/Clinical Unit:

Interpreter Information/Language Line

Preferred Name:

Diagnosis:

Allergies:

Reason for Admission:

Current Surgery:

Persons To Contact & Next of Kin if different: please write two contact names
Please state if persons to contact/next of kin wish to be contacted at night or in an emergency

Name:

Name:

Relationship To Patient:

Relationship To Patient:

Address:

Address:

Tel. No. Home:

Tel. No. Home:

Tel. No. Work:

Tel. No. Work:

Date Of Admission:

Date Of Discharge:

Height:
cms

Weight
kg

Named Nurse:

Relevant Medical History (includes infectious diseases - MRSA, VRE, hepatitis, tuberculosis, measles, chickenpox):

Symptoms:

Medications:
Any difficulty taking medications ?   ☐ Yes ☐ No
If Yes, give details:

Does the patient self administer their medications ?   ☐ Yes ☐ No

If Yes, does the patient want to continue to self administer their medications in hospital ?   ☐ Yes ☐ No

Valuables/ Property:

Has The Patient Brought Valuables In To The Hospital With Them ? ☐ Yes ☐ No If Yes tick appropriate boxes and sign

The patient has retained custody of the valuables   ☐   Date: Signature:

The patient has been offered, and has accepted, that the valuables be kept in safe custody by the hospital   ☐   Date: Signature:

Valuables sent to Cashier's office   ☐   Date: Signature:

Valuables returned to the patient   ☐   Date: Signature:

Is The Patient Able To Care For Their Own Property ? ☐ Yes ☐ No
If No, please state arrangements:

F16

Physical Assessment Vital Signs: T P B/P Resps.:		
Respiratory	**Elimination**	
Neurological & Sensory	**Mobility/Manual Handling Needs**	
	Pressure Sore Audit Tool ☐ tick if completed	
Nutrition	**Wounds/Dressings/Appliances/Pressure Areas**	
Oral & Personal Hygiene	**Sleep & Rest**	

Psychological & Social Assessment	
Family & Social Situation (includes child care/finances)	
Community & Social Services on admission	
Psychological, Body Image & Sexual Issues	
Religious, Spiritual & Cultural Needs/Issues	
<u>Admitting Nurse Signature:</u> _____	<u>Date:</u> _____

Figure 1.1   The Royal Marsden Hospital Multidisciplinary Care Plan and Patient Assessment Form.

COMMUNITY SERVICES

	Required or N/A	Date of Referral	Name and Contact Number	Letter Complete	Letter Sent/Fax	Date of Visit
District Nurse						
Equipment						
Macmillan/ Hospice Home Care Team						
Hospice or Respite Care Admission						
Social Services						
Other e.g. Physio., Stoma care, Marie Curie						

Transport: Required ☐ Yes ☐ No   walker/chair/escort/stretcher/oxygen

Booked for (date): _____

DISCHARGE PLANNING

Predicted New Problems for Discharge:

Is a Social Services Referral Form Required ? ☐ Yes ☐ No

Planned Discharge Date: _____

Discharge Plan
Agreed and discussed with the patient ☐ Yes   Patient informed of date ☐ Yes
Agreed and discussed with the family/carer ☐ Yes   Family/carer informed of date ☐ Yes
State date discussed and with whom etc. in evaluation   State date discussed and with whom etc. in evaluation

HOSPITAL SERVICES

	Date Referred	Date Assessed	Community Needs Required
Occupational Therapist			
Physiotherapist			
Dietitian			
Social Services			
Community Liaison Nurse Specialist			

DATE	DISCHARGE PLANNING CONTINUOUS EVALUATION AND REVIEW	SIGNATURE

THE ROYAL MARSDEN HOSPITAL
DAY UNIT ASSESSMENT

Relevant Health History

State whether patient has :

Diabetes
MRSA
VRE
Hepatitis
Tuberculosis
Measles
Chicken Pox

Pre-Treatment Assessments

State any toxicities from previous treatment (including any side effects)

State if no problems

Any problems with :
Sight
Hearing
Changes in sensation or consciousness
Nutrition
Personal hygiene
Elimination
Mobility
Sleep or fatigue
Any worries or concerns

Other Needs (activities in daily living)

State difficulties in :
Shopping
Cooking
Dependants
Accommodation
Work
Finance - income
Benefits
Community services

Referrals

Physio
Community
OT
Dietician
Hospice/Macmillan nurse
Social Services
Nurse specialist
GP

Evaluation of Care

State circumstances of patient intervention
State any problems with the event and state solutions

Discharge/Transfer

TTOs
OPD appt.
Transport - own or hospital
Information booklets
Carer/relative informed
Discharged home
Transferred to ward (which one)

DATE	COMMUNICATION & SUMMARY OF WARD ROUNDS	SIGNATURE

NAME: **HOSPITAL NO.:**

CARE CHECKLIST - Activities of Daily Living (ADLs)
Write if assistance required (e.g. 1 or 2 nurses etc.) and any equipment needed
Assess DAILY or Set Review Date/Time if appropriate: Evaluate as ADLs on evaluation sheet

Nutrition	Oral & Personal Hygiene	Elimination	Mobility & Manual Handling
			Date:
			Signature:
			Review date:
			Date:
			Signature:
			Review date:

PROBLEMS/AREAS OF CARE

NUMBER Each Problem. Assess DAILY or Set Review Date/Time if appropriate:

No	No	No	No	Areas of Care: Please state and number each area of care.
				Date:
				Signature:
				Review date:
				Date:
				Signature:
				Review date:

Figure 1.1 The Royal Marsden Hospital Multidisciplinary Care Plan and Patient Assessment Form *(cont'd)*

NAME: **HOSPITAL NO.:**

Worries & Concerns:
Identify the patient's main worries & concerns including their understanding of their diagnosis and treatment and those worries & concerns of the family & carer(s)

DISCHARGE PLANNING

Predicted New Problems for Discharge (If COMPLEX discharge - use complex discharge sheet):

Identify if any changes/difficulties with Community Services since the last admission - please describe

Is a Social Services Referral Form Required ? ☐ Yes ☐ No

Discharge Plan

		Planned Discharge Date:	
Agreed and discussed with the patient	☐ Yes	**Patient informed of date**	☐ Yes
Agreed and discussed with the family/carer	☐ Yes	**Family/carer informed of date**	☐ Yes
State date discussed and with whom etc: in evaluation		State date discussed and with whom etc: in evaluation	

Transport: **Required**   ☐ Yes   ☐ No
Booked for (date): _____ walker/chair/escort/stretcher/oxygen

Referrals: **Identify any referrals made on this admission**

Valuables/ Property:
Has The Patient Brought Valuables In To The Hospital With Them ? ☐ Yes ☐ No If YES tick appropriate boxes and sign

The patient has retained custody of the valuables	☐	Date: Signature:
The patient has been offered, and has accepted, that the valuables be kept in safe custody by the hospital	☐	Date: Signature:
Valuables sent to Cashier's office	☐	Date: Signature:
Valuables returned to the patient	☐	Date: Signature:

Is the patient able to care for their own property ? ☐ Yes ☐ No
If No, please state arrangements:

Admitting Nurse Signature: _____ **Date:** _____

HOSPITAL NO.:

RE-ADMISSION ASSESSMENT

NAME:

Identify Changes Since The Last Admission. Indicate New And Ongoing Areas Of Care.
Complete the patient's Activities of Daily Living (ADL's), their manual handling needs & identify problems/areas of care on the Care Checklist.

Patient Information Details Checked ☐ (Tick when checked)

Date Of Admission:	**Date Of Discharge:**

Reason for Admission:

(Check Allergies)

Observations: T, P, Resps & B/P (if appropriate)

Height:	**Weight**	**Named Nurse:**
cms	kg	

Medications
Any difficulty taking medications ?   ☐ Yes ☐ No
If Yes, give details.

Does the patient self administer their medications ?   ☐ Yes ☐ No

If Yes, does the patient want to continue to self administer their medications in hospital ?   ☐ Yes ☐ No

Physical Assessment
Identify if the patient has any concerns/difficulties about the following since their last admission ? If YES please describe:

Symptoms or Side effects/ Toxicities	☐ yes ☐ no
Sight, Hearing	☐ yes ☐ no
Changes in Sensation Drowsiness/Confusion	☐ yes ☐ no
Nutrition	☐ yes ☐ no
Personal Hygiene	☐ yes ☐ no
Elimination	☐ yes ☐ no
Mobility	☐ yes ☐ no
Sleep & Fatigue	☐ yes ☐ no

Social Assessment
Identify if the patient has any concerns/difficulties about the following since their last admission ? If YES please describe:

Your Home Life e.g. Shopping, Cooking, Housework, Driving or Child care, dependants (child/adult)	☐ yes ☐ no
Your Accommodation	☐ yes ☐ no
Your Work	☐ yes ☐ no
Finances e.g. income, benefits	☐ yes ☐ no

F19

The Royal Marsden Hospital - Short Stay Admission

Attach Patient Label

Name: Hospital No.:   G. P. Name:

DOB: Marital Status: Address:

Address: Religion: Tel:

Tel. No.:   **Communication: (sight/hearing/speech/language)**

Age: Consultant/Clinical Unit: **Interpreter Information &/or language line**

Preferred Name:

Diagnosis: Allergies:

Reason for Admission:

Medications
Any difficulty taking medications ?   ☐ Yes ☐ No
If Yes, give details:

Does the patient self administer their medications ?   ☐ Yes ☐ No

If Yes, does the patient want to continue to self administer their medications in hospital ?   ☐ Yes ☐ No

Persons To Contact & Next of Kin if different: please write two contact names
Please state if persons to contact/next of kin wish to be contacted at night or in an emergency

Name: Name:

Relationship To Patient: Relationship To Patient:

Address: Address:

                                Tel. No.: Home:

Tel. No.: Home: Tel. No.: Work:

Tel. No.: Work:

Date Of Admission: Date Of Discharge:

Height: Weight   Named Nurse:
       cms   kg

Observations: T, P, Resps & B/P (if appropriate)

Relevant Medical History (includes infectious diseases - MRSA, VRE, hepatitis, tuberculosis, measles, chickenpox):

Symptoms:

Physical Assessment
Identify if the patient has any concerns/difficulties about the following ? If YES please describe:

Symptoms or Side effects/ Toxicities	☐ yes	☐ no
Sight, Hearing	☐ yes	☐ no
Changes in Sensation Drowsiness/Confusion	☐ yes	☐ no
Nutrition	☐ yes	☐ no
Personal Hygiene	☐ yes	☐ no
Elimination	☐ yes	☐ no
Mobility	☐ yes	☐ no
Sleep & Fatigue	☐ yes	☐ no

Social Assessment
Identify if the patient has any concerns/difficulties about the following ? If YES please describe:

Your Home Life e.g. Shopping, Cooking, Housework, Driving or Child care, dependants (child/adult)	☐ yes	☐ no
Your Accommodation	☐ yes	☐ no
Your Work	☐ yes	☐ no
Finances e.g. income, benefits	☐ yes	☐ no

Worries & Concerns:
Identify the patient's main worries & concerns including their understanding of their diagnosis and treatment and those worries & concerns of the family & carer(s)

F31

Figure 1.1   The Royal Marsden Hospital Multidisciplinary Care Plan and Patient Assessment Form (cont'd)

DISCHARGE PLANNING, COMMUNICATION & SUMMARY OF WARD ROUNDS CONTINUOUS EVALUATION AND REVIEW

DATE	SIGNATURE

NAME: _____   HOSPITAL N0.: _____

DATE	AREA OF CARE	No.:	SIGNATURE

ANTICIPATED OUTCOME:

ACTION:

DISCHARGE PLANNING

Predicted New Problems for Discharge (If COMPLEX discharge - use complex discharge sheet):

Identify if any changes/difficulties with Community Services since the last admission - please describe

Is a Social Services Referral Form Required ? ☐ Yes ☐ No

Discharge Plan   **Planned Discharge Date:** _____
Agreed and discussed with the patient   ☐ Yes   Patient informed of date   ☐ Yes
Agreed and discussed with the family/carer   ☐ Yes   Family/carer informed of date   ☐ Yes
State date discussed and with whom etc. in evaluation   State date discussed and with whom etc. in evaluation

Transport: Required   ☐ Yes   ☐ No
Booked for (date): _____   walker/chair/escort/stretcher/oxygen

Referrals - Hospital & Community (tick, & date, identify reason for referral in evaluation):

Social Worker	☐	District Nurse	☐ ....
Welfare Rights	☐	Macmillan Nurse or Hospice Home Care	☐ ....
Community Liaison Nurse Specialist (bleep no. _____)	☐	Nurse Specialist (please state who & bleep no.)	☐ ....
Dietician	☐	Research Nurse (please state who & bleep no)	☐ ....
Physiotherapist	☐		
Occupational Therapist	☐		

Valuables/ Property:
Has The Patient Brought Valuables In To The Hospital With Them ? ☐ Yes ☐ No
If Yes tick appropriate boxes and sign

The patient has retained custody of the valuables	☐	Date:	Signature:
The patient has been offered, and has accepted, that the valuables be kept in safe custody by the hospital	☐	Date:	Signature:
Valuables sent to Cashier's office	☐	Date:	Signature:
Valuables returned to the patient	☐	Date:	Signature:

Is the patient able to care for their own property ? ☐ Yes ☐ No
If No, please state arrangements:

Admitting Nurse Signature: _____   **Date:** _____

THE ROYAL MARSDEN HOSPITAL
OPD Nurse Documentation Information Sheet

Name:

Hospital No.:

G. P. Name:

Address:

DOB:

Age:

Marital Status:

Tel:

Address:

COMMUNICATION:
Sight - good ☐ yes ☐ no   Speech - good ☐ yes ☐ no
Hearing - good ☐ yes ☐ no   Language - English ☐ yes ☐ no

Tel:

If no, please describe:
glasses ☐   contact lenses ☐   hearing aid ☐

Religion:

Interpreter Information &/or language line ☐

Preferred Name:

Diagnosis:

Allergies:

Medical History:
(includes infectious diseases - MRSA, VRE, hepatitis, Tuberculosis, measles, chickenpox)

Observations:

Ht .... cms   Wt .... kg   TPR & B/P (if appropriate)

Worries & Concerns:
Identify the patient's main worries & concerns including their understanding of their diagnosis and treatment and those worries & concerns of the family & carer(s)

Physical Assessment
Has the patient any concerns/difficulties about the following ? If yes, please describe:

Symptoms or
Side effects/ Toxicities   ☐ yes ☐ no

Sight, Hearing	☐ yes	☐ no
Changes in Sensation Drowsiness/Confusion	☐ yes	☐ no
Nutrition	☐ yes	☐ no
Personal Hygiene	☐ yes	☐ no
Elimination	☐ yes	☐ no
Mobility	☐ yes	☐ no
Sleep & Fatigue	☐ yes	☐ no

Social Assessment
Have you any changes/difficulties with the following ? If yes, please describe

Your Home Life
e.g. Shopping, Cooking,
Housework, Driving or Child
care, dependants (child/adult)   ☐ yes ☐ no

Your Accommodation   ☐ yes ☐ no

Your Work   ☐ yes ☐ no

Finances   ☐ yes ☐ no
e.g. income, benefits

Community Services   ☐ yes ☐ no

Referrals (tick & date):

Dietician	☐	District Nurse ☐ ....
Occupational Therapist	☐	Macmillan Nurse or Hospice Home Care ☐ ....
Physiotherapist	☐	GP Liaison ☐ ....
Nurse Specialist (please state who & bleep no.)	☐	Community Liaison Nurse ☐ ....
IV Team/Day Care	☐	Other Referrals/Tests (please state who & bleep no. if appropriate)
Research Nurse (please state who & bleep no.)	☐	
Social Worker	☐	
Welfare Rights	☐	

Signature ....   Date ....

Figure 1.1   The Royal Marsden Hospital Multidisciplinary Care Plan and Patient Assessment Form (cont'd)

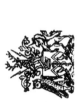

The Royal Marsden Hospital

Multidisciplinary Care Plan

1 Assessment (*to be completed within 24 hours*)
2 Discharge Planning and Evaluation
3 Communication and Summary of Ward Rounds
4 Care Checklist
  Activities of Daily Living (ADLs) – the patient's self-care
  abilities and manual handling needs
  Problem identification and Care Plans (core care plans if
  appropriate)
5 Problem Evaluation

CARE CHECKLIST – a quick reference of current care

- Complete activities of daily living and manual handling daily or set a review date: date, time and sign each entry and print your name and if appropriate your agency name
- Number care plans and refer to the number in the continuous evaluation
- Update care plans – cross through 'actions' that have changed with a single black line, date and sign and add new actions at the bottom of the plan, date, time and sign accordingly. Start new care plan if care changed greatly. Ensure that you have updated the care checklist in addition to the care plan, stating the rationale for the change in the problem evaluation section

Re-admission Assessment

- Complete re-admission assessment on each admission and complete a care checklist for the activities of daily living and manual handling assessment
- If a patient has complex needs or has major changes in his or her condition since the last admission, complete an initial assessment

Short Stay Admission Sheet

- May be used for an admission of 24–48 hours only or if the assessment required is not complex. If the notes are missing and patient information details are required on a re-admission, use the short stay sheet if appropriate

Communication and Summary of Ward Rounds

- Identify and document any changes in treatment and patient care following consultations and the content of any discussions with the family or patient

Discharge Planning and Evaluation

- Discharge planning assessment to be made on each admission and throughout admission
- Discuss with the patient and family/carer the discharge plan and expected date of discharge
- Document any discussion with the patient or family/carer(s) or the community team in the discharge planning evaluation section

Medical History

- Document *relevant* medical history including infectious diseases, e.g. MRSA, VRE, hepatitis, tuberculosis, measles, chicken pox, or latex sensitivity and any symptoms patient may have
- Has patient had any childhood illnesses, major illnesses or operations relevant to this admission? Has patient had any previous cancer treatments or care or is this treatment/care ongoing?
- Clarify other health problems, e.g. diabetes, hypertension, arthritis, epilepsy

Medications

- Check that patient's medications are correctly prescribed by the doctor on the drug chart
- Clarify whether patient has difficulty taking his or her medications and if patient wishes to self administer his or her drugs during the hospital stay

Information Sheet

Patient Information

- Complete patient information details as requested
- Check if there are any allergies including drug, food or latex sensitivities
- Enter reason for admission and details for the current surgery when patient's operation has taken place
- State if patient has communication needs/difficulties, e.g. double or blurred vision, blindness, glasses or contact wearer, deafness, tinnitus, speech disorders, use of voice aids
- State if patient has language difficulties – state interpreter information or use of language line
- Please enter two names for person to contact in event of an emergency
- Indicate who patient would like information about his or her illness or hospitalization to be given to and what information patient would like shared with him or her

Valuables and Property

- State if patient has been offered and has accepted that valuables be kept in safe custody by the hospital, or valuables sent to the cashier's office. State when valuables returned to patient and sign accordingly
- State clearly the arrangement for patient's property if patient is confused or unconscious

Figure 1.2 Guidelines and flowcharts for the Royal Marsden Hospital Multidisciplinary Care Plan.

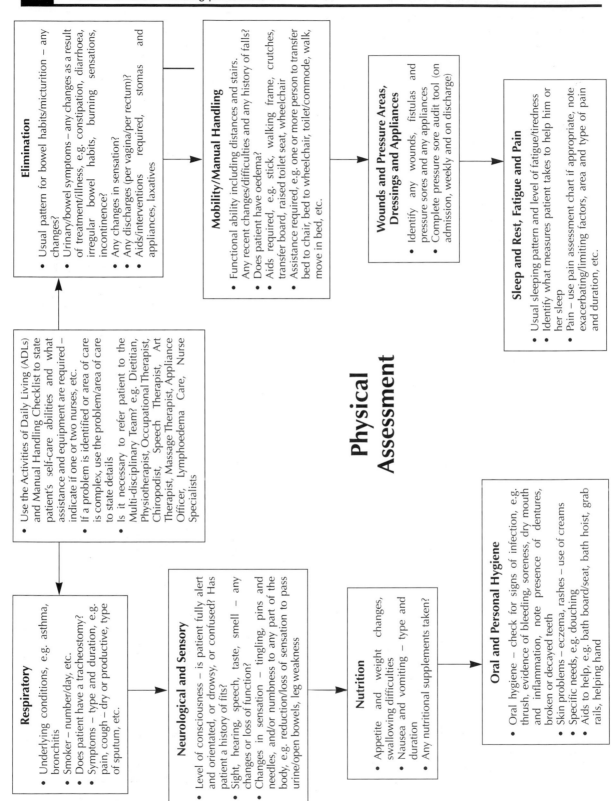

Physical Assessment

Elimination

- Usual pattern for bowel habits/micturition – any changes?
- Urinary/bowel symptoms – any changes as a result of treatment/illness, e.g. constipation, diarrhoea, irregular bowel habits, burning sensations, incontinence?
- Any changes in sensation?
- Any discharges (per vagina/per rectum)?
- Aids/interventions required, stomas and appliances, laxatives

Mobility/Manual Handling

- Functional ability including distances and stairs.
- Any recent changes/difficulties and any history of falls?
- Does patient have oedema?
- Aids required, e.g. stick, walking frame, crutches, transfer board, raised toilet seat, wheelchair
- Assistance required, e.g. one or more person to transfer bed to chair, bed to wheelchair, toilet/commode, walk, move in bed, etc.

Wounds and Pressure Areas, Dressings and Appliances

- Identify any wounds, fistulas and pressure sores and any appliances
- Complete pressure sore audit tool (on admission, weekly and on discharge)

Sleep and Rest, Fatigue and Pain

- Usual sleeping pattern and level of fatigue/tiredness
- Identify what measures patient takes to help him or her sleep
- Pain – use pain assessment chart if appropriate, note exacerbating/limiting factors, area and type of pain and duration, etc.

- Use the Activities of Daily Living (ADLs) and Manual Handling Checklist to state patient's self-care abilities and what assistance and equipment are required – indicate if one or two nurses, etc.
- If a problem is identified or area of care is complex, use the problem/area of care to state details
- Is it necessary to refer patient to the Multi-disciplinary Team? e.g. Dietitian, Physiotherapist, Occupational Therapist, Chiropodist, Speech Therapist, Art Therapist, Massage Therapist, Appliance Officer, Lymphoedema Care, Nurse Specialists

Respiratory

- Underlying conditions, e.g. asthma, bronchitis
- Smoker – number/day, etc.
- Does patient have a tracheostomy?
- Symptoms – type and duration, e.g. pain, cough – dry or productive, type of sputum, etc.

Neurological and Sensory

- Level of consciousness – is patient fully alert and orientated, or drowsy, or confused? Has patient a history of fits?
- Sight, hearing, speech, taste, smell – any changes or loss of function?
- Changes in sensation – tingling, pins and needles, and/or numbness to any part of the body, e.g. reduction/loss of sensation to pass urine/open bowels, leg weakness

Nutrition

- Appetite and weight changes, swallowing difficulties
- Nausea and vomiting – type and duration
- Any nutritional supplements taken?

Oral and Personal Hygiene

- Oral hygiene – check for signs of infection, e.g. thrush, evidence of bleeding, soreness, dry mouth and inflammation, note presence of dentures, broken or decayed teeth
- Skin problems – eczema, rashes – use of creams
- Specific needs, e.g. douching
- Aids to help, e.g. bath board/seat, bath hoist, grab rails, helping hand

Psychological and Social Assessment

Family and Social Situation

Include family tree, child care, and finances

- Does patient or carer require advice on support services in the community?
- Is it necessary to complete a social services referral form or refer to the welfare rights officer?

- Does patient have any concerns during his or her hospital stay or after treatment regarding the following: accommodation, work, shopping, cooking, housework, child care arrangements – school journeys, effect of illness on the children, driving, travel to and from hospital, and finances – income or benefits
- Accommodation problems – identify number of stairs, number of floors, situation of kitchen/bathroom facilities, sheltered housing, etc.
- Consider:
  - type of work and ability to work, job security re. sickness
  - financial concerns, current benefits
  - who does washing, housework and shopping

- Does patient have any dependants, especially children under 18 years and vulnerable adults? Does patient live alone? Consider: family, carer(s), friends, neighbour support, who is significant to patient (family tree if appropriate)
- Who does patient live with, e.g. if patient cares for elderly or disabled relative, etc., what is the proximity and support of family/neighbours, friends?

Community and Social Services on Admission

- What professional help does patient/carer have?
District Nurse: name and contact number, how often visits, and current reason for visits
Macmillan Nurse: name and contact number, and how well known to patient
Social Services: carer for personal care, meals on wheels, home help – include name and contact number

Religious/Spiritual and Cultural Needs/Issues

- Does patient have any specific beliefs?
- Do they practise any religion?
- What is important to them, e.g. hobbies, music, etc.?
- Do they have any specific cultural issues, e.g. dress, food?

Psychological, Body Image and Sexual Issues

Document patient/family/carer's specific concerns

- Ask about patient's perceptions of diagnosis and treatment – what are their worries and concerns? What has helped them cope in the past? What are their usual ways of coping? What is helping them to cope at the moment? Give opportunity for patient and family to discuss their concerns and what they may expect following treatment or how their illness may affect them
- Ask about how their illness or treatment has affected the way they feel. Have their relationships been affected since their diagnosis and/or treatment?
- Advise re. opportunities to discuss issues with relevant health care professional, e.g. clinical nurse specialist, relevant support groups, information services, etc.
- Would patient or his/her family welcome the opportunity to talk with the Social Worker?

Discharge Planning:

Evaluate on white discharge planning and evaluation sheet

- Predict new problems for discharge
Identify new problems, e.g. wound care, hickman line care, deteriorating condition, mobility problems, shopping etc.
- Hospital services
Clarify need for hospital referrals – identify date of referral, multidisciplinary team to document when assessed patient and community needs required
- Community services
Clarify need for community referrals – document when made and letters completed and sent, etc.
Identify when community team are to make the first visit to the patient
Document discussion in the discharge planning evaluation
- Transport
Check type of transport required – 24/48 hours necessary (check eligibility)
Check patient has drugs, equipment and future appointments on discharge

Figure 1.2 Guidelines and flowcharts for the Royal Marsden Hospital Multidisciplinary Care Plan (cont'd)

in decreased anxiety, decreased pain levels, a reduced number of complications and side-effects of treatment, improved compliance, an enhanced coping ability and an increased speed of convalescence (Wilson-Barnett 1982; Watson 1983; Meissner et al. 1990; Schapiro et al. 1992; Pruitt et al. 1993; Poroch 1995). It is unsurprising, therefore, that patients with cancer have been found to consistently rank information/communication highly when asked to consider which nursing activities are most important to them (Larson 1984; Borgers et al. 1993; Hughes 1993).

Enormous scope exists for improving the contribution of nurses to the care and support of families of people with cancer (Yates 1999). It is important to recognize that partners or families may also have communication needs (Bluglass 1991; Northouse et al. 1991). They are often responsible for the majority of care given to the cancer patient in the community and may wish to talk to the doctor or nurse but may not receive the information they require through inhibition or uncertainty (Macleod Clark & Sims 1988).

The value to patients of communication activities, that is whether they are regarded as positive or negative, may depend on the degree of importance that this holds for them in the clinical environment and the context in which they are produced (Mallett 1997). For example, information giving can only be considered therapeutic when it meets the patient's needs, while in other situations it may be inappropriate and therefore not therapeutic. It could be suggested, therefore, that no such activity can be considered therapeutic for all patients in a given setting or for one patient all of the time (Mallett 1997). Further research into what constitutes and defines therapeutic communication is indicated.

Verbal and non-verbal communication

Communication is complex and involves more than the spoken word. It is also about listening to patients and attempting to understand their knowledge, fears and expectations in relation to proposed investigations and treatments (Jarman 1995). Both verbal and non-verbal activity are integral to the process of communication and should be given consideration whenever nurse–patient interactions are studied (Mallett 1997). Factors such as voice tone, volume and inflection form vocal content. However, the research into communication in nursing is often deductive, precategorized and plays little attention to the organization of naturally occurring verbal and, particularly, non-verbal communication. This may result in a lack of consideration of the importance of factors such as gaze and gestures in nurse–patient interactions (Mallett 1997).

Body movements and touch are examples of non-verbal communication that may be crucial in assessing patients' needs (Porchet-Munro 1991). This author states that 'body language gives away our uncertainties' and 'unmasks words'. Thus, in a clinical situation it may be possible to give one verbal message whilst transmitting an incongruous non-verbal one. For example, a nurse may adopt an inappropriate, cheerful expression while conveying bad news to a relative. Touch is another important aspect of non-verbal communication that can be directed and used in a meaningful manner. However, McCann & McKenna (1993) indicate that most of nursing touch may be task orientated rather than expressive in nature, but some patients may not perceive any touch positively. Touch that is perceived as inappropriate to the patient is not therapeutic.

It is important to recognize the differences in non-verbal communication across different cultures as non-verbal cues may not be universal in their meaning. Pease (1981) suggests that we do not necessarily have to look to other continents or countries to find differences; people from rural communities have variances in their behaviour from city dwellers. Non-verbal expressions may also be specific to the situation as well as to the culture. Other differences may also arise due to social background, family upbringing, sexuality, gender and past experience (Davitz et al. 1976).

Skills of communication

There is a clear distinction to be made between communication that could be considered therapeutic and skilled communication, as the two are not necessarily synonymous (Mallett 1989). The following section focuses on those skills that may be considered central to effective communication in nursing care.

Considering first the more elementary skills, some examples of these are clarification, reflection, silence, probing and summarizing (Macleod Clark & Sims 1988; Burton 1991; Burton & Watson 1998). For example, clarification can be illustrated as:

Patient: 'I don't think I can cope with chemotherapy.'
Nurse: 'What would be most difficult about the chemotherapy for you to cope with?'

Here the nurse is seeking to understand more specifically what the patient means. Reflection may be used to communicate understanding, to check accuracy and to invite the patient to elaborate, such as:

Patient: 'I'm finding things really hard at the moment.'
Nurse: 'Really hard?'

Silence, although uncomfortable at times, can also be a powerful communication skill used to encourage the patient to reflect on what has been said (Faulkner & Maguire 1984; Burnard 1990). At times probing may be employed to invite the patient to expand on a particular issue and clarify any vagueness, for example:

Nurse: 'You mentioned you were having trouble sleeping. Can you tell me more about that?'

Summarizing helps the nurse and the patient draw the main issues of the interaction together. It is especially useful to help the patient and nurse focus and move on and also allows for clarification of mutual understanding (Hargie et al. 1987). It can be done at a number of points throughout an encounter and can be particularly helpful as a method of closing the session (Burton & Watson 1998).

The use of open questions can be considered one of the simplest and yet most effective means of encouraging patients to communicate, as many research studies confirm (Hargie *et al.* 1987; Macleod Clark & Sims 1988; Burnard 1990). Open questions are useful to try and identify as much information as possible in a limited time, to show understanding and, it is hoped, to help more effectively and give more relevant information (Ramirez *et al.* 1994). An open question is prefixed by words such as 'When', 'What' or 'How', and will help to discourage a 'Yes' or 'No' response. In this way open communication may be facilitated. Questions beginning with the word 'Why', while sometimes appropriate, may be perceived as threatening or provocative (Brennan & Swan 1995).

Some advanced skills that require more practice and self-awareness are listening, challenging, empathy and unconditional positive regard (Rogers 1967, 1980; Egan 1994). Listening has been described as giving full attention and involves following very intently what the patient is saying in order to hear and understand (Nichols 1993). Thus listening effectively allows nurses to respond more completely to patients' needs (Metcalf 1998).

Challenging is defined by Egan (1994) as 'an invitation to examine internal or external behaviour that seems to be self-defeating, harmful to others or both and to change the behaviour if it is found to be so'. It may involve confronting evasiveness or inconsistencies.

Rogers (1980) said of empathy that it 'means entering the private perceptual world of the other and becoming thoroughly at home in it'. Burton & Watson (1998) suggest empathy is the ability to sense the other person's world of felt meanings, as if they were one's own. However confusion arises from the distinction between empathy as a way of being and empathy as a communication process or skill (Egan 1994). Rogers' phrase 'unconditional positive regard' (Rogers 1967) means that the patient is viewed with dignity and value as a worthwhile human being. The regard is offered without preconditions or demand for reciprocity and so involves a deep and positive feeling for the person.

Debate exists as to whether communication skills can be taught (Brereton 1995). While it was once assumed that good communicators are born, not made, others consider health care professionals can learn and develop such skills with appropriate preparation and training (Bannister & Kagan 1985; Macleod Clark & Sims 1988; Razavi & Delvaux 1997; Fallowfield *et al.* 1998; Wilkinson *et al.* 1998).

Counselling could also be viewed as an advanced skill. However, Macleod Clark *et al.* (1991) indicate that nurses using advanced communication skills may not be counselling in the formal sense. Some required conditions for counselling are undergoing a recognized training programme and having appropriate supervision. The definition of counselling is given by the British Association for Counselling (1989a) as:

> An interaction in which one person offers another person time, attention and respect, with the intention of helping that person to explore, discover and clarify ways of living more resourcefully and toward greater well-being.

Skills of counselling differ from listening skills or formal counselling and can be summarized in the following quote from the British Association for Counselling (1989b):

> What distinguishes the use of counselling skills from these other two activities are the intentions of the user, which are to enhance the performance of their functional role and the recipient will, in turn, perceive them in that role.

Thus it can be deduced that for nurses to be formally counselling they have to be perceived by patients to be in that role and must be adequately prepared. Counselling must not be seen as a panacea but may be a preferred option for consenting patients or family members who will need to be referred to suitably qualified staff. If the person referred has refused to consent then they are unlikely to be able to engage in the counselling process. Egan (1994), who provides one model of counselling, states that outcomes depend on the competence and motivation of the helper and client and that the client has to be willing to take part.

There are some patient groups who may not be appropriate for counselling, for example severely brain-damaged patients or those with psychotic symptoms. This stresses the importance of assessment of the patient's individual needs and the implications for nurses to consider referral to appropriate agencies if necessary. Nurses need to communicate with every patient, but only a few patients will require formal counselling. Therefore there is a clear distinction to be made between good communication and formal counselling.

Barriers to communication

It would appear that a strong relationship exists between effectiveness of communication and overall satisfaction with care (Lack & Holloway 1992), so much so that patients tend to be more dissatisfied with poor communication than with any other aspect of their care. It has been suggested that 'without failures in communication, there would be a dramatic fall in the number of complaints received' (Health Service Commissioner Report 1992).

Dissatisfaction with regard to information received is an all too common theme pervading research into the needs of patients with cancer (Corney *et al.* 1992; Wong & Bramwell 1992; Crockford *et al.* 1993; Suominen *et al.* 1994). Somewhat alarmingly, both nursing and medical staff have been found to be less than proficient in the area of communication skills (Faulkner 1986; Ricketts 1996; Razavi & Devaux 1997; Burton & Watson 1998; Fallowfield *et al.* 1998). Many studies have continued to produce evidence of poor communication between staff and patients, suggesting that this can often be accredited to nurses who may lack essential communication skills.

It has been suggested that nurses' communication skills with cancer patients have not improved over the past 20 years (Wilkinson 1999), and remain superficial, routinized, task related (Hewison 1995) or highly technical (Dennison 1995) and that nurses frequently use blocking tactics to prevent patients divulging their problems (Wilkinson

1991). However, it is important to bear in mind that communication is a two-way process and a criticism of some such studies is that the influence of the patient on the communication process is missing (Mallett 1997). Future research needs to consider both patients' and nurses' contributions to nurse–patient communication (Jarrett & Payne 1995). In an earlier report Webster (1981) describes how nurses avoid communicating with dying patients in seven different ways such as an abrupt change of the subject of conversation and withdrawing from a stressful situation. Although some studies highlight a requirement for nurses to be more aware of the importance of communication skills, greater self-awareness may in itself lead to increased emotional needs (Vachon 1995; Naish 1996; Wilkinson 1999). This may then necessitate further support from their peers and/or colleagues.

Nurses are expected to be able to cope with their own emotional reactions as well as those of patients and families. In communicating with patients there is always the risk that difficult issues may arise, and nurses may not feel equipped to deal with them effectively or fear that they themselves may become affected. Burton & Watson (1998) suggest that professionals may use distancing techniques if they are concerned about becoming too emotionally involved with patients. These may include avoiding eye contact, discouraging questions and focusing on the physical illness and symptoms. Parle *et al.* (1997) and Maguire (1985) also highlight barriers such as distancing, giving false reassurance and selective attention used by staff to prevent them getting close to patients' psychological suffering. They suggest that regular psychological support, opportunities for taking time out and models for training may enable staff to relinquish these distancing tactics. Although avoidance and distancing are natural defence mechanisms in stressful situations, nurses who develop increased self-awareness may recognize those obstructive defence mechanisms employed in their everyday work (Burnard 1990).

Burnard (1990) defines self-awareness as:

> the gradual and continuous process of noticing and exploring aspects of the self, whether behavioural, psychological or physical, with the intention of developing personal and interpersonal understanding.

He goes on to argue that the benefits of increased self-awareness extend outwards to facilitate meaningful relationships with others.

Avoidance behaviours may also be employed by patients and family members, either by choice or as a consequence of denial. They may wish not to have information regarding, for instance, the extent of the disease. This highlights the need for an individual approach. Glaser & Strauss (1965) studied terminally ill patients and identified four awareness contexts which may apply to patients and those close to them:

- Closed
- Suspected
- Mutual pretence and
- Open awareness.

With closed and suspected awareness there is an imbalance of information as the family, nursing or medical staff act as custodians of information that the patient does not have. There is more potential for misunderstandings and distress to all parties than when communication is open and mutual. It is important to recognize that these categories are not absolute; the patient and family may move between levels of awareness at different stages of the illness experience and may be influenced by their perceived ability to cope at the time. The nurse's role is to recognize the difficulties that may arise from misunderstandings between the people involved and offer clarification and support where required (Macleod Clark & Sims, 1988).

Awareness and recognition of the patient's emotional adjustment to cancer may enable nurses to communicate more effectively with them. Factors such as the stage of illness, available support, physical symptoms and so on will affect the fluctuation between adjustment styles (Moorey & Greer 1989). The primary role of the nurse in communication is to assess, identify and help prioritize the needs of patients and families as well as facilitating their expression of feelings (catharsis) and building a relationship in which care can take place. Moorey & Greer (1989) state that the thought process of the person with cancer incorporates three key factors:

- The view of the diagnosis
- Perceived control and
- The view of the prognosis.

In addition, there are five adjustment styles identified by Greer & Watson (1987) which indicate how patients may react to the experience of cancer. These are:

1 Fighting spirit
2 Avoidance or denial
3 Fatalism
4 Helplessness and hopelessness
5 Anxious preoccupation.

In the first of these, the diagnosis is seen as a challenge, the person can exert some control over the stress and the prognosis is seen as optimistic. With avoidance or denial the threat from the diagnosis is minimal, the issue of control is irrelevant and the prognosis is seen as good. For the fatalist, the diagnosis represents a relatively minor threat, there is no control that can be exerted over the situation and the consequences of lack of control can and should be accepted with equanimity. In the fourth adjustment style, the diagnosis is seen as a major threat, no control can be exerted over the situation and the inevitable negative outcome is experienced as if this has already come about. With anxious preoccupation, where the person compulsively searches for reassurance, the diagnosis represents a major threat and there is uncertainty over the possibility of exerting control over the situation or the future. Similar to the awareness contexts, patients may change adjustment styles according to their circumstances and there is a danger in assuming patients may fall into specific categories. The adjustment styles are perhaps most helpful in enabling the nurse to assess patients' emotional reactions over time.

There may be many barriers to effective communication between the nurse and patient besides denial. Examples of these attributable to patients include fear of appearing ignorant, a reluctance to question professionals, a hesitancy to take up too much time, not knowing what to ask, embarrassment about discussing delicate/sensitive issues and fear of hearing bad news (Meissner *et al.* 1990; Corney *et al.* 1992; Borgers *et al.* 1993; Suominen *et al.* 1994). In addition emotional anguish, anxiety, depression or the presence of physical symptoms such as pain may impair the ability of the patient to retain information. Where possible the nurse should endeavour to minimize or eliminate physical discomfort prior to giving information or conducting a meaningful conversation.

There are also many factors in the hospital setting that may inhibit therapeutic communication such as noise, excessive heat, harsh lighting, interruptions and lack of privacy (Naish 1996). It is helpful if the patient and/or family can be seen in a private room where an engaged sign on the door can minimize interruptions and the telephone is silenced. Screens around the patient's bed are not sufficient as they only provide visual privacy.

Communication needs of children with cancer

Children with cancer have special communication needs highlighted by several factors given in the literature. There are different fears at different ages for the child. Sepion (1988) states that for young children, fears of abandonment and isolation are most prevalent while for the teenager, peer group rejection may be the greatest fear (Thompson 1988). There is an intensified need to truth-tell to avoid confusion arising out of myths and secrecy (Sepion 1988). Bluebond-Langner (1978) substantiates this by demonstrating that if parents and children resist communicating the mutual pretence used as a defence mechanism may deny children the opportunity to express their fears. Also, there may be iatrogenic educational problems for the child and physical and emotional disruption for siblings (Lansdown & Goldman 1991). It can be seen from this that there is a need to involve the whole family in the treatment of the child which gives a greater sense of control for each family member (Lansdown & Goldman 1991). Readers are referred to more specialized texts which explore these issues in greater depth (Koocher & O'Malley 1991; Last & VanVeldhuizen 1992; Muller *et al.* 1992; Douglas 1993; Eiser 1993).

Genetic counselling

There has been a recent impetus in the study of genetic predisposition to cancer and this has led to the establishment of cancer family history clinics which are increasing in number (Eeles 1995). The role of such clinics is to obtain a detailed family history and to make an accurate assessment of the risk of developing cancer so that families can be advised accordingly. Screening can be arranged where appropriate and information can be provided on the availability of genetic tests and studies relating to the prevention of cancer if indicated (Eeles *et al.* 1994; Eeles 1995; Gogas & Sacks 1996). To facilitate this there has been a parallel growth in genetic counselling services. An initial assessment of the person's perceived risk and the basis for it is a prerequisite of the genetic counselling process. Goals of an education and counselling session should include objective assessment of risk, increased understanding about the natural history of cancer, knowledge regarding appropriate lifestyle changes and recommendations for screening. Predictive gene testing should only be performed after full genetic counselling, as the implications of a positive test result for carriers are considerable (Ardern-Jones & Eeles 1997). Patients may visit for counselling several times and specialist nurses are ideally placed to liaise closely with the patient throughout, providing support and demonstrating sound understanding of potentially complex issues.

Opportunity to address those psychological needs which have been reported following cancer risk assessment, including fear, anger, denial, guilt, grief and the implications of feeling continually threatened by the disease, should also be provided (Josten *et al.* 1985; Smith 1992). It is important to spend time counselling individuals, thus providing the opportunity for them to initiate their own health promoting strategies (Gray 1995).

Increasing availability of cancer genetics counselling highlights a number of issues with regard to the process of giving information about an individual's risk of developing cancer. The effectiveness of genetic counselling is very much dependent on the attendee's comprehension of risk, the level of reassurance they may derive from counselling and their willingness to adhere to suggested recommendations (Lloyd *et al.* 1996). Studies are being conducted to examine the best way to present genetic information so that it is easily understood by patients and is retained (Gray 1995). All cancer family clinics should conduct a prospective evaluation of emotional state and provide integrated psychological counselling for gene carriers, non-carriers and their partners/families if required (Watson *et al.* 1996). Nurses are clearly in a position to provide support and assistance to patients and their families but must be aware of the complexities of such communication and the somewhat unique psychological support these patients may need.

Summary

Communication can be seen to be a vital part of nursing care. It is hoped that this brief review will highlight the most salient concerns for the nurse wishing to explore the use of effective communication skills. It can be seen that there are complex difficulties when researching communication, but this remains essential in order to promote this key aspect of care. Patients are individuals with unique needs that may be addressed through careful assessment and with the use of therapeutic communication. However, promotion of a patient focused approach inevitably gives rise to moral and ethical dilemmas which require consideration and debate. In the final part of this chapter, some such dilemmas will be explored in the context of consent to examination and treatment.

Consent to examination and treatment

Consent is an individual's freely given agreement to examination, treatment or an act of care based on information about, and an understanding of, what is proposed. In order to give consent, a person must be deemed to be competent (Kennedy & Grubb 1994). Obtaining valid consent prior to a clinical procedure is both a legal and an ethical imperative. The process requires sophisticated assessment and communication skills, together with a profound respect for the rights of the individual. The health care professional, in order to demonstrate their respect for another person, the patient, and to avoid committing a civil wrong in law, must obtain that individual's consent prior to any procedure.

The nurse's responsibilities towards patients are clearly laid down in the *Code of Professional Conduct* (UKCC 1992) and *Exercising Accountability* (UKCC 1989). These are essential reading for all practitioners and form a useful introduction to the detailed information presented here. First, consideration is given to a possible ethical framework to be applied to the consent process. Second, the law is examined to determine what is required of the practitioner. Finally, a brief mention is made of consent in a research setting, with provision of further references.

An ethical basis for consent

The law and the Department of Health (DoH) in its documents *Patient Consent to Examination or Treatment* (1990) and *The Patient's Charter* (1995) use the language of rights to describe a patient's claims on, or expectations of, health care. 'Rights' is also a term which has been used widely by society in general in the 1990s. It is necessary to consider the nature of these rights, particularly in relationship to the health care professional's duties.

Health care professionals have a special relationship with their patients. On entering this relationship the practitioner assumes certain special duties towards the patient, over and above those which ordinary human beings have to each other, such as a duty not to kill them, a duty to keep a promise or a duty not to tell a lie. The features of this relationship are described generally as a duty of care which contains the following:

- A duty to respect the patient's autonomy
- A duty to act in the patient's best interests
- A duty to promote health and prevent harm (UKCC 1992).

The patient can then be said to have certain rights, as mirror images of those duties, that is the right to expect the practitioner to respect their autonomy, the right to expect the practitioner to act in their best interests and the right to expect the practitioner to promote their health and not cause them harm.

There also exists on behalf of the practitioner a duty to advise the patient and to inform them of what is proposed. This duty may be seen as part of the duty to respect autonomy as the information imparted will enable the patient to determine what action should be taken, or it could be viewed by the practitioner as part of their duty to act in the best interests of the patient, in which case only selected information may be forthcoming (Speechley 1992).

Duties, and therefore rights, may be ordered in more than one way and this order is dependent on the opinion of the individual practitioner – one duty may be given greater or lesser weight in a particular circumstance. Respect for autonomy may be overridden in order to act in the best interests, or vice versa. The professional is in control and, therefore, the patient's rights are restructured in order of importance by them. Consideration of rights from this perspective loses much of the force normally given to the term, as the patient's rights are decided and prioritized by another. Because rights mirror duties, they are negative rights which the patient does not own or have control of; for example they may not be waived or alienated. The right may only be exercised in one way, the way determined by the professional. For example, information to the patient may be controlled so that the action (choice of treatment) is what the practitioner regards as in the patient's best interests (the most medically efficacious) (Speechley 1992).

The humanist principles of biomedical ethics formulated and developed by Beauchamp & Childress (1994) contain similar elements to those embodied within a duty of care – respect for autonomy, nonmaleficence, beneficence – plus the concept of justice. Justice may be applied on an individual basis as fair, equitable and appropriate treatment or at a societal level as fair, equitable and appropriate distribution of health care in society. These principles may also be ranked in different orders, so that once again the respect for autonomy may not be uppermost.

Of the three components of valid consent, information is the one which can be best used to illustrate the different ways in which the duty of care and the principle of respect for autonomy can be used. Selective information giving is justified using a number of possible arguments.

- In seeking help, the patient has demonstrated a willingness to undergo the recommended treatment and explicit consent, demanded as a respect for autonomy, is not required.

- The patient, given their vulnerability and anxiety, is not autonomous and, therefore, cannot rationally decide between treatment options. There is no autonomy to be respected.

- Withholding information is in the patient's best interests as full knowledge of the situation and/or treatment may cause distress and may even lead to the patient refusing the recommended treatment.

- The patient will not be able to understand the rationale and complexities of the treatment given that she/he has not had the training and experience of the professional and there is not sufficient time to explain the intricacies of therapy, if the desired outcome is to be achieved.

- Full disclosure, particularly of any uncertainty, will cause confusion and distress resulting in loss of trust and confidence and, once again, cannot be considered as compatible with a duty of care.

The theory of positive patients' rights to make a valid consent to examination, treatment or act of care originates from the North American doctrine of the informed consent theorists (Beauchamp & Childress 1994), which is supported in part by law. The assertion that patients have a prima facie right to make an informed choice about treatment is grounded in the principle of autonomy or self-determination and levels a positive duty to inform upon the professional.

There are several practical difficulties within informed consent theory due to the burden which it places on the professional or that which rests with the patient. However, it is a useful concept within which to consider what rights are exercised during the consent process and what kind of rights they are. In order for a competent person to make a voluntary decision two rights need to be exercised:

- The right to self determination
- The right to information to enable autonomous action.

Rights-based moral theorists adopt slightly differing views depending on whether those rights are grounded in autonomy (Hart 1984) or equal respect (Dworkin 1984). The autonomy-based theorist proposes that a natural right is discretionary, that is it may be exercised as we please within the limits of the rights of others. Discretionary rights are alienable in that they can be waived temporarily or relinquished permanently provided only that the decision to do this is fully informed, well considered and fully voluntary.

When equal respect is used as the central premise, rights are again regarded as discretionary but inalienable, that is always retained. However, that to which the right pertains is alienable. For example, the right to life is discretionary and inalienable, to live or die as we choose within the boundaries of autonomy. However, that to which we have the right is alienable, that is life. Therefore the right to life may be exercised as the right to die, unimpeded by others.

Both these views of rights place control firmly with the individual and, in addition, allow them to decide to what extent they wish to control a situation such as information giving or decision making. The individual is further respected if one incorporates the view of Mackie (1984) that rights provide a 'persistent defence of . . . certain vital interests of people', which are largely determined by that person to protect the 'choice of how to live [one's life]'.

All rights-based theories stress autonomy and therefore can only be valid in circumstances where the individual is, or has been, autonomous (legally competent). However, if autonomous, the individual's wishes are paramount and should be respected even if they appear to conflict or lack congruence with the health care professional's opinions, or current thought. Difficulties may also arise due to the nature of our multicultural society where, in some instances, responsibility for decision-making is routinely delegated to the professional, a family member or is dictated by societal

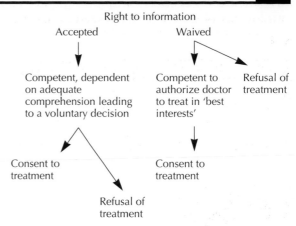

Figure 1.3 The right to information and self-determination: treatment (Speechley 1992).

norms for example collective decision-making (Boston 1993; Wilkins 1993). The consent process requires careful assessment of the person's needs and use of verbal and non-verbal communication skills to elicit the degree of control they wish to exercise and how much information is desired (Hansson 1998), and to acknowledge respect for this.

This model provides a flexible framework in which the patient always leads but which is not onerous to themselves or the practitioner, and also enables joint or negotiated decision making to occur. A schematic representation is shown in Fig. 1.3 (Speechley 1992). The concept has been further developed in public in the late 1990s (Kings Fund 1997) and several papers have considered both shared decision-making and patients' rights and responsibilities (Buetow 1998).

Lack of autonomy, refusal of treatment and advance directives

Problems arise, however, when an individual is not, or has never been, autonomous as they are accorded no rights. In this situation an autonomous proxy may enter consent on behalf of a minor using a 'best interests' approach as required by law, or the incompetent adult may be treated within the health care professional's duty of care using the same criteria (Law Commission 1995).

If a patient has been autonomous but is no longer, the right to self-determination may be exercised using an advance directive. The ethical issues surrounding the right to anticipatory decision making, particularly related to refusal of treatment and rejection of life-prolonging procedures, have been widely discussed but mainly in the context of actively withdrawing treatment (Scowen 1993, 1994; Craig 1994; Ashby & Stoffell 1995; Dunlop et al. 1995) or with people who have AIDS (Schlyter 1992), including 'do not resuscitate' orders.

An instruction by the patient fits comfortably within a rights-based theoretical framework and this view has recently been accepted in English law (*Re T* 1992; *Re C*

1993). Although these cases dealt primarily with refusal of treatment in both instances, advance directives are acknowledged and commented upon.

In *Re T* Lord Donaldson, Master of the Rolls, states that the patient must express his wishes 'in clear terms', preferably in writing. It is Grubb's opinion (1992) that *Re T* had 'undoubtedly given the "green light" for advance directives in the form of "living wills"'.

In *Re C* this stance was reinforced as C did not just wish to prevent amputation of his leg at the time he was competent but also in the future when he might become incompetent. Once again Grubb's view (1993) is that 'The injunction granted by Thorpe, J. only gave court backing to what was already legally binding upon the doctors'. Competency (autonomy) was an issue in this case and Grubb welcomes the three stage approach adopted by Mr Justice Thorpe as 'it is important . . . that the law does not make the hurdle of competence too onerous otherwise the law will effectively deprive all but the most "comprehending" of their right of self determination'.

Nevertheless, this view is disputed by some (Stauch 1995) and endorsed by others, namely the Law Commission in its report on mental incapacity (1995). This includes a section on advance statements in health care which 'embraces anticipatory decision-making by the person while competent to make arrangements for future incapacity'.

Summary

Exploration of moral theory and principles enables the discovery of an approach which places the patient at the centre of decision-making, but in a flexible and pragmatic way. Rights emerge as positive claims which are enduring. The non-autonomous (legally incompetent) individual is protected within the professional's duty of care.

Conflict between the wishes of the patient, the professional and occasionally the relatives may be resolved more easily within this framework and the process of allocating pre-eminence to one duty or principle unnecessary.

The legal basis for consent

> A patient has the right under common law to give or withhold consent prior to examination or treatment. . . . This is one of the basic principles of health care. (DoH 1990).

English common law identifies three components of a valid consent:

1 Competency
2 Information
3 Voluntariness.

If an examination, procedure or treatment is carried out without these requirements being fulfilled then a civil action may be brought in the tort of battery, which protects a person from unwanted touching, or in the tort of negligence, where harm results directly from the procedure. It is the health care professional's duty to ensure that a person is competent to consent, has sufficient information on which to base their decision and that the decision is voluntary and uncoerced (DoH 1990).

Competency

Competency or capacity to consent to a procedure must be considered in all situations. It should not be assumed that an adult or a child is competent, or incompetent, without a full assessment of that individual. The law provides some guidance here.

Minors, that is children under the age of 16 years: following *Gillick* v. *West Norfolk and Wisbech AHA* (1986), in which the lawfulness of prescribing contraceptives to a minor was considered, a competent child is defined as one who '. . . is capable of understanding what is proposed, and of expressing his or her wishes . . .' (Lord Justice Fraser). In practice, most children are accompanied by their parents or legal guardians who will formally consent after discussion with the child and health care professional. In the case of a child who is not competent, a parent will usually offer a proxy consent on behalf of their child. Others who may be empowered to act as proxy for a child are laid down in the Children Act 1989 [in Scotland, the Age of Legal Capacity (Scotland) Act 1991]. All proxies must adopt a 'best interests' approach, that is they act in the child's best interests, inherent in which is that the examination, procedure or treatment is therapeutic and intended to benefit the particular individual. However, there is a view developing in health care research that actions which would 'not be against the interests of the child' may also be acceptable (Grubb 1997).

Persons between the ages of 16 and 18 years: The Family Law Reform Act 1969 states in section 8 (1) that:

> The consent of a minor who has attained the age of sixteen years to any surgical, medical or dental treatment which, in the absence of consent, would constitute a trespass to his person, shall be as effective as it would be if he were of full age; and where a minor has by virtue of this section given an effective consent to any treatment it shall not be necessary to obtain any consent for it from his parent or guardian.

If a person between 16 and 18 years is not competent, using the 'Gillick' definition, a proxy consent will be appropriate, as for minors.

Although statute law and common law indicate who is competent to consent, there is a contradiction regarding competency to refuse treatment. Recent cases, *Re R* (a minor) (wardship: medical treatment) 1991 and *Re W* (minor: refusal of treatment) 1992, one concerning a child under 16 and one over (Grubb 1993), have given both a parent and a court the power to override a refusal of treatment by a competent child.

Adults: when considering if an adult is competent to consent to a clinical procedure, an individual approach is, once again, necessary as Lord Donaldson, Master of the Rolls, pointed out (*Re T* 1992) that:

> . . . every adult is presumed to have . . . capacity [to consent], but it is a presumption which can be rebutted.

This was stated in a contrasting way by Skegg (1984):

> The fact that a person is suffering from a mental disorder, as defined in the Mental Health Act 1983, does not in itself preclude that person from giving a legally effective consent.

There are several circumstances within health care, and more specifically cancer care, where capacity to consent may be wrongly perceived to be present or absent. Examples include:

1 Persons with mental disabilities or learning disorders, where capacity may be dependent solely on the communication skills of the health care professional.
2 Patients with cerebral tumours where a physical disability or speech impediment does not necessarily indicate an impairment of comprehension.
3 Patients who are in pain, emotionally distressed or shocked and temporarily lacking competency which may by restored by pain relief, time, patience and psychological support.

Competency, as defined by the courts and for the purposes of this section, is based on the capability of a person to understand and express a view. Therefore, all measures to assist this process must be employed, such as provision of interpreters, including those proficient in British sign language, and the involvement of speech and language therapists for people with communication difficulties. Examples of legal, health and social services cases where choices have been influenced by communication can be found in *Access to Justice* (Nuffield Foundation 1993).

With regard to proxy consent on behalf of an incompetent adult, the view put forward by Professor Skegg is that

> ... there is no general doctrine whereby a spouse or near relative is empowered to give legally effective consent to medical procedures to be carried out on an adult.

The common law appears to support this view and Lord Goff (*Re F* 1990, in Kennedy & Grubb 1994), concerning sterilization, uses the principle of necessity to solve the practical problems related to this. He says '. . . the doctor must then act in the best interests of his patient, just as if he had received his patient's consent to do so'. However, the decision will most frequently be taken after discussion with relatives, carers and other health care professionals. In cases of conflicting views or doubt, the courts should be consulted.

Information

> Patients are entitled to receive sufficient information in a way that they understand about proposed treatments, the possible alternatives and any substantial risks, so that they can make a balanced judgement. (DoH 1990)

As Kennedy & Grubb point out (1994):

> The aphorism 'informed consent' has entered the language as being synonymous with valid consent. . . . The requirement that consent be informed is only one, albeit a very important

ingredient of valid consent. Furthermore, the expression informed consent begs all the necessary questions . . . for example, how informed is informed?

So how much information is required by English law to be given to the patient? Various medical negligence cases provide a background to the current requirements and some clarification of the Department of Health's statement which opens this section. These legal cases also provide the definition of the standard of care which patients may expect from all health care professionals carrying out procedures such as those contained in this manual.

In *Hills v. Potter* (1984) Mr Justice Hirst states:

> . . . on any view English law does require the surgeon to supply to the patient information to enable the plaintiff to decide whether or not to undergo the operation.

He continues:

> . . . In my judgement, McNair, J. in *Bolam v. Friern Barnet Hospital Management Committee* (1957) applied the medical standard to advice prior to an operation, as well as to diagnosis and to treatment. . . . In every case the court must be satisfied that the standard contended for on their behalf accords with that upheld by a substantial body of medical opinion, and that this body of medical opinion is both respectable and responsible, and experienced in this particular field of medicine.

The amount and quality of information became the point at issue once again in *Sidaway v. Board of Governors of the Bethlem Royal Hospital* (1985). The majority judgement in the House of Lords confirmed the view expressed in *Hills v. Potter*. However, two new elements were identified in Sidaway. First was the need to warn of risk which Lord Bridge described as a 'substantial risk of grave adverse consequences'. Lord Templeman offered a similar but slightly more specific definition:

> There is no doubt that a doctor ought to draw the attention of a patient to a danger which may be special in kind or magnitude or special to the patient.

Despite these statements it was acknowledged that this remains an area where clinical judgement is the prime determinant.

Second was the duty to answer questions which, again, was addressed by Lord Bridge who said:

> when questioned specifically by a patient of apparently sound mind about the risks involved in a particular treatment proposed, the doctor's duty must, in my opinion, be to answer both truthfully and as fully as the questioner requires.

The importance of assessment – what is important, or likely to be important, to the patient – and communication of information is reinforced here. Sometimes the content of an answer may not be in doubt but the means of communicating it may be vital to understanding, and the subsequent decision.

There have been several 'failure to warn' cases since Sidaway in the mid-1980s, all of which have supported the views expressed by one or other of their Lordships. However, courts in other common law jurisdictions have challenged the judgement in Sidaway, notably Australia in 1992 (Kirby 1995).

In 1994 three cases of actions for negligence addressed the issue of information in the English courts. In *Smith v. Barking, Havering and Brentwood Health Authority*, the surgeon was found to be negligent in having failed to warn of the risks inherent in the operation and failing to inform the plaintiff of the possible consequences of not having the operation (Stern 1995). Also in *Smith v. Salford Health Authority* the surgeon was found to be negligent in his pre-operative assessment of the patient and his explanation of the risks of both treatment and non-treatment (Stern 1995). However, in neither instance did the actions succeed on the basis of this alone, as in both it was found that even if given the appropriate information, the patients would have consented to the operations and, therefore, the outcome would have been unchanged. In the third case, *Smith v. Tunbridge Wells Health Authority* (1994) negligence was proven based on non-disclosure of information. Mr Justice Morland considered that the patient would have been acting reasonably in refusing to follow the surgeon's advice and have the operation if he had known of the risk of impotence associated with it. Therefore, the harm was caused by lack of information.

Provision of information to patients to achieve a valid consent to examination, treatment and care requires the health care professional to use their clinical judgement:

- To assess the amount of information needed by the patient and carers
- To explain the procedure clearly and accurately
- To provide honest answers to the patient's questions in a sympathetic manner.

These require considerable communication skills and, perhaps most important of all, time.

Kirby (1995) concludes with a criticism of the differing standards of information between England and other countries, saying

> ... at the heart of the difference is an attitude to the fundamental rights of the particular patients. Those rights should take primacy both in legal formulae and in medical practice.

There is an indication that the English courts may become more prescriptive in determining the standard of care, and therefore the standard of information required, in the future (Lewis 1998).

Voluntariness

> Consent to treatment must be given freely and without coercion ... (DoH 1990).

In the USA the President's Commission report on making health care decisions (1983) (in Kennedy & Grubb 1994) considered voluntariness in decision making thus:

> The patient's participation in the decision making process and ultimate decision regarding care must be voluntary. A choice that has been coerced, or that resulted from serious manipulation of a person's ability to make an intelligent and informed decision, is not the person's own free choice. This has long been

recognised in law: a consent forced by threats or induced by fraud or misrepresentation is legally viewed as no consent at all.

Within this statement three issues are identified – force, coercion and manipulation.

The nature of cancer, the vulnerability of an individual faced with an unfamiliar and frightening environment and the disproportionate amount of power and perceived inequality between health care professional and patient may all, to varying degrees, intrude into the decision making process.

Force is not a concept normally associated with health care. However, the subtle features of this are explained by the President's Commission (1983) (in Kennedy & Grubb 1994):

> Although it is typically not viewed as forced treatment, a good deal of routine care ... is provided without explicit and voluntary consent by patients. The expectation on the part of professionals is that patients, once in such a setting, will simply go along with such routine care.

This far-reaching report included a survey of treatment refusals and observational studies in care settings where the communications which accompanied the care offered no choice, compliance was expected and enforced. In addition the routine tests or acts of care were those most likely to be refused.

Coercion is

> ... when the person is credibly threatened by another individual, either explicitly or by implication, with unwanted and avoidable consequences unless the patient accedes to the specified course of action. (President's Commission 1983 in Kennedy & Grubb 1994)

Coercion is typically perceived to be associated with an imbalance of power between professional and patient, and this may indeed be so. However, the motivation may be benevolent when conflicts arise as to the best course of action to be taken but, even so, this cannot be condoned.

Pressure may also be exerted by family or carers, acting with the patient's best interests in mind or from an ulterior motive to further their own ends. All members of the caring team need to be aware of this possibility and, if the situation arises, support the patient and assist them to overcome such pressure.

Manipulation is often a more subtle way of influencing the voluntary nature of choice. For example, while on one hand information may be withheld or distorted, alternatives may not be presented and risks may be minimized, on the other hand '... a professional's careful choice of words or nuances of tone and emphasis might present the situation in a manner calculated to heighten the appeal of a particular course of action' (President's Commission 1983).

Many legal cases relate to institutional settings where it could be said that there is no freedom to exercise choice. However in *Re T* (adult: refusal of treatment) 1992 Lord Donaldson offered guidance as to what could be considered undue influence by English law:

> ... (t)he doctors have to consider whether the decision is really that of the patient ... (d)oes the patient really mean what he says or is he merely saying it for a quiet life, to satisfy

someone else, or because the advice and persuasion to which he has been subjected is such that he can no longer think and decide for himself?'

Lord Donaldson went on to say that consideration should also be given to the strength of will of the patient and the relationship between the patient and the persuader, whether personal or professional. In *Re T* it was found that using these criteria T's decision (to refuse a blood transfusion) was not her own but that of her mother.

In cancer care health professionals have several responsibilities related to the voluntary nature of decision making:

- To recognize the vulnerability of patients and to be alert to circumstances when undue influence may be exerted by colleagues or relatives.
- To gain consent for all investigations, treatment or acts of care and not to assume that 'routine' procedures will be carried out automatically.
- To communicate effectively and impartially with patients to enable them to reach a voluntary decision, and to offer support for that decision.

Since voluntariness is one of the foundation stones of . . . consent, professionals have a high ethical obligation to avoid coercion and manipulation of their patients. The law penalises those who ignore the requirements of consent or who directly coerce it. (President's Commission 1983 in Kennedy & Grubb 1994).

Summary

'The ethical principle that each person has a right to self determination finds its expression in law through the concept of consent' (Kennedy & Grubb 1994). The authors go on to quote the definitive statement of Mr Justice Cardoza in *Schloendorff* v. *Society of New York Hospitals* (1914):

Every human being of adult years and sound mind has a right to determine what shall be done with his own body; and a surgeon who performs an operation without his patient's consent commits an assault . . .

The scope of this statement has now been expanded as health care has become increasingly sophisticated and personnel performing invasive procedures have become multidisciplinary. The consent procedure is formalized and explicit and continuing consent should be obtained throughout all stages of management.

Issues relating to consent

Waiver

Within the rights-based ethical framework outlined, rights are perceived as discretionary and, therefore, can be waived or relinquished. There is little opinion expressed in English law regarding the legal validity of waiver. Kennedy & Grubb (1994) are of the view that:

while the patient may waive the right to information as to risks or whatever, it would be against public policy to allow him to waive the right to be informed of the 'nature and purpose' of the proposed procedure.

The North American view was expressed by the President's Commission (1983) (in Kennedy & Grubb 1994) as follows:

it is questionable whether patients should be permitted to waive the professional's obligation to disclose fundamental information about the nature and implications of certain procedures (such as, 'when you wake up, you will learn that your limb has been amputated' or 'that you are irreversibly sterile'). In the absence of explicitly legal guidance, health care professionals should be quite circumspect about allowing or disallowing, encouraging or discouraging, a patient's use of waiver.

However, within its report it also comments

The impact of the waiver exception is that if a waiver is properly obtained the patient remains the ultimate decision maker, but the content of his decision is shifted . . . from the equivalent of 'I want this treatment (or that treatment or no treatment)' to 'I don't want any information about the treatment' . . .

which allows the patient to exercise his rights. As previously described, the health care professional may proceed with treatment using the 'best interests' approach.

Treatment without consent

As is clear from both the legal and ethical basis for consent, treatment without consent is only permissible in an emergency situation where there is no explicit refusal, oral or written, which has been entered by the patient.

Emergency treatment has been defined as that which is both necessary and cannot be reasonably delayed. Lord Goff in *Re F* states

Where, for example, a surgeon performs an operation without his consent on a patient temporarily rendered unconscious in an accident, he should do no more than is reasonably required, in the best interests of the patient, before he recovers consciousness. I can see no practical difficulty arising from this requirement, which derives from the fact that the patient is expected before long to regain consciousness and can then be consulted about longer term measures.

In many situations the relatives may be consulted but the onus is on the health care professional to assess the need for examination or treatment and proceed accordingly.

The more troublesome issue of what is permissible when a secondary condition is discovered during the course of an operative procedure – whether a surgeon should proceed with treatment or await the patient's recovery and gain consent – requires the practitioner to differentiate between necessity and convenience.

The form and scope of consent

Consent may be implied or explicit. Implied consent may be illustrated by a patient who rolls up their sleeve to allow their blood pressure to be measured or a blood sample to be taken. This is regarded by many commentators as unsatisfactory (Kennedy & Grubb 1994) and at best should be

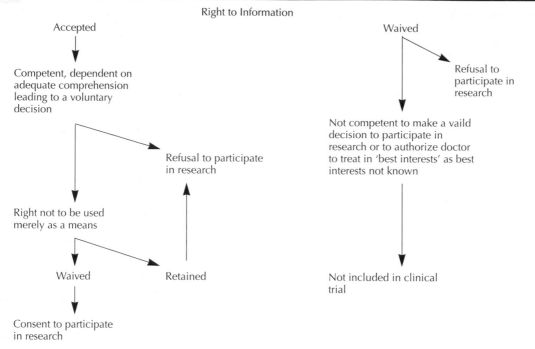

Figure 1.4 The right to information and self-determination: research (Speechley 1992).

regarded only as the absence of any objection. This form of consent may only be acceptable if a procedure is negligible in terms of risk and non-invasiveness.

Explicit or express consent may be verbal or, more commonly, written. Which form is employed will depend on the relationship between professional and patient, the nature of the procedure – invasiveness, degree of physical or psychological risk or harm – and local policy. The Department of Health has extended the necessity to obtain written consent from operative procedures alone to examinations, investigations and non-surgical treatments. Written consent is increasingly becoming the norm in most areas of clinical practice.

However, a written consent form is merely evidence of what was agreed between practitioner and patient. The process by which that consent was obtained is by far the more important dimension, as discussed previously. Moreover, consent can be said to be valid only at the time at which it is given. It is the professional's responsibility to reaffirm that the patient has not changed his mind between the signature being placed on the form and the procedure occurring. This is particularly important when a series of treatments (or course of treatment), investigations or procedures is embarked upon, often with intervals of days or weeks in between each one.

Research

The clinical procedures within this book may be carried out in either a treatment or research setting. The research

will usually be therapeutic but it is not the sole intention to benefit the patient, the demands of science are also served. There is currently no statute law which governs the conduct of research generally, but considerable guidance has been produced in recent years (Foster 1997) and regulatory bodies exist to consider research proposals and advise NHS bodies (DoH 1991). Consent to research is of equal importance with consent to treatment, and many would argue more so, but it is not within the brief of this chapter to discuss these issues in detail. Consent to research, however, must be explicit and well informed. From the legal perspective a health care professional cannot justify any action without this by using a 'best interests' defence when these are unknown. From an ethical point of view the patient is asked to consent not only to therapy but to agree to be used as a means to the ends of research. Briefly these are just two of the differences between consent to treatment and consent to research which require greater debate and are fully discussed in other references (Baum 1990; Botros 1990; Williams 1992; Hansson 1998). A schematic representation is shown in Fig. 1.4 (Speechley 1992).

Conclusion

The procedures in this book affect the whole person. They range from those which are observational and physically non-invasive to those involving intrusion into both the physical body and the psychological persona. The intent also varies; some are diagnostic, others therapeutic and some are supportive with the aim of increasing well-being. Finally, there are those where the purpose is to resuscitate the individual or to prolong their life.

This introductory chapter has emphasized, and reiterated, the need for the patient to be the central focus, whatever the situation and whatever the procedure or activity. Assessment is the starting point, to ascertain the patient's attitudes, beliefs and values, and to discover their needs – the amount of involvement they wish to have in their care, how much information they require and what is acceptable to them, particularly as their disease experience progresses.

Assessment is impossible without the ability to communicate, using both verbal and non-verbal skills to explore, and allow expression of, the patient's feelings. Fear of many of the procedures described here may exist – because they are unknown, because of previous experiences or because of what may be revealed. Good, clear communication may be able to allay fears, minimize discomfort and enable individual adjustment.

The nature and complexity of the consent process, required for all procedures, relies greatly on both assessment and communication skills in order to be conducted in a responsible manner. Both the ethical and legal background emphasize the need for dynamic assessment and the importance of not making assumptions or dismissing what the patient says or expresses.

Conflicts due to lack of congruence between professionals' and patients' beliefs or priorities are not uncommon and can be painful for both parties, for example leading to refusal of treatment. It is hoped that this chapter will help to avoid, minimize or resolve such dilemmas.

References

Alderson, P. (1993) *Children's Consent to Surgery*. Open University Press, Buckingham.

Alfaro-Lefevre, R. (1994) *Applying Nursing Process*, 3rd edn. J.B. Lippincott, Philadelphia.

Allen, D. (1998) Record-keeping and routine nursing practice: the view from the wards. *J Adv Nurs*, **27**, 1223–30.

Ardern-Jones, A. & Eeles, R. (1997) Predictive gene testing for breast cancer. *Trends Urol Gynaecol Sexual Health*, Jan/Feb, 1–2.

Ashby, M. & Stoffell, B. (1995) Artificial hydration and alimentation at the end of life: a reply to Craig. *J Med Ethics*, **21**(3), 135–40.

Bannister, P. & Kagan, C. (1985) The need for research into interpersonal skills in nursing. In: *Interpersonal Skills in Nursing: Research and Applications* (ed. C. Kagan). Croom Helm, Beckenham.

Barnett, D. (1997) Clinical applications. *Inf Tech Nurs*, **9**(1), 7–8.

Baum, M. (1990) The ethics of clinical research. In: *Ethics and Law in Health Care and Research* (ed. P. Byrne). Wiley, Chichester.

Beauchamp, T.L. & Childress, J.F. (1994) *Principles of Biomedical Ethics*, 4th edn. Oxford University Press, Oxford.

Bluebond-Langner, M. (1978) *The Private Worlds of Dying Children*. Princeton University Press, New Jersey.

Bluglass, K. (1991) Care of the cancer patient's family. In: *Cancer Patient Care: Psychosocial Treatment Methods* (ed. M. Watson). BPS Books and Cambridge University Press, Cambridge.

Borgers, R., Mullen, P., Meertens, R. *et al.* (1993) The information-seeking behaviour of cancer outpatients: a description of the situation. *Patient Educ Counsel*, **22**(1), 35–46.

Boston, P. (1993) Culture and cancer: the relevance of cultural orientation within cancer education programmes. *Eur J Cancer Care*, **2**, 72–6.

Botros, S. (1990) Equipoise, consent and the ethics of randomised clinical trials. In: *Ethics and Law in Health Care and Research* (ed. P. Byrne). Wiley, Chichester.

Bowling, A. (1997) *Measuring Health – A Review of Quality of Life Measurement Scales*, 2nd edn. Open University Press, Buckingham.

Brennan, W. & Swan, T. (1995) *Managing Violence and Aggression. Royal College of General Practitioners, Members' Reference Book*, pp. 443–5. Sabrecrown, London.

Brereton, M. (1995) Communication in nursing: the theory–practice relationship. *J Adv Nurs*, **21**, 314–24.

British Association for Counselling (1989a) *BAC Training Directory*. BAC, Rugby.

British Association for Counselling (1989b) *Code of Ethics and Practice for Counselling Skills*. BAC, Rugby.

Buetow, S. (1998) The scope for the involvement of patients in their consultations with health professionals: rights, responsibilities and preferences of patients. *J Med Ethics*, **24**, 243–7.

Burnard, P. (1990) *Learning Human Skills: An Experiential Guide for Nurses*, 2nd edn. Heinemann Nursing, Oxford.

Burton, M. (1991) Counselling in routine care: a client-centred approach. In: *Cancer Patient Care: Psychosocial Treatment Methods* (ed. M. Watson). BPS Books and Cambridge University Press, Cambridge.

Burton, M. & Watson, M. (1998) *Counselling People with Cancer*. John Wiley, Chichester.

Carpenito, L.J. (1993) *Nursing Diagnosis. Application to Clinical Practice*, 5th edn. J.B. Lippincott, Philadelphia.

Chin, S., Kucuk, O., Peterson, R. & Ezdinli, E. (1992) Variables contributing to anticipatory nausea and vomiting in cancer chemotherapy. *Am J Clin Oncol*, **15**(3), 262–7.

Corney, R., Everatt, H., Howells, A. *et al.* (1992) The care of patients undergoing surgery for gynaecological cancer: the need for information, emotional support and counselling. *J Adv Nurs*, **17**(6), 667–71.

Craig, G.M. (1994) On withholding nutrition and hydration in the terminally ill: has palliative medicine gone too far? *J Med Ethics*, **20**(3), 139–43.

Crockford, E., Holloway, I. & Walker, J. (1993) Nurses' perceptions of patient' feelings about breast surgery. *J Adv Nurs*, **18**, 1710–18.

Davies, S., Laker, S. & Ellis, L. (1997) Promoting autonomy and independence for older people within nursing practice: a literature review. *J Adv Nurs*, **26**, 408–417.

Davitz, L. *et al.* (1976) Suffering as viewed in six different cultures. *Am J Nurs*, **76**(8), 1296–7.

Dennison, S. (1995) An exploration of the communication that takes place between nurses and patients whilst cancer chemotherapy is administered. *J Clin Nurs*, **4**(4), 227–33.

DoH (1990) *Patient Consent to Examination or Treatment*. HC (90)22. Stationery Office, London.

DoH (1991) *Local Research Ethics Committees*. HSG 91(5). Stationery Office, London.

DoH (1995) *The Patient's Charter*. Stationery Office, London.

Douglas, J. (1993) *Psychology and Nursing Children*, (ed. D. Muller). BPS Books, Leicester.

Dunlop, R.J., Ellershaw, J.E. & Baines, M.J. (1995) On withholding nutrition and hydration in the terminally ill: has palliative medicine gone too far? A reply. *J Med Ethics*, **21**(3), 141–3.

Dworkin, R. (1984) Rights as trumps. In: *Theories of Rights* (ed. J. Waldron). Oxford University Press, Oxford.

Eeles, R. (1995) Developments in the study of familial breast cancer. *Nurs Times*, **91**(5), 29–33.

Eeles, R., Stratton, M., Goldgar, D. *et al.* (1994) The genetics of familial breast cancer and their practical implications. *Eur J Cancer*, **30a**(9), 1383–90.

Egan, G. (1994) *The Skilled Helper: A Systematic Approach to Effective Helping*, 5th edn. Brooks/Cole, Belmont, California.

Ehrenberg, A., Ehnfors, M. & Thorell-Ekstrand, I. (1996) Nursing documentation in patient records: experience of the use of the VIPS model. *J Adv Nurs*, **24**, 853–67.

Eilers, J., Berger, A.M. & Petersen, M.C. (1988) Development, testing, and application of the oral assessment guide. *Oncol Nurs Forum*, **15**(3), 325–30.

Eiser, C. (1993) *Growing Up with a Chronic Disease: The Impact on Children and Their Family*. J. Kingsley, London.

Fallowfield, L., Lipkin, M. & Hall, A. (1998) Teaching senior oncologists communication skills: results from phase 1 of a comprehensive longitudinal program in the United Kingdom. *J Clin Oncol*, **16**(5), 1961–8.

Faulkner, A. (1986) Talking to patients. Human interest. *Nurs Times*, **82**(33), 33–4.

Faulkner, A. & Maguire, P. (1984) Teaching assessment skills. In: *Recent Advances in Nursing 7, Communication* (ed. A. Faulkner). Churchill Livingstone, Edinburgh.

Fawcett, J. (1995) *Analysis and Evaluation of Conceptual Models for Nursing*, 3rd edn. F.A. Davis, Philadelphia.

Foster, C. (1997) *Manual for Research Ethics Committees*, 5th edn. Centre for Medical Law and Ethics, King's College, London.

Frank-Stramborg, M. & Olsen, S.J. (1997) *Instruments for Clinical Health Care – Research*, 2nd edn. Jones and Bartlett, London.

George, J.B. (1995) *Nursing Theories, the Base for Professional Nursing Practice*, 4th edn. Prentice Hall, London.

Gillick v. West Norfolk and Wisbech AHA (1986) AC 112, 1985 3 All ER 402, 1985 2 BMLR 11 (HL). In: *Medical Law: Text with Materials*, 2nd edn. (I. Kennedy & A. Grubb), p. 111. Butterworths, London, Dublin and Edinburgh.

Glaser, B. & Strauss, A. (1965) *Awareness of Dying*. Weidenfeld and Nicolson, London.

Gogas, H. & Sacks, N. (1996) Familial breast cancer. *Cancer J*, **9**(3), 115–17.

Goossen, W.T.F., Epping, P.J.M.M. & Dassen, T. (1997) Criteria for nursing information systems as a component of the electronic patient record. *Comput Nurs*, **15**(6), 307–315.

Gordon, M. (1994) *Nursing Diagnosis, Process and Application*. Mosby, Missouri.

Gray, S. (1995) Role of the Research nurse. *Nurs Times*, **91**(5), 33–5.

Greer, S. & Watson, M. (1987) Mental adjustment to cancer: its measurement and prognostic importance. *Cancer Surveys*, **6**, 439–53.

Grubb, A. (1992) Refusal of medical treatment I – the competent adult. *Dispatches*, **3**(1), 1–4.

Grubb, A. (1993) Refusal of medical treatment II – the competent child. *Dispatches*, **3**(2), 6–8.

Grubb, A. (1997) The law relating to consent. In: *Manual for Research Ethics Committees*, 5th edn. (ed. C. Foster). Centre for Medical Law and Ethics, King's College, London.

Hansson, M.O. (1998) Balancing the quality of consent. *J Med Ethics*, **24**, 182–7.

Hardwick, S. (1998) Clarification of nursing diagnosis from a British perspective. *Assign – Ongoing Work Health Care Stud*, **4**(2), 3–9.

Hargie, O. *et al.* (1987) *Social Skills in Interpersonal Communication*, 2nd edn. Routledge, London.

Hart, H.L.A. (1984) Are there any natural rights? In: *Theories of Rights* (ed. J. Waldron). Oxford University Press, Oxford.

Hayward, K. (1998) Patient-held oncology records. *Nurs Stand*, **12**(35), 44–6.

Health Service Commissioner for England, Scotland and Wales (1992–1993) *Annual Report*. Stationery Office, London.

Heartfield, M. (1996) Nursing documentation and nursing practice: a discourse analysis. *J Adv Nurs*, **24**, 98–103.

Heath, H. (1998) Reflection and patterns of knowing in nursing. *J Adv Nurs*, **27**, 1054–9.

Hewison, A. (1995) Nurses' power in interactions with patients. *J Adv Nurs*, **21**(1), 75–82.

Hills v. Potter (1984) 1 WLR 641n. In: *Medical Law: Text with Materials*, 2nd edn. (I. Kennedy & A. Grubb), pp. 172–3. Butterworths, London, Dublin and Edinburgh.

Hocking, J. & Shamash, J. (1998) Poor record keeping harms patient care, says report. *Nurs Stand*, **12**(21), 5.

Hogston, R. (1997) Nursing diagnosis and classification systems: a position paper. *J Adv Nurs*, **26**, 496–500.

Hughes, K. (1993) Decision making by patients with breast cancer: the role of information in treatment selection. *Oncol Nurs Forum*, **20**(4), 623–8.

Hunter, M. (1998) Rehabilitation in cancer care: a patient focused approach. *Eur J Cancer Care*, **7**, 85–7.

Jarman, F. (1995) Communication problems: a patient's view. *Nurs Times*, **91**(18), 30–31.

Jarrett, N. & Payne, S. (1995) A selective review of the literature on nurse–patient communication: has the patients' contribution been neglected? *J Adv Nurs*, **22**(1), 72–8.

Jenner, E.A. (1998) A case study analysis of nurses' roles, education and training needs associated with patient focused care. *J Adv Nurs*, **27**, 1087–95.

Josten, D., Evans, A. & Love, R. (1985) The cancer prevention clinic: a service program for cancer-prone families. *J Psychosoc Oncol*, **3**, 5–20.

Katoaka-Yahirom & Saylor C. (1995) Critical thinking in nursing. In: Hardwick, S. (1995) Clasification of nursing diagnosis from a British perspective. *Assign – Ongoing Work Health Care Stud*, **4**(2), 3–9.

Kemp, N. & Richardson, E. (1994) *The Nursing Process and Quality Care*. Edward Arnold, London.

Kennedy, I. & Grubb, A. (1994) *Medical Law: Text with Materials*, 2nd edn. Butterworths, London, Dublin and Edinburgh. (See subject of 'Waiver', pp. 232–3; 'Implied Consent', p. 101; 'Making Health Care Decisions', pp. 233–5.)

Kings Fund (1997) Promoting patient choice together. *Conference Proceedings*. Kings Fund, London.

Kirby, M. (1995) Patients' rights – why the Australian courts have rejected *Bolam*. *J Med Ethics*, **21**, 5–8.

Koocher, G. & O'Malley, J. (1991) *The Damocles Syndrome*. McGraw Hill, New York.

Lack, L. & Holloway, I. (1992) Post surgical hormone replacement therapy: information needs of women. *J Clin Nurs*, **1**, 323–7.

Lambe, N. (1995) The law on mental incapacity: a major overhaul. *Dispatches*, **5**(3), 3–5.

Lansdown, R. & Goldman, A. (1991) Children with cancer. In: *Cancer Patient Care: Psychosocial Treatment Methods* (ed. M. Watson). BPS Books and Cambridge University Press, Cambridge.

Larson, P. (1984) Important nurse caring behaviours perceived by patients with cancer. *Oncol Nurs Forum*, **11**, 46–50.

Larsson, G., Widmark Peterson, V., Lampic, C. *et al.* (1998) Cancer patient and staff ratings of the importance of caring behaviours and their relations to patient anxiety and depression. *J Adv Nurs*, **27**, 855–64.

Last, B. & VanVeldhuizen, A. (1992) *Developments in Paediatric Oncology*. Taylor and Francis, Washington DC.

Lauri, S., Lepisto, M. & Kappeli, S. (1997) Patients' needs in hospital: nurses' and patients' views. *J Adv Nurs*, **25**, 339–46.

Law Commission (1995) Report on mental incapacity. *Bull Med Ethics*, **106**, 13–18.

Leih, P. & Salentijn, C. (1994) Nursing diagnosis: a Dutch perspective. *J Clin Nurs*, **3**, 313–20.

Lev, E., Munro, B.H. & McCorkle, R. (1993) A shortened version of an instrument measuring bereavement. *Int J Nurs Stud*, **30**(3), 213–26.

Lewis, P. (1998) Law notes. *Dispatches*, **8**(2/3), 7–9.

Lloyd, S., Watson, M., Waites, B. *et al.* (1996) Familial breast cancer: a controlled study of risk perception, psychological morbidity and health beliefs in women attending for genetic counselling. *Br J Cancer*, **74**, 482–7.

McCann, K. & McKenna, H. (1993) An examination of touch between nurses and elderly patients in a continuing care setting in Northern Ireland. *J Adv Nurs*, **18**, 838–46.

Mackie, J.L. (1984) Can there be a right-based moral theory? In: *Theories of Rights* (ed. J. Waldron). Oxford University Press, Oxford.

Macleod Clark, J. & Sims, S. (1988) Communication with patients and relatives. In: *Oncology for Nurses and Health Care Professionals*, Vol. 2 (eds R. Tiffany & P. Webb), 2nd edn. Harper and Row, Beaconsfield.

Macleod Clark, J. *et al.* (1991) Progression to counselling. *Nurs Times*, **87**(8), 41–3.

Maguire, P. (1985) Barriers to psychological care of the dying. *Br Med J*, **291**, 1711–13.

Mallett, J. (1989) Taking patients round. *Nurs Times*, **85**(38), 37–9.

Mallett, J. (1997) *Nurse–patient haemodialysis sessions: orchestrated institutional communication and mundane conversations*. PhD thesis, Open University.

Meissner, H., Anderson, D. & Odenkirchen, J. (1990) Meeting information needs of significant others: use of the cancer information service. *Patient Educ Counsel*, **15**(2), 171–9.

Metcalf, C. (1998) Stoma care: exploring the value of effective listening. *Br J Nurs*, **7**(6), 311–15.

Moorey, S. & Greer, S. (1989) *Psychological Therapy for Patients with Cancer: A New Approach*. Heinemann Medical, Oxford.

Motyka, M., Motyka, H. & Wsolek, R. (1997) Elements of psychological support in nursing care. *J Adv Nurs*, **26**, 909–912.

Muller, D., Harris, P. & Wattley, L. (1992) *Nursing Children: The Psychology, Research and Practice*, 2nd edn. Chapman & Hall, London.

Naish, J. (1996) The route to effective nurse–patient communication. *Nurs Times*, **93**(17), 27–30.

Nichols, K. (1993) *Psychological Care in Physical Illness*, 2nd edn. Chapman & Hall, London.

Northhouse, L., Cracchiolo-Caraway, A. & Pappas Appel, C. (1991) Psychologic consequences of breast cancer on partner and family. *Semin Oncol Nurs*, **7**(3), 216–33.

Nuffield Foundation (1993) *Access to Justice: Non-English Speakers in the Legal System*. Nuffield Interpreter Project, Nuffield Foundation, London.

O'Neill, E.S. & Dluhy, N.M. (1997) A longitudinal framework for fostering critical thinking and diagnostic reasoning. *J Adv Nurs*, **26**, 825–32.

Orem, D.E. (1991) *Nursing: Concepts of Practice*, 4th edn. Mosby, St Louis.

Parle, M., Maguire, P. & Heaven, C. (1997) The development of a training model to improve health professionals' skills, self-efficacy and outcome expectancies when communicating with cancer patients. *Soc Sci Med*, **44**(2), 231–40.

Pease, A. (1981) *Body Language: How to Read Others' Thoughts by their Gestures*. Sheldon Press, London.

Peplau, H.E. (1992) Interpersonal relations: a theoretical framework for application in nursing practice. *Nurs Sci Q*, **5**, 13–18.

Piper, B.F. (1997) Measuring fatigue. In: *Instruments for Clinical Health Care Research*, 2nd edn. (eds M. Frank-Stromborg & S.J. Olsen), pp. 482–96. Jones and Bartlett, Massachusetts.

Porchet-Munro, S. (1991) Aspects of non-verbal communication. *Recent Results Cancer Res*, **121**, 313–20.

Poroch, D. (1995) The effect of preparatory patient education on the anxiety and satisfaction of cancer patients receiving radiation therapy. *Cancer Nurs*, **18**(3), 206–14.

Pruitt, B., Walgora-Serafin, B., McMahon, T. *et al.* (1993) An educational intervention for newly diagnosed cancer patients undergoing radiotherapy. *Psycho-Oncol*, **2**, 55–62.

Ramirez, A., Richardson, M., Rees, G. *et al.* (1994) Effective communication in oncology. *J Cancer Care*, **3**, 84–93.

Razavi, D. & Delvaux, N. (1997) Communication skills and psychological training in oncology. *Eur J Cancer*, Suppl. **6**, S15–21.

Re C (Adult: refusal of treatment) (1993) in Law update. *Dispatches*, **4**(1), 10–12.

Re T (Adult: refusal of treatment) (1992). 4 All English (law) Reports 649 (CA).

Richardson, A. & Wilson Barnett, J. (eds) (1995) *Nursing Research in Cancer Care*. Scutari Press, London.

Ricketts, T. (1996) General satisfaction and satisfaction with nursing communication on an adult psychiatric ward. *J Adv Nurs*, **24**(3), 478–87.

Roebuck, A. (1998) Critical pathways: an aid to practice. *Nurs Times*, **94**(35), 50–51.

Rogers, C. (1967) *On Becoming a Person*. Constable, London.

Rogers, C. (1980) *A Way of Being*. Houghton Mifflin, Boston.

Schapiro, D., Boggs, R., Melamed, B. *et al.* (1992) The effect of varied physician affect on recall, anxiety and perceptions in women at risk for breast cancer: an analogue study. *Health Psychol*, **11**(1), 61–6.

Schlyter, C. (1992) *Advance Directives and AIDS*. Centre for Medical Law and Ethics, King's College, London.

Scowen, E. (1993) The case of Anthony Bland – reflections. *Dispatches*, **4**(1), 1–4.

Scowen, E. (1994) The case of Anthony Bland – further reflections. *Dispatches*, **4**(2), 10–11.

Scullion, J.E. & Henry, C. (1998) A multidisciplinary approach to managing breathlessness in lung cancer. *Int J Palliat Nurs*, **4**(2), 65–9.

Sepion, B. (1988) Children with cancer. In: *Oncology for Nurses and Health Care Professionals*, Vol. 2 (eds R. Tiffany & P. Webb), 2nd edn. Harper and Row, Beaconsfield.

Sidaway v. Board of Governors of the Bethlem Royal Hospital (1985) AC 871; 1985 1 All ER 643. In: *Medical Law: Text with Materials*, 2nd edn. (I. Kennedy & A. Grubb), pp. 173–84. Butterworths, London, Dublin and Edinburgh.

Skegg, P.D.G. (1984) Law ethics and medicine. In: *Medical Law: Text with Materials*, 2nd edn. (I. Kennedy & A. Grubb), p. 116. Butterworths, London, Dublin and Edinburgh.

Smith v. Tunbridge Wells Health Authority (1994) 5 Med LR 334. In: Law Notes. *Dispatches*, **5**(3), 8–10.

Smith, G., Sr & Richardson, A. (1996) Development of nursing documentation for use in the outpatient oncology setting. *Eur J Cancer Care*, **5**, 225–32.

Smith, P. (1992) Familial breast and ovarian cancers. *Semin Oncol Nurs*, **8**(4), 258–64.

Speechley, V. (1992) *Provision of an information service for people with cancer: legal and ethical issues*. MA thesis, King's College, London.

Stauch, M. (1995) Rationality and the refusal of medical treatment: a critique of the recent approach of the English courts. *J Med Ethics*, **2**(3), 162–5.

Stern, K. (1995) What might have happened? Causation in cases of negligent medical ommission. *Dispatches*, **5**(2), 1–3.

Suominen, T., Leino-Kilpi, H. & Laippala, P. (1994) Nurses' role in informing breast cancer patients: a comparison between patients' and nurses' opinions. *J Adv Nurs*, **19**, 6–11.

The Age of Legal Capacity (Scotland) Act 1991. Stationery Office, London.

The Children Act 1989. Stationery Office, London.

The Family Law Reform Act 1969. Stationery Office, London.

The Mental Health Act 1983. Stationery Office, London.

Thompson, J. (1988) Adolescents with cancer. In: *Oncology for Nurses and Health Care Professionals* (eds R. Tiffany & P. Webb), Vol. 2, 2nd edn. Harper and Row, Beaconsfield.

Tierney, A.J. (1998) Nursing models: extant or extinct? *J Adv Nurs*, **28**(1), 77–85.

United Kingdom Central Council for Nursing, Midwifery and Health Visiting (1989) *Exercising Accountability*. UKCC, London.

United Kingdom Central Council for Nursing, Midwifery and Health Visiting (1992) *Code of Professional Conduct*. UKCC, London.

United Kingdom Central Council for Nursing, Midwifery and Health Visiting (1993) *Standards for Records and Record Keeping*. UKCC, London.

Vachon, M. (1995) Staff stress in hospice/palliative care: a review. *Palliat Med*, **9**, 91–122.

Walker, V.A. *et al.* (1987) Pain Assessment Chart in the management of chronic pain. *Palliat Med*, **1**, 111–16.

Watson, M. (1983) Psychosocial interventions with cancer patients: a review. *Psychol Med*, **13**, 839–46.

Watson, M., Lloyd, S. & Eeles, R. (1996) Psychological impact of testing for the BRCA 1 breast cancer gene: an investigation of two families in the research setting. *Psycho-Oncol*, **5**, 233.

Webster, M. (1981) Communicating with dying patients. *Nurs Times*, 4 June, 999–1002.

Wilkins, H. (1993) Transcultural nursing: a selective review of the literature 1985–1991. *J Adv Nurs*, **18**, 602–612.

Wilkinson, S. (1991) Factors which influence how nurses communicate with cancer patients. *J Adv Nurs*, **16**, 677–88.

Wilkinson, S. (1992) Effective communication: learning from ourselves. In: *Proc 7th Int Conf Cancer Nurs* (ed. C. Bailey), pp. 62–7. Rapid Communications, Oxford.

Wilkinson, S. (1995) The changing pressures for cancer nurses 1986–93. *Eur J Cancer Care*, **4**, 69–74.

Wilkinson, S. (1999) Schering Plough clinical lecture communication: it makes a difference. *Cancer Nurse*, **22**(1), 17–20.

Wilkinson, S., Roberts, A. & Aldridge, J. (1998) Nurse–patient communication in palliative care: an evaluation of a communication skills programme. *Palliat Med*, **12**, 13–22.

Williams, C. (ed.) (1992) *Introducing New Treatments for Cancer: Practical, Ethical and Legal Problems*. Wiley, Chichester.

Williams, C. *et al.* (1994) A framework for patient assessment. *Nurs Stand*, **8**(38), 29–33.

Wilmoth, M.C. (1994) *Development and testing of the sexual behaviours questionnaire*. Department of Nursing, Central Missouri State University, Missouri.

Wilson-Barnett, J. (1982) Studies evaluating patient teaching: implications for practice. *Int J Nurs Stud*, **20**(1), 33–44.

Wong, C. & Bramwell, L. (1992) Uncertainty and anxiety after mastectomy for breast cancer. *Cancer Nurs*, **15**(5), 363–71.

Yates, P. (1999) Family coping: issues and challenges for cancer nursing. *Cancer Nurse*, **22**(1), 63–71.

Abdominal Paracentesis

Definition

Abdominal paracentesis is the puncture of the abdominal wall with an abdominal trochar and cannula, which is inserted into the peritoneal cavity (Hoerr & Osol 1956; Oliver 1996). This is usually for the relief of ascites and the management of symptoms (Eriksonn & Redlin Frazier 1997). The cannula may also be used for the administration of solutions into the peritoneal cavity.

Indications

Abdominal paracentesis is indicated under the following circumstances:

1 To obtain a specimen of fluid for analysis
2 To relieve the symptoms associated with ascites, both physical and psychological
3 To administer substances such as radioactive gold colloid or cytotoxic drugs (e.g. bleomycin, cisplatin) into the peritoneal cavity, to achieve regression of serosae deposits responsible for fluid formation.

Reference material

Abdominal ascites is an 'abnormal accumulation of serous (oedematous) fluid within the peritoneal cavity'. It can be caused by non-malignant conditions such as advanced congestive heart failure, chronic pericarditis and cirrhosis of the liver, or by malignant conditions such as metastatic cancer of the ovary, stomach, colon or breast (Kehoe 1991; Preston 1995). It is accompanied by debilitating symptoms of breathlessness, indigestion, alteration in bowel habit, fatigue, ankle oedema, reduced mobility, loss of appetite, nausea and vomiting, abdominal swelling, pain and change in body image (Preston 1995; Parsons et al. 1996). For some patients, minimal ascites can cause great distress through the effect upon their body image and the meaning of the symptoms to the individual (Preston 1997).

Symptomatic paracentesis is still the mainstay of treatment for patients with malignant ascites, giving good, although temporary, relief of symptoms in about 90% of patients (Ross et al. 1989). Analysis of ascitic fluid is required to establish cause, however it has been suggested that only 50% of patients have their fluid analysed for malignant cells (Kehoe 1991; Parsons et al. 1996; Preston 1997).

Abdominal paracentesis is not undertaken lightly because of the risk of inducing hypovolaemia, hypokalaemia or hyponatraemia (Kehoe 1991). Because ascitic fluid contains proteins, repeated paracentesis may cause protein depletion (Zehner & Hoogstraten 1985; Preston 1997). The serum albumin may also be lowered substantially (Parsons et al. 1996). Occasional complications include perforation of the bowel, which can be reduced by ultrasound guided paracentesis (Ross et al. 1989; Preston 1997; Eriksonn & Redlin Frazier 1997). The introduction of infection during insertion of the ascitic drain can be reduced by following aseptic technique (Kehoe 1991). Up to 13% of patients may develop an abdominal wall metastasis at the puncture site following abdominal paracentesis and, depending upon the size of the abdominal wall metastasis, radiotherapy may be required (Krutiwagen et al. 1996). Ascitic fluid may become loculated in the peritoneal cavity, making it difficult to drain the ascitic fluid. Large amounts of fluid in the peritoneal cavity cause an increase in intra-abdominal pressure. There may be pain as a result of pressure on internal structures. Gastric pressure may cause anorexia, indigestion or hiatus hernia. Intestinal pressure may result in constipation, bowel obstruction or decreased bladder capacity. Pressure on the diaphragm decreases the intrathoracic space and causes shortness of breath.

The relief of symptoms following paracentesis can be dramatic. Many cancer patients with ascites have a prognosis of only a few months (Zehner & Hoogstraten 1985), and the procedure is often justified by the relief offered. The insertion of cytotoxic agents such as bleomycin or cisplatin may delay or prevent recurrence of malignant effusions (Ostrowski 1986; Howell 1988).

Nursing care

Nursing care of patients with abdominal ascites is aimed at relief of the suffering caused by the symptoms. Care of the patient undergoing abdominal paracentesis is directed at prevention of discomfort and complications. It is an invasive procedure performed by a doctor assisted by a nurse at the patient's bedside.

There is much debate about whether it is safe to drain large volumes of fluid rapidly from the abdomen. Profound hypotension may follow because of the sudden release of intra-abdominal pressure and consequent possible vasodilation. Kearney (1990) recommends a rate of 1 litre every 2 hours up to a maximum of 4 litres, and states that removing large amounts of ascitic fluid from frail patients can be debilitating, suggesting that a 'partial' paracentesis may be enough to relieve symptoms. Regnard & Mannix (1989) state that it is usual to drain to dryness over 6 hours.

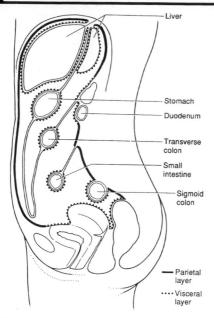

Figure 2.1 Peritoneum of female in lateral view.

1 Parietal layer – this covers the abdominal and pelvic walls and the under surface of the diaphragm
2 Visceral layer – this lines and supports the abdominal organs and the parietal peritoneum (Fig. 2.1).

Fluid is produced from the capillaries lining the peritoneal cavity and is drained by lymphatic vessels under the diaphragm. The fluid is collected by the right lymphatic duct which drains into the vena cava. However, in patients with malignant ascites, this balance of production and drainage is disrupted, and ascitic fluid collects in the peritoneal cavity. The increased production of fluid in the peritoneal cavity in the presence of a tumour is due to increased permeability (Hirabayashi & Graham 1970).

The ascitic fluid accumulated is called exudate and is protein rich (Preston 1997). It has been demonstrated that patients with malignant ascites have a marked decrease in flow from the peritoneal cavity due to blockage of the diaphragmatic lymphatics (Bronskill *et al.* 1977). A separate cause is compression of the hepatic portal vein by a tumour, leading to fluid being forced into the peritoneal cavity. Fluid produced as a result of mechanical obstruction is called a transudate and is low in protein concentration (Preston 1997).

Functions of the peritoneum

1 The peritoneum is a serous membrane which enables the abdominal contents to glide over each other without friction.
2 It forms partial or complete cover for the abdominal organs.
3 It forms ligaments and mesenteries which help keep the organs in position.
4 The mesenteries contain fat and act as a store for the body.
5 The mesenteries can move to engulf areas of inflammation and this prevents the spread of infection.
6 It has the power to absorb fluids and exchange electrolytes.

Smith & Powles (1993) recommend that no more than 2 litres are drained initially, then 1 litre every 4 hours for 24 hours, and finally free drainage. They also recommend that if ascitic protein content exceeds 20 g/l, protein should be replaced by intravenous infusion of 4.5% human albumin. Speed of drainage has not been evaluated in malignant ascites with drainage regimens ranging from 1 litre per hour to 1 litre per 24 hours (Preston 1997). Clinical practice at The Royal Marsden Hospital reflects a drainage pattern of 1 litre every 4 hours depending on the medical condition of the patient. Albumin replacement is not common in the treatment of malignant ascites.

Nursing interventions for patients undergoing abdominal paracentesis include education about the nature of the procedure, about what results can realistically be expected, and about the importance of diet and fluid intake to replace proteins and fluid lost in the ascitic fluid. Consideration must be given at this point to quality of life and what expectations the patient and her family have, with full knowledge of the course of disease (Eriksson & Redlin Frazier 1997). Regular observations must be carried out to detect early signs of shock and infection, which can then be treated quickly. Drainage of the fluid must be monitored regularly, volumes recorded and blockages detected and managed. Patients may require assistance to move and position themselves, and may experience pain requiring careful repositioning or appropriate analgesia (see the Nursing Care Plan).

Anatomy and physiology

The peritoneum is a semi-permeable serous membrane consisting of two separate layers:

References and further reading

Bronskill, M., Bush, R. & Ege, G. (1977) A quantitative measurement of peritoneal drainage in malignant ascites. *Cancer* **40**, 2375–80.
Eriksson, J. & Redlin Frazier, S. (1997) Epithelial cancers of the ovary and fallopian tube. In: *Women and Cancer; a Gynaecologic Oncology Nursing Perspective* (ed. G.J. Moore). Prentice Hall, London, pp. 232–4.
Hirabayashi, K. & Graham, J. (1970) Genesis of ascites in ovarian cancer. *Am J Obstet Gynaecol*, **106**, 492–7.
Hoerr, N. & Osol, A. (eds) (1956) *Blakiston's New Gould Medical Dictionary*. McGraw Hill, New York.
Howell, S.B. (1988) Intraperitoneal chemotherapy for ovarian cancer. *J Clin Oncol*, **6**, 1673–5.
Kearney, M. (1990) Gynaecologic malignancy: care of the terminally ill. In: *Clinical Gynaecological Oncology* (eds J.H. Shepherd & J.M. Monaghan), 2nd edn. Blackwell Scientific Publications, Oxford.
Kehoe, C. (1991) Malignant ascites: etiology, diagnosis and treatment. *Oncol Nurs Forum*, **18**, 523–30.

Krutiwagen, R. et al. (1996) Incidence and effect on survival of abdominal wall metastases at trocar of puncture sites following laparoscopy or paracentesis in women with ovarian cancer. *Gynaecol Oncol*, **60**, 233–7.

Lifschitz, S. (1982) Ascites: pathophysiology and control measures. *Int J Radiat Oncol Biol Phys*, **8**, 1423–6.

Marieb, E.N. (1989) *Human Anatomy and Physiology*. The Benjamin/Cummings Publishing Co Inc, Redwood City.

Maxwell, M.B. (1997) Malignant effusions and edemas. In: *Cancer Nursing: Principles and Practice* (eds S.L. Groenwald, M. Hansen Frogge, M. Goodman, et al.). Jones & Bartlett, London, pp. 721–41.

Oliver, G. (1996) Gynaecological tumors. In: *Nursing the Patient with Cancer* (ed V. Tschudin). Prentice Hall, London, pp. 17–281.

Ostrowski, M. (1986) An assessment of the long-term results of controlling the reaccumulation of malignant effusions using intracavity bleomycin. *Cancer*, **57**, 721–7.

Parsons, S.L., Lang, M.W. & Steele, R.J. (1996) Malignant ascites: a two year review from a teaching hospital. *Eur J Surg Oncol*, **22**, 237–9.

Parsons, S.L., Watson, S.A. & Steele, R.J. (1996) Malignant ascites: review. *Br J Surg*, **83**, 6–14.

Preston, N. (1995) New strategies for the management of malignant ascites. *Eur J Cancer Care*, **4**, 178–83.

Preston, N. (1997) Current practice in the management of malignant ascites. *J Cancer Care*, **13**, 144–6.

Regnard, C. & Mannix, K. (1989) Management of ascites in advanced cancer: a flow diagram. *Palliative Medicine*, **4**, 45–7.

Regnard, C. & Tempest, S. (1992) *A Guide to Symptom Relief in Advanced Cancer*, 3rd edn. Haigh & Hochland, Manchester.

Ross, G., Kessler, H., Clair, M. et al. (1989) Sonographical guided paracentesis for palliation of symptomatic malignant ascites. *Am J Roentgenol*, **153**, 1309–11.

Sears, W. & Winwood, R. (1985) *Anatomy and Physiology for Nurses*, 6th edn. Edward Arnold, London.

Smith, I.E. & Powles, T.J. (1993) Specific medical problems: effusions, brain, spinal and meningeal disease. In: *Medical Management of Breast Cancer* (eds T.J. Powles & I.E. Smith). Dunitz, London.

Twycross, R.G. & Lack, S.A. (1990) *Therapeutics in Terminal Cancer*, 2nd edn. Churchill Livingstone, Edinburgh.

Zehner, L.C. & Hoogstraten, B. (1985) Malignant effusions and their management. *Semin Oncol Nurs*, **1**(4), 259–68.

GUIDELINES · Abdominal paracentesis

Equipment

1 Sterile abdominal paracentesis set containing forceps, scalpel blade and blade holder, swabs, towels, suturing equipment, trocar and cannula (or other approved catheter and introducer), connector to attach to the cannula and guide fluid into the container.

2 Sterile dressing pack.

3 Sterile receiver.

4 Sterile specimen pots.

5 Local anaesthetic.

6 Needles and syringes.

7 Chlorhexidine 0.5% in 70% alcohol.

8 Adhesive dressing.

9 Large sterile drainage bag or container (with connector if appropriate to attach to cannula).

10 Gate clamps.

11 Sterile gloves.

12 Weighing scales if appropriate.

13 Tape measure if appropriate.

Procedure

Action

1 Explain and discuss the procedure with the patient.

2 Ask the patient to void bladder.

3 Weigh patient before and after procedure and record if appropriate

4 Ensure privacy.

5 Measure patient's girth around umbilicus before and after procedure and record if appropriate.

6 The patient should lie supine in bed with the head raised 45–50 cm with a back rest.

Rationale

To ensure that the patient understands the procedure and gives his/her valid consent.

If the bladder is full there is a chance of it being punctured when the trocar is introduced.

To assess if weight changes due to the fluid loss.

This provides an indication of fluid shift and how much fluid has reaccumulated.

Normally the pressure in the peritoneal cavity is no greater than atmospheric pressure, but, when fluid is present, pressure becomes greater than atmospheric pressure. This position will then aid gravity in the removal of fluid and the fluid will drain of its own accord until the pressure is equalized.

Guidelines • *Abdominal paracentesis (cont'd)*

Action	Rationale
7 The procedure is performed by a doctor assisted by a nurse throughout:	To reduce the risk of local and/or systemic infection. The peritoneal cavity is normally sterile.
(a) The abdomen is prepared aseptically and draped with sterile towels. Local anaesthetic is administered.	
(b) Once the anaesthetic has taken effect the doctor makes an incision.	To minimize pain during the procedure and thus maximize patient comfort and facilitate cooperation.
(c) The trocar and cannula are inserted via the incision.	
(d) The trocar is removed.	
8 Ascitic fluid is collected (20–100 ml as instructed by the doctor) and sent for cytology.	In order to diagnose the cause of ascites.
9 If the cannula is to remain in position, sutures will be inserted.	To ensure cannula remains in situ. To reduce risk of trauma to the patient.
10 A closed drainage system is now attached to the cannula using a connector if appropriate. A supportive dry dressing applied and taped firmly in position.	A sterile container with a non-return valve is necessary to maintain sterility. To reduce local and/or systemic infection.
11 Monitor the patient's blood pressure, pulse and respirations and observe the rate and nature of the drainage. A clamp should be available on the tubing to reduce the flow of fluid if necessary.	To observe for signs of shock and/or infection, and to ensure unobstructed drainage.
12 Monitor the patient's fluid balance. Encourage a high-protein and high-calorie diet.	After removal of large amounts of peritoneal fluid, fluid moves from the vascular space and reaccumulates in the peritoneal cavity. Ascitic fluid contains protein in addition to sodium and potassium. Problems of dehydration and electrolyte imbalance may be present.
13 When the cannula is withdrawn, apply a sterile dressing to the wound.	To maintain asepsis and protect the wound.

GUIDELINES • Removal of an intraperitoneal drain (short term)

Equipment

1 Sterile dressing pack.
2 Sterile gloves.
3 Stitch cutter (if drain has a suture holding it in place).
4 Adhesive tape.

5 Transparent dressing.
6 Gauze (low linting).
7 Bactericidal alcohol hand rub (if appropriate).

Procedure

This procedure is usually carried out by a member of the nursing team who has been instructed in the removal of intraperitoneal drains.

Action	Rationale
1 Explain and discuss the procedure with the patient.	To ensure the patient understands the procedure and gives his/her valid consent.
2 Establish that the patient is comfortable, and is not in pain or allergic to the tape to be used.	To reduce unnecessary discomfort and to ensure the patient will not have a local reaction to the tape.
3 Wash hands with bactericidal soap and water or bactericidal alcohol hand rub.	To reduce the risk of infection.

4 Prepare equipment using aseptic technique. Apply gloves.

To minimize the risk of contamination.

5 Remove the old dressing.

To allow access to the relevant area.

6 Cut the knot from the purse-string suture (if present).

To allow mobility of the suture.

7 Cut the suture holding the drain in place. A second nurse may be required to hold the drain in place.

To free the drain and prevent it falling out.

8 Tie the purse-string suture loosely at skin level.

To enable rapid tightening of the suture when the drain is removed.

9 Instruct patient to breathe normally, explain that you are about to take the drain out and steadily pull the drain out.

To ensure that the patient is fully aware of what is about to happen so as not to cause unnecessary distress.

10 As the drain leaves the skin, tighten the purse-string suture and tie a firm double knot.

To prevent leakage of fluids.

11 Place gauze over the site and secure it firmly. A transparent dressing may also be used to provide a seal.

To prevent leakage of fluids.

12 Explain to the patient that the procedure is complete and that there may be some temporary leakage. In the event of this occurring, the dressing will be changed or a stoma bag may be placed over the site for a short period of time.

To reduce the risk of and prevent the patient becoming distressed if there is leakage and to reduce risk of contamination to clothes.

13 Ensure the patient is comfortable and clear the equipment away.

To reduce the risk of cross-infection.

14 Wash hands with bactericidal soap and water.

To reduce the risk of cross-infection.

15 Measure fluid drained and record in appropriate document.

To provide an accurate record.

16 Record vital signs and document procedure done.

To ascertain that the patient is stable and to promote continuity of care and for future reference.

Nursing care plan

Problem	Cause	Suggested action
Patient exhibits shock.	Major circulatory shift of fluid or sudden release of intra-abdominal pressure, vasodilatation and subsequent lowering of blood pressure.	Clamp the drainage tube with a gate clamp to prevent further fluid loss. Record the patient's vital signs. Refer to the medical staff for immediate intervention.
Cessation of drainage of ascitic fluid.	Abdomen is empty of ascitic fluid.	Check with the total output of ascitic fluid given on the patient's fluid balance chart. Measure the patient's girth; compare this measurement with the pre-abdominal paracentesis measurement. Suggest to medical staff that the cannula should be removed. Discontinue the drainage system.
	Patient's position is inhibiting drainage.	Change the patient's position, i.e. move the patient upright or onto his/her side to encourage flow by gravity.

Problem	Cause	Suggested action
	The ascitic fluid has clotted in the drainage system.	'Milk' the tubing. If this is unsuccessful, change the drainage system aseptically.
Signs of local or systemic infection.	Bacterial invasion at site of abdominal paracentesis cannula.	Obtain a swab from the site of the cannula for cultural review. Apply a dry dressing. Refer to the medical staff.
Cannula becomes dislodged.	Ineffective sutures or trauma at the puncture site.	Apply a dry dressing. Inform the medical staff.
Pain.	Pressure of ascites or position of drain.	Identify cause. Anchor drain securely to avoid pulling at insertion site or movement within abdomen. Assist patient with repositioning. Administer appropriate prescribed analgesic, monitor the patient's response and inform medical staff.

Aseptic Technique

3

Definition

Aseptic technique is the effort taken to keep the patient as free from hospital micro-organisms as possible (Crow 1989). It is a method used to prevent contamination of wounds and other susceptible sites by organisms that could cause infection. This can be achieved by ensuring that only sterile equipment and fluids are used during invasive medical and nursing procedures. Potter & Perry (1992) suggest that there are two types of asepsis: medical and surgical asepsis. Medical or clean asepsis reduces the number of organisms and prevents their spread; surgical or sterile asepsis includes procedures to eliminate microorganisms from an area and is practised by nurses in operating theatres and treatment areas.

Indications

Patients have a right to be protected from preventable infection and nurses have a duty to safeguard the well-being of their patients (King 1998). An aseptic technique should be implemented during any invasive procedure that bypasses the body's natural defences, e.g. the skin and mucous membranes, or when handling equipment such as intravenous cannulae and urinary catheters that have been used during these procedures. However, it is difficult to maintain sterility. A study to evaluate contamination during routine aseptic techniques found contamination ranging from 0 to 11.3% with an overall rate of 2.7% in theatre, whilst tests conducted in conditions of industrial sterility standards, showed a contamination rate of 0.16% (Klapes et al. 1987). Briggs et al. (1996) suggest assessment of the individual patient's circumstances before each procedure. By predicting and planning for potential problems asepsis can be maintained.

Reference material

Hospital acquired infection (also called nosocomial infection) is defined as infection occurring in patients after admission to hospital that was neither present nor incubating at the time of admission. Infections acquired in hospital but not manifest until after the patient is discharged are included in the definition (Ayliffe et al. 1992). Crowe & Cooke (1998) reviewed the case definition for nosocomial infections, finding areas of concensus and variation which made comparisons of infection rates difficult.

The cost of infection is high, both to the patient and the hospital. Nosocomial infections increase mortality and morbidity and cause an increase in pain and suffering experienced by the patients (Sproat & Inglis 1992). The patient may be inconvenienced by a prolonged period of hospitalization, which can cause economic and social hardships to the whole family. The hospital will have increased waiting lists and increased hospital costs. It is essential that when aseptic techniques are used as a method of preventing infection that these procedures are sound in theory and are carried out correctly.

The cost of nosocomial infections to the NHS in 1992 was an estimated £110 million (Chapman et al. 1993). Health authorities recognize the significance of nosocomial infections and employ infection control teams to:

1 Reduce the likelihood of patients being exposed to infectious micro-organisms while in hospital.
2 Provide adequate care for patients with communicable infections.
3 Minimize the likelihood of employees, visitors and communicable contacts being exposed to infectious micro-organisms.
4 Develop policies for appropriate management of patients with communicable infections.
5 Provide surveillance systems which give adequate feedback to appropriate staff.
6 Provide education in techniques to prevent the emergence and spread of infection.

A 10-year study in the USA found that an infection control team reduced the incidence of nosocomial infection by up to 32%. Hospitals in the study with no infection control programme experienced an increase in infection rates of up to 18% (Haley et al. 1985a). A 3-year study reported a reduction in the infection rate from 10.5 to 5.6% following the introduction of an infection control team (French et al. 1989). It has been estimated that a reduction by one fifth of the UK nosocomial infection rate of 5% would save the NHS £15.6 million, even if the costs of infection control teams and programmes are taken into account (Chaudhuri 1993).

A survey of factors which influence compliance with infection control procedures highlighted lack of knowledge, lack of time and shortage of staff and the standard set by senior staff including surgeons and nurses (Sherwood 1995) as relevant indicators. It was suggested that greater emphasis and knowledge may motivate staff to make time for correct compliance with infection control procedures. The importance of the ward sister being convinced of the need for strict asepsis and insisting medical and nursing staff adhere to hospital policy has also been emphasized (Krakowska 1986).

When cross-infection does occur the cost of investigating and controlling even a small outbreak is high. It has been estimated that an infected patient has an average increased hospital stay of 17 days and average increased costs of £2220 (O'Donaghue & Allen 1992), emphasizing how important it is to prevent infection. The Infection Control Standards Working Party has prepared standards for practice to make prevention, detection and control of infection in hospitals as effective as possible (Infection Control Standards Working Party 1993). Surgical wound infections are the second most common nosocomial infection in England and Wales, which is directly related to wound contamination at the time of operation (Table 3.1) (Cruse & Foord 1980).

Similarly, urinary tract infections continue to be the most common hospital acquired infections. The prevalence study in 1980 by the Public Health Laboratory showed that urinary tract infection caused 30.3% of all infections; of the 8.6% of patients catheterized, 21.2% had infections, compared with 2.9% in non-catheterized patients (Meers *et al.* 1981), illustrating the association between invasive procedure and infection.

The diagnosis of infection relies on classic signs of inflammation such as local redness, swelling and pain, although decreased numbers of neutrophils produce minimal or atypical clinical signs of infection (Candell & Whedon 1991). These local signs and symptoms can precede a further sequence of events, which can be lymphangitis, lymphadenitis, bacteraemia and septicaemia which, if not promptly recognized and treated, can result in death (Laurence 1991).

A study to assess nurses' adherence to aseptic techniques revealed an unanticipated high number of errors (McLane *et al.* 1983). The nurses' heavy workload was a contributing factor in poor compliance to aseptic techniques, which suggests that unnecessary time consuming aspects of an aseptic technique should be avoided (Kelso 1989). This view is supported by Bree-Williams & Waterman's (1996) study, which highlighted that the practice of aseptic technique has become ritualistic and complex, and simpler practices are easier, cheaper and are not detrimental to the patients.

Gwyther (1988) discusses how most teaching occurs on the hospital ward and questioned whether this teaching was based on knowledge of the principles of, for example, wound care, or simply on experience. Jenks & Ferguson (1994) reviewed the discrepancy between what is taught in the classroom and what nurses experience in the clinical setting. This suggested that collaboration is needed between education and service staff to integrate learning within the nursing curricula. Thomlison (1990) emphasizes the importance of replacing infection control procedures which involve unnecessary ritual with sound, cost efficient and environmentally responsible practices to encourage a greater understanding of the principles of asepsis. These authors highlight a continuing problem and it has been suggested that the principles of aseptic techniques need to be re-established (Lund & Caruso 1993), to ensure nurses understand the importance of prevention of infection (Davey 1997).

Principles of asepsis

Infection is caused by organisms which invade the host's immunological defence mechanisms, although susceptibility to infection may vary from person to person (Gould 1994b). The risk of infection is increased if the patient is immunocompromised (Hart 1990) by:

1 Age. Neonates and the elderly are more at risk due to their less efficient immune systems.
2 Underlying disease. For example, those patients with severe debilitating or malignant disease.
3 Prior drug therapy, such as the use of immunosuppressive drugs or the use of broad-spectrum antimicrobials.
4 Patients undergoing surgery or instrumentation.

The following factors must be considered when nursing immunocompromised patients (Trester 1982):

1 Classic signs and symptoms of infection are often absent.
2 Untreated infection may disseminate rapidly.
3 Infections may be caused by unusual organisms or organisms which, in most circumstances, are non-pathogenic.
4 Some antibiotics are less effective in immunocompromised patients.
5 Repeated infections may be caused by the same organism.
6 Superimposed infection is a frequent occurrence requiring nursing care of the highest standard to prevent infection (Gurevich *et al.* 1986), which includes strict adherence to aseptic techniques.

Sproat & Inglis (1992) suggest that a basic principle of infection control for all patients is to assess the risk of infection from one patient to another and to plan nursing care accordingly before action is taken. Haley *et al.* (1985b) add that if each patient is evaluated individually it is possible to focus more closely on those patients who are most susceptible to infection. The most usual means for spread of infection include:

1 Hands of the staff involved
2 Inanimate objects, e.g. instruments and clothes
3 Dust particles or droplet nuclei suspended in the atmosphere.

Hand washing

Hand washing is well researched and uncontroversial (Briggs *et al.* 1996), having been found to be the single

Table 3.1 Category of wound and infection rate.

Category of wound	Infection rate (%)
Clean	1.5
Clean contaminated	7.7
Contaminated	15.2
Dirty	40.0

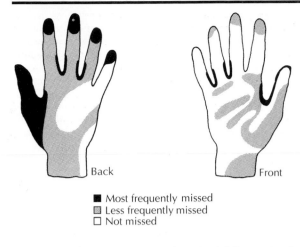

■ Most frequently missed
▨ Less frequently missed
☐ Not missed

Figure 3.1 Areas most commonly missed following hand washing. (Reproduced by kind permission of *Nursing Times*, where this article first appeared in 1978.)

most important procedure for preventing nosocomial infection as hands have been shown to be an important route of transmission of infection (Casewell *et al.* 1977). Even brief contact can transmit 10 000 colony-forming units to hands (Gould 1993), and wearing rings increases the number of micro-organisms on the hands (Jacobson *et al.* 1985). However, studies have shown that hand washing is rarely carried out in a satisfactory manner (Taylor 1978a), with the most important factor inhibiting hand washing being busyness (Larson *et al.* 1982) or inaccessible sinks (Albert *et al.* 1981). Studies have shown that up to 89% of staff miss some part of the hand surface during hand washing (Taylor 1978a) (Fig. 3.1).

Taylor (1978b) and Phillips (1989) use Feldman's criteria for hand washing, which include the following:

1 Roll up sleeves, remove rings and wrist watches.
2 Use soap.
3 Use continuously running water.
4 Position hands to avoid contaminating arms.
5 Avoid splashing clothing or floor.
6 Rub hands together vigorously.
7 Use friction on all surfaces.
8 Rinse hands thoroughly with hand held down to rinse.
9 Dry hands thoroughly.

Hand washing should be undertaken after patient contact and before an aseptic technique is performed (Centre for Disease Control 1986).

Gould (1993) pointed out that *Klebsiella* could survive 150 minutes on nurses' hands during normal duty. Transient bacteria can be almost completely removed from the hands by soap and water washing (Lowbury *et al.* 1974a). Conversely, soap and water do not reduce the number of resident bacteria by any significant amount. Resident skin flora, such as *Staphylococcus aureus*, are removed most effectively by rubbing the hands with a bactericidal alcoholic solution of chlorhexidine. Lowbury *et al.* (1974b) showed that rinsing the hands with alcoholic chlorhexidine

0.5% removed more resident skin flora than did washing the hands with a chlorhexidine 4% detergent wash. Alcoholic hand rubs are as effective as the more time consuming, conventional antiseptic detergent hand wash method (Pereira *et al.* 1997). Alcoholic hand rub also reduces the shedding of bacteria and skin squames after handwashing (Meers & Yeo 1978). Kampf *et al.*'s (1998) study showed that a chlorhexidine based alcoholic hand rub was more effective against MRSA than the conventional chorhexidine detergent.

It is suggested that a preparation such as chlorhexidine 4% detergent wash is used for cleaning physically dirty or contaminated hands, while a bactericidal alcoholic hand rub should be used for disinfecting clean hands immediately before carrying out an aseptic technique. A dispenser of alcoholic hand rub should be placed on the lower shelf of all trolleys used for aseptic techniques, to allow hands to be cleaned during the aseptic technique. A nurse with 'socially clean' hands will not need to wash them during the aseptic procedure, but should use a bactericidal alcoholic hand rub whenever disinfection is required, e.g. after opening the outer wrappers of dressings. It is unlikely that nurses' hands will become soiled with blood or body fluids as long as blood and body fluid precautions are adopted at all times (Hart 1991). The use of a hand rub will also remove the need for the nurse to leave the patient during the procedure to wash the hands at the nearest basin, during which time contamination (Kelso 1989) or cooling of the wound may occur which can inhibit healing (Johnson 1987).

Paper towels have been shown to be a quick, convenient and reliable method of drying hands (Blackmore 1987) and are preferable to a roller towel which could be a source of cross-infection (Rowland & Alder 1972). Hot air dryers which dry hands slowly and, in some cases, inadequately (Matthews & Newman 1987), may discourage some people from washing their hands (Blackmore 1987).

One study found that electric air dryers were very effective in removing *Escherichia coli* and rotaviruses from washed hands (Ansari *et al.* 1991), while Matthews & Newman (1987) found no difference between paper or air dryers in the reduction of bacteria on hands following hand washing. However, electric hand dryers can disperse bacteria for about 1 m around the dryer, which suggests that dryers are unsuitable for use in critical patient care areas (Ngeow *et al.* 1989). This view is supported by Gould (1994a).

No-touch technique

A no-touch technique is essential to ensure that hands, even though they have been washed, do not contaminate the sterile equipment or the patient. This can be achieved either by the use of forceps or sterile gloves (Lascelles 1982). However, it must be remembered that gloves can become damaged and allow the passage of bacteria (Rowland *et al.* 1985; Reingold *et al.* 1988), while forceps may damage tissue (David 1991).

The availability of gloves and antibiotics has given a false sense of security when providing wound care. It has been reported that prolonged glove use can produce occlusion conditions which encourage the rapid growth of skin flora on nurses' hands (Pereira *et al.* 1997). It is, therefore, essential to wash hands following removal of gloves.

Inanimate objects

All instruments, fluids and materials that come into contact with the wound must be sterile if the risk of contamination is to be reduced. Crow (1994) suggests four principles of asepsis which are, know what is sterile, and what is not sterile, keep these two types of items separate and replace contaminated items immediately. The sterile supplies department should normally provide all sterile instruments. The manufacturer's recommendations for all clinical supplies must be followed at all times. The reuse of single use items must not occur and could result in legal, economic and ethical consequences (Medical Devices Agency 1995). In the event of supplies being short in an emergency, it is acceptable to disinfect a clean instrument, such as a pair of scissors, by immersing it completely in 70% ethanol alcohol for 10 minutes. This will destroy vegetative bacteria, mycobacteria and viruses but not bacteria spores (Ayliffe *et al.* 1984).

Forceps can be used to arrange the dressing pack, and then to remove the used dressing before the forceps are discarded (Kelso 1989). Alternatively the washed hands can be inserted into the polythene waste bag to arrange the pack before removing the used dressing and then inverting the bag containing the used dressing before attaching the bag to the dressing trolley. Any equipment that becomes contaminated during a procedure must be discarded. On *no* account should it be returned to the sterile field. Care must also be taken to ensure that equipment and lotions are sterile and that packaging is undamaged before use.

While following aseptic techniques, it is also important to evaluate the whole procedure to ensure the principles are being followed during the whole process; errors such as taking adhesive tape from a contaminated roll (Oldman 1987) or using dressings left over from a previous dressing (Roberts 1987) must be avoided.

The dressing trolley

Most disinfectants are not sporicidal and have a limited antimicrobial spectrum and must be used only on clean surfaces or equipment, e.g. instruments, as they may fail to penetrate blood or pus (Ayliffe *et al.* 1984). Therefore it is essential that equipment such as trolleys are cleaned daily and, when contaminated, with a detergent solution and dried carefully with paper towels. This will remove a high proportion of micro-organisms, including bacterial spores (Ayliffe *et al.* 1992). Prior to use for aseptic technique, trolleys should be wiped over with chlorhexidine in 70% ethanol alcohol using a clean paper towel (Ayliffe *et al.* 1984). Trolleys used for aseptic procedures must not be used for any other purpose.

Protective clothing

Protective clothing may be worn for a variety of reasons, including the need to proclaim the identity of the wearer (Sparrow 1991). Generally, however, protective clothing is worn for the following reasons:

1 To prevent the user's clothing becoming contaminated with pathogenic micro-organisms which may subsequently be transferred to other patients in their care.
2 To prevent the user's clothing becoming soiled, wet or stained during the course of their duties.
3 To prevent transfer of potentially pathogenic micro-organisms from user to patient.
4 To prevent the user acquiring infection from the patient (Ayton *et al.* 1984).

There is evidence that transfer of organisms can occur from one room to another on clothing (Hambraeus 1973). An impermeable apron offers better protection than a cotton gown, which allows bacteria and moisture to pass through because of the weave (Mackintosh *et al.* 1980). It is therefore recommended that a disposable plastic apron, which is impermeable to bacteria, is worn during aseptic procedures. Aprons should be changed or removed after each dressing.

Surgical masks are an integral part of theatre clothing. The data do not support the use of a mask to protect patients and health care workers during aseptic techniques from airborne bacteria (Ransjon 1986; McCluskey 1996). Masks must be worn as part of routine universal precautions when there is a risk of airborne aerosol of blood or body fluids, administration of toxic drugs or contact with patients who are smear positive with drug resistant tuberculosis. These masks must comply with The Control of Substances Hazardous to Health (COSSH) 1988 regulations. Studies have shown that not wearing a mask does not alter infection rates (Orr 1981) and that masks contribute little or nothing to the protection of people in wards. Therefore the routine use of masks for aseptic ward procedures is unnecessary (Taylor 1980). However, there is some justification for wearing masks when giving prolonged close care to major burn patients (Ayton *et al.* 1984).

Patient hygiene

The patient's skin flora is an important source of infection following invasive procedures (Goodinson 1990). Patient hygiene will reduce this hazard (Mackenzie 1988). Studies comparing washing with soap or chlorhexidine solution demonstrated a marked decrease in bacteriuria in patients washing with chlorhexidine (Sanderson 1990). Other research has shown that the use of chlorhexidine solution for bathing or showering pre- and postoperatively reduces the incidence of wound infections (Randall *et al.* 1984).

Studies to establish whether the incidence of infection or prolonged or delayed healing occurred when stitches became wet during washing showed that getting stitches wet was not detrimental to wound healing (Noe *et al.*

1988). Therefore, a patient with, for example, an indwelling intravenous central catheter, while showering with stitches still in situ should wear a protective dressing, to protect the wound and stitches from being disturbed during the bath or shower, and after showering any non-waterproof dressing should be changed immediately (Mitchell 1984). The use of a transparent film dressing allows continuous inspection and more secure anchorage as well as protecting against wetting during showering (Ward *et al.* 1997).

Airborne contamination

The spread of airborne infection is most likely to occur following procedures such as bed making and cleaning, which can disperse organisms into the air. Ideally such activities should cease 30 minutes before a dressing is to be undertaken. To reduce further the risk of airborne contamination of open wounds curtains should be drawn round the bed 10 minutes before the dressing is to be changed and the wound should be exposed for as short a time as possible (Ayliffe *et al.* 1992). Dirty dressings should be placed carefully in a yellow clinical waste bag, which is sealed before disposal (Lowbury *et al.* 1981). Clean wounds should be dressed before contaminated wounds. Colostomies and infected wounds should be dressed last of all to minimize environmental contamination and cross-infection.

Air movement should be kept to a minimum during the dressing. This means that adjacent windows should be closed and the movement of personnel within the area discouraged.

References and further reading

Albert, R.K. *et al.* (1981) Handwashing patterns in medical intensive care units. *New Engl J Med*, **304**, 1465–6.

Ansari, S.A. *et al.* (1991) Comparison of cloth, paper and warm air drying in eliminating viruses and bacteria from washed hands. *Am J Infect Control*, **19**(5), 243–9.

Ayliffe, G.A.J. *et al.* (1984) *Chemical Disinfection in Hospitals*, pp. 7–8. Public Health Laboratory Service, London.

Ayliffe, G.A.J. *et al.* (1992) *Control of Hospital Infection. A Practical Handbook*, 3rd edn. Chapman & Hall Medical, London.

Ayton, M. *et al.* (1984) *Report of a Working Party on Ward Protective Clothing*. Infection Control Nurses Association, London.

Blackmore, M. (1987) Hand drying methods. *Nurs Times*, **83**(37), 71–4.

Bree-Williams, E.J. & Waterman, H. (1996) An examination of nurses' practices when performing aseptic technique for wound dressing. *J Adv Nurs*, **23**, 48–54.

Briggs, M., Wilson, S. & Fuller, A. (1996) The principles of aseptic technique in wound care. *Prof Nurse*, **11**(12), 805–8.

Candell, K.A. & Whedon, M.B. (1991) Haematopoietic complications found in bone marrow transplantation. In: *Principles, Practices and Nursing Insight* (ed. M.B. Whedon), pp. 135–57. Jones & Bartlett, Boston.

Casewell, M. *et al.* (1977) Hands as route of transmission for *Klebsiella* species. *Br Med J*, **2**, 1315–17.

Centre for Disease Control (1986) Guidelines for handwashing and hospital environmental control. *Infect Control*, **7**(4), 233–5.

Chapman, R. *et al.* (1993) Surveillance and feedback of hospital acquired infection rates in the USA. *Public Health Lab Serv Microbiol Dig*, **11**(1), 35–7.

Chaudhuri, A.K. (1993) Infection control in hospitals: has its quality enhancing and cost effective role been appreciated? *J Hosp Infect*, **25**, 1–6.

Crow, S. (1989) Asepsis: an indispensable part of the patient's care plan. *Crit Care Nurse Questions*, **11**(4), 11–15.

Crow, S. (1994) Asepsis: a prophylactic technique. *Semin Perioper Nurs*, **3**(2), 93–100.

Crowe, M.J. & Cooke, E.M. (1998) Review of case definition for nosocomial infection – towards a consensus. Presentation by nosocomial infection surveillance unit to hospital infection liaison group, subcommittee of Federation of Infection Societies. *J Hosp Infect*, **39**(1), 3–11.

Cruse, P.J.E. & Foord, R. (1980) The epidemiology of wound infection – a 10-year prospective study of 62 939 wounds. *Surg Clin N Am*, **60**(1), 27–40.

Davey, J.G. (1997) Discvering nursing students' understanding about aseptic technique. *Int J Nurs Pract*, **3**(2), 105–10.

David, J. (1991) Letters. *Wound Manag*, **1**(2), 15.

French, G.L. *et al.* (1989) Repeated prevalence surveys for monitoring effectiveness of hospital infection control. *Lancet*, **11**, 1021–3.

Goodinson, S.M. (1990) Keeping the flora out. *Prof Nurse*, **5**(11), 572–5.

Gould, D. (1993) Assessing nurses' hand decontamination performance. *Nurs Times*, **89**(25), 47–50.

Gould, D. (1994a) The significance of hand-drying in the prevention of infection. *Nurs Times*, **90**(47), 33–5.

Gould, D. (1994b) Understanding the nature of bacteria. *Nurs Stand*, **8**(28), 29–31.

Gurevich, I. *et al.* (1986) The compromised host deficit specific infection and the spectrum of prevention. *Cancer Nurs*, **9**, 263–75.

Gwyther, J. (1988) Skilled dressing. *Nurs Times*, **84**(19), 60–61.

Haley, R.W. *et al.* (1985a) The efficiency of infection surveillance and control programmes in preventing nosocomial infections in US hospitals. *Am J Epidemiol*, **121**, 182–205.

Haley, R.W. *et al.* (1985b) Identifying multivariate index of patients' susceptibility and wound contamination. *Am J Epidemiol*, **121**(2), 206–15.

Hambraeus, A. (1973) Transfer of *Staphylococcus aureus* via nurses' uniform. *J Hyg*, **71**, 799–814.

Hart, S. (1990) The immunosuppressed patient in infection control. In: *Guidelines for Nursing Care* (eds M.A. Worsley *et al.*), pp. 15–20. Surgikos Ltd.

Hart, S. (1991) Blood and body precautions. *Nurs Stand*, **5**(25), 25–8.

Infection Control Standards Working Party (1993) *Standards in Infection Control in Hospitals*. HMSO, London.

Jacobson, G. *et al.* (1985) Handwashing: ring-wearing and number of microorganisms. *Nurs Res*, **34**(3), 186–8.

Jenks, A.M. & Ferguson, K.E. (1994) Intergrating what is taught with what is practised in the nursing curriculum, a multidimensional model. *J Adv Nurs*, **20**, 687–95.

Johnson, A. (1987) Wound care: packing wound cavities. *Nurs Times*, **83**(36), 59–62.

Kampf, G., Jarosch, R. & Ruden, H. (1998) Limited effectiveness of chlorhexidine based hand disinfectants against methicillin resistant *Staphylococcus aureus* (MRSA). *J Hosp Infect*, **38**, 297–303.

Kelso, H. (1989) Alternative technique. *Nurs Times*, **85**(23), 68–72.

King, S. (1998) Decontamination of equipment and the environment. *Nurs Stand*, **12**(52), 57–63.

Klapes, N.A., Greene, V.W. & Langholz, A.C. (1987) Microbial contamination associated with routine aseptic practice. *J Hosp Infect*, **10**(3), 299–304.

Krakowska, G. (1986) Practice versus procedure. *Nurs Times*, **82**(49), 64–9.

Larson, E. *et al.* (1982) Factors influencing handwashing behaviour of patients' care personnel. *Am J Infect Control*, **10**(3), 93–9.

Lascelles, I. (1982) Wound dressing technique. *Nursing*, **2**(8), 217–19.

Laurence, C. (1991) Bacterial infection of wounds. *Wound Manag*, **1**(1), 13–15.

Lowbury, E.J. *et al.* (1974a) Disinfection of hands: removal of transient organisms. *Br Med J*, **2**, 230–33.

Lowbury, E.J. *et al.* (1974b) Preoperative disinfection of surgeons' hands: use of alcoholic solutions and effects of gloves on skin flora. *Br Med J*, **4**, 369–72.

Lowbury, E.J. *et al.* (1981). *Control of Hospital Infection – A Practical Handbook*, 2nd edn. Chapman & Hall, London.

Lund, C. & Caruso, R. (1993) Nursing perspective: aseptic technique in wound care. *Dermatol Nurs*, **5**(3), 2215–16.

McCluskey, F. (1996) Does wearing a face mask reduce bacterial wound infection? A literature review. *Br J Theatre Nurs*, **6**(5), 18–20.

Mackenzie, I. (1988) Pre-operative skin preparation and surgical outcome. *J Hosp Infect*, Suppl. B, 27–32.

Mackintosh, C.A. *et al.* (1980) The evaluation of fabric in relation to their use as protective garments in nursing and surgery. *J Hyg*, **85**, 393–403.

McLane, C. *et al.* (1983) A nursing practice problem: failure to observe aseptic techniques. *Am J Infect Control*, **11**(5), 178–82.

Matthews, J.A. & Newman, S.W. (1987) Hot air electric hand dryers compared with paper towels for potential spread of airborne bacteria. *J Hosp Infect*, **9**(1), 85–8.

Medical Devices Agency (1995) *The Reuse of Medical Devices Supplied for Single Use Only*. DB 9501. Department of Health, London.

Meers, P.D. & Yeo, G.A. (1978) Shedding of bacteria and skin squames after handwashing. *J Hyg*, **81**, 99–105.

Meers, P.D. *et al.* (1981) Report on the National Survey of Infection in Hospital 1980. *J Hosp Infect*, **2**(Suppl), 1–53.

Mitchell, N.J. (1984) Whole-body disinfection with chlorhexidine in shower bathing more effective than bathing. *J Hosp Infect*, **5**, 96–9.

Ngeow, Y.F., Ong, H.W. & Tan, P. (1989) Dispersal of bacteria by an electric air hand dryer. *Malay J Pathol*, **11**, 53–6.

Noe, J.M. *et al.* (1988) Can stitches get wet? *Plast Reconstruct Surg*, **81**(1), 82–4.

O'Donoghue, M.A.T. & Allen, K.D. (1992) Cost of an outbreak of wound infections in an orthopaedic ward. *J Hosp Infect*, **22**, 73–9.

Oldman, P.M. (1987) An unkind cut. *Nurs Times*, **83**(48), 71–4.

Oldman, P. (1991) A sticky situation – microbiological study of adhesive tape used to secure IV cannulae. *Prof Nurse*, Feb, 265–9.

Orr, N.W.M. (1981) Is a mask necessary in the operating theatre? *Ann R Coll Surg*, **63**, 390–92.

Pereira, L.J., Lee, G.M. & Wade, K.J. (1997) An evaluation of five protocols for surgical handwashing in relation to skin condition and microbial counts. *J Hosp Infect*, **36**, 49–65.

Phillips, C. (1989) Hand hygiene. *Nurs Times*, **85**(37), 76–9.

Potter, P.A. & Perry, A.G. (1992) *Fundamentals of Nursing*, 3rd edn. Mosby, London.

Randall, P.E. *et al.* (1984) Prevention of wound infection following vasectomy. *Br J Urol*, **57**, 227–9.

Ransjon, U. (1986) Mask: a ward investigation and review of the literature. *J Hosp Infect*, **7**(3), 289–94.

Reingold, A.L., Kane, M.A. & Hightower, A.W. (1988) Failure of gloves and other protective devices to prevent transmission of hepatitis B virus to oral surgeons. *JAMA*, **259**(17), 2558–60.

Roberts, J. (1987) Pennywise, pound foolish. *Nurs Times*, **83**(37), 68–9.

Rowland, A.J. & Alder, V.G. (1972) Transmission of infection through towels. *Commun Med*, **5**, 71–3.

Rowland, C. *et al.* (1985) In the surgeons' hands. *Nurs Times*, Suppl., 5–7.

Sanderson, P.J. (1990) A comparison of the effect of chlorhexidine antisepsis, soap and antibiotics on bacteriuria, perineal colonization and environmental contamination in spinally injured patients. *J Hosp Infect*, **15**, 235–43.

Sherwood, E. (1995) Motivation, the key factor. *Nurs Times*, **91**(20), 65–6.

Sparrow, S. (1991) An exploration of the role of the nurses' uniform through a period of non-uniform wear on an acute medical ward. *J Adv Nurs*, **16**, 116–22.

Sproat, L.J. & Inglis, T.J.J. (1992) Preventing infection in the intensive care unit. *Br J Intens Care*, September, 277–85.

Stronge, V.L. (1984) Principles of wound care. *Nursing*, **2**(26), Suppl., 7–10.

Taylor, L. (1978a) An evaluation of handwashing techniques 1. *Nurs Times*, **74**(2), 54–5.

Taylor, L. (1978b) An evaluation of handwashing techniques 2. *Nurs Times*, **74**(3), 108–10.

Taylor, L.J. (1980) Are masks necessary in operating theatres and wards? *J Hosp Infect*, **1**, 173–4.

Thomlinson, D. (1990) Time to dispense with the rituals. *Prof Nurse*, May, 421–4.

Trester, A. (1982) Nursing management of patients receiving cancer chemotherapy. *Cancer Nurs*, **6**, 206–10.

Ward, V., Wilson, J., Taylor, L. *et al.* (1997) *Preventing Hospital Acquired Infection. Clinical guidelines* pp. 19–21. Publie Health Laboratory Service, London.

Webster, M. (1986) Control measures. *Nurs Times*, **82**(5), 26–8.

GUIDELINES · Aseptic technique

Equipment

1 Sterile dressing pack* containing gallipots or an indented plastic tray, low-linting swabs and/or medical foam, disposable forceps, gloves, sterile field, disposable bag.

2 Fluids for cleaning and/or irrigation.

Any other material will be determined by the nature of the dressing: special features of a dressing should be referred to

3 Hypo-allergenic tape.

4 Appropriate dressing (see Chap. 47, Wound management).

5 Appropriate hand hygiene preparation.

in the patient's nursing care plan.

Procedure

Action

1 Explain and discuss the procedure with the patient.

2 Clean trolley with chlorhexidine in 70% spirit with a paper towel.

3 Place all the equipment required for the procedure on the bottom shelf of a clean dressing trolley.

4 Take the patient to the treatment room or screen the bed. Position the patient comfortably so that the area to be dealt with is easily accessible without exposing the patient unduly.

5 If the procedure is a dressing and the wound is infected or producing copious amounts of exudate, put on a disposable plastic apron.

6 Take the trolley to the treatment room or patient's bedside, disturbing the screens as little as possible.

7 Loosen the dressing tape

8 Wash your hands with bactericidal soap and water or a bactericidal alcohol hand rub.

9 Check the pack is sterile (i.e., the pack is undamaged, intact and dry. If autoclave tape is present, check that it has changed colour from beige to beige and brown lines) open the outer cover of the sterile pack and slide the contents onto the top shelf of the trolley.

10 Open the sterile field using only the corners of the paper.

11 Check any other packs for sterility and open, tipping their contents gently onto the centre of the sterile field.

12 Wash hands with a bactericidal alcohol rub.

13 Place hand in disposable bag, arrange contents of dressing pack.

14 Remove used dressing with hand covered with the disposable bag, invert bag and stick to trolley.

15 Where appropriate, swab along the 'tear area' of lotion sachet with chlorhexidine in 70% spirit/swab saturated with 70% isopropyl alcohol. Tear open sachet and pour lotion into gallipots or on indented plastic tray (see Table 47.3).

16 Put on sterile gloves, touching only the inside wrist end.

Rationale

To ensure that the patient understands the procedure and gives his/her valid consent.

To provide a clean working surface.

To maintain the top shelf as a clean working surface.

To allow dust and airborne organisms to settle before the sterile field (and in the case of a dressing, the wound) is exposed. Maintain the patient's dignity and comfort.

To reduce the risk of spreading infection.

To minimize airborne contamination.

To make it easier to remove the dressing.

To reduce the risk of wound infection.

To ensure that only sterile products are used.

So that areas of potential contamination are kept to a minimum.

To prepare the equipment and, in the case of a wound dressing, reduce the amount of time that the wound is uncovered. This reduces the risk of infection and a drop in temperature of the wound which will delay wound healing (Stronge 1984).

Hands may become contaminated by handling outer packets, etc.

To maintain sterility of pack.

To minimize risk of contamination, by containing dressing in bag.

To minimize risk of contamination of lotion.

To reduce the risk of infection. Gloves provide greater sensitivity than forceps and are less likely to cause trauma to the patient.

Carry out procedure

17 Make sure the patient is comfortable.

Guidelines • Aseptic technique (cont'd)

Action	Rationale
18 Dispose of waste in yellow plastic clinical waste bags.	To prevent environmental contamination. Yellow is the recognized colour for clinical waste.
19 If necessary, draw back curtains or, if appropriate, help the patient back to the bed area and ensure the patient is comfortable.	
20 Check that the trolley remains dry and physically clean. If necessary, wash with liquid detergent and water and dry throughly with a paper towel.	To reduce the risk of spreading infection.
21 Wash hands with soap and water.	To reduce the risk of spreading infection.

* Please note that for some procedures it may be more appropriate to use different types of sterile packs (e.g. intravenous packs). Since usage of these will vary locally reference is generally made to 'sterile dressing pack'.

Barrier Nursing: Nursing the Infectious or Immunosuppressed Patient

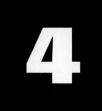

4

Barrier nursing

Definition

Barrier nursing is the use of infection control practices aimed at controlling the spread of, and destroying, pathogenic organisms. These practices may require the setting up of mechanical barriers to contain pathogenic organisms within a specified area.

Indications

Barrier nursing includes:

1 Source isolation to segregate infected patients in single rooms to prevent the spread of infection.
2 Cohort source isolation to segregate a number of patients with the same infection in one ward when there are inadequate number of single rooms, to prevent the spread of infection (Working Party 1998).
3 Protective isolation (reverse barrier nursing) to segregate immunosuppressed patients to protect them from acquiring an exogenous infection.
4 Strict source isolation to segregate patients infected with a serious contagious disease, e.g. viral haemorrhagic fever, in isolation units to prevent the spread of infection (DoH 1998).

Reference material

A recent study of infection among hospitalized patient in the UK and Republic of Ireland found a 9% (range 2–29%) overall prevalence. The four major sites of infection were urinary tract (23.2% of patients), surgical wounds (10.7%), lower respiratory tract (22.9%) and skin infections (9.6%). The incidence of nosocomial (hospital acquired) infections in neutropenic patients is significantly higher, with a 48.3% infection rate reported by one author (Carlisle et al. 1993). Infection is the major cause of morbidity and mortality in the neutropenic patient with leukemia (Oniboni 1990). However, the risk of infection depends on the patient's ability to respond to infection, rather that the number of neutrophils in the peripheral blood (Dale et al. 1998). A careful patient medical history and physical examination provides an initial assessment of the patient's susceptibility to infection.

Most precautions against transferring infection demand more effort, take more time and cost more when neutropenic patients are cared for, than the comparable procedures in normal circumstances. However, the cost of an outbreak of infection can be far more. In 1991, 175 patients developed nosocomial *Clostridium difficile* diarrhoea. As a direct result 17 patients died and the organism was a contributing factor in a further 43 deaths. The cost of managing the outbreak was at least £75 000 (Worsley 1993).

For the infected patient the consequences can be considerable and may include the following:

1 Delayed or prevented recovery.
2 Increased pain, discomfort and anxiety.
3 Extended hospitalization, which has implications for the patient, the family and the hospital.
4 Psychological stress as a result of long periods spent in isolation (Knowles 1993).

One study of the psychological effects of hospitalization and source isolation found that isolated patients were significantly more anxious and depressed than other hospitalized patients. The fear of the unknown, of further spread and contamination to others and feelings of guilt were linked to uncertainty and loss of control as patients experienced lack of clarity, ambiguity and lack of information from staff (Gammon 1998).

Sources of infection

Self-infection (endogenous infection)

Self-infection results when tissues become infected from other sites in the patient's body. The normal microbial flora of the human body consists largely of the organisms in the alimentary tract, upper respiratory tract and female genital tract and on the skin. This flora may include versatile pathogens (e.g. *Staphylococcus aureus*) that may cause disease in almost any tissue, as well as others (e.g. micrococcus species and diphtheroids) which are usually of very low pathogenicity, and rarely cause infection. Many organisms exist with capabilities between these extremes (Mims et al. 1993).

Cross-infection (exogenous infection)

Cross-infection may be caused by infection from patients, hospital staff or visitors who are suffering from the relevant disease (cases) or who are symptomless carriers. Food and the environment may also be factors in cross-infection

(Wall *et al.* 1996a; Public Health Laboratory Service Communicable Disease Surveillance Centre 1999).

Routes and reservoirs of infection

A reservoir of infection is anywhere where organisms can survive and multiply. For infection to occur there has to be a route of transmission between the reservoir and the susceptible host. Routes of spread include:

Direct contact

Organisms can be transmitted directly to susceptible people by contaminated equipment or by the hands of health care workers (Casewell *et al.* 1977). Hand washing has been shown to reduce the spread of infection (Ward *et al.* 1997). However, studies of hand washing by nurses and others have shown that this procedure is generally not carried out efficiently (Gidley 1987). Washing with soap removes transient micro-organisms, whilst the use of a bactericidal soap removes both transient and resident skin micro-organisms (Ward *et al.* 1997). In clinical areas washing in running water is essential. Basins should be deep enough to contain any splashing water and should be plugless. Taps should not be operated by hand but by remote control, elbow, knee or foot, as appropriate.

A quick, convenient and effective disinfectant for clean hands, without the use of soap and water, is an alcoholic hand rub containing 70% isopropyl and a bactericidal agent such as chlorhexidine, with the addition of enough glycerine to prevent excessive drying of the skin (Lee *et al.* 1988). Such solutions may not be effective against some viruses, therefore if contamination is likely, for example when leaving a source isolation room, washing the hands with a bactericidal soap and water before using the alcoholic hand rub is advised (Ayliffe *et al.* 1992).

Hands must be washed using a bactericidal soap before and after direct patient contact or contact with contaminated material, e.g. toys, bed linen etc., and before contact with susceptible patients (Gidley 1987), and dried thoroughly using a good quality disposable paper towel (Rowland 1972) (see Chap. 3, Aseptic Technique).

Particular types of soap, a higher number of hand washes per shift and a greater number of times gloves were worn were associated with increase in skin damage (Larson *et al.* 1997). The use of alcoholic hand rubs reduces skin damage in comparison to soap (Newman & Seitz 1990).

Airborne

Organisms can be transmitted in dust or skin scales carried by air. This is likely to occur during procedures such as bed making, when particles may land directly on open wounds or puncture sites (Glenister 1983). Airborne infection may also occur through droplets. Water from nebulizers or humidifiers may be contaminated by *Pseudomonas* species (Redding *et al.* 1980). Fine droplet spray from ventilation cooling towers or showers contaminated with *Legionella pneumophila* has also been shown to be a hazard (Alderman 1988).

Food borne

Food poisoning occurs when contaminated foods are ingested, with *Salmonella* species being one of the most common causes (Wall *et al.* 1996b).

Blood borne

Blood, or blood-stained material, is potentially hazardous, transmitting infection through inoculation accidents, existing breaks in the skin, gross contamination of mucous membranes, sexual activity or, prenatally, from mother to baby (Hart 1991).

Vector borne (an insect or animal carrier/transmitter of disease)

International movement of people and products is associated with the emergence of infectious diseases (Ostroff & Kozarsky 1998) by introducing infectious agents into areas in which they had previously been absent (Gratz 1999). Research on vaccines, environmentally safe insecticides, vector control and training programmes for health care workers can assist in disease control (Gubler 1998). Although disease transmitted by biting insects is not a major problem in the UK, insects such as cockroaches can carry pathogenic organisms on their bodies and in their digestive tracts. This may infect the hospital environment, which includes food and sterile supplies (Burgess 1979). Storage of supplies in dry, clean, well ventilated areas is therefore essential.

Types of barrier nursing

1 Source isolation
2 Protective isolation

Source isolation is designed to prevent the spread of pathogenic micro-organisms from an infected patient to other patients, hospital personnel and visitors. The need for isolation is determined by the ease with which the disease can be transmitted in hospital and, if it is transmittable, by its severity. As infectious diseases are transmitted by different routes, isolation procedures must, in order to be effective, provide appropriate barriers to the route of transmission. In addition, the procedures imposing these barriers must be adhered to universally by all hospital staff entering the isolation unit.

Protective isolation protects the patient from the hospital environment. Protective isolation techniques have also been referred to as reverse barrier nursing and reverse isolation, and include laminar air flow rooms (Caudell & Bakitas Whedon 1991) (see 'Protective isolation', below).

Source isolation

Definition

Source isolation is a process of care whereby an infectious patient and any material that has been in contact with them or eliminated by them is isolated from others to prevent the spread of infection.

Indications

The decision to isolate a patient will be influenced by the availability of facilities as well as by the physical condition of the area where the isolation is to take place. In determining the most suitable area, a number of criteria need to be met. Among these are the relative cleanliness of the ward, the standard of domestic services support, the microbiological infectious or the immune status of the other patients and the anticipated length of the isolation.

Reference material

Source isolation may be achieved by:

1 Purpose-built infectious disease wards
2 Plastic isolators found in strict source isolation units and used only for infections such as viral haemorrhagic fever (Bowell 1986)
3 Single rooms on general wards.

Transmission rates of bacteria causing infections have been seen to be transmitted more easily between patients in the same ward compared to those patients in separate single rooms (Fryklund *et al.* 1997). The bed around infected patients can often be contaminated with the infecting organism (Green *et al.* 1998).

Effective source barrier nursing practice is achieved most easily by isolating the patient in a single room with the following:

1 An anteroom area for protective clothing
2 Hand washing facilities
3 Toilet facilities.

However, with good technique, an area in the ward away from especially vulnerable patients can be used. In some instances where cross-infection has occurred it may be more appropriate to cohort nurse these patients together in a small ward with designated staff, so containing the infection to one area, rather than using side rooms on different wards (Duckworth 1990). Uninfected patients must not be admitted into this area until all the infected patients have been discharged and the area thoroughly cleaned.

General principles of source isolation

The main emphasis for successful source isolation nursing procedures, is on hand washing and protection of clothes. Several general principles need to be adhered to if effective barrier nursing is to occur. Every effort must be made to ensure that instructions are kept simple and realistic. Regular assessment and evaluation of the situation must take place to ascertain whether barrier nursing continues to remain the most appropriate form of care.

Protective clothing

Gowns or aprons

The wearing of a protective gown or apron is an accepted part of barrier nursing technique to prevent the spread of micro-organisms from one patient to the next on clothing (Callaghan 1998b).

Disposable plastic aprons are cheap, impermeable to bacteria and water (Babb *et al.* 1983), are easy to put on, protect the probable area of maximum contamination and are preferable to cotton gowns, which provide increased cover but are *readily penetrated* by moisture and bacteria (Mackintosh 1982). Isolation gowns are assumed to protect the wearer from contamination. However one study indicated that commercially available gowns were not effective against microbial contamination (Lovitt *et al.* 1992). The authors suggested that isolation gowns provide a false sense of security. Another investigation found that uniforms and plastic aprons were heavily contaminated with bacteria (Callaghan 1998b) and the author recommended that nurses are provided with a clean uniform each day (Callaghan 1998a).

Caps

Although the wearing of disposable caps while nursing infected patients is still practised, hair that is clean and tidy has not been implicated in cross-infection. Therefore, unless heavy contamination or splashing is present, the wearing of caps is not justified (Gaya 1980).

Masks

Masks are sometimes worn to protect the patient, for example when a large burn is being dressed. Studies indicate that masks are generally of little value outside the operating theatre (see Chap. 30, Peri-operative care), while the improper use of a mask can increase hand contamination (Ayton 1984). Masks can also be worn to protect the wearer, for example when caring for patients with untreated meningococcal meningitis. The organism which causes meningococcal meningitis is found at the back of the throat, and can be passed from person to person by droplet spread from the mouth and nose (DHSS 1987a). Masks should be worn by all persons providing regular and prolonged close contact with patients suspected or confirmed to be tuberculosis smear positive, particularly during bronchoscopy and other cough inducing procedures (Interdepartmental Working Group on Tuberculosis 1998). Masks must be worn during all procedures likely to cause splashing of body substances into the face (Ward *et al.* 1997). If a mask needs to be worn it must be a filter type and fit the face closely.

Overshoes

The floors of hospital wards become easily contaminated by large numbers of bacteria (Ayliffe *et al.* 1967). However, the wearing of overshoes has little value and there could even be an increased risk of cross-infection by contaminating the hands while putting on overshoes, making it necessary for the hands to be washed after putting on or taking them off (Jones *et al.* 1988).

If airborne transmission of micro-organisms is a potential risk, a dry dust control mat placed at the patient's door, which is vacuumed daily and washed weekly, will be an effective means of limiting spread of infection by feet and trolley wheels (Meddick 1977).

Gloves

Boxed, clean non-sterile gloves are adequate for routine non-invasive nursing care (Rossoff *et al.* 1993). Clean gloves must be worn when handling blood or body fluids, or cleaning (Hart 1991), but are not a substitute for hand washing, as gloved hands can become contaminated during as many as 13% of all contacts with patients' mucous membranes (Bolsen *et al.* 1993). Gloves must be changed between patients, and hands must be washed with bactericidal soap and water or bactericidal alcohol hand rub after removing gloves.

Cleaning

Scrupulous daily cleaning of the barrier nursing room is essential. All furniture must be damp dusted to remove organisms dispersed into the air from bed making. The floor must be either vacuum cleaned with a machine fitted with a filter or damp mopped with hot, soapy water (the mop head must be laundered daily). Dry dusting or the use of a broom should be forbidden as studies have shown this method of cleaning simply redisperses the organisms into the air (Ayliffe 1982). The cleaning equipment must be kept for this patient's sole use.

Patient hygiene

The numbers of micro-organisms on the skin will be reduced by using an antiseptic detergent for skin and hair washing (Mitchell 1984) and this has been shown to be effective in eradicating the carriage of MRSA (Duckworth 1990). The antiseptic should be applied directly to the flannel and rinsed off thoroughly.

Studies comparing standard baths with shower baths showed no overall significant difference between the two bathing techniques. However, one study indicated that shower baths were more effective in disinfecting axillae, and standard baths more efficient in reducing microbes in the perineum (Mitchell 1984). Assessment and evaluation of the patients must be made to establish which patients will benefit most from a standard bath and which patients will benefit from a shower bath.

It is essential that baths are cleaned and dried between patients with a non-abrasive cleaning agent, ideally incorporating a hypochlorite (Austin 1988), as viable organisms can survive in bath scum (Ayliffe *et al.* 1975). Bathing and showering are preferable to bed baths, as organisms can be redistributed over the body during bed bathing (Greaves 1985). If bed bathing is unavoidable the patient should be supplied with their own bowl which is washed and dried after use and stored at the bedside to prevent cross-infection.

Waste

Infected rubbish must be disposed of in yellow clinical waste bags. Full bags must be sealed securely within the room before being sent for incineration (Health and Safety Commission 1982). Sharps must be placed immediately into a sharps disposal box (DHSS 1983) which, when full, must be sealed before being sent for incineration (Health and Safety Commission 1982).

Linen

Infected linen must be placed in a red alginate polythene bag. The bag is tied shut and then placed in a red linen bag to be sent in a safe manner to the laundry for barrier washing. This entails placing the full alginate bag in the washing machine where it dissolves, allowing the hot water to wash and disinfect the linen. In this way staff and the environment are protected from contamination (DHSS 1987b).

Cutlery, crockery

Crockery and cutlery can become contaminated with pathogenic organisms. Hands must be washed after handling utensils used by patients (Redpath & Farrington 1997). All crockery must be machine washed in a dishwasher with a final rinse of 82°C to disinfect it (Collins 1981). Disposable crockery and cutlery are needed only when gross contamination has occurred or if a dishwasher is not available.

Urine, faeces and vomit

These are to be disposed of immediately down a heat-disinfecting bedpan washer.

Notification of infection

If a patient develops signs and symptoms of infection or if bacteriological analysis identifies an organism which necessitates barrier nursing, swift communication and action are needed to instigate this. Any problems may be discussed with the infection control team.

Informing the patient and visitors

Giving careful explanation to the patient is essential so that he/she can cooperate fully with the restrictions. (Wilson-Barnett *et al.* 1983). The nurse should be sensitive to the psychological implications of being labelled 'infectious' and of being confined in isolation (Gammon 1998). Wilkins *et al.* (1988) examined the psychological effects of being admitted to a barrier nursing room, and found that patients were unlikely to have significant psychological problems unless there was a previous history of mental illness. Fortunately, many patients in fact preferred a single room, and adapted well to any subsequent loneliness and boredom. Other research has indicated that patients' needs are sometimes neglected when they are barrier nursed (Knowles 1993). The patient's visitors must also be told why the barrier nursing restrictions are necessary. Visitors will generally be allowed into the room at the discretion of the infection control team. They must be taught to observe the correct procedures for entering and leaving the room. As children are more susceptible to infection than adults, any visit by a child should be discussed with the infection control team.

Domestic staff

The domestic manager must be informed as soon as barrier nursing is commenced. He or she will then provide the ward domestic with written instructions.

The ward domestic staff must understand clearly why barrier nursing is required and should be instructed on the correct procedure. The nursing staff must check that the ward domestics understand and are following their instructions correctly. If the patient is in a single room, a mop (laundered daily), bucket (washed and dried after use), cleaning fluid and disposable cloths should be used solely for this patient's use. If the patient is in a general ward, special care must be taken with the cleaning so that potentially infectious material is not transferred from the area around the infected patient to other patient areas. The infected patient's area must be cleaned last and separately.

Staff allocation

A minimum number of staff should be involved with an infected patient. The nurse concerned with the infected patient should not also attend to other susceptible patients. If barrier nursing is for an infectious disease such as chicken pox, it is preferable that only personnel who have already had the disease should attend this patient.

The protection of staff against the risk of infection is one of the main functions of the occupational health department. This department offers an immunization and counselling service.

References and further reading

Alderman, C. (1988) The cooler culprits. *Nurs Stand*, **2**(33), 22.

Austin, L. (1988) The salt bath myth. *Nurs Times*, **84**(9), 79–83.

Ayliffe, G.A.J. (1982) Airborne infection in hospital. *J Hosp Infect*, **3**, 217–40.

Ayliffe, G.A.J. *et al.* (1967) Ward floors and other surfaces as reservoirs of hospital infection. *J Hyg*, **65**, 515–36.

Ayliffe, G.A.J. *et al.* (1975) Disinfection of baths and bath water. *Nurs Times*, **71**(37), 22–3.

Ayliffe, G.A.J. *et al.* (1992) *Control of Hospital Infection: A Practical Handbook*. Chapman & Hall, London.

Ayton, M. (1984) Protective clothing: what do we use and when? *Nurs Times*, **80**(19), 68–70.

Babb, J.R. *et al.* (1983) Contamination of protective clothing and nurses' uniforms in an isolation ward. *J Hosp Infect*, **4**, 149–57.

Bolsen, R.J. *et al.* (1993) Examination gloves as barriers to hand contamination in clinical practice. *JAMA*, **270**(3), 350–53.

Bowell, B. (1992) Protecting the patient. *Nurs Times*, **88**(13), 32–5.

Bowell, E. (1986) Nursing the isolated patient; Lassa fever. *Nurs Times*, **82**(33), 72–81.

Burgess, N.R.H. (1979) Cockroaches and the hospital environment. *Nurs Times*, **75**(11) (Contact), 5–7.

Callaghan, I. (1998a) Bacterial contamination of nurse's uniform: a study. *Nurs Stand*, **13**(1), 37–42.

Callaghan, I. (1998b) Implementing change: influencing the process. *Nurs Stand*, **13**(2), 37–42.

Carlisle, P.S. *et al.* (1993) Nosocomial infections in neutropenic cancer patients. *Infect Control Hosp Epidemiol*, **14**(6), 320–24.

Casewell, M. *et al.* (1977) Hands as route of transmission of *Klebsiella* species. *Br Med J*, **2**, 1315–17.

Caudell, K.A. & Bakitas Whedon, B. (1991) Hematopoietic complications. In: *Bone Marrow Transplantation* (ed. M. Bakitas Whedon). Jones and Bartlett, Boston.

Collins, B. (1981) Infection and the hospital environment. *Nursing*, **1**, Suppl., 1–3.

Dale, D.C. *et al.* (1998) How many neutrophils are enough? *Lancet*, **351**, 1752–3.

DHSS (1983) *Containers for the Disposal of Used Needles and Sharp Instruments*. TSS/8/330. DHSS, London.

DHSS (1987a) *Meningococcal Meningitis*. DA(87)26. DHSS, London.

DHSS (1987b) *Hospital Laundry Arrangements for Used and Infected Linen*. HC(87)30. DHSS, London.

DoH (1998) *Management and Control of Viral Haemorrhagic Fevers. Summary of Guidance from the Advisory Committee on Dangerous Pathogens*. 12491 HP 14k 1P Mar 98 (MUL). Stationery Office, London.

Duckworth, G. (1990) Revised guidelines for the control of epidemic methicillin-resistant *Staphylococcus aureus*. *J Hosp Infect*, **16**, 351–77.

Fryklund, B. *et al.* (1997) Transmission of urinary bacterial strains between patients with indwelling catheters nursing in the same room and in separate rooms compared. *J Hosp Infect*, **36**, 147–53.

Gammon, J. (1998) Analysis of the stressful effects of hospitalization and source isolation on coping and psychological constructs. *Int J Nurs Pract*, **4**, 84–96.

Gaya, H. (1980) Questions and answer section. Is it necessary for staff and visitors in an intensive care unit to wear masks, hats, gowns and overshoes? *J Hosp Infect*, **1**, 369–71.

Gidley, C. (1987) Now wash your hands. *Nurs Times*, **83**(29), 40–42.

Glenister, H. (1983) The passage of infection. *Nurs Mirror*, **79**(12 Jan), 28–30.

Gratz, N.G. (1999) Emerging and resurging vector-borne diseases. *Annu Rev Entomol*, **44**, 51–75.

Greaves, A. (1985) We'll just freshen you up, dear. . . . *Nurs Times*, **81**(9), Suppl., 3–8.

Green, J. *et al.* (1998) The role of environmental contamination with small round structured viruses in a hospital outbreak investigated by reverse transcriptase polymerase chain reaction assay. *J Hosp Infect*, **39**, 39–45.

Gubler, D.J. (1998) Resurgent vector borne diseases as a global health problem. *Emerg Infect Dis*, **4**(3), 442–50.

Hambraeus, A. (1973) Transfer of *Staphylococcus aureus* via nurses' uniform. *J Hyg*, **71**, 799–814.

Hart, S. (1991) Blood and body fluid precautions. *Nurs Stand*, **5**(25), 25–8.

Health and Safety Commission (1982) *The Safe Disposal of Clinical Waste*. HMSO, London.

Interdepartmental Working Group on Tuberculosis (1998) *The Prevention and Control of Tuberculosis in the United Kingdom*. Stationery Office, London.

Joint Tuberculosis Committee of the British Thoracic Society (1983) Control and prevention of tuberculosis: a code of practice. *Br Med J*, **287**, 1118–21.

Joint Tuberculosis Committee of the British Thoracic Society (1994) Control and Prevention of Tuberculosis in the United Kingdom: Code of Practice. *Thorax*, **49**, 1193–1200.

Jones, M. *et al.* (1988) Over-estimating overshoes. *Nurs Times*, **84**(41), 66–71.

Knowles, H.E. (1993) The experience of infectious patients in isolation. *Nurs Times*, **89**(30), 53–6.

Larson, E. *et al.* (1997) Prevalence and correlates of skin damage on the hands of nurses. *Heart Lung*, **26**(5), 404–12.

Lee, M.G. *et al.* (1988) A comparison of two bactericidal hand-washing agents containing chlorhexidine. *J Hosp Infect*, **12**, 59–63.

Lovitt, S.A. *et al.* (1992) Isolation gowns a false sense of security. *Am J Infect Control*, **20**(4), 185–91.

Mackenzie, I. (1988) Pre-operative skin preparation and surgical outcome. *J Hosp Infect* **II**, Suppl. B, 27–32.

Mackintosh, C.A. (1982) A testing time for gowns. *J Hosp Infect*, **3**, 5–8.

Mayon-White, R.T. *et al.* (1988) An international survey of the prevalence of hospital acquired infection. *J Hosp Infect*, **11**, Suppl. A, 43.

Meddick, H.M. (1977) Bacterial contamination. Control mats: – a comparative study. *J Hyg*, **79**, 133–40.

Medcraft, J.W. *et al.* (1987) Potential hazard from spray cleaning of floors in hospital wards. *J Hosp Infect*, **9**(2), 151–7.

Meers, P.D. *et al.* (1981) Report on the national survey of infection in hospital, 1980. *J Hosp Infect*, Suppl. **2**, 1–51.

Mims, C.A. *et al.* (1993) *Medical Microbiology*. Mosby, London.

Mitchell, N.J. (1984) Whole-body disinfection with chlorhexidine in shower bathing more effective than bathing. *J Hosp Infect*, **5**, 96–9.

Munir, A.K., Einarsson, R. & Dreborg, S.K. (1993) Vacuum cleaning decreases the level of mite allergen in house dust. *Pediatr Allergy Immunol*, **4**(3), 136–43.

Newman, J.L. & Seitz, J.C. (1990) Intermittent use of an antimicrobial hand gel for reducing soap induced irritation of health care personnel. *Am J Infect Control*, **18**(3), 194–200.

Ostroff, S.M. & Kaozarsky, P. (1998) Emerging infectious diseases and travel medicine. *Infect Dis Clin North Am*, **12**(1), 231–41.

Oniboni, A.C. (1990) Infection in the neutropenic patient. *Semin Oncol Nurs*, **6**(1), 50–60.

Public Health Laboratory Service Communicable Disease Surveillance Centre (1999) Surveillance of waterborne disease and water quality: January to June 1999, and summary of 1998. *Commun Dis Rep*, **9**(34), 305–307.

Redding, R.J. *et al.* (1980) *Pseudomonas fluorescens* cross-infection due to contaminated humidifier water. *Br Med J*, **281**, 26 July, 275.

Redpath, C. & Farnington, M. (1997) Dispose of disposables. *J Hosp Infect*, **35**(4), 313–17.

Rossoff, L.J. *et al.* (1993) Is the use of boxed gloves in an intensive care unit safe? *Am J Med*, **94**, 602–607.

Rowland, A.J. (1972) Transmission of infection through towels. *Commun Med*, 5 May, 71–2.

Suzuki, A., Namba, Y., Matsuura, M. *et al.* (1984) Bacterial contamination of floors and other surfaces in operating rooms: a five year survey. *J Hyg (Lond)*, **93**(3), 559–66.

Wall, P.G. *et al.* (1996a) Outbreak of salmonellosis in hospitals in England and Wales: 1992–1994. *J Hosp Infect*, **33**, 181–90.

Wall, P.G. *et al.* (1996b) Food poisoning: notification, laboratory reports and outbreaks – where do the statistics come from and what do they mean? *Commun Dis Rep*, **6**(7), R93–100.

Ward, V., Wilson, J., Taylor, L. *et al.* (1997) *Preventing Hospital Acquired Infection*, pp. 5–9. Public Health Laboratory Service, London.

Wilkins, E.G.L. *et al.* (1988) Does isolation of patients with infection induce mental illness? *J Infect*, **17**, 43–7.

Wilson-Barnett, J. *et al.* (1983) Studies evaluating patient teaching implication for practice. *Int J Nurs Stud*, **20**(1), 33–40.

Working Party (1998) Revised guidelines for the control of methicillin resistant *Staphylococcus aureus* infection in hospitals. *J Hosp Infect*, **39**, 253–90.

Worsley, M.A. (1993) A major outbreak of antibiotic associated diarrhoea. *Pub Health Lab Serv Microbiol Dig*, **10**(2), 97–9.

GUIDELINES · Source isolation

Equipment

1 Isolation suite if possible.
2 All items required to meet the patient's nursing needs during the period of isolation, e.g. instruments to assess vital signs.

Procedure

Preparation of the isolation room

Action

1 Place a barrier nursing sign outside the door.

2 List requirements for personnel before entering and after leaving the isolation area.

Rationale

To inform anyone intending to enter the room of the situation.

To decrease entries and exits to the room.

| **3** Remove all non-essential furniture. The remaining furniture should be easy to clean and should not conceal or retain dirt or moisture either within or around it. | To minimize the risk of furniture harbouring microbial spores or growth colonies. |

| **4** Stock the hand basin with a suitable bactericidal soap preparation and paper towels for staff use. | Facilities for hand washing within the infected area are essential for effective barrier nursing. |

| **5** Place yellow clinical waste bag in the room on a foot-operated stand. The bag must be sealed before it is removed from the room. | For containing contaminated rubbish within the room. Yellow is the recognized colour for clinical waste. |

| **6** Place a container for 'sharps' in the room. | To contain contaminated 'sharps' within the infected area. |

| **7** When the 'sharps' container is two-thirds full it must be firmly shut and sent for incineration. | To minimize the risk of leakage from the 'sharps' container. |

| **8** Keep the patient's personal property to a minimum. Advise him/her to wear hospital clothing. All belongings taken into the room should be washable, cleanable or disposable. | The patient's belongings may become contaminated and cannot be taken home unless they are washable or cleanable. Anything else may have to be destroyed. |

| **9** Provide the patient with his/her own thermometer and sphygmomanometer, and all items necessary for attending to personal hygiene. | Equipment used regularly by the patient should be kept within the infected area to prevent the spread of infection. |

| **10** Keep dressing solutions, creams and lotions, etc. to a minimum and store them within the room. | All partially used materials must be discarded when barrier nursing ends (sterilization is not possible), therefore unnecessary waste should be avoided. |

| **11** Set up a trolley outside the door to hold plastic aprons and bactericidal alcoholic hand rub (this is contraindicated if the trolley causes an obstruction or is a hazard to staff and others). | Staff are more likely to use the equipment if it is readily available. |

Entering the room

Action	*Rationale*
1 Collect all equipment needed.	To avoid entering and leaving the infected area unnecessarily.
2 Roll up long sleeves to the elbow.	To allow hand washing to take place.
3 Put on a disposable plastic apron.	A plastic apron is inexpensive, quick to put on and protects the front of the uniform which is the most likely area to come in contact with the patient.
4 Put on a disposable, impermeable gown for close work (e.g. lifting, nursing neonates).	To protect clothing from contamination to shoulders, arms and back. Cotton gowns are an ineffective barrier against bacteria, particularly when wet.
5 Put on a disposable well-fitting mask if there is a risk of airborne contamination, i.e. (a) Meningococcus meningitis. (b) Blood and body fluids.	To reduce the risk of inhaling organisms and to comply with safe techniques and practices.
6 Safety glasses, visors and goggles should be put on when it is likely that aerosolized droplets of blood or body fluids are present in the air.	To give protection to the conjunctiva from blood and body fluid splashes.
7 Rinse hands with bactericidal hand rub.	Hands must be cleaned before and after patient contact to reduce the risk of cross-infection.
8 Put on disposable gloves only if you are intending to deal with blood, excreta or contaminated material.	To reduce the risk of hand contamination.

Guidelines • Source isolation (cont'd)

Action	Rationale
9 Enter the room, shutting the door behind you.	To reduce the risk of airborne organisms leaving the room.

Attending to the patient

Action	Rationale
1 *Meals*. Meals only need to be served on disposable crockery and eaten with disposable cutlery if deemed necessary by the infection control team. Disposables and uneaten food should be discarded in the appropriate bag.	Contaminated crockery is a potential disease vector.
2 *Non-disposable crockery and cutlery* must be washed in a dishwasher with a hot disinfecting cycle.	Water at 80°C for 1 minute in a dishwasher will disinfect crockery and cutlery.
3 *Excreta*. Ideally, a toilet should be kept solely for the patient's use. If neither this nor disposable items are available, a separate bedpan or urinal and commode should be left in the patient's room. Gloves must be worn by staff when dealing with excreta. Bedpans and urinals should be bagged in the isolation room, emptied and then washed in a bedpan washer, then dried and returned immediately to the patient's room. On discharge of the patient, bedpans/urinals must be sent to SSD for disinfection.	To minimize the risk of infection being spread from excreta, e.g. via a toilet seat or a bedpan.
4 *Accidental spills*. Any suspected contaminated fluids must be mopped up immediately and the area cleaned with disinfectant.	Damp areas encourage microbial growth and increase the risk of spread of infection.
5 *Bathing*. An infected patient must be bathed last on the ward. Clean and dry the bath after the previous patient and after the infected patient.	Leaving the bath dry after disinfection reduces the risk of microbes surviving and infecting others. Bacteria will not easily grow on clean, dry surfaces.
6 *Dressings*. Aseptic technique must be used for changing all dressings. Waste materials and dirty dressings should be discarded in the appropriate bag. Used lotions, creams, etc. must be kept in the room and not used for other patients.	Aseptic procedure minimizes the risk of cross-infection. Lotions and creams can become easily contaminated.
7 *Linen*. Place infected linen in a red alginate polythene bag, which must be secured tightly before it leaves the room. Just outside the room, place this bag into a red linen bag which must be secured tightly and not used for other patients. These bags should await the laundry collection in a safe area.	Placing infected linen in a red alginate polythene bag confines the organisms and allows staff handling the linen to recognize the potential hazard.
8 *Waste*. Yellow clinical waste bags should be kept in the room for disposal of all the patient's rubbish. The bag's top should be sealed and labelled with the name of the ward or department before it is removed from the room.	Yellow is the international colour for clinical waste.

Leaving the room

Action	Rationale
1 If wearing gloves, remove and discard them in the yellow clinical waste bag. Wash hands with an appropriate bactericidal detergent	To remove pathogenic organisms acquired during contact with patient before removing gown, so preventing contamination of uniform.
2 Remove apron and discard it in the appropriate bag. Wash hands again with an appropriate bactercidal solution.	Hands may be contaminated by a dirty gown.

3	Used gowns should not be re-used.	To reduce the risk of cross-infection by contaminated uniforms, as staff find it hard to distinguish the inside/outside of a gown. If the gown is worn inside out, uniforms can be contaminated.
4	Leave the room, shutting the door behind you.	To reduce the risk of airborne spread of infection.
5	Rub hands with a bactericidal alcoholic hand rub.	To remove pathogenic organisms acquired from such items as the door handle.

Cleaning the room

Action   *Rationale*

1	Domestic staff must understand why barrier nursing is required and should be instructed on the correct procedure.	To reduce the risk of mistakes and to ensure that barrier nursing is maintained.
2	The area where barrier nursing is being carried out must be cleaned last.	To reduce the risk of the transmission of organisms.
3	Separate cleaning equipment must be kept for this area.	Cleaning equipment can easily become infected. Cross-infection may result from shared cleaning equipment.
4	Members of the domestic services staff must wear gloves and plastic aprons.	To reduce the risk of cross-infection.
5	*Floor* (hard surface). This must be washed daily with a disinfectant as appropriate. All excess water must be removed.	Daily cleaning will keep bacterial count reduced. Organisms, especially Gram-negative bacteria, multiply quickly in the presence of moisture (Suzuki *et al.* 1984).
6	Cleaning solutions must be freshly diluted and the spray container emptied, cleaned and dried daily.	Cleaning fluid can easily become contaminated (Medcraft *et al.* 1987).
7	After use, the bucket must be cleaned and dried.	Bacteria will not easily survive on clean dry surfaces.
8	Mop heads should be laundered in a hot wash daily.	Mop heads become contaminated easily.
9	*Floor* (carpet). An infected patient may have been admitted into a room with a carpet. A vacuum cleaner should be used which is fitted with an efficient filter. After use the dust bag must be changed and the brush head washed and dried.	Vacuum cleaning reduces the dust thus reducing organisms (Munir *et al.* 1993).
10	On discharge, the carpet must be steam cleaned.	Bacteria can survive in dust trapped in the carpet fibres. The heat of the steam will kill these bacteria.
11	Furniture and fittings should be damp dusted using a disposable cloth and a detergent solution or a disinfectant if appropriate.	To remove any organisms.
12	The toilet, shower and bathroom area must be cleaned at least once a day using a non-abrasive hypochlorite powder or cream. A disinfectant will only be required if soiling of the area has occurred.	Non-abrasive powders or creams preserve the integrity of the surfaces. These areas recontaminate rapidly after cleaning and routine chemical disinfection is of little value and should be saved for terminal cleaning following discharge of the patient.

Transporting infected patients outside the source isolation area

Action   *Rationale*

| **1** | Inform the department concerned about the diagnosis. | To allow other departments time to make their own arrangements. |

Guidelines • Source isolation (cont'd)

Action

2 Arrange for the patient to have the last appointment of the day.

3 Any porters involved must be instructed carefully. The trolley or chair should be cleaned after use.

4 It may be necessary for the nurse to escort the patient.

Rationale

The department concerned, the hospital corridors, lifts etc., will be less busy and will allow more time for special cleaning and disinfecting.

Protection and reassurance of porters are necessary to allay fear and to minimize the risk of the infection being spread to them.

To ensure the necessary precautions are maintained.

Discharging the patient

Action

1 Inform the infection control team when the patient is due for discharge.

2 The room should be stripped and aired. All textiles must be changed and curtains sent to the laundry.

3 Impervious surfaces, e.g. lockers, stools, blinds and thermometer holders, should be washed with soap and water.

4 The floor must be washed and dried thoroughly.

5 The room can be reused as soon as it has been correctly and thoroughly cleaned.

Rationale

The infection control team will advise on any special precautions.

Curtains readily become colonized with bacteria.

Wiping of surfaces is the most effective way of removing contaminants. Relatively inaccessible places, e.g. ceilings, may be omitted; these are not generally relevant to any infection risk.

To remove any organisms present.

Most organisms will survive in the environment for long periods of time. Effective cleaning will remove these organisms. Once cleaning has been completed, the room is ready to admit another patient.

Protective isolation

Definition

Protective isolation is a process of care which provides a safe environment for patients who are susceptible to infection by isolating them as far as possible from the risk of infection from all exogenous sources.

Indications

Protective isolation can be an appropriate form of care for many patients, e.g. burns patients, children with immunodeficiency disease and patients receiving bone marrow transplantation. The aim of protective isolation is to prevent and treat infection until the period of immunosuppression is past.

Immunosuppression is a generalized depression of the immune system, which increases the risk of acquiring an infection. This necessitates protecting immunosuppressed patients from micro-organisms carried in the environment, on health care workers providing care, on visitors and on other patients.

Immunosuppression can be caused by many factors including:

1 Primary disease such as leukaemia, lymphoma (Field *et al.* 1977), acquired immune deficiency syndrome (AIDS) (Centre for Disease Control 1988), severe combined immunodeficiency disease (SCID) (Hill 1989).
2 Secondary disease, such as diabetes, which may complicate primary disease (Reeves 1980).
3 Drugs, in particular cytotoxic drugs and corticosteroids (Reheis 1985; Carlisle *et al.* 1993).
4 Antimicrobial therapy causing changes in the patient's microbial flora (Hahn *et al.* 1978).
5 Irradiation therapy: the degree of immunosuppression is related directly to the area being treated (Strober *et al.* 1981).
6 Trauma (Maclean *et al.* 1975) and burns (Miller *et al.* 1979).
7 Age (Leonard 1986).

A careful clinical history and physical examination will provide an initial assessment of the patient's susceptibility to infection (Dales & Liles 1998).

The risk of infection will be increased by breaches in the body's natural defence mechanisms, for example:

1 Skin by, for example, indwelling catheters, repeated venepuncture, pressure ulcers (Wade *et al*. 1982; Yuen *et al*. 1998).
2 Mucous membranes, from oral ulceration (Richardson 1987; Yuen *et al*. 1998).
3 Body cavities by urinary catheters or endotracheal tubes (Ward *et al*. 1997).

Nursing care of the highest standard is required when involved in such procedures to reduce the risk of infection as much as practically possible (Buchsel & Kelleher 1989). It has been suggested that the risk of infection depends on the patient's ability to respond to infection rather than the actual number of neutrophils in the peripheral blood (Dales & Liles 1998). However, infection rates have been seen to be related to the absolute level of circulating granulocytes (Bodey *et al*. 1966) with the frequency of infection rising as the granulocytes count drops below 0.5×10^9/litre, with a dramatic increase as the granulocyte count reaches zero (Schimpff *et al*. 1978). Granulocytopenia, occurring rapidly, is more likely to be associated with an increased risk of infection than is a slow decline or a stable granulocytopenia (Dale *et al*. 1979).

Some patients have an increased risk of infection due to a combination of immunosuppressive factors (Yuen *et al*. 1998). For example, a patient with leukaemia who is undergoing bone marrow transplantation and who develops graft-versus-host disease (GVHD) may require treatment with increased doses of immunosuppressive drug (Van Der Meer 1994).

In the 1970s and 1980s trials to evaluate the effectiveness of protective isolation were undertaken. For example Yates *et al*.'s (1973) study found no difference in infection rates in the first 21 days following admission. However, after this time patients experienced fewer infections if they were being cared for in protective isolation rooms. Others have demonstrated that protective isolation with topical and non-absorbable antibiotics and low microbial diet significantly reduced the number of infections, but did not affect long term survival (Levine *et al*. 1973; Ribas-Mundom *et al*. 1981). It has also been suggested that protective isolation reduces the incidence of GVHD in patients with aplastic anaemia (Storb *et al*. 1983), although in contrast Petersen *et al*.'s (1987) study suggested that incidence of GVHD was not affected. Nevertheless, the results of Petersen *et al*.'s project indicated that infection rates were significantly reduced in patients in protective isolation compared to those patients in conventional hospital rooms. The Center for Disease Control in the USA (Garner & Simmons 1983) highlights that expensive isolation precautions do not prevent endogenous infections and therefore do not appear to be warranted for most compromised patients. This view is supported by Grifiths-Jones (1998), who points out that the majority of infections will be endogenous and will have very little to do with the environment. In addition it has been suggested that reducing rigid isolation techniques to only washing hands on entering and leaving the room would reduce costs, inconvenience and stress to patients, and would more than compensate for those infections that did occur in standard

single rooms (Russell *et al*. 1992). A survey of 91 bone marrow transplantation units in the USA found that while all units used some type of protective environment practice, these varied between units. The researchers recommended that national standards for protective isolation needed to be compiled, which could be used to rationalize nursing care (Poe *et al*. 1994).

The British Committee for Standards in Haematology (BCS 1995) defines four levels of care required for the management of adult patients with haematological malignancies and bone marrow failure as:

1 Level 1 for patients with transient severe neutropenia. This involves rooms designated for neutropenic patients, which have skilled staff over the 24 hour period. Expert advice and support are available from a nurse specialist.
2 Level 2 for patients requiring induction chemotherapy for leukaemia.
3 Level 3 for patients undergoing autologous transplantation. Levels 2 and 3 management require single rooms with en suite facilities. Level 2 requires experienced nurses with recognized certificates in haematology.
4 Level 4 for patients undergoing related allogeneic and autologous transplantation. Care at level 4 requires single rooms, en suite facilities, laminar airflow or positive filtered air conditioning and a designated kitchen area. Levels 3 and 4 require nurses who are experienced, with at least 25% of nurses having certificates in haematology or oncology. The BSC (1995) highlights the stresses experienced by nurses caring for bone marrow transplantation (BMT) patients and recommends the provision of staff support.

Reference material

Protective isolation may be achieved by:

1 Purpose-built units (Borley 1982)
2 Plastic isolators (Bergerat *et al*. 1978; Bowell 1986)
3 Single rooms on a general ward (Nauseef *et al*. 1981)
4 Shared rooms within a controlled environment on a general ward.

Purpose-built units

A purpose-built unit will include:

1 Filtered air supply
2 Single rooms with integral toilet, shower, a hatch system for the aseptic transfer of equipment into the room, an entry area for visitors and staff where protective clothing can be donned and hands washed
3 Facilities to provide pathogen-free food
4 Gastrointestinal decontamination (Jameson *et al*. 1971).

These units are expensive to build, maintain and staff.

Plastic isolators

An isolator consists of a framework erected around a bed from which a PVC tent is suspended (Trexler 1975). The tent has an air supply attached which keeps the whole apparatus inflated. A positive air pressure is usually maintained within the isolator. In some cases, for example when nursing patients with Lassa fever, the pressure within the isolator is slightly below atmospheric pressure, which prevents the escape of any infected particles. Although patients may feel a strong sense of containment within the isolator (Ransjo 1978), this system does have the advantage of achieving high standards of bacteriological control, and it can be assembled and dismantled rapidly.

Single rooms and shared rooms in general wards

The decision to isolate a patient will be influenced by the availability of facilities coupled to the general condition of the ward area where the isolation is to take place. In determining the most suitable area, a number of criteria need to be met. Among these are the relative cleanliness of the ward, the standard of domestic services support, the microbiological status of the other patients and the anticipated length of the isolation. This less vigorous method of protective isolation is unlikely to greatly reduce the acquisition of potential pathogens, as only person-to-person transfer of infection is prevented, since facilities such as clean air and pathogen-free food are not usually available on general wards (Hann et al. 1984).

Protective isolation environment

The prevention of exogenous transmission of infection is important and can be achieved by careful monitoring of the environment to remove items which could predispose to infection, for example flowers (Taplin et al. 1973). Scrupulous cleaning with special attention to furniture and equipment within the room will also prevent transmission (Crane 1980; Boden 1999). All surfaces must be cleanable, especially items such as chairs (Custovic et al. 1998), with excess equipment removed to make the cleaning process easier and more effective (King 1998). The patient area must be well maintained. This was highlighted by Loach (1997), who discussed how her experience of protective isolation was badly affected by a shower being broken. In addition, contaminated plumbing can be an infection risk, which can be reduced by routine servicing (Ferroni et al. 1998).

Patient hygiene

Studies have highlighted the overwhelming fatigue experienced by patients with leukaemia and lymphoma. Fatigue hinders patient ability to take care of themselves and demonstrates the importance of expert nursing intervention and assessment (Persson et al. 1997).

The limiting of endogenous transmission of infection, which is the major cause of infection in immunosuppressed patients (Schimpff et al. 1970; Selden et al. 1971) is difficult but good patient hygiene and restriction of invasive devices and procedures are useful.

Infection

The most common areas of early infection include the lung, pharynx, anorectal area, skin and subcutaneous tissue (Reheis 1985). Unfortunately, signs and symptoms of infection are often absent in immunosuppressed patients (Sickles et al. 1975). As progression of infection in the immunosuppressed patient may be rapid and widespread, the earliest signs of infection must be looked for (see Chap. 28, Observations). When fever appears, diagnostic and therapeutic measures must be instigated immediately (Klastersky 1993). When infections are left untreated, fatality rate ranging from 18% to 40% can occur within the first 48 hours (Schimpff 1977). Patient survival depends upon prompt recognition of problems and instigation of medical and nursing intervention (Shaffer & Wilson 1993). Investigations to establish the cause of infection include chest X-ray, bacteriological and viral culture of blood, urine and sputum and swabs obtained from any suspicious lesion. Riley (1998) discusses the value of surveillance cultures in predicting causative organisms of infection, suggesting they should be limited to weekly samples from nose, throat and stool samples (see Chap. 37, Specimen collection).

Bacterial infections are generally caused by Gram-negative organisms, such as *Pseudomonas* species, *Escherichia coli* and *Klebsiella* species, normally found in the gastrointestinal tract. Gram-positive organisms causing infections are commonly *Staphylococcus epidermidis*, which is generally a skin contaminant (Bodey 1975). The most common fungal infection is by *Candida albicans*, which is most usually found in the oral cavity, but which may affect the oesophagus, bowel or vagina and cause systemic infection, pneumonia and septicaemia (Edwards 1995). *Aspergillus* infection, particularly associated with nearby building work, has also been seen (see the aspergillosis section later in this chapter). Viral infections, particularly by cytomegalovirus and herpes zoster, may occur (see the section on herpes viruses, later in this chapter).

Hand washing

Immunosuppressed patients are at increased risk of nosocomial infection, and bacteria that cause infection are particularly easily disseminated by health care workers' hands (Larson 1988). Strict hand washing before and after patient contact, can reduce rates of infection (Gould 1993) (see 'Aseptic techniques' in Chap. 3). Hand washing can be said to be the most important means of infection control (Bowell 1992). Compliance with hand washing can be poor; one study found only 56% of clinicians and 86% of nurses complied with hand washing policy requirements (Lai et al. 1998).

Diet

Food is a potential source of infection (Correa et al. 1991) and good food hygiene practice is essential (Barrie 1996). Generally, if non-absorbable gut antibiotics are prescribed, pathogen-free food must be provided (Patterson 1993). This includes thoroughly cooked foods, canned foods and foods known to be pathogen-free such as cereal. Reheated food is not likely to be pathogen-free and should not be used. If pathogen-free food is unavailable the diet should consist only of food that has been well cooked, with foods known to have high bacterial counts avoided (Roberts 1982). Foods known to have an increased risk of being contaminated, for example fresh cream, shellfish, soft cheeses, pâté, raw vegetables, salads and fruit that cannot be washed and peeled, must be eliminated from the diet. Infection from ice can also occur from contamination within the ice maker or from staff, patients or visitors. Surveys of hospital ward ice machines demonstrated a wide range of potentially opportunistic pathogenic micro-organisms (Wilson et al. 1997), and that only one machine fully complied with the cleaning policy (Anson & Allen 1997). It should be noted that microwave cookers have been found to be an unreliable means of heating food (Gearge 1997) and therefore should not be used in these circumstances.

Well-nourished people undergoing BMT have a better survival rate and shorter hospital stay than undernourished patients (Henry 1997). Food provided for patients must be prepared following recognized food safety regulations (General Food Hygiene Regulations 1995), including thorough hand washing. Food cooked and brought in from home must be avoided as this may not have been prepared according to good food hygiene practices. Visitors should be encouraged to bring in pre-packaged food such as biscuits and crisps or tinned items (McCulloch 1998) which will have been manufactured to the necessary food hygiene standards. A review of practice related to clean diets found evidence of a move away from stringent sterile diets towards more relaxed regimes with rational, justifiable food hygiene guidelines (Patterson 1993).

Psychological issues

Protective isolation can cause increased stress for patients (Gaston-Johnson et al. 1992), and they should be prepared before they enter isolation (Bater 1989; Collins et al. 1989). Nurses can reduce anxiety by assisting patients to learn about their situation and about health promoting activities (Belec 1992). It is important that health care workers are aware of the impact of protective isolation on patients (Gaskill et al. 1997), and it has been suggested that patients should only be offered a BMT if anticipated physical and psychological benefits outweigh the risk (Collins et al. 1989). Other studies suggest that patients view protective isolation as a temporary inconvenience rather than a stressor (Zerbe et al. 1994). A study of long-term adult BMT survivors found that despite lingering side-effects these patients were leading full and meaningful lives (Haberman et al. 1993). However, one patient's view of isolation highlighted the stifling confined environment, loss of bodily freedom and the shock of physical deterioration (Loach 1997).

Nursing care

Orientation, education and training for new and existing staff are essential (Lin et al. 1993), to allow nurses to keep up with developments and to ensure optimum patient care (Porter 1998). Larson et al.'s (1993) study describes the lack of nurses' perception of the patient's distress during hospitalization for BMT. Other studies highlight the importance of BMT nurses' training, which should include specific psychosocial strategies to delineate psychosocial needs of patients and families (Winters et al. 1994).

It is suggested that nursing on a protective isolation unit, particularly with patients undergoing BMT, increases the stress suffered by nurses themselves (Borley 1985; Collins et al. 1989). This can result in burn-out, producing symptoms such as fatigue, anxiety, depression and poor concentration (Scully 1980), which can be detrimental to nurses, their colleagues and the patients in their care. Nursing managers of intensive care units such as protective isolation units need to be aware of this risk and provide support and a treatment plan if burn-out does occur (McElroy 1982).

Nurses must recognize the factors which increase the risk of infection and must not contribute to this risk (McCulloch 1998). Pettinger & Nettleman's (1991) study investigating compliance with isolation precautions found that non-compliance with protective isolation procedures was widespread, although visitors were more compliant than health care workers.

References and further reading

Anson, J.J. & Allen, K.D. (1997) Hospital ice machines. J Hosp Infect, 37(4), 335–6.
Barrie, D. (1996) The provision of food and catering services in hospital. J Hosp Infect, 33, 13–33.
Bater, M. (1989) Preparing for bone marrow transplantation. Nurs Times, 85(7), 46–7.
Belec, R.H. (1992) Quality of life: perception of long-term survivors of bone marrow transplantation. Oncol Nurs Forum, 19(1), 31–7.
Bergerat, J.P. et al. (1978) Use of plastic isolators in the prevention of infection in high risk patients with hematologic diseases. Sem Hosp, 54(37–40), 1137–343.
Boden, M. (1999) Contamination in moving and handling equipment. Prof Nurse, 14(7), 484–7.
Bodey, C.P. et al. (1966) Quantitative relationships between circulating leukocytes and infection in patients with acute leukaemia. Ann Int Med, 64, 328–40.
Bodey, C.P. (1975) Infections in cancer patients. Cancer Treat Rev, 2, 89–128.
Borley, D. (1982) A protected environment for bone marrow transplantation. Pict Nurs Med Educ, 6, 156–8.
Borley, D. (1985) Bone marrow patients can plant extra stress on nurses. Nurs Mirror, 160(8), 6.
Bowell, B. (1992) Protecting the patient at risk. Nurs Times, 88(3), 32–5.
Bowell, E. (1986) Nursing the isolated patient. Nurs Times, 82(33), 72–81.
British Committee for Standards in Haematology (BSC) (1995) Guidelines on the provision of facilities for the care of adult patients with haematological malignancies (including leukaemia and lymphoma and severe bone marrow failure). Clin Lab Haem, 17, 3–10.
Buchsel, P.C. & Kelleher, J. (1989) Bone marrow transplantation. Nurs Clin North Am, 24(4), 907–38.
Carlisle, P.S., Gucalp, R. & Wiernik, P.H. (1993) Nosocomial infections on neutropenic cancer patients. Infect Control Hosp Epidemiol, 14(6), 320–24.

Center for Disease Control (1988) Revision of CDC surveillance case definition of AIDS. *Morb Mort Week Rep*, **36**, 1–15.

Collins, C., Upright, C. & Aleksich, J. (1989) Reverse isolation: what patients perceive. *Oncol Nurse Forum*, **16**(5), 675–9.

Correa, C.M.C. *et al.* (1991) Vegatables as a source of infection with *Pseudomonas aeruginosa* in a university and oncology hospital of Rio de Janeiro. *J Hosp Infect*, **18**, 301–306.

Crane, L.R. (1980) Prevention of infection on the oncology unit. *Nurs Clin North Am*, **15**(4), 843–55.

Custovic, A. *et al.* (1998) Domestic allergens in public places. *Clin Exp Allergy*, **28**(1), 53–9.

Dale, D.C. *et al.* (1979) Chronic neutropenia. *Medicine*, **58**, 128–44.

Dale, D.C. & Liled, C. (1998) How many neutrophils are enough? *Lancet*, **351**(9118), 1752–3.

DoH (1995) *General Food Hygiene Regulations*. Stationery Office, London.

Edwards, J.E. (1995) *Candida* species, 4th edn. In: *Principles and Practice of Infectious Diseases* (eds G.L. Mandell, J.E. Bennett & R. Dolin). Churchill Livingstone, New York.

Emmerson, A.M. *et al.* (1996) The second national prevalence survey of infection in hospital – overview of the results. *J Hosp Infect*, **32**(3), 175–90.

Evans, H.S. *et al.* (1998) General outbreaks of infectious intestinal disease in England and Wales, 1995–1996. *Commun Dis Public Health*, **1**(3), 165–71.

Ferroni, A. *et al.* (1998) Outbreak of nosocomial urinary tract infections due to *Pseudomonas aeruginosa* in a paediatric surgical unit associated with tap water contamination. *J Hosp Infect*, **39**, 301–307.

Field, R. *et al.* (1977) Infections in patients with malignant lymphoma treated with combination chemotherapy. *Cancer*, **39**, 1018–77.

Garner, J.S. & Simmons, B.P. (1983) CDC guidelines for isolation precautions in hospital. *Infect Control*, **4**(4), 325.

Gaskill, D., Henderson, A. & Fraser, M. (1997) Exploring the everyday world of the patient in isolation. *Oncol Nurse Forum*, **24**(4), 695–700.

Gaston-Johnson, F. *et al.* (1992) Pain and psychological distress in patients undergoing autologous bone marrow transplantation. *Oncol Nurs Forum*, **19**(1), 41–7.

George, R.H. (1997) Killing activity of microwaves in milk. *J Hosp Infect*, **35**, 319–26.

Gould, D. (1993) Assessing nurses' hand decontamination performance. *Nurs Times*, **90**(25), 47–50.

Griffiths-Jones, A. (1998) Infection control Isolation precautions. *Health Serv Risks Spec Rep*, **25**, 1–7.

Haberman, M. *et al.* (1993) Quality of life of adult long term survivors of bone marrow transplantation: a quantitative analysis of narrative data. *Oncol Nurs Forum*, **20**(10), 1545–53.

Hahn, D.M. *et al.* (1978) Infection in acute leukaemia patients receiving oral, non-absorbable antibiotics. *Antimicrob Agents Chemother*, **13**, 958–64.

Hann, I.M. *et al.* (1984) Infection prophylaxis in the patient with bone marrow failure. *Clin Haem*, **13**(3), 523–46.

Henry, L. (1997) Immunocompromised patients and nutrition. *Prof Nurse*, **12**(9), 655–9.

Henry, L. & Souchon, V. (1998) Nutritional support. In: *The Clinical Practice of Stem Cell Transplantation* (eds J. Barrett & J. Treleaven) ISIS Med Media, Oxford, **2**(53), 812–25.

Hill, H.R. (1989) Infection complicating congenital immunodeficiency syndromes. In: *Clinical Approaches to Infection in the Compromised Host* (eds R.H. Rubin & L.S. Young), 2nd edn, pp. 407–32. Plenum Medical, London.

Jameson, B. *et al.* (1971) Five-year analysis of protective isolation. *Lancet*, **1**, 1034–40.

King, S. (1998) Decontamination of equipment and the environment. *Nurs Stand*, **12**(52), 57–63.

Klastersky, J. (1993) Febrile neutropenia. *Support Care Cancer*, **1**(5), 233–9.

Lai, K.K. *et al.* (1998) Failure to eradicate vancomycin resistant enterococci in a university hospital and the cost of barrier precautions. *Infect Control Hosp Epidemiol*, **19**(9), 647–52.

Larson, E. (1988) A causal link between hand washing and risk of infection. *Infect Control Hosp Epidemiol*, **9**, 28–35.

Larson, P.J. *et al.* (1993) Comparison of perceived symptoms of patients undergoing bone marrow transplant and the nurses caring for them. *Oncol Nurs Forum*, **20**(1), 81–8.

Leonard, M. (1986) Handling infection. *Nurs Times*, **82**(33), 81–4.

Levine, A.S., Siegal, S.E. & Schrieber, A.D. (1973) Protected environment and prophylactic antibiotics. A perspective controlled study of their utility in the therapy of acute leukaemia. *New Engl J Med*, **288**, 477–83.

Lin, E.M., Tierney, D.K. & Stadtmauer, E.A. (1993) Autologous bone marrow transplantation. A review of the principles and complications. *Cancer Nurs*, **16**(3), 204–13.

Loach, L. (1997) Blue days. *Nurs Times*, **93**(32), 31–2.

Lovitt, S.A. *et al.* (1992) Isolation gowns, a false sense of security. *Am J Infect Control*, **20**(4), 185–91.

Maclean, L.D. *et al.* (1975) Host resistance in sepsis and trauma. *Ann Surg*, **182**, 207–15.

McCulloch, J. (1998) Infection control: principles for practice. *Nurs Stand*, **13**(1), 49–52.

McElroy, A. (1982) Burn-out: a review of the literature with application to cancer nursing. *Cancer Nurs*, **3**(6), 211–17.

Meers, P.D. *et al.* (1981) Report on the Natural Survey of Infections in Hospitals, 1980. *J Hosp Infect*, (Suppl.) **2**, 1–53.

Meyer, I.D. (1986) Infection in bone marrow transplant recipients. *Am J Med*, **81**, 27–8.

Miller, C.L. *et al.* (1979) Changes in lymphocyte activity after thermal injury. *J Clin Invest*, **63**, 202–210.

Mims, C.A. *et al.* (1993) *Medical Microbiology*. Mosby, London.

Nauseef, W.M. *et al.* (1981) A study of the value of simple protective isolation in patients with granulocytopenia. *New Engl J Med*, **304**(8), 448–53.

Patterson, A.J. (1993) Review of current practices in clean diets in the UK. *J Hum Nutr Diet*, **6**, 3–11.

Persson, L., Hallberg, I.R. & Ohlsson, O. (1997) Survivors of acute leukaemia and highly malignant lymphoma – retrospective views of daily life problems during treatment and when in remission. *J Adv Nurs*, **25**, 68–78.

Petersen, F.B. *et al.* (1987) Infectious complications in patients undergoing marrow transplantation: a prospective randomized study of the additional effects of contamination and laminar air flow isolation among patients receiving prophylactic systemic antibiotics. *Scand J Infect Dis*, **19**(5), 559–67.

Pettinger, A. & Nettleman, M.D. (1991) Epidemiology of isolation precautions. *Infect Control Hosp Epidemiol*, **12**(5), 303–307.

Poe, S.S. *et al.* (1994) A national survey of infection prevention practices on bone marrow transplant units. *Oncol Nurs Forum*, **21**(10), 1687–93.

Porter, H. (1998) Nursing management in the BMT unit. In: *The Clinical Practice of Stem-Cell Transplantation* (eds J. Barrett & J. Treleaven). ISIS Medical Media, Oxford, **2**(59), 879–89.

Ransjo, U. (1978) Isolation care of infection prone burn patients. *Scand J Infect Dis*, (Suppl.), **11**, 1–46.

Redpath, C. & Farrington, M. (1997) Dispose of disposables. *J Hosp Infect*, **35**, 313–17.

Reeves, W.G. (1980) Immunology of diabetes and insulin therapy. *Rec Adv Clin Immunol*, **2**, 183–7.

Reheis, C.E. (1985) Neutropenia causes complications: treatment and resulting nursing care. *Nurs Clin North Am*, **20**(1), 219–25.

Ribas-Mundom, M., Granena, A. & Rozman, C. (1981) Evaluation of a protective environment in the management of granulocytopenic patients. A comparative study. *Cancer*, **48**, 419–24.

Richardson, A. (1987) A process standard for oral care. *Nurs Times*, **83**(32), 38–40.

Riley, U. (1998) Bacterial infections. In: *The Clinical Practice of Stem Cell Transplantation* (eds J. Barrett & J. Treleaven). ISIS Medical Media, Oxford, **2**(43), 690–97.

Roberts, D. (1982) Factors contributing to outbreaks of food poisoning in England and Wales, 1970–1979. *J Hyg*, **89**, 491.

Rubin, R.H. *et al.* (1990) Therapy, both immunosuppressive and antimicrobial for the transplant patient in the 1990s. In: *Organ Transplantation – Current Clinical and Immunological Concepts* (eds L. Brent & R. Sells), pp. 71–89. Baillière Tindall, Eastbourne.

Russell, J.A. *et al.* (1992) Allogeneic bone marrow transplantation without protective isolation in adults with malignant disease. *Lancet*, **339**(8784), 38–40.

Schimpff, S.C. (1977) Therapy for infection in patients with granulocytopenia. *Med Clin North Am*, **61**, 1101–18.

Schimpff, S.C. *et al.* (1970) Relationship of colonization with *Pseudomonas aeruginosa* to development of *Pseudomonas* bacteraemia in cancer patients. *Antimicrob Chemother*, **10**, 240–44.

Schimpff, S.C. *et al.* (1978) Infection prevention in acute leukaemia. *Leuk Res*, **2**, 231–40.

Scully, R. (1980) Stress in the nurse. *Am J Nurs*, **80**(5), 912–15.

Selden, R. *et al.* (1971) Nosocomial *Klebsiella* infections. Intestinal colonization as a reservoir. *Ann Int Med*, **74**, 675–84.

Shaffer, S. & Wilson, J.N. (1993) Bone marrow transplantation. Critical Care nurses. *Clin North Am*, **5**(3), 531–50.

Sickles, E.A. *et al.* (1975) Clinical presentation of infection in granulocytopenia patients. *Arch Int Med*, **135**, 715–19.

Storb, R. *et al.* (1983) GVHD and survival in patients with aplastic anaemia treated by bone marrow grafts with HLA identifiable siblings. *New Engl J Med*, **308**, 302–307.

Strober, S. *et al.* (1981) Immunosuppressive and tolerogenic effect of whole-body total lymphoid regional irradiation. In: *Immunosuppressive Therapy* (ed. J.R. Salaman). MTP Press, Lancaster.

Strom, T.B. (1990) Immunosuppression in graft rejection. In: *Organ Transplantation – Current Clinical and Immunological Concepts* (eds L. Brent & R. Sells), pp. 44–56. Baillière Tindall, Eastbourne.

Taplin, D. *et al.* (1973) Flower vases in hospital as reservoirs of pathogens. *Lancet*, **11**, 1279–81.

Trexler, P.C. (1975) Microbial isolators for use in the hospital. *Biomed Eng*, **10**(2), 63–7.

Van Der Meer, J.W.N. (1994) Defects in the host immune mechanisms. In: *Clinical Approaches to Infection in the Compromised Host* (eds R.H. Rubins & L.S. Young), 3rd edn. Plenum Medical, London.

Wade, J.C. *et al.* (1982) *Staphylococcus epidemidis*, an increasingly but frequently recognised cause of infection in granulocytopenia. *Ann Int Med*, **97**, 503–508.

Wilson, I.G., Hogg, G.M. & Barr, J.G. (1997) Microbiological quality of ice in hospital and community. *J Hosp Infect*, **36**, 171–80.

Ward, V., Wilson, J., Taylor, L. *et al.* (1997) *Preventing Hospital Acquired Infection*, pp. 25–35. Public Health Laboratory Service, London.

Winters, G. *et al.* (1994) Provisional practice: the nature of psychosocial bone marrow transplant nursing. *Oncol Nurs Forum*, **21**(7), 1147–54.

Yates, J.W. *et al.* (1973) A controlled study of isolation and endogenous microbial suppression in acute myelocytic leukaemia patients. *Cancer*, **32**, 1490–8.

Yuen, K.Y. *et al.* (1998) Unique risk factors for bacteraemia in allogeneic bone marrow transplant recipients before and after engraftment. *Bone Marrow Transpl*, **21**(11), 1137–43.

Zerbe, M.B., Parkerson, S.G. & Spitzer, T. (1994) Laminar air flow versus reverse isolation: nurses' assessment of moods, behaviours, and activity levels in patients receiving bone marrow transplants. *Oncol Nurs Forum*, **21**(3), 565–8.

GUIDELINES · Nursing the neutropenic patient

Procedure

Preparation of the room and maintenance of general cleanliness

Action	Rationale
1 A single room should be used if possible.	To reduce airborne transfer of micro-organisms.
2 A toilet to be kept for the sole use of the patient.	To reduce the risk of cross-infection.
3 Area to be cleaned meticulously before the patient is admitted.	To reduce the risk of infection.
4 Equipment and supplies to be kept for the sole use of the patient. (This must also include any cleaning equipment used by domestic staff.)	To reduce the risk of cross-infection. Cleaning equipment can easily become colonized with micro-organisms which may cause cross-infection.
5 Surfaces and furniture to be damp dusted daily using disposable cleaning cloths and detergent solution.	Damp dusting and mopping removes micro-organisms without distributing them into the air.
6 Floor to be mopped daily using soap and water.	To reduce the risk of cross-infection.

Guidelines • Nursing the neutropenic patient (cont'd)

Action	Rationale
7 Mop head to be laundered daily.	As above.
8 Bucket and mop handle to be cleaned and dried.	As above.

Nursing procedure

Entering room

Action	Rationale
1 Hands must be washed thoroughly with bactericidal soap and water or bactericidal alcohol hand rub.	Hands are regarded as the principle source of transfer of micro-organisms. (For further information see Chap. 3, Aseptic technique.)
2 A disposable plastic apron should be worn when in contact with the patient.	To protect staff clothing from becoming contaminated, which could transfer organisms to the other patients in their care.
3 Door of room to be kept closed. Ideally the air in the room should be under slightly positive pressure. The air flow should be from the room into the corridor.	To reduce the risk of airborne transmission of infection from other areas of the ward.

Visitors

Action	Rationale
1 The patient should be asked to nominate close relatives and friends who may then, after instruction, visit freely. The patient or his or her representative should inform casual acquaintances or non-essential visitors that they should avoid visiting during the period of neutropenia.	The incidence of infection increases in proportion to the number of people visiting. Large numbers of visitors are difficult to screen and educate. Unlimited visiting by close relatives and friends diminishes the sense of isolation that the patient may experience.
2 Any visitor with an infection or who has been in contact with infection should be excluded.	Neutropenic patients are susceptible to infection.
3 Children, unless very close relatives, should be discouraged.	Children are more likely to have been in contact with infectious diseases which can have serious consequences if transmitted to a neutropenic patient.

Diet

Action	Rationale
1 Educate the patient to choose only cooked food from the hospital menu and avoid raw fruit, salads and uncooked vegetables, whether on the menu or brought in by visitors.	Uncooked foods are often heavily colonized by micro-organisms, particularly Gram-negative bacteria.
2 Food brought into the hospital by visitors must be restricted and: (a) Obtained from well-known, reliable firms (b) In undamaged, sealed tins and packets (c) Within the expiry date.	Correctly processed and packaged foods are more likely to be of an acceptable food hygiene standard.
3 Water may be filtered or boiled and allowed to cool in a covered jug.	Tap water is safe to drink but can become colonized by organisms, particularly Gram-negative organisms found in the plug hole of sinks or overflow outlet when the water is being filled.
4 Sealed packets of fruit juice (long shelf-life varieties, particularly those rich in vitamins) are suitable. It should be poured directly into a clean jug and drunk the same day.	These juices have been pasteurized and remain pathogen-free until they are opened.

Discharging the patient

Action	Rationale
1 Crowded areas, for example shops, cinemas, pubs and discos, should be avoided.	Although the patient's white cell count is usually high enough for discharge, the patient remains immunocompromised for some time.
2 Pets should not be allowed to lick the patient, and new pets should not be obtained.	Pets are known carriers of infection (Mims *et al.*1993).
3 Certain foods, for example take-away meals, soft cheese and pâté, should continue to be avoided.	Take-away meals are subject to handling by a large number of individuals and are stored for longer periods, both of which increase the likelihood of contamination.
4 Salads and fruit should be washed carefully, dried and, if possible, peeled.	To remove as many pathogens as possible.
5 Any sign or symptoms of infection should be reported immediately to the patient's general practitioner or to the discharging hospital.	Any infection may continue to have serious consequences if left unlocated.

Acquired immune deficiency syndrome (AIDS)

Definition

Acquired immune deficiency syndrome (AIDS) is a state of immunosuppression caused by the human immunodeficiency viruses 1 (HIV 1) and 2 (HIV 2), which causes a chronic, progressive disruption of the immune system (Stine 1993). As no overall description can be made for AIDS, an internationally agreed case definition has been made (Public Health Laboratory Service Communicable Disease Centre 1987) and includes the following:

1 Certain opportunistic infections
2 Certain cancers
3 Wasting syndrome
4 Encephalopathy

AIDS-defining cancers include

1 Kaposi sarcoma which is decreasing in prevalence
2 Primary CNS lymphoma
3 Non-Hodgkins lymphoma (Burkitt's or immunoblastic)
4 Invasive cervical cancer

The outlook for the latter three cancers is poor. Goedert *et al.* (1998) investigated the relationship of HIV and cancer and found that AIDS leads to immunological failure which predisposes to a significant increase in the risk of cancers; this risk increases with longer survival.

The definition was revised in 1992. This definition provides uniform, simple criteria for categorizing HIV conditions to facilitate evaluation of treatment and care of persons with HIV (Center for Disease Control 1992).

Reference material

Since 1989 several investigators have independently reported cases of unexplained severe immunodeficiency without evidence of infection with HIV 1 or 2 (Pankhurst & Peakman 1989; Jowitt *et al.* 1991; Laurence *et al.* 1992). In an extensive search for such cases, initiated in the USA by the Center for Disease Control (CDC), 80 widely scattered cases were identified. A review of these cases, however, did not reveal any epidemiological links between them. Other investigators have concluded that cases of unexplained severe immunodeficiency without HIV infection are rare, and that the available data do not show that unexplained severe immunodeficiency without HIV is endemic (WHO 1993).

A relatively small number of people claim that HIV does not cause AIDS (Stine 1993). Duesberg (1991), for example, states that the disease is caused by 'lifestyle'. This explanation has been discounted by others (Weiss & Jaffe 1990).

Up to 1996 there were nearly 30 million HIV infections and 8 million AIDS cases in the world, with 95% of new infections occurring in the developing world (Davison & Nicoll 1997). In the UK there were 16 426 AIDS cases by July 1999 (Public Health Laboratory Service Communicable Disease Surveillance Centre 1999). It is estimated that only 1% of AIDS cases and 3% of HIV infection routes of transmission have not been identified (Hughes 1997).

There are two HIV 1 subgroups, namely M (major) and O (outlier). Within the M subgroup there are 10 recognized subgroups (A–J), with subgroup B predominating in USA and Western Europe. The greatest number of subtypes are found in Africa. Recently a new strain of HIV has been identified in France which has been classified as N strain (Gottlieb 1998). This new strain has only been found in Cameroonians, but there is always the risk that it could spread and cause a new pandemic.

Many patients diagnosed with HIV infection in the UK receive care at centres outside their own health authority of residence, with the Thames regions caring for the largest number of resident and non-resident cases in need of treatment (Molesworth 1998).

Serological tests are used to diagnose HIV infection. Recent advances in HIV testing technology include simple rapid tests (Kassler 1997) using finger stick blood, oral fluids, urine (Hashida *et al.* 1997) and saliva dried on filter paper (Ishikawa 1996). Concerns have been raised related to the reliability of the enzyme linked immunosorbent assay (ELISA) blood test, used for first line screening for HIV, as other illnesses can produce a false positive test (Harrison & Corbett 1999). The Department of Health and Social Security (DHSS 1985) recommended that patients should not be tested for HIV antibodies without their consent, and that counselling should be offered to the patient before and after the test. During this counselling the patient should be informed about how HIV is transmitted and the significance of a negative and positive test. In 1996 further Department of Health guidelines provided a framework for counselling as there was a lack of consistency in the content of pre-test counselling. Hospitals involved in anonymous HIV antibody screening must ensure that patients are aware of the ongoing research project. No post-test counselling is possible in these circumstances.

The major disadvantage of diagnosis based on serology is the window period before IgG antibodies are produced in response to the HIV infection. Earlier diagnosis can be obtained by the use of IgM antibody screening. The presence of IgM indicates recent infection, which will help narrow the window period. Diagnosis can also be aided by the use of the HIV 1 p24 antigen assay (Erb & Matter 1998). p24 antigen is present in serum samples prior to and following seroconversion, when the antibody screening test is negative or indeterminate (Weber *et al.* 1998). p24 antigen tests can be used for diagnosis of HIV from the time of seroconversion until late stages of disease (Hashida *et al.* 1996). Viral load in peripheral blood can be measured and used for diagnostic, prognostic and monitoring of antiviral therapy purposes (Erb & Matter 1998).

Transmission

HIV has been isolated in the blood (Gallo *et al.* 1984), semen (Zagury *et al.* 1984), tears and saliva (Fujikawara *et al.* 1985), breast milk (Thiry *et al.* 1985), genital secretions of women (Wofsy *et al.* 1986) and cerebrospinal fluid and the brain (Levy 1985). Sexual intercourse between men accounts for 70% of all UK AIDS cases, with over 60% of HIV reports involving bisexual and homosexual men (Macdonald 1997). It has been reported that this figure is not likely to improve as unsafe sexual behaviour has increased among homosexual men since 1990 (Sadiq *et al.* 1998). It has been found, however, that skill-based sexual risk reduction interventions for women lead to safer sex practices (Belcher *et al.* 1998) and education intervention raises awareness to the risk of HIV infection (James *et al.* 1998). Heterosexual intercourse accounts for 15% of AIDS cases and 19% of HIV infection (McGarrigle *et al.* 1997). The remaining AIDS cases include injecting drug misusers (IVDU) 6% (Madden *et al.* 1997), infected blood, tissue or blood components 5% and mother to child transmission 2% (Molesworth & Tookey 1997).

It is expected that heat treatment of blood products, and increased risk awareness through donation and donor screening, will virtually eliminate new infections through blood products transfusion and transplantation (Mortimer & Spooner 1997). These factors, coupled with more conservative use of blood, should result in a decrease in the transmission of HIV infection by blood transfusion (Lackritz 1998). However, debate continues with regard to the value of including viral antigen tests in the screening tests applied to all blood donations (Korelitz *et al.* 1996).

Unusual HIV transmissions have occurred, for example by fighting, removal of bleeding bodies from railway lines and deliberate self-inoculation with known HIV positive blood (Gilbert *et al.* 1998). However, studies of prolonged social contact with HIV infection have failed to show that transmission has occurred, unless the transmission routes already mentioned are present (Jason *et al.* 1986). There have been exceptions to this, including from a child to a mother who was providing health care (Center for Disease Control 1986), and transmission between children living in the same house (Center for Disease Control 1993).

HIV is not a notifiable disease, although partner notification is encouraged. Most patients do cooperate in notifying some of their sex partners, who are generally receptive to being notified although they are often unaware of the HIV risks; these sex partners are often found to have high rates of HIV infection (West & Stark 1997).

Women and children

HIV disease in women disproportionately affects minorities (Nicoll *et al.* 1998), being associated with IVDUs, ethnic minorities and those with medical problems and associated conditions. Women appear to have a more rapid course of illness after diagnosis, but this is probably associated with differences in health care seeking behaviour. Although Madges *et al.* (1998) found 81% of HIV positive women were registered with a general practitioner, 83% of GPs were aware of their HIV positive status.

Perinatal transmission of HIV from mother to foetus can occur during intra-uterine, intrapartum and postpartum periods. During the postpartum period it is mainly through breast feeding, as HIV has been found in both colostrum and breast milk. The risk of the transmission of HIV via breast milk has to be balanced against the effect of early weaning on infant mortality, morbidity and maternal fertility (Leroy *et al.* 1998). The incidence of vertical transmission varies in different continents and is more likely to occur in Africa (Kotler 1998). Risk factors for transmission include: maternal immune status, this risk increases as maternal immune status decreases; increased maternal viral load (concentration of HIV 1 RNA in plasma); obstetrical risk factors; long duration of ruptured membranes; factors such as bleeding during pregnancy and amniocentesis; maternal drug use during pregnancy; and the presence of sexually transmitted diseases (Nourse & Butler 1998). High viral load is also associated with premature delivery (O'Shea *et al.* 1998). These research findings can be used to reduce the risk of transmission for infants born of HIV 1 infected women (Goedert *et al.* 1991).

There are advantages in testing pregnant women for HIV (Lindgren *et al.* 1998), since this has implications in terms of avoiding breast feeding, administration of Zidovu-dine (AZT), avoiding invasive procedures and provision of counselling. In addition, some women may wish to terminate the pregnancy and make informed decisions about further pregnancies (Mercey 1998). However Gibb *et al.* (1998) report that uptake of HIV testing is unacceptably low in pregnant women and new approaches are urgently required to improve uptake. Women who are made aware of their HIV diagnosis have been seen to act to reduce the risk of transmission to their infants (Lyall *et al.* 1998). HIV negative women who are identified as being at risk should be counselled about reducing their risk behaviour and retested in 6 months (Samson & King 1998). Seven studies reviewing the effects of pregnancy in women infected with HIV found HIV progression was significantly more common in developing countries, compared to the developed countries, where there did not appear to be an association between pregnancy and HIV progression (French & Brocklehurst 1998).

AZT, given during pregnancy, has been seen to decrease vertical transmission of HIV. Noone & Goldberg's (1997) study found a reduction from 25% to 8%, while the European collaborative study data indicated a reduction from 15% to 9% (Sperling *et al.* 1998). No problems have been identified from AZT taken during pregnancy (Sperling *et al.* 1998). Other anti-retroviral agents have not been seen to offer protection to the foetus. Although a substantial proportion of HIV infected children develop AIDS very early in life, an increasing percentage survive into adolescence without developing AIDS (Pliner *et al.* 1998). Kuhn *et al.*'s (1998) USA study found that between 36% and 61% of children survived to age 13 years. However, there is an urgent need to strengthen paediatric HIV/AIDS care in developing countries (Lepage *et al.* 1998). The strain and stress of HIV infection in a family are high (Howe 1998) and affect the entire family (Hansell *et al.* 1998), especially if the mother is also infected with HIV (Terriff & Synoground 1998). Coordination of care between the various health care workers in these situations is imperative (Thorne *et al.* 1998).

Clinical presentation

The window period generally occurs within 3 to 6 months of exposure, although longer window periods have been reported (Center for Disease Control 1996). An acute glandular fever-like illness may occur during this time. Following seroconversion an HIV antibody test will become positive, and the incubation period begins. Estimates to measure incubation periods vary; Bailey's (1997) revised assessment suggested 12.8 years. The UK register of HIV Seroconverters Steering Committee (1998) suggests that a person aged 16 years and over has a 60.2% risk of progressing to AIDS in 10 years. Significant variations are seen, for example a boy aged 4 years developed AIDS 4.5 months after receiving infected blood; this short incubation period was attributed to a large innoculum of HIV virus in the transfusion (Chuansumrit *et al.* 1996). Grant *et al.* (1997) suggest that, due to poor health care provision, progression

to AIDS and survival with AIDS will be shorter in developing countries compared to industrialized countries.

An AIDS diagnosis is when an HIV antibody positive person fulfils the case definition described above. The medical management of HIV and AIDS has improved, with the duration of survival following an AIDS diagnosis improving with time. There is a median survival of 10.6 months in cases diagnosed before 1987 and 18.4 months for those diagnosed each year since then (Rogers *et al.* 1997). There are reports of fewer opportunistic infections, admissions to hospital and deaths in industrial countries (De Cock 1997). However, opportunistic infections continue to be a relatively frequent complication of HIV disease (Moore & Chaisson 1996). The incidence of HIV related encephalopathy has also decreased (Pratt 1998).

It is clear that an AIDS diagnosis increases mortality significantly (Stover & Way 1998). Prognostic factors can be used to predict survival times of people with advance disease (Chene *et al.* 1997). Those patients with good performamce status will have a longer survival rate (Apolonio *et al.* 1995), while those patients with low body weight and neurological manifestations will have a reduced survival rate (Gerard *et al.* 1996). High plasma viral load levels and a low CD4+ T lymphocyte count (CD4 is the antigenic marker of helper T cells) are the best predictors of progression to AIDS and death (Mellors *et al.* 1997). These predictions allow the patient and the clinician to make informed decisions about therapy (Brettle *et al.* 1997). In addition, identification of survival patterns allows planning of health care resources (Colford *et al.* 1994).

Treatment

A wider understanding of the biology of HIV, improved methods of monitoring and early institution of appropriate combinations of newly available antiviral therapies have improved patient outcome (Carpenter *et al.* 1998). The National Institute of Health (1998) provides specific recommendations for the treatment of HIV infection. These include the recommendation that anti-retroviral therapy should be started before the immune system is irrevocably compromised. In cases with falling CD4 counts and deteriorating clinical conditions therapy should be urgently considered (Brettle *et al.* 1997). Aggressive therapy can reduce HIV RNA below the level of detection, which may delay or prevent the emergence of resistant viruses. Patient compliance with therapy is essential (Coffin 1996). HIV resistant strains have been found in previously untreated patients, which highlights the need for continuing education to prevent transmission of HIV (Wainberg & William Cameron 1998).

The use of combination anti-retroviral therapy has largely replaced monotherapy for HIV infection. The advantages of combination chemotherapy include synergistic interaction among some drugs, reduction or delay in the emergence of drug resistance and targeting of different cell types or tissue (Pillay 1998). Changes in therapy are necessary when there is treatment failure, unacceptable toxicity or intolerance, non-adherence and current use of suboptimal therapy. Factors that will need to be considered when changing therapy include the patient's previous anti-retroviral history, options available and the patient's physical status (Hirsch *et al.* 1998). Treatment for a few HIV positive patients has been to receive a bone marrow transplantation (Contu *et al.* 1993; Cooper *et al.* 1993; Gabarre *et al.* 1996). Medication for HIV infected patients includes anti-retroviral, opportunistic infection treatments and prophylaxis, adjunctive therapies, supportive care medications, alternative medications and investigative drugs. These can produce problems with some drugs needing to be taken before food, while others must be taken with food, spacing of medications, drug interactions, compliance, cost and confusion with drug names. Strategies to increase compliance with medications are essential.

With the improvement in combination therapy, many people who thought their time was limited are beginning to think about returning to work and leading improved lives (Rabkin 1997).

Vaccine

Containment of HIV will require an effective vaccine (Letvin 1998). Such a vaccine will need to be preventive to protect HIV negative people and therapeutic to reduce infectivity in those already found to be HIV positive. Considerable effort is now being focused on evaluating different approaches in developing a vaccine (Baltimore & Heilman 1998). Vaccine formation will need to take into consideration the special needs and problems of the developing world (Smith *et al.* 1998), since lack of resources and the ability to vaccinate large numbers of people in developing countries create particular difficulties.

Confidentiality

AIDS raises many ethical issues (Reisman 1988). Mindel (1987) discusses the importance of confidentiality when dealing with any antibody positive patient. This was supported by the United Kingdom Central Council for Nursing, Midwifery and Health Visiting (1986) and the DHSS (1990) which also states that health care workers dealing with known or suspected seropositive patients or specimens must be made fully aware of the risk.

Psychological support

Anxiety is a universal problem for people with AIDS (Phillips & Morrow 1998). Katz's (1997) study explored the feelings of HIV positive people and highlighted the enormous stress of an HIV diagnosis. The study found that disclosure to family and friends was considered traumatic, although family members generally overcame these feelings and provided valuable help and support. This suggested that the initial emotional distress at the time of disclosure was worthwhile. Depression is not an inevitable consequence of HIV disease, being neither common nor expectable (Rabkin 1997), and feelings of unhappiness, anger, grief or diminished future expectations are often accompanied by or intermingled with positive emotions

and a fighting spirit. AIDS counsellors have been identified as the main source of psychosocial help for people with HIV/AIDS (Burnard 1992).

HIV palliative care offers disease specific therapy and comfort with symptom oriented treatment throughout the clinical course of the disease not just at the end of life. Issues such as treatment choices and resuscitation need to be discussed early and whenever physical status changes.

Infection control

There is a legal requirement for employers under the general duties of the *Health and Safety at Work etc. Act 1975*, Management of Health and Safety at Work Regulations 1992 and the Control of Substances Hazardous to Health Regulations 1994 to safeguard employees and others against occupational risk. This includes risk posed by blood borne infection (Wilcox 1997). Strategies must be in place to reduce the incidence of exposure to HIV (McKee 1996). The risk of HIV infection in health care workers can be reduced by strict adherence to universal precautions (Reyes & Legg 1997). Employees have a responsibility to adopt universal precautions for all patients (Ward *et al.* 1997). Factors such as fatigue, stress, levels of training, skill and experience affect safe practices. If nurses are willing to care for infected patients they are entitled to the safest environment that can reasonably be created (Hanrahan & Reutter 1997).

HIV infection alone does not affect a person's ability to continue with regular employment (Department of Employment – Health and Safety Executive 1987), unless injury to the worker could result in blood contaminating a patient's open tissues (DoH 1991). Therefore HIV infected health care workers must not perform exposure prone procedures. In addition, these workers must receive regular medical and occupational health supervision while they provide clinical care to patients (DoH 1998).

In the UK the Department of Health has issued guidance for health care workers (DoH 1991) and procedures to be followed when health care workers involved in invasive procedures are found to be HIV antibody positive (DoH 1993). One paper discusses how three cases of doctors found to be HIV positive were followed up very differently, with lessons learnt from each incident (Pell *et al.* 1996). In such circumstances the patient should be informed of the low risk and encouraged to have an HIV test.

The risk of acquiring HIV infection following a needle stick injury is 3 per 1000 injuries. The risk of acquiring HIV through mucous membrane exposure is even less at 1 in 1000 (DoH 1997). As many as 286 reports of occupationally acquired HIV infection in the world have been received (Public Health Laboratory Service AIDS and STD Centre 1997). In the UK, to June 1997, four people were known to have developed HIV following a documented accident, with eight others who may have occupationally acquired HIV (Local Collaborators 1998). The Chief Medical Officer's Expert Advisory Group on AIDS advises that post exposure prophylaxis is offered following exposure to a patient known or strongly suspected to be infected with HIV; accidents leading to exposure include percutaneous injury, contamination of broken skin and exposure of mucous membrane including the eye (DoH 1997).

Concerns have been raised related to the possibility of drug resistant HIV being transmitted to health care workers who have received a significant inoculation accident (Veenstra *et al.* 1995), to sexual partners (Carlon *et al.* 1994) or by vertical transmission (Frenkel *et al.* 1995).

The risk of patients acquiring HIV from HIV positive health care workers is low. Two HIV infected health care workers, a dentist in Florida and an orthopaedic surgeon in France, have transmitted HIV infection during exposure prone procedures. Similarly, patients may be at risk by inadequate infection control practices, an example being child transmission through exposure to HIV positive needles in a sharps bin (Public Health Laboratory Service AIDS and STD Centre 1997). Post exposure to HIV prophylaxis is now available following high risk unprotected anal or vaginal intercourse (Katz & Gerberding 1997).

Nursing care

Nursing problems associated with HIV include pain, confusion, depression, anxiety, fatigue, fever, dyspnea, nausea and vomiting, diarrhoea, wasting and dehydration (Kemp & Stepp 1995). Nutrition is a significant issue; early detection and intervention can decrease problems (Davidhizar & Dunn 1998). Good care is essential for persons with HIV/AIDS, although surveys have indicated that patients are not universally satisfied with the care they are receiving (McDonald *et al.* 1998), the quality of care received by the overwhelming majority of patients being only adequate (Siminof *et al.* 1998). This was supported by a recent study which indicated that health care workers' knowledge of HIV was poor and there was a reluctance to care for HIV positive patients (Brusaferro *et al.* 1997). Whitehead (1996) suggests specialist nurses can coordinate and facilitate care. This was highlighted by an audit which indicated a large number of staff incorrectly thought isolation necessary for patients infected with blood borne viruses (Perry & Gore 1997). Similarly, reports of excessive or selective infection control practices due to discriminatory attitudes and anxiety have been identified (Bermingham & Kippax 1998). In addition, most surgeons were found to underestimate the risk of blood borne pathogens, and protective clothing was not used correctly (Patterson *et al.* 1998). McCann & Sharkey (1998) stress that education can improve knowledge, attitudes and willingness to care. Tillett (1991) supports this view, stating that HIV related anxiety and conflicts can be reduced by education programmes.

The Public Health (Infectious Diseases) Regulations (1985) make certain provisions to safeguard public health related to a person with AIDS. It is stressed that these provisions are to be used only in exceptional circumstances where transmission of HIV may occur. One study has indicated that HIV remains viable for a considerable time in a cadaver. It is important, therefore, that careful procedures to avoid contamination are maintained after the death of an infected person (Ball *et al.* 1991).

Prevention of hospital acquired infection relies on the availability of resources for cleaning and, where necessary, sterilization of both equipment and the environment (Mims *et al.* 1993). Patients' accommodation can be vacuum cleaned and washed with hot soapy water (Ayliffe *et al.* 1992), unless contamination with blood or body fluids has occurred. In these circumstances, the statutory regulations require cleaning with fresh hypochlorite solution or granules (Health and Safety Commission 1988). When nondisposable equipment is used, autoclaving is the method of choice for sterilization (Ayliffe *et al.* 1992). Equipment likely to be damaged by autoclaving can be disinfected with glutaraldehyde in the manner specified by the 1988 Control of Substances Hazardous to Health (COSHH) guidelines. Glutaraldehyde inactivates vegetative bacteria, mycobacteria, spores and viruses (Ayliffe *et al.* 1984).

Nurses must keep up to date with improved, earlier diagnosis of AIDS with better treatments and the increased use of prophylaxis. They must be ready to adapt to these changes and be prepared and able to provide good care. This process will be achieved only by good education (Armstrong-Esther *et al.* 1990) and management support.

References and further reading

Apolonio, E.G. *et al.* (1995) Prognostic factors in HIV positive patients with CD 4+ lymphocyte count below 50 microlitres. *J Infect Dis*, **171**(4), 829–36.

Armstrong-Esther, C. *et al.* (1990) The effect of education on nurses' perception of AIDS. *J Adv Nurs*, **15**, 638–51.

Ayliffe, G.A.J. *et al.* (1984) *Chemical Disinfection in Hospitals.* Public Health Laboratory Service, London.

Ayliffe, G.A.J. *et al.* (1992) *Control of Hospital Infection. A Practical Handbook.* Chapman & Hall, London.

Bailey, N.T. (1997) A revised assessment of the HIV/AIDS incubation period, assuming a very short early period of high infectivity and using San Francisco public health data on prevalence and incidence. *Stat Med*, **16**(21), 2447–58.

Ball, J. *et al.* (1991) Long lasting viability of HIV after patient's death. *Lancet*, **338**, 63.

Baltimore, D. & Heilman, C. (1998) HIV vaccine: prospects and challenges. *Sci Am*, **279**(1), 98–103.

Belcher, L. *et al.* (1998) A randomized trial of a brief HIV risk reduction counseling intervention for women. *J Consult Clin Psychol*, **66**(5), 856–61.

Bermingham, S. & Kippax, S. (1998) Infection control and HIV related discrimination and anxiety. Glove use during venipuncture. *Aust Fam Physician*, **27**, Suppl. 2, S60–65.

Brettle, R.P. *et al.* (1997) British HIV Association guidelines for antiretroviral treatment of HIV seropositive individuals. *Lancet*, **349**, 1837–8.

Brusaferro, S. *et al.* (1997) Epidemiological study on knowledge, attitudes and behaviour of health care workers with respect to HIV infection. *Med Lav*, **88**(6), 495–506.

Bulterys, M. & Lepage, P. (1998) Mother to child transmission of HIV. *Curr Opin Pediatr*, **10**(2), 143–50.

Burnard, P. (1992) Nurse training needs in AIDS counselling. *Nurs Stand*, **6**(34), 34–9.

Carlon, C.P., Klenerman, P., Edwards, A. *et al.* (1994) Heterosexual transmission of HIV type 1 variants associated with zidovudine resistance. *J Infect Dis*, **169**, 411–15.

Carpenter, C.C. *et al.* (1998) Antiretroviral therapy for HIV infection in 1998: updated recommendations of the international AIDS Society – USA panel. *J Am Med Assoc*, **280**(1), 78–86.

Center for Disease Control (1986) Apparent transmission of human T-lymphotropic type 111/lymphadenopathy associated virus from a child to a mother providing health care. *Morb Mort Week Rep*, **35**, 76–9.

Center for Disease Control (1992) Revised classification system for HIV infection and expanded surveillance case definition for AIDS among adolescents and adults. *Morb Mort Week Rep*, **41**, 1–19.

Center for Disease Control (1993) HIV transmission between children at home. Public Health Laboratory Service Communicable Disease Surveillance Centre, London. *Commun Dis Rep*, **3**(52), 1.

Center for Disease Control (1994) Recommendations of the US Public Health Service Task Force on the use of zidovudine to reduce perinatal transmission of human immunodeficiency virus. *Morb Mort Week Rep*, **43**, RR-11.

Center for Disease Control (1996) Persistent lack of detectable HIV-1 antibody in a person with HIV infection, Utah, 1995. *Morb Mort Week Rep*, **454**(8), 181–5.

Chene, G. et al. (1997) Long term survival in patients with advanced immunodeficiency. *AIDS*, **11**(2), 209–16.

Chuansumrit, A. et al. (1996) Transfusion-transmitted AIDS with blood negative for anti HIV and HIV antigen. *Vox Sang*, **71**(1), 64–5.

Coffin, J.M. (1996) HIV viral dynnamics. *AIDS*, **10**, Suppl. 3, S75–84.

Colford, J.M., Ngo, L. & Tager, I. (1994) Factors associated with survival in HIV infected patients with very low CD4 counts. *Am J Epidemiol*, **139**(2), 206–18.

Contu, L. et al. (1993) Allogeneic bone marrow transplantation combined with multiple anti-HIV-1 treatment in the case of AIDS. *Bone Marrow Transplant*, **12**(6), 669–71.

Cooper, M.H. et al. (1993) HIV infection in autologous and allogeneic bone marrow transplant patients: a retrospective analysis of the Marseille bone marrow transplant population. *J Acq Immun Defic Syndr*, **6**(3), 277–84.

Davidhizar, R. & Dunn, C. (1998) Nutrition and the client with AIDS. *J Pract Nurs*, **48**(1), 16–25.

Davison, K. & Nicoll, A. (1997) The changing global epidemiology of HIV infection and AIDS. *CDC Rev*, **7**(9), R134–46.

De Cock, K.M. (1997) Guidelines for managing HIV infection. *Br Med J*, **315**, 1–2.

Department of Employment – Health and Safety Executive (1987) *AIDS and Employment*. Central Office of Information, London.

DHSS (1985) *The Public Health (Infectious Diseases) Regulations 1985 (HC(85)17) (LAC(85)10)*. Stationery Office.

DHSS (1990) *Advisory Committee on Dangerous Pathogens. HIV. The Causative Agent of AIDS and Related Conditions. Second Revision of Guidelines HN(90)4*. Stationery Office, London.

DoH (1991) *AIDS and HIV-Infected Health Care Workers: Occupational Guidance for Health Care Workers, their Physicians and Employers*. Stationery Office, London.

DoH (1993) *AIDS-HIV Infected Health Care Workers: Practical Guidance on Notifying Patients*. Stationery Office.

DoH (1996) *Guidelines for Pre-Test Discussion on HIV Testing*. Stationery Office, London.

DoH (1997) *Guidelines on Post-Exposure Prophylaxis for Health Care Workers Occupationally Exposed to HIV*. PL/CO[97]. Stationery Office, London.

DoH (1998) AIDS/HIV infected health care workers: guidance on the management of infected health care workers and patient notification. Stationery Office, London.

Duesberg, P.H. (1991) AIDS epidemiology: inconsistencies with human immunodeficiency virus and with infectious disease. *Proc Natl Acad Sci USA*, **88**(4), 1575–9.

Erb, P. & Matter, L. (1998) HIV diagnosis 1998. *Ther Umsch*, **55**(5), 279–84.

European Collaborative Study (1998) Therapeutic and other interventions to reduce the risk of mother-to-child transmission of HIV-1 in Europe. *Br J Obstet Gynaecol*, **105**(7), 704–709.

French, R. & Brocklehurst, P. (1998) The effects of pregnancy on survival in women infected with HIV: a systematic review of the literature and meta analysis. *Br J Obstet Gynaecol*, **105**(8), 827–35.

Frenkel, L.M. et al. (1995) Effects of zidovudine use during pregnancy on resistance and vertical transmission of HIV type 1. *Clin Infect Dis*, **20**, 1321–6.

Fujikawara, L.S. et al. (1985) Isolation of human T lymphotropic virus type 111 from tears of patients with AIDS. *Lancet*, **2**, 529–30.

Gabarre, J. et al. (1996) Autologous bone marrow transplantation in relapsed HIV related non-Hodgkin's lymphoma. *Bone Marrow Transplant*, **18**(6), 1195–7.

Gallo, R.C. et al. (1984) Frequent detection and continuous production of cytopathic retroviruses (HTLV III) from patients with AIDS. *Science*, **224**, 497–500.

Gerard, L. et al. (1996) Life expectancy in hospitalised patients with AIDS: prognostic factors on admission. *J Palliat Care*, **12**(1), 26–30.

Gibb, D.M. et al. (1998) Factors affecting uptake of antenatal HIV testing in London: results of a multicentre study. *Br Med J*, **316**, 259–61.

Gilbert, V.L. et al. (1998) Unusual HIV transmission through blood contact: analysis of cases reported in the UK. To December 1997. *Commun Dis Public Health*, **1**(2), 108–13.

Goedert, J.J. et al. (1991) High risk of HIV-1 infection for first born twins. The international registry of HIV exposed twins. *Lancet*, **338**, 1471–5.

Goedert, J.J. et al. (1998) Spectrum of AIDS associated malignant disorders. *Lancet*, **351**, 1833–9.

Gottlieb, S. (1998) New HIV strain may be resistant to drugs. *Br Med J*, **317**(7151), 100.

Grant, A.D. Djomand, G. & De Cock, K.M. (1997) Natural history and spectrum of disease in adults with HIV/AIDS in Africa. *AIDS*, **11**, Suppl. B, S43–54.

Hanrahan, A. & Reutter, L. (1997) A critical review of the literature on sharps injuries: epidemiology, management of exposure and prevention. *J Adv Nurs*, **25**, 144–54.

Hansell, P.S. et al. (1998) The effect of a social support boosting intervention on stress, coping, and social support in caregivers of children with HIV/AIDS. *Nurs Res*, **47**(2), 79–86.

Harrison, R. & Corbett, K. (1999) Screening of pregnant women for HIV: the case against. *Practis Midwife*, **2**(7), 24–9.

Hashida, S. et al. (1996) Shortening of the window period in diagnosis of HIV-1 infection by simultaneous detection of p24 antigen and antibody IgG to p17 and reverse transcriptase in serum with ultrasensitive enzyme immunoassay. *J Virol Method*, **62**(1), 43–53.

Hashida, S. et al. (1997) More reliable diagnosis of infection with HIV. *J Clin Lab Anal*, **11**(5), 267–86.

Health and Safety Commission (1994) *Control of Substances Hazardous to Health (COSHH) Approved Code of Practice*. Stationery Office, London.

Hirsch, M.S. et al. (1998) Antiretroviral drug resistance testing in adults with HIV infection: implications for clinical management. International AIDS Society. US Panel. *JAMA*, **279**(24), 1984–91.

Hoover, D.R. et al. (1992) The progression of untreated HIV-1 infection prior to AIDS. *Am J Public Health*, **82**(11), 1538–41.

Howe, J. (1998) HIV. *Prim Health Care*, **8**(2), 18–24.

Hughes, G. (1997) An overview of the HIV and AIDS epidemic

in the United Kingdom. *Commun Dis Rep CDR Rev*, **7**(9), R121–2.

Ishikawa, S. *et al.* (1996) Whole saliva dried on filter paper or diagnosis of HIV-1 infection by detection of antibody IgG to HIV-1 with ultrasensitive enzyme immunoassay using recombinant reverse transcriptase as antigen. *J Clin Lab Anal*, **10**(1), 35–41.

James, N.J., Gilles, P.A. & Bignell, C.J. (1998) Evaluation of a randomized controlled trial of HIV and sexually transmitted disease prevention in a genitourinary medicine clinic setting. *AIDS*, **12**(10), 1235–42.

Jason, J.M. *et al.* (1986) HTLV III/LAV antibody and immune status of household contacts and sexual partners of persons with haemophilia. *J Am Med Assoc*, **155**, 212.

Jowitt, S.N. *et al.* (1991) CD4 lymphocytopenia without HIV in patients with cryptococcal infection. *Lancet*, **337**, 500–501.

Kassler, W.J. (1997) Advances in HIV testing technology and their potential impact on prevention. *AIDS Educ Prev*, **9**(3 Suppl.), 27–40.

Katz, A. (1997) 'Mom, I have something to tell you'. Disclosing HIV infection. *J Adv Nurs* **25**, 139–43.

Katz, M.H. & Gerberding, J.L. (1997) Postexposure treatment of people exposed to HIV through sexual contact or injection–drug use. *New Engl J Med*, **336**, 1097–1100.

Kemp, C. & Stepp, L. (1995) Palliative care for patients with acquired immunodeficiency syndrome. *Am J Hosp Palliat Care*, **12**(6), 14, 17–27.

Korelitz, J.J., Busch, M.P. & Williams, A.E. (1996) Antigen testing for HIV and the magnet effect: will the benefit of a new HIV test be offset by the number of higher risk, test seeking donors attracted to blood centers? Retrovirus Epidemiology Donor Study. *Transfusion*, **36**(3), 203–208.

Kotler, D.P. (1998) HIV in pregnancy. *Gastroenterol Clin North Am*, **27**(1), 269–80.

Kuhn, L., Thomas, P., Singh, T. *et al.* (1998) Long term survival of children with HIV infection in New York City; estimate on population based surveillance data. *Am J Epidemiol*, **147**(9), 846–54.

Lackritz, E.M. (1998) Prevention of HIV transmission by blood transfusion in the developing world: achievements and continuing challenges. *AIDS*, **12**, Suppl A, S81–6.

Laurence, J. *et al.* (1992) AIDS without evidence of infection with HIV-1 and 2. *Lancet*, **340**, 273–4.

Lemp, G.F. (1990) Survival trends for patients with AIDS. *J Am Med Assoc*, **263**, 402–406.

Lepage, P. *et al.* (1998) Care of HIV infected children in developing countries. International Working Group on mother to child transmission of HIV. *Pediatr Infect Dis J*, **17**(7), 581–6.

Leroy, V. *et al.* (1998) International multicentre pooled analysis of late postnatal mother to child transmission of HIV-1 infection. Ghent International Working Group on mother to child transmission of HIV. *Lancet*, **352**(9128), 597–600.

Letvin, N.L. (1998) Progress in the development of an HIV 1 vaccine. *Science*, **280**, 1875–80.

Levy, J.A. (1985) Isolation of AIDS-associated retroviruses from cerebrospinal fluid and brain of patients with neurological symptoms. *Lancet*, **2**, 586–8.

Lindgren, S. *et al.* (1998) Pregnancy in HIV infected women. Counseling and care. 12 years' experiences and results. *Acta Obstet Gynecol Scand*, **77**(5), 532–41.

Local Collaborators (1998) Occupational acquisition of HIV infection among health care workers in the UK: data to June 1997. *Commun Dis Public Health*, **1**(2), 103–107.

Lyall, E.G.H. *et al.* (1998) Review of uptake of intervention to reduce mother-to-child transmission of HIV by women aware of their HIV status. *Br Med J*, **316**(16), 268–70.

Macdonald, N.D. (1997) AIDS and HIV infection acquired

through sexual intercourse between men. *Commun Dis Rep*, **7**(9), R123–4.

Madden, P.B. *et al.* (1997) The HIV epidemic in injecting drug users. *CDR Rev*, **7**(9), R128–30.

McCann, T.V. & Sharkey, R.J. (1998) Education intervention with international nurses and changes in knowledge, attitudes and willingness to provide care to patients with HIV/AIDS. *J Adv Nurs*, **27**(2), 267–73.

McDonald, R. *et al.* (1998) Client preferences for HIV inpatient care delivery. *AIDS Care*, **10**, Suppl. 2, S123–35.

McGarrigle, C., Gilbert, V. & Nicoll, A. (1997) AIDS and HIV infection acquired heterosexually. *Commun Dis Rep*, **7**(9), R125–7.

McKee, J.M. (1996) Human immunodeficiency virus. Healthcare workers' safety issues. *J Intraven Nurs*, **19**(3), 132–40.

Madges, S. *et al.* (1998) Do women with HIV infection consult with their GPs? *Br J Gen Pract*, **48**(431), 1329–30.

Mellors, J.W. *et al.* (1997) Plasma viral load and CD 4+ lymphocytes as prognostic markers of HIV-1 infection. *Ann Intern Med*, **126**(12), 946–54.

Mercey, D. (1998) Antinatal HIV testing. *Br Med J*, **316**, 241–2.

Mims, C.A., Playfair, J.H.L., Roitt, I.M. *et al.* (1993) *Medical Microbiology*. Mosby, London.

Mindel, A. (1987) Management of early HIV infection. *Br Med J*, **294**, 1145–7.

Molesworth, A. (1998) Results of a survey of diagnosed HIV infections prevalent in 1996 in England and Wales. *Commun Dis Public Health*, **1**(4), 271–5.

Molesworth, A. & Tookey, P. (1997) Paediatric AIDS and HIV infection. *CDR Rev*, **7**(9), R132–4.

Moore, R.D. & Chaisson, R.E. (1996) Natural history of opportunistic disease in an HIV-infected urban clinical cohort. *Ann Intern Med*, **124**(7), 633–42.

Mortimer, J.Y. & Spooner, R.J.D. (1997) HIV infection transmitted through blood product treatment, blood transfusion, and tissue transplantation. *CDR Rev*, **7**(9), R130–32.

National Institute of Health (1998) Report of the NIH panel to define principles of therapy of HIV infection. *Ann Intern Med*, **128**(12, Part 2), 1057–78.

Nicoll, A. *et al.* (1998) Epidemiology and detection of HIV-1 among pregnant women in the UK: results from national surveillance 1988–1996. *Br Med J*, **316**, 253–8.

Noone, A. & Goldberg, D. (1997) Antinatal HIV testing: what now? *Br Med J*, **314**, 1429–30.

Nourse, C.B. & Butler, K.M. (1998) Perinatal transmission of HIV and diagnosis of HIV infection in infants: a review. *Irish J Med Sci*, **167**(1), 28–32.

O'Shea, S. *et al.* (1998) Maternal viral load, CD4 count and vertical transmission of HIV-1. *J Med Virol*, **54**(2), 113–17.

Owens, D.K., Edwards, D.M. & Shachter, R.D. (1998) Population effects of prevention and therapeutic HIV vaccines in early and late stage epidemics. *AIDS*, **12**(9), 1057–66.

Pankhurst, C. & Peakman, M. (1989) Reduced CD4 T-cells and severe candidiasis in absence of HIV infection. *Lancet*, **1**, 672.

Patterson, J.M. *et al.* (1998) Surgeon's concern and practices of protection against bloodborne pathogens. *Ann Surg*, **228**(2), 266–72.

Pell, J. *et al.* (1996) Management of HIV infected health care workers: lessons from three cases. *Br Med J*, **312**(7039), 1150–53.

Perry, C. & Gore, J. (1997) Now, wash your hands please. *Nursing Times*, **93**(19), 64–8.

Phillips, K.D. & Morrow, J.H. (1998) Nursing management of anxiety in HIV infection. *Issues Ment Health Nurs*, **19**(4), 375–97.

Pillay, D. (1998) Emergence and control of resistance to antiviral drugs in resistance in herpes viruses, hepatitis B, and HIV. *Commun Dis Public Health*, **1**(1), 5–13.

Pliner, V. et al. (1998) Incubation period of HIV-1 perinatally infected children. New York City perinatal HIV transmission collaborative study group. *AIDS*, **12**(7), 759–66.

Pratt, R.R. (1998) HIV related encephalopathy. *Nurs Stand*, **13**(7), 38–40.

Public Health Laboratory Service AIDS and STD Centre (1997) Occupational transmission of HIV. PHLS, London.

Public Health Laboratory Service Communicable Disease Surveillance Centre (1999) AIDS and HIV infection in the United Kingdom: monthly report. *Commun Dis Rep*, **9**(31), 277–80.

Rabkin, J. (1997) Meeting the challenge of depression in HIV. *Treatment Issues*, **11**(10), 6–11.

Reisman, E.C. (1988) Ethical issues confronting nurses. *Nurs Clin North Am*, **23**(4), 789–801.

Reyes, E.M. & Legg, J.J. (1997) Prevention of HIV transmission. *Prim Care*, **24**(3), 469–77.

Rogers, P.A. et al. (1997) Survival of adults with AIDS in the UK. *Commun Dis Rep*, **7**(7), R93–100.

Sadiq, S.T., Copas, A.J. & Johnson, A.M. (1998) Factors associated with gonorrhoea in men aware of being positive for HIV infection: case-control study. *Br Med J*, **317**, 1052–3.

Samson, L. & King, S. (1998) Evidence-based guidelines for universal counselling and offering of HIV testing in pregnancy in Canada. *CMAJ*, **158**(11), 1449–57.

Siminoff, L.A., Erlen, J.A. & Sereika, S. (1998) Do nurses avoid AIDS patients? Avoidance behaviours and the quality of care of hospitalized AIDS patients. *AIDS Care*, **10**(2), 147–63.

Smith, T.L., Van Rensburg, E.J. & Engelbrecht, S. (1998) Neutralization of HIV-1 subtypes: implication for vaccine formations. *J Med Virol*, **56**(3), 264–8.

Sperling, R.S. et al. (1998) Safety of the maternal–infant zidovudine regimen utilized in the pediatric AIDS Clinical Trial Group 076 study. *AIDS*, **12**(14), 1805–13.

Stine, G.J. (1993) *AIDS Update 1993*. Prentice Hall, New Jersey.

Stover, J. & Way, P. (1998) Projecting the impact of AIDS on mortality. *AIDS*, **12**, Suppl. 1, S29–39.

Terriff, C.M. & Synoground, G. (1998) Antiretroviral therapy for pediatric and adolescent HIV. *J School Nurs*, **14**(2), 36–46.

Thiry, L. et al. (1985) Isolation of AIDS virus from cell-free breast milk of three healthy virus carriers. *Lancet*, **1**, 891–2.

Thorne, C., Newell, M.L. & Peckham, C. (1998) Social care of children born to HIV-infected mothers in Europe. European Collaborative Study. *AIDS Care*, **10**(1), 7–16.

Tillett, G. (1991) HIV and occupational health. *Aust J Adv Nurs*, **8**(4), 18–25.

United Kingdom Central Council for Nursing, Midwifery and Health Visiting (1986) *Confidentiality – An Elaboration of Clause 9 of the Second Edition of the UKCC's Code of Professional Conduct*. UKCC, London.

UK Register of HIV Seroconverters Steering Committee (1998) The AIDS incubation period in the UK estimated from a national register of HIV seroconverters. *AIDS*, **12**(6), 659–67.

Veenstra, J. et al. (1995) Transmission of zidovudine-resistant HIV type 1 variants following deliberate injection of blood from a patient with AIDS. Characteristics and natural history of the virus. *Clin Infect Dis*, **21**, 536–60.

Wainberg, M.A. & William Cameron, D. (1998) HIV resistance to antiviral drugs: public health implications. *Drug Resistant Updates*, **1**, 104–108.

Ward, V., Wilson, J. & Taylor, L. (1997) Guidelines for routine blood and body substances precautions. In: *Preventing Hospital Acquired Infection. Clinical Guidelines*, pp. 11–16. Public Health Laboratory Service, London.

Weber, B. et al. (1998) Reduction of diagnostic window by new fourth-generation HIV screening assays. *J Clin Microbiol*, **36**(8), 2235–9.

Weiss, R.A. & Jaffe, H.W. (1990) Duesberg, HIV and AIDS. *Nature*, **345**, 659–60.

West, G.R. & Stark, K.A. (1997) Partner notification for HIV prevention: a critical reexamination. *AIDS Educ Pre*, **9**(Suppl. 3), 68–78.

Whitehead, C.M. (1996) The specialist nurse in HIV/AIDS medicine. *Postgrad Med J*, **72**(846), 211–13.

WHO (1990) *WHO Weekly Epidemiology Record*, 20 July. WHO, Geneva.

WHO (1993) *Global Programme on AIDS. The HIV/AIDS Pandemic: 1993 Overview*. GPA/CNP/EVA 93.1. WHO, Geneva.

WHO (1993) *Report of a Scientific Meeting on Unexplained Severe Immunodeficiency Without Evidence of HIV Infection*. GPA/RES/93.3. WHO, Geneva.

Wilcox, M.H. (1997) Bloodborne viruses. *Croner's Health Service Risks*, **9**, 2–7.

Wofsy, C.B. et al. (1986) Isolation of AIDS associated retrovirus from genital secretions of women with antibodies to the virus. *Lancet*, **1**, 527–9.

Zagury, D. et al. (1984) HTLV III cells culture from semen in two patients with AIDS. *Science*, **226**, 449–51.

Human immunodeficiency virus 2 (HIV 2)

Definition

HIV 2 is closely related to HIV 1 but is antigenically distinct and demonstrates distinct replication and cytopathic characteristics (Albert et al. 1990).

Reference material

HIV 2 was first recognized in 1986 (Clavel et al. 1986), although evidence that HIV 2 infections were present in many West Africans as far back as 1966 (Karamura et al. 1989) has been disputed (Mohammed et al. 1989). Sero-logical evidence supporting the existence of a second HIV was published in 1985 (Barin et al. 1985). HIV 2 is not as widely prevalent in most countries as HIV 1 (Solomon et al. 1998), except in many West African countries, where it is the more common cause of AIDS than HIV 1 (Naucler et al. 1989).

In the UK, screening of blood donors and people attending genitourinary medicine clinics shows that the occurrence of HIV 2 infection is rare. A few HIV 2 infections have been reported in many European countries, and 18 HIV 2 infections have been reported in the USA. Of these, over two-thirds of patients had contact with, or were from, Africa (Evans et al. 1991).

Transmission of HIV 2 follows the same pattern as HIV 1 (Kroegal et al. 1987), although the rate of vertical transmission from mother to child is uncertain, with some studies suggesting that it might be low (Morgan *et al.* 1990). De Cock *et al.* (1994) investigated effects of maternal HIV 1 and HIV 2 on outcome of pregnancy, infant mortality and child survival in Abidjan and found that spontaneous abortion was similar in both groups, while vertical transmission and infant mortality were lower in children borne of HIV 2 infected mothers, suggesting that maternal HIV 2 infection has less influence on child survival than HIV 1 infection.

Despite the high prevalence of HIV 2 infections in West Africa, there have been far fewer reported AIDS cases compared with East and Central Africa, where HIV 1 predominates, implying HIV 2 is less pathogenic than HIV 1 (Romieu *et al.* 1990). Whittle *et al.*'s (1994) study found that mortality rate in HIV 2 infected patients was approximately two-thirds of that for HIV 1 infected patients. An 8 year prospective study to determine and compare disease progression in women infected with HIV 1 and HIV 2 found that women infected with HIV 1 had a 67% probability of AIDS free survival 5 years after seroconversion, compared with 100% for HIV 2 infected women (Marlink *et al.* 1994). In contrast, Van der Ende *et al.*'s (1996) study of 12 West European residents, nine of West African descent, found that disease progression was the same for HIV 1 and HIV 2 infected persons. Whittle *et al.* (1998) suggest that HIV 2 is less pathogenic and less transmissible than HIV 1, which may be associated with T cell recognition, and control of viral load replication may be more efficient in HIV 2 infection than in HIV 1 infection. Albert *et al.*'s (1990) study found that HIV 2 isolated could be divided into two groups: a rapid/high group found in patients with symptoms and a slow/low group found in asymptomatic individuals. HIV 2 infected individuals living with an infected spouse had significantly higher mortality than those living with an uninfected spouse (Poulsen 1997).

The range of opportunistic infections and malignancies and the wasting and dementia associated with progressive HIV 1 infections are also present in HIV 2 disease, although *Pneumocystis carinii* pneumonia (Clavel *et al.* 1987) and active tuberculosis may be less common in HIV 2 infected people than in those infected with HIV 1. However, this may represent a difference in prevalence of opportunistic pathogens rather than being a direct effect of HIV infection (Kanki 1989; Soro *et al.* 1993).

In May 1989 the AIDS laboratory diagnostic working group advised combined screening in diagnostic laboratories in the UK (Evans *et al.* 1991). In July 1990, combined anti-HIV 1/HIV 2 testing of all donations of blood was introduced in the UK Blood Transfusion Service. Of the first 250 000 donations, only one HIV 2 infected donor was detected.

Since there is no difference in the method of transmission and symptoms between HIV 1 and HIV 2, prevention and nursing care are the same.

References and further reading

Albert, J. *et al.* (1990) Replicative capacity of HIV-2 like HIV-1, correlates with severity of immunosuppression. *AIDS*, **4**(4), 291–5.

Ayliffe, G.A.J. *et al.* (1992) *Control of Hospital Infection. A Practical Handbook*, 3rd edn. Chapman & Hall Medical, London.

Barin, F. *et al.* (1985) Serological evidence for virus related to Simian T-lymphotropic retrovirus III in residents of West Africa. *Lancet*, **2**, 1387–9.

Clavel, F. *et al.* (1986) Isolation of a new human retrovirus from West African patients with AIDS. *Science*, **233**, 343–6.

Clavel, F. *et al.* (1987) Human immunodeficiency virus type 2 infection associated with AIDS in West Africa. *New Engl J Med*, **316**, 1180–85.

De Cock, K.M. *et al.* (1994) Retrospective study of maternal HIV-1 and HIV-2 infections and child survival in Abidjan, Cote d'Ivoire. *Br Med J*, **308**(6926), 441–3.

Evans, B.G. *et al.* (1991) HIV 2 in the United Kingdom. A review. *Commun Dis Rep*, **1**(2), R19–232.

Horton, R. & Parker, L. (1997) *Informed Infection Control Practice*. Churchill Livingstone, New York.

Kanki, P.J. (1989) Clinical significance of HIV 2 infection in West Africa. *AIDS Clin Rev*, 95–108.

Karamura, M. *et al.* (1989) HIV 2 in West Africa in 1966. *Lancet*, **1**, 385.

Kroegal, C. *et al.* (1987) Routes of HIV 2 transmissions in Western Europe. *Lancet*, **1**, 1150.

Marlink, R. *et al.* (1994) Reduced rates of disease development after HIV 2 infection as compared to HIV 1. *Science*, **265**(5178), 1587–90.

Mohammed, I. *et al.* (1989) HIV 2 West Africa in 1966. *Lancet*, **1**, 385.

Morgan, G. *et al.* (1990) AIDS following mother to child transmission of HIV 2. *AIDS*, **4**, 879–82.

Naucler, A. *et al.* (1989) HIV 2-associated AIDS and HIV 2 seroprevalence in Bissau, Guinea-Bissau. *J AIDS*, **2**, 88–93.

Poulsen, A.G. *et al.* (1997) Nine-year HIV-2 associated mortality in an urban community in Bissau, West Africa. *Lancet*, **349**(9056), 911–14.

Pratt, R. (1991) *AIDS: A Strategy for Nursing Care*. Edward Arnold, London.

Romieu, I. *et al.* (1990) HIV 2 link to AIDS in West Africa. *J AIDS*, **3**, 220–30.

Solomon, S. *et al.* (1998) Prevalence and risk factors of HIV 1 and HIV 2 infection in urban and rural area in Tamil Nadu, India. *Int J STD AIDS*, **9**(2), 98–103.

Soro, B.N., Gershy-Damet, G.M. & Rey, J.L. (1993) The pathogenicity of the human immunodeficiency virus HIV 2 as seen by epidemiologists. *Med Trop*, **53**(1), 45–53.

Van der Ende, M.E. *et al.* (1996) HIV-2 infection in 12 European residents: virus characteristics and disease progression. *AIDS*, **10**(4), 1649–55.

Whittle, H. *et al.* (1994) HIV-2 infected patients survive longer than HIV-1 infected patients. *AIDS*, **8**(11), 1617–20.

Whittle, H.C., Ariyoshi, K. & Rowland-Jones, S. (1998) HIV-2 and T cell recognition. *Curr Opin Immunol*, **10**(4), 382–7.

Wilson, J. (1995) *Infection Control in Clinical Practice*. Baillière Tindall, London.

GUIDELINES • Acquired immune deficiency syndrome in a general ward

Procedure

Action	Rationale
1 All staff should read and be familiar with government guidelines on AIDS and their own hospital's codes of practice.	To ensure all staff are aware of, and take, the necessary precautions.
2 Hospital staff should cover any broken skin with a waterproof dressing.	To prevent the entry of infectious material.
3 Immunodeficient-compromised staff, either through illness or therapy, should not nurse patients who are HIV antibody positive.	HIV antibody positive patients who present with generalized infection could put this category of staff at risk.
4 Staff suffering from eczema should not nurse patients who are HIV antibody positive.	Any break in staff members' skin should be covered with a waterproof dressing to prevent entry of HIV. This would be difficult to accomplish with eczema lesions and would exacerbate the eczema.
5 Accidental inoculations must be avoided at all cost.	Serious inoculation accidents have been seen to be a means of transmission of HIV.
6 In the event of gross contamination of intact skin the affected area must be washed thoroughly with soap under warm water. A scrubbing brush must not be used.	Intact skin is a natural barrier against infection. By thorough washing the infectious material can be removed. Scrubbing brushes can cause skin damage which allows infection to enter.
7 Puncture wounds or cuts must be made to bleed freely and washed under hot running water.	To flush out infectious material.
8 A waterproof dressing must be applied and medical advice sought for large wounds.	To prevent further infection to the wound.
9 An accident form must be completed immediately and taken to bacteriology, the occupational health physician or other medical advisor as appropriate.	It is important to have accurate records of all accidents and incidents in order to monitor events.
10 HIV post exposure prophylaxis should be considered for all significant exposure to HIV.	HIV post exposure prophylaxis antiviral therapy has been shown to prevent seroconversion following significant exposure to HIV (DoH 1997).

Low-risk, HIV positive individuals (i.e. patients who are not bleeding, incontinent, confused or infected with a contagious disease)

Nursing assessment of the risk of contamination of the environment with pathogenic organisms, blood or body fluids from a patient known to be HIV antibody positive allows care to be more accurately planned.

Action	Rationale
1 If the patient is not bleeding, incontinent, confused or infected with a contagious disease, he/she is considered to be of low risk of transmitting infection to others and can be nursed on an open ward using all the patients' facilities as normal.	HIV cannot be transmitted by social contact that occurs in hospital wards.
2 If a low-risk, HIV positive individual develops an infection, is undergoing invasive procedures or becomes incontinent nursing care will commence as for high-risk, HIV positive persons.	Incontinent, bleeding HIV antibody positive patients have the potential risk of transmitting the HIV virus to others.

Increased risk, HIV positive individuals

Action

1 Known or strongly suspected HIV antibody positive
patients who are bleeding, incontinent, infected with a
contagious disease or receiving invasive procedures should
be nursed in a single room with its own toilet and handwashing facilities.

Rationale

To minimize the risk of transmitting infection. HIV can be
transmitted via blood and body fluid.

Entering the room

Action

1 When the patient is not bleeding, coughing,
incontinent or receiving procedures, protective clothing
is not required.

2 When the patient is incontinent, bleeding or
undergoing invasive procedures, disposable well-fitting
gloves and a plastic apron are needed.

3 If there is a possibility of airborne contamination, a
correctly fitting mask and safety spectacles should
be worn.

Rationale

Transmission of HIV is not possible from general contact in
the absence of blood and blood stained body fluids.

Transmission of HIV is possible from body fluids.

Transmission of HIV is possible if contaminated material is
allowed to contaminate mucous membrane.

Liquid waste

Action

1 All liquid waste from HIV positive patients must be
disposed of in a bedpan washer immediately, taking
care to avoid splashing.

2 Areas without bedpan washers will need to use the
slop hopper. Great care must be taken to pour waste
slowly and carefully down the hopper to avoid splashing.

Rationale

To prevent contamination of the environment.

To prevent contamination of the environment.

Non-disposable equipment

Action

1 Cleaning of non-disposable equipment needs to be
performed thoroughly and in a safe manner.

2 Gloves/aprons must be worn, together with
masks/eye protection if appropriate, when
cleaning non-disposable equipment.

3 Before disinfection, equipment must be cleaned with
soap and water, avoiding splashing.

4 The equipment must then be dried carefully.

5 If equipment will not be damaged by immersion in
freshly activated 2% glutaraldehyde for 30 minutes,
this is the method of choice.

6 If the equipment will be damaged by immersion in the
glutaraldehyde solution, or is too big to fit into the
disinfection container, these items must be first washed
thoroughly with soap and water and dried, followed by
washing and drying with a hypochlorite 1% solution.

Rationale

Careless cleaning, immersion, drying, etc. can increase
contamination of the environment.

To prevent self-contamination.

Disinfectants cannot completely penetrate organic matter.

Wet objects would alter the disinfectant's strength and
could inactivate the solution if soap and soiling were still
present.

Glutaraldehyde's bacteriostatic action is completely
effective against the AIDS retrovirus.

Hypochlorite 1% solution has a non-corrosive action for
delicate equipment and is less toxic to staff than
glutaraldehyde.

Guidelines • Acquired immune deficiency syndrome in a general ward (cont'd)

Action	Rationale
7 If the equipment will be damaged by glutaraldehyde or hypochlorite solution, these items must be first washed thoroughly with soap and water and dried, and immersed in 70% ethanol.	70% ethanol is virucidal against most categories of viruses, but does not penetrate organic matter and is inflammable.
8 If the equipment can be autoclaved it must be placed in a sterile supplies department (SSD) bag, taped shut with biohazard tape and marked with a biohazard label. The bag must then be taken to SSD.	Autoclaving is the most effective sterilization method. Correct bagging and transportation of the equipment will prevent contamination of the environment.
9 Expensive, delicate items which have had prolonged, close contact with the patient, i.e. a ventilator, will require ethylene oxide disinfection.	Ethylene oxide disinfection is the second process of choice after autoclaving (Ayliffe *et al*. 1992).
10 Before the ethylene oxide disinfection process, these items must have all their disposable parts, filters, etc. removed and the whole item cleaned completely and thoroughly with hypochlorite 1% solution and dried carefully.	To prevent contamination of the environment.
11 The transportation and ethylene oxide process will take some time. Thought must be given beforehand to the use of this equipment for actively bleeding, incontinent patients.	Ethylene oxide disinfection involves lengthy airing of equipment after the process to ensure it is safe to re-use. During this time other patients may be deprived of the item.
12 All staff handling contaminated equipment and disinfectants must comply with the Control of Substances Hazardous to Health Regulations (COSHH) 1988.	These regulations are designed to protect people against risks to their health including hazardous substances such as disinfectants and micro-organisms.

Other hospital departments

Action	Rationale
1 It is essential that all request cards for items such as specimens, have the biohazard label attached.	To ensure all departments are informed that the sample is potentially dangerous.
2 All specimens must have the biohazard label attached and be double bagged in a specimen polythene biohazard bag with a biohazard label attached to the bag.	To ensure the laboratory is aware of potential risk and that the specimen is correctly contained to prevent cross-infection. (For further information see Chap. 37, Specimen collection.)
3 The specimen should be taken to the laboratory in a washable, covered container.	To prevent contamination of the environment. If leakage does occur, it can be simply contained and cleaned up.
4 A nurse should accompany an antibody-positive patient to other departments. If there is not a departmental nurse available, the ward nurse should remain with the patient.	To give help and advice.
5 The patient will normally be given the last appointment of the day if invasive procedures are planned.	The department will be less crowded and busy, thus allowing time for appropriate precautions to be taken.

Domestic staff

Action	Rationale
1 The room must be cleaned daily. (For further information see Guidelines. Source isolation, above.)	To minimize the risk of cross-infection.
2 A nurse must check the patient's room to establish that it is suitable for the domestic staff to clean.	To ensure the room is not contaminated with blood or body fluids.
3 If contamination of the environment with blood or body fluids occurs it must be treated with a	To prevent cross-infection.

hypochlorite solution or granules containing 10 000 ppm available chlorine.

Terminal cleaning of the room

Action

1 The room must be cleared of all equipment in appropriate manner (see above) before it is cleaned.

2 The carpet must be steam cleaned if contamination by blood or excreta has occurred.

3 The walls should only be cleaned if contamination is known to have occurred.

4 The curtains must be changed if contamination has occurred.

Rationale

It is impossible to clean thoroughly if potentially contaminated items are in the room.

Organisms have been known to survive in carpets. Heat is the best method of decontamination.

HIV does not survive on intact walls.

Discretion and assessment need to be used. If the room has only been used for a short time for a patient who has not contaminated the environment, curtains would not need changing.

The patient

Action

1 As soon as possible, the probable/known diagnosis must be discussed with the patient and the hospital policy explained.

2 Psychological support is essential.

3 It is necessary that all nurses caring for antibody positive patients are familiar with treatment and care procedures.

4 Staff should adopt a non-judgemental approach in their dealings with antibody positive patients.

5 It may be appropriate to recommend voluntary agencies to antibody positive patients.

Rationale

It is essential that the patient understands fully the reason for these restrictions which, while protecting contacts, also protect the patient from further risks of infection.

Psychological dysfunction is likely and should be recognized and treated early to alleviate and contain the mental distress which an AIDS patient may experience.

To ensure appropriate nursing care is delivered.

It is the responsibility of all health professionals to care for patients and not to pass moral judgements.

Support groups have knowledge and experience which can help HIV antibody positive individuals.

Visiting

Action

1 Visitors should be encouraged.

2 The diagnosis of AIDS is confidential and should not be disclosed.

Rationale

To prevent isolation.

To maintain confidentiality.

Discharging the patient

Action

1 Almost all patients with AIDS will require community services at some time during their illness.

2 If an AIDS patient requires community services, the patient must have given consent for HIV antibody positive diagnosis to be given to the general practitioner and community care personnel.

Rationale

AIDS patients will need to be admitted to hospital for the treatment of clinical illness, but will be encouraged to resume their normal activities when at home.

Confidentiality must not be breached without the patient's consent. However, health care workers such as ambulance men and women and district nurses will need to take precautions if bleeding, incontinence or infections are present.

Guidelines • Acquired immune deficiency syndrome in a general ward (cont'd)

Disposal of waste in the community

Action

1 Excreta and infected fluids can be discarded into the toilet in the normal manner.

2 Infected waste such as dressings, gloves and aprons, must be burned or placed in yellow clinical waste bags and the local authority asked to collect them.

3 Sharps must be placed in a sharps box and stored in a safe place when full, and collected by the local health authority.

Rationale

To prevent contamination of the environment.

Yellow is the international colour for infected waste bags, and they are available on request from the local authority.

To prevent inoculation accidents.

Laundry in the community

Action

1 Clothes and linen which are heavily soiled or bloodstained should be washed separately by washing machine using a hot wash cycle 71°C for 3 minutes. Wash as above if using a public launderette.

2 If the person is not fit enough, infected linen should be placed in red alginate polythene bags and the local authority asked to arrange collection and laundering.

Rationale

Heat inactivation combined with the considerable dilution factor found in a washing machine renders linen safe for reuse (Horton & Parker 1997).

Red alginate polythene bags are recognized internationally for infected linen.

Crockery and cutlery

Action

1 Ideally, crockery and cutlery should be washed in a dishwasher with a final rinse temperature of at least 80°C.

2 There is no need to keep a separate store of crockery and cutlery if washed appropriately.

Rationale

Heat is effective in destroying the HIV.

Crockery and cutlery present no risk of contamination if washed in a dish washer with a final rinse temperature of at least 80°C.

Protective clothing in the community

Action

1 Disposable apron and gloves need be worn only when blood or excreta are being handled.

2 Disinfectants are required only if blood or excreta spillage has occurred. A strong hypochlorite solution (1 part household bleach to 10 parts water) is recommended.

Rationale

There is no risk of acquiring infection from general social contact.

Unnecessary use of disinfectants is expensive and may be potentially hazardous to staff and the environment (Health and Safety Commission 1994).

Visitors in the community

Action

1 Visitors should be encouraged.

2 The patient should be encouraged to resume social activities.

Rationale

There is no risk of acquiring infection from social contact.

To minimize effects of boredom and loneliness (Pratt 1991).

Prevention of further infection

Action	Rationale
1 The patient should be encouraged to stay away from individuals with infections.	AIDS patients are susceptible to infections.
2 If the patient develops any signs and symptoms of ill health, the general practitioner or hospital must be informed immediately.	Early treatment of symptoms will enhance the chances of containing the disease.

(For further details on discharge planning see Chap. 11.)

Death

Action	Rationale
1 The body should be laid out as described in the Procedure, Last offices (Chap. 22). In addition, the nurse should wear gloves and a plastic apron.	To prevent contamination.
2 All orifices must be packed.	The body continues to secrete fluids after death has occurred. Any leakage may contaminate the environment.
3 Any wounds, intravenous sites or skin breakages must be sealed with waterproof dressing.	To prevent leakage of contaminated fluids.
4 All documentation relating to this procedure must have a biohazard label attached.	To alert administration, portering and mortuary staff of the infection risks.
5 Once the body has been laid out and the room made presentable, family and friends may view the body.	Once the body has left the ward or home, viewing will be difficult if the funeral director adheres strictly to infectious diseases regulations.
6 The body must be placed in a cadaver bag and sealed securely with biohazard tape.	The cadaver bag will prevent leakage and ensures infectious diseases regulations are complied with.
7 Porters must be given help and support.	There is no infection risk when the body is sealed in a cadaver bag unless the bag becomes torn or damaged in transportation. Gloves and aprons will prevent contamination of the staff handling the body.

Funeral arrangements

Action	Rationale
1 Ideally, the hospital administration should have a list of funeral directors who will attend to an HIV antibody positive patient.	It is important that the bereaved relatives are given every help and support to prevent unnecessary distress.

Antibiotic-resistant organisms

Definition

The term *antibiotic resistance* denotes a strain of organism not killed or inhibited by antimicrobial agents to which the species is generally sensitive.

Reference material

The importance of antibiotic-resistant organisms cannot be overemphasized. The increasing resistance of organisms to antibiotics brings the prospects of a return to the pre antibiotic era (Cookson 1997). The Standing Medical Advisory Committee (1998) points out that micro-organisms are getting ahead and therapeutic options are narrowing. This is because since the 1980s only improvements of antimicrobial agents, rather than the development of new drugs, has occurred. Emphasis on antibiotic resistance has shifted from recognition to prevention (Burke & Pestotnik 1996). In addition, research has been aimed at improving understanding of resistance and transmissibility of resistant organisms (Huovinen & Cars 1998). The widespread and often indiscriminate use of antibiotics for prophylactic and veterinary purposes, as well as the inappropriate selection of these antibiotics, is believed to be an important factor in the development of resistant forms of bacteria (Swan Joint Committee 1969; Garrod 1972). Wise et al. (1998) suggest that 50% of antibiotics are used for humans and the rest for agriculture. As much as 75% of usage is of questionable therapeutic value. For example, antibiotics are commonly prescribed for respiratory infections where the majority are caused by viral infections (Wise et al. 1998). This type of misuse leads to resistance (Monnet 1998). However, recent evidence indicates that there has been a reduction in the use of antibiotics for minor illnesses such as sore throats (Standing Medical Advisory Committee 1998).

The transmission of genetic material between bacteria by conjugation has been well documented (Jaffe et al. 1980; Mendoza 1985) and this conjugation accounts in part for the rapid spread of resistance, with mutation, transformation and transduction also being involved (Sande & Mandell 1980). The possibility of vancomycin resistant enterococci (VRE) transferring the vancomycin resistance gene to methicillin resistant Staphylococcus aureus (MRSA) is a real concern (Bates 1997). The consequences of a patient being infected with a resistant form of bacteria are demanding in terms of increased length of stay in hospital, costs of care and treatment (Granzebrook 1986). Resistance to antiviral drugs has also been seen. Of 15 antiviral drugs now available for clinical use in the UK, resistance has been documented to most (Pillay 1998). Person to person transmission of drug resistant viruses has also been reported (Gedded 1996). Patients who are immunocompromised, debilitated or have open wounds are at particular risk and deaths have occurred (Cox et al. 1995).

Dennesen et al. (1998) stress that compliance with infection control measures and restrictive use of antibiotics are the key measures to prevent epidemics of multiresistant bacterial infection. The potential risk of patients suing hospitals for hospital acquired infections has been highlighted; while the number of cases is currently small, they can be costly – some cases settled out of court have cost £13 500 and £17 000 (Moore 1997).

Theoretically, any organism can develop antibiotic resistance. In practice MRSA, Staphylococcus epidermidis, Streptococcus pneumoniae, VRE and coliforms cause particular problems (Mimms et al. 1993).

Gram-negative bacteria

Gram-negative bacteria normally inhabit the gut, but can cause infections in the urinary tract, respiratory tract and wounds. Outbreaks of resistant forms have been reported (Casewell 1982; Dance 1987), which may be the consequence of excessive use of broad-spectrum antibiotics. Pseudomonas species may cause particular problems (Jarvis & Martone 1992), being ubiquitous in the hospital environment (Laa Poh & Yeo 1993). Resistance in many Gram-negative bacteria is caused by the beta-lactamase production enzyme, which can inactivate antibacterial agents (Thornsberry 1995). These organisms can multiply in warm, moist conditions and have been identified in eye drops, soap solutions, lotions and in the tubing used for ventilators and incubators. This is particularly difficult because of the shortage of drugs which are effective against resistant forms of Pseudomonas species (Mimms et al. 1993). Risk factors for spread include overcrowded wards, lapses in hygiene and poor infection control practices. Spread is primarily by direct or indirect person to person contact (Rae 1998), especially by busy hospital staff (Flaherty & Weinstein 1996). However, contamination of equipment such as humidifiers and nebulizers has also been implicated in spread (Rae 1998). Outbreaks of multiple resistant Klebsiella have occurred, causing life threatening infections (Hobson et al. 1996). Investigation of a multi-resistant Klebsiella outbreak found that the strain could be easily isolated from the environment, from inadequately cleaned and disinfected equipment (Jumaa & Chattopadhyay 1994) and from the hands of medical and nursing staff and visitors (Coovadia et al. 1992). These organisms can persist endemically in the ward environment (Branger et al. 1997).

Gram-negative bacteraemia is associated with septic shock (Ferguson 1991), which occurs primarily in debilitated, hospitalized patients who are the group that also develop the resistant form of Gram-negative bacteraemia (Bryant et al. 1971). The major problem regarding Gram-negative-resistant organisms is that shock progresses before antibiotic sensitivities are known, producing increased clinical manifestations of infection, which can result in death (Glauser et al. 1991; Truett 1991).

Gram-positive bacteria

Methicillin resistant Staphylococcus aureus (MRSA) (coagulase positive Staphylococcus aureus)

Staphylococcus aureus is part of the normal human flora, with large numbers of the organism being found on the skin and mucosa. Colonization or infection by MRSA is therefore more likely to occur in the nose, lesions and sites of abnormal skin, and in indwelling devices such as catheters and tracheostomies (Ayliffe 1986). Soon after the introduction of benzyl penicillin in the 1940s incidences of resistance were seen. With penicillin usage, the prevalence of resistant strains increased. In the 1960s methicillin was introduced and MRSA was soon reported (Jevons 1961). S. aureus resistance to methicillin results from the expression of cell wall synthesizing enzyme, which has a low affinity for all β-lactams (Johnson 1998). In 1981 the first epidemic strains of MRSA (EMRSA) were reported. Since then

EMRSA strains 1 to 16 have been detected. EMRSA can also be resistant to other antimicrobial agents. Until recently all MRSA continued to be susceptible to vancomycin; now reports of vancomycin resistant MRSA termed VRSA have been reported in Japan (Hiramatsu *et al.* 1997) and the USA (Center for Disease Control 1997). One USA patient developed VRSA following 6 months' intermittent use of vancomycin for MRSA bacteraemia (Turco *et al.* 1998). Hiramatsu (1998) stresses the importance of being aware of VRSA, and the need to develop new therapeutic measures to prevent the 'final day of antibiotic chemotherapy'. As resistance accelerated so will the adverse clinical consequences of infection caused by MRSA (Linden 1998).

Resistance to mupirocin cream which is used to irradicate MRSA colonization from nose, skin and wounds is also occurring (Marples *et al.* 1995; Eltringham 1997). It is anticipated that the situation will increase with the use of mupirocin (Miller *et al.* 1996), and may contribute to the failure of MRSA control (Casewell 1995). Other products such as fusidic acid, bacitracon (Irish *et al.* 1998) and tea tree oil are being evaluated (Chan & Loudon 1998) for irradication of MRSA colonization. Fortunately, disinfectant agents used for hand washing and cleaning remain equally effective against sensitive and antibiotic strains of bacteria if manufacturers' recommendations are followed (Payne *et al.* 1998). Revised guidelines for the control of MRSA in hospital (Working Party Report 1998) and the community (DoH 1996) have been compiled. The guidelines for hospitals suggest the cost of not controlling MRSA is higher than that of control and that prevention and control are worthwhile. Others do not agree, suggesting that trying to control MRSA cause more problems than it solves, arguing that resources used for MRSA control could be put to better use (Barrett *et al.* 1998).

While rates of patients colonized with MRSA appear to be greater than those infected with MRSA, these infections are significant due to the difficulties in treating systemic infection and the ability of the organism to spread and colonize debilitated patients. It is reported that 21% of all *S. aureus* isolated from cerebrospinal fluid and blood culture is MRSA (Speller *et al.* 1997). Statistical analysis indicates that MRSA is independently associated with death, with the risk of death three times higher among MRSA infected patients compared to those infected with methicillin sensitive *S. aureus* (Romero-Vivas *et al.* 1995).

Risk factors for MRSA include previous hospitalization, particularly in high dependency units, presence of IV catheters, tracheotomies, wounds and pressure ulcers, underlying disease and recent antibiotics (Maslow *et al.* 1995). Colonization with MRSA has been seen to be a risk factor for acquiring a hospital infection (Cookson *et al.* 1997). Actively seeking and treating carriers has been seen to lead to a reduction in MRSA. Screening specimens include nose, throat, axilla, groin and wounds (Working Party Report 1998). Delay in initiation of effective therapy has been shown to be a significant morbidity factor (French *et al.* 1990).

MRSA infection results in increased length of stay in hospital with associated costs, in particular IV antibiotics.

The cost of an outbreak of MRSA involving 400 patients in Kettering was estimated to be £400 000 (Cox *et al.* 1995). In addition, the detrimental effects on patients, their family and friends, such as pain, anxiety and depression, are a vital consideration. In one study, five patients being barrier nursed due to MRSA infection expressed feelings of loneliness, stigma, monotony and issues of control (Oldman 1998). Kennedy & Hamilton's (1997) study indicated that patients felt their rehabilitation was affected positively by their MRSA, although nurses in the same study recognized their patients' problems. None of these nurses were worried about acquiring MRSA, which contrasted to an earlier investigation, where the nurses thought they were at risk of acquiring an infection (Knowles 1993).

Screening

Patients transferred from hospitals and countries known to have an MRSA problem should be screened on admission, and treated as suspect until the results of screening specimens are known (Duckworth 1990). These restrictions may be minimal, with nursing care involving good hand washing following patient contact. However, if the patient is obviously ill, for example with a discharging wound, then this would necessitate source isolation nursing (see the beginning of this chapter). Any patients in contact with infected patients must be screened to detect cross-infection. This would include nose swabs and swabs from skin lesions and urinary and intravenous catheters (Cox *et al.* 1995). If cross-infection occurs it may be necessary to close a ward to new admissions, particularly to surgical or intensive care patients. Once patients have been discharged, the ward must be cleaned thoroughly before patients are readmitted (Duckworth 1990).

All staff in contact with the infected patient should be screened, including medical, nursing, paramedical and domestic staff. There is no evidence that MRSA poses a risk to healthy staff, but staff may become colonized and could transmit MRSA to other patients (Locksley 1982).

In patients known to be colonized with MRSA, signs of infection must be treated as significant, with MRSA considered to be the possible cause. Early investigations, appropriate specimen collection and treatment is essential (see Chap. 37, Specimen collection). Relapses may occur, especially in debilitated patients and particularly in sites such as tracheotomies (Cox *et al.* 1995). This means that source isolation must be maintained even after three negative cultures have been obtained. The presence of MRSA should be documented in the patient's records in order to alert staff should readmission be necessary (Cookson *et al.* 1986).

Transmission

MRSA is mainly spread by hands (Phillips & Young 1996), therefore hand hygiene is the most important factor in controlling an outbreak of MRSA (Crowcroft *et al.* 1996). Environmental cleanliness is also important (Schmitz *et al.* 1998). The airborne route can be a means of spread, particularly during bed making when particles carrying MRSA can be widely dispersed leading to contamination of the environment (Marshall *et al.* 1998), to areas as diverse as television sets (Stacey *et al.* 1998), floors, beds and mattresses (Kumari *et al.* 1998). Patients with large wounds, eczema or respiratory tract infection with a productive cough will be heavy dispersers of MRSA and are often responsible for spread. Faulty ventilation systems (Cotterill *et al.* 1996; Kumari *et al.* 1998) and crowded conditions have also been implicated in the spread of MRSA (Kibbler *et al.* 1998). Source isolation in a single room with the door closed is required (Jernigan *et al.* 1996).

When there are a large number of MRSA infected/colonized patients, cohort nursing in one ward is an effective means of controlling outbreaks. Other measures include:

1 Correctly performed hand washing before and after patient contact. A bactericidal alcoholic hand rub can be used when hands are clean (Kampf *et al.* 1998).
2 High standard of ward cleaning, as inanimate surfaces near affected patients are commonly contaminated with MRSA (Boyce *et al.* 1997).
3 Careful containment and disposal of waste.
4 Careful segregation, containment and laundering of used linen.
5 Careful education of the patient and their visitors to ensure compliance to policy, as familial carriage and subsequent infection have been reported (Hollis *et al.* 1995).
6 Planned cleaning of the ward, e.g. curtains.
7 Ward closure may be necessary when the above control measures fail to prevent spread (Working Party Report 1998).
8 Appropriate investigation and treatment of health care workers. While MRSA rarely causes infection in healthy persons, healthcare workers can become colonized with MRSA and go on to transmit MRSA to their patients (Cox & Conquest 1997). Investigation and treatment of healthcare workers is the responsibility of the occupational health department, with the help of the infection control team (Working Party Report 1998).

In areas where MRSA is endemic a risk assessment may need to be undertaken. The Working Party (1998) advises that patients' needs can be prioritized by dividing them into groups:

1 Non-acute – long stay care of elderly, psychiatric and psychogeriatric patients.
2 Low risk areas – medical, general, acute care of the elderly and non-neonatal paediatrics.
3 Moderate risk areas – general, surgical, urological, gynaecologic, obstetric and dermatologic.
4 High risk areas – all special units and intensive care.

Unfortunately, those patients in non-acute areas may subsequently require intensive care (Dennesen *et al.* 1998). Following discharge from hospital untreated carriers of MRSA create a new reservoir of colonized patients (Casewell 1995).

Community care

Inter-hospital movement should be restricted to the absolute minimum. If the patient must be transferred to another hospital the receiving hospital must be informed in plenty of time for the necessary arrangements to be made. The ambulance service should be notified if it is being used to transfer an MRSA patient, mainly to prevent another patient being placed in the same vehicle before it is cleaned. Hand washing by the ambulance service staff and cleaning of local areas of patient contact, i.e. chair or stretcher, is all that is required after transport of an affected patient.

People colonized with MRSA do not present a risk to healthy people in the community, and should live their lives without restrictions. However in residential homes where other residents may have postoperative wounds, strict attention to hand washing, environmental cleanliness and compliance with aseptic techniques is important, making segregation unnecessary (DoH 1996).

Staphylococcus epidermidis *(coagulase negative staphylococci)*

Staphylococcus epidermidis is part of the body's normal commensal flora and an important cause of infection, particularly in immunosuppressed patients or those with invasive devices such as IV catheters. Significant levels of resistance are seen, reflecting antibiotic usage (Burnie & Loudon 1997). Cross-infection can occur and is associated with hospitalization longer than 6 days (Kotilainen *et al.* 1995). Thurn *et al.* (1992) indicate that the incidence of resistant *S. epidermidis* in patients will become more like that found in health care professionals with whom they are in contact. Patrick *et al.*'s (1992) study supports this view as 62% of the nurses were found to be colonized with resistant *S. epidermidis*.

Streptococcus pneumoniae

Resistant *Streptococcus pneumoniae* was recognized in the 1960s, but was not seen in the UK until 1976 in a patient with a history of foreign travel (Meers & Matthews 1978). Since this time, resistance to penicillin has been increasing (Johnson 1998) with a marked ability to cause cross-infection (Johnson 1998). The increased incidence of *S. pneumoniae* infection has led to the increase use of vaccine. These vaccines are based on the serotype antigen of the *pneumoniae*, therefore the serotype of the organism needs to be known to ensure the appropriate vaccine is given. Currently there are available multivalent vaccines which contain the antibiotic resistant serotypes (George *et al.* 1997).

Vancomycin resistant enterococci *(VRE)*

Enterococcus species were once considered normal bacterial flora which occasionally acted as opportunistic pathogens. Now *Enterococcus faecalis* and *faecium* are an important cause of nosocomial infection (Hunt 1998). The origin of VRE may be due to selection of VRE by the use of vancomycin, or introduced into the hospital by patients already colonized with VRE due to acquisition from animals or via the food chain.

VRE infection and colonization is associated with previous vancomycin use and/or broad-spectrum antibiotic therapy, severe underlying disease, immunosuppression, intra-abdominal surgery and prolonged hospitalization (Gopal *et al.* 1997), particularly in HDUs (Bonten *et al.* 1998). Most VRE infections are endogenous, however transmission from patient to patient or by direct contact, particularly by unwashed hands or contamination of equipment or the environment frequently occurs (Hospital Infection Control Practices Advisory Committee (HICPAC) 1995).

The food chain, especially raw minced meat, is thought to be responsible for the increased incidence of VRE in humans, due to use of the glycopeptide avoparcin as a food additive. However, a large German study of raw minced meat and pork failed to demonstrate a connection between 8% of meat samples positive for VRE and patients' clinical isolates, which were of different resistance patterns (Klein *et al.* 1998). A great cause of concern is the appearance of transferable high-level glycopeptide resistance in enterococci, producing some strains that are now resistant to all available antibiotics. Enterococci readily colonize the bowel, spread rapidly among hospital patients and transfer their antibiotic resistance widely among themselves and other Gram-positive species (French 1998). Carriage of VRE can be prolonged (Brennen *et al.* 1998). While VRE is not particularly pathogenic, with many infections resolving without specific therapy (Quale *et al.* 1996), the potential to transfer their resistance gene to more pathogenic Gram-positive bacteria would produce major problems (Moellering 1998).

Contamination of the environment readily occurs (Murrey 1998). This was demonstrated in a recent study which followed cancer patients in an outpatients department. Environmental cultures from clinic rooms before and after patient care showed widespread contamination which was not removed by superficial cleaning (Smith *et al.* 1998). Byers *et al.* (1998) suggest that conventional cleaning took an average of 2.8 cleans to eradicate VRE from a hospital room. VRE can survive temperatures of 71°C for 10 minutes or 80°C for 3 minutes (Bradley & Fraise 1996); it can survive in 150 ppm available chlorine for 5 minutes (Kearnes *et al.* 1995) and in the environment for more than 3 days (Weber *et al.* 1997).

Thorough cleaning of the environment and equipment, and strict attention to hand washing before and after patient contact are essential. Patients must wash their hands after visiting the toilet and before meals. While universal precautions are generally adequate for caring for VRE positive patients, when patients have diarrhoea or cannot comply with infection control policies barrier nursing is required, particularly if other patients in the area are immunocompromised (Bowler *et al.* 1998).

References and further reading

Ayliffe, G.A.J. (1986) Guidelines for the control of epidemic methicillin-resistant *Staphylococcus aureus*. *J Infect*, **7**, 193–201.

Baquero, F. (1997) Gram-positive resistance: challenge for the development of new antibiotics. *J Antimicrob Chemother*, **39**(Suppl. A), 1–6.

Barrett, S.P., Mummery, R.V. & Chattopadhyay, B. (1998) Trying to control MRSA causes more problems than it solves. *Hosp Infect*, **39**, 85–93.

Bartzokas, C.A. *et al.* (1984) Control and eradication of methicillin-resistant *Staphylococcus aureus* on a surgical unit. *New Engl J Med*, **311**, 1422–5.

Bates, J. (1997) Epidemiology of vancomycin resistant enterococci in the community and the relevance of farm animals to human infection. *J Hosp Infect*, **37**, 89–101.

Beedle, D. (1993) Beating the bug. *Nurs Times*, **89**(45), *J Infect Control Nurs*, Suppl., i–vi.

Bonten, M.J. *et al.* (1998) The role of 'colonization pressure' in the spread of vancomycin resistant enterococci: an important infection control variable. *Arch Intern Med*, **158**(10), 1127–32.

Bowler, I.C.J.W. *et al.* (1998) Guidelines for the management of patients colonised or infected with vancomycin resistant enterococci. *J Hosp Infect*, **39**, 75–82.

Boyce, J.M. *et al.* (1997) Environmental contamination due to methicillin resistant *Staphylococcus aureus*: possible infection control implications. *Infect Control Hosp Epidemiol*, **18**(9), 622–7.

Bradley, C.R. & Fraise, A.P. (1996) Heat and chemical resistance of enterococci. *J Hosp Infect*, **34**, 191–6.

Branger, C., *et al.* (1997) Epidemiology typing of extended-spectrum beta-lactamase producing *Klebsiella* pneumoniae isolates responsible for five outbreaks in a university hospital. *J Hosp Infect*, **36**(1), 23–36.

Brennen, C., Wagener, M.M. & Muder, R.R. (1998) Vancomycin resistant *Enterococcus faecium* in a long term care facility. *Am Geriatr Soc*, **46**(2), 157–60.

Bryant, R.E. *et al.* (1971) Factors affecting mortality of Gram-negative rod bacteraemia. *Arch Int Med*, **127**, 120.

Burke, J.P. & Pestotnik, S.L. (1996) Breaking the chain of antibiotic resistance. *Curr Opin Infect Dis*, **9**, 253–5.

Burnie, J.P. & Loudon, K.W. (1997) Ciprofloxacin resistant *Staphylococcus epidermidis* and hands. *Lancet*, **349**, 649–50.

Byers, K.E. *et al.* (1995) New theatres in the control of methicillin resistant *Staphylococcus aureus*. *J Hosp Infect*, **30**, Suppl., 465–571.

Byers, K.E. *et al.* (1998) Disinfection of hospital rooms contaminated with vancomycin resistant *Enterococcus faecium*. *Infect Control Hosp Epidemiol*, **19**(4), 261–4.

Casewell, M.W. (1982) The role of multiply resistant coliforms in hospital acquired infection. *Recent Adv Infect*, **2**, 31–50.

Casewell, M.W. (1995) New threats to the control of methicillin-resistant *Staphylococcus aureus*. *J Hosp Infect*, **30**(Suppl), 465–71.

Center for Disease Control (1997) *Staphylococcus aureus* with reduced susceptibility to vancomycin, United States. *Morb Mort Week Rep*, **46**, 765–6.

Chan, C.H. & Loudon, K.W. (1998) Activity of tea tree oil on methicillin resistant *Staphylococcus aureus* (MRSA). *J Hosp Infect*, **39**(3), 244.

Coello, R. *et al.* (1997) Risk factors for developing clinical infection with methicillin resistant *Staphylococcus aureus* (MRSA) amongst hospital patients initially only colonised with MRSA. *J Hosp Infect*, **37**(1), 39–46.

Cookson, B. (1997) How to resist? *Health Serv J*, October 30, 9–11.

Cookson, B.D. *et al.* (1986) A hospital computer system as a tool for infection control. In: *Current Perspectives in Health Care Computing* (eds J. Bryant, J. Roberts & P. Windson), pp. 126–31. British Computer Society Health Information, Specialist Group, and *Br J Health Care Comput*, London.

Cookson, B.D. *et al.* (1989) Staff carriage of epidemic methicillin-resistant *Staphylococcus aureus*. *J Clin Microbiol*, **27**, 1471–6.

Cookson, B.D., Morrison, D. & Marples, R.R. (1997) Nosocomial gram positive infection. *J Med Microbiol*, **6**, 439–42.

Coovadia, Y.M., Johnson, A.P., Bhana, R.H., *et al.* (1992) Multiresistant *Klebsiella pneumoniae* in a neonatal nursery: the importance of maintenance of infection control policies and procedures in the prevention of outbreaks. *J Hosp Infect*, **22**(3), 197–205.

Cotterill, S., Evans, R. & Fraise, A.P. (1996) An unusual source of an outbreak of methicillin resistant *Staphylococcus aureus* on an intensive therapy unit. *J Hosp Infect*, **32**(3), 207–16.

Cox, R.A. & Conquest, C. (1997) Strategies for the management of health care staff colonized with epidemic methicillin resistant *Staphylococcus aureus*. *J Hosp Infect*, **35**(2), 117–27.

Cox, R.A. *et al.* (1995) A major outbreak of methicillin-resistant *Staphylococcus aureus* caused by a new phage-type (EMRSA-16). *J Hosp Infect*, **29**, 87–106.

Crowcroft, N. *et al.* (1996) Methicillin resistant *Staphylococcus aureus*: investigations of a hospital outbreak using a case-control study. *J Hosp Infect*, **34**, 301–309.

Cunnery, R.J. *et al.* (1993) Failure of teicoplanin therapy in *Staphylococcus* septicaemia. *J Hosp Infect*, **3**, 325–7.

Dance, D.A.B. (1987) A hospital outbreak caused by a chlorhexidine and antibiotic resistant *Proteus mirabilis*. *J Hosp Infect*, **10**, 10–16.

Dennesen, P.J., Bonten, M.J. & Weinstein, R.A. (1998) Multiresistant bacteria as a hospital epidemic problem. *Ann Med*, **30**(2), 176–85.

DoH (1996) Guidelines on the control of infection in residential and nursing homes. Stationery Office, London.

Duckworth, G. (1990) Revised guidelines for the control of epidemic methicillin-resistant *Staphylococcus aureus*. *J Hosp Infect*, **16**, 351–77.

Eltringham, I. (1997) Mupirocin resistance and methicillin resistant *Staphylococcus aureus* (MRSA). *J Hosp Infect*, **35**(1), 1–8.

Ferguson, J. (1991) Septic shock in the critically ill patient. *Surg Nurse*, **4**(2), 21–4.

Flaherty, J.P. & Weinstein, R.A. (1996) Nosocomial infection caused by antibiotic-resistant organisms in the intensive-care unit. *Infect Control Hosp Epidemiol*, **17**(4) 236–48.

French, G. *et al.* (1990) Hong Kong strains of methicillin resistant and methicillin sensitive *Staphylococcus aureus* have similar virulence. *J Hosp Infect*, **15**, 117–25.

French, G.L. (1998) Enterococci and vancomycin resistance. *Clin Infect Dis*, **27**(Suppl. 1), S75–83.

Garrod, L.P. (1972) Causes of failure in antibiotic treatment. *Br Med J*, **4**, 473–6.

Gedded, A.M. (1996) Antiviral drug resistance. *Br Med J*, **313**, 503–504.

George, R.C. *et al.* (1997) Serogroups/types and antibiotic resistance of referred isolates of *Streptococcus pneumoniae*, 1993–1995. *CDR Rev*, **7**, R159–64.

Glauser, M.P. *et al.* (1991) Septic shock: pathogenesis. *Lancet*, **338**, 732–5.

Gopal Rao, G., Ojo, F. & Kolokithas, D. (1997) Vancomycin resistant gram positive cocci: risk factors for faecal carriage. *J Hosp Infect*, **35**, 63–9.

Granzebrook, J. (1986) Counting the cost of infection. *Nurs Times*, **83**(6), 24–6.

Hill, R.L.R. *et al.* (1988) Elimination of nasal carriage of methicillin-resistant *Staphylococcus aureus* with mupirocin during a hospital outbreak. *J Antimicrob Chemother*, **22**, 377–84.

Hiramatsu, K. (1998) Vancomycin resistance in staphylococci. *Drug Resist Updates*, **1**, 135–50.

Hiramatsu, K. *et al.* (1997) Methicillin resistant *Staphylococcus aureus* clinical strain with reduced vancomycin susceptibility. *Chemotherapy*, **40**, 135–6.

Hobson, R.P., MacKenzie, F.M. & Gould, I.M. (1996) An outbreak of multiply resistant *Klebsiella pneumoniae* in the Grampian region of Scotland. *J Hosp Infect*, **33**(4), 249–62.

Hollis, R.J. *et al.* (1995) Familial carriage of methicillin resistant *Staphylococcus aureus* and subsequent infection in a premature neonate. *Clin Infect Dis*, **21**(2), 328–32.

Hughes, W.T. (1971) Fatal infections in childhood leukaemia. *Am J Dis Childhood*, **122**, 283–7.

Hunt, C.P. (1998) The emergence of enterococci as a cause of nosocomial infection. *Br J Biomed Sci*, **55**, 149–56.

Huovinen, P. & Cars, O. (1998) Control of antimicrobial resistance: time for action. *Br Med J*, **317**, 613.

Irish, D. *et al.* (1998) Control of an outbreak of an epidemic methicillin resistant *Staphylococcus aureus* also resistant to mupirocin. *J Hosp Infect*, **39**, 19–26.

Jaffe, H.W. *et al.* (1980) Identity and interspecific transfer of gentamicin resistant plasmids in *Staphylococcus aureus* and *Staphylococcus epidermidis*. *J Infect Dis*, **141**, 738.

Jarvis, W.R. & Martone, W.J. (1992) Predominant pathogen in hospital infection. *J Antimicrobiol Chemother*, **29**(Suppl. A), 19–24.

Jernigan, J.A. *et al.* (1996) Effectiveness of contact isolation during a hospital outbreak of methicillin resistant *Staphylococcus aureus*. *Am J Epidemiol*, **143**(5), 496–504.

Jevons, M.P. (1961) Celberin resistant staphylococci. *Br Med J*, **1**, 124–5.

Johnson, A.P. (1998) Antibiotic resistance among clinically important gram positive bacteria in the UK. *J Hosp Infect*, **40**, 17–26.

Johnson, A.P. *et al.* (1996) Prevalence of antibiotic resistance and serotype in pneumococci in England and Wales: results of observational surveys in 1990 and 1995. *Br Med J*, **312**, 1454–6.

Jumaa, P. & Chattopadhyay, B. (1994) Outbreak of gentamicin, ciprofloxacin resistant *Pseudomonas aeruginosa* in an intensive care unit, traced to contaminated quivers. *J Hosp Infect*, **28**(3), 209–18.

Kampf, G., Jarosch, R. & Ruden, H. (1998) Limited effectiveness of chlorhexidine based hand disinfectants against methicillin-resistant *Staphylococcus aureus* (MRSA). *J Hosp Infect*, **38**, 297–303.

Kearns, A.M., Freeman, R. & Lightfoot, N.F. (1995) Nosocomial enterococci; resistance to heat and sodium hypochlorite. *J Hosp Infect*, **30**, 193–9.

Kennedy, P. & Hamilton, L.R. (1997) Psychological impact of the management of methicillin resistant *Staphylococcus aureus* (MRSA) in patients with spinal cord injury. *Spinal Cord*, **35**(9), 617–19.

Kibbler, C.C., Quick, A. & O'Neil, A.M. (1998) The effect of increased bed numbers on MRSA transmission in acute medical wards. *J Hosp Infect*, **39**, 213–19.

Klein, G., Pack, A. & Reuter, G. (1998) Antibiotic resistance patterns of enterococci and occurrence of vancomycin-resistant enterococci in raw minced beef and pork in Germany. *Appl Environ Microbiol*, **64**(5), 1825–30.

Knowles, H.E. (1993) The experience of infectious patients in isolation. *Nurs Times*, **89**(30), 53–6.

Kotilainen, P. *et al.* (1995) Epidemiology of the colonization of out-patients and inpatients with ciprofloxacin resistant coagulase-negative staphylococci. *Clin Infect Dis*, **21**(3), 685–7.

Kumari, D.N. *et al.* (1998) Ventilation grilles as a potential source of methicillin resistant *Staphylococcus aureus* causing an outbreak in an orthopaedic ward at a district general hospital. *J Hosp Infect*, **39**(2), 127–33.

Laa Poh, C. & Yeo, C.C. (1993) Recent advances in typing *Pseudomonas aeruginosa*. *J Hosp Infect*, **24**, 175–81.

Linden, P.K. (1998) Clinical implications of nosocomial gram-positive bacteremia and superimposed antimicrobial resistance. *Am J Med*, **104**(5A), 24S–33S.

Locksley, R.M. (1982) Multiple antibiotic resistant *Staphylococcus aureus*: introduction, transmission and evaluation of nosocomial infection. *Ann Intern Med*, **97**, 317–24.

Marples, R.R., Speller, D.C. & Cookson, B.D. (1995) Prevalence of mupirocin resistance in *Staphylococcus aureus. J Hosp Infect*, **29**(2), 153–5.

Marshall, B. *et al.* (1998) Environmental contamination of a new general surgical ward. *J Hosp Infect*, **39**(3), 242–3.

Maslow, J.N., Brecher, S. & Gunn, J. (1995) Variation and persistence of methicillin resistant *Staphylococcus aureus* strains among individual patients over extended periods of time. *Eur J Clin Microbiol Infect Dis*, **14**, 282–90.

Mayet, F. (1989) The microbe file. *Nurs Stand*, **3**, 57–8.

Meers, P.D. & Matthews, R.B. (1978) Multiply-resistant pneumococcus. *Lancet*, **ii**, 219.

Mendoza, M.C. (1985) Evidence for the dispersion and evolution of R. plasmids from *Serratia marcescens* in hospital. *J Hosp Infect*, **6**, 147–53.

Miller, M.A., Dascal, A., Portnoy, J. *et al.* (1996) Development of mupirocin resistance among methicillin resistant *Staphylococcus aureus* after widespread use of nasal mupirocin ointment. *Infect Control Hosp Epidemiol*, **17**(12), 811–13.

Mims, C.A. *et al.* (1993) *Medical Microbiology*. Mosby, London.

Moellering, R.C. (1998) Vancomycin resistant enterococci. *Clin Infect Dis*, **26**(5), 1196–9.

Monnet, D.L. (1998) Methicillin resistant *Staphylococcus aureus* and its relationship to antimicrobial use: possible implications for control. *Infect Control Hosp Epidemiol*, **19**(8), 552–9.

Moore, A. (1997) Hospital bugbear. *Health Serv J*, October 30, 1–5.

Molyneux, R. & Chadwick, C. (1997) Vancomycin resistant enterococci: implications for infection control. *Prof Nurse*, **12**(9), 641–4.

Murrey, B.E. (1998) Diversity among multidrug-resistant enterococci. *Emerg Infect Dis*, **4**(1), 37–47.

Oldman, T. (1998) Isolated cases. *Nurs Times*, **94**(11), 67–71.

Patrick, C.H. *et al.* (1992) Relatedness of strains of methicillin resistant coagulase negative *Staphylococcus* colonizing hospital personnel and producing bacteremias in the neonatal intensive care unit. *Pediatr Infect Dis*, **11**(11), 935–40.

Payne, D.N., Gibson, S.A. & Lewis, R. (1998) Antiseptics: a forgotten weapon in the control of antibiotic resistant bacteria in hospital and community setting. *J R Soc Health*, **18**(1), 18–22.

Peters, G. *et al.* (1983) Antibacterial activity of teichomycin – a new glycopeptide antibiotic in comparison to vancomycin. *J Antimicrob Chemother*, **11**, 94–5.

Phillips, E. & Young, T. (1996) Methicillin resistant *Staphylococcus aureus* and wound management. *Br J Nurs*, **4**(22), 1345–9.

Pillay, D. (1998) Emergence and control of resistance to antiviral drugs in resistance in herpes viruses, hepatitis B virus and HIV. *Commun Dis Public Health*, **1**(1), 5–13.

Quale, J. *et al.* (1996) Experience with a hospital-wide outbreak of vancomycin resistant enterococci. *Am J Infect Control*, **24**(5), 372–9.

Rae, G.G. (1998) Risk factors for the spread of antibiotic-resistant bacteria. *Drugs*, **55**(3), 323–30.

Richardson, J.F. *et al.* (1988) Another strain of methicillin-resistant *Staphylococcus aureus* epidemic in London. *Lancet*, **2**, 748–9.

Romero-Vivas, J. *et al.* (1995) Mortality associated with nosocomial bacteraemia due to methicillin resistant *Staphylococcus aureus. Clin Infect Dis*, **21**, 1417–23.

Rossi, T. *et al.* (1996) Eradication of the long term carriage of methicillin resistant *Staphylococcus aureus* in patients wearing dentures; a follow up of 10 patients. *J Hosp Infect*, **34**, 311–20.

Sande, M.A. & Mandell, G.L. (1980) Chemotherapy of microbial diseases. In: *The Pharmacological Basis of Therapeutics* (eds L.S. Goodman *et al.*). Macmillan, London.

Schmitz, F.J. *et al.* (1998) Impact of hygienic measures on the development of methicillin resistance among staphylococci between 1991 and 1996 in a university hospital. *J Hosp Infect*, **38**(3), 237–40.

Selkon, J.B. *et al.* (1980) The role of an isolation unit in the control of hospital infection with multi-resistant *Staphylococcus aureus. J Hosp Infect*, 1, 41–6.

Simpson, S. (1992) Methicillin resistant *Staphylococcus aureus* and its implications for nursing practice. A literature review. *Nurs Pract*, **5**(2), 2–7.

Smith, S.M. *et al.* (1989) Ciprofloxacin therapy for methicillin-resistant *Staphylococcus aureus* infection or colonizations. *Antimicrob Agents Chemother*, **33**, 181–4.

Smith, T.L., Iwen, P.C., Olson, S.B. *et al.* (1998) Environmental contamination with vancomycin-resistant enterococci in an outpatient setting. *Infect Control Hosp Epidemiol*, **19**(7), 515–18.

Sparling, F.P. *et al.* (1976) Antibiotic resistance in the gonococcus. In: *Microbiology* (ed. D. Schlessinger). American Society of Microbiology, New York.

Speller, D.C.E. *et al.* (1997) Resistance to methicillin and other antibiotics in isolates of *Staphylococcus aureus* from blood and cerebrospinal fluid. England and Wales 1989–1995. *Lancet*, **350**, 323–5.

Stacey, A. *et al.* (1998) Contamination of television sets by methicillin resistant *Staphylococcus aureus* (MRSA). *J Hosp Infect*, **39**(3), 243–4.

Standing Medical Advisory Committee (1998) The path of least resistance. Department of Health, Wetherby.

Swan Joint Committee (1969) *Use of Antibiotics in Animal Husbandry and Veterinary Medicine*. HMSO, London.

Thornsberry, C. (1995) Trends in antimicrobial resistance among today's bacterial pathogens. *Pharmacotherapy*, **15**(1, Part 2), 3SD–8S.

Thurn, J.R., Crossley, K.B., Gerdts, A. *et al.* (1992) Dynamics of coagulase negative staphylococcal colonization in patients and employees in a surgical intensive care unit. *J Hosp Infect*, **20**(4), 247–55.

Truett, L. (1991) The septic syndrome. *Cancer Nurs*, **14**(4), 175–80.

Tuffnall, C. (1988) MRSA: isolating the patients and nurses. *N Z Nurs J*, 1, 21–3.

Turco, T.F., Melko, G.P. & Williams, J.R. (1998) Vancomycin intermediate resistant *Staphylococcus aureus. Ann Pharmacother*, **32**(7–8), 758–60.

Weber, J.D. & Rutala, W.A. (1997) Role of environmental contamination in the transmission of vancomycin resistant enterococci. *Infect Control Hosp Epidemiol*, **18**, 306–309.

Wise, R. *et al.* (1998) Antimicrobial resistance. *Br Med J*, **317**, 609–610.

Working Party Report (1998) Revised guidelines for the control of methicillin-resistant *Staphylococcus aureus* infection in hospitals. *J Hosp Infect*, **39**, 253–90.

Aspergillosis

Definition

An infection caused by a fungus of the genus *Aspergillus*, causing inflammatory granulomatous lesions on, or in, any organ (Bennett 1995).

Reference material

Aspergillus species are common saprophytic moulds, easily recognized by their conidiophores, which are swollen ends of hyphae, from which radiate large numbers of sterigmata which end in short chains of spores. Each *Aspergillus* conidiospore releases thousands of spores, which remain suspended in the air for long periods and are viable for many months in dry locations. They are among the most buoyant of fungal spores and are present in all unfiltered air (Rhame 1991). Over 200 species of *Aspergillus* have been characterized, but fewer than 20 are reported as being pathogenic to man, the most common species causing allergic and invasive disease being A. *fumigatus* (Warren *et al.* 1982). In recent years A. *flavus* has also emerged as an important pathogen, particularly in invasive disease of immunosuppressed patients (Bennett 1995).

Aspergillus spores are commonly found in soil, decaying vegetation, spices, potted plants and dried flowers. Cases of allergic and invasive disease have been reported among individuals working in close contact with such substances and who inhale large numbers of *Aspergillus* spores. Examples include fungus inhalation during building work (Hodgson *et al.* 1998), continual prolonged exposure, such as farmers exposed to mouldy hay (Patterson *et al.* 1974), and factory workers exposed to the spores derived from manufacturing materials (Jensen *et al.* 1993).

Generally, aspergillosis has been associated with building renovation, when large numbers of spores are often liberated into the environment (Arnow *et al.* 1978). These spores are then inhaled and deposited in the lungs. Ear, cutaneous, sinus and dental infections have also been known to occur. Other reported modes of transmission include airborne spread, which is associated with indwelling catheters, implants and contaminated bandages (Anaissie 1992), and food borne spread. A. *flavus* can generate a carcinogenic substance called aflatoxin in foodstuffs (Rhame 1991).

Normal healthy people rarely develop invasive disease. Although incidence of infection in healthy people has been seen (see above), aspergillosis is primarily an infection of severely immunocompromised patients. The major predisposing factor of infection includes prolonged neutropenia, chronic administration of steroids, insertion of prosthetic devices and tissue damage due to prior infection or trauma (Khardoni 1989). In addition, patients on broad-spectrum antibiotics are susceptible (Siberry *et al.* 1997).

The incidence of invasive aspergillosis has risen as a consequence of the widespread use of aggressive chemotherapy, increased transplantation and AIDS disease (Manuel & Kibbler 1998). Significant infection has been reported among patients receiving heart and lung (Anteby *et al.* 1997), liver (Singh *et al.* 1997) and bone marrow transplants (Verschraegen *et al.* 1997). Transmission of invasive aspergillosis from the infected donor to three organ recipients has occurred (Keating *et al.* 1996). A retrospective analysis of 48 bone marrow transplantation patients with documented or probable invasive aspergillosis found that 33% had recurring aspergillosis, with a mortality rate of 88% (Offner *et al.* 1998). The organism is capable of invasion across all natural barriers, including cartilage and bone, and has a propensity for invading blood vessels, causing thrombosis and infection. The major concern is the potential for severe haemorrhage, which may cause death and which occurs in about 10% of patients. Generally, infection is chronic, causing symptoms directly related to the site of infection. Infections requiring surgical treatment have been seen among transplantation patients (Heinz *et al.* 1996).

Diagnosis

Diagnosis is difficult, as isolation of *Apergillus* may be due to contamination of the specimen from environmental *Aspergillus*. Diagnosis relies on demonstration of *Aspergillus* by culture and microscopy along with consideration of the patient's clinical condition. Lack of sensitivity of serological antigen tests reduces their clinical usefulness (Bennett 1995).

Treatment

Therapy for invasive aspergillosis has been less than satisfactory, with amphotericin B being the antifungal agent with established activity against the infection (Pizzo *et al.* 1982). The availability of new drugs and alternative forms of amphotericin B has increased treatment options (White & Santamauro 1995). The outcome of aspergillosis is likely to depend on the extent of underlying pulmonary disease, delays in diagnosis and commencement of effective therapy (Saraceno *et al.* 1997).

Prevention

Control measures are essential in preventing *Aspergillus* infection. Air conditioning systems must be functioning and well maintained, and the environment kept scrupulously clean, with emphasis placed on vacuuming, damp dusting and mopping. Instruments, dressings, equipment and linen must always be stored properly to prevent contamination by *Aspergillus*. This highlights the importance of removing wound dressings for the shortest period of time possible before dressing changes to prevent contamination of open wounds.

During constructive or renovation projects in hospital, infection control teams must identify the infection risks posed by each project and plan ways to minimize the risk (Carter & Barr 1997). The use of barriers to prevent *Aspergillus* spores entering patient areas is essential (Overberger *et al.* 1995). Ideally, relocation of immune suppressed patients to unaffected areas is advisable, and thorough cleaning of work areas before the return of patients is imperative (Arnow *et al.* 1978). Antifungal prophylaxis during building work has been seen to reduce the incidence of aspergillosis (Lamy *et al.* 1998).

Person to person spread has not been demonstrated, and therefore barrier nursing is not required. However, sputum should be disposed of carefully and patients encouraged to cover the mouth and nose when coughing.

One outbreak of aspergillosis was found to be due to contamination of a ward kitchen area, including fridge, ice machine, microwave and tea caddy (Loudon *et al.* 1996). This highlights that scrupulous cleaning and maintenance of the environment is essential.

References and further reading

Anaissie, E. (1992) Opportunistic mycoses in the immunocompromised host: experience at a cancer centre and review. *Clin Infect Dis*, **14**(Suppl. 1), S43–S53.

Anteby, I. *et al.* (1997) Necrotizing choroiditis-retinitis as presenting symptom of disseminated aspergillosis after lung transplantation. *Eur J Ophthalmol*, **7**(3), 294–6.

Arnow, P.M. *et al.* (1978) Pulmonary aspergillosis during hospital renovation. *Am Rev Resp Dis*, **118**, 49–53.

Bennett, J.F. (1995) *Aspergillus* species, 4th edn. In: *Principles and Practice of Infectious Diseases* (eds G.L. Mandell, J.E. Bennett & R. Dolan). Churchill Livingstone, New York. Chap. 238, 2306–11.

Carter, C.D. & Barr, B.A. (1997) Infection control issues in construction and renovation. *Infect Control Hosp Epidemiol*, **18**(8), 587–96.

Heinz, T. *et al.* (1996) Soft-tissue fungal infections: surgical management of 12 immunocompromised patients. *Plast Reconstr Surg*, **97**(7), 1391–9.

Hodgson, M.J. *et al.* (1998) Building associated pulmonary disease from exposure to *Stachybotrys chartarum* and *Aspergillus versicolor*. *J Occup Environ Med*, **40**(3), 241–9.

Jensen, P.A. *et al.* (1993) Evaluation and control of workers exposed to fungi in a beet sugar refinery. *Am Ind Hyg Assoc J*, **54**, 742–8.

Keating, M.R. *et al.* (1996) Transmission of invasive aspergillosis from a subclinically infected donor to three different organ transplant recipients. *Chest*, **109**(4), 119–24.

Khardoni, N. (1989) Host–parasite interactions in fungal infections. *Eur J Clin Microbiol Infect Dis*, **8**, 331–52.

Lam, T. *et al.* (1998) Prophylactic use of itraconazole for the prevention of invasive pulmonary aspergillosis in high risk neutropenic patients. *Leuk Lymphoma*, **30**(1–2), 163–74.

Loudon, K.W. *et al.* (1996) Kitchens as a source of *Aspergillus niger* infection. *J Hosp Infect*, **32**, 191–8.

Manuel, R.J. & Kibbler, C.C. (1998) The epidemiology and prevention of aspergillosis. *J Hosp Infect*, **39**(2), 95–109.

Offner, F. *et al.* (1998) Impact of previous aspergillosis on the outcome of bone marrow transplantation. *Clin Infect Dis*, **26**(5), 1098–103.

Overberger, P.A., Wadowsky, R.M. & Schaper, M.M. (1995) Evaluation of airborne particulates and fungi during hospital building renovation. *Am Ind Hyg Assoc J*, **56**(7), 706–712.

Patterson, R., Sommers, H. & Fink, J.N. (1974) Farmer's lung following inhalation of *Aspergillus flavus* growing in mouldy hay. *Clin Allegy*, **4**, 79–86.

Pizzo, P.A. *et al.* (1982) Empiric antibiotic and antifungal therapy for cancer patients with prolonged fever and granulocytopenia. *Am J Med*, **72**, 101–111.

Rhame, F.S. (1991) Prevention of nosocomial aspergillosis. *J Hosp Infect*, **18**(Suppl. A), 466–72.

Saraceno, J.L. *et al.* (1997) Chronic necrotizing pulmonary aspergillosis: approach to management. *Chest*, **112**(2), 542–8.

Siberry, G.K., Costarangos, C. & Cohen, B.A. (1997) Destruction of the nasal septum by *Aspergillus* infection after autologous bone marrow transplantation. *New Engl J Med*, **337**(4), 275–6.

Singh, N. *et al.* (1997) Invasive aspergillosis in liver transplant recipients in the 1990s. *Transplantation*, **64**(5), 716–20.

Verschraegen, C.F. *et al.* (1997) Invasive *Aspergillus* sinusitis during bone marrow transplantation. *Scand J Infect Dis*, **29**(4), 436–8.

Warren, R.E. *et al.* (1982) Clinical manifestations and management of aspergillosis in the compromised patient. In: *Fungal Infections in the Compromised Patient* (eds D.W. Warnock & M.D. Richardson), pp. 119–53. John Wiley, New York.

White, D.A. & Santamauro, J.T. (1995) Pulmonary infections in immunosuppressed patients. *Curr Opin Pulm Med*, **1**(3), 202–208.

Clostidium difficile

Definition

Clostridium difficile is a slender, Gram-positive anaerobic rod which is spore forming and motile and is capable of surviving in the environment for prolonged periods (Cunha 1998). Bacteria of this type may be a normal component of gut flora and flourish when other gut organisms are eradicated by antibiotics (Zadik & Moore 1998).

Reference material

Clostridium difficile was first recognized in the late 1970s when it was identified as the causative organism for pseudomembranous colitis (PMC). In the 1980s it was identified as a major cause of antibiotic associated diarrhoea (AAD) (Duerden *et al.* 1994). Numbers of infections continue to rise (Wilcox & Smyth 1998). It is now one of the most commonly detected enteric pathogens and an important cause of nosocomial infection in nursing homes and hospitals (Zadik & Moore 1998).

Diarrhoea can be caused by disruption of the normal flora of the gut by antibiotics which allow *C. difficile* to multiply. The colonic mucosa becomes covered with a characteristic fibrinous pseudomembrane. Signs and symptoms can be relatively mild, resolving when antibiotics are discontinued, or more severe, as in cases of pseudomembranous colitis, which may require surgical resection of parts of the colon and is associated with a significant mortality rate.

About 5% of healthy adults carry *C. difficile* in their faeces, usually in small numbers. The elderly are at particular risk and appear to develop more serious symptoms compared with younger patients (Melillo 1998). This causes considerable mortality and morbidity among elderly people, costing the Health Service millions of pounds each year (Brazier & Duerden 1998). During an outbreak in Ireland 9.6% of elderly patients died (Kyne et al. 1998). Infants are more likely to carry the organisms but are less likely to develop colitis (Fekety & Shah 1993).

Data suggest that an average size general hospital will have 100 cases of C. difficile each year, with an extra annual cost of £4 000 000 and 2100 lost bed days (Spencer 1998).

Diagnosis

Diagnosis is based on clinical findings, endoscopy and laboratory evaluation. Clinical findings range from profuse, watery, green, foul smelling or bloody diarrhoea, with cramping abdominal pains, tenderness and high fever, to hypovolaemic shock and overwhelming sepsis. Endoscopy may reveal effects similar to those seen in non-specific colitis, or may show the yellow–white raised plaques which go on to form a membrane on the intestinal mucosa (Kofsky et al. 1991).

Laboratory diagnosis

Clostridium difficile is difficult to isolate in ordinary culture because of overgrowth by other organisms. To overcome this a selective culture medium is used. The presence of C. difficile in culture is not by itself an indication of infection, it simply marks the organism's presence. Infection or disease is indicated by the presence of toxins produced by the organism which can be identified using screening tests (Cleary 1998). Pathogenic strains of C. difficile produce two protein exotoxins, toxin A (enterotoxin) and toxin B (cytotoxin) (Brazier 1998). Clostridium difficile toxin A induces detachment of human epithelial cells from the basement membrane and subsequent death by apoptosis (Mahida et al. 1998). This process may be asymptomatic or cause mild diarrhoea or it can lead to pseudomembranous colitis (Kelly & LaMont 1998). Recurrence is common (Do et al. 1998) ranging from 5 to 42% of patients (Zimmerman et al. 1997).

Treatment

Initial treatment involves discontinuing antibiotics and providing supportive care (Wei et al. 1997). However, significant infection can be treated with metronidazole or vancomycin (Cunha 1998). In extreme cases of pseudomembranous colitis surgery will be required, which may include resectional or diversion procedures (Viswanath & Griffiths 1998), but death can occur even when diagnosis is made early and appropriate therapy is given (Kavan et al. 1998). Patients susceptible to C. difficile reinfection need to be protected from exposure until their bowel flora recovers (Wilcox 1998).

Transmission

Pseudomembranous colitis develops from overgrowth of C. difficile already present in the gut, or from exogenous organisms acquired via the person to person contact or the faecal-oral route. C. difficile can be transmitted on the hands of hospital personnel (McFarland et al. 1989), and outbreaks in hospital have resulted in the deaths of a number of elderly people (Duerden et al. 1994). One such outbreak affected 39 elderly patients, five of whom died. In this instance the ward was closed for thorough cleaning to eliminate the infection (Snell 1992). Worsley (1993) describes a prolonged outbreak of C. difficile involving 175 patients in three hospitals. The infection caused 17 deaths directly and contributed to a further 43. In addition to an estimated financial cost of £75 000, there was a loss of public confidence and an increase in staff sick leave. Bignardi (1998) identified nine risk factors which appear to influence the chance of acquiring C. difficile; these were increasing age, severity of underlying disease, non-surgical gastrointestinal procedures, presence of nasogastric tube, antiulcer medication, stay in ITU, duration of hospital stay, duration of antibiotic therapy and administration of multiple antibiotics.

Antibiotic use was shown to be statistically significantly associated with both diarrhoea and carriage of C. difficile. Risks include type of antibiotic, route of administration and dose. Accurate identification of risk factors allows for appropriate decisions to be made to reduce risk and thereby reduce incidence. High risk patients can be monitored closely to facilitate early detection of infection, commencement of treatment and infection control precautions.

Prevention of spread and management of infection

Reducing the risk of an outbreak of C. difficile relies on restriction of the use of those antibiotics associated with the highest risk, reducing the duration of antibiotic courses and the length of stay in hospital (Bignardi 1998). Prevention of epidemics relies on careful hand washing (Worsley 1998), environmental decontamination (Surawicz 1998) and isolation of symptomatic patients (Wilcox et al. 1998). Cross-infection has been seen to be reduced by thorough cleaning of the environment and the use of clean equipment for each patient (Worsley 1998). For example, the use of tympanic thermometers instead of oral and rectal thermometers appears to reduce the incidence of C. difficile (Brooks et al. 1998). Johnson et al. (1990) demonstrated a decrease in the incidence of infection following the introduction of gloves for staff in contact with patients infected with C. difficile. When an infected patient is discharged, the ward must be thoroughly cleaned before other patients are allowed into the area.

Nursing care

Careful barrier nursing is required for all patients with toxin producing C. difficile or unexplained diarrhoea. Segregation from other patients must continue until stool cultures are clear of infectious organisms.

References and further reading

Brazier, J.S. (1998) The diagnosis of *Clostridium difficile* associated disease. *J Antimicrob Chemother*, **41** (Suppl. C), 29–40.

Brazier, J.S. & Duerden, B.I. (1998) Guidelines for optimal surveillance of *Clostridium difficile* infection in hospitals. *Commun Dis Public Health*, **1** (4), 229–30.

Bignardi, G.E. (1998) Risk factors for *Clostridium difficile* infection. *J Hosp Infect*, **40**, 1–15.

Brooks, S. *et al.* (1998) Reduction in vancomycin resistant enterococcus and *Clostridium difficile* infections following change to tympanic thermometers. *Infect Control Hosp Epidemiol*, **19** (5), 333–6.

Cleary, R.K. (1998) *Clostridium difficile*-associated diarrhoea and colitis: clinical manifestations, diagnosis and treatment. *Dis Colon Rectum*, **41** (11), 1435–49.

Cunha, B.A. (1998) Nosocomial diarrhoea. *Crit Care Clin*, **14** (2), 329–38.

Do, A.N. *et al.* (1998) Risk factors for early recurrent *Clostridium difficile* associated diarrhoea. *Clin Infect Dis*, **26** (4), 954–9.

Duerden, B.I. *et al.* (1994) Report of the PHLS *Clostridium difficile* working party. *Public Health Lab Serv Microbiol Dig*, **11** (1), 22–4.

Fekety, R. & Shah, A.B. (1993) Diagnosis and treatment of *Clostridium difficile* colitis. *J Am Med Assoc*, **269** (1), 71–5.

Johnson, S. *et al.* (1990) Prospective controlled study of vinyl glove use to interrupt *Clostridium difficile* transmission. *Am J Med*, **88**, 137–40.

Kavan, P. *et al.* (1998) Pseudomembraneous *Clostridium* after autologous bone marrow transplantation. *Bone Marrow Trans*, **21** (5), 521–3.

Kelly, C.P. & LaMont, J.T. (1998) *Clostridium difficile* infection. *Annu Rev Med*, **49**, 375–90.

Kim, K.H. *et al.* (1981) Isolation of *Clostridium difficile* from the environment and contacts of patients with antibiotic associated colitis. *J Infect Dis*, **143**, 42–4.

Kofsky, P. *et al.* (1991) *Clostridium difficile*: a common and costly colitis. *Dis Colon Rectum*, **34** (3), 244–8.

Kyne, L. *et al.* (1998) Simultaneous outbreak of two strains of toxigenic *Clostridium difficile* in a general hospital. *J Hosp Infect*, **38** (2), 101–112.

McFarland, L.V. *et al.* (1989) Nosocomial acquisition of *Clostridium difficile* infection. *New Engl J Med*, **320** (4), 204–210.

Mahida, Y.R. *et al.* (1998) Effect of *Clostridium difficile* toxin A on human colonic lamina propria cells: early loss of macrophages followed by T cell apoptosis. *Infect Immunol*, **66** (11), 5462–9.

Melillo, K.D. (1998) *Clostridium difficile* and older adults: what primary care providers should know. *Nurse Pract*, **23** (7), 25–6.

Public Health Laboratory Service Communicable Disease Surveillance Centre (1993) Typing service for *Clostridium difficile*. *Commun Dis Rep*, **3** (53), 1.

Snell, J. (1992) Old die in *Clostridium* outbreak. *Nurs Times*, **88** (3), 6.

Spencer, R.C. (1998) Clinical impact and associated costs of *Clostridium difficile*-associated disease. *J Antimicrob Chemother*, **41** (Suppl. C), 5–12.

Surawicz, C.M. (1998) *Clostridium difficile* disease: diagnosis and treatment. *Gastroenterologist*, **6** (1), 60–65.

Viswanath, Y.K. & Griffiths, C.D. (1998) The role of surgery in pseudomembranous enterocolitis. *Postgrad Med J*, **74** (870), 2216–19.

Wei, S.C. *et al.* (1997) Diagnostic role of endoscopy, stool culture, and toxin A in *Clostridium difficile*-associated disease. *J Formos Med Assoc*, **96** (11), 879–83.

Wilcox, M.H. & Smyth, E.T. (1998) Incidence and impact of *Clostridium difficile* infection in the UK, 1993–1996. *J Hosp Infect*, **39** (3), 181–7.

Wilcox, M.H. (1998) Treatment of *Clostridium difficile* infection. *J Antimicrob Chemother*, **41** (Suppl. C), 41–6.

Wilcox, M.H. *et al.* (1998) Recurrence of symptoms in *Clostridium difficile* infection; relapse or reinfection? *J Hosp Infect*, **38** (2), 93–100.

Worsley, M. (1993) A major outbreak of antibiotic associated diarrhoea. *Public Health Lab Serv Microbiol Dig*, **10** (2), 97–9.

Worsley, M.A. (1998) Infection control and prevention of *Clostridium difficile* infection. *J Antimicrob Chemother*, **41** (Suppl. C), 59–66.

Zadik, P.M. & Moore, A.P. (1998) Antimicrobial association of an outbreak of diarrhoea due to *Clostridium difficile*. *J Hosp Infect*, **39** (3), 189–93.

Zimmerman, M.J., Bak, A. & Sutherland, L.R. (1997) Review article: treatment of *Clostridium difficile* infection. *Aliment Pharmacol Ther*, **11** (6), 1003–1012.

Cryptosporidiosis

Definition

Cryptosporidium is a protozoan coccidian parasite, first isolated in 1907. Human infection is usually caused by *Cryptosporidium parvum* (DoH 1990).

Reference material

Cryptosporidium species were initially considered a cause of severe protracted diarrhoea (Navin *et al.* 1984) in immunocompromised patients (Wolfson *et al.* 1985). *Cryptosporidium* is now being increasingly recognized as the cause of self-limiting enteritis in otherwise healthy people, with sporadic and epidemic cryptosporidiosis most commonly recorded in young children (Holley *et al.* 1986).

Transmission

Cryptosporidium infects livestock, particularly calves and lambs, whose faecal matter infects water supplies, which then can infect man (Tzipori 1983). Based on epidemiological evidence, consumption of certain foods (especially undercooked sausages, offal and unpasteurized milk) appears to be a risk factor (Casemore 1987). Infection can also occur following direct contact with animals by hand to mouth route, and is easily transmitted from one person to another (DoH 1990; Ungar 1995). This latter route is probably the main mode of transmission in urban populations. Only a small inoculum of organism appears to be required to cause infection.

Two outbreaks of cryptosporidiosis traceable to swimming baths have been reported: in one case the cause was contamination of water in the pool by a swimmer, in the other a plumbing defect allowed sewage to enter the water circulating system (Hunt *et al.* 1994).

Cryptosporidium is unaffected by chlorine in the concentrations that can be used in the treatment of drinking water, and is inactivated only by being frozen or heated to temperatures of 65–85°C for 5 to 10 minutes or by exposure to boiling water. Prevention relies on compliance with safe practices by water companies and health authorities in water treatment processes.

Routine water disinfection by chlorination is ineffective in controlling the organism except in small numbers. Therefore all domestic water supplies are filtered to remove harmful pathogens. As 30% of all public water supplies in England and Wales comes from ground water, contamination of the water supply generally occurs when heavy rains follow drought (Peeters *et al.* 1989), causing leakage of effluent or slurry into treated water. The public water supplies in the UK are generally of a very high standard (Casemore 1998), with outbreaks of cryptosporidiosis due to contamination of mains tap water in the UK being uncommon. However, 14 outbreaks have occurred between 1992 and 1995 and were associated with public water and swimming pools (Furtado *et al.* 1998). Outbreaks can be very disruptive. In 1997 a large outbreak involving 345 people occurred in North Thames, London, 746 000 local people needed to boil their drinking water for 3 weeks. Long periods of illness were seen, including diarrhoea, abdominal pain, fever, vomiting and flu-like symptoms; 26 people were admitted to hospital, two died, although cryptosporidiosis was not thought to be the main reason for all admissions or the two deaths (Willocks *et al.* 1998). Infection can also be acquired from ice cubes and contaminated drinking water, eating food that has been cleaned and inadequately cooked in contaminated water and from milk (Ravin *et al.* 1991).

The time from ingestion of oocysts to the development of symptoms can range from 5 to 28 days (Ungar 1995). *Cryptosporidium* infection in the immune competent person generally causes a self-limiting gastroenteritis. Symptoms include watery stools, vomiting and weight loss (Casemore *et al.* 1994), fever, nausea, vomiting and weakness (Ungar 1995). Recovery involves an intact humoral and cellular immune response. Excretion of oocysts can continue after symptoms have ceased (Ungar 1995). During an outbreak involving water in 1991, 85 immunocompetent cases were involved, 10% of the cases required hospital admission and symptoms lasted an average of 13 days (Aston *et al.* 1991). For severely immunocompromised patients, particularly those with AIDS and bone marrow transplant recipients, infection is protracted, severe and sometimes life threatening (Gardner 1994). Severity reflects the level of immunosuppression (Petersen 1992). Symptoms include a debilitating cholera-like diarrhoea and vomiting which, when found in terminal AIDS patients, is particularly distressing. Remission and relapse of cryptosporidiosis probably reflects fluctuation in immune status (Casemore *et al.* 1994).

Respiratory tract involvement has been described either through aspiration of oocysts during vomiting or through haematogenous spread. Coughing can result in aerosol transmission of oocysts to others. Rare presentations include cholecystitis, hepatitis, pancreatitis and reactive arthritis (Ungar 1995).

Prevention

Immune competent people who swim in or drink water may be regularly exposed to infection, and may have higher levels of immunity to infection. The Third Report of the Group of Experts on *Cryptosporidium* in Water Supplies (1998) states that there is a strong correlation between outbreaks of infection and inadequacy in the treatment of water supplies or where there is overloading of the treatment process. This group and others recommend that immunocompromised persons should:

1 Boil all tap and bottled water used for drinking.
2 Avoid contact with infected animals and people (Heathcock *et al.* 1998).
3 Avoid contaminated water during recreational activities (Kramer *et al.* 1998).
4 Avoid uncooked food that may have been washed in contaminated water.
5 Avoid exposure to young farm animals and pets, and avoid acquiring new young pets, as young animals are particularly susceptible to crytosporidiosis (Current 1987).
6 Filter domestic water supplies. Currently water companies regularly monitor water supplies; increased continuous sampling is being considered (Casemore 1998). If contamination occurs users are informed and told to boil all drinking water; supplies are not turned off as water is needed for flushing toilets and fighting fires, etc.

Treatment

The host immune response prevents initial infection and facilitates clearance of infection; prolonged infection is seen in immunocompromised persons. There is no reliable curative treatment for cryptosporidiosis (Ungar 1995).

Nursing care

Oocysts are shed in large numbers during infection and only a small number of oocysts are required to cause infection. Strict barrier nursing is required while diarrhoea persists, with segregation from other patients continuing until clear specimens of stool cultures are obtained.

Special attention to hand washing is essential. Nurses were found to develop infection from a very ill, demented patient who had severe diarrhoea and vomiting. In this instance infection control practices were good, however it was thought that cross-infection occurred by both the faecal-oral and aerosol routes (O'Mohony *et al.* 1992). Any sign of cross-infection must be pursued vigorously to prevent further spread. This will include close cooperation with health and local authorities, with the appropriate water companies and between the outbreak control team and the authority.

References and further reading

Aston, R., Mawer, S. & Casemore, D. (1991) *Report of the Out-break Control Group to Coordinate the Investigation and Control of the Outbreak of cryptosporidiosis in North Humberside.* Formal report to the local authorities of Beverley and Kingston-upon-Hull, UK.

Casemore, D.P. (1987) Cryptosporidiosis PHLS. *Microbiol Dig*, **4**, 1–5.

Casemore, D.P. (1998) *Cryptosporidium* and the safety of our water supplies. *Commun Dis Public Health*, **1**(4), 218–19.

Casemore, D.P., Gardner, C.A. & O'Mahony, C.O. (1994) Cryp-tosporidial infection, with special reference to nosocomial trans-mission of *Cryptosporidium parvum*: a review. *Folia Parasitol*, **41**, 17–21.

Current, W.L. (1987) *Cryptosporidium*: its biology and potential for environmental transmission. *CRC Crit Rev Environ Control*, **17**, 21–51.

DoH (1990) *Report of the Group of Experts on Cryptosporidium in Water Supplies* (Chairman Sir John Badenock). Stationery Office, London.

Furtado, C. *et al.* (1998) Outbreaks of waterborne infectious disease in England and Wales 1992–5. *Epidemiol Infect*, **121**(1), 109–119.

Gardner, C. (1994) An outbreak of hospital acquired cryp-tosporidiosis. *Br J Nurs*, **3**(4), 154–8.

Heathcock, R. *et al.* (1998) Survey of food safety awareness among HIV positive individuals. *AIDS Care*, **10**(2), 237–41.

Holley, H.P. *et al.* (1986) Cryptosporidiosis – a common cause of parasitic diarrhoea in otherwise healthy individuals. *J Infect Dis*, **153**, 365–7.

Hunt, D.A. *et al.* (1994) Cryptosporidiosis associated with a swim-ming pool complex. *Commun Dis Rep*, **4**(2), R20–22.

Kramer, M.H. *et al.* (1998) First reported outbreak in the United States of cryptosporidiosis associated with a recreational lake. *Clin Infect Dis*, **26**(1), 27–33.

Navin, T.R. *et al.* (1984) Cryptosporidiosis – clinical, epidemiolog-ical and parasitologic review. *Rev Infect Dis*, **6**, 313–27.

O'Mohony, C., Gardner, C. & Casemore, D.P. (1992) Hospital acquired cryptosporidiosis. *Public Health Lab Serv Commun Dis Rep*, **3**(2), R18–19.

Peeters, J.E. *et al.* (1989) Effects of disinfection of drinking water with ozone or chlorine dioxide on survival of *Cryptosporidium parvum* oocysts. *Appl Microbiol*, **55**(6), 1519–22.

Petersen, C. (1992) *Cryptosporidium* in patients infected with HIV. *Clin Infect Dis*, **15**, 903–909.

Ravin, P., Lundgren, J.D. & Kjaeldgaard, P. (1991) Nosocomial outbreak of *Cryptosporidium* in AIDS patients. *Br Med J*, **302**, 277–80.

Soave, R. *et al.* (1986) *Cryptosporidium* and cryptosporidiosis. *Rev Infect Dis*, **8**, 1012–23.

Third Report of the Group of Experts (1998) *Cryptosporidium* in water supplies. Department of the Environment, Transport and the Regions, and Department of Health, London.

Tzipori, S. (1983) Cryptosporidiosis in animals and humans. *Microbiol Rev*, **47**, 84–96.

Ungar, B.L.P. (1995) *Cryptosporidium*. In: *Principles and Practices of Infectious Disease*, 4th edn. (eds G.L. Mandell, J.E. Bennett & R. Dolan). Churchill Livingstone, New York. Vol. 2, Chap. 262, 2500–2510.

Willocks, L. *et al.* (1998) A large outbreak of cryptosporidiosis associated with a public water supply from a deep chalk bore-hole. *Commun Dis Public Health*, **1**(4), 239–44.

Wolfson, J.S. *et al.* (1985) Cryptosporidiosis in immunocompetent patients. *New Engl J Med*, **312**, 1278–82.

Hepatitis

Hepatitis may be caused by a variety of agents including viruses and certain chemicals, and it may be secondary to other illnesses. Nurses need to be aware of the epidemiol-ogy, modes of transmission and prevention of hepatitis.

Hepatitis A

Definition

Hepatitis A is an enterically transmitted Picornaviridae virus, which causes an acute, self-limiting infection of the liver (Battegay *et al.* 1995).

Reference material

HAV is a small, symmetrical RNA virus (enterovirus type 72) (Melnick 1982). The virus is unusually stable, resisting heat at 60°C for 1 hour, at 25°C for 3 months, indefinite cold storage (5°C), acidic conditions (pH 3) and non-ionic detergents (Siegl *et al.* 1984; Sorbey *et al.* 1988). It can survive for several months in sewage and the environment. However, HAV can be inactivated after 4 minutes at 70°C,

after 5 seconds at 80°C and instantly at 85°C (Battegay *et al.* 1995).

HAV is spread predominantly by the faecal-oral route, and viral replication probably occurs in the jejunum before transmission via the portal vein to the liver (Siegl 1988). HAV has been associated with the following:

1 Contaminated water, milk and food. Any uncooked food and drink could be responsible for infection. However, particular problems are due to contamination at the time of harvesting and packaging of uncooked frozen foods which are then thawed and used (Ramsey *et al.* 1989).

2 Poor general hygiene and low economic status (Ayoola 1988), contact with children in day centres (Hadler *et al.* 1986) and neonatal intensive care units (Azimi *et al.* 1986). Outbreaks of HVA at school were associated with lack of toilet paper, soap and hand towels (Rajaratnam *et al.* 1992) and school toilets (Leoni *et al.* 1998).

3 Foreign travel to countries where HAV is endemic (Skinhof *et al.* 1981).

4 Blood transfusions (Noble *et al.* 1984). Documented evi-dence that HVA has been transmitted by factor VIII concentrate (Soucie *et al.* 1998).

5 Contact with a case of hepatitis A in the home (Maguire *et al.* 1995).

7 Sexual contact. HAV can be reduced among homosexual men by HAV vaccination (Center for Disease Control 1998).

8 Perinatal transmission of hepatitis A is extremely uncommon (Duff 1998), although an instance of an infant being infected by his mother before or during birth has been reported (Watson *et al.* 1993).

9 Intravenous drug misusers. Needle sharing practices contribute to the spread of HVA (Stene-Johansen *et al.* 1998).

Diagnosis of acute HAV infection is usually confirmed serologically, by detecting immunoglobulin M (IgM) antibodies to HA antigen (Ag) which appear in serum 2–7 weeks after oral inoculation, and may persist for some time, occasionally for more than a year (Lemon *et al.* 1980). Evidence of past infection, and therefore immunity which can persist for life (Lemon 1985), is obtained by detecting serologically the presence of IgG antibody to HAAg.

HAV has an incubation period of 2–7 weeks. HAAg can be detected in stools early in the course of illness. HAAg levels decline rapidly with the onset of symptoms but can remain detectable for up to 2 weeks after the onset of clinical hepatitis (Coulepis *et al.* 1980).

HAV usually causes a minor illness in children and young adults, with as few as 5% of cases being symptomatic (Eddleston 1990). The illness often presents as an upper respiratory infection with the following signs and symptoms: anorexia, malaise, weight loss, pyrexia, diarrhoea and vomiting (Wright *et al.* 1985), dark urine and jaundice. Complications of HVA include cholestasis, prolonged or relapsing disease, extrahepatic disease and fulminant hepatitis (Bategay *et al.* 1995).

Control and prevention of HAV relies on provision of good sanitation facilities, clean drinking water and supervision of food handlers. Passive immunization with intramuscular normal pooled immunoglobulin (HNIg) gives protection against clinical hepatitis for about 3 months in most people. However, it is probable that passive immunization allows HAV infection with greatly attenuating effects which could lead to life-long immunity (Gust *et al.* 1988). Post exposure prophylaxis is advisable for household contacts during outbreaks of HAV infection (DoH 1996).

Hepatitis A vaccine is available and immunization has been seen to be effective (Werzberger *et al.* 1998). One dose provides protection for one year, a booster dose at 6–12 months provides immunity for up to 10 years. The vaccine should be administered to those travelling in developing countries (Dick 1998), in areas of moderate or high HAV endemicity, particularly where sanitation and food hygiene are poor, but it is not an alternative to preventive behaviours (Birthistle 1998). The Department of Health (1992) has recommended that sewage workers, military personnel and foreign diplomats should be considered for vaccination. In institutions for the care of the mentally ill, and in children's centres where the children are not toilet trained, vaccination policy should be formulated according to local circumstances (DoH 1992). However a study by Maguire *et al.* (1995) showed no clear evidence

that health care workers are at increased occupational risk of acquiring hepatitis A.

A combined hepatitis A and B vaccine is also available (Zuckerman 1998). Human normal immunoglobulin (HNIG) offers short term protection for up to 4 months and can be given to people who have been in close contact with infected cases and to those travelling to where the disease is endemic (DoH 1996).

HAV infection does not generally require hospital treatment. Strict barrier nursing in a single room with en suite toilet would be required (Pearse 1992). Two outbreaks of HVA among health care workers were attributed to inadequate hand washing and eating on the ward (Doebbeling *et al.* 1993; Hanna *et al.* 1996).

References and further reading

Ayoola, E.A. (1988) Viral hepatitis in Africa. In: *Viral Hepatitis and Liver Disease* (ed. A.J. Zuckerman), pp. 161–9. Alan R. Liss, New York.

Azimi, P.H. *et al.* (1986) Transfusion-acquired hepatitis A in a premature infant with second nosocomial spread in an intensive care nursery. *Am J Dis Childhood*, **140**, 23–7.

Battegay, M., Gust, I.D. & Feinstone, S.M. (1995) Hepatitis A virus. In: *Principles and Practice of Infectious Diseases*, 4th edn. (eds G.L. Mandell, J.E. Bennett & R. Dolin). Churchill Livingstone, New York. Vol. 2, Chap. 150, 1636–66.

Birthistle, K. (1998) New combined hepatitis A and B vaccine. New vaccine is an adjunct, not an alternative to preventive behaviors. *Br Med J*, **316**(7140), 1317.

Center for Disease Control (1998) Hepatitis A vaccination of men who have sex with men. Atlanta Georgia, 1996–1997. *Morb Mort Week Rep*, **47**(34), 708–11.

Coulepis, A.C. *et al.* (1980) Detection of hepatitis A virus in the faeces of patients with naturally acquired infection. *J Infect Dis*, **141**, 151–6.

DoH (1996) *Immunisation Against Infectious Diseases*. Stationery Office, London.

Dick, L. (1998) Travel medicine: helping patients prepare for trips abroad. *Am Fam Physician*, **58**(2), 383–98.

Doebbeling, B.N., Li, N. & Wenzel, R.P. (1993) An outbreak of hepatitis A among health care workers: risk factors for transmission. *Am J Public Health*, **83**(12), 1679–84.

Duff, A. (1998) Hepatitis in pregnancy. *Semin Perinatal*, **22**(4), 277–83.

Eddleston, A. (1990) Modern vaccines. Hepatitis. *Lancet*, **335**, 1142–5.

Gust, I.D. *et al.* (1988) Prevention and control of hepatitis A. In: *Viral Hepatitis and Liver Disease* (ed. A.J. Zuckerman), pp. 77–80. Alan R. Liss, New York.

Hadler, S.C. *et al.* (1986) Hepatitis in day care centres. Epidemiology and prevention. *Rev Infect Dis*, **8**, 548–57.

Hanna, J.N. *et al.* (1996) An outbreak of hepatitis A in an intensive care unit. *Anaesth Intensive Care*, **24**(4), 440–44.

Lemon, S.M. (1985) Type A viral hepatitis. New developments in an old disease. *New Engl J Med*, **313**, 1059–67.

Lemon, S.M. *et al.* (1980) Specific immunoglobulin A response to hepatitis A virus determined by solid phase radioimmunoassay. *Infect Immunol*, **28**, 927–36.

Leoni, E. *et al.* (1998) An outbreak of intrafamiliar hepatitis A associated with clam consumption: epidemic transmission to a school community. *Eur J Epidemiol*, **14**(2), 187–92.

Maguire, H.C. *et al.* (1995) A collaboration case control study of sporadic hepatitis A in England. *Commun Dis Rep*, **5**(3), R33–40.

Melnick, J.-L. (1982) Classification of hepatitis A virus as enterovirus type 72 and of hepatitis B virus as hepadnovirus type 1. *Intervirology*, **18**, 105–106.

Noble, R.C. *et al.* (1984) Post-transfusion hepatitis A in a neonatal intensive care unit. *J Am Med Assoc*, **252**, 2711–15.

Pearse, J. (1992) Infection control. Nursing management of a patient with hepatitis A and B. *Nurs RSA*, **7**(5), 28–9.

Rajaratnam, G. *et al.* (1992) An outbreak of hepatitis A: school toilets as a source of transmission. *J Public Health Med*, **14**(1), 72–7.

Ramsey, C.N. *et al.* (1989) Hepatitis A and frozen raspberries. *Lancet*, **1**, 43–4.

Siegl, G. *et al.* (1984) Stability of hepatitis A virus. *Intervirology*, **22**, 218–26.

Siegl, G. (1988) Virology of hepatitis. In: *Viral Hepatitis and Liver Disease* (ed. A.J. Zuckerman), pp. 3–7. Alan R. Liss, New York.

Skinhof, P. *et al.* (1981) Travellers' hepatitis: origin and characteristics of cases in Copenhagen, 1976–1978. *Scand J Infect Dis*, **13**, 1–4.

Sorbey, M.D. *et al.* (1988) Survival and persistence of hepatitis A virus in environmental samples. In: *Viral Hepatitis and Liver Disease* (ed. A.J. Zuckerman), pp. 121–4. Alan R. Liss, New York.

Soucie, J.M. *et al.* (1998) Hepatitis A virus infection associated with clotting factor concentrate in the United States. *Transfusion*, **38**(6), 573–9.

Stene-Johansen, K. *et al.* (1998) A unique hepatitis A virus strain caused an epidemic in Norway associated with intravenous drug abuse. The Hepatitis A study group. *Scand J Infect*, **30**(1), 35–8.

Watson, J.C. *et al.* (1993) Vertical transmission of hepatitis A resulting in an outbreak in a neonatal intensive care unit. *J Infect Dis*, **167**(3), 567–71.

Werzeberger, A., Kuter, B. & Nalin, B. (1998) Six years following after hepatitis A vaccination. *New Engl J Med*, **338**(16), 1160.

Wright, R. *et al.* (1985) Acute viral hepatitis. In: *Liver and Biliary Disease* (eds R. Wright *et al.*), pp. 677–767. Baillière Tindall, London.

Zuckerman, J.N. (1998) New combined hepatitis A and B vaccine. Risks of viral hepatitis related to travel. *Br Med J*, **316**(7140), 1317.

GUIDELINES • Hepatitis A

Outpatient

Action	Rationale
1 It is not usually necessary to admit the individual to hospital.	Self-limiting disease.
2 Patient education is essential and must include advice on good personal hygiene and careful hand washing.	Limits the spread of the virus. Careful hand washing removes contamination from hands.
3 Separate soap, flannel and towel must be provided.	To minimize the risk of infection being spread via equipment used for hygiene purposes.
4 Meticulous cleaning of bath, wash basin and toilet with a cream cleaner and hot water.	To remove contamination.
5 Bath and wash basin must be allowed to dry after use.	Viruses will not survive on clean dry surfaces.
6 Soiled bed linen and underclothing should be washed.	To remove contamination.
7 Patient should refrain from intimate kissing and sexual intercourse while symptoms are present.	To reduce risk of cross-infection.
8 People with hepatitis A should avoid contact with susceptible people, i.e. very young, old or those with debilitating illness.	To reduce the likelihood of infection.
9 Crockery and cutlery must be washed and rinsed in hot water.	Heat destroys the virus.

Inpatient

Action	Rationale
1 Whenever possible, the patient should have medical or surgical treatment postponed until he/she is symptom free.	Medical and surgical treatment will debilitate the patient further and recovery will be slower.
2 Ideally, the patient should be discharged.	Cross-infection is less likely to occur at home.

Guidelines • Hepatitis A (cont'd)

Action	Rationale

3 A single room with separate toilet should be made available for the patient, although barrier nursing is not necessary.

In general patients are no longer excreting the virus once they have become symptomatic, however there are always exceptions.

4 Blood, secretions and excreta (particularly faeces) must be disposed of immediately in a heat-disinfecting bedpan washer.

To prevent cross-infection.

5 Careful hand washing after patient contact.

To prevent cross-infection.

Hepatitis B

Definition

Hepatitis B is a serious infectious disease caused by the hepatitis B virus (HBV), which produces an inflammatory condition of the liver characterized by jaundice, hepatomegaly, anorexia, abdominal and gastric discomfort, abnormal liver function, clay-coloured stools and dark urine (Hsu *et al.* 1995).

Reference material

HBV is a 42-nm double-shelled particle, inside which is a 27-nm inner core particle which contains the viral nucleic acid and represents the intact infectious virion (Lau & Wright 1993). HBV was termed initially 'Dane particle' after its discoverer (Dane *et al.* 1970).

Corrarino (1997) suggests HBV is the most common chronic infectious disease in the world, with 2000 million HBV infected persons alive today and 350 million persons chronically infected carriers of HBV (Kane 1995). Outbreaks continue to occur in developing countries due to inadequate infection control policies (Singh *et al.* 1998). Prevention of HBV includes vaccination, prophylaxis and improved infection control and safer sex practices (Alexander 1998).

Epidemiology

HBV may be found in virtually all body secretions and excreta of patients with acute hepatitis B and carriers of the virus. Blood, semen and vaginal fluids are mainly implicated in the transmission of infection, which occurs by:

1 Sexual transmission, both vaginal and anal (Brook 1988).
2 Accidental inoculation of blood following, for example, a sharps injury, or by drug addicts sharing used needles and syringes (Shattock *et al.* 1985).
3 Contamination of mucous membranes, eye, nose or mouth (Reed *et al.* 1993).
4 Contamination of non-intact skin (Bowden *et al.* 1993).
5 Perinatal route at or about the time of birth (Ramsay *et al.* 1998).

6 Blood transfusion. The frequency of post-transfusion HBV infection has decreased significantly since the exclusion of hepatitis B surface antigen (HBsAg) seropositive blood donors in Britain (O'Grady *et al.* 1988); one example involved an HBsAg negative donor who later proved to be HBc positive (Parry *et al.* 1997). The risk of transmitting HBV infection by screened blood is very small (Schreiber *et al.* 1996) due to improved donor selection and screening criteria (Gresens & Holland 1998). Transfusions abroad are still implicated as sources of infection (Papaevangelou *et al.* 1984).

High rates of infection occur in narcotic drug addicts, promiscuous homosexuals and prostitutes (Durante & Heptonstall 1995). A high prevalence of HBV infection has been reported in areas of the world where socioeconomic conditions are poor, and in individuals requiring repeated transfusions of blood or blood products, in institutions for those with learning difficulties and in some semi-closed institutions (Follett 1987). Perinatal acquisition of HBV is the major cause of infection in infants and children (Corrarino 1997). Perinatal transmission of HBV occurs in a high percentage of infants born to mothers with HBV at the time of delivery. The majority of infants who acquire HBV during the perinatal period become HBV carriers with no clinical symptoms (Tong 1989). HBV infection acquired during infancy and early childhood has a high likelihood of progressing to chronic infection, which can lead to chronic hepatitis, cirrhosis and primary hepatocellular carcinoma (Shapiro & Margolis 1992). Without vaccine during infancy 90% of infants born to HBV positive mothers will become lifelong carriers (Corrarino 1997). Tang *et al.*'s (1998) study found that those babies who were hepatitis positive at birth, even though they received immunoglobulin prophylaxis, were more likely to become carriers.

The prevalance of HBV infection in the UK is low, with many infections appearing to be acquired outside the UK (Gay *et al.* 1999).

Clinical response

HBV infection is clinically extremely variable, with the incubation period varying from 4 weeks to as long as 6 months. Clinical signs of HBV occur in about 50% of adults and only 5% of children (Zimmerman *et al.* 1997). Approximately 60% of adult cases produce a subclinical infection with only mild symptoms such as fatigue and malaise, which often go unnoticed. Acute infection occurs in about 40% of adults, with spontaneous recovery usually within one month, although prolonged recovery can occur and is accompanied by post-viral depression. Ninety per cent of adults recover completely from HBV while 90% of children 4 years and under develop chronic infection (Gitlin 1997). HBV plays an important part in hepatocarcinogenesis (Abe *et al.* 1998). Ikeda *et al.*'s (1998) study found that the risk of hepatocellular carcinoma in chronic hepatitis increases with time: 2.1% at 5 years, 4.9% at 10 years and 18.8% at 15 years. Omata (1998) suggests cumulative survival is significantly higher among patients in whom HBeAg is eliminated, than in those patients who remain seropositive. However, the risk of developing hepatocellular carcinoma may increase when HBV becomes quiescent.

The incidence of chronic infection is higher in those in whom there is a relative deficit of T cell function, the young, the aged, those with Down's syndrome, those with malignancy and those receiving immunosuppressive or cytotoxic therapy (Alexander 1990). HBV reactivation can occur in patients following allogeneic bone marrow transplantation and has been reported as 20.5% of cases (Dhedin *et al.* 1998). Ter-Borg *et al.* (1998) suggest this is due to enhanced immunological responses to hepatocytes harbouring reactivated HBV.

Infectivity

The progress of HBV can be monitored by serological testing. HBsAg is detected in the blood approximately 3 to 4 weeks after exposure, with antibodies to hepatitis B core (HBc) antigen (HBcAg) developing about 2 weeks after HBsAg occurs. Anti-HBc will eventually be replaced by anti-HBs, the antibody to HBsAg, which marks the end of high infectivity and the development of immunity to subsequent HBV infection (Lau & Wright 1993). The antigen HBeAg is an internal component of the core of HBs and is an indicator of high infectivity; it will be replaced eventually by anti-HBe, which correlates with loss of viral replication (Tedder 1980). HBV is capable of surviving for at least 1 week in the environment (Trevelyan 1991).

Diagnosis

Diagnosis is confirmed by a virological blood test with regular monitoring of antigen and antibody status to evaluate progress (Teo 1992).

Screening policy for HBsAg

Screening of the entire hospital patient population would be an effective way to identify hepatitis B infection, but this would be costly and time consuming in terms of the benefits derived. It is important, however, to screen patients before their admission to a transplant or renal unit (Tedder 1980).

In general, the best compromise is to test those patients belonging to groups in which there is a high prevalence of hepatitis B. These include the following people:

1 All new admissions who currently live or were born in countries where there is a high prevalence of hepatitis B, such as the developing countries.
2 Drug addicts.
3 Promiscuous persons (i.e. individuals who frequently change sexual partners).
4 Institutionalized persons with learning difficulties.
5 Multiple transfusion patients.
6 All patients acutely or recently jaundiced.

Transmission of HBV in the health care setting

Studies of health care workers who have sustained inoculation accidents involving HBsAg positive blood indicate the risk of transmission to be approximately 20%, where the potential source of infection is an HBeAg positive patient or carrier (Werner *et al.* 1982). Most carriers can be classified as low risk where blood contains anti-HBe. The chance of transmission from these patients is approximately 0.1%; overall, the chance of transmission of infection is probably of the order of 5%.

There is no evidence of transmission of HBV by inhalation of droplets, neither has faecal-oral transmission been demonstrated (DoH 1990). However, one study estimated that up to 94% of HBV infections among health care workers may have been acquired without any inoculation injury (Callender *et al.* 1982).

Immunization and vaccination

Passive protection against hepatitis B

Specific hepatitis B immunoglobulin (HBIG), prepared from pooled plasma with a high titre of hepatitis B surface antibody, is available for passive protection and is usually used in combination with hepatitis B vaccine to confer passive/active immunity under certain defined conditions (DoH 1996), including:

1 Persons who have an inoculation, ingestion or splashing accident with HBsAg-infected blood.
2 Babies of mothers with hepatitis B. In these cases babies should receive HBIG no later than 48 hours after birth.
3 Sexual partners and, in some cases, family contacts judged to be high risk, or individuals suffering from acute hepatitis B and who are seen within one week of onset of jaundice.

Active immunization

Active immunization is by hepatitis B vaccine. Hepatitis B vaccine is a genetically engineered vaccine prepared from yeast cells using recombinant DNA technology. The HBsAg is absorbed onto aluminium hydroxide adjuvant. The plasma derived vaccine is no longer marketed in the UK (DoH 1996). The basic regimen consists of three doses of vaccine over 6 months, with a booster dose every 5 years. An accelerated schedule of three doses over 3 months with a booster at 12 months and then every 5 years can be given when rapid acquisition of immunity is required. Approximately 80 to 90% of vaccinated individuals respond to the vaccine.

Risk groups which include health care workers who have direct contact with blood and body fluids are recommended to be immunized against HBV. Their response to the vaccine must be checked: levels of 100 IU/ml and above indicate immunity; levels of 10–100 IU/ml indicate the need for a booster dose of vaccine; levels below 10 IU/ml indicate no response. Between 10 and 20% of those receiving vaccine will not respond at all to hepatitis B vaccine. Lack of response is more common in people aged 40 years and over and in people who are immunocompromised (DoH 1996).

Health care workers involved in exposure prone procedures (EPP), including theatre nurses, are required to be immunized against HBV. This means theatre nurses will have to provide evidence of HBV vaccination prior to employment. Those who fail to respond to vaccine have to be tested for HBV every 6 months to prove their continuing non-carrier status (Fox 1996).

Indications for immunization include:

1 Personnel including teaching, training and nursing staff directly involved over a period of time in patient care where there is a high prevalence of HBV or where blood and blood products are handled regularly.
2 Laboratory workers.
3 Dentists, dental personnel.
4 Medical and surgical personnel.
5 Health care personnel on secondment to work in areas of the world where there is a high prevalence of HBV.
6 Patients on entry to residential institutions where there is a high prevalence of HBV.
7 Patients treated by maintenance haemodialysis.
8 Sexual contacts of patients with acute HBV or carriers of HBV.
9 Infants born to mothers who are HBsAg positive.
10 Health care workers who receive an inoculation accident from a needle used on a patient who is HBsAg positive, either used alone or in combination with hepatitis B immunoglobulin.

In addition, HBV vaccine is offered to selected high risk populations, this includes homosexual men attending genitourinary clinics, as studies indicate they are at the greatest risk of acquiring HBV. Gilson et al.'s (1998) study found 38.7% of homosexual men, 5.9% of heterosexual men and 3.5% of women attending a London genitourinary clinic had evidence of HBV infection. It has been suggested that there is no need to extend HBV vaccination programmes to include other risk groups besides homosexual men (El Dalil et al. 1997). Unfortunately vaccination uptake is poor, and is likely to remain low (Mangtani et al. 1998), with transmission of HBV remaining a problem (Goldberg & McMenamin 1998).

A recent review evaluated that mass HBV immunization would not be cost effective in the UK, while the selective immunization strategy needs to be properly implemented (Edmunds 1998). A combined HBV and HAV vaccine is now available (Zuckerman 1998) which has been seen to be safe and well tolerated (Reutter et al. 1998).

Prevention of hepatitis B in health care workers

Dienstag & Ryan (1982) have shown that nurses are at no greater risk of acquiring hepatitis B than the general population. However, it is important that health care workers adopt safe techniques when in contact with blood and body fluids of all patients, regardless of their hepatitis status.

Avoiding inoculation accidents is an essential component of safe techniques. Resheathing needles accounts for 15–41% of all needlestick injuries and must not be undertaken (McCormick et al. 1981). Resheathing commonly occurs as a result of trying to ensure safe transit to a disposal sharps bin (Edmond et al. 1990), suggesting that sharps bins should be either attached to trolleys or placed at the bedside (Hart 1990).

Vickers et al. (1994) reviewed an outbreak of hepatitis B which involved three volunteers at a residential drug trial unit where blood samples were taken by staff who did not wash their hands after each patient contact, and whose hands, gloves, and equipment were visibly contaminated with blood. Such incidents demonstrate the importance of written policies that are regularly reviewed and updated.

Employment of HBsAg carriers

Tedder (1980) discusses the problem of carriers of HBsAg who want to return to full-time employment, particularly those whose carrier state lasts for many years or possibly for the rest of their lives. Prentice et al. (1992) report that between 1975 and 1990 there was on average one outbreak a year of hepatitis B which could be attributed to transmission from hospital staff to patients. Heptonstall's (1991) study indicates that infected surgical health care staff were associated with these outbreaks. New guidelines issued in 1993 by the Department of Health recommend that health care workers who are HBeAg positive must not carry out procedures in which there is a risk that injury to the health care worker could result in their blood contaminating the open tissues of patients. Previously all HBsAg positive staff were excluded from working on a renal dialysis units, now only HBeAg positive staff are excluded (DoH 1993).

Death of patients with hepatitis B

When infected patients die, their bodies are no more hazardous than when they were alive, providing that appropriate precautions against contamination with blood and body fluids are maintained (Young & Healing 1995). Guidelines recommend that bodies of patients known to be infected with hepatitis B, C or non-A and non-B should be placed in a body bag. Relatives and significant others should be permitted to view, touch and spend time with the deceased person. However, embalming should not be undertaken (Healing *et al.* 1995). The first fatal outcome resulting from transmission of hepatitis B from surgeon to patient was reported in 1996 (Sundkvisst *et al.* 1998).

Patient education

The DHSS (1984) recommends that individuals found to be HBsAg carriers should be educated about the ways in which hepatitis B may spread and the precautions which can be taken to reduce the risk to others. It is stressed that unnecessary restrictions and precautions may cause distress and should be avoided.

Antiviral therapy

Interferon-alpha is the treatment of choice for HBV, although long term remission is only 25–40%. Combination therapies are being evaluated (Marques *et al.* 1998).

References and further reading

Abe, K. *et al.* (1998) In situ detection of hepatitis B, C, and G virus nucleic acid in human hepatocellular carcinoma tissues from different geographic regions. *Hepatology*, **28**(2), 568–72.

Alexander, G.J.M. (1990) Immunology of hepatitis B virus infection. *Br Med Bull*, **46**(2), 354–67.

Alexander, I.M. (1998) Viral hepatitis: primary care diagnosis and management. *Nurse Pract*, **23**(10), 13–14.

Bowden, F.J., Pollett, B., Birrell, F. *et al.* (1993) Occupational exposure to the human immunodeficiency virus and other blood borne pathgens. A six year prospective study. *Med J Aust*, **158**(12), 810–12.

Brook, M.G. (1998) Sexual transmission and prevention of the hepatitis viruses A-E and G. *Sex Transm Infect*, **74**(6), 395–8.

Callender, M.E. *et al.* (1982) Hepatitis B virus infection in medical and health care personnel. *Br Med J*, **284**, 423–6.

Corrarino, J.E. (1997) Perinatal hepatitis B. Update and recommendations. *Am J Matern Child Nurs*, **23**(5), 246–52.

Dane, D.S. *et al.* (1970) Virus-like particle in serum of patients with Australian antigen-associated hepatitis. *Lancet*, **1**, 695–8.

Deinhardt, F.D. *et al.* (1985) Immunization against hepatitis B. Report of a WHO meeting on viral hepatitis in Europe. *J Med Virol*, **17**, 209–17.

Dhedin, N. *et al.* (1998) Reverse seroconversion of hepatitis B after allogeneic bone marrow transplantation: a retrospective study of 37 patients with pretransplant anti HBs and anti HBc. *Transplantation*, **66**(5), 616–19.

DHSS (1981) *Hepatitis B and NHS Staff. CMO (81)11*. Stationery Office, London.

DHSS (1984) *Guidance for Health Service Personnel Dealing with Patients Infected with Hepatitis B Virus. CMO (84)11, CNO (84)7*. Stationery Office, London.

DHSS (1996) *Immunisation Against Infectious Disease*. Stationery Office, London.

Dienstag, J.L. & Ryan, D.M. (1982) Occupational exposure to hepatitis B virus in hospital personnel; infection or immunization. *Am J Epidemiol*, **115**, 22–9.

DoH (1990) *Guidance for Clinical Health Care Workers; Protection Against Infection with HIV and Hepatitis Viruses*. Stationery Office, London.

DoH (1993) *Protecting Health Care Workers and Patients from Hepatitis B. HSG (93) 40*. Department of Health, London.

DoH (1996) *Immunisation Against Infectious Diseases*. Stationery Office, London.

Durante, A.J. & Heptonstall, J. (1995) How many people in England and Wales risk infection from injecting drug use? *Commun Dis Rep*, **5**(3), R40–44.

Edmond, M. *et al.* (1990) Effects of bedside needle disposal units on needle recapping frequency and needlestick injury. *Can Intraven Nurs Assoc J*, **6**(1), 10–11.

Edmunds, W.J. (1998) Universal or selective immunization against hepatitis B virus in the United Kingdom? A review of recent cost-effective studies. *Commun Dis Public Health*, **1**(4), 221–8.

El-Dalil, A.A. *et al.* (1997) Hepatitis B markers in heterosexual patients attending two genitourinary medicine clinics in the West Midlands. *Genitourin Med*, **73**(2), 127–30.

Follett, E. (1987) Psychiatric hospitals and the mentally handicapped – a special case. *R Coll Nurs Wembley Conf Rep*, 7, 8, 16. Mark Allen Publishing, London.

Fox, J.A. (1996) Hepatitis B and the theatre nurse. *Br J Theatre Nurs*, **6**(7), 26–9.

Gay, N.J. *et al.* (1999) The prevalence of hepatitis B infection in adults in England and Wales. *Epidemiol Infect*, **122**(1), 133–8.

Gilson, R.J. *et al.* (1998) Hepatitis B virus infection in patients attending a genitourinary medicine clinic: risk factors and vaccine coverage. *Sex Transm Infect*, **74**(2), 110–15.

Gitlin, N. (1997) Hepatitis B: diagnosis, prevention and treatment. *Clin Chem*, **43**(8, Part 2), 1500–1506.

Goldberg, D. & McMenamin, J. (1998) The United Kingdom's hepatitis B immunization strategy – where now? *Commun Dis Public Health*, **1**(2), 79–83.

Gresens, C.J. & Holland, P.V. (1998) Current risks of viral hepatitis from blood transfusions. *J Gastroenterol Hepatol*, **13**(4), 443–9.

Hart, S. (1990) Clinical hepatitis B; guidelines for infection control. *Nurs Stand*, **4**(45), 24–7.

Healing, T.D. *et al.* (1995) The infection hazards of human cadavers. *Commun Dis Rep*, **5**, R61–9.

Heptonstall, J. (1991) Outbreak of hepatitis B virus infection associated with infected surgical staff. *Commun Dis Rep*, **1**(8), R81–5.

Hsu, H.H., Feinstone, S.M. & Hoofnagle (1995) Acute viral hepatitis. In: *Principles and Practices of Infectious Diseases*, 4th edn. (eds G.L. Mandell, J.E. Bennett & R. Dolin). Churchill Livingstone, New York. Vol. 1, Chap. 96, 1137–53.

Ikeda, K. *et al.* (1998) Disease progression and hepatocellular carcinogenesis in patients with chronic viral hepatitis: a prospective observation of 2215 patients. *J Hepatol*, **28**(6), 930–938.

Kane, M. (1995) Globule programme for control of hepatitis B infection. *Vaccine*, **13**(Suppl. 1), S47–9.

Lau, J.Y.N. & Wright, T.L. (1993) Molecular virology and pathogenesis of hepatitis B. *Lancet*, **342**, 1335–9.

McCormick, R.D. *et al.* (1981) Epidemiology of needlestick injuries in hospital personnel. *Am J Med*, **70**, 928–32.

Mangtani, P., Heptonstall, J. & Hall, A.J. (1998) Enhanced surveillance of acute symptomatic hepatitis B in England and Wales. *Commun Dis Public Health*, **1**(2), 114–20.

Marques, A.R. *et al.* (1998) Combination therapy with famciclovir and interferon-alpha for the treatment of chronic hepatitis B. *J Infect Dis*, **178**(5), 1483–7.

Medical Research Council and Public Health Laboratory Service (1980) The incidence of hepatitis B infection after accidental exposure and anti-HBs immunoglobulin prophylaxis. *Lancet*, **1**, 6–8.

O'Grady, J.G. *et al.* (1988) Early indicators of prognosis in acute liver failure and their applications of patients for orthotopic liver transplantation. *Gastroenterology*, **94**, A578.

Omata, M. (1998) Treatment of chronic hepatitis B infection. *New Engl J Med*, **339**(2), 114–15.

Papaevangelou, G. *et al.* (1984) Etiology of fulminant viral hepatitis in Greece. *Hepatology*, **4**, 369–72.

Parry, C.M. *et al.* (1997) A case of hepatitis B in a haemodialysis unit. *J Hosp Infect*, **37**(1), 65–9.

Polakoff, S. (1989) *Acute Viral Hepatitis B in Laboratory Reports 1985–1988. Communicable Disease Report 89/92 3–6*. Stationery Office, London.

Prentice, M.S. *et al.* (1992) Infection with hepatitis B virus after open heart surgery. *Br Med J*, **304**, 761–4.

Ramsay, M. *et al.* (1998) Control of hepatitis B in the United Kingdom. *Vaccine*, **16**(Suppl.), S52–5.

Reed, E. *et al.* (1993) Occupational infectious disease exposure in EMS personnel. *J Emerg Med*, **11**(1), 9–16.

Reutter, J. *et al.* (1998) Production of antibody to hepatitis A and hepatitis B surface antigen measured after combined hepatitis A/hepatitis B vaccination in 242 adult volunteers. *J Viral Hepat*, **5**(3), 205–211.

Schreiber, G.B. *et al.* (1996) The risk of transfusion transmitted viral infections. The retrovirus epidemiology donor study. *New Engl J Med*, **334**(26), 1685–90.

Shapiro, C.N. & Margolis, H.S. (1992) Impact of hepatitis B virus infection on women and children. *Infect Dis Clin North Am*, **6**(1), 75–96.

Shattock, A.C. *et al.* (1985) Increased severity and morbidity of acute hepatitis in drug abusers with simultaneously acquired hepatitis B and hepatitis D infection. *Br Med J*, **290**, 1377–80.

Singh, J. *et al.* (1998) Outbreak of viral hepatitis B in rural community in India linked to inadequately sterilized needles and syringes. *Bull World Health Organ*, **76**(1), 93–8.

Stevens, C.F. *et al.* (1975) Vertical transmission of hepatitis B antigen in Taiwan. *New Engl J Med*, **292**, 771–4.

Sundkvisst, T. *et al.* (1998) Fatal outcome of transmission of hepatitis B from an e antigen negative surgeon. *Commun Dis Public Health*, **1**(1), 48–50.

Tang, J.R. *et al.* (1998) Hepatitis B surface antigenemia at birth: a long-term follow-up study. *J Pediatr*, **133**(3), 374–7.

Tedder, R.S. (1980) Hepatitis B in hospitals. *Br J Hosp Med*, **23**(3), 266–79.

Teo, C.G. (1992) The virology and serology of hepatitis: an overview. *Commun Dis Rep*, **2**(10), R109–113.

Ter Borg, F. *et al.* (1998) Recovery from life threatening, corticosteroid-unresponsive, chemotherapy-related reactivation of hepatitis B associated with lamivudine therapy. *Dig Dis Sci*, **43**(10), 2267–70.

Tong, M.J. (1989) Hepatitis B vaccination of neonates and children. *Am J Med*, **87**(3A), 33S–5S.

Trevelyan, J. (1991) Hepatitis B – who is at risk? *Nurs Times*, **87**(5), 26–9.

Vickers, V. *et al.* (1994) Hepatitis B outbreak in a drug trials unit: investigations and recommendations. *Commun Dis Rep*, **4**(1), R1–4.

Werner, B.G. *et al.* (1982) Accidental hepatitis B surface-antigen-positive inoculations. *Ann Int Med*, **97**, 367–9.

Young, S.E.J. & Healing, T.D. (1995) The management of the deceased with known or suspected infectious disease. *Commun Dis Rep*, **5**, R69–73.

Zimmerman, R.K., Ruben, F.L. & Ahwesh, E.R. (1997) Hepatitis B virus infection, hepatitis B vaccine and hepatitis B immune globulin. *J Fam Pract*, **45**(4), 295–315.

Zuckerman, A.J. (1990) Immunization against hepatitis B. *Br Med Bull*, **46**(2), 383–98.

Zuckerman, J.N. (1998) New combined hepatitis A and B vaccine. Risks of viral hepatitis related to travel. *Br Med J*, **316**(7140), 1317.

GUIDELINES • Hepatitis B

Procedure

Action

1 The patient may be nursed on an open ward using all the patients' facilities as normal unless there is a high risk of blood contamination of the ward environment.

2 The patient must be assessed daily to establish accurately any sites of bleeding. Changes in the patient's condition should be recorded in the care plan.

3 Used sharps must be correctly disposed of in a sharps bin.

4 A yellow clinical waste bag should be kept on a regular holder with a lid for the patient's disposable waste. When full this should be securely closed, and sent for incineration.

5 The patient's personal hygiene equipment must be kept at the bedside.

6 Used linen that is not bloodstained is placed in the ward linen bags in the usual way.

Rationale

If adequate precautions can be adhered to on an open ward, there is no need to isolate the patient.

Sites of bleeding must be identified in order that the appropriate precautions can be taken.

Contaminated sharps are a potential inoculation hazard to others, so particular caution must be taken in handling them. Overloaded sharps containers may cause needles to pierce the walls of the container or even protrude through the top.

To confine potentially contaminated material, e.g. bloodstained tissues. Yellow to the internationally recognized colour for clinical waste.

To prevent accidental use of equipment by others.

Linen free from blood stains is not contaminated and may be dealt with in the normal manner.

7 During venepuncture or other procedures likely to cause bleeding, furniture, bedding and clothing in the adjacent area should be protected with polythene sheeting.

To prevent contamination of the environment with spilled blood.

8 All staff involved with the patient should cover any cuts or grazes on their hands with waterproof dressings.

Broken skin provides a portal of entry for the hepatitis virus in the event of contact with the patient's blood.

9 Routine daily cleaning procedures may be carried out as normal. As part of universal safe technique and practices, domestic staff will be aware of the potential hazard associated with any blood contamination.

Education is necessary so the domestic staff can understand the hazards involved.

Accidental inoculation or spillage of blood

Action

Rationale

1 Any accident involving skin penetration or heavy contamination of abraded skin or mucosal surfaces of staff should be recorded on an accident form and this taken to bacteriology immediately. Occupational health must be informed, who will make an assessment for the need of HBV vaccine or HBV IgG.

To protect personnel. To comply with legal and/or hospital requirements (DoH 1993).

2 Blood spillage onto unbroken skin should be washed off with soap and running water. A scrubbing brush should not be used as this could break the skin. Complete an accident form, as above and inform occupational health.

To remove the source of potential contamination. To comply with legal and/or hospital requirements.

3 Accidental inoculation sites should be cleaned under running water, encouraged to bleed freely and then cover with waterproof plaster. Complete an accident form, as above.

Bleeding helps to expel the inoculated virus from the site. To comply with legal and/or hospital requirements.

4 Blood spilled on hard surfaces must be wiped up immediately with paper towels and the area washed well with a solution such as hypochlorite.

To prevent viral spread. Dried blood remains infectious for several days.

5 Linen stained with blood should be treated as infected linen and placed in red alginate polythene bag before being placed in a red linen bag.

Bloodstained linen is highly infectious. All linen in red alginate polythene bags will be washed in a barrier wash at the laundry.

Precautions if bleeding is present

Action

Rationale

1 If bleeding is present in the mouth:
   (a) Use disposable crockery and cutlery and, with any contaminated food, dispose of as clinical waste.
   (b) Keep a personal food tray and water jug at the bedside.
   (c) Disposable mouth-care equipment, sputum pot and tissues should be kept at the bedside.

The sputum may be contaminated with blood from the mouth, therefore precautions must include avoiding contact with the patient's sputum.

2 If haematuria or melaena is present:
   (a) Wear plastic gowns and gloves when handling excreta.
   (b) Keep a toilet and handbasin for the patient's sole use, if practicable.
   (c) If a toilet is not available for the patient's sole use, bedpans or urinals must be used. These should be washed in the usual manner in the bedpan washer

Blood present in the urine or faeces makes the patient's excreta a potential source of hepatitis B contamination.

Guidelines • Hepatitis B (cont'd)

Action	Rationale
and dried carefully. They should then be placed in the appropriate bag, marked 'high risk', stapled securely and sent to the sterile supplies department for autoclaving. Disposable bedpans are dealt with in the routine manner.	
3 If the patient has a wound or a break in the skin: (a) Cover the area adequately so that there is no seepage. (b) Used dressings should be sealed securely in a plastic bag before being disposed of as clinical waste. (c) All tapes, lotions and creams are kept solely for the patient's use. (d) The dressing trolley must be cleaned carefully before re-use. (e) Non-disposable equipment should be emptied and wiped clean, placed in a central sterile supplies department bag, securely stapled shut, marked 'high risk', and sent to the sterile supplies department in a safe manner, to be resterilized.	To prevent the spread of the virus from dried or fresh blood. Dried blood can remain infectious for several days.

Other hospital departments

Action	Rationale
1 All departments and staff involved with the patient must be made aware of the diagnosis.	To allow them to make their own precautionary arrangements.
2 All request cards to be labelled appropriately.	To alert the receiving department of the diagnosis.
3 All specimens to be labelled appropriately and correctly bagged. (For further information on specimen collection see Chapter 37.)	To alert the receiving department of the diagnosis and prevent contamination of the environment.
4 If a patient who is bleeding has to be transported elsewhere, the porter involved should be provided with the following: (a) Disposable gloves and aprons. (b) Cleaning equipment for the trolley or chair before use by the next patient.	To prevent the contamination of the porter or other patients.

Discharging the patient

Action	Rationale
1 The majority of precautions can cease.	Discharge normally implies that the risk of cross-infection is no longer present.
2 The patient should be advised not to share razors, toothbrushes or similar personal property likely to be contaminated by blood.	To reduce the risk of cross-infection.
3 If bleeding occurs, the patient clears up the blood himself/herself and disposes safely of such items as contaminated tissues by burning, flushing down the toilet or sealing in a polythene bag for routine council rubbish collection. If regular persistent bloodstained waste is generated, the health authority must be requested to make special collections.	To reduce the risk of cross-infection.

4 If emergency treatment or dental care is required, the patient must inform the health care worker of the fact that he/she has a recent history of hepatitis B infection.

To allow the correct precautions to be taken.

Death of a patient with hepatitis B

Action

Rationale

1 There should be minimal handling of the body.

To reduce the risk of infecting the nursing staff.

2 Nurses should wear disposable plastic aprons and gloves when handling the body.

3 The body should be totally enclosed in a cadaver bag specifically designed for infected patients.

To reduce the risk of infecting the nursing staff.

4 The mortuary staff should be informed of the diagnosis.

To ensure that all staff are aware of the infection risk.

5 If the relatives want to view the body, they must be supervised. The cadaver bag can be opened by a nurse to allow viewing.

To prevent contamination.

Non-A non-B hepatitis

Definition

Due to major advances in knowledge concerning hepatitis, hepatitis A, B, C, D, E, F and G have been distinguished. There remains the theoretical possibility of further hepatitis types being reported. Until this time, the hepatitis virus non-A non-B (NANB) is the term given to all clinical hepatitis that does not fall into the above-mentioned categories (Editorial 1990). The etiology of non-A non-B hepatitis remains unclear (Fukai *et al.* 1998).

Reference material

There are no accepted serological tests for NANB. Diagnosis is achieved by excluding infections associated with NANB (Main *et al.* 1992). These include symptoms associated with hepatitis A, B and C, cytomegalovirus, Epstein-Barr virus, toxic and drug-induced liver injury (including alcoholic liver disease), circulatory abnormalities, shock, sepsis, biliary tract disease and metabolic liver disease (Dienstag 1983; Hsu *et al.* 1995). As new hepatitis viruses are discovered, studies involving retesting patients previously diagnosed as NANB hepatitis continue to highlight patients who fall into none of the known hepatitis categories (Wejstal *et al.* 1997). A search for yet another hepatitis virus continues (Crow & Ng 1997).

Non-A non-B hepatitis has been shown to occur in patients who have received:

1 Blood transfusions (Dienstag *et al.* 1977)
2 Clotting factors for coagulation disorders
3 Haemodialysis
4 Outbreaks of epidemics in tropical areas (Wong *et al.* 1980)
5 Sporadic cases with no identifiable cause.

Transmission appears to be similar to that of hepatitis B, i.e. principally through blood and blood products. There is an increased incidence in drug addicts due to the sharing of contaminated needles and syringes (Bamber *et al.* 1983). There is evidence, however, of sporadic cases with no obvious contributory factors (Farrow *et al.* 1981).

The incubation period is estimated at 6–8 weeks followed by clinical features similar to hepatitis B, although as a rule acute illness tends to be less severe. Rochling *et al.*'s (1997) study found that patients with NANB hepatitis have been seen to have a more acute illness than those with HCV infection. Despite its relatively mild, often asymptomatic and anicteric presentation during acute infection, approximately 20% of people infected with NANB will develop cirrhosis and may die from hepatic-related death such as hepatocellular carcinoma (Lefkowitch *et al.* 1987). Assessment of treatment protocols for chronic NANB hepatitis has been hindered by the lack of viral markers (Ellis 1990).

Recombinant interferon is showing promising results in the management of NANB hepatitis (Hoofnagle *et al.* 1986). Generally, treatment involves responding to the signs and symptoms as they occur. Liver transplantation is the treatment for patients with liver failure (Dusheiko 1990).

It is essential that safe techniques are used at all times when in contact with blood and body fluids. Human immunoglobulin should be given prophylactically following a previous history of needlestick injuries.

References and further reading

Bamber, M. *et al.* (1983) Acute type A, B and non-A non-B hepatitis in a hospital population in London: clinical and epidemiological features. *GUT*, **24**(6), 561–4.

Crow, W.C. & Ng, H.S. (1997) Hepatitis C, E and G virus – three new viruses identified by molecular biology techniques in the last decade. *Ann Acad Med Singapore*, **26**(5), 682–6.

Dienstag, J.L. (1983) Non-A non-B hepatitis recognition epidemiology and clinical features. *Gastroenterology*, **85**, 439–62.

Dienstag, J.L. *et al.* (1977) Non-A non-B post transfusion hepatitis. *Lancet*, **1**, 560–62.

Dusheiko, G.M. (1990) Hepatocellular carcinoma associated with chronic viral hepatitis. Aetiology, diagnosis and treatment. *Br Med Bull*, **46**(2), 492–511.

Editorial (1990) The A to F of viral hepatitis. *Lancet*, **336**, 1158–60.

Ellis, M.E. (1990) Non-A non-B hepatitis; quandaries in serological testing and treatment. *J Infect*, **21**, 235–40.

Farrow, L.J. *et al.* (1981) Non-A non-B hepatitis in west London. *Lancet*, **1**, 982–4.

Fukai, K., Yokosuka, O., Fujiwara, K. *et al.* (1998) Etiologic considerations of fulminant non-A/non-B viral hepatitis in Japan: analysis by nucleic acid amplification method. *J Infect Dis*, **178**(2), 325–33.

Hoofnagle, J.H. *et al.* (1986) Treatment of chronic non-A non-B hepatitis with recombinant human alpha interferon. *New Engl J Med*, **315**, 1575–8.

Hsu, H.Y. *et al.* (1995) Precore mutant of hepatitis B virus in childhood fulminant hepatitis B: an infrequent association. *J Infect Dis*, **171**(4), 776–81.

Inarson, S. *et al.* (1973) Multiple attacks of hepatitis in drug addicts. *J Infect Dis*, **12**, 165–9.

Lefkowitch, J.H. *et al.* (1987) Liver cell dysplasia and hepatocellular carcinoma in non-A non-B hepatitis. *Arch Path Lab Med*, **III**, 170–73.

Main, J. *et al.* (1992) The diagnosis and management of viral hepatitis. *Commun Dis Rep*, **2**(10), R117–20.

Rochling, F.A., Jones, W.F., Chau, K. *et al.* (1997) Acute sporadic non-A, non B, non-C, non-D, non-E hepatitis. *Hepatology*, **25**(2), 478–83.

Wejstal, R., Norkrans, G. & Widell, A. (1997) Chronic non-A, non-B, non-C: is hepatitis G/GBV-C involved? *Scand J Gastroenterol*, **32**(10), 1046–51.

Wong, O.C. *et al.* (1980) Epidemic and endemic hepatitis in India: evidence for a non-A non-B hepatitis virus aetiology. *Lancet*, **2**, 876–8.

GUIDELINES • Non-A non-B hepatitis

The procedure should be as for hepatitis B (see above).

Hepatitis C virus (HCV)

Definition

Hepatitis C is an acute infectious disease caused by hepatitis C virus (HCV), which is a single-stranded RNA virus, and a member of the Flaviviridae (Forns & Bukh 1998).

Reference material

HCV was discovered in 1989, and is a major health problem. It is estimated that the global prevalence of HCV ranges from 0.1 to 5% in different countries (Consensus Statement 1999), with about 150 million chronic HCV carriers throughout the world. The prevalence of hepatitis C in the UK is estimated to be between 0.1 and 1% of the general population (DoH 1995). Hepatitis C virus is transmitted primarily through contact with blood and blood products (Crowe 1994). One important means of transmission is misuse of intravenous drugs and sharing of needles (DoH 1995). Between 1992 and 1996, 5232 cases of HCV were reported in England and Wales, 41% of these were asymptomatic and 59% had signs and symptoms of disease, which included chronic liver disease and heptocellular carcinoma (Ramsay *et al.* 1998). In industrial countries, HCV causes 20% of cases of acute hepatitis, 70% of cases of chronic hepatitis, 40% of end stage cirrhosis, 60% of hepatocellular carcinoma and 30% of liver transplants (Consensus Statement 1999).

Clinical response

The incubation period following infection varies from 6 to 8 weeks (Teo 1992). The clinical manifestations of hepatitis C infection are non-specific and include fatigue, malaise and nausea, with only about 5% of patients developing acute jaundice (Girakar *et al.* 1993). The disease may be mild and go unnoticed by the infected person (Griffiths-Jones 1994), with patients recovering spontaneously and completely (Smith 1993). However, up to 50% of patients develop chronic active hepatitis and 20% progress to cirrhosis. Infection with hepatitis C also appears to be associated with cancer of the liver (Mims *et al.* 1993). The risk of developing hepatocellular carcinoma in chronic HCV increases with time: 4.8% at 5 years, 13.6% at 10 years and 26% at 15 years. This risk is increased in HCV compared with HBV (Ikeda *et al.* 1998). Studies to determine the prevalence of HVC in liver tissue from hepatocellular carcinoma found a high incidence of HVC: 61.5% in Japanese, 60% in Spanish and 41.5% in American patients (Abe *et al.* 1998). Alcohol misuse presents an increased risk of hepatic complications associated with HCV (Booth 1998).

Transmission

HCV can also be sexually transmitted (Buzby 1996). In homosexual men the prevalence of HCV increases with age, lifetime numbers of sexually transmitted diseases and genitourinary clinic reattenders (Gilson *et al.* 1998). Education and counselling appear to reduce the risk of sexually transmitted HCV (Weinstock *et al.* 1993; Buzby 1996). The possibility of intrafamilial transmission appears low, one study found that only 6% of cases of acute HCV transmitted to sexual or household contacts of an infected person (Alter *et al.* 1992). The risk of perinatal transmission of HCV infection appears to be low except in women with co-infection with HIV (Freitag-Koontz 1996) or in those with high HCV viral titres (Duff 1998): 0–10% of pregnancies compared to 5–36% if co-infected with HIV (Hardie & Hamilton 1999).

Transfusion services in the UK began to screen for antibodies to HCV in September 1991 (DoH 1995). The screening programme was estimated to have a considerable positive effect on the prevention of post-transfusion HCV infection (Teo 1992). It is estimated that 1 in 2000 blood donors in the UK may have been anti-HCV positive when screening was introduced (Communicable Disease Report 1995). The risk of an HCV infected donation entering the blood supply is 1 in more than 200 000 (Ramsay *et al.* 1998). The prevalence of HCV was higher in blood transfusion recipients transfused before 1995 (2.6%) compared with those transfused after 1995 (1%) (Ramsay *et al.* 1998). Recipients of blood or blood components from donors now known to be carriers of HVC are being traced with the view to providing counselling, testing and referral to a specialist, if appropriate.

Transmission of HCV following percutaneous exposure to blood has been documented (Marranconi *et al.* 1992). Follow-up care for health care workers who report accidents involving patients with HCV includes anti-HCV testing 3 and 6 months after the exposure. Routine anti-HCV testing of patients whose HCV status is not known is not recommended unless a significant percutaneous incident has occurred. The routine use of human immunoglobulin or hepatitis B immunoglobulin as prophylaxis for HCV infection is not recommended, as there is no published evidence to suggest that such prophylaxis is of value, and documented instances exist where it has failed to prevent the spread of HCV infection (Public Health Laboratory Service Hepatitis Sub-committee 1993).

Diagnosis

Diagnosis of acute hepatitis C infection is established by the presence of antibodies to hepatitis C (anti-HCV IgG) in the blood. Results are confirmed by recombinant immunoblot assay (DoH 1995).

Treatment

Cases should be referred to a specialist in liver disease for evaluation, close observation and care (Consensus Statement 1999). This may involve liver biopsy and liver function tests. Interferon-alpha is the proven treatment for HCV infection (Vakil & McCaughan 1998); less than one third of patients have a sustained response (Forns & Bukh 1998). Patients who have failed to respond or relapsed after interferon therapy alone, and in some cases interferon-naïve patients, may have an improved outcome with interferon/ribavarin combination therapy (Hardie & Hamilton 1999).

Nursing care

Since there is no vaccine for HVC it is critical for health care workers to work safely to prevent exposure to HCV (Lanphear 1997). Watson's (1997) survey of nurses' knowl-edge of HCV found that their understanding of HCV was poor and that the majority felt that they were not provided with adequate protection against HCV while at work.

Nursing care for the patient infected with hepatitis C is the same as for patients with hepatitis B (see Guidelines • Hepatitis B, above).

References and further reading

Abe, K. *et al.* (1998) In situ detection of hepatitis B, C and G virus nucleic acid in human hepatocellular carcinoma tissues from different geographic regions. *Hepatology*, **28**(2), 568–72.

Alter, M.J. *et al.* (1992) The natural history of community acquired hepatitis C in the United States. *N Engl J Med*, **325**, 1325–32.

Booth, J.C. (1998) Chronic hepatitis C: the virus, its discovery and the natural history of the disease. *J Viral Hepat*, **5**(4), 213–22.

Bresters, D. *et al.* (1993) Sexual transmission of hepatitis C. *Lancet*, **342**, 210–11.

Buzby, M. (1996) Viral hepatitis C: a sexually transmitted disease. *Nurse Pract Forum*, **7**(1), 10–15.

Consensus Statement (1999) EASL international consensus conference on hepatitis C. *J Hepatol*, **30**, 956–61.

Crowe, H.M. (1994) Forum: a perspective on hepatitis. *Asepsis*, **16**(2), 13–17.

DoH (1995) *Hepatitis C and Blood Transfusion Look Back*. PL CMO *(95)1*. Stationary Office, London.

Duff, P. (1998) Hepatitis in pregnancy. *Semin Perinatal*, **22**(4), 277–83.

Forns, X. & Bukh, J. (1998) Methods for determining the hepatitis C virus genotype. *Viral Hep Rev*, **4**(1), 1–19.

Freitag-Koontz (1996) Prevention of hepatitis B and C transmission during pregnancy and the first year of life. *J Perinat Neonatal Nurs*, **10**(2), 40–55.

Gilson, R.J. *et al.* (1998) Hepatitis B virus infection in patients attending a genitourinary medicine clinic; risk factors and vaccine coverage. *Sex Trans Infect*, **74**(2), 110–15.

Girakar, A. *et al.* (1993) Hepatitis C virus: when to suspect, how to detect. *J Crit Illness*, **8**, 1287–95.

Goldberg, D., Cameron, S. & McMenamin, J. (1998) Hepatitis C virus antibody prevalence among drug injecting users in Glasgow has fallen but remains high. *Commun Dis Public Health*, **1**(2), 95–7.

Griffiths-Jones, A. (1994) Hepatitis revisited. *Nurs Times*, **90**(46), 54–62.

Hardie, R. & Hamilton, G. (1999) *Hepatitis C. Information pack*. Public Health Laboratory Service Communicable Disease Surveillance Centre, London.

Ikeda, K. *et al.* (1998) Disease progression and hepatocellular carcinogenesis in patients with chronic viral hepatitis: a prospective observation of 2215 patients. *J Hepatol*, **28**(6), 930–38.

Kamitsukasa, H. *et al.* (1989) Interfamilial transmission of hepatitis C virus. *Lancet*, **1**, 987.

Lanphear, B.P. (1997) Transmission and control of blood borne viral hepatitis in health care workers. *Occup Med*, **12**(4), 717–30.

Marranconi, F. *et al.* (1992) HCV infection after accidental needlestick injury in health care workers. *Infections*, **20**, 111.

Mims, C.A. *et al.* (1993) *Medical Microbiology*, Mosby, London.

Neal, K.R., Dornan, J. & Irving, W.L. (1997) Prevalence of hepatitis C antibodies among health care workers in two teaching hospitals. Who is at risk? *Br Med J*, **314**, 179–80.

Public Health Laboratory Service Communicable Disease Surveillance Centre (1995) Hepatitis C and blood transfusion. *Commun Dis Rep*, **5**(3), 1.

Public Health Laboratory Service Hepatitis Sub-committee (1993) Hepatitis C virus: guidance on the risks and current management of occupational exposure. *Commun Dis Rep Rev*, 3(10), R135–9.

Ramsay M.E. *et al.* (1998) Laboratory surveillance and hepatitis C virus infection in England and Wales. *Commun Dis Public Health*, 1(2), 89–94.

Smith, J.P. (1993) Hepatitis C: a major public health problem. *J Adv Nurs*, 18(3), 503–506.

Teo, C.G. (1992) The virology and serology of hepatitis: an overview. *Commun Dis Rep*, 2(10), R109–114.

Vakil, D. & McCaughan, G. (1998) Update on the management of hepatitis C. *Aust Fam Physician*, 27(9), 780–86.

Watson, C. (1997) Hepatitis C: it's in the blood. *Nurs Times*, 93(19), 68–9.

Weinstock, H.S. *et al.* (1993) Hepatitis C virus infection among patients attending a clinic for sexually transmitted diseases. *JAMA*, 269(3), 392–4.

Hepatitis D

Definition

Hepatitis D virus (HDV), also referred to as delta virus, is a very small RNA virus (Mims *et al.* 1993). HDV is always associated with hepatitis B virus (HBV) and causes both fulminant hepatitis and the accelerated progression of pre-existing HBV hepatitis (Monjardino *et al.* 1990). HDV can only multiply in a cell which is infected with hepatitis B as it is dependent on HBV for its surface antigens (Barbara & Contreras 1990).

Reference material

Hepatitis D is uncommon in the UK and USA, but common in parts of South America and Africa. Worldwide it is present in about 5% of HBV carriers (Mims *et al.* 1993). HDV is transmitted in the same way as HBV (Crowe 1994). Huang *et al.* (1998) evaluated the correlation of HDV antibody levels, in particular IgM with HDV viraemia, and found that an anti-HDV titre of 100 or over could be considered to be a marker for acute HDV. Chronic HDV is defined as HDV viraemia for more than 6 months (Huang *et al.* 1998).

HDV has a relatively short incubation period of 3–6 weeks (Teo 1992). Infection with HBV and HDV results in a more severe and symptomatic illness than infection with HBV alone (Crowe 1994).

Diagnosis

Diagnosis relies on the detection of HDV antibody in serum (Center for Disease Control 1990).

Prevention

Prevention is based on vaccination (Mims *et al.* 1993) as HBV vaccine is also effective against HDV (Duff 1998).

Treatment

It has been suggested that high dose interferon-alpha may be beneficial in chronic HDV infection, although relapses can occur (Farci *et al.* 1994). Children with HBV and associated HDV progress to liver cirrhosis within 15 to 20 years. While interferon-alpha reduces viral replication and activity of HBV it has no effect on the concurrent HDV infection (Scneider *et al.* 1998). Liver transplantation for delta cirrhosis has proved to be a successful treatment for HDV cirrhosis, with few reinfections of the grafted liver (Hadziyannis 1997).

Presenting symptoms and nursing care are the same as for hepatitis B (see hepatitis B, above).

References

Barbara, J.A.J. & Contreras, M. (1990) Infectious complications of blood transfusions. *Br Med J*, 300, 450–53.

Center for Disease Control (1990) Protection against viral hepatitis. *Morb Mort Week Rep*, 39(RR2), 1–26.

Crowe, H.M. (1994) Forum: perspective on hepatitis. *Asepsis*, 16(2), 13–17.

Duff, P. (1998) Hepatitis in pregnancy. *Semin Perinatal*, 22(4), 277–83.

Farci, P. *et al.* (1994) Treatment for chronic hepatitis D with interferon alpha-2a. *New Engl J Med*, 330, 88–94.

Hadziyannis, S.J. (1997) Review: hepatitis delta. *J Gastroenterol Hepatol*, 12(4), 289–98.

Huang, Z.S. & Wu, H.N. (1998) Identification and characterization of the RNA chaperone activity of hepatitis delta antigen peptides. *J Biol Chem*, 273(41), 26455–61.

Mims, C.A. *et al.* (1993) *Medical Microbiology*. Mosby, London.

Monjardino, J.P. *et al.* (1990) Delta hepatitis. The disease and the virus. *Br Med Bull*, 46(2), 399–407.

Schneider, A. *et al.* (1998) Alpha-interferon treatment in HbeAg positive children with chronic hepatitis B and associated hepatitis D. *Klin Padiatr*, 210(5), 363–5.

Teo, C.G. (1992) The virology and serology of hepatitis: an overview. *Commun Dis Rep*, 2(10), R109–14.

Hepatitis E

Definition

Hepatitis E is caused by an acute icteric virus leading to self-limiting disease. HEV is a member of the Calicivirus family (Balayan 1997).

Reference material

HEV is a faeco-orally transmitted hepatitis virus which has many features similar to HAV (Skidmore 1997). Major outbreaks have occurred due to consumption of contaminated food and water (Clayson *et al.* 1998), although person to person transmission is rarely seen (Rab *et al.*

1997). Travelling to endemic areas carries a risk of HEV infection (Wu *et al.* 1998). HEV is widely spread in many tropical and subtropical countries (Balayan 1997), and is also found in sewage in Spain. This has implications for contamination of the environment and shellfish (Pina *et al.* 1998). Cases of HEV have been seen in England, but have been associated with patients returning from the Indian subcontinent (Hussaini *et al.* 1997).

Experimental data suggest HEV may be a zoonosis as HEV is pathogenic for some domestic and wild animals (Balayan 1997). Pigs in the USA have been found to be infected with swine HEV which is closely related to human HEV; there is experimental evidence that cross-species infection with swine HEV can occur (Meng *et al.* 1998). Parenteral (Duff 1998), intrauterine and perinatal routes of spread, while uncommon, have been implicated in the spread of HEV (Irshad 1997).

The incubation period ranges between 2 and 9 weeks, with an average of 6 weeks (Teo 1992). The virus is eliminated from the body on recovery, which prevents carriage of the virus (Mims *et al.* 1993). HEV has been associated with other hepatotropic viruses and can induce fulminant hepatitis with or without the simultaneous presence of other viruses (Irshad 1997). In areas with endemic HEV acute liver failure is found secondary to HEV infection (Hussaini *et al.* 1997). HEV is common in pregnancy and associated with a mortality rate of up to 20% (Hussaini *et al.* 1997).

Chauhan *et al.* (1998) investigated the effectiveness of HEV antibodies in humans and found they offered little protection from further infection. In India preparations of immune serum globulin were evaluated in pregnant women; some patients went on to develop HEV (Arankalle *et al.* 1998).

Diagnosis

Diagnosis is made by detecting HEV antibody in serum (Tilton 1994). Serologic tests for HEV vary in different laboratories (Ghabrah *et al.* 1998).

Vaccination

There is no vaccine for HEV prevention (Moyer & Mast 1998).

Nursing care

Barrier nursing is necessary for patients with hepatitis E infection.

References and further reading

Arankalle, V.A. *et al.* (1998) Role of immune serum globulin in pregnant women during an epidemic of hepatitis E. *J Viral Hepat*, **5**(3), 199–204.

Balayan, M.S. (1997) Epidemiology of hepatitis E virus infection. *J Viral Hepat*, **4**(3), 155–65.

Chauhan, A. *et al.* (1998) Role of long-persisting human hepatitis E virus antibodies in protection. *Vaccine*, **16**(7), 755–6.

Clayson, E.T. *et al.* (1998) Association of hepatitis E virus with an outbreak of hepatitis at a military training camp in Nepal. *J Med Virol*, **54**(3), 178–82.

Duff, P. (1998) Hepatitis in pregnancy. *Semin Perinatal*, **22**(4), 277–83.

Ghabrah, T.M. *et al.* (1998) Comparison tests for antibody to hepatitis E virus. *J Med Virol*, **55**(2), 134–7.

Hussaini, S.H. *et al.* (1997) Severe hepatitis E infection during pregnancy. *J Viral Hepat*, **4**(1), 51–4.

Irshad, M. (1997) Hepatitis E virus: a global view of its seroepidemiology and transmission pattern. *Trop Gastroenterol*, **18**(2), 45–9.

Meng, X.J. *et al.* (1998) Genetic and experimental evidence for cross-species infection by swine hepatitis E virus. *J Virol*, **72**(12), 9714–21.

Mims, C.A. *et al.* (1993) *Medical Microbiology*. Mosby, London.

Moyer, L.A. & Mast, E.E. (1998) Hepatitis A through E. *J Intraven Nurs*, **21**(5), 286–90.

Pina, S. *et al.* (1998) Characterization of a strain of infectious hepatitis E virus isolated from sewage in an area where hepatitis E is not endemic. *Appl Environ Microbiol*, **64**(11), 4485–8.

Rab, M.A. *et al.* (1997) Water-borne hepatitis E virus epidemic in Islamabad, Pakistan: a common source outbreak traced to the malfunction of a modern water treatment plant. *Am J Trop Med Hyg*, **57**(2), 151–7.

Skidmore, S.J. (1997) Tropical aspects of viral hepatitis: hepatitis E. *Trans R Soc Trop Med Hyg*, **91**(2), 125–6.

Teo, C.G. (1992) The virology and serology of hepatitis: an overview. *Commun Dis Rep*, **2**(10), R109–14.

Tilton, R.C. (1994) Forum: a perspective on hepatitis. *Asepsis*, **16**(2), 18–22.

Wu, J.C. *et al.* (1998) The impact of traveling to endemic areas on the spread of hepatitis E virus infection: epidemiological and molecular analyses. *Hepatology*, **27**(5), 1415–20.

Hepatitis B genotype F

Definition

Hepatitis B genotype F is the name given to a recently discovered virus causing hepatitis (Uchida *et al.* 1994a). This virus is commonly referred to as hepatitis B virus genotype F (Norder *et al.* 1994), as immunodiffusion experiments show that this virus is a serotype of the hepatitis B virus (Magnius & Norder 1995).

Reference material

HBV genotype F is regarded as indigenous to the American Indian population of the New World (Arauz-Ruiz *et al.* 1997). It appears to cause acute and chronic liver disease (Uchida *et al.* 1994b) and is associated with serious disease, with outbreaks of hepatitis B genotype F causing significant morbidity and mortality (Casey *et al.* 1996). Much remains to be learned about this virus. Nursing care is as for hepatitis B.

References

Arauz-Ruiz, P. et al. (1997) Genotype F prevails in HBV infected patients of hispanic origin in Central America and may carry the precore stop mutant. *J Med Virol*, **51**(4), 305–312.

Casey, J.L. et al. (1996) Hepatitis B virus (HBV)/hepatitis D virus coinfection in outbreaks of acute hepatitis in the Peruvian Amazon basin: the role of HDV genotype III and HBV genotype F. *J Infect Dis*, **174**(5), 920–6.

Casey, J.L. et al. (1997) Genotype F prevails in HBV infected patients of hispanic origin of Central America and may carry the precore stop mutant. *J Med Virol*, **51**(4), 305–12.

Magnius, L.O. & Norder, H. (1995) Subtype, genotypes and molecular epidemiology of the hepatitis B virus reflected by sequence variability of the S-gene. *Intervirology*, **38**(1–2), 24–34.

Norder, H. et al. (1994) Complete genomes, phylogenetic relateness, and structural proteins of six strains of the hepatitis B virus, four of which represent two new genotypes. *Virology*, **198**(2), 489–503.

Uchida, T. et al. (1994a) Silent hepatitis B virus mutants are responsible for non-A, non-B, non-C, non-D, non-E hepatitis. *Microbiol Immunol*, **38**(4), 281–5.

Uchida, T. et al. (1994b) Pathology of livers infected with silent hepatitis B virus mutant. *Liver*, **14**(5), 251–6.

Hepatitis G

Definition

Hepatitis G (HGV) is a recently identified member of the Flaviviridae family (Guilera et al. 1998), and is a positive, single stranded RNA virus, distantly related to HCV (Miyakawa & Mayumi 1997). HGV causes acute and chronic liver disease (De Medina et al. 1998) and fulminant hepatitis (Sheng et al. 1998).

Reference material

HGV was first described in Egypt and Indonesia, but has also been found in the Americas, Europe and Australia (Corwin et al. 1997). HGV route of transmission is similar to hepatitis B and C, and HIV (Bonacini et al. 1998). Patients infected with HGV have been found to be concurrently infected with hepatitis B, C and/or D (Wu et al. 1998). Frider et al.'s (1998) study highlighted that the route of community acquired HGV infection is not fully understood. Transmission has occurred via inoculation. In one study of Spainish patients, half used illicit intravenous drugs (Saiz et al. 1997). In addition, Muller et al. (1997) found that HGV was associated with blood transfusions. HGV has also been seen to be transmitted by sexual contact after two patients developed HGV after sexual contact with a prostitute (Tanaka et al. 1998). These reports are supported by a study which found 32.6% of transfused patients and 5% of blood donors in Thailand were HGV positive (Poovorawan et al. 1998). Mother to child transmission is frequent and occurs antenatally; infection persists for long lengths of time without evident disease (Je Martino et al. 1998). HGV RNA levels are suppressed but not eradicated by interferon-alpha and are unaffected by ribavirin treatment. Spontaneous loss of HGV RNA occurs over time in a proportion of patients (Marrone et al. 1997). Much remains to be learned about HGV. Nursing care is as for hepatitis B.

References and furthur reading

Bonacini, M. et al. (1998) Prevalence of hepatitis G virus RNA in the sera of patients with HIV infection. *J Acquir Immune Defic Syndr Hum Retrovirol*, **19**(1), 40–43.

Corwin, A.L. et al. (1997) Short report: evidence of worldwide transmission of hepatitis G virus. *Am J Trop Med Hyg*, **57**(4), 455–6.

De Medina, M. et al. (1998) Prevalence of hepatitis C and G virus infection in chronic hemodialysis patients. *Am J Kidney Dis*, **31**(2), 224–6.

Diamantis, I.D. et al. (1997) Influence of hepatitis G virus infection on liver disease. *Eur J Clin Microbiol Infect Dis*, **16**(12), 916–19.

Frider, B. et al. (1998) Detection of hepatitis G virus RNA in patients with acute non-A–E hepatitis. *J Viral Hepat*, **5**(3), 161–4.

Guilera, M., Saiz, J.C., Lopez-Labrador, F.X. et al. (1998) Hepatitis G virus infection in chronic liver disease. *Gut*, **42**(1), 107–111.

Je Martino, M. et al. (1998) Hepatitis G virus infection in HIV type-1 infected mothers and children. *J Infect Dis*, **178**(3), 862–5.

Marrone, A. et al. (1997) Prevalence of hepatitis G virus in patients with hepatocellular carcinoma. *J Viral Hepat*, **4**(6), 411–14.

Miyakawa, Y. & Mayumi, M. (1997) Hepatitis G virus. A true hepatitis virus or an accidental tourist? *New Engl J Med*, **336**(11), 795–6.

Muller, C. et al. (1997) Prevalence of hepatitis G virus in patients with hepatocellular carcinoma. *J Viral Hepat*, **4**(6), 411–14.

Poovorawan, Y. et al. (1998) High prevalence of hepatitis G virus infection in multiply transfused children with thalassaemia. *J Gastroenterol Hepatol*, **13**(3), 253–6.

Saiz, J.C. et al. (1997) Hepatitis G virus infection in fulminant hepatic failure. *Gut*, **41**(5), 696–9.

Sheng, L. et al. (1998) Hepatitis G virus infection in acute fulminant hepatitis: prevalence of HGV infection and sequence analysis of a specific viral strain. *J Viral Hepat*, **5**(5), 301–306.

Tanaka, E. et al. (1998) Two patients with acute hepatitis B with suspected sexual transmission of hepatitis G virus. *J Gastroenterol*, **33**(3), 419–23.

Wu, J.C. et al. (1998) Prevalence, implication, and viral nucleotide sequence analysis of GB virus-c/hepatitis G virus infection in acute fulminant and nonfulminant hepatitis. *J Med Virol*, **56**(2), 118–22.

The herpes viruses

There are four human herpes viruses which cause infection. These are detected more frequently in immunocompromised people than in immunologically intact individuals (Kedzierski 1991). The four types are:

1 Cytomegalovirus (CMV)
2 Epstein–Barr virus (EBV)
3 Herpes simplex virus (HSV)
4 Varicella zoster virus (VZV)

Cytomegalovirus (CMV)

Definition

Cytomegalovirus (CMV) is a member of the herpes virus family.

Reference material

Primary CMV infection in a immunocompetent person causes a transient infectious mononucleosis-like illness, often in childhood (Horowitz *et al.* 1986), but it can occur throughout life in an non-immune person. Following primary infection CMV persists in a latent state in leukocytes where they can reactivate later in life, particularly when a person is immunosuppressed. Secondary CMV infection occurs when a previously immune person is infected with a new strain of CMV or through reactivation with the person's latent endogenous strain of CMV (Prentice *et al.* 1998). Clinical disease can occur from both primary and secondary infection, although primary infection appears to cause more severe infection (Ho 1995). In the immunosuppressed, e.g. immature neonate, patients who are receiving a transplant and in HIV positive patients primary CMV causes significant infection (Ho 1995).

CMV is distributed widely throughout the world. There are many strains of CMV, with identical strains found in individuals connected with one another. Babies born with congenital CMV infection, for example, have the same strain as their mother (Griffiths 1991).

CMV infection can be acquired by intrauterine, perinatal (Stagno *et al.* 1986), intrafamilial and sexual transmission (Handfield *et al.* 1985) as well as following blood transfusion (Hersman *et al.* 1982) or transplantation (Peterson *et al.* 1980). Approximately 50% of the population in the UK carry the antibody to CMV. Consequently, many people are capable of transmitting the infection through blood donation. Those most recently infected appear to be more likely to do so (Barbara 1990).

During primary infection, the virus can be isolated from saliva, tears, urine, breast milk, blood, semen and cervical secretions (Pomeroy *et al.* 1987). After initial infection the virus establishes a latent infection thought to be in the lymphocytes. The latent infection may subsequently reactivate with production of infectious virions. Reactivation is generally controlled by the host's cell mediated immune response. Hence CMV infection is common in immunocompromised people (Meyers *et al.* 1986), particularly patients with AIDS (Weller 1993). Approximately 1% of all babies have congenital CMV infection, and 90–95% of these infants are asymptomatic. Some infants with asymptomatic symptoms at birth may have sensorineural hearing loss (Stagno *et al.* 1977) and others may have mild learning disabilities (Hanshaw *et al.* 1976). Clinical manifestation of congenital infection includes jaundice, hepatosplenomegaly, rash, multiple organ involvement including the central nervous system. CMV-associated morbidity has been seen in both full-term (Kumar *et al.* 1984) and pre-term infants (Yeager *et al.* 1983). Postnatally acquired CMV infection is less acute and multiple organ infection is rare.

Patients with malignancies, or those receiving chemotherapeutic therapies, transplantation of kidney (Chou 1986), heart (Hofflin *et al.* 1987) or bone marrow (Meyers 1988), have a high risk of contracting CMV disease.

Infection in healthy adults is mild and the prognosis is good. However, infection in the immunosuppresed can be severe and be a major cause of mortality and morbidity, with interstitial pneumonitis, hepatitis, Guillain-Barre syndrome, meningoencephalitis, myocarditis, colitis, thrombocytopenia and haemolytic anemia, plus retinitis in patients with AIDS (Ho 1995).

Patients with acute leukemia treated with high dose chemotherapy and bone marrow transplantation are at high risk of CMV infection (Reusser 1998). The incidence of CMV infection among allogeneic bone marrow transplants was significant higher in patients who received HLA matched unrelated donations compared to those from human histocompatibility complex (HLA) matched sibling donors (Takenaka *et al.* 1997). A significant increase in the incidence of graft versus host disease has been noted in the CMV positive group compared to the CMV negative group (Matthes-Martin *et al.* 1998). The use of CMV-free blood is recommended for CMV seronegative patients with newly diagnosed malignant disease, for whom a bone marrow transplant is a future treatment option (Preiksaitis *et al.* 1997). CMV infection should be suspected if CMV seropositive patients with leukaemia have unexplained fever, drop in blood count, lung infiltrates or gastrointestinal symptoms (Singhal *et al.* 1997). Treatment should be commenced early and the disease monitored.

HIV positive patients with CMV infection have an increased risk of death independently of CD4 cell counts (Chaisson *et al.* 1998). The use of HIV protease inhibitors in combination antiretroviral therapy has been associated with a marked increase in the survival of patients with CMV retinitis, with median survival increasing from 256 days before 1995 to 720 days in 1996 (Walsh *et al.* 1998).

Diagnosis

The diagnosis of CMV requires laboratory confirmation and cannot be made on clinical evidence alone. Laboratory tests include demonstration of the virus or serological antibody screening. CMV is readily found in urine, mouth swabs and buffy coat of blood (Ho 1995), bronchoalveolar lavage fluid, biopsy and autopsy specimens (Prentice *et al.* 1998).

Treatment

Antiviral treatment with ganciclovir and foscarnet have been seen to reduce mortality from CMV infection (Anders *et al.* 1998). Newer antiviral drugs continue to be evaluated and may be active against certain strains of virus resistant CMV (Kendle & Fan-Havard 1998; Reusser 1998). Continuing CMV viraemia after 7 to 10 ganciclovir treatments suggests drug resistance; foscarnet is the drug of second choice. The IV antibiotics have been safely administered in the community, which has significantly reduced length of hospital stay as well as improving patient satisfaction (Kayley *et al.* 1996).

Prevention

Prevention relies on decreasing the risk of virus acquisition and reactivation. Therefore, blood products used should either derive from CMV seronegative donors or be free from viable leucocytes, which can be achieved by irradiating or washing the blood product (Pamphilon *et al.* 1999).

Transmission of CMV within the hospital setting from seropositive patients to seronegative patients (Spector 1983) and staff (Lipscomb *et al.* 1984) has been seen but is thought to be low (Adler 1986; Adler *et al.* 1986). Routine blood and body fluid precautions are essential to maintain these numbers at their low level.

Patients with CMV infection generally do not require barrier nursing as they feel ill and do not mix closely with other patients. Therefore, patient to patient transmission is unlikely.

References and further reading

Adler, S.P. (1986) Nosocomial transmission of cytomegalovirus. *Pediat Infectious Disease*, **5**(2), 239–46.

Adler, S.P. *et al.* (1986) Molecular epidemiology of cytomegalovirus in a nursery: lack of evidence for nosocomial transmission. *J Pediat*, **108**, 117–23.

Anders, H.J. *et al.* (1998) Ganciclovir and foscarnet efficacy in AIDS related CMV polyradiculopathy. *J Infect*, **36**(1), 29–33.

Barbara, J. (1990) Microbiology in the national blood transfusion service. *Public Health Lab Serv Microbiol Dig*, **7**(1), 4–7.

Chaisson, R.E. *et al.* (1998) Impact of opportunistic disease on survival in patients with HIV infection. *AIDS*, **12**(1), 29–33.

Chou, S. (1986) Acquisition of donor strains of cytomegalovirus by renal transplant recipients. *New Engl J Med*, **314**, 1418–23.

Griffiths, P.D. (1991) Advances in the prevention and treatment of cytomegalovirus infection in hospital patients. *J Hosp Infect*, **18**(Suppl. A), 330–34.

Handfield, H.N. *et al.* (1985) Cytomegalovirus infection in sex partners – evidence for sexual transmission. *J Infect Dis*, **151**, 344–8.

Hanshaw, J.B. *et al.* (1976) School failure and deafness after silent congenital cytomegalovirus infection. *New Engl J Med*, **295**, 468–70.

Hersman, J. *et al.* (1982) The effect of granulocyte transfusion on the incidence of CMV infection after allogenic marrow transplantation. *Ann Int Med*, **96**, 149–52.

Ho, M. (1995) Cytomegalovirus. In: *Principles and Practice of Infectious Disease*, 4th edn. (eds G.L. Mandell, J.E. Bennett & R. Dolin). Churchill Livingstone, New York. Vol. 2, Chap. 117, pp. 1351–64.

Hofflin, J.M. *et al.* (1987) Infectious complications in heart transplant recipients receiving cyclosporine and corticosteroids. *Ann Int Med*, **106**, 209–16.

Horowitz, C.A. *et al.* (1986) Clinical and laboratory evaluation of cytomegalovirus in previously healthy individuals. *Medicine*, **65**, 124–33.

Kayley, J. *et al.* (1996) Safe intravenous antibiotic therapy at home: experience of a UK based programme. *J Antimicrob Chemother* **37**(5), 1023–9.

Kedzierski, M. (1991) Diseases of the herpes viruses. *Nurs Stand*, **5**(31), 28–32.

Kendle, J.B. & Fan-Havard, P. (1998) Cidofovir in the treatment of CMV. *Ann Pharmacother*, **32**(11), 1181–92.

Kumar, M.L. *et al.* (1984) Postnatally acquired cytomegalovirus infection in infants of CMV-excreting mothers. *J Paediat*, **104**, 669.

Lipscomb, J.A. *et al.* (1984) Prevalence of cytomegalovirus antibody in nursing personnel. *Infect Control*, **5**(11), 513–18.

Matthes-Martin, S. *et al.* (1998) CMV-viraemia during allogenic bone marrow transplantation in paediatric patients: association with survival and graft-versus-host disease. *Bone Marrow Transplant*, **21**(Suppl. 2), S53–6.

Meyers, J.D. (1988) Management of cytomegalovirus infection. *Am J Med*, **85**(2A), 102–106.

Meyers, J.D. *et al.* (1986) Risk factors for cytomegalovirus infection after human marrow transplantation. *J Infect Dis*, **153**, 478–88.

Pamphilon, D.H. *et al.* (1999) Prevention of tranfusion – transmuted cytomegalovirus infection. *Transfus Med*, **9**(2), 115–23.

Peterson, P.K. *et al.* (1980) Cytomegalovirus disease in renal allograft recipients: a prospective study of the clinical features, risk factors and impact on renal transplantation medicine. *Medicine*, **59**, 283–300.

Pillay, D. (1998) Emergence and control of resistance to antiviral drugs in resistant herpes viruses, hepatitis B virus and HIV. *Commun Dis Public Health*, **1**(1), 5–13.

Pomeroy, C. *et al.* (1987) Cytomegalovirus epidemiology and infection control. *Am J Infect Control*, **15**, 107–19.

Preiksaitis, J.K. *et al.* (1997) Transfusion and community acquired CMV infection in children with malignant disease: a prospective study. *Transfusion*, **37**(9), 941–6.

Prentice, G., Grundy, J.E. & Kho, P. (1998) Cytomegalovirus. In: *The Clinical Practice of Stem Cell Transplantation* (eds J. Barrett & J. Treleaven). ISIS Medical Media, Oxford, **2**(44), 698–707.

Reusser, P. (1998) Current concepts and challenges in the prevention and treatment of viral infections in the immunocompromised cancer patients. *Support Care Cancer*, **6**(1), 39–45.

Singhal, S. *et al.* (1997) Cytomegaloviremia after autografting for leukemia: clinical significance and lack of effect on engraftment. *Leukemia*, **11**(6), 835–8.

Spector, S.A. (1983) Transmission of cytomegalovirus among infants in hospital documented by restriction-endonuclease-digestion analyses. *Lancet*, **2**, 378–81.

Stagno, S. *et al.* (1977) Auditory and visual defects resulting from symptomatic and subclinical congenital cytomegalovirus and toxoplasma infections. *Paediatrics*, **59**, 669–78.

Stagno, S. *et al.* (1986) Primary cytomegalovirus infection in pregnancy. *J Am Med Assoc*, **256**, 1904–1908.

Takenaka, K. *et al.* (1997) Increased incidence of CMV infection and CMV associated disease after allogeneic bone marrow transplantation from unrelated donors. The Fukuoko bone marrow transplantation group. *Bone Marrow Transplant*, **19**(3), 241–8.

Walsh, J.C. *et al.* (1998) Increasing survival in AIDS patients with CMV retinitis treated with combination antiretroviral therapy including HIV protease inhibitors. *AIDS*, **12**(6), 613–18.

Weller, B. (1993) AIDS focus. HIV roundup. *Nurs Stand*, **7**(39), 54.

Weller, I.V.D. (1993) Treatment and infections and antiviral agents. In: *ABC of AIDS* (ed. M.W. Adler), 3rd edn. British Medical Journal Publishing Group, London.

Yeager, A.S. *et al.* (1983) Sequelae of maternally derived cytomegalovirus infection in premature infants. *J Paediat*, **102**, 918.

Epstein–Barr virus

Definition

Epstein–Barr virus (EBV) is a herpes virus which causes infectious mononucleosis. EBV is generally a self-limiting infection characterized by fever, malaise, headache, anorexia, pharyngitis and adenopathy, which resolves spontaneously in 2 to 3 weeks (Peter & Ray 1998).

Reference material

EBV primary infection in childhood is usually asymptomatic, although occasional cases have been seen to resemble chronic active hepatitis (Lloyd-Still *et al.* 1986). In adolescence, approximately 50% of cases are accompanied by fever, malaise, pharyngitis and lymphadenopathy (Hoagland 1960), while in adults over age 40, fever, jaundice and hepatomegaly can commonly occur (Axelrod & Finestone 1990).

EBV can persist in the host and reactivate at a later time, particularly during immunosuppression (Crawford *et al.* 1981), commonly following transplantation (Strauch *et al.* 1974) or in people with cancer or leukaemia (Lange *et al.* 1978). Immunosuppression decreases EBV specific immune function, which results in increased EBV load in peripheral blood and in the oropharynx (Haque *et al.* 1997). Initially, EBV replication appears to take place in epithelial cells of the nasopharynx (Sixbey *et al.* 1984) followed by infection of B lymphocytes. The incubation period between exposure and clinical manifestation in normal people varies from 30 to 50 days.

EBV is found in the saliva (Sixbey *et al.* 1984) and on the cervix (Sixbey *et al.* 1986), and can be transmitted by kissing and sexual contact, and rarely by blood transfusion (McMonigal *et al.* 1983). Diagnosis relies on serological methods that detect the presence of IgG and IgM antibodies to EBV viral capsid antigen (Wielaard *et al.* 1988).

EBV infection in healthy people is generally self-limiting with spontaneous recovery. Management consists of basic supportive care (Peter & Ray 1998) as the use of antiviral agents and corticosteroids in the treatment of EBV remains limited (Scooley 1995). Barrier nursing is not necessary for EBV infection, but the patient should avoid kissing and sexual contact while symptoms persist. The patient's personal hygiene articles must not be shared.

References and further reading

Axelrod, P. & Finestone, A.J. (1990) Infectious mononucleosis in older adults. *Am Fam Physician*, **42**(6), 1599–1606.

Crawford, D.H. *et al.* (1981) Long-term T cell-mediated immunity to Epstein-Barr virus in renal allograft recipients receiving cyclosporin A. *Lancet*, **1**, 10–13.

Haque, T. *et al.* (1997) A prospective study in heart and lung transplant recipients correlating persistent Epstein-Barr virus infection with clinical events. *Transplantation*, **64**(7), 1028–34.

Hirsch, M.S. (1988) Herpes group virus infections in the compromised host. In: *Clinical Approach to Infection in the Compromised Host* (eds R.H. Rubin & L.S. Young), pp. 347–66. Plenum Medical, New York and London.

Hoagland, R.J. (1960) The clinical manifestation of infectious mononucleosis. A report of 200 cases. *Am J Med Sci*, **240**, 55–63.

Lange, B. *et al.* (1978) Longitudinal study of Epstein-Barr virus antibody titre and excretion in paediatric patients with Hodgkin's disease. *Int J Cancer*, **22**, 521–7.

Lloyd-Still, J.D. *et al.* (1986) The spectrum of Epstein-Barr virus hepatitis in children. *Paediat Pathol*, **5**, 337–51.

McMonigal, K. *et al.* (1983) Post-perfusion syndrome due to Epstein-Barr virus. Report of two cases and review of the literature. *Transfusion*, **23**, 331–5.

Peter, J. & Ray, C.G. (1998) Infectious mononucleosis. *Pediatr Rev*, **19**(8), 276–9.

Scooley, R.T. (1995) Epstein-Barr virus (infectious mononucleosis). In: *Principles and Practice of Infectious Disease* (eds G.L. Mandell, J.E. Bennett & R. Dolin). Churchill Livingstone, New York. Vol. 2, Chap. 118, pp. 1364–77.

Sixbey, J.W. *et al.* (1984) Epstein-Barr virus replication in oropharyngeal epithelial cells. *New Engl J Med*, **310**, 1225–30.

Sixbey, J.W. *et al.* (1986) A second site for Epstein-Barr virus shedding the uterine cervix. *Lancet*, **2**, 1122–4.

Strauch, J.W. *et al.* (1974) Oropharyngeal excretion of Epstein-Barr virus by renal transplant recipient and other patients treated with immunosuppressive drugs. *Lancet*, **1**, 234–7.

Wielaard, F. *et al.* (1988) Development of an antibody-capture IgM enzyme-linked immunosorbent assay for diagnosis of acute Epstein-Barr virus infection. *J Virol Meth*, **21**, 105–15.

Herpes simplex virus (HSV)

Definition

Herpes simplex virus (HSV) is a herpes virus which causes a range of infections, from painful vesicular lesions (cold sores) to life-threatening illness in the immunocompromised patient (Goodall 1992). It has an affinity for the skin and nervous system.

Reference material

HSV has two presentations:

1 HSV 1 infections (oral herpes or cold sores) tend to occur on the face or lips. However, primary infection can occur in the conjunctiva, where it causes conjunctivitis and keratitis; in the fingers, where it causes herpetic whitlow; and in the mouth where it causes herpes gingivomatitis (Arvin & Prober 1991). The HSV 1 incubation period is 2–12 days.
2 HSV 2 infections (herpes genitalis or genital herpes) are usually limited to the genital region (Corey et al. 1983a). However, both types of herpes can be contracted either genitally or orally. The HSV 2 incubation period is 2–7 days.

Herpes simplex infections are worldwide in distribution. HSV 1 usually infects children between the ages of 2 and 10 years. Latent infection is then lifelong (Kedzierski 1991). Transmission is primarily by contact with oral secretions. HSV 1 is chiefly responsible for perioral, ocular and encephalitic infections in adults. HSV 2 is spread by genital contact. Statistical information about HSV 2, and a number of other sexually transmitted diseases, is passed to the Department of Health by clinics specializing in these diseases (Barlow & Sherrard 1992). HSV 2 is the major cause of penile vesicular lesions, cervicovaginitis and proctitis, as well as neonatal disseminated disease (Hirsch 1988).

Recurrent infection occurs frequently, generally as a result of reactivation of the virus, since HSV 1 may become latent within the trigeminal sensory nerve ganglion, and HSV 2 within the corresponding sacral ganglion (Mims & White 1984). Infection or reactivation in the normal host tends to be a mild, self-limiting disease (Kedzierski 1991). The reactivated disease tends to be less severe than the primary infection (Williams 1994). In most cases there are prodromal symptoms such as burning and tingling sensations before blisters appear (Goodall 1992).

Individuals who are immunocompromised are susceptible to more severe presentations of HSV infections. Examples include: organ transplant recipients (Rubin 1993); patients receiving cytotoxic chemotherapy for cancer (Muller et al. 1972); people with congenital or acquired cellular immune defects (Seigal et al. 1981); burns patients (Foley et al. 1970); people with skin disorders (Wheeler et al. 1966); and people with AIDS (Drew et al. 1988). In an individual with no other cause of underlying immunodeficiency, but with laboratory evidence of the presence of HIV, chronic mucocutaneous HSV infection for longer than one month is diagnostic of AIDS (Center for Disease Control 1987).

HSV infection in immunosuppressed patients can produce large, chronic ulcerated lesions (herpes phagenda). In addition, HSV 2 can cause severe perianal and rectal damage (although this is primarily found in homosexual men with AIDS) (Stine 1993), diffused interstitial pneumonitis and oesophagitis. The liver, adrenals (Hirsch 1988), gastrointestinal tract and central nervous system can be involved and lesions may persist for some months to years (Hirsch 1988).

HSV transmission can occur both from asymptomatic and symptomatic excretors (Woolley 1997). One means of minimizing the risk of infection is to avoid contact with infected lesions. Gloves are essential for all health care staff in direct contact with lesions. The use of condoms is advisable to minimize the risk of transmission during sexual intercourse (Corey et al. 1983b).

Caesarean section for women with clinically apparent cervical or genital infection prevents transmission of the infection to the infant (Corey et al. 1983b), provided that effective infection control measures are adopted by the mother when handling the child. Caesarean section should be performed before the rupture of the membranes (Kedzierski 1991).

Diagnosis

Mucocutaneous HSV infections are often easily recognizable. Visceral involvement is more difficult to identify. Confirmation of diagnosis is obtained by isolation of the virus in cell culture, and by an increase in antibody levels (Mims et al. 1993).

Treatment

The majority of infections in normal hosts resolve spontaneously. For the immunocompromised patient, prompt treatment with antiviral chemotherapy reduces morbidity and the risk of serious complications. Oral, intravenous and topical preparations of acyclovir are available. Women at greatest risk of transmitting HSV 2 to their neonates are those who developed HSV 2 late in pregnancy. Infected neonates have localized skin, eye and mucosal lesions, invasive central nervous infection or disseminated disease, therefore prevention of HSV 2 infection during pregnancy is very important (Riley 1998). The choice of route of administration, dose and duration of treatment depends on the nature and severity of the infection (Mims et al. 1993). Acyclovir resistance occurs in approximately 0.1 to 0.6% of immunocompetent individuals, whether or not they had previously received treatment, while the prevalence of resistance in previously treated immunocompromised persons is approximately 6% (Clayton et al. 1998). Foscarnet would be an alternative treatment (Darville et al. 1998).

Nursing care

Barrier nursing is essential in cases of extensive infection with herpes virus. Counselling (Kinghorn 1993) and psychological support may also be required (Williams 1994). Studies have shown that 50% of people with recurrent herpes infection experience depression, 15% have suicidal thoughts and 10% avoid sexual relationships (Chandiok 1992). Goodall (1992) suggests that these effects may be a result of insufficient information and understanding of the true nature of HSV infection.

References and further reading

Arvin, A.M. & Prober, C.G. (1991) Herpes simplex viruses. In: *Manual of Clinical Microbiology* (eds A. Balows *et al.*), 5th edn., pp. 822–8. American Society for Microbiology, Washington.

Barlow, D. & Sherrard, J. (1992) Sexually transmitted diseases. *Public Health Lab Serv Microbiol Dig*, **9**(3), 129–31.

Center for Disease Control (1987) Revision of the CDC surveillance case definition for acquired immunodeficiency syndrome. *Morb Mort Week Rep*, **36**, 15.

Clayton, C.J. *et al.* (1998) Survey of resistance of herpes simplex virus to acyclovir in northwest England. *Antimicrob Agents Chemother*, **42**(4), 868–72.

Corey, L. *et al.* (1983a) Genital herpes simplex virus infection. Clinical manifestations, cause and complications. *Ann Intern Med*, **98**, 958–72.

Corey, I. *et al.* (1983b) Genital herpes simplex virus infection. Current concepts in diagnosis, therapy and prevention. *Ann Intern Med*, **98**, 973–83.

Chandiok, S. (1992) The GP's role in the management of viral STDs. *J Sex Health*, **1**(1), 32–3.

Darville, J.M. *et al.* (1998) Acyclovir-resistant herpes simplex virus infection in a bone marrow transplant population. *Bone Marrow Transplant*, **22**(6), 587–9.

Drew, W.L. *et al.* (1988) Herpes virus infections. In: *The Management of AIDS* (eds M.A. Sande & P.A. Volberding). W.B. Saunders, London.

Foley, F.D. *et al.* (1970) Herpes virus infection in burns patient. *New Engl J Med*, **282**, 652–6.

Goodall, B. (1992) A recurring problem. *Nursing*, **5**(5), 23–4.

Hirsch, M.S. (1988) Herpes group virus infection in the compromised host. In: *Clinical Approach to Infection in the Compromised Host* (eds R.H. Rubin & L.S. Young), 2nd edn., pp. 347–66. Plenum Medical, New York and London.

Kedzierski, M. (1991) Diseases of the herpes viruses. *Nurs Stand*, **5**(31), 28–32.

Kinghorn, G.R. (1993) Genital herpes natural history and treatment of acute episodes. *J Med Virol* (Suppl), **1**, 33–8.

Mims, C.A. & White, D.O. (1984) *Viral Pathogenesis and Immunology*. Blackwell Scientific Publications, Oxford.

Mims, C.A. *et al.* (1993) *Medical Microbiology*, Mosby, London.

Muller, S.A. *et al.* (1972) Herpes simplex infections in hematologic malignancies. *Am J Med*, **52**, 102–14.

Riley, E. (1998) Herpes simplex virus. *Semin Perinatal*, **22**(4), 284–92.

Rubin, R.H. (1993) Infectious disease complications of renal transplantation. *Kidney Int*, **44**, 221–36.

Seigal, E.P. *et al.* (1981) Severe acquired immunodeficiency in male homosexuals, manifested by chronic perianal ulcerative herpes simplex lesions. *New Engl J Med*, **305**, 1439–44.

Stine, G.J. (1993) *AIDS Update 1993*. Prentice Hall, New Jersey.

Wheeler, C.E. *et al.* (1966) Eczema herpeticum: primary and recurrent. *Arch Dermatol*, **93**, 162–73.

Williams, K. (1994) Fact or fiction? *Nur Times*, **90**(3), 38–41.

Woolley, P. (1997) Genital herpes: recognizing the problem. *Medscape Women's Health*, **2**(5), 2.

Woolley, P.D. & Chandiok, S. (1996) Survey of the management of genital herpes in general practice. *Int J STD AIDS*, **7**(3), 206–11.

Varicella zoster virus (VZV)

Definition

Initial infection with varicella zoster virus (VZV) causes varicella (chicken pox). Following clinical recovery, the virus persists in the latent form in the dorsal root ganglia of nerves; reactivation of the latent VZV causes zoster (shingles) (Gershon 1996). Viral reactivation appears as cellular immunity wanes (Weller 1996). Between 80 and 90% of adults in the UK have had chicken pox (Jones *et al.* 1997), but there is a constant immigration of non-immune adults who will be susceptible to acquiring varicella from a person with varicella or zoster infection (Weller 1996).

Reference material

Varicella

The varicella incubation period is 11–21 days. Varicella is characterized by fever, viraemia and scattered vesicular lesions of the skin. Neuralgia often precedes the onset of herpes zoster (shingles), which is a localized, painful, vesicular rash involving one or adjacent dermatomes (Arvin 1996). Chronic pain may persist after the rash has healed and is referred to as postherpetic neuralgia (PHN), which can often be severe and refractory to many forms of treatment. In elderly patients the incidence of PHN varies from 27 to 68% (Schmader 1998). PHN is probably related to neuronal inflammation induced by the replicating VZV (Wood 1991). VZV viraemia occurs in patients with varicella and zoster (Mainka *et al.* 1998).

VZV is a highly infectious virus; transmission is by airborne route for chicken pox, and via infected vesicle fluid in shingles. People who have not been infected with VZV can acquire varicella from individuals infected with varicella or zoster. However, there is little evidence to support the view that in healthy people zoster can be contracted by exposure to zoster or varicella (Dolin *et al.* 1978). A person is infectious 2–3 days before the chicken pox rash appears and until the lesions crust (Jones & Reeves 1997). Immunosuppressed patients have been known to develop chicken pox when they are within 20–30 m of an infected patient (Jones *et al.* 1997). Air samples from hospital rooms of patients with VZV found that the virus was detectable 1.2–5.5 m from the bed and for up to 6 days following the onset of the rash (Sawyer *et al.* 1994).

Following local replication, the virus will be carried by the bloodstream to other sites (Arvin 1996). It is thought that infected lymphocytes persist in the circulation and can go on to carry virus to major organs, causing pneumonia, hepatitis or other life-threatening complications (Arvin et al. 1996). Both chicken pox and shingles can lead to neurological infection and disease. The virus reaches the nervous system either through the bloodstream or by direct spread from sensory ganglia. The most frequent manifestations include cerebral ataxia, neuralgia, acute encephalitis, aseptic meningitis and myelitis (Echevarria et al. 1997). Recovery from varicella in a fit adult is usually spontaneous and without sequelae (Mims et al. 1993) but can result in serious life-threatening complications in healthy children (Phuah et al. 1998).

Immunocompromised patients with VZV infection are at greater risk for dissemination and development of complications than the immunocompetent person (Rolston et al. 1998), and can be associated with serious morbidity and significant mortality (Stover & Bratcher 1998). In the immunocompromised adult or child, a much more serious presentation occurs, with a high mortality rate for untreated varicella (Rowland et al. 1995). Visceral dissemination and death is not uncommon in children with cancer. When peripheral blood lymphocyte counts are below 500/mm^3, the mortality rate is 7–30% following infection (Feldman et al. 1975). In the immunocompromised patient visceral involvement involving the lung usually occurs 3 to 7 days after the onset of skin lesions. Neurological complications occur less commonly and generally present 4–8 days after the onset of rash, and often indicate a poor prognosis. The liver is less commonly involved (Hirsch 1989).

Zoster

Every year, about 4 in every 1000 people suffer an attack of zoster (Milbourn 1989). It is thought that zoster appears when cell mediated immunity fails to curtail virus reactivation. This may happen as a result of age, the side-effects of drugs, or disease. The virus reactivates randomly in the nerve ganglion and spreads down the peripheral nerve producing vesicular skin lesions at the site supplied by the affected neurons (Mims et al. 1993). Cancer patients are particularly susceptible to zoster, which is more common during advanced stage disease and develops more frequently at areas of regionalized tumour and/or localized radiotherapy. Most cases of zoster occur within the first year after the diagnosis of cancer, although no single chemotherapeutic regimen or agent has been consistently implicated (Dolin et al. 1978).

Patients with AIDS or AIDS-related complex (ARC) appear to be at increased risk of zoster; the incidence of zoster in an HIV antibody positive person appears to be a sign for the development of AIDS (Melbye et al. 1987). VZV is particularly severe in patients with AIDS (Stewart 1995). Rapidly progressive VZV herpetic retinal necrosis can occur (Ormerod et al. 1998). Clinical presentation includes mild to moderate ocular or periorbital pain, foreign body sensation and a red eye; visual symptoms include hazy vision, floaters and decreased vision. If left untreated permanent damage can result (Spires 1992). Early diagnosis and aggressive therapy may enable return of useful vision (Lee et al. 1998).

Chicken pox during the first year of life predisposes to zoster infections in childhood. The incidence of childhood zoster is five times greater following infection with varicella at 0–2 months (Baba et al. 1986). This is presumed to be a result of immunological immaturity (Craddock-Watson 1990). A small number of cases of childhood zoster occur in children who themselves have no history of varicella, but whose mothers had the disease during the third to seventh months of pregnancy (Brunell Kotchmar 1981). Maternal varicella immediately pre- and postpartum can lead to neonatal varicella, in most cases a mild clinical form of the disease (Craddock-Watson 1990). More than 30 cases of infants with major abnormalities following varicella in the first 20 weeks of pregnancy have been described (Kiga et al. 1987).

Diagnosis

The diagnosis of chicken pox can usually be made from the characteristic pattern of vesicles. Confirmation is possible by culture of vesicle fluid or by serological antibody tests (Whitley 1995). Neuralgia often proclaims the onset of zoster and can occur several days before skin signs occur. Erythematous patches are the first sign. They progress to macules then to papules and finally to vesicles. New outbreaks of vesicles continue in untreated persons for some time (Couillard-Getreuer 1982). Fever, headaches and malaise can accompany the rash (Mims et al. 1993). The vesicles generally correspond in distribution to one or more sensory nerves. Secondary bacterial infection of the lesions can develop (Hirsch 1988). To minimize the risk of infection, care must be taken not to break the vesicles. Daily hygiene must be meticulous. Dissemination of zoster in an immunosuppressed patient generally occurs 6–10 days after the onset of localized lesions and is usually limited to cutaneous involvement, with occasional involvement of the central nervous system (CNS), lung, heart or gastrointestinal tract (Jemsek 1983).

Treatment

Treatment of varicella is normally only necessary for immunosuppressed patients, and involves the use of antiviral agents such as acyclovir, which reduces the time of new lesion formation, fever and visceral complications. The sequential use of IV followed by oral acyclovir has been shown to be effective and results in reduction of IV therapy and hospitalization (Carcao et al. 1998). Oral acyclovir administered to healthy people who have been exposed to varicella can effectively prevent or modify clinical varicella (Lin et al. 1997). Failure to respond to 7–10 days of acyclovir suggests drug resistance (Pillay 1998); in such cases foscarnet (Wutzler 1997) or ganciclovir would be the drug of choice (Reusser et al. 1996).

Prevention

Pregnant women who have not had chicken pox should be counselled to avoid contact with people with chicken pox (Chapman 1998), as infants born to women who acquire varicella during or shortly after pregnancy are at high risk of infection (Weller 1996). Varicella embryopathy is rare, occurring in 1–2% of maternal infections, particularly in the first half of pregnancy. Varicella of the newborn is a life-threatening illness which may occur when birth is within 5 days of the onset of maternal illness, or due to post delivery exposure to varicella (Chapman 1998).

Immunosuppressed patients without a history of varicella and, in some cases, patients with a history of varicella, but who are currently on high dose chemotherapy, should receive varicella zoster immunoglobulin (VZIg) when exposed to varicella or zoster. To be effective, VZIg must be administered as soon after exposure as possible (Wisnes 1978), which will give protection for approximately 4 weeks. Second cases of chicken pox in healthy people are extremely rare. However, among the immunosuppressed, second cases have been seen to occur and are often referred to as atypical disseminated zoster or varicelliform zoster. They do not have dermatomal distribution (Dolin et al. 1978).

A varicella vaccine is available and has been seen to be safe and effective (Stover & Bratcher 1998). Studies evaluating the costs and benefits of vaccinating varicella susceptible health care workers suggest there are cost benefits (Tennenberg et al. 1997). Health care workers should be screened for VZV immunity (Weber et al. 1996). Non-immune health care workers exposed to varicella infection should be removed from patient contact during the 10–21 day incubation period to prevent them infecting patients if they were to develop chicken pox (Swinker 1997).

Nursing care

Nurses must identify those patients at increased risk of VZV infection, and plan and implement interventions to decrease this risk to prevent outbreaks of VZV among patients (Kavaliotis et al. 1998). Only staff who have had varicella should have contact with patients with varicella or zoster. Source isolation is essential (see the beginning of this chapter). The door of the room must be kept closed to minimize airborne transmission of the virus (Josephson & Gombert 1988).

References and further reading

Arvin, A.M. (1996) Varicella-zoster virus. *Clin Microbiol Rev*, **9**(3), 361–81.

Arvin, A.M., Moffat, J.F. & Redman, R. (1996) Varicella-zoster virus: aspects of pathogenesis and host response to natural infection and varicella vaccine. *Adv Virus Res*, **46**, 263–309.

Baba, K. et al. (1986) Increased incidence of herpes zoster in normal children infected with varicella zoster during infancy. *J Pediat*, **108**, 372–7.

Brunel, I.P.A. & Kotchmar, G.S. (1981) Zoster in infancy: failure to maintain virus latency following intrauterine infection. *J Pediat*, **98**, 71–3.

Carcao, M.D. et al. (1998) Sequential use of intravenous and oral acyclovir in the therapy of varicella in immunocompromised children. *Pediatr Infect Dis J*, **17**(7), 626–31.

Chapman, S.J. (1998) Varicella in pregnancy. *Semin Perinatal*, **22**(4), 339–46.

Couillard-Getreuer, D.L. (1982) Herpes zoster in the immuno-compromised patient. *Cancer Nurs*, **10**, 361–70.

Craddock-Watson, J.E. (1990) Chickenpox in pregnancy. *Pub Health Lab Service Microbiol Dig*, **7**(2), 40–5.

Dolin, R. et al. (1978) Herpes zoster-varicella infection in immunosuppressed patients. *Ann Intern Med*, **89**, 375–88.

Echevarria, J.M., Casas, I. & Martinez-Martin, A. (1997) Infection of the nervous system caused by varicella zoster virus: a review. *Intervirology*, **40**(2–3), 72–84.

Feldman, S., Hughes, W.T. & Daniel, C.B. (1975) Varicella in children with cancer. Seventy seven cases. *Pediatrics*, **56**, 388–97.

Gershon, A.A. (1996) Epidemiology and management of postherpetic neuralgia. *Semin Dermatol*, **15**(Suppl. 1), 8–13.

Hirsch, M.S. (1988) Herpes group virus infection in the compromised host. In: *Clinical Approach to Infection in the Compromised Host* (eds R.H. Rubin & L.S. Young), 2nd edn, pp. 347–66. Plenum Medical Books, New York and London.

Jemsek, J. (1983) Herpes zoster-associated encephalitis: clinico-pathologic report of 12 cases and review of the literature. *Medicine*, **62**(2), 81–97.

Jones, E.M. & Reeves, D.S. (1997) Controlling chickenpox in hospital. *Br Med J*, **314**, 4–5.

Jones, E.M. et al. (1997) Control of varicella-zoster infection on renal and other specialist units. *J Hosp Infect*, **36**, 133–40.

Josephson, A. & Gombert, M. E. (1988) Airborne transmission of nosocomial varicella from localized zoster. *J Infect Dis*, **158**(1), 238–41.

Kavaliotis, J. et al. (1998) Outbreak of varicella in a pediatric oncology unit. *Med Pediatr Oncol*, **31**(3), 166–9.

Kiga, K. et al. (1987) Varicella-zoster virus infection during pregnancy: hypothesis concerning the mechanisms of congenital malformation. *Obstet Gynecol*, **69**(2), 214–22.

Lee, M.S. et al. (1998) Varicella zoster virus retrobulbar optic neuritis preceding retinitis in patients with acquired immune deficiency syndrome. *Ophthalmology*, **105**(3), 467–71.

Lin, T.Y. et al. (1997) Oral acyclovir prophylaxis of varicella after intimate contact. *Pediatr Infect Dis*, **16**(12), 1162–5.

Mainka, C. et al. (1998) Characterization of viremia at different stages of varicella-zoster virus infection. *J Med Virol*, **56**(1), 91–8.

Melbye, M. et al. (1987) Risk of AIDS after herpes zoster. *Lancet*, **1**, 728–31.

Milbourn, S. (1989) Caring for patients with herpes zoster ophthalmicus. *Prof Nurse*, January, 186–7.

Mims, C.A. et al. (1993) *Medical Microbiology*. Mosby, London.

Ormerod, L.D. et al. (1998) Rapidly progressive herpetic retinal necrosis: a blinding disease charcteristic of advanced AIDS. *Clin Infect Dis*, **26**(1), 34–45.

Pawlik, K.M. (1998) Varicella zoster infection in the immunocompromised child. *J Soc Pediatr Nurs*, **3**(1), 13–20.

Phuah, H.K. et al. (1998) Complicated varicella zoster infection in eight paediatric patients and review of literature. *Singapore Med J*, **39**(3), 115–20.

Pillay, D. (1998) Emergence and control of resistance to antiviral drugs in resistance in herpes viruses, hepatitis B virus, and HIV. *Commun Dis Public Health*, **1**(1), 5–14.

Reusser, P. et al. (1996) European survey of herpes virus resistance to antiviral drugs in bone marrow transplant recipients. Infectious Diseases Working Party of the European Group for Blood and Marrow Transplantation (EBMT). Bone Marrow Transplant, **17**(5), 813–17.

Rolston, K.V. et al. (1998) Ambulatory management of varicella-zoster virus infection in immunocompromised cancer patients. Support Care Cancer, **6**(1), 57–62.

Rowland, P. et al. (1995) Progressive varicella presenting with pain and minimal skin involvement in children with acute lymphoblastic leukemia. J Clin Oncol, **13**(7), 1697–703.

Sawyer, M.H. et al. (1994) Detection of varicella-zoster virus DNA in air samples from hospital rooms. J Infect Dis, **169**, 91–4.

Schmader, K. (1998) Post-therapeutic neuralgia in immunocompetent elderly people. Vaccine, **16**(18), 1768–70.

Spires, R. (1992) Acute retinal necrosis syndrome. J Ophthalmic Nurs Technol, **11**(3), 103–108.

Steward, J.A. et al. (1995) Herpesvirus infection in persons infected with HIV. Clin Infect Dis, **21**(Suppl. 1), S114–20.

Stover, B.H. & Bratcher, D.F. (1998) Varicella-zoster virus: infection, control and prevention. Am J Infect Control, **26**(3), 369–81.

Swinker, M. (1997) Occupational infection in health care workers: prevention and intervention. Am Fam Physician, **56**(9), 2291–300.

Tennenberg, A.M. et al. (1997) Varicella vaccination for health care workers at a university hospital: an analysis of costs and benefits. Infect Control Hosp Epidemiol, **18**(6), 405–11.

Weber, D.J., Rutala, W.A. & Hamilton, H. (1996) Prevention and control of varicella-zoster infections in healthcare facilities. Infect Control Hosp Epidemiol, **17**(10), 694–705.

Weller, T.H. (1996) Varicella: historical perspective and clinical overview. J Infect Dis, **174**(Suppl. 3), S306–309.

Whitley, R. (1995) Varicella-zoster virus. In: Principles and Practice of Infectious Diseases, 4th edn. (eds G.L. Mandell, J.E. Bennett & R. Dolin). Churchill Livingstone, New York. Vol. 2, Chap. 116, pp. 1345–50.

Wisnes, R. (1978) Efficacy of zoster immunoglobulin in prophylaxis of varicella in high-risk patients. Acta Paediatr Scand, **67**, 77–82.

Wood, M.J. (1991) Herpes zoster and pain. Scand J Infect Dis Suppl, **80**, 53–61.

Wutzler, P. (1997) Antiviral therapy of herpes simplex and varicella-zoster virus infections. Intervirology, **40**(5–6), 343–56.

Legionnaires' disease

Definition

Legionnaires' disease is an acute bacterial pneumonia caused by infection with Legionella pneumophila. This is responsible for about 90% of infection caused by the Legionella family. Legionella is a Gram-negative, aerobic, non-spore-forming unencapsulated bacillus (Yu 1995).

Reference material

In the summer of 1976 an outbreak of pneumonia occurred among about 5000 people who had attended an American Legion convention in Philadelphia. There were 182 cases and 29 deaths. The epidemic aroused enormous public interest. Epidemiological investigations showed that the focus was the lobby of a famous hotel, but the cause remained unidentified for months until a small Gram-negative organism was found, which subsequently became known as Legionella pneumophila (Fraser et al. 1977).

There are more than 30 species of the Legionella family, with more than 50 serotypes (Yu 1995) which have been isolated from a range of environmental sites including lakes, rivers, soils and man-made water systems such as cooling towers and water distribution systems (Cooper 1991). The latter two sites have been responsible for numerous outbreaks of legionnaires' disease which have occurred mainly during June to October (Center for Disease Control 1978). Since 1987, countries in Europe have collaborated in surveillance of legionnaires' disease. Over 50 clusters of travel related disease have been reported. Many cases are associated with Mediterranean countries, reflecting the large numbers of holidaymakers from across Europe who visit the area (Public Health Laboratory Service Communicable Disease Surveillance Centre 1994).

Up to 30% of sporadic cases of hospital acquired pneumonia are caused by Legionella (Hart & Makin 1991). The pattern of infection is unique. The outbreaks are site specific and associated with factors which predispose to infection, including water systems contaminated with the organism. Legionella pneumophila is a thermophile which flourishes at temperatures from 25 to 42°C and can survive a range of temperatures from 5 to 58°C. However, it is unusual for this organism to proliferate in temperatures of below 20°C (Health and Safety Executive 1991). The most critical temperature is 36°C. Every effort should be made to avoid stagnant water conditions and to store and supply water outside this critical temperature (Harper 1986). The quality of cold water can be improved by a dedicated supply direct from the incoming mains, and circulating hot water should be kept at a temperature of 60°C (Patterson et al. 1997).

Legionella is ubiquitous in surface water. The major route of infection is by aerosol dispersion and inhalation of the bacteria from, for example, shower heads (Alderman 1988), or more commonly from air conditioning systems. Contaminated shower heads and tap water aerosolize low numbers of the organisms during use. The aerosols are small enough to penetrate the lower respiratory system and cause infection (Bollin et al. 1985). Effective maintenance of water systems is essential to minimize the risk of Legionella infection (NHSE 1994). Removal of 'dead legs' in plumbing systems where sludge has formed, which predisposes to proliferation of the organisms, plus regular flushing of water systems not in regular use, reduce legionellae to below detectable levels (Makin & Hart 1990). In air-conditioning systems the organism may multiply in the water of cooling towers. When water from this source evaporates, droplets containing Legionella may be drawn into the air intakes of the building or fall on people passing by (Health and Safety Executive 1991).

Legionnaires' disease is not a notifiable disease, but since 1977 the Communicable Disease Surveillance Centre has maintained a surveillance programme of cases reported voluntarily by medical microbiologists. Between 1980 and 1990 an average of 188 cases were seen each year (Health and Safety Executive 1992). Since then, in 1994 (Public Health Laboratory Service Communicable Disease Surveillance Centre 1995), 1995 (Public Health Laboratory Service Communicable Disease Surveillance Centre 1996), 1996 (Public Health Laboratory Service Communicable Disease Surveillance Centre 1997) and 1997 (Joseph *et al.* 1998) there were 160 cases with 27 deaths, 160 cases with 20 deaths, 201 cases with 24 deaths and 226 cases with 29 deaths, and 89, 90, 101 and 114 were associated with travel, respectively.

Virulence is coupled to a susceptible host. The disease tends to affect males, by a factor of 2 or 3 to 1. Those who smoke or consume excess alcohol, people who are already immunocompromised and the elderly are all predisposed to infection (Stout 1987).

The incubation period is about 2–10 days following first exposure. The signs and symptoms include malaise, general aches and headache, diarrhoea and vomiting, followed by high temperature, cough, rigors and respiratory distress. Immunosuppressed patients may have fever without any other symptoms of infection despite radiographic abnormalities (Muder & Yu 1995). Some patients do not develop pneumonia but progress to profound septicaemia with symptoms of diplopia and mental confusion (Potterton 1985). Pneumonia is the most common presentation of *Legionella* infection, but wound infections have followed immersion in contaminated water (Brabender *et al.* 1993). Fatality rates are about 10% (Rowbotham 1998).

Diagnosis

Diagnosis relies on laboratory diagnosis by:

1 Isolation of the causative organism
2 Demonstration of the presence of the organism, its antigen or its products in the patient's body fluids or tissues (Harrison 1985)
3 Demonstration of specific antibodies directed against the organism, its antigens or its products (Harrison 1985).

The above are coupled to the clinical picture and chest X-ray findings.

Treatment

Historically, treatment has included the antibiotic erythromycin (Center for Disease Control 1978), although newer antibiotics are being used (Yu 1995). Supportive therapy is also required for complications as they arise, which may include pulmonary failure, shock and acute renal failure. Person to person spread has never been demonstrated (Hart & Makin 1991) and therefore barrier nursing is not required. However, careful disposal of sputum and encouraging patients to cover their mouth and nose when coughing are necessary precautions.

Prevention

Prevention relies on regular inspection and maintenance of the water system, including planning, installation and commissioning (Finch 1988). Each case of nosocomial legionnaires' disease must be investigated to ensure that the outbreak has been contained (Fallon 1994).

References and further reading

Alderman, C. (1988) The cooler culprits. *Nurs Stand*, **2**(33), 22.
Bollin, G.E. *et al.* (1985) Aerosols containing *Legionella pneumophila* generated by shower heads and hot water faucets. *Appl Environ Microbiol*, **50**(5), 1128–31.
Brabender, W., Hinthorn, D.R. & Asher, M. (1993) *Legionella pneumophila* wound infection. *JAMA*, **250**, 3091–5.
Centers for Disease Control (1978) Legionnaires' disease, diagnosis and management. *Ann Intern Med*, **88**, 363–5.
Cooper, J. (1991) Positive discrimination. *Lab Pract*, **40**(1), 16–17.
Fallon, R.J. (1994) How to prevent an outbreak of legionnaires' disease. *J Hosp Infect*, **27**, 247–56.
Finch, R. (1988) Minimizing the risk of Legionnaires' disease. *Br Med J*, **296**, 1343–5.
Fraser, D.W. *et al.* (1977) Legionnaires' disease: description of an epidemic of pneumonia. *New Engl J Med*, **297**, 1189–97.
Harper, D. (1986) Legionnaires' disease: prevention better than cure. *Health Safety Work*, March, 41–6.
Harrison, T.G. (1985) A nasty family from Philadelphia. *Med Lab World*, September, 19–23.
Hart, C.A. & Makin, T. (1991) Legionella in hospitals: a review. *J Hosp Infect*, **18**(Suppl. A), 481–9.
Health and Safety Executive (1991) *The Control of Legionellosis including Legionnaires' Disease*. Stationery Office, London.
Health and Safety Executive (1992) *Joint Health and Safety Executive and Department of Health Working Group on Legionellosis*. Stationery Office, London.
Joseph, C.A. *et al.* (1998) Legionnaires' disease in residents of England and Wales 1997. *Commun Dis Public Health*, **1**(44), 252–8.
Makin, T. & Hart, C.A. (1990) The efficacy of control measures for eradicating legionellae in showers. *J Infect Control*, **16**(1), 1–7.
Muder, R.R. & Yu, V.L. (1995) Other legionella species. In: *Principles and Practices of Infectious Disease*, 4th edn. (eds G.L. Mandell, J.E. Bennett & R. Dolin). Churchill Livingstone, New York. Vol. 2, Chap. 212, pp. 2097–103.
National Health Service Executive (NHSE) (1994) *The control of legionellae in Health Care Premises*, Health Technical Memorandum 2040, Code of Practice NHS Estates. Stationery Office, London.
Patterson, W.J. *et al.* (1997) Colonization of transplant unit water supplies with legionella and protozoa: precautions required to reduce the risk of legionellosis. *J Hosp Infect*, **37**(1), 7–17.
Potterton, D. (1985) Mystery of the organism. *Nurs Times*, **82**(22), 20–21.
Public Health Laboratory Service Communicable Disease Surveillance Centre (1994) European surveillance of legionnaires' disease associated with travel. *Commun Dis Rep*, **4**(6), 25.
Public Health Laboratory Service Communicable Disease Surveil-

lance Centre (1995) Legionnaires' disease surveillance: England and Wales 1994. *Commun Dis Rep*, **5**(12), R180–83.

Public Health Laboratory Service Communicable Disease Surveillance Centre (1996) Legionnaires' disease surveillance: England and Wales 1995. *Commun Dis Rep*, **6**(11), R151–5.

Public Health Laboratory Service Communicable Disease Surveillance Centre (1997) Legionnaires' disease surveillance: England and Wales 1996. *Commun Dis Rep*, **7**(11), R153–9.

Rowbotham, T.J. (1998) Legionellosis associated with ships 1977–1997. *Commun Dis Public Health*, **1**(3), 146–51.

Stout, J.E. (1987) Legionnaires' disease acquired within the homes of two patients. *J Am Med Assoc*, **257**(9), 1215–17.

Yu, V.L. (1995) *Legionella pneumophila* (legionnaires' disease). In: *Principles and Practices of Infectious Disease*, 4th edn. (eds G.L. Mandell, J.E. Bennett & R. Dolin). Churchill Livingstone, New York. Vol. 2, Chap. 211, 2087–97.

Listeriosis

Definition

Listeriosis is an infectious disease caused by *Listeria monocytogenes*, a Gram-negative bacterium, and is a serious life-threatening infection (Riviera *et al.* 1993).

Reference material

Listeria has a widespread distribution in the environment, including in soil, dust and vegetation (Watkins *et al.* 1981). It also inhabits the gastrointestional tract of animals and humans who may remain symptomless (Botsen-Moller 1972). The genus *Listeria* includes many types which are non-pathogenic to man. *Listeria monocytogenes* is recognized as being the cause of listeriosis in man (Lamont *et al.* 1988). Infection in immunocompromised adults varies from a mild, chill-like illness to bacteraemia, septicaemia and meningitis (Limaye *et al.* 1998). *Listeria* was initially isolated and described in 1992 (Low & Donachie 1997), with most cases arising from ingestion of contaminated food (Low & Donachie 1997). A USA study found that at least one food specimen in the refrigerators of infected patients grew *Listeria* (Pinner *et al.* 1992). Gilot *et al.* (1997), however, suggest that most cases of listeriosis occur sporadically and can rarely be linked with consumption of a specific food.

Growth of this organism is optimal at 37°C, but it will survive and multiply at a range of 26–42°C and is not easily inactivated by environmental influences such as freezing, thawing and strong sunlight (Gray 1963).

Instances of human infection are increasing (McLauchlin 1988), particularly among immunocompromised people. A review of 776 cases of central nervous system infection found the highest number among haematological malignancy and kidney transplantation patients, while 36% of patients had no underlying disease (Mylonakis *et al.* 1998). Immunocompetent patients are more likely to survive than immunocompromised patients (Skogberg *et al.* 1992). Adult and paediatric cancer patients are equally at risk (Mora *et al.* 1998), while infection among AIDS patients is relatively uncommon (Decker *et al.* 1991; Cooper & Walker 1998).

Transmission, particularly among the immunocompromised patients (Hung *et al.* 1995) and pregnant women (McLauchin 1990), causes bacteremia and meningitis, and in pregnant women premature delivery and often fetal death (Armstrong 1995). The fetus and the newborn are especially prone to infection due to the immaturity of their immune systems. In the UK, there is about one incidence in every 9700 of perinatal listeriosis births (McLauchlin 1987). Maternal symptoms are often absent, and neonatal listeriosis presents as meningitis or occasionally as septicaemia (Gill 1988). In cases where the mother presented with decreased fetal movement, diagnosis was made by ultrasound examination (Quinlivan *et al.* 1998; Miyakoshi *et al.* 1998). Abortion and stillbirths due to listeriosis have been reported (MacNaughton 1962).

Treatment

Early diagnosis and prompt administration of appropriate antibiotics is essential (Jones & MacGowan 1995), even so deaths will still occur (Chang *et al.* 1995). Ampicillin or penicillin is usually regarded as the drug of choice (Trautman *et al.* 1985), often in combination with gentamicin (Azimi *et al.* 1979). However, even with prompt antibiotic therapy, mortality may be as high as 30% in patients with other serious underlying conditions (Rouquette & Berche 1996).

Transmission

Contaminated food is the most important as a vehicle of spread (McLaughlin & Gilbert 1990). Of 822 shop bought food specimens, 136 soil and 692 faecal specimens cultured for *Listeria* species 19.7% of the food, 93.9% of the soil and 14.7% of the faecal specimens were found to be positive (MacGowan *et al.* 1994). There are increasing reports of *Listeria* found in raw meat, fruit and vegetables which predispose to contamination of, for example, coleslaw. An outbreak involving coleslaw prepared from contaminated cabbage involved seven adults and 34 newborn babies in Canada (Schlech *et al.* 1983). Prepared mixed salads have a much higher rate of contamination than individual salad ingredients, probably because prepared salads are contaminated during the chopping, mixing and packaging process (Valani & Robert 1990).

Prevention entails scrupulous preparation of cooked food for immunocompromised people and the avoidance of uncooked foods. Person to person transmission during normal contact is unlikely. However, careful disposal of blood and body fluids and thorough hand washing after contact with the patient is essential.

References and further reading

Armstrong, D. (1995) *Listeria monocytogenes*. In: *Principles and Practice of Infectious Diseases* (eds G.L. Mandell, J.E. Bennett & R. Dolin). Churchill Livingstone, New York. Vol. 2, Chap. 185, pp. 1880–85.

Azimi, P.H. *et al.* (1979) *Listeria monocytogenes*. Synergistic effects of ampicillin and gentamicin. *Am J Clin Pathol*, **72**, 974–7.

Botsen-Moller, J. (1972) Human listeriosis, diagnostic epidemiological and clinical studies. *Acta Pathol Microbiol Scand*, **229**(Suppl.), 1–57.

Chang, J. *et al.* (1995) Listeriosis in bone marrow transplant recipients: incidence, clinical features, and treatment. *Clin Infect Dis*, **21**(5), 1289–90.

Cooper, J. & Walker, R.D. (1998) Listeriosis. *Vet Clin North Am Food Anim Pract*, **14**(1), 113–25.

Decker, C.F. *et al.* (1991) *Listeria monocytogenes* infection in patients with AIDS: report of five cases and review. *Rev Infect Dis*, **13**(3), 413–17.

Gill, P. (1988) Is listeriosis often a food-borne illness? *J Infect*, **17**, 1–5.

Gilot, P. *et al.* (1997) Sporadic case of listeriosis associated with the consumption of a *Listeria monocytogenes*-contaminated 'Camembert' cheese. *J Infect*, **35**(2), 195–7.

Gray, M.L. (1963) Epidemiological aspects of listeriosis. *Am J Public Health*, **53**, 554–63.

Hung, C.C. *et al.* (1995) Antibiotic therapy for *Listeria monocytogenes* bacteremia. *J Formos Med Assoc*, **94**(1–2), 19–22.

Jones, E.M. & MacGowan, A.P. (1995) Antimicrobial chemotherapy of human infection due to *Listeria monocytogenes*. *Eur J Clin Microbiol Infect Dis*, **14**(3), 165–75.

Lamont, R.J. *et al.* (1988) *Listeria monocytogenes* and its role in human infection. *J Infect*, **17**, 7–28.

Limaye, A.P., Perkins, J.D. & Kowdley, K.V. (1998) Listeria infection after liver transplantation: report of a case and review of the literature. *Am J Gastroenterol*, **93**(10), 1942–4.

Low, J.C. & Donachie, W. (1997) A review of *Listeria monocytogenes* and listeriosis. *Vet*, **153**(1), 9–29.

MacGowan, A.P., Bowker, K., McLauchlin, J. *et al.* (1994) The occurrence and seasonal changes in the isolation of *Listeria* spp. in shop bought foodstuff, human faeces, sewage and soil from urban sources. *Int J Food Microbiol*, **21**(4), 325–43.

McLauchlin, J. (1987) *Listeria monocytogenes*: recent advances in the taxonomy and epidemiology of listeriosis in humans. *J Appl Bacteriol*, **63**, 1–11.

McLauchlin, J. (1988) Listeriosis and food-borne transmission. *Lancet*, **1**, 177–8.

McLauchlin, J. (1990) Human listeriosis in Britain. *Epidemiol Infect*, **104**, 181–90.

McLaughlin, J. & Gilbert, R.J. (1990) Listeria in food. *Public Health Lab Serv Microbiol Dig*, **7**(3), 54–5.

MacNaughton, M.C. (1962) *Listeria monocytogenes* in abortion. *Lancet*, **11**, 484.

Miyakoshi, K., Tanaka, M., Miyazaki, T. *et al.* (1998) Prenatal ultrasound diagnosis of small bowel torsion. *Obstet Gynecol*, **91**(5, Part 2), 802–803.

Mora, J., White, M. & Dunkel, I.J. (1998) Listeriosis in pediatric oncology patients. *Cancer*, **83**(4), 817–20.

Mylonakis, E., Hohmann, E.L. & Calderwood, S.B. (1998) Central nervous system infection with *Listeria monocytogenes*. 33 years' experience at a general hospital and review of 776 episodes from the literature. *Medicine (Baltimore)*, **77**(5), 313–36.

Pinner, R.W. *et al.* (1992) Role of food in sporadic listeriosis. Microbiologic and epidemiologic investigation. The listeria study group. *JAMA*, **267**(15), 2046–50.

Quinlivan, J.A., Newnham, J.P. & Dickinson, J.E. (1998) Ultrasound features of congenital listeriosis. A case report. *Prenat Diag*, **18**(10), 1075–8.

Riviera, L., Dubini, F. & Bellotti, M.G. (1993) *Listeria monocytogenes* infections: the organism, its pathogenicity and antimicrobial drugs susceptibility. *New Microbiol*, **16**(2), 189–203.

Rouquette, C. & Berche, P. (1996) The pathgenosis of infection by *Listeria monocytogenes*. *Microbiologia*, **12**(2), 245–58.

Ruutu, P. & Valtonen, V. (1992) Clinical presentation and outcome of listeriosis in patients with and without immunosuppressive therapy. *Clin Infect Dis*, **14**(4), 815–21.

Schlech, W.F. *et al.* (1983) Epidemic listeriosis. Evidence of a transmission by food. *New Engl J Med*, **308**, 203–206.

Skogberg, K., Syrjanen, J., Jahkola, M. *et al.* (1992) Clinical presentation and outcome of listeriosis in patients with and without immunosuppressive therapy. *Clin Infect Dis*, **14**(4), 815–21.

Trautman, M. *et al.* (1985) Listeria meningitis: report of 10 cases and review of current therapeutic recommendations. *J Infect*, **10**, 107–14.

Valani, S. & Robert, D. (1990) *Listeria monocytogenes* and other *Listeria* spp. in pre-packed mixed salads and individual salad ingredients. *Public Health Lab Serv Microbiol Dig*, **8**(1), 21–2.

Watkins, J. *et al.* (1981) Isolation and enumeration of *Listeria monocytogenes* from sewage, sewage study and river water. *J Appl Bacteriol*, **5**, 1–9.

Pneumocystosis

Definition

Pneumocystosis is an infection caused by the organism *Pneumocystis carinii* (PC), which is closely related to fungi (Mandell *et al.* 1995).

Reference material

Pneumocystis carinii was first discovered in 1909 and was associated with outbreaks of pneumonia in people subjected to malnutrition and overcrowding (Radman 1973). PC is an organism that is widely distributed in the environ-ment and most children demonstrate that they have been harmlessly exposed to PC at an early age (Walzer 1995). PC can be detected in hospital and community areas with and without infected patients being present (Bartlet *et al.* 1997). It is thought that acquisition of PC is from the environment (Olsson *et al.* 1998). Person to person transmission has not been recognized (Bartlet *et al.* 1997).

The organism has been recognized as being an important cause of pneumonia in the immunocompromised host for over 20 years. Three types of patients have been particularly affected:

1 Patients of all ages receiving immunosuppressive agents for the treatment of cancer and during organ transplantation (Walzer *et al.* 1973).

2 Children and infants with primary immunodeficiency disorders, particularly severe combined immunodeficiency (SCID) (Gajdusek 1957).
3 Patients with acquired immune deficiency syndrome (AIDS), particularly in patients whose blood CD4 T lymphocytes are below 200/mm^3 of blood (Phair et al. 1990). PC remains the most frequently reported serious opportunistic infection in AIDS patients and the second highest cause of mortality among people with AIDS (Moorman et al. 1998). In addition, the occurrence of PC is significantly associated with the death of HIV positive people (Chaisson et al. 1998). PC is commonest among those who are unaware of their HIV positive status or who have declined prophylaxis despite knowing they are HIV positive (Miller 1998). The incidence of PC among IV drug misusers, heterosexual and homosexual men is very similar, while subsequent survival is lowest among IV drug misusers, possibly due to the lower uptake of antiretrovirals in this group (Laing et al. 1997). PC prophylaxis for HIV positive patients has been seen to be cost effective (Freedberg et al. 1998). Studies evaluating efficacy and toxicity rates for prophylaxis regimens are ongoing (Wynia et al. 1998). PC may still occur despite appropriate prophylaxis (Massie et al. 1998).

Most epidemiological studies have focused on clusters of cases within hospitals, orphanages or private clinics. All have common denominators of overcrowding, protein calorie malnutrition, prematurity or immunosuppressive disease, predisposing to Pneumocystis carinii pneumonia (PCP). These studies give the impression of outbreaks of infection, when no spread has actually occurred; rather the disease probably occurred from reactivation of latent infection triggered by immunosuppression (Dutz 1970).

Watanable and colleagues (1965) reported a cluster of infection in a family of three. A healthy woman developed fatal PCP several days before her husband, who had acute lymphatic leukaemia and who also died. Their 7-year-old daughter had had a typical respiratory disease 2 months before her parents' illness. Although she recovered, she may have transmitted the disease to her non-immune parents, suggesting that person to person or airborne transmission is possible among immunologically naive subjects.

PC infections associated with deprivation in children are reported to be slow and insidious in onset, with initial non-specific signs of restlessness, lethargy, poor feeding over a period of weeks, resulting in tachypnoea, severe dyspnoea, use of accessory muscles for breathing, marked cyanosis and exhausting non-productive cough (Perera et al. 1970). Children and adults with underlying disease such as neoplasm often experience an abrupt onset of illness, with high fever, tachypnoea and cough, which can progress to a fatal outcome even with treatment (Walzer 1970).

Diagnosis

It is possible, using polymerase chain reaction (PCR) tests, to detect PC in specimens containing low numbers of PC where conventional microscopic staining failed to do so (Lundgren & Wakefield 1998).

Fibreoptictic bronchoscopy or bronchial washings are now favoured because of the increase of PC infection among AIDS patients, where large numbers of organisms are generally present in bronchial secretions, sputum and transtrachial aspirations. Unfortunately, if such specimens yield negative results, open lung biopsy may have to be undertaken expeditiously before the patient deteriorates further. Survival is related directly to the aggressiveness with which the diagnosis is pursued in the early stages of disease and with the early institution of appropriate therapy (Young 1984).

Treatment

Trimethoprim-sulphamethoxazole is the treatment of choice (Barnes 1998), but can be toxic and may fail, resulting in treatment changes (Deresinski 1997). Pentamidine, clindamycin-primaquine and atovaquone are suitable for those patients unable to tolerate trimethoprim-sulphamethoxazole (Barnes 1998). Aerosolized pentamidine prophylaxis has significantly improved the prognosis for patients with AIDS (Miller et al. 1989). Therefore, patients receiving aerosolized prophylaxis must be monitored carefully for signs of disseminated disease (Dubé & Sattler 1993).

Nursing care

Hospitalized patients who develop PCP may well be cared for in areas where there are large concentrations of immunosuppressed patients. Due to the reports of clustering of this disease and the difficulty of identifying whether this represents person to person spread, patients with a productive cough should be placed in a single room until the cough improves. Precautions other than careful hand washing following patient contact are unnecessary.

References and further reading

Barnes, R.A. (1998) Fungal infections. In: *The Clinical Practice of Stem Cell Transplantation* (eds J. Barrett & J. Treleaven). ISIS Medical Media, Oxford, **2**(46), 724–40.

Bartlet, M.S. et al. (1997) Detection of Pneumocystis carinii DNA in air samples: likely environmental risk to susceptible persons. *J Clin Microbiol*, **35**(10), 2511–13.

Carter, T.-R. et al. (1988) Pneumocystis carinii infection of the small intestine in a patient with acquired immunodeficiency syndrome. *Am J Clin Pathol*, **89**, 679–83.

Chaisson, R.E. et al. (1998) Impact of opportunistic disease on survival in patients with HIV infection. *AIDS*, **12**(1), 29–33.

Deresinski, S.C. (1997) Treatment of Pneumocystis carinii pneumonia in adults with AIDS. *Semin Respir Infect*, **12**(2), 9–97.

Dubé, M. & Sattler, F.R. (1993) Prevention and treatment of opportunistic infections. *Curr Opin Infect Dis*, **6**, 230–36.

Dutz, W. (1970) Pneumocystis carinii pneumonia. *Path Ann*, **5**, 309.

Freedberg, K.A. et al. (1998) The cost effectiveness of preventing AIDS related opportunistic infections. *JAMA*, **279**(2), 130–36.

Friedberg, D.-N. et al. (1990) Asymptomatic dissemination of Pneumocystis carinii infection detected by ophthalmoscopy. *Lancet*, **2**, 1256–7.

Gajdusek, D.C. (1957) *Pneumocystis carinii* etiologic agent of interstitial plasma cell pneumonia of young and premature infants. *Paediatrics*, **19**, 543.

Galland, J.E. (1988) *Pneumocystis carinii* thyroiditis. *Am J Med*, **84**, 303–306.

Gherman, C.R. (1988) *Pneumocystis carinii* otitis media and mastoiditis as the initial manifestation of the acquired immunodeficiency syndrome. *Am J Med*, **85**, 250–52.

Laing, R., Brettle, R., Leen, C. *et al.* (1997) Features and outcome of *Pneumocystis carinii* pneumonia according to risk category for HIV infection. *Scand J Infect Dis*, **29**(1), 57–61.

Lundgren, B. & Wakefield, A.E. (1998) PCR for detecting *Pneumocystis carinii* in clinical or environmental samples. *Immunol Med Microbiol*, **22**(1–2), 97–101.

Massie, R.J. *et al.* (1998) *Pneumocystis carinii* pneumonia: pitfalls of prophylaxis *J Paediatr Child Health*, **43**(5), 477–9.

Miller, R. (1998) Clinical aspects of pneumocystis pneumonia in HIV infected patients 1997. *Immunol Med Microbiol*, **22**(1–2), 103–105.

Miller, R.F. *et al.* (1989) Nebulized pentamidine as treatment for *Pneumocystis carinii* pneumonia in the acquired immunodeficiency syndrome. *Thorax*, **44**, 565–9.

Moorman, A.C. (1998) *Pneumocystis carinii* pneumonia incidence and chemoprophylaxis failure in ambulatory HIV infected patients. HIV Out Study (HOPS) Investigators. *J AIDS Hum Retrovirol*, **19**(2), 182–8.

Olsson, M. *et al.* (1998) Identification of *Pneumocystis carinii* f. sp. *Hominis* gene sequences in filtered air in hospital environment. *J Clin Microbiol*, **36**(6), 1737–40.

Pearson, R.D. *et al.* (1985) Pentamidine for the treatment of *Pneumocystis carinii* pneumonia and other protozoan diseases. *Ann Intern Med*, **103**, 782–6.

Perera, D.R. *et al.* (1970) *Pneumocystis carinii* pneumonia in a hospital for children. *J Am Med Assoc*, **214**, 1074–8.

Phair, J. *et al.* (1990) The risk of *Pneumocystis carinii* pneumonia among men infected with human immune deficiency virus type 1. *New Engl J Med*, **322**, 161–5.

Pilon, V.A. *et al.* (1987) *Pneumocystis carinii* infection in AIDS. *New Engl J Med*, **316**, 1410–11.

Poblete, R.B. *et al.* (1989) *Pneumocystis carinii* hepatitis in the acquired immunodeficiency syndrome. *Am J Intern Med*, **110**, 737–8.

Radman, J.C. (1973) *Pneumocystis carinii* pneumonia in an adopted Vietnamese infant. *J Am Med Assoc*, **230**, 1561–3.

Ruskin, J. (1989) Parasitic disease in the compromised host. In: *Clinical Approaches to Infection in the Compromised Host* (eds R.H. Rubin & L.S. Young), 2nd edn. Plenum Medical, London.

Walzer, P.D. (1970) *Pneumocystis carinii* infection. Review article. *Southern Med J*, **70**(11), 1330–33.

Walzer, P.D. (1995) *Pneumocystis carinii*. In: *Principles and Practices of Infectious Diseases*, 4th edn. (eds G.L. Mandell, J.E. Bennett & R. Dolin). Churchill Livingstone, New York. Vol. 2, Chap. 258, pp. 2475–86.

Walzer, P.D. *et al.* (1973) *Pneumocystis carinii* pneumonia and primary immune deficiency disease in infancy and childhood. *J Paediatr*, **82**, 416–22.

Watanable, J.M. (1965) *Pneumocystis carinii* pneumonia in a family. *J Am Med Assoc*, **193**, 113.

Wharton, M. *et al.* (1986) Trimethoprim sulphamethoxazole or pentamidine for *Pneumocystis carinii* pneumonia in the acquired immunodeficiency syndrome. *Ann Intern Med*, **105**, 37–44.

Wynia, M.K., Ioannidis, J.P. & Lau, J. (1998) Analysis of life-long strategies to prevent *Pneumocystis carinii* pneumonia in patients with variable HIV progression rates. *AIDS*, **12**(11), 1317–25.

Young, L.S. (1984) Clinical aspects of pneumocystosis in man. In: *Pneumocystis carinii Pneumonia* (ed. L.S. Young), pp. 139–74. Marcel Dekker, New York.

Tuberculosis

Definition

Tuberculosis (TB) is a destructive infectious disease caused by *Mycobacterium tuberculosis*, which is an acid fast bacillus. Other species of *Mycobacterium* which cause infection are referred to as 'atypical' mycobacteria (Mims *et al.* 1993).

Reference material

Mycobacterium tuberculosis is defined as an acid-fast bacillus because of a waxy material in the cell wall, which resists simple laboratory staining techniques unless treated with hot carbol fuchsin, which allows impregnation by the dye. This is retained despite attempts to decolourize it with acid or alcohol (Mims *et al.* 1993). Mycobacteria are distributed widely throughout the world, but only a few species are pathogenic to man. This includes M. *tuberculosis*, whose main host is man, and M. *bovis* (the bovine type of tubercle bacillus), which is pathogenic to man as well as to cattle. Outbreaks of infection in humans due to M. *bovis* have been reported (Guerrero *et al.* 1997).

There are also atypical mycobacteria associated with patients who are severely immunocompromised due to human immunodeficiency virus (HIV) infection. These are

M. *avium intracellulare*, M. *malmoense*, M. *xenopi* and M. *kansasii* (Lamden *et al.* 1996). In the past, these types rarely caused disease in man, but now cause a disease which quickly disseminates to most organs in the body (Young 1996), and do not respond as readily to established tuberculosis drugs (Chaisson 1993). Atypical mycobacteria are not highly adapted to humans like M. *tuberculosis* and are not transmitted from person to person, but can survive in the environment and pass to human hosts.

TB causes characteristically chronic granulamatous lesions, mainly in the lungs, but the glands, bones, joints, brain and meninges and other internal organs may be affected (Alvarez *et al.* 1984). Infection in immunocompromised adults varies from a mild, chill-like illness to bacteraemia, septicaemia and meningitis.

Epidemiology

The incidence of TB in the world is expected to increase from 8.8 million cases in 1995 to 10.2 million cases by the year 2000. Three million deaths occurred in 1995 and 3.5 are expected in the year 2000 (Pilheu 1998). In the UK a steady decline in the number of TB notifications ceased in the mid 1980s, when slight increases were seen (DoH 1998). The number of TB notifications increased by 7% between 1996 and 1997. Respiratory TB increased by 13% while non-respiratory TB decreased by 6% (Public Health

Laboratory Service Communicable Disease Surveillance Centre Supplement 1998a). Initially, increases were attributed to minority subgroups, in particular immigrants (Public Health Laboratory Service Communicable Disease Surveillance Centre 1998b). Ormerod (1996) suggests a 25-fold increased incidence in immigrant subgroups. The Center for Disease Control (1998a) outlines how linguistic, cultural and health service barriers impeded the provision of TB preventative therapy. The effects of poverty, homelessness and the HIV epidemic also account for the increase in infections (Mangtani et al. 1995). Transmission between families occurs (Quigley 1997). Some authors suggest badgers infect cattle in the UK (Mairtin et al. 1998).

Certain conditions predispose to the development of tuberculosis, including general physical debilitation and lowered resistance due to disease, immunosuppressive drugs and alcoholism (Washington & Miller 1998). Among 4360 patients with AIDS, 200 were reported to have TB in 1991 (Watson et al. 1993). TB has the potential to cause progression of HIV disease (Perneger et al. 1995), with HIV positive people being more likely to progress to active disease than an immunocompetent person (DoH 1998).

Transmission

The mode of spread for tuberculosis is occasionally by ingestion, for example by drinking infected milk, but principally by inhalation of small droplets produced by coughing. These droplets are probably the most effective vehicle of spread since they dry rapidly in the air to yield droplet nuclei of less than 5 nm in diameter which, when inhaled, can reach the alveoli. The organism can survive in moist or dried sputum for up to 6 weeks, but is killed by a few hours' exposure to direct sunlight (Loudon et al. 1969).

Special attention must be given to equipment contaminated with Mycobacterium species. Thorough cleaning followed by autoclaving is the sterilization method of choice. As certain equipment such as endoscopes can be damaged by autoclaving, disinfection must be used. A greater resistance by the organism to glutaraldehyde solution has been seen, and so thoroughly precleaned equipment must be totally immersed for 20 minutes in a freshly prepared glutaraldehyde solution before use and between cases (DHSS 1986; Working Party 1998). Other disinfectants such as peracetic acid are alternatives to glutaraldehyde (Griffiths et al. 1999). An audit of the disinfection of fibreoptic bronchoscopes showed that many units do not adhere to guidelines related to disinfection procedures and staff safety (Honeybourne & Neumann 1997). Transmission of TB has occurred due to inadequately cleaned bronchoscopes (Michele et al. 1997).

Diagnosis

Tuberculosis should be suspected in all people with a cough with or without cause, which lasts more than 3 weeks, with or without weight loss, anorexia, fever, night sweats or haemoptysis (DoH 1998). A provisional diagnosis can be based on microscopical findings of acid-fast bacilli in, for example, sputum, tissue, urine or cerebrospinal fluid. This is termed 'smear positive'. Confirmation and species identification by culture may take several weeks and is termed 'culture positive' (Drobniewski et al. 1994). Newer methods are now available which reduce the time required for identification, making it possible to carry out an antibiotic assay more rapidly (Ginesu et al. 1998; Drobniewski 1998; DoH 1998).

Patients with smear-positive pulmonary disease are infectious, those with smear-negative or non-pulmonary disease are not. Once appropriate combination chemotherapy has commenced (Joint Tuberculosis Committee of the British Thoracic Society 1994) smear-positive people are considered non-infectious after 2 weeks of treatment (Subcommittee of the Joint Tuberculosis Committee of the British Thoracic Society 1990) and when three consecutive good quality sputum samples are found to be smear-negative (DoH 1998).

Treatment

Until the 1960s, treatment included bed rest and attention to diet, but chemotherapy is now the preferred treatment. It involves the use of combination drugs designed to reduce viable bacteria as rapidly as possible in order to minimize the risk of ineffective treatment in those patients infected by drug-resistant bacteria (Cooke 1985). A 3 to 6 month regimen with four standard drugs in the initial phase, for all forms of TB excluding meningitis (which may need to be treated for a longer period (Ormerod 1990)), supervised by physicians with full training and care provided by nurse specialists, is recommended in the UK (Joint Tuberculosis Committee of the British Thoracic Society 1998).

An increase in multidrug-resistant TB (MDR-TB) is a major cause for concern (Hayward et al. 1995). In the USA, cases have been reported of transmission of Mycobacterium tuberculosis to patients and staff, including multidrug-resistant strains (Pitchenik et al. 1990; Center for Disease Control 1990). TB resistance to isoniazid and rifampicin is termed multiple drug-resistant tuberculosis (MDR-TB) (Drobniewski 1998). Outbreaks of hospital acquired MDR-TB have been associated with mortality rates of 72–89% (Beck-Sage et al. 1992). Deaths have occurred among health care staff in the USA who are believed to have contracted tuberculosis at work (Di Perri et al. 1992). Resistance to drugs in the UK remains low but is rising. Alternative drugs are available but are less effective and are more often associated with side-effects than standard drug regimens (DoH 1998). Rates of MDR-TB in the UK remain low (DoH 1998). If the resistant pattern is extensive there may be no suitable treatment that the patient can tolerate. Outbreaks of MDR-TB have occurred in London; one involved seven HIV positive patients where the index case and two contacts died. Cross-infection was due to the index patient being cared for in a positive pressure single room (Breathnach et al. 1998).

European evaluation of treatment outcomes is ongoing (Veen et al. 1998). Transmission of MDR-TB to health care workers has been seen (Center for Disease Control 1990). Respiratory protection is an important element of TB infection control, especially important during procedures such as bronchoscopy and autopsy (Nicas 1998). The recent increase in MDR-TB has meant that health care workers should wear a dust/mist respirator mask rather than a surgical mask (McCullough *et al.* 1997) when caring for smear-positive TB patients where there is a risk of MDR-TB (Chen *et al.* 1994).

Coker (1998) explains how failure of treatment compliance is the basis of a drug-resistant TB epidemic. In New York by 1989, the proportion of patients completing their treatment programme was as low as 60%. This meant that patients remained infectious, relapses were more frequent and drug resistance flourished. Vagrants, alcoholics and patients with learning difficulties would be among those expected to be non-compliant patients. Simple urine tests are available to check for the patient's adherence to treatment (Ormerod 1990). Improvement was only seen when infection control improved, services were coordinated and observed therapy programmes were implemented.

TB continues to be a notifiable disease (DoH 1995). It is the responsibility of the Medical Officer for Environmental Health to follow up all contacts of infected people. This has proved to be a valuable and worthwhile procedure (British Thoracic and Tuberculosis Association 1978). Contact tracing involves identifying the index case, plus those who may have become infected. As transmission requires prolonged close contact with a smear-positive case, contact tracing is generally limited to those from the same household or equivalent. If transmission is shown to have occurred among this close contact group a wider contact tracing may be required, including family, friends and work colleagues (DoH 1998). TB is found in 1% of contacts; about 10% of notified cases each year are found through contact tracing (Ejidokun *et al.* 1998). Only contacts of smear-positive TB infected persons are followed up as the transmission from smear-negative persons is very low. One study evaluated 85 young children who had been closely and regularly in contact with a smear-negative child care assistant, and no evidence of transmission was found (Millership *et al.* 1998). The infection control doctor with the consultant in communicable disease will evaluate whether hospital contacts will be followed up; generally this will only involve immunocompromised patients and health care workers. Contact tracing is likely to start from the date one month before the patient became symptomatic. In cases without symptoms it may be necessary to look back over 3 months (DoH 1998). Advice on handling outbreaks of TB is available (National Health Service Executive 1993, 1995).

The World Health Organization and the International Union Against Tuberculosis and Lung Disease have published two joint statements, one on the prevention of TB in people infected with HIV and one on the prevention of the transmission of TB in health care settings in developing countries (WHO 1993a, 1993b). Guidance in these statements reflects advice published by the Joint Tuberculosis Committee of the British Thoracic Society in 1990 and 1994.

Prevention

The priorities for TB control are early detection of cases, examination of contacts, barrier nursing if appropriate and immunization of people with a negative tuberculin skin test, with Bacillus Calmette-Guérin vaccine (BCG). BCG vaccine contains a live attenuated strain derived from *Mycobacterium bovis*. Since 1953, children are immunized before they leave school. The vaccine has been shown to be 70 to 80% effective in protecting against TB, with protection lasting at least 15 years. It is recommended that all health care workers who have not had BCG and may have contact with infectious patients or specimens are immunized with BCG. A tuberculin skin test must be carried out before BCG immunization. The test assesses the person's sensitivity to tuberculin protein – the greater the reaction the more likely the individual is to have active disease. Those with a strongly positive test need to be referred to a chest clinic for assessment (DoH 1996). BCG is less effective in HIV positive persons and, being a live vaccine, is not recommended in the UK. Any immunity from a previous BCG can be expected to reduce as the CD4 count falls (DoH 1998).

Certain professions, for example those working in hospitals, prisons, care of older people homes and schools, should be screened on employment. This may include a tuberculin test and chest radiography (Jachuck 1988) for staff who have not received a BCG vaccination in the past. TB can be transmitted from patients to health care workers, but in areas of low incidence where infection control practices are good the risk of transmission is negligible (Riley *et al.* 1997). Transmission from health care worker to patient rarely occurs (Menzies *et al.* 1995). There are four recorded incidences of hospital staff being diagnosed with smear-positive pulmonary TB. All relevant patients and staff who had had close contact were followed up, but no cases of TB were found (National Health Service Executive 1998). However, outbreaks involving children in a hospital nursery where infection and active disease developed relatively quickly have been seen (Nivin *et al.* 1998).

Staff in contact with untreated, smear-positive patients for a week or more should be reported to the occupational health department, and a chest X-ray arranged for 6 months' time. However, if the employee develops suspicious symptoms such as an unexplained cough lasting longer than 3 weeks, persistent fever or weight loss, then a full examination must be undertaken.

The World Health Organization advises that control of TB relies on consideration of the type of TB, presence of concomitant infection with HIV and patient characteristics (Maher & Nunn 1998). Van Buynder (1998) suggests that control in developed countries must focus on the groups at risk of TB, which includes ethnic minorities, the homeless and those with impaired immunity. Singleton *et al.* (1997) state that patients with TB who are non-adherent to therapy or who have complicated medical and social problems pose a threat to public health. Therefore, specialized medical management for patients to complete therapy in a safe and supportive environment is essential.

Patients infected with HIV predispose to develop TB (Haramati & Jenny-Avital 1998). Preventive treatment against TB in adults infected with HIV has been seen to reduce the incidence of infection (Wilkinson *et al.* 1998). TB is more likely to be diagnosed in patients unaware of their HIV diagnosis and therefore not offered prophylaxis (Porter *et al.* 1996). Early diagnosis and effective treatment of TB among HIV infected patients is critical for curing and minimizing the negative effects of TB on HIV progression (Center for Disease Control 1998b), as TB increases the risk of death among HIV positive persons independently of CD4 cell counts (Chaisson *et al.* 1998).

Nursing care

Patients do not necessarily require admission to hospital but can be investigated and treated on an outpatient basis. Generally, home contacts will have already been exposed and will be routinely contacted and investigated (DoH 1998). Segregation while undergoing tests or routine visits to the outpatient department is required to prevent more people being exposed.

Evaluation of infectivity will be necessary. Sputum smear-positive people are considered infectious and those whose results are not yet known are treated as potentially positive. People who have smear-negative culture-positive pulmonary disease, plus non-pulmonary disease, are considered not to be infectious (DoH 1998). Infectious and potentially infectious patients should be cared for in a single room with the door closed. Patients being cared for with immunocompromised persons must be placed in a negative pressure room which is continuously and automatically monitored. All patients with known or suspected MDR-TB must be placed in a negative pressure single room with the door closed. If the patient is HIV antibody positive this room should be near, but physically separated from, the HIV ward (DoH 1998).

Patients require careful explanation to ensure they and their visitors comply with the barrier nursing precautions. Initially visitors should be restricted to those who have already had contact. Visitors who themselves are immunocompromised should only visit after careful discussion with and agreement by their own physician. Paediatric facilities and restrictions should be the same as the adults' (Kellerman *et al.* 1998).

Patients must be taught to cover their mouths when coughing to prevent droplet spread, and to wash their hands after coughing. Patients must expectorate into sputum pots with tight fitting lids, and the pots must be changed frequently. As compliance to therapy can be poor, patients must be encouraged and, if necessary, supervised to ensure compliance with the drug treatment. Unconscious patients will need to have their drugs administered via a nasogastric tube, intravenously or intramuscularly (Ormerod 1990).

Legislation

Patients with TB who are non-adherent to therapy or who have complicated medical and social problems may pose a threat to others (Singleton *et al.* 1997). Sections 37 and 38 of the *Public Health (Control of Disease Act 1984)* provide legal powers to control infected patients who refuse to comply with treatment and pose a threat to public health. The Control of Substances Hazardous to Health (COSHH) Regulations 1994 include issues such as TB and disinfectants. These guidelines requires a risk assessment, and the provision of adequate information, instruction and training to be carried out where an employee is exposed to substances hazardous to health.

References and further reading

Alvarez, S. *et al.* (1984) Extrapulmonary tuberculosis revisited. A review of experience at Boston City and other hospitals. *Medicine (Baltimore)*, **63**, 25.

Ayliffe, G.A.J. *et al.* (1984) *Chemical Disinfection in Hospital*, p. 3. Public Health Laboratory Service, London.

Beck-Sage, C. *et al.* (1992) Hospital outbreak of multidrug resistant *Mycobacterium tuberculosis* infection: factors in transmission to staff and HIV-infected patients. *J Am Med Assoc*, **268**, 1280–86.

Breathnach, A.S. *et al.* (1998) An outbreak of multi drug resistant tuberculosis in a London teaching hospital. *J Hosp Infect*, **39**(2), 111–17.

British Thoracic and Tuberculosis Association (1975) Tuberculosis among immigrants related to length of residence in England and Wales. *Br Med J*, **3**, 698–9.

British Thoracic and Tuberculosis Association (1978) A study of standardized contact procedure in tuberculosis. *Tubercle*, **59**, 245–59.

Center for Disease Control (1990) Guidelines for preventing the transmission of tuberculosis in health care settings with special focus on HIV-related issues. *Morb Mort Week Rep*, **39**, Suppl RR-17, 1–29.

Center for Disease Control (1993) Estimates of future global tuberculosis morbidity and mortality. *Morb Mort Week Rep*, **42**, 961–4.

Center for Disease Control (1998a) Recommendations for prevention and control of tuberculosis among foreign-born persons. Report of the working group on tuberculosis among foreign born persons. *Morb Mort Week Rep*, **47**(RR-16), 1–29.

Center for Disease Control (1998b) Prevention and treatment of tuberculosis among patients infected with HIV: principles of therapy and revised recommendations. *Morb Mort Week Rep*, **47**(RR-20), 1–51.

Chaisson, R. (1993) Mycobacterial infections and AIDS. *Curr Opin Infect Dis*, **6**, 237–43.

Chaisson, R.E. *et al.* (1998) Impact of opportunistic disease on survival in patents with HIV infection. *AIDS*, **12**(1), 29–33.

Chen, S.K. *et al.* (1994) Evaluation of single use mask and respirators for protection of health care workers against mycobacterial aerosols. *Am J Infect Control*, **22**(2), 65–74.

Coker, R. (1998) Lessons from New York's tuberculosis epidemic, *Br Med J*, **317**, 616.

Cooke, N.J. (1985) Treatment of tuberculosis. *Br Med J*, **291**, 497–8.

Cowle, R. (1995) TB: cure, care and control. *Nurs Times*, **91**(38), 29–30.

DHSS (1986) *Safety Information Bulletin 28*. DHSS, London.

Di Perri, G. *et al.* (1992) Transmission of HIV associated tuberculosis of health care workers. *Lancet*, **340**(8820), 682.

DoH (1995) *Hospital Infection Control. Guidance on the control of infection in hospitals*. Lancashire Health Publications Unit, 2383 IP 25K, February 1995.

DoH (1996) *Immunisation Against Infectious Disease.* Stationery Office, London.

DoH (1998) *The Prevention and Control of Tuberculosis in the United Kingdom. HSC 1998/196.* Stationery Office, London.

Drobniewski, F.A. (1998) Diagnosing multidrug resistant tuberculosis in Britain. *Br Med J*, **317**, 1263–4.

Drobniewski, F.A. *et al.* (1994) Molecular biology in the diagnosis and epidemiology of tuberculosis. *J Hosp Infect*, **28**, 249–63.

Ejidokun, O.O., Ramaiah, S. & Sandhu, S. (1998) A cluster of tuberculosis cases in a family. *Commun Dis Public Health*, **1**(4), 259–62.

Ginesu, F. *et al.* (1998) Microbiological diagnosis of tuberculosis: a comparison of old and new methods. *J Chemother*, **10**(4), 295–300.

Goldsmith, M.F. (1993) New reports make recommendations, ask for resources to stem TB epidemic. *J Am Med Assoc*, **269**(2), 187–8, 191.

Guerrero, A. *et al.* (1997) Nosocomial transmission of *Mycobacterium bovis* resistant to 11 drugs in people with advanced HIV-1 infection. *Lancet*, **350**(9093), 1738–42.

Haramati, L.B. & Jenny-Avital, E.R. (1998) Approach to the diagnosis of pulmonary disease in patients infected with the human immunodeficiency virus. *J Thorac Imaging*, **13**(4), 247–60.

Hayward, C.M., Herrman, J.L. & Griffin, G.E. (1995) Drug resistant tuberculosis: mechanisms and management. *Br J Hosp Med*, **54**(10), 494–500.

Honeybourne, D. & Neumann, C.S. (1997) An audit of bronchoscopy practice in the United Kingdom: a survey of adherence to national guidelines. *Thorax*, **52**(8), 709–13.

Jachuck, S.J. (1988) Is a pre-employment chest radiograph necessary for NHS employees? *Br Med J*, **296**, 1187–8.

Joint Tuberculosis Committee of the British Thoracic Society (1990) Control and prevention of tuberculosis in Britain: an updated code of practice. *Br Med J*, **300**, 995–9.

Joint Tuberculosis Committee of the British Thoracic Society (1994) Control and prevention of tuberculosis in the United Kingdom: Code of Practice 1994. *Thorax*, **49**, 1193–200.

Joint Tuberculosis Committee of the British Thoracic Society (1998) Chemotherapy and management of tuberculosis in the United Kingdom. *Thorax*, **53**(7), 536–48.

Kellerman, S.E. *et al.* (1998) APIC and CDC survey of *Mycobacterium tuberculosis* isolation and control practices in hospitals caring for children. Part 2: environmental and administrative controls. *Am J Infect Control*, **26**(5), 483–7.

Lamden, K. *et al.* (1996) Opportunist mycobacteria in England and Wales 1982–1994. *Commun Dis Rep CDR Rev*, **6**(11), R147–51.

Loudon, R.G. *et al.* (1969) Cough frequency and infectivity in patient with pulmonary tuberculosis. *Am Rev Resp Dis*, **99**, 109–11.

McCullough, N.V. *et al.* (1997) Collection of three bacterial aerosols by respirator and surgical mask filters under varying conditions of flow and relative humidity. *Ann Occup Hyg*, **41**(6), 677–90.

Maher, D. & Nunn, P. (1998) Evaluation and determinants of outcome of tuberculosis treatment. *Bull World Health Organ*, **76**(3), 307–308.

Mairtin, D.O. *et al.* (1998) The effect of a badger removal programme on the incidence of tuberculosis in an Irish cattle population. *Pre Vet Med*, **34**(1), 47–56.

Mangtani, P. *et al.* (1995) Socioeconomic deprivation and notification rates for tuberculosis in London during 1987–1991. *Br Med J*, **310**, 963–6.

Menzies, D. *et al.* (1995) Review article: current concepts: tuberculosis among health care workers. *N Engl J Med*, **332**, 92–8.

Michele, T.M. *et al.* (1997) Transmission of *Mycobacterium tuberculosis* by a fiberoptic bronchoscope. Identification by DNA fingerprinting. *JAMA*, **278**(13), 1093–5.

Millership, S., Roberts, C.M. & Irwin, D.J. (1998) Screening child playgroup contacts of an adult with smear negative tuberculosis. *Commun Dis Pub Health*, **1**(4), 283–4.

Mims, C.A. *et al.* (1993) *Medical Microbiology.* Mosby, London.

National Health Service Executive (1993) *Public Health: Responsibilities of the NHS and the Roles of Others. HSG (93) 56.* Stationery Office, London.

National Health Service Executive (1995) *Hospital Infection Control: Guidance on the Control of Infection in Hospitals. HSG (95) 10 1995.* Stationery Office, London.

National Health Service Executive (1998) *Communicable Disease Control in the Thames Regions in 1997*, pp. 8–11. Department of Health, London.

Nicas, M. (1998) Assessing the relative importance of the components of an occupational tuberculosis control program. *J Occup Environ Med*, **40**(7), 648–54.

Nivin, B. *et al.* (1998) A continuing outbreak of multidrug-resistant tuberculosis, with transmission in a hospital nursery. *Clin Infect Dis*, **26**(2), 303–307.

Ormerod, L.P. (1990) Chemotherapy and management of tuberculosis in the United Kingdom: recommendations of the Joint Tuberculosis Committee of the British Thoracic Society. *Thorax*, **45**, 403–408.

Ormerod, L.P. (1996) Tuberculosis and immigration. *Br J Hosp Med*, **56**(5), 209–12.

Perneger, T.V. *et al.* (1995) Does the onset of tuberculosis in AIDS predict shorter survival? Results of a cohort study in 17 European countries over 13 years. *Br Med J*, **311**, 1468–71.

Pilheu, J.A. (1998) Tuberculosis 2000: problems and solutions. *Int J Tuberc Lung Dis*, **2**(9), 696–703.

Pitchenik, A.E. *et al.* (1990) Outbreaks of drug-resistant tuberculosis to health care workers and HIV infected patients in urban hospitals. *Morb Mort Week Rep*, **39**, 718–22.

Porter, K. *et al.* (1996) AIDS: defining disease in the UK. The impact of PCP prophylaxis and twelve years of change. *Int J STD AIDS*, **7**(4), 252–7.

Public Health Laboratory Service Communicable Disease Surveillance Centre Supplement (1998a) Infectious diseases in England and Wales: April 1966 to June 1997. *Commun Dis Rep*, **8**(2), S3.

Public Health Laboratory Service Communicable Disease Surveillance Centre (1998b) National survey of tuberculosis in England and Wales 1998. *Commun Dis Rep*, **8**(24), 209.

Quigley, C. (1997) Investigation of tuberculosis in an adolescent. The outbreak control team. *Commun Dis Rep CDR Rev*, **7**(8), R113–16.

Riley, M. *et al.* (1997) Tuberculosis in health care service employees in Northern Ireland. *Respir Med*, **91**(9), 546–50.

Singleton, L. *et al.* (1997) Long term hospitalization for tuberculosis control. Experience with a medical-psychosocial inpatient unit. *JAMA*, **278**(10), 838–42.

Subcommittee of the Joint Tuberculosis Committee of the British Thoracic Society (1990) Control and prevention of tuberculosis in Britain. An updated code of practice. *Br Med J*, **300**, 995–9.

Van Buynder, P. (1998) Enhanced surveillance of tuberculosis in England and Wales: circling the wagons. *Commun Dis Public Health*, **1**(4), 219–20.

Veen, J. *et al.* (1998) Standardized tuberculosis treatment outcome monitoring in Europe. *Eur Resp*, **12**(2), 505–10.

Washington, L. & Miller, W.T. (1998) Mycobacterial infection in immunocompromised patients. *J Thorac Imag*, **13**(4), 271–81.

Watson, J.M. *et al.* (1993) Tuberculosis and HIV estimates of the overlap in England and Wales. *Thorax*, **48**, 199–203.

WHO (1993a) Tuberculosis preventive therapy in HIV-infected

individuals. A joint statement of the World Health Organization Tuberculosis Programme and the Global Programme on AIDS, and the International Union Against Tuberculosis and Lung Disease. *Week Epidemiol Rec*, **68**(49), 361–4.

WHO (1993b) Control of tuberculosis transmission in health care settings. A joint statement of the World Health Organization Tuberculosis Programme and the International Union Against Tuberculosis and Lung Disease. *Week Epidemiol Rec*, **68**(50), 369–71.

Wilkinson, D., Squire, S.B. & Garner, P. (1998) Effect of preventive treatment for tuberculosis in adults infected with HIV. *Br Med J*, **317**(7159), 625–9.

Working Party (1998) Cleaning and disinfection of equipment for gastrointestinal endoscopy. Report of a Working Party of the British Society of Gastroenterology Endoscopy Committee. *Gut*, **42**(4), 585–93.

Young, L.S. (1996) Mycobacterial infection in immunocompromised patients. *Curr Opin Infect Dis*, **9**, 240–45.

Bladder Lavage and Irrigation

Definitions

Lavage

Bladder lavage is the washing out of the bladder with sterile fluid.

Irrigation

Bladder irrigation is the continuous washing out of the bladder with sterile fluid.

Indications

Bladder lavage or irrigation is indicated for the following reasons:

Lavage

1 To clear an obstructed catheter.
2 To remove the potential souces of obstruction, e.g. blood clots or sediment from infection.

Irrigation

1 To prevent the formation and retention of blood clots, e.g. following prostatic surgery.
2 On rare occasions to remove heavily contaminated material from a diseased urinary bladder.

Reference material

Solutions used for lavage and irrigation

A number of solutions are available for cleansing the bladder and the selection of a particular solution will depend on its therapeutic properties in relation to the patient's needs.

0.9% sodium chloride is the agent most commonly recommended for lavage and irrigation and should be used in every case unless an alternative solution is prescribed. It is isotonic so it does not affect the body's fluid or electrolyte levels, therefore large volumes may be used as necessary. Three litre bags of 0.9% sodium chloride are available for irrigation purposes.

Careful monitoring of bladder irrigation is essential for, although not a common complication, absorption of irrigation fluid can occur. This leads to electrolyte imbalance and circulatory overload, producing a potentially critical situation. Absorption is most likely to occur in theatre where irrigation fluid, devoid of sodium or potassium, is forced under pressure into the prostatic veins (Fillingham & Douglas 1997), but the risk remains while irrigation continues. 0.9% sodium chloride is not used during surgery as the electrolytes it contains interfere with the diathermy therefore glycine is used (Gilbert & Gobbi 1989).

Water should never be used to irrigate the bladder as it will be readily absorbed by the process of osmosis. Water may be used as a purely mechanical means to flush out catheters for patients at home (Blannin & Hobden 1980).

The use of bladder wash-outs is an area where there is considerable confusion and controversy (Getliffe 1996; Rew 1999). Poor levels of knowledge have been found among nurses with regard to the type of wash-out fluid to use in specific circumstances and also the frequency of administration (Bailey 1991). Bladder lavage has been used in the management of catheter associated infections, catheter encrustation and blockage (Getliffe 1996).

A number of pre-packed sterile wash-out solutions are available; these include the following:

1 0.9% sodium chloride is used for mechanical flushing to remove tissue debris and small blood clots.
2 Chlorhexidine 0.02% is used to prevent or reduce bacterial growth, in particular *Escherichia coli* and *Klebsiella*.
3 Mandelic acid (1%) is used to prevent the growth of urease-producing bacteria by acidifying the urine.
4 6% citric acid solution, 'solution R', is used to dissolve persistent crystallization in the catheter or bladder.
5 3.23% citric acid and magnesium oxide solution, 'Suby G', is used to prevent, and dissolve, crystallization in the catheter or bladder.

Catheter-associated infection

Catheter-associated urinary tract infections are a common complication occurring in over 90% of patients within 4 weeks of catheterization (Jewes *et al.* 1988). Antibiotics will not prevent infection in long-term catheterized patients and their use is not recommended unless systemic symptoms are present (Kennedy & Brocklehurst 1982; Kunin 1987). Bladder wash-outs using antibiotic or antiseptic solutions in order to prevent, reduce or treat urinary tract infections have been commonly used, but these have been found to be ineffective.

Chlorhexidine has been shown to be ineffective against a number of commonly occurring pathogens. It may, in fact, remove sensitive bacteria in the normal urethral flora, allowing subsequent colonization by resistant organisms (Davies *et al.* 1987; Stickler *et al.* 1987; King & Stickler 1992). Other solutions reviewed include noxythiolin, providone iodine, acetic acid and a range of antibiotics (Gopal Roa & Elliott 1988). These have also been shown not to be effective. Therefore their use in long-term catheterized patients is not advocated (Stickler & Chawla 1987; Stickler 1990).

Catheter associated urinary infections are difficult to treat as bacteria adhere to the surface of the catheter in the form of a biofilm. Bacteria in this biofilm are generally less susceptible to antimicrobial agents than their free-living counterparts (Gristina *et al.* 1987). Bacteria in the urine may be successfully killed but may persist in the biofilm and restart the cycle of infection (Stickler *et al.* 1987). As yet there is no catheter material that resists biofilm formation in the clinical setting (Getliffe 1996).

Catheter encrustations and blockages

Recurrent catheter encrustation and blockage is a common problem with approximately 50% of catheterized patients being susceptible (Kohler-Ockmore 1992; Getliffe 1994a). Catheter blockage may occur as the result of detrusor spasm, twisted drainage tubing or constipation, but the most common reason is the formation of encrustation on the catheter surface and within its lumen (Getliffe 1996).

Catheter encrustations commonly consist of magnesium, ammonium phosphate and calcium phosphate (Hedelin *et al.* 1984; Cox *et al.* 1987) which precipitate from urine when it becomes alkaline during infection from urease-secreting micro-organisms (Mobley & Warren 1987; Getliffe 1996). The urease producers implicated most commonly in catheter encrustations are of the *Proteus* species (Getliffe 1996).

The development of catheter encrustations may lead to:

1 Blockage of the catheter lumen
2 Bypassing of urine
3 Retention of urine
4 Pain
5 Recatheterization

(Rew 1999).

Getliffe's (1994a) study attempted to identify characteristics of patients who were at greater risk of obstructing their catheters. Patients who 'blocked' their catheters were found to have high urinary pH and ammonia concentrations. High ammonia concentration and alkaline urine are found when urine is infected with urease producing microorganisms, such as *Proteus mirabilis*. Significantly more females were classed as 'blockers', this may be due to the greater risks females have of developing catheter associated urinary infections (Kennedy *et al.* 1983), as the shorter female urethra may allow more rapid colonization. 'Blockers' were also found to be significantly less mobile than 'non-blockers'. There was no significant relationship noted between non-blockers and high average daily fluid intake; this study therefore does not support the advice conventionally given to 'drink plenty' to reduce mineral precipitation.

There have been very few clinical studies of the use of bladder wash-outs. 0.9% sodium chloride has been shown to have no effect in dissolving encrustations but may, through the mechanical effect of flushing, dislodge debris (Flack 1993).

A study carried out by Kennedy *et al.* (1992) showed that citric acid solution with (Suby G) and without magnesium oxide (solution R) administered twice weekly for 3 weeks did not have a demonstrable effect in preventing crystal formation. However, 6% citric acid solution R has been shown to dissolve fragments of struvite renal calculi following lithotripsy (Holden & Rao 1991). Catheter encrustations may be dissolved using this solution but potential inflammatory tissue reactions limit its use (Getliffe 1996). Getliffe (1996) suggests it may be used prior to catheter removal to dissolve external encrustations, which cause pain and tissue trauma on withdrawal of the catheter. Getliffe's (1994b) *in vitro* study suggested that mandelic acid solution may be particularly effective in reducing encrustation.

Mandelic acid 1% has been shown to be effective in removing *Pseudomonas* species from the urine of catheterized patients, although it needs to be used twice a day for a long period (on average 19 days). It has also shown to be a biocidal agent against some biofilms of single or mixed bacterial species (Stickler & Hewitt 1991). This agent is thought to have a dual role, first in reducing urinary pH and second in dissolving struvite and calcium phosphate deposits. However, tissue reactions to mandelic acid 1% in clinical situations have yet to be demonstrated, as does its efficacy in the presence of urinary elements such as mucin and organic debris (Getliffe 1996; Rew 1999).

Potential risks to the bladder urothelium associated with bladder lavage solutions have raised concerns. Dilute acid solutions have been shown to remove the surface layer of mucus in the bladder (Parsons *et al.* 1970) and an increased shedding of urethelial cells has been observed following wash-outs (Elliot *et al.* 1989). Reassessment of bladder irrigation methods and the indication for their use is therefore called for.

To date there has been no research to advise on the frequency with which wash-outs should be used or the volumes of solution needed. Recently it has been suggested that 'mini' wash-outs regularly performed would be effective at reducing encrustations and minimizing irritant effects on the bladder (Getliffe 1994a; Getliffe & Dolman 1997). A catheter lumen holds 4–5 ml of fluid, therefore smaller volumes of 10–20 ml would still completely fill the catheter lumen and bathe the catheter tip. Therefore the bladder mucosa would not be exposed to large volumes of wash-out solution. Getliffe (1994a) suggests that wash-outs could then be performed more frequently without increasing the risk of tissue damage. The researchers working in this area identify the need for further work to be carried out in the whole area of bladder lavage.

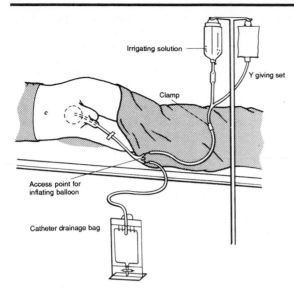

Irrigating solution

Y giving set

Clamp

Access point for
inflating balloon

Catheter drainage bag

Figure 5.1 Closed urinary drainage system with provision
for intermittent or continuous irrigation.

Patient assessment

There are a number of risks associated with bladder lavage
and the procedure should not be undertaken lightly.
Patients should be assessed and a catheter history should
be noted before the decision to use bladder wash-outs.
Assessment of all aspects of catheter care should be taken,
including:

1 Patient activity and mobility
2 Diet and fluid intake
3 Standards of patient hygiene
4 Patients' and/or carers' ability to care for the catheter

(Getliffe 1996; Rew 1999).

Newly catheterized patients should be monitored to
ascertain how long the catheter remains in situ before
showing signs of blockage, without any interference with
prophylactic wash-outs. A catheter history should be
established, and documented, to enable future care to be
planned (Rew 1999). Norberg et al. (1983) suggest that
three to five consecutive catheters should be observed
before treatment, if needed, is instigated.

In patients where a pattern can be established, scheduled catheter changes prior to likely blockages are an
important aspect of their management (Getliffe 1996).
In patients where no clear pattern emerges, or for whom
frequent catheter changes are traumatic, acidic bladder
lavages can be beneficial in reducing catheter encrustations (Getliffe 1996; Rew 1999).

Cytotoxic agents given intravesically

For details on the administration of cytotoxic agents, see
Chap. 10, Cytotoxic Drugs, Guidelines • Intravesical
instillation of cytotoxic drugs.

Catheters used for irrigation

A three-way urinary catheter must be used for irrigation in
order that fluid may simultaneously be run into, and
drained out from, the bladder. This catheter is commonly
passed in theatre when irrigation is required, e.g. after
prostatectomy (Maxfield et al. 1994). Occasionally if a
patient is admitted with a heavily contaminated bladder,
e.g. blood clots, bladder irrigation may be started on the
ward. If the patient has a two-way catheter, this must be
replaced with a three-way type (Fig. 5.1).

It is recommended that a three-way catheter is passed if
frequent intravesical instillations of drugs or antiseptic
solutions are prescribed and the risk of catheter obstruction is not considered to be very great. In such cases the
most important factor is minimizing the risk of introducing
infection and maintaining a closed urinary drainage
system, for which the three-way catheter allows.

References and further reading

Bailey, S. (1991) Using bladder washouts. *Nurs Times*, **87**(24),
75–6.
Baillie, L. (1987) Chlorhexidine resistance among bacteria iso-
lated from urine of catheterised patients. *J Hosp Infect*, **10**, 83–6.
Blannin, J. & Hobden, J. (1980) The catheter of choice. *Nurs
Times*, **76**, 2092–3.
Brocklehurst, J.C. & Brocklehurst, S. (1978) Management of
indwelling catheters. *B J Urol*, **50**, 102–105.
Bruce, A.W. et al. (1974) The problem of catheter encrustation.
Can Med Assoc J, **111**, 238–41.
Cox, A.J. et al. (1987) Calcium phosphate in catheter encrusta-
tion. *Br J Urol*, **59**, 159–63.
Cox, A.J., Harries, J.E., Hukins, D.W.L. et al. (1987) Calcium
phosphate in catheter encrustation. *Br J Urol*, **59**, 159–63.
Datta, P.K. (1981) The post-prostatectomy patient. *Nurs Times*,
77, 1759–61.
Davies, A.J. et al. (1987) Does instillation of chlorhexidine into
the bladder of catheterised geriatric patients help reduce bacteriuria? *J Hosp Infect*, **9**, 72–5.
Dudley, M.N. & Barriere, S.L. (1981) Antimicrobial irrigations in
the prevention and treatment of catheter-related urinary tract
infections. *Am J Hosp Pharm*, **38**, 59–65.
Elliott, T. (1990) Disadvantages of bladder irrigation (in catheter-
ized patients. Brief research report). *Nurs Times*, **86**, 52.
Elliott, T.S. et al. (1989) Bladder irrigation or irritation? *Br J Urol*,
64, 391–4.
Ferrie, B.G. et al. (1979) Long-term urethral catheter drainage. *Br
Med J*, **279**, 1046–7.
Fillingham, S. & Douglas, J. (1997) *Urological Nursing*. Baillière
Tindall, London.
Flack, S. (1993) Finding the best solution. *Nurs Times*, **11**, 68–74.
Getliffe, K.A. (1994a) The characteristics and management of
patients with recurrent blockage of long-term urinary catheters.
J Adv Nurs, **20**, 140–49.
Getliffe, K.A. (1994b) The use of bladder wash-outs to reduce
urinary catheter encrustation. *Br J Urol*, **73**, 696–700.
Getliffe, K.A. (1996) Bladder instillations and bladder washouts in
the management of catheterized patients. *J Adv Nurs*, **23**,
548–54.
Getliffe, K.A. & Dolman, M. (1997) *Promoting Continence: A
Clinical and Research Resource*. Baillière Tindall, London.
Gilbert, V. & Gobbi, M. (1989) Bladder irrigation (principles and
methods). *Nurs Times Nurs Mirror*, **85**, 40–42.

Gopal Rao, G. & Elliott, T.S.J. (1988) Bladder irrigation. *Age Ageing*, **17**, 373–8.

Griffith, D.P. & Musher, O.N. (1976) Urease: the primary cause of infection induced urinary stones. *Invest Urol*, **13**(5), 346–82.

Gristina, A.G., Hobgood, C.D., Webb, L.X. & Myrvik, Q.N. (1987) Adhesive colonisation of biomaterials and antibiotic resistance. *Biomaterials*, **8**, 423–6.

Harper, W. (1981) An appraisal of 12 solutions used for bladder irrigation or instillation. *Br J Urol*, **53**, 433–8.

Harper, W. & Matz, L. (1975) The effect of chlorhexidine irrigation of the bladder in the rat. *Br J Urol*, **47**, 539–43.

Harper, W. & Matz, L. (1976) Further studies on effects of irrigating solutions on rat bladders. *Br J Urol*, **48**, 463–7.

Hedelin, H., Eddeland, A., Larsson, L. et al. (1984) The composition of catheter encrustations, including the effects of allopurinol treatment. *Br J Urol*, **56**, 250–54.

Holden, D. & Rao, P.N. (1991) Management of staghorn stones using a combination of lithotripsy, percutaneous nephrolithotomy and solution R irrigation. *Br J Urol*, **67**, 13–17.

Jewes, L.A., Gillespie, W.A., Leadbetter, A. et al. (1988) Bacteriuria and bacteraemia in patients with long-term indwelling catheters: a domiciliary study. *J Med Microbiol*, **26**, 61–5.

Kennedy, A. (1984) Trial of new bladder washout system. *Nurs Times*, **80**, 48–51.

Kennedy, A.P. & Brocklehurst, J.C. (1982) The nursing management of patients with long-term indwelling catheters. *J Adv Nurs*, **7**, 411–17.

Kennedy, A.P. et al. (1983) Factors relating to the problems of long-term catheterization. *J Adv Nurs*, **8**, 207–12.

Kennedy, A.P. et al. (1992) Assessment of the use of bladder washouts/instillations in patients with long term indwelling catheters. *Br J Urol*, **70**, 610–15.

King, J.B. & Stickler, D.J. (1992) The effects of repeated instillations of antiseptics on catheter-associated urinary tract infections. *Urol Res*, **20**, 403–407.

Kohler-Ockmore, J. (1992) Urinary catheter complications. *J District Nurs*, **10**(8), 18–20.

Kunin, C.M. (1987) *Detection, Prevention and Management of Urinary Tract Infections*, 4th edn. Lea and Febiger, Philadelphia.

Lowthian, P. (1991) Using bladder syringes sparingly. *Nurs Times*, **87**(10), 61–4.

Macaulay, D. (1994) Urinary drainage systems. In: *Urological Nursing* (ed. C. Laker). Scutari Press, Harrow.

Martindale, W. (1982) *The Extra Pharmacopoeia*, 28th edn. Pharmaceutical Press, London.

Maxfield, J. et al. (1994) Prostatic problems. In: *Urological Nursing* (ed. C. Laker). Scutari Press, Harrow.

Mobley, H.L.T. & Warren, J.W. (1987) Urease positive bacteriuria and obstruction of long-term urinary catheters. *J Clin Microbiol*, **25**, 2216–17.

Norberg, B., Norberg, A. & Parkhede, U. (1983) The spontaneous variation in catheter life in long-stay geriatric patients with indwelling catheters. *Gerontology*, **29**, 332–5.

Parsons, C.L., Mulholland, S.G. & Anwar, H. (1970) Antibacterial activity of bladder surface mucin duplicated by exogenous glycosaminoglycan (heparin). *Infect Immun*, **25**, 552–4.

Rew, M. (1999) Use of catheter maintenance solutions for long-term catheters. *Br J Nurs*, **8**(11), 708–15.

Roe, B.H. (1989) Use of bladder washouts: a study of nurses' recommendations. *J Adv Nurs*, **14**(6), 494–500.

Roe, B. (1990) The basis for sound practice. *Nur Stand*, **4**, 25–7.

Slade, N. & Gillespie, W.A. (1985) *The Urinary Tract and the Catheter – Infection and Other Problems*. John Wiley, Chichester.

Stickler, D.J. (1990) The role of antiseptics in the management of patients undergoing short term indwelling bladder catheterisation. *J Hosp Infect*, **16**, 89–108.

Stickler, D.J. & Chawla, J.C. (1987) The role of antiseptics in the management of patients with long term indwelling bladder catheters. *J Hosp Infect*, **10**, 219–28.

Stickler, D.J. & Hewitt, P. (1991) Activity of antiseptic against biofilms of mixed bacterial species growing on silicone surfaces. *Eur J Microbiol Infect*, **10**, 416–21.

Stickler, D.J., Clayton, C.L. & Chawla, J.C. (1987) The resistance of urinary tract pathogens to chlorhexidine bladder washouts. *J Hosp Infect*, **10**, 28–39.

Stickler, D.J. et al. (1981) Some observations on the activity of three antiseptics used as bladder irrigants in the treatment of UTI in patients with indwelling catheters. *Paraplegia*, **19**, 325–33.

Waghorn, D.J. et al. (1988) Urinary catheters. *Br Med J*, **296**, 1250.

Walker, E.M. & Lowes, J.A. (1985) An investigation into in vitro methods for the detection of chlorhexidine resistance. *J Hosp Infect* **6**, 389–97.

Warren, J. et al. (1978) Antibiotic irrigation and catheter-associated urinary tract infection. *New Engl J Med*, **299**, 570–73.

GUIDELINES • Bladder lavage

Equipment

1 Sterile dressing pack.
2 Sterile bladder syringe, 60 ml.
3 Sterile jug.
4 Antiseptic solution.
5 Bactericidal alcohol hand rub.

6 Clamp.
7 New catheter bag (for balloon two-way catheter) or sterile spigot (for three-way catheter).
8 Sterile receiver.
9 Sterile solution for lavage.

Procedure

Action

1 Explain and discuss the procedure with the patient.

2 Screen the bed. Ensure that the patient is in a comfortable position allowing access to the catheter.

Rationale

To ensure that the patient understands the procedure and gives his/her valid consent.

For the patient's privacy and to reduce the risk of cross-infection. Curtains are drawn at this stage so that

	dust and airborne organisms disturbed by the curtains do not settle on the sterile field.
3 Perform the procedure using an aseptic technique.	To minimize the risk of infection. (For further information on aseptic technique see Chap. 3.)
4 If necessary, draw up solutions using a 60 ml syringe, preferably with needle adapter. Cap the syringe and place it in a sterile receiver.	It is easier to draw up solutions from vials in the clinical area than at the bedside.
5 Take the trolley to the bedside, disturbing the screens as little as possible. Open the outer wrappings of packs and put them on the top shelf of the trolley.	To minimize airborne contamination. To begin to prepare equipment for procedure.
6 Prepare the sterile field. Pour the lavage solution into the sterile jug.	To prepare equipment for procedure.
7 Wash hands with a bactericidal alcohol hand rub.	To reduce the risk of infection.
8 Clamp the catheter. Place a sterile paper towel under the junction of the catheter and the tubing of the drainage bag and disconnect them.	To prevent leakage when the catheter is disconnected. To create a sterile field and reduce the risk of cross-infection. When the patient has a three-way catheter the drainage bag will not need disconnecting as the washout fluid is injected through the side-arm of the catheter. This should be spigotted off after use and the fluid remaining in the bladder will drain into the catheter bag.
9 Clean gloved hands with a bactericidal alcohol hand rub. Clean around the end of the catheter with sterile low-linting gauze and an antiseptic solution.	To remove surface organisms from gloves and catheter and thus reduce the risk of introducing infection into the catheter.
10 Draw up the irrigating fluid into the bladder syringe and insert the nozzle into the end of the catheter.	To prepare syringe for lavage.
11 Release the clamp on the catheter and gently inject the contents of the syringe into the bladder, trying not to inject air.	Rapid injection of fluid could be uncomfortable for the patient. Large volumes of air in the bladder cause distension and discomfort.
12 Remove the syringe and allow the bladder contents to drain by gravity into a receiver placed on a sterile towel.	To allow catheter to drain gently. To reduce risk of cross-infection.
13 Repeat steps 11 and 12 of the procedure until the washout is complete or the returning fluid is clear.	To ensure bladder is free of contaminants.
14 If the fluid does not return naturally, aspirate gently with the syringe.	Gentle suction is sometimes required to remove obstructive material from the catheter. If suction is applied too forcefully the urothelium may be sucked into the eyes of the catheter, preventing drainage and causing pain and trauma which may predispose to infection (Lowthian, 1991; Macaulay, 1994).
15 Connect a new catheter bag or sterile spigot if a three-way catheter is in place, and allow the remaining fluid to drain out.	A closed drainage system must be re-established as soon as possible to reduce the risk of bacterial invasion through the catheter.
16 If the solution is to remain in the bladder, the catheter should be clamped when all the fluid has been injected and the clamp released after the desired period.	To allow solution to act on bladder mucosa/catheter.
17 Measure the volume of washout fluid returned and compare it with the volume of fluid injected. Record any discrepancies of volume in the appropriate documents.	To keep an accurate record of urinary output and to observe for catheter obstruction.
18 Make the patient comfortable, remove equipment, clean the trolley, and wash hands.	To reduce the risk of cross-infection.

Guidelines • Bladder lavage (cont'd)

As an alternative to the use of bladder syringe and irrigating solution, a pre-packed filled reservoir with sterile catheter adaptor called Uro-tainer is now available. Kennedy (1984) found that the use of Uro-tainer compared with traditional 0.9% sodium chloride washout procedure produced a reduced incidence of urinary tract infection.

GUIDELINES • Continuous bladder irrigation

Equipment

1 Sterile dressing pack.
2 Antiseptic solution.
3 Bactericidal alcohol hand rub.
4 Clamp.
5 Sterile irrigation fluid.
6 Disposable irrigation set.
7 Infusion stand.
8 Sterile jug.

Procedure

Commencing bladder irrigation

Action	Rationale
1 Explain and discuss the procedure with the patient.	To ensure that the patient understands the procedure and gives his/her valid consent.
2 Screen the patient and ensure that he or she is in a comfortable position allowing access to the catheter.	For the patient's privacy and to reduce the risk of cross-infection. Curtains are drawn at this stage so that dust and airborne organisms disturbed by the curtains do not settle on the sterile trolley.
3 Perform the procedure using an aseptic technique.	To minimize the risk of infection. (For further information on aseptic technique, see Chap. 3.)
4 Open the outer wrappings of the pack and put it on the top shelf of the trolley.	To prepare equipment.
5 Insert the end of the irrigation giving set into the fluid bag and hang the bag on the infusion stand. Allow fluid to run through the tubing so that air is expelled.	To prime the irrigation set so that it is ready for use. Air is expelled in order to prevent discomfort from air in the patient's bladder.
6 Clamp the catheter.	To prevent leakage of urine through irrigation arm when spigot is removed.
7 Clean hands with a bactericidal alcohol hand rub. Put on gloves.	To minimize the risk of cross-infection.
8 Place a sterile paper towel under the irrigation inlet of the catheter and remove the spigot.	To create sterile field. To prepare catheter for connection to irrigation set.
9 Discard the spigot.	To prevent re-use and reduce risk of cross-infection.
10 Clean gloved hands with a bactericidal alcohol hand rub. Clean around the end of the irrigation arm with sterile low linting gauze and an antiseptic solution.	To remove surface organisms from gloves and catheter and to reduce the risk of introducing infection into the catheter.
11 Attach the irrigation giving set to the irrigation arm of the catheter. Keep the clamp of the irrigation giving set closed.	To prevent overdistension of the bladder, which can occur if fluid is run into the bladder before the drainage tube has been unclamped.
12 Release the clamp on the catheter tube and allow any accumulated urine to drain into the catheter bag. Empty the urine from the catheter bag into a sterile jug.	Urine drainage should be measured before commencing irrigation so that the fluid balance may be monitored more accurately.
13 Discard the gloves.	These will be contaminated, having handled the cathether bag.

	Action	Rationale
14	Set irrigation at the required rate and ensure that fluid is draining into the catheter bag.	To check that the drainage system is patent and to prevent fluid accumulating in the bladder.
15	Make the patient comfortable, remove unnecessary equipment and clean the trolley.	To reduce the risk of cross-infection.
16	Wash hands.	To reduce the risk of cross-infection.

Care of the patient during irrigation

Action

Rationale

1 Adjust the rate of infusion according to the degree of haematuria. This will be greatest in the first 12 h following surgery (average fluid input is 6–9 litres during the first 12 h, falling to 3–6 litres during the next 12 h). The aim is to obtain a drainage fluid which is rosè in colour.

To remove blood from the bladder before it clots and to minimize the risk of catheter obstruction and clot retention.

2 Check the volume in the drainage bag frequently when infusion is in progress, e.g. half-hourly or hourly, or more frequently as required.

To ensure that fluid is draining from the bladder and to detect blockages as soon as possible, also to prevent over-distension of the bladder and patient discomfort. To empty catheter drainage bags before they reach capacity.

3 Using rubber-tipped 'milking' tongs, 'milk' the catheter and drainage tube, as required.

To remove clots from within the drainage system and to maintain an efficient outlet.

4 Record the fluid balance chart accurately. The fluid balance of all patients having bladder irrigation must be monitored.

So that urine output is known and any related problems, e.g. renal dysfunction, may be detected quickly and easily.

Bladder irrigation recording chart

The bladder irrigation recording chart (Fig. 5.2) is designed to provide an accurate record of the patient's urinary output during the period of irrigation.

Procedure for use of chart

Record the time (column A) and the fluid volume in each bag of irrigating solution (column B) as it is put up.

When the irrigating fluid has all run from the first bag into the bladder, record the original volume in the bag in column C. Record the corresponding time in column A. Do not attempt to estimate the fluid volume run in while a bag is in progress as this will be inaccurate. If, however, a bag is discontinued, the volume run in can be calculated by measuring the volume left in the bag and deducting this from the original volume. This should be recorded in column C.

The catheter bag should be emptied as often as is necessary, the volume being recorded in column D and the corresponding time in column A. The catheter bag must also be emptied whenever the bag of irrigating fluid is empty, and the volume recorded in column D.

When each bag of fluid has run through, add up the total volume drained by the catheter in column D, and write this in red. Subtract from this the total volume run in (column C) to find the urine output (D − C = E). Write this in column E. Draw a line across the page to indicate that this calculation is complete and continue underneath for the next bag.

Patient name:　　　　　　　　　　Hospital no:

(A) Date and time	(B) Volume put up	(C) Volume run in	(D) Total volume out	(E) Urine	(F) Urine running total
10/7/96 10.00	2000				
10.30			700		
11.10			850		
11.40		2000	600		
			2150	150	150
11.45	2000				
12.30			500		
13.15			700		
14.20		2000	800		
			2400	400	550
14.25	2000				
15.30			850		
17.00	Irrigation stopped	1200	800		
			1650	450	1000

Figure 5.2 Bladder irrigation recording chart.

Nursing care plan

Problem	Cause	Suggested action
Fluid retained in the bladder when the catheter is in position.	Fault in drainage apparatus, e.g.	
	Blocked catheter.	'Milk' the tubing. Wash out the bladder with 0.9% sodium chloride.
	Kinked tubing.	Straighten the tubing.
	Overfull drainage bag.	Empty the drainage bag.
	Catheter clamped off.	Unclamp the catheter.
Distended abdomen related to an overfull bladder during the irrigation procedure.	Irrigation fluid is infused at too rapid a rate.	Slow down the infusion rate.
	Fault in drainage apparatus.	Check the patency of the drainage apparatus.
Leakage of fluid from around the catheter.	Catheter slipping out of the bladder.	Insert the catheter further in. Decompress balloon fully to assess the amount of water necessary. Refill balloon until it remains in situ, taking care not to overfill beyond safe level (see manufacturer's instructions).
	Catheter too large or unsuitable for the patient's anatomy.	If leakage is profuse or catheter is uncomfortable for the patient, replace the catheter with one of smaller size.
Patient experiences pain during the lavage or irrigation procedure.	Volume of fluid in the bladder is too great for comfort.	Reduce the fluid volume within the bladder.
	Solution is painful to raw areas in the bladder.	Inform the doctor. Administer analgesia as prescribed.
Retention of fluid with or without distended abdomen, with or without pain.	Perforated bladder.	Stop irrigation. Maintain in recovery position. Call medical assistance. Monitor vital signs. Monitor patient for pain, tense abdomen.

For further details, see Chap. 43, Urinary Catheterization, Nursing care plan with catheter in place.

Bowel Care

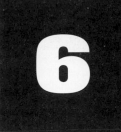

Definitions

Diarrhoea

Diarrhoea results when the balance among absorption, secretion and intestinal motility is disturbed (Hogan 1998). It has been defined as an 'abnormal increase in the quantity, frequency and fluid content of stool and associated with urgency, perianal discomfort and incontinence' (Basch 1987).

Constipation

Constipation results when there is a delayed movement of intestinal content through the bowel (Watson 1987). It is characterized by infrequent, hard, dry stools, which may be difficult to pass (Norton 1996a; Winney 1998).

General introduction

It should be borne in mind that many patients are too embarrassed to talk about bowel function and will often delay reporting the problem until it has been present for a few days. Generally, complaints will be either that the patient has diarrhoea or is constipated. Both diarrhoea and constipation should be seen as symptoms of some underlying disease or malfunction, and managed accordingly.

The nurse's priority in either case is immediate resolution of the problem and re-education of the patient to avoid such problems in the future. However, it is necessary to assess what the patient means by the terms diarrhoea and constipation as well as to assess the cause.

Reference material

Anatomy and physiology

The main events of digestion and absorption occur in the small intestine. The small intestine begins at the pyloric sphincter of the stomach, coils through the abdomen and opens into the large intestine at the ileocaecal junction. It is approximately 6.4 m in length and is divided into three segments: the duodenum, jejunum and ileum. The mucosal surface of the small intestine is covered with finger-like processes called villi, which increase the surface area available for absorption and digestion. A number of digestive enzymes are also secreted by the small intestine (Tortora & Grabowski 1993).

Movement through the small bowel is divided into two types, segmentation and peristalsis. Segmentation refers to the localized contraction of the intestine, which mixes the intestinal contents and brings particles of food into contact with the mucosa for absorption. Intestinal content usually remains in the small bowel for 3–5 hours and it is moved along by peristaltic action. These actions are controlled by the autonomic nervous system (Tortora & Grabowski 1993).

Absorption of nutrients, electrolytes and water occur by diffusion, facilitated diffusion, osmosis and active transport. Water can move across the intestinal mucosa in both directions (Tortora & Grabowski 1993). There are differences in the water and sodium absorption between the jejunum, ileum and colon. The sodium concentration in the intraluminal contents of the jejunum is kept at approximately 90 mmol/l by the ready absorption and secretion of sodium through the loose intracellular junctions of the jejunal mucosa. Water absorption is controlled by the osmolarity of the intraluminal fluid. Sodium absorption, in the ileum, takes place against a concentration gradient and the absorption of water results in only about a litre of effluent passing through into the colon (Woods 1996).

From the ileocaecal sphincter to the anus the colon is approximately 1.5 m in length. Its main function is to eliminate the waste products of digestion by the propulsion of faeces towards the anus. In addition, it produces mucus to lubricate the faecal mass, thus aiding its expulsion. Other functions include the absorption of fluid and electrolytes, the storage of faeces and the synthesis of vitamins B and K by bacterial flora (Tortora & Grabowski 1993).

Faeces consist of the unabsorbed end products of digestion, bile pigments, cellulose, bacteria, epithelial cells, mucus and some inorganic material. They are normally semi-solid in consistency and contain about 70% water (Tortora & Grabowski 1993).

The movement of faeces through the colon towards the anus is by peristaltic action. Three to four times a day there is a strong peristaltic wave. This wave begins at the middle of the transverse colon and quickly drives the colonic contents into the rectum. This is known as the *gastrocolic reflex*, and it is initiated by food in the stomach (Tortora & Grabowski 1993). The colon absorbs about 2 litres of water in 24 hours. If faeces are not expelled they will, therefore, gradually become hard due to dehydration and will be difficult to expel. If there is insufficient roughage (fibre) in the faeces, colonic stasis occurs. This leads to continued water absorption and the faeces will harden still further.

Faeces normally remain in the sigmoid colon until the

stimulus to defaecate occurs. This stimulus varies in individuals according to habit. The stimulus can be controlled by conscious effort. After a few minutes the stimulus disappears and does not return for several hours. If these natural reflexes are inhibited on a regular basis they are eventually suppressed and reflex defaecation is inhibited. The result is that the individual becomes severely constipated. In response to the stimulus faeces move into the rectum (Tortora & Grabowski 1993; Norton 1996b; Taylor 1997).

The rectum is very sensitive to rises in pressure, even of 2–3 mm Hg, and distension will cause a perineal sensation with a consequent desire to defaecate. A coordinated reflex empties the bowel from mid-transverse colon to the anus. During this phase the diaphragm, abdominal and levator ani muscles contract and the glottis closes. Waves of peristalsis occur in the distal colon and the anal sphincter relaxes, allowing the evacuation of faeces (Tortora & Grabowski 1993).

Diarrhoea

Diarrhoea can be characterized according to its onset and duration (acute or chronic) or by type (secretory, osmotic or mixed). Sudden onset acute diarrhoea is very common, it is usually self-limiting and lasts less than 2 weeks. It often requires no investigation or treatment. Chronic diarrhoea generally last longer than 2 weeks and may have more complex origins (Hogan 1998). The causes of acute diarrhoea include:

1 Dietary indiscretion (eating too much fruit, alcohol abuse)
2 Allergy to food constituents
3 Infective:
   (a) Traveller's diarrhoea
   (b) Viral gastroenteritis
   (c) Food poisoning

Chronic causes include:

1 Inflammatory bowel disease (ulcerative colitis, Crohn's disease)
2 Malabsoption (coeliac disease, tropical sprue)
3 Organic disease (neoplasms, diverticulitis)
4 Endocrine disorders (thyrotoxicosis, diabetes, VIPoma, carcinoid tumours)
5 Miscellaneous colitis (drug therapy, gut reaction, pseudomembranous colitis, blind loop syndrome, radiation enteritis)

(Taylor 1997).

Diarrhoea can have profound physiological and psychosocial consequences on a patient. Severe or extended episodes of diarrhoea may result in dehydration, electrolyte imbalance and malnutrition. Patients not only have to cope with increased frequency of bowel movement but may have abdominal pain, cramping, proctitis and anal or perianal skin breakdown. Food aversions may develop or patients may stop eating altogether as they anticipate subsequent diarrhoea following intake. Consequently this leads to weight loss and malnutrition. Fatigue, sleep disturbances, feelings of isolation and depression are all common for those who may have uncontrolled diarrhoea (Roberts 1993; Hogan 1998).

Assessment

The cause of diarrhoea needs to be identified before effective treatment can be instigated. Ongoing nursing assessment of a patient is essential for ensuring individualized management and care. Assessment should include:

1 History of onset, frequency and duration of diarrhoea
2 Consistency and colour of stool: presence of blood, fat, mucus
3 Symptoms associated with diarrhoea, i.e. pain, nausea, vomiting, fatigue, weight loss, fever
4 Recent lifestyle changes, emotional disturbances, or travel abroad
5 Dietary history including any cause and effect relationships between food consumption and bowel action
6 Normal medication including recent antibiotics, laxatives or chemotherapy
7 Effectiveness of antidiarrhoeal medication (dose and frequency)
8 Significant past medical history, i.e. bowel resection, pancreatitis, pelvic radiotherapy
9 Hydration status (i.e. evaluation of mucus membranes and skin turgor)
10 Perianal or peristomal skin integrity

(Taylor 1997; Hogan 1998).

Management

Once the cause of diarrhoea has been established management should be focused on resolving the cause of the diarrhoea and providing physical and psychological support for the patient. Most cases of chronic diarrhoea will resolve once the underlying condition is treated, e.g. drug therapy for Crohn's disease, or with dietary management, e.g. for coeliac disease. Episodes of acute diarrhoea generally require little treatment and management is centred on symptom management and the prevention of complications (Taylor 1997).

The prevention and/or correction of dehydration is the first step in managing an episode of diarrhoea. Simple steps to encourage patients to drink include:

1 Providing drinks to suit individual taste preferences
2 Adding ice to drinks
3 Ice-lollies
4 Using china cups or glass instead of plastic or polystyrene cups.

Dehydration can be corrected by using oral rehydration solutions, for example WHO oral rehydration salts, or by intravenous fluids and electrolytes.

Preserving the patient's privacy and dignity is essential during episodes of diarrhoea. It is important that the patient has easy access to clean toilet and washing facilities; the use of bedside commodes may be helpful. After every bowel action it is recommended that the anal area is bathed with warm water and patted dry with a soft cloth or disposable wipe. The use of soap and alcohol wipes should be discouraged as they may dry the skin (Roberts 1993; Taylor 1997).

All episodes of acute diarrhoea must be considered potentially infectious until proved otherwise. The risk of spreading the infection to others can be reduced by adopting universal precautions such as wearing of gloves, aprons and gowns, disposing of all excreta immediately and, ideally, nursing the patient in a side room with access to their own toilet. Advice should be sought from infection control teams.

Antimotility drugs, such as loperamide, codeine phosphate and co-phenotrope may be useful in some cases, for example in blind loop syndrome and radiation enteritis. It is important to rule out any infective agent as the cause of diarrhoea before using any of these drugs as they may make the situation worse by slowing the clearance of the infective agent (Taylor 1997).

Constipation

Constipation occurs when there is a failure of colonic propulsion (slow transit), or a failure to evacuate the rectum or a combination of these problems (Norton 1996a). Constipation is a symptom which affects up to 10% of the population (Norton 1996a). Its management is dependent on its cause. There are many possible causes and many patients may be affected by more than one causative factor (see Fig. 6.1).

There is no one universally accepted definition of constipation; it is open to individual interpretation, which can lead to confusion. There are a range of symptoms which are commonly characterized as constipation. These include:

1 Reduced or infrequent defecation
2 Difficulty in defecation
3 Hard stools
4 Bulky stools
5 Pellet-sized stools
6 A feeling of incomplete emptying of rectal contents

(Maestri-Banks 1996; Norton 1996a; Winney 1998).

Constipation is associated with abdominal pain or cramps, feelings of general malaise or fatigue and feelings of bloatedness. Nausea, anorexia, headaches, confusion, restlessness, retention of urine, faecal incontinence and halitosis may also be present in some cases (Maestri-Banks 1996; Norton 1996b). While constipation is not life-threatening it does cause a great deal of distress and discomfort.

The myth of daily bowel evacuation being essential to healthy living has persisted through the centuries. This myth has resulted in laxative abuse becoming one of the commonest types of drug abuse in the Western world. An individual's bowel habit is dictated by their diet, lifestyle and environment. The notion of what is a 'normal' bowel habit varies considerably. Studies reveal that in the USA and UK 95% of people pass three stools per week (Bartolo & Wexner 1995). Normal bowel movement has been defined as ranging between three times a day to three times a week (Roberts 1987). Given that there is such a wide normal range it is important to establish the patient's usual bowel habit and the changes that have occurred.

Assessment

Assessment and the identification of the underlying cause and/or identification of any contributory cause are instrumental to the successful management of constipation. There are many factors which may affect normal bowel functioning. These include:

1 Change in diet
2 Change in fluid intake
3 Lack of exercise
4 The use of drugs, e.g. analgesics, antacids, iron preparations, antidepressants
5 Lack of privacy, e.g. having to use shared toilet facilities, commodes or bedpans
6 Change in patient's normal routine
7 Disease process or symptoms, e.g. neoplasm, vomiting
8 X-ray investigation of the bowel involving the use of barium.

A careful history of a patient's bowel habits should be taken, with particular note taken of the following:

1 Any changes in the patient's usual bowel activity. How long have these changes been present and have they occurred before?
2 Frequency of bowel action
3 Volume, consistency and colour of the stool
4 Presence of mucus, blood, undigested food or offensive odour
5 Presence of pain or discomfort on defaecation
6 Use of oral or rectal medication to stimulate defaecation and their effectiveness.

The assessment should also include a dietary history (including fluid intake), significant medical history and present medical situation, current medication, recent lifestyle changes such as decrease in mobility/physical activity or change in home circumstances, and psychological status, e.g. depression. A digital rectal examination should also be performed to assess the contents of the rectum and to identify conditions which may cause discomfort such as haemorrhoids or anal fissure (Taylor 1997; Winney 1998).

Management

The effective treatment of constipation relies on the cause being identified. Constipation can be categorized as either primary or secondary. Factors that lead to the development of primary constipation include:

1 An inadequate diet (low fibre)
2 Poor fluid intake
3 A lifestyle change
4 Ignoring the urge to defecate.

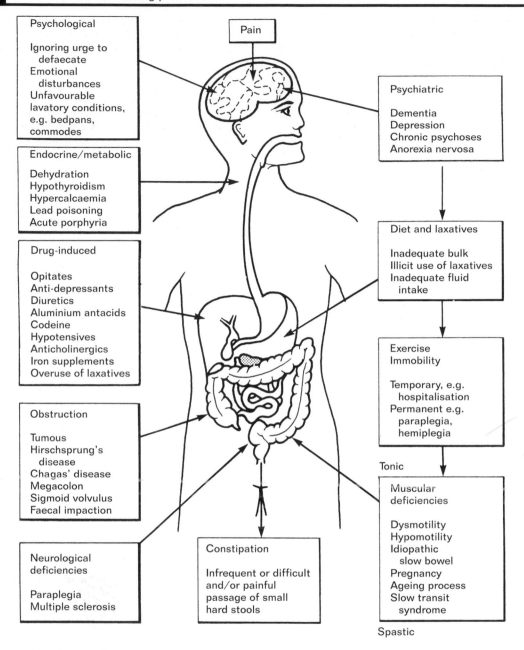

Psychological

Ignoring urge to
  defaecate
Emotional
  disturbances
Unfavourable
lavatory conditions,
e.g. bedpans,
commodes

Endocrine/metabolic

Dehydration
Hypothyroidism
Hypercalcaemia
Lead poisoning
Acute porphyria

Drug-induced

Opitates
Anti-depressants
Diuretics
Aluminium antacids
Codeine
Hypotensives
Anticholinergics
Iron supplements
Overuse of laxatives

Obstruction

Tumous
Hirschsprung's
  disease
Chagas' disease
Megacolon
Sigmoid volvulus
Faecal impaction

Neurological
deficiencies

Paraplegia
Multiple sclerosis

Pain

Psychiatric

Dementia
Depression
Chronic psychoses
Anorexia nervosa

Diet and laxatives

Inadequate bulk
Illicit use of laxatives
Inadequate fluid
  intake

Exercise
Immobility

Temporary, e.g.
  hospitalisation
Permanent e.g.
  paraplegia,
  hemiplegia

Tonic

Muscular
deficiencies

Dysmotility
Hypomotility
Idiopathic
  slow bowel
Pregnancy
Ageing process
Slow transit
  syndrome

Spastic

Constipation

Infrequent or difficult
and/or painful
passage of small
hard stools

Figure 6.1 Classification of constipation – combined sources.

Constipation that is attributed to a disease process or surgical and/or medical conditions such as anal fissures, colonic tumours or hypercalcaemia is classified as secondary constipation. Constipation of unknown cause must be investigated before treatment is instigated (Stilwell 1992; Taylor 1997).

Dietary manipulations may help to resolve mild constipation, although it is much more likely to help prevent constipation from recurring. Increasing dietary fibre increases stool bulk, which in turn improves peristalsis and stool transit time. This results in a softer stool being delivered to the rectum (Norton 1996b). The UK average daily fibre intake of 12–13 g could be usefully doubled to help improve bowel health. However, care should be taken to increase dietary bran intake gradually as bloating and abdominal discomfort can result from a sudden increase (Cummings 1994; Norton 1996b). Other sources of dietary laxatives should be encouraged, for example prunes contain diphenylisatin and onions contain indigestible sugars (Norton 1996b).

Dietary changes need to be taken in combination with other lifestyle changes. Daily fluid intake should be between 2 and 2.5 litres (Hanham 1990; Taylor 1997). Fruit juices such as orange and prune juice can help stimulate bowel activity (Winney 1998) and coffee is thought to increase colonic motility and thus has a mild laxative effect (Brown *et al.* 1990). Patients should be advised not to ignore the urge to defaecate and to allow sufficient time for defaecation (Norton 1996b).

It is important that the correct posture for defaecation is adopted. Crouching or a 'crouch like' posture is considered anatomically correct (Taylor 1997). The use of a foot stool by the toilet may enable patients to adopted a better defecation posture (Norton 1996b). The use of the bedpan should always be avoided if possible. The poor posture adopted while using a bedpan has been shown to cause extreme straining during defecation (Lewin 1976; Taylor 1997). Patients should be supported with pillows to enable them to achieve an upright position if the use of a bedpan is unavoidable.

Laxatives are the most commonly used treatment for constipation (Table 6.1). In general they should be used as a short-term measure to help relieve an episode of constipation as long-term use can perpetuate constipation and a dependence on laxatives can develop (Butler 1998).

Laxatives

Weller (1989) defines laxatives as medicine that loosens bowel contents and encourages evacuation. A laxative with a mild or gentle effect is also known as an aperient and one with a strong effect is referred to as a cathartic or a purgative. Purgatives should be used only in exceptional circumstances, i.e. where all other interventions have failed, or when they are prescribed for a specific purpose. Wherever possible the most natural means of bowel evacuation should be employed.

The many different types of laxatives available may be grouped into four types according to the action they have (Table 6.1).

Stool softeners

These act by lowering the surface tension of faeces which allows water to penetrate and soften the stool. They may also have a weak stimulatory effect (Barrett 1992), but drugs of this type are often given in combination with a chemical stimulant. Softening agents take 24–48 hours to work (Martindale 1993).

Liquid paraffin acts as a lubricant as well as a stool softener by coating the faeces and allowing easier passage. However, its use should be avoided as there are a number of problems associated with this preparation. The use of liquid paraffin interferes with the absorption of fat-soluble vitamins. Accidental inhalation of droplets of liquid paraffin may result in lipoid pneumonia (Barrett 1992; Taylor 1997).

Osmotic agents

These may be divided into two subgroups: lactulose and magnesium preparations. Lactulose is a synthetic disaccharide which exerts an osmotic effect in the small bowel. Distension of the small bowel induces propulsion which in turn reduces transit time. Colonic bacteria metabolize lactulose into a short chain organic salt which is then absorbed; therefore the osmotic effect does not continue throughout the colon (Barrett 1992). This process of metabolism also produces gas which in turn stimulates colonic movements and increases bacterial growth. This results in increased stool weight and thus colonic transit time is shortened (Spiller 1994). Bowel action may occur 3 hours after administration or up to 48 hours later (Taylor 1997). Flatulence, cramps and abdominal discomfort are associated with high dosages. Magnesium preparations also exert an osmotic effect on the gut and additionally they stimulate the release of cholecystokinin. This encourages intestinal mobility and fluid secretion (Nathan 1996). They have a rapid effect, working within 2–6 hours. Fluid intake is important with these preparations as patients may easily become dehydrated (Martindale 1993). These preparations should be avoided in patients with renal or hepatic impairment (Taylor 1997).

Stimulant laxatives

These stimulate the nerve plexuses in the gut wall causing irritation and increased peristalsis in the small and large bowel (Barrett 1992; Nathan 1996). Abdominal cramping may be increased if the stool is hard and a stool softener

Table 6.1 Types of laxatives

Type of laxative	Example	Brand names and sources
Stool softeners	Synthetic surface active agents, liquid paraffin	Agarol, Dioctyl, Petrolager, Milpar
Osmotic agents	Sodium, potassium and magnesium salts	Magnesium sulphate, milk of magnesia, lactulose
Stimulant laxatives	Sodium picosulphate, glycerin	Senna, Senokot, bisacodyl, Dulcolax, co-danthrusate, Picolax, glycerol
Bulk producers	Dietary fibre Mucilaginous polysaccharides Methylcellulose	Bran, wholemeal bread, Fybogel (ispaghula), Normacol (sterculia)

may be used in combination with this group of drugs (Taylor 1997; ABPI 1999). Long-term use of these laxatives should be avoided, except for patients on long-term opiates, as they may lead to impaired bowel function such as atonic non-functioning colon (Taylor 1997; ABPI 1999).

Preparations containing Danthron are restricted to certain groups of patients, i.e. the elderly, the terminally ill and some cardiac patients, as some rodent studies have indicated a potential carcinogenic risk (Taylor 1997; ABPI 1999). Danthron preparations should not be used for incontinent patients especially those with limited mobility as prolonged skin contact will colour the skin pink or red and superficial sloughing of the discoloured skin will occur (Taylor 1997; ABPI 1999).

Bulking agents

These work by retaining water and promoting microbial growth in the colon. This increases faecal mass production which stimulates peristalsis. Ispaghula husk (Isogel, Regulan) and sterculia (Normacol) both trap water in the intestine by the formation of a highly viscous gel which softens faeces, increases weight and reduces transit time (Butler 1998). These agents need plenty of fluid in order to work (2–3 litres per day) (Taylor 1997). They take a few days to exert their effect so are not suitable to relieve acute constipation. They are not suitable for use in patients who have bowel obstruction or reduced muscle tone. Increasing the bulk may worsen impaction, lead to increased colonic faecal loading or even intestinal obstruction (Norton 1996b), and may also increase the risk of faecal incontinence (Ardron & Main 1990). Other potentially harmful effects include malabsorption of minerals, calcium, iron, and fat-soluble vitamins, and reduced bioavailability of some drugs (Taylor 1997). Another problem initially is that bulk laxatives tend to distend the abdomen, often making the patient feel full and uncomfortable. Sometimes this leads to temporary anorexia (Taylor 1997).

Studies have now shown that there are a number of types and components of 'dietary fibre', which makes this too imprecise a term for health care professionals to use: its closest, more exact description is now 'non-starch polysaccharides'. A more detailed discussion of this area can be found in *Dietary Reference Values for Food Energy and Nutrients for the United Kingdom* (DoH 1991).

Enemas

Definition

An enema is the introduction into the rectum or lower colon of a stream of fluid for the purpose of producing a bowel action or instilling medication (Clarke 1988).

Indications

Enemas may be prescribed for the following reasons:

1 To clean the lower bowel before surgery; X-ray examination of the bowel using contrast medium; before endoscopy examination or in cases of severe constipation.
2 To introduce medication into the system.
3 To soothe and treat irritated bowel mucosa.
4 To decrease body temperature (due to contact with the proximal vascular system).
5 To stop local haemorrhage.
6 To reduce hyperkalaemia (calcium resonium).
7 To reduce portal systemic encephalopathy (phosphate enema).

Contraindications

Enemas are contraindicated under the following circumstances:

1 In paralytic ileus.
2 In colonic obstruction.
3 Where the administration of tap water or soap and water enemas may cause circulatory overload, water intoxication, mucosal damage and necrosis, hyperkalaemia and cardiac arrhythmias.
4 Where the administration of large amounts of fluid high into the colon may cause perforation and haemorrhage.
5 Following gastrointestinal or gynaecological surgery, where suture lines may be ruptured (unless medical consent has been given).
6 The use of micro-enemas and hypertonic saline enemas in patients with inflammatory or ulcerative conditions of the large colon.

Reference material

Types of enemas

Evacuant enemas

An evacuant enema is a solution introduced into the rectum or lower colon with the intention of its being expelled, along with faecal matter and flatus, within a few minutes. The following solutions are used:

1 Phosphate enemas with standard or long rectal tubes in single-dose disposable packs.
2 Dioctyl sodium sulphosuccinate 0.1%, sorbitol 25% in single-dose disposable packs.
3 Sodium citrate 450 mg, sodium alkysulphoacetate 45 mg, sorbic acid 5 mg in single-dose disposable packs.

Enemas containing dioctyl sodium sulphosuccinate lubricate and soften impacted faeces. Phosphate enemas are useful in bowel clearance before X-ray examination and surgery.

Retention enemas

A retention enema is a solution introduced into the rectum or lower colon with the intention of being retained for a specified period of time. Three types of retention enema are in common use:

1 Arachis oil (may be obtained in a single-dose disposable pack)
2 Olive oil
3 Prednisolone.

Enemas containing olive oil or arachis oil will soften and lubricate impacted faeces. These work by penetrating faeces, increasing the bulk and softness of stools. They work most effectively when warmed, to body temperature, and retained for as long as possible (Clarke 1988). Retention enemas given to administer medications will be prescribed by the doctor. The product must be checked with the prescription before its administration.

Suppositories

Definition

A suppository is a solid or semi-solid pellet introduced into the anal canal for medicinal purposes.

Indications

The use of suppositories is indicated under the following circumstances:

1 To empty the bowel before certain types of surgery.
2 To empty the bowel to relieve acute constipation or when other treatments for constipation have failed.
3 To empty the bowel before endoscopic examination.
4 To introduce medication into the system.
5 To soothe and treat haemorrhoids or anal pruritus.

Contraindications

The use of suppositories is contraindicated when one or more of the following pertain:

1 Chronic constipation, which would require repetitive use
2 Paralytic ileus
3 Colonic obstruction
4 Following gastrointestinal or gynaecological operations, unless on the specific instructions of the doctor.

Reference material

Administration of suppositories

The use of suppositories dates back to about 460 BC. Hippocrates recommended the use of cylindrical suppositories of honey smeared with ox gall (Hurst 1970). Several types are now commonly available.

Lubricant suppositories, e.g. glycerine, should be inserted directly into the faeces and allowed to dissolve to enable softening of the faecal mass. However, stimulant types, such as bisacodyl, must come into contact with the mucus membrane of the rectum if they are to be effective. Other types, such as sodium bicarbonate and anhydrous sodium acid phosphate, exert their influence by releasing carbon dioxide, causing rectal distension when they contact water or mucous membrane.

Manual evacuation

Manual evacuation of the rectum should be avoided if possible; it should only be performed if all other methods of relieving constipation have failed. It is a distressing, often painful and potentially dangerous procedure for the patient. If the procedure proves unavoidable, it may be necessary to sedate the patient before carrying it out. It should only be performed by a nurse who has been properly trained in the procedure (Norton 1996a).

To resolve faecal impaction a course of disposable enemas (phosphate if the stool is soft and dioctyl if hard) over a period of 7–10 days, or until there is no further return, is the best method (Norton 1996a). Impaction is often extensive, therefore a single enema is rarely sufficient even if an apparently good result is obtained. The first enema only clears the lowest portion of the bowel.

Managing bowel problems such as constipation and prolonged bowel evacuation in patients following spinal cord injury requires a multimodality approach. This includes dietary fibre, digital stimulation, enemas, suppositories, stool softeners and abdominal massage (Amir *et al.* 1998). Digital stimulation is a method of initiating the defaecation reflex by dilating the anus, either by a finger or an anal dilator (Norton 1996a). This approach is only useful if the rectum is full.

Rectal lavage

Definition

Rectal lavage is the washing out of the rectum using large volumes of non-sterile fluid.

Indications

Rectal lavage is performed for the following purposes:

1 To clear the lower bowel before investigation by barium enema and thus enable good images to be obtained.
2 To assist in clearing the lower bowel before major abdominal surgery and thus decreasing the risk of infection and aiding satisfactory healing.
3 To clear the lower bowel of residual faecal matter following previous surgery, e.g. formation of colostomy.

Contraindications

Rectal lavage is contraindicated in patients who have a history of any one of the following:

1 Severe or prolapsed haemorrhoids
2 Anal fissure

3 Inflammatory bowel disease
4 Large tumour in the rectum or sigmoid colon
5 Post-radiation proctitis
6 Internal fistulae
7 Pelvic radiotherapy
8 Recent bowel surgery
9 Congestive cardiac failure
10 Impaired renal function.

In points 1 to 8 of the contraindications listed above, the reason for employing caution is because of the damage that could be inflicted by the mechanical aspects of rectal lavage. When the bowel has already been traumatized there is a greater potential risk of causing irritation or, in extreme cases, perforation while inserting the catheter and running large volumes of fluid in and out of the rectum.

With the last two contraindications the potential risk lies with the possibility of large amounts of fluid and/or electrolytes becoming absorbed through the bowel. (Generally speaking, with the amounts and type of fluid used and the relatively short time that it stays in the bowel, this should not present a major problem.)

Caution should be exercised when giving tap water lavage to infants or patients with altered kidneys or cardiac reserve, but otherwise tap water is the solution of choice.

Reference material

Choice of fluid

Several solutions can be used to clear the bowel.

Hypertonic solutions

Hypertonic solutions, e.g. sodium phosphate and sodium acid phosphate in solution, act by drawing water from the intestinal cells by osmosis. This increases the fluid in the faecal mass, causing first distension then contraction and defaecation.

For patients who have a large amount of faecal matter to evacuate, small volumes of these solutions are very effective. Hypertonic solutions should not be given to patients whose capacity to utilize sodium is affected, as some sodium may be absorbed. These solutions are available as commercially prepared enemas but are not suitable for administration in large volumes.

Tap water

Rectal lavage is a procedure that is normally used in combination with other methods of clearing the bowel, e.g. oral aperients and dietary restrictions. In this situation, it can be anticipated that there will be very little residue remaining in the lower bowel. What is needed, therefore, is a simple, non-sterile solution that can be used with relative safety in large volumes to wash out the residual faecal matter. The solution which fulfils these criteria ideally is tap water.

Rectal lavage using tap water is not without risk as large volumes of this hypotonic solution can upset the patient's electrolyte balance. Water is drawn by osmosis into the intestinal cells and water intoxication can result, with symptoms of weakness, sweating, pallor, vomiting, coughing and dizziness. However, this is a relatively rare complication and generally tap water is very well tolerated.

The other advantages of tap water are as follows:

1 It is cheap and easily available.
2 It can be easily warmed to the correct temperature (37°C).
3 It is non-irritant to the bowel mucosa.
4 It does not cause excessive peristalsis with resulting cramps and colic.

Isotonic saline

An isotonic saline solution can be substituted for patients with compromised electrolyte status. This is prepared by adding 2 level teaspoons of salt to 1 litre of plain water. Its effect on the bowel is similar to that of water in that it stimulates peristaltic action by distending the intestinal walls. With isotonic saline, however, there is less danger of electrolyte imbalance.

Choice of catheter

Several manufacturers produce rectal catheters. The criteria for selection should be as follows:

1 The catheter should be of an adequate length. Most are approximately 30 cm long.
2 The lumen should be large enough to allow the free drainage of particulate matter, i.e. a minimum Charrière gauge of 24.
3 The tip of the catheter should be open ended or have large opposed eyelets to minimize the possibility of blockage.
4 The catheter should be made from a soft flexible material; rubber or plastic is suitable.

References and further reading

Abd-El-Maeboud, K.H., El-Naggar, T. & El-Hawi, E.M.M. (1991) Rectal suppositories: commonsense mode of insertion. *Lancet*, **338**, 798–800.
ABPI (1999) *ABPI Compendium of Data Sheets and Summaries of Product Characteristics 1999–2000*. Datapharm Publications.
Amir, I., Sharma, R., Bauman, W.A. *et al.* (1998) Bowel care for the individual with spinal cord injury: comparison of four approaches. *Spinal Med*, **21**(1), 21–4.
Ardron, M.E. & Main, A.N.H. (1990) Management of constipation. *Br Med J*, **300**, 1400.
Barrett, J.A. (1992) Faecal incontinence. In: *Clinial Nursing Practice. The Promotion and Management of Continence* (ed. B. Roe). Prentice Hall, New York.
Bartolo, D.G.C. & Wexner, S.D. (1995) *Constipation, its Etiology, Evaluation and Management*. Butterworth Heinemann, Philadelphia.
Basch, A. (1987) Symptom distress changes in elimination. *Semin Oncol Nurs*, **3**(4), 287–92.
Booth, S. & Booth, B. (1986) Aperients can be deceptive. *Nurs Times*, **82**(39), 38–9.

British Medical Association/Pharmaceutical Society of Great Britain (1988) *British National Formulary*. BMA, London.

Brown, S.R., Cann, P.A. & Read, N. (1990) Effect of coffee on distal colon function. *Gut*, **31**, 450–53.

Butler, M. (1998) Laxatives and rectal preparations. *Nurs Times*, **94**(3), 56–8.

Clarke, B. (1988) Making sense of enemas. *Nurs Times*, **84**(30), 40–44.

Cummings, J.H. (1994) Non-starch polysaccharides (dietary fibre) including bulk laxatives in constipation. In: *Constipation* (eds M.A. Kamm & J.E. Lennard-Jones). Wrightson Biomedical, Petersfield.

DoH (1991) *Report on Health and Social Subjects 41, Dietary Reference Values for Food Energy and Nutrients for the United Kingdom*, pp. 61–71. Stationery Office, London.

Donowitz, M., Kokke, F.T. & Saidi, R. (1995) Evaluation of patients with chronic diarrhea. *New Engl J Med*, **332**, 725–9.

Emly, M. (1993) Abdominal massage. *Nurs Times*, **89**(3), 34–9.

Evans, L., Barnett, C. & McTurk, K. (1996) Movement through change. *Nurs Times*, **92**(2), 30–31.

Greenwood, J. (1955) Treatment with dignity. *Nurs Times*, **91**(17), 65–7.

Hanham, S. (1990) Management of constipation. *Nursing*, **4**(17), 28–31.

Hogan, C.M. (1998) The nurse's role in diarrhoea management. *Oncol Nurs Forum*, **25**(5), 879–86.

Hurst, Sir A. (1970) *Selected Writings of Sir Arthur Hurst* (1989–1944). Spottiswode, Ballantyne.

Kamm, M.A. & Lennard-Jones, J.E. (1994) *Constipation*. Wrightson Biomedical, Petersfield.

Kendall, L. & Munchiando, J. (1993) Comparison of two bowel programmes for CVA patients. *Rehab Nurs*, **18**(3), 168–9.

Lewin, D. (1976) Care of the constipated patient. *Nurs Times*, **72**, 444–6.

Maestri-Banks, A. (1996) Assessing constipation. *Nurs Times*, **92**(21), 28–30.

Martindale, W. (1993) *The Extra Pharmacopia*, 30th edn. (ed. J.E.F. Reynolds). Pharmaceutical Press, London.

Murray, B. (1997) Preventing constipation. *J Commun Nurs*, **5**, 1250–52.

Murray, F.E. (1992) Constipation; an update on a common problem. *Geriat Med*, **55**, 58.

Nathan, A. (1996) Laxatives. *Pharm J*, **257**, 52–5.

Nazarko, L. (1996) Preventing constipation in older people. *Prof Nurse*, **11**(12), 816–18.

Norton, C. (1996a) *Nursing for Continence*, 2nd edn. Beaconsfield, Beaconsfield.

Norton, C. (1996b) The causes and nursing management of constipation. *Br J Nurs*, **5**(20), 1252–8.

Portenoy, R.K. (1987) Constipation in the cancer patient: causes and management. *Med Clin North Am*, **71**(2), 303–311.

Roberts, A. (1987) Systems of life, no. 146. *Nurs Times*, **83**(5), 47–8.

Roberts, M.F. (1993) Diarrhoea: a symptom. *Hol Nurse Pract*, **7**(2), 73–80.

Robinson, B. (1993) Be alert to an avoidable problem: management and prevention of antibiotic-aquired diarrhoea. *Prof Nurse*, **8**(8), 510–12.

Robinson, Z. (1996) Bowel management and nursing's hidden work. *Nurs Times*, **92**(21), 26–8.

Sadler, C. (1988) The power of purgatives. *Commun Outlook*, June, 11–12.

Smith, S. (1987) Drugs and the gastrointestinal tract. *Nurs Times*, **83**(26), 50–52.

Spiller, R.C. (1994) *Diarrhoea and Constipation*. Libra Pharm, Petroc Press.

Stilwell, B. (1992) Skills update: assessing the adult with constipation. *Commun Outlook*, **2**(9), 26–7.

Taylor, C. (1997) Constipation and diarrhoea. In: *Gastroenterology* (eds L. Bruce & T.M.D. Finlay). Churchill Livingstone, Oxford.

Tortora, G.J. & Grabowski, S.R. (1993) *Principles of Anatomy and Physiology*. Harper Collins, New York.

Watson, J.E. & Royle, J.R. (1987) *Watson's Medical-Surgical Nursing and Related Physiology*, 3rd edn. Baillière Tindall, London.

Weller, B. (1989). *Encyclopaedic Dictionary of Nursing and Health Care*. Baillière Tindall, Eastbourne.

White, T. (1995) Dealing with constipation in terminal illness. *Nurs Times*, **91**(14), 57–8.

Wieck, L. et al. (1986) *Illustrated Manual of Nursing Techniques*, 3rd edn. J.B. Lippincott, Philadelphia.

Winney, J. (1998) Constipation. *Nurs Stand*, **13**(11), 49–56.

Woods, S. (1996) Nutrition and the short bowel syndrome. In: *Stoma Care Nursing: A Patient-centred Approach* (ed. C. Myres). Edward Arnold, London.

GUIDELINES • Administration of enemas

Equipment

1 Disposable incontinence pad.
2 Disposable gloves.
3 Topical swabs.
4 Lubricating jelly.

5 Rectal tube and funnel (if not using a commercially prepared pack).
6 Solution required or commercially prepared enema.
7 Bath thermometer.

Procedure

Action

1 Explain and discuss the procedure with the patient.

2 Ensure privacy.

3 Allow patient to empty bladder first if necessary.

Rationale

To ensure that the patient understands the procedure and gives his/her valid consent.

To avoid unnecessary embarrassment to the patient.

A full bladder may cause discomfort during procedure.

Guidelines • Administration of enemas (cont'd)

Action	Rationale
4 Ensure that a bedpan, commode or toilet is readily available.	In case the patient feels the need to expel the enema before the procedure is completed.
5 Warm the enema to the required temperature by immersing in a jug of hot water, testing with a bath thermometer. A temperature of 40.5–43.3°C is recommended for adults. Oil retention enemas should be warmed to 37.8°C.	Heat is an effective stimulant of the nerve plexi in the intestinal mucosa. An enema temperature of body temperature or just above will not damage the intestinal mucosa. The temperature of the environment, the rate of fluid administration and the length of the tubing will all have an effect on the temperature of the fluid in the rectum.
6 Assist the patient to lie in the required position, i.e. on the left side, with knees well flexed, the upper higher than the lower one, and with the buttocks near the edge of the bed.	This allows ease of passage into the rectum by following the natural anatomy of the colon. In this position gravity will aid the flow of the solution into the colon. Flexing the knees ensures a more comfortable passage of the enema nozzle or rectal tube.
7 Place a disposable incontinence pad beneath the patient's hips and buttocks.	To reduce potential infection caused by soiled linen. To avoid embarrassing the patient if the fluid is ejected prematurely following administration.
8 Wash hands with bactericidal soap and water or bactericidal alcohol hand rub, and put on disposable gloves.	To minimize the risk of cross-infection.
9 Place some lubricating jelly on a topical swab and lubricate the nozzle of the enema or the rectal tube.	To prevent trauma to the anal and rectal mucosa by reducing surface friction.
10 Expel excessive air and introduce the nozzle or tube slowly into the anal canal while separating the buttocks. (A small amount of air may be introduced if bowel evacuation is desired.)	The introduction of air into the colon causes distention of its walls, resulting in unnecessary discomfort to the patient and increases peristalsis. The slow introduction of the lubricated tube will minimize spasm of the intestinal wall. (Evacuation will be more effectively induced due to the increased peristalsis.)
11 Slowly introduce the tube or nozzle to a depth of 10–12.5 cm.	This will bypass the anal canal (2.5–4 cm in length) and ensure that the tube or nozzle is in the rectum.
12 If a retention enema is used, introduce the fluid slowly and leave the patient in bed with the foot of the bed elevated by 45° for as long as prescribed.	To avoid increasing peristalsis. The slower the rate at which the fluid is introduced the less pressure is exerted on the intestinal wall. Elevating the foot of the bed aids in retention of the enema by force of gravity.
13 If an evacuant enema is used, introduce the fluid slowly by rolling the pack from the bottom to the top to prevent backflow, until the pack is empty or the solution is completely finished.	The faster the rate of flow of the fluid the greater the pressure on the rectal walls. Distention and irritation of the bowel wall will produce strong peristalsis which is sufficient to empty the lower bowel.
14 If using a funnel and rectal tube, adjust the height of the funnel according to the rate of flow desired.	The forces of gravity will cause the solution to flow from the funnel into the rectum. The greater the elevation of the funnel, the faster the flow of fluid.
15 Clamp the tubing before all the fluid has run in.	To avoid air entering the rectum and causing further discomfort.
16 Slowly withdraw the tube or nozzle.	To avoid reflex emptying of the rectum.
17 Dry the patient's perineal area with a gauze swab.	To promote patient comfort and avoid excoriation.
18 Ask the patient to retain the enema for 10–15 minutes before evacuating the bowel.	To enhance the evacuant effect.
19 Ensure that the patient has access to the nurse call system, is near to the bedpan, commode or toilet, and has adequate toilet paper.	To enhance patient comfort and safety. To minimize the patient's embarrassment.

20 Remove and dispose of equipment.

To minimize risk of cross-infection.

21 Wash hands.

To minimize risk of cross-infection.

22 Record in the appropriate documents that the enema has been given, its effects on the patient and its results (colour, consistency, content and amount of faeces produced).

To monitor the patient's bowel function.

Nursing care plan

Problem	Cause	Suggested action
Unable to insert the nozzle of enema pack or rectal tube into the anal canal.	Tube not adequately lubricated.	Apply more lubricating jelly.
	Patient in an incorrect position.	Ask the patient to draw knees up further towards the chest.
	Patient apprehensive and embarrassed about the situation.	Ensure adequate privacy and give frequent explanations to the patient about the procedure.
	Patient unable to relax anal sphincter.	Ask the patient to take deep breaths and 'bear down' as if defaecating.
Unable to advance the tube or nozzle into the anal canal.	Spasm of the canal walls.	Wait until spasm has passed before inserting the tube or nozzle more slowly, thus minimizing spasm. Ask patient to take slow deep breaths to help to relax.
Unable to advance the tube or nozzle into the rectum.	Blockage by faeces.	Withdraw tubing slightly and allow a little solution to flow and then insert the tube further.
	Blockage by tumour.	If resistance is still met, stop the procedure and inform a doctor.
Patient complains of cramping or the desire to evacuate the enema before the end of the procedure.	Distension and irritation of the intestinal wall produce stong peristalsis sufficient to empty the lower bowel.	Temporarily stop the infusion of fluid by clamping the tubing or lowering the funnel until the patient says the feeling has subsided. If the feeling does not subside, stop procedure and allow patient to evacuate bowel.
Patient unable to open bowels after an evacuant enema and the fluid has not returned.	Reduced neuromuscular response in the bowel wall.	Insert a rectal tube and try to siphon the fluid off. Measure and record the amount. If this is not successful, perform rectal lavage. (For further information, see Rectal lavage, above.) Measure and record the amount returned.

GUIDELINES · Administration of suppositories

Equipment

1 Disposable incontinence pad.
2 Disposable gloves.
3 Topical swabs or tissues.

4 Lubricating jelly.
5 Suppository(ies) as required (check prescription before administering a medicinal suppository, e.g. aminophylline).

Guidelines • Administration of suppositories (cont'd)

Procedure

Action	*Rationale*
1 Explain and discuss the procedure with the patient. If you are administering a medicated suppository, it is best to do so after the patient has emptied his/her bowels.	To ensure that the patient understands the procedure and gives his/her valid consent. To ensure that the active ingredients are not impeded from being absorbed by the rectal mucosa or that the suppository is not expelled before its active ingredients have been released.
2 Ensure privacy.	To avoid unnecessary embarrassment to the patient.
3 Ensure that a bedpan, commode or the toilet is readily available.	In case of premature ejection of the suppositories or rapid bowel evacuation following their administration.
4 Assist the patient to lie in the required position, i.e. on the left side, with the knees flexed, the upper higher than the lower one, with the buttocks near the edge of the bed.	This allows ease of passage of the suppository into the rectum by following the natural anatomy of the colon. Flexing the knees will reduce discomfort as the suppository is passed through the anal sphincter.
5 Place a disposable incontinence pad beneath the patient's hips and buttocks.	To avoid unnecessary soiling of linen, leading to potential infection and embarrassment to the patient if the suppositories are ejected prematurely or there is rapid bowel evacuation following their administration.
6 Wash hands with bactericidal soap and water or bactericidal alcohol hand rub, and put on gloves.	To reduce the risk of cross-infection.
7 Place some lubricating jelly on the topical swab and lubricate the blunt end of the suppository if it is being used to obtain systemic action. Separate the patient's buttocks and insert the suppository blunt end first, advancing it for about 2–4 cm. Repeat this procedure if a second suppository is to be inserted.	Lubricating reduces surface friction and thus eases insertion of the suppository and avoids anal mucosal trauma. Research has shown that the suppository is more readily retained if inserted blunt end first (Abd-El-Maeboud *et al.* (1991). (For further information see Suppositories, above.) The anal canal is approximately 2–4 cm long. Inserting the the suppository beyond this ensures that it will be retained.
8 Once suppository(ies) has been inserted, clean any excess lubricating jelly from the patient's perineal area.	To ensure the patient's comfort and avoid anal excoriation.
9 Ask the patient to retain the suppository(ies) for 20 minutes, or until he or she is no longer able to do so. If medicated suppository given remind patient that its aim is not to stimulate evacuation and to retain suppository for at least 20 minutes or as long as possible.	This will allow the suppository to melt and release the active ingredients.
10 Remove and dispose of equipment. Wash hands.	To reduce risk of infection.
11 Record that the suppository(ies) have been given, the effect on the patient and the result (amount, colour, consistency and content) in the appropriate documents.	To monitor the patient's bowel function.

GUIDELINES • Administration of rectal lavage

Equipment

1 Rectal lavage pack containing a large funnel, rubber tubing, straight connector, 1 litre jug and rectal catheter (Charrière gauge 24). (Commercial packs are also available.)
2 Non-sterile topical swabs.
3 Lubricating jelly.
4 Disposable gloves.
5 Disposable incontinence pad.
6 Plastic sheet and draw sheet.
7 Large non-sterile jug.
8 Bucket.
9 Gate clip or clamp.

10 Toilet paper or tissues.

11 Disposable plastic apron.

12 Large disposable bag.

13 Measured volume of warm tap water (37–40 °C).

Procedure

Action	*Rationale*
1 Explain and discuss the procedure with the patient.	To ensure that the patient understands the procedure and gives his/her valid consent.
2 Prepare the area, i.e. the patient's bed or a couch. Protect the bed or couch with plastic sheet and draw sheet. Place a disposable incontinence pad on the floor.	To prevent non-disposable equipment becoming contaminated with faecal matter, thus minimizing the risk of cross-infection.
3 Wash hands with bactericidal soap and water or bactericidal alcohol hand rub, and dry hands, clean the trolley and prepare the equipment for the procedure by opening the pack and laying out the contents on the top of the shelf.	Although this is not an aseptic procedure, care must be taken to avoid unnecessary contamination.
4 Attach a large disposable bag to the trolley.	To provide a suitable receptacle for safe disposal of potentially large amounts of contaminated waste.
5 Fill a large non-sterile jug with a measured volume of warm (37–40 °C) tap water. Check the temperature with a lotion thermometer. Place the filled jug on the lower shelf of the trolley. Put a bucket for receiving effluent by the side of the bed or couch.	As the bowel is not sterile, there is no need to use sterile fluid. A large volume needs to be available for use, up to a maximum of six litres, although the total amount used will vary with each patient and may be much less. If the solution is too warm, the intestinal mucosa may be damaged; if too cold, unnecessary cramping may occur.
6 Assist the patient to lie in the required position, i.e. on the left side, with the knees well flexed, the upper higher than the lower one, and with the buttocks near the edge of the bed. Tilt the foot of the bed slightly upwards if possible.	This position allows ease of access for insertion of the catheter into the rectum, follows the natural anatomy of the colon and aids gravity in promoting the flow of fluid into the sigmoid and descending colon. Tilting the bed also aids the flow.
7 Check that the patient's clothing is tucked out of the way and that both the patient and the bed are adequately protected. Ensure that the patient is as comfortable as possible before continuing with the procedure.	As the procedure can be lengthy and is potentially messy, the patient needs to be as relaxed and well protected as possible.
8 Wash hands with bactericidal soap and water or bactericidal alcohol hand rub, and put on disposable gloves and a disposable plastic apron.	To reduce the risk of cross-infection.
9 Connect up the funnel, tubing and rectal catheter, using a straight connector between the latter two items. Fix a gate clamp or clip in position approximately 15 cm from the end of the rectal catheter.	To allow the tubing and the catheter to be primed and filled with fluid, thus preventing the entry of air into the rectum and discomfort to the patient.
10 Using non-sterile topical swab lubricate the last 15 cm of the rectal catheter with a generous amount of lubricating jelly.	To aid insertion and minimize patient discomfort and trauma to the rectal mucosa.
11 Fill a small jug with one litre from the measured volume of warm tap water.	A small jug is more manageable and allows measurement of the amount of fluid used each time.
12 Prime the catheter and the tubing.	To prepare equipment.
13 Gently insert 7.5–10 cm of the catheter into the rectum.	The rectum is approximately 12.5 cm long and the anal canal 2.5 cm. Inserting the catheter 7.5–10 cm ensures that the rectum will be adequately filled with the minimum trauma to the patient.
14 Encourage the patient to take deep breaths.	Deep breathing relaxes the anal sphincter.

Guidelines • Administration of rectal lavage (cont'd)

Action	Rationale
15 Check that the patient is comfortable.	
16 Fill the funnel with approximately 400 ml of fluid from the jug.	The rectum will hold 200–400 ml without causing trauma.
17 Hold the funnel about 30 cm above the rectum, release the clamp and allow the fluid to run into the rectum, holding the catheter in position.	Aqueous solution exerts pressure of 0.225 kg for every 30 cm of elevation. The pressure should not exceed 0.45 kg as this may cause cramping or even rupture of the intestinal wall.
18 Ask the patient to rock gently from side to side.	To ensure efficient lavage of the bowel lumen.
19 Before the funnel is completely empty, invert it over the bucket to allow the lavage fluid and faecal matter to drain out.	To prevent unnecessary amounts of air entering the rectum and causing the patient discomfort.
20 Refill the funnel with another measure of fluid, keeping the tubing pinched or clamped and the funnel at patient level until it is filled.	To prevent entry of air into rectum and discomfort to the patient.
21 Repeat the last two procedures until: (a) The effluent runs clear (b) A maximum volume of 6 litres has been used.	If the bowel is not clear after this volume, other methods need to be employed.
22 Note how much fluid was used during the procedure.	To ensure that not more than 6 litres are used to reduce the risk of circulatory fluid overload.
23 At the end of the procedure: (a) Measure the amount of effluent obtained and compare it with the volume run in. (b) Clear away and dispose of equipment. (c) Ensure that the patient is clean and tidy.	To ensure that the patient has not absorbed fluid in such a quantity that will carry the risk of fluid overload. To minimize risk of cross-infection.
24 Settle the patient into bed, on an incontinence pad and with a bedpan or commode at hand.	To minimize risk of infection caused by soiled linen.

Nursing care plan

Problem	Cause	Suggested action
Fluid will not run in freely.	Catheter is pressed against the bowel wall.	Gently manoeuvre the catheter around in the rectum.
	Catheter is blocked with faecal material.	Remove the catheter and unblock. Reinsert and recommence procedure.
	Insufficient gravity flow.	Raise the funnel slightly but not above a height of 50 cm.
Leakage of fluid around the catheter.	Poor positioning of the catheter or displacement following insertion. Poor tone of the anal sphincer muscles.	Check that the catheter is 7–10 cm into the rectum. Hold it gently in position. Ask the patient to try and tighten muscles as fluid is run in. Elevate the foot of the bed to aid flow.
Discomfort and/or cramping when the fluid is run in.	Fluid is too cold.	Check the temperature of the fluid and warm to a temperature of 37–40°C.

	Pressure of the fluid entering the rectum is too high.	Lower the funnel to stop fluid from running until the spasm passes, but leave the catheter in to relieve distension.
	Extreme tension and anxiety.	When the spasm has passed, gradually raise the funnel and allow fluid to enter very slowly. Encourage deep breathing through the mouth to relax the abdominal muscles and decrease colonic pressures.
	Perforation of the rectum.	Stop the procedure immediately. Check the patient's vital signs. Inform a doctor.
Severe pain accompanied by perspiration, pallor and tachycardia.	Perforation of the gut around the site of a large tumour due to increased peristalsis.	Check the patient's vital signs. Inform a doctor. Do not allow the patient to eat or drink until seen by a doctor as patient may require emergency surgery.
Blood is returned in the effluent.	Insertion of the catheter has caused internal haemorrhoids to bleed.	Stop the procedure and inform a doctor. Record the appropriate amount of blood that has been passed and observe further bowel motions.
	Trauma to rectal mucosa.	
Large discrepancy between amount of fluid run in and the effluent obtained.	Excessive leakage on to pads during the procedure.	Try to estimate the amount of fluid on pads, etc.
	Patient has retained a certain amount of fluid that may be passed later.	Measure carefully all subsequent bowel actions.
	Patient has absorbed the excess fluid.	Check the patient's vital signs. Record further intake and output carefully. Inform a doctor.
Sudden onset of pallor, perspiration, vomiting, coughing and dizziness.	Water intoxication due to absorption of water from the rectum.	Stop the procedure immediately. Inform a doctor. Check the patient's vital signs.

Breast Aspiration

7

Definition

Breast aspiration is the insertion of a needle into the breast to obtain cells for cytological examination or to remove fluid to drain a cyst. It is usually carried out using a fine needle and so is often referred to as fine needle aspiration or FNA.

Reference material

Anatomy and physiology

The breast is a glandular organ designed to produce milk in women (Fig. 7.1). Each breast contains 12–20 lobes, each of which branches into hundreds of tiny lobules where milk is produced when a woman breast feeds (Chaplin 1996). The lobules are connected to the nipple by a ductal system. Male and female breasts have a similar rudimentary duct system until puberty. The female breast develops further after puberty due to hormonal influences, whereas the male breast remains unchanged (Tucker 1993). The entire breast is enclosed by two layers of fibrous tissue called the fascia. The superficial fascia is thinner and lies between the breast and the skin. The deep fascia, the thicker layer, lies underneath the breast, separating it from the pectoralis major and the pectoralis minor (the muscles of the chest wall) (Baum et al. 1995). Most of the normal breast is composed of fat. Less than 5% is made up of duct epithelial cells. The vast majority of breast cancers and most benign conditions arise in these cells (Dixon 1995).

Breast tissue in women is highly sensitive to hormonal changes that occur naturally, for example during the menstrual cycle or in pregnancy. Hormonal control of normal physiological change is largely determined by oestrogen and progesterone. As a result of their influence, the breasts are subject to constant change that may result in the development of nodularity. This nodularity or lumpiness is more pronounced in some women than in others (Tucker 1993; Baum et al. 1995). Cyclical nodularity is so common that it can be regarded as physiological rather than pathological. Focal breast nodularity or lumpiness is the most common cause of a breast lump and is seen in women of all ages (Dixon 1995).

Breast cancer

Breast cancer is a disease that affects 34 500 women in the UK every year (Cancer Research Campaign 1996). Inva-

sive ductal carcinoma is the most common type of breast cancer accounting for over 70% of cases. Invasive lobular carcinoma forms the next biggest group, although only 9% are of this histological type. The remainder are made up of less common tumours such as Paget's disease, inflammatory carcinoma, mucinous carcinoma, medullary carcinoma, tubular carcinoma and very rare types such as lymphomas or sarcomas of the breast (Dixon & Sainsbury 1997; Brogi & Harris 1999; Diab et al. 1999; Pederson et al. 1999). Most breast cancers are invasive, i.e. the cells have spread through the linings of the ducts into surrounding tissues, but a few may be non-invasive or in situ. Not all breast malignancies become invasive. However, as yet, it is not known what proportion of cancers will progress, or how long they may take to do so (Baum et al. 1995).

Most lumps in the breast are found by patients themselves and these are far more likely to represent a benign condition such as a cyst or a fibroadenoma. Nine out of every ten breast lumps investigated in the hospital setting are benign (DoH 1993; Galea 1994). Consequently the majority of women are undergoing investigations to exclude malignancy. It is therefore important to find a

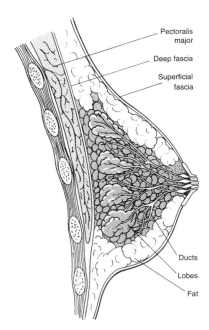

Figure 7.1   Anatomy of the breast.

Pectoralis major

Deep fascia

Superficial fascia

Ducts

Lobes

Fat

simple, non-invasive test that can determine malignancy within given resources at minimal inconvenience to the patient.

Diagnostic methods

When a lump is found in the breast it is necessary to differentiate between benign and malignant disease in order to provide the appropriate treatment and care. Historically, where breast cancer was suspected diagnosis was made by surgical excision of a tumour (known as excision biopsy) under general anaesthetic and then examination of the tumour by a histopathologist. The patient was given the results and subsequently, if positive, needed further excision requiring a second anaesthetic. Alternatively, histopathological examination was carried out rapidly using a frozen section of the tumour while the patient was anaesthetized. Where the tumour was shown to be malignant, further excision or even mastectomy was carried out at the time. While this had the advantage of giving the patient only one anaesthetic, the disadvantage was that patients frequently went to theatre not knowing whether they had cancer or indeed whether they would undergo mastectomy. Nowadays diagnosis is facilitated by triple assessment, a correlation of clinical examination, mammogram and/or ultrasound and FNA cytology. Combining all three leads to a marked improvement in diagnostic accuracy (National Cancer Institute 1997; British Association of Surgical Oncologists 1998) and enables a definitive diagnosis to be made in the vast majority of patients (Dixon & Sainsbury 1997). Consequently patients will know the diagnosis prior to any surgical intervention and can be prepared and informed beforehand. Health care professionals are also less reliant on surgery in the first instance, at a time when chemotherapy and endocrine therapy are increasingly used as primary treatments for breast cancer.

An alternative method of biopsy is trucut biopsy. This is where an incision is made in the breast under local anaesthetic and a wide bore needle used to take a core of breast tissue. This also gives the patient the diagnosis before surgery, but is more invasive and more painful than FNA. However unlike tissue removed by FNA, tissue gathered using this method can be used to distinguish between invasive or non-invasive tumours. Many other prognostic markers can now be measured from FNAs. In conjunction with immunocytochemistry it is possible to measure oestrogen receptor, progesterone receptor and other markers such as the p53 enzyme (Trott 1991).

Fine needle aspiration cytology

Accuracy

Although aspiration cytodiagnosis has been possible since the nineteenth century, the first report of its widespread use (3479 patients) was in 1968 in Scandinavia (Franzen & Zajicek 1968). It is now possible to obtain very high accuracy rates in diagnosing breast cancer with FNA cytology. Both sensitivity (the number of cancers reported as cancer) and specificity (the number of benign lesions reported as benign) with this technique are reported as between 90 and 98% (Dixon 1995; Rocha et al. 1997; Arisio et al. 1998). Recent data suggest that most centres report false positive rates (i.e. mistaken diagnosis of cancer) of less than 0.5% (Dixon 1995) and false negative rates of about 5% (Layfield et al. 1993). False negative readings can occur when insufficient cells are obtained for analysis or when cancer cells are missed. Therefore accuracy is largely dependent on the expertise of the individuals performing the aspiration and interpreting the results (Shumate 1996). It is essential that people undertaking this procedure are adequately trained, have been assessed as competent (Koss 1993) and practise several times a week to ensure consistent results (Ljung et al. 1994).

Application

Advantages of FNA are that it is quick, relatively non-invasive and can be performed in the outpatient department. It also enables solid and cystic lesions to be differentiated. If the lump is a cyst then the fluid will drain out on aspiration and the lump will disappear. Clear fluid aspirated from breast cysts need not have cytologic examination unless the lump has not disappeared. Discoloured or cloudy fluid, either blood stained or green, should be sent to the laboratory for examination as carcinoma can, on rare occasions, be associated with a cyst (Trott 1991).

Preparation of sample

Once obtained the aspirate is expressed onto microscope slides and sent to the cytology department. Two main staining techniques are used for the visualization of the slides. The Papanicolaou stain requires fixing in spirit (95% ethanol) before it dries so it is suitable for a thick smear of cells. The Romanovsky technique using the May-Grunwald Giemsa stain requires the cells to dry almost instantaneously in order to achieve good staining and therefore is better when the smear is scanty. Ideally both stains should be made for each specimen as different lesions are more easily identifiable using the different techniques (Trott 1991). Special preparation of material may be required for measuring prognostic markers, for example cytospins. This technique is more costly but enables high quality preparations to be made (National Cancer Institute 1997). The cytologist will also find it useful to be given a description of what is felt in the breast when the needle is inserted. Cancers often feel more gritty and benign lesions feel more rubbery.

Reporting

Reports are usually descriptive and have a numerical score or 'C score' (standing for cytology): C5 confirms malignancy; C4 indicates the cells are highly suspicious for malignancy (70–90% of these will eventually turn out to be malignant); C3 is reported when atypical cells are seen, but the majority of these will still be benign; C2 indicates benign cells only with no atypical features; C1 is usually reported when only scanty material has been obtained, which is insufficient for a diagnosis to be made (Dixon & Sainsbury 1997).

The patient's experience

Many patients undergoing this procedure may be highly anxious due to concern over the possible diagnosis of cancer. Anxiety may increase the perceived pain of the procedure and if the patient is restless due to anxiety they may move when the needle is inserted. If the patient moves then the FNA may not be accurate and the chances of pneumothorax and haematoma are increased. It is hypothetically possible to pierce the lung and cause pneumothorax so care should be taken when performing aspiration in those areas of the breast where there is little breast tissue. However, the risk from this is considered negligible (Trott 1991). Tumours are often vascular so there is a risk of haematoma formation if care is not taken. This in turn can cause distortion of a mammogram and therefore difficulty in interpretation, which may delay the time a patient has to wait to receive a definitive diagnosis and perpetuates further anxiety.

The process of aspiration can be uncomfortable or even painful for some. Local anaesthetic is not normally used because this may distort the area to be needled and decrease the accuracy. From general experience most people find the administration of the local anaesthetic to be as painful as the FNA itself.

It is essential that patients receive explanations about each step of the procedure and are given a chance to discuss it or ask questions as required. Information delivered at a pace and in a language the patient can understand may result in decreased anxiety, decreased pain levels and improved compliance (Meissner et al. 1990; Schapiro et al. 1992; Poroch 1995).

Conclusion

FNA is cost effective and accurate (Koss 1993) and causes less discomfort and emotional distress than open biopsy (Layfied et al. 1993). With the proviso that experienced personnel undertake the procedure and examination of cells, for the majority of centres this is now the preferred method of diagnosis in breast cancer.

References and further reading

Arisio, R., Cuccorese, C., Accinelli, G. et al. (1998) Role of fine-needle aspiration biopsy in breast lesions: analysis of a series of 4110 cases. *Diagn Cytopathol*, **18**(6), 462–7.

Baum, M., Saunders, C. & Meredith, S. (1995) *Breast Cancer – A Guide for Every Woman*. Oxford University Press, Oxford.

British Association of Surgical Oncologists (1998) Guidelines for surgeons in the management of symptomatic breast disease in the UK (revision) *Eur J Surg Oncol*, **24**, 464–76.

Brogi, E. & Harris, N. (1999) Lymphomas of the breast: pathology and clinical behaviour. *Semin Oncol*, **26**(3), 357–64.

Cancer Research Campaign (1996) *Factsheet 6. Breast Cancer*. Cancer Research Campaign, London.

Chaplin, B. (1996) Breast cancer: knowledge for practice. *Nurs Times*, Prof Dev Suppl, **92**(10), 1–4.

Diab, S., Clark, G., Osborne, C. et al. (1999) Tumour characteristics and clinical outcome of tubular and mucinous breast carcinomas. *J Clin Oncol*, **17**(5), 1442–8.

Dixon, J. (1995) *ABC of Breast Diseases*. BMJ Publishing Group, London.

Dixon, M. & Sainsbury, R. (1997) *Handbook of Diseases of the Breast*, 2nd edn. Churchill Livingstone, London.

DoH (1993) *Breast Cancer*. Stationery Office, London.

Franzen, S. & Zajicek, J. (1968) Aspiration biopsy in diagnosis of palpable lesions of the breast: critical review of 3479 consecutive biopsies. *Acta Radiol*, **7**, 241–62.

Galea, M. (1994) Breast disease. *Matern Child Health*, 386–91.

Koss, L. (1993) The palpable breast nodule: a cost-effectiveness analysis of alternate diagnostic approaches. *Cancer*, **72**(5), 1499–1502.

Layfield, L. et al. (1993) The palpable breast nodule: a cost-effectiveness analysis of alternate diagnostic approaches. *Cancer*, **72**(5), 1642–51.

Ljung, B.-M. et al. (1994) Fine needle aspiration techniques for the characterization of breast cancers. *Cancer*, **74**, 1000–1005.

Miessner, H., Anderson, D. & Odenkirchen, J. (1990) Meeting information needs of significant others and the use of the cancer information service. *Patient Educ Counsel*, **15**(2), 171–9.

National Cancer Institute (1997) The uniform approach to breast fine needle aspiration biopsy. *Am J Surg*, **174**(4), 371–85.

Pederson, L., Holck, S., Mouridsen, H. et al. (1999) Prognostic comparison of three classifications for medullary carcinoma of the breast. *Histopathology*, **34**(2), 175–8.

Poroch, D. (1995) The effect of preparatory patient education on the anxiety and satisfaction of cancer patients receiving radiation therapy. *Cancer Nurs*, **18**(3), 206–14.

Rocha, P., Nadkarni, N. & Menezes, S. (1997) Fine needle aspiration biopsy of breast lesions and histopathological correlation. An analysis of 837 cases in 4 years. *Acta Cytol*, **41**(3), 705–12 .

Schapiro, D., Boggs, R., Melamed, B. et al. (1992) The effect of varied physician effect on recall, anxiety and perceptions in women at risk for breast cancer: an analogue study. *Health Psychol*, **11**(1), 61–6.

Shumate, C. (1996) Surgical evaluation and treatment of breast cancer. In: *Diagnosis and Management of Breast Disease* (eds R. Blackwell & J. Grotting). Blackwell Science, Massachusetts.

Trott, P. (1991) Aspiration cytodiagnosis of the breast. *Diag Oncol*, **1**, 79–87.

Tucker, A.K. (1993) *Textbook of Mammography*. Churchill Livingstone, London.

Walker, S. (1998) A randomized controlled trial comparing a 21G needle with a 23G needle for fine needle aspiration of breast lumps. *J R Coll Surg*, **43**(5), 322–3.

GUIDELINES • Breast aspiration

Equipment

1 70% isopropyl alcohol swabs.
2 Sterile syringes (10 or 20 ml).
3 Sterile needles 21 or 23 g.
4 Microscope slides.
5 Universal container.
6 Slide tray.
7 Fixative (ethanol).
8 Low-linting gauze.
9 Plaster/surgical tape.
10 Sharps container.
11 Cytology request form.
12 Microscope slide holders.

Procedure

Action	Rationale
1 Explain and discuss the procedure with the patient.	To ensure that the patient understands the procedure and gives his/her valid consent.
2 Place slides on a tray.	In preparation for breast aspirate.
3 Prepare syringe by introducing 2 ml of air into the barrel.	To prevent aspirated material being sucked into the syringe.
4 Choose appropriate size needle and attach to the syringe.	Usually 23 g, but for a large breast or deep lesion 21 g may be necessary (Walker 1998).
5 Clean area of patient's skin with single use sterile swab saturated with 70% isopropyl alcohol.	To reduce the risk of infection.
6 Firmly fix breast lump or area of clinical interest between the fingers of one hand.	To stabilize the area before introducing the needle to ensure the correct area sampled.
7 Warn the patient that a needle is about to be inserted.	To reduce the risk of the patient moving.
8 Push the needle tip into the centre of the lump or area of clinical interest. Note consistency (Fig. 7.2).	To obtain specimen from appropriate area. Consistency can be a diagnostic indicator, i.e. gritty (malignant) or rubbery (benign). This information is of use to the cytologist.

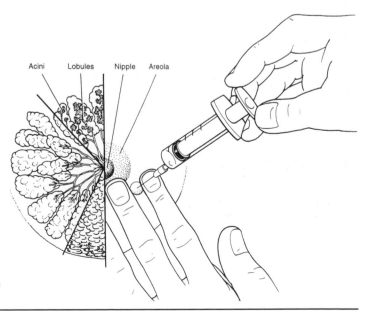

Acini   Lobules   Nipple   Areola

Figure 7.2 Performing fine needle aspiration of the breast.

Guidelines • Breast aspiration (cont'd)

Action	Rationale
9 If the lump is thought to be cystic be careful not to move the needle whilst withdrawing fluid. Withdraw the needle when no further fluid appears in the syringe. If the fluid is discoloured send for cytological examination.	The needle must be kept in place in the cyst sack whilst withdrawing fluid to enable complete drainage of the cyst and reduce chances of it refilling. Clear fluid is indicative of a cyst only. Anything else should be sent to the laboratory to exclude malignancy.
10 Aspirate a solid lesion or area of clinical interest using the maximum amount of suction moving the tip of the needle back and forth and in different directions without withdrawing the needle through the skin.	To enable sampling of different areas and to obtain an adequate sample for transferring to the slide. There is no evidence that tumour cells can be disseminated along the needle tract.
11 After aspiration, allow the barrel of the syringe to return to 2 ml before withdrawing the needle to eliminate any negative pressure in the syringe.	To avoid the contents of the needle being sucked into the syringe.
12 After withdrawal of the needle from the breast, express the aspirate on to the slides. If the aspirate is thick then more slides will be required. Smear the cells evenly on the slides, usually with a second slide.	To prepare the cells for cytodiagnosis. A monolayer is required because if the smear is blood stained or there is too much material on the slide staining can be a problem and the cytologist cannot make a diagnosis.
13 Low linting swab should be placed over the puncture site and pressure applied for at least one minute or until bleeding has stopped.	To reduce the risk of haematoma formation.
14 Leave one slide to dry in the air and add fixative to the other as required by the cytologist. Label appropriately.	When such a small amount of material is available the cytologist will require different staining techniques for accurate diagnosis.
15 If the aspirate is lost into the barrel of the needle 5 ml of 0.9% sodium chloride should be drawn into the syringe through the same needle and the resultant suspension placed in a universal container.	So that the sample can be recovered by centrifugation and then stained as normal. A large percentage of the cells will still be lost.
16 Dispose of needle and syringe in sharps container.	To reduce risk of injury and infection to staff.
17 Label slides with name, number and which breast.	To ensure correct identification of specimen.
18 Apply a plaster or non-allergenic dressing to puncture site.	To protect clothing.
19 Complete cytology forms with full details.	To ensure correct identification and most accurate information for diagnosis.
20 Place slides in slide holder. Slide holder and cytology forms to be placed in plastic specimen bag.	To ensure safe transfer to laboratory.

Cardiopulmonary Resuscitation

8

Definition

Cardiac arrest can be defined as the abrupt cessation of cardiac function which is potentially reversible. Respiratory and cardiac arrest may produce similar signs but there is one important difference: cardiac arrest – no arterial pulse; respiratory arrest – arterial pulse is present.

The three arrhythmias that cause cardiac arrest are:

1 Asystole
2 Ventricular fibrillation
3 Electromechanical dissociation.

For the purposes of resuscitation guidelines, these three are now divided into:

1 Ventricular fibrillation
2 Pulseless ventricular tachycardia (VT)
3 Non-VF/VT.

Indications

Indications of cardiac arrest are as follows:

1 The patient rapidly loses consciousness, becoming pale and cyanosed with absent pulses in major vessels (carotid and femoral arteries).
2 Respiration is absent or slow and stertorous.

Reference material

Principles

The primary objective of cardiopulmonary resuscitation is to prevent irreversible cerebral damage due to anoxia by restoring effective circulation within 4 minutes.

Resuscitation is the emergency treatment of any condition in which the brain fails to receive enough oxygen. The basic technique involves a rapid simple assessment of the patient followed by the ABC of resuscitation (Fig. 8.1). This is known as Basic Life Support.

Assessment

There are two stages of assessment:

1 An immediate assessment by the first-responder to ensure that cardiopulmonary resuscitation may safely proceed (i.e. checking there is no immediate hazard to the first responder from any hazard, for example electrical power supply).

2 Assessment by the first-responder of the likelihood of injury sustained by the patient, particularly injury to the cervical spine. Although there may be no external evidence of injury, the immediate situation may provide the necessary evidence. For example trauma to the cervical spine should be suspected in an accelerating/decelerating injury such as a road traffic accident with a motorbike travelling at speed.

Check the patient's level of consciousness by eliciting a response (1) to verbal stimuli then (2) to painful stimuli, i.e. digital pressure on the ear lobe or fingernail. If there is no response to either verbal or painful stimuli, the first aider should commence the basic life support assessment (Fig. 8.2) immediately.

Note: if the patient is being monitored, for example in Accident and Emergency, Coronary Care or Intensive Care then as soon as an arrest arrhythmia is seen a precordial thump may be used. The precordial thump is a single thump with the closed fist onto the mid to lower third of the sternum. It is used once only. If used immediately it can sometimes convert the cardiac rhythm from asystole or ventricular tachycardia back to sinus rhythm (Colqhhoun *et al.* 1995).

Basic Life Support

Basic Life Support is sometimes known as the 'ABC'.

Airway

The rescuer should look in the mouth and, where possible, remove any obstruction. The most likely obstruction in an unconscious person is the tongue. The airway therefore needs to be extended by tilting back the head which will result in moving the tongue from blocking the oropharynx.

Note: if there is any suspicion of cervical spine injury (see note above) particular care must be taken during handling and resuscitation to maintain alignment of the head, neck and chest in a neutral position. Any head tilt should be the minimum that allows unobstructed ventilation or intubation (Handley *et al.* 1997).

Breathing

The first responder should assess the breathing by placing their cheek close to the patient's mouth while looking down the chest for any movement. As soon as it has been

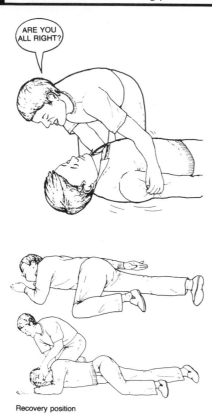

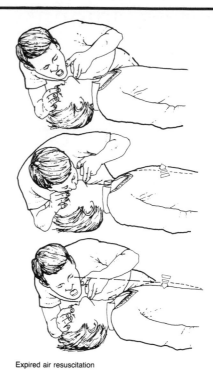

Expired air resuscitation

Figure 8.1b If patient is not breathing, expired air resuscitation must be started immediately.

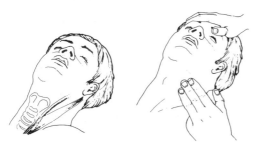

Recovery position

Figure 8.1a The ABC of resuscitation, Rapid, simple assessment of patient, and placement in the recovery position.

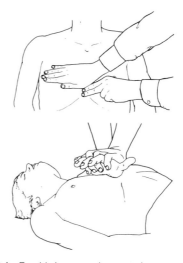

Figure 8.1c If patient does not have a pulse in a major artery (carotid), or if there is a neck injury, the femoral artery may be felt. Circulation must then be established with compression.

Figure 8.1d Establishing circulation with compression. Note fingers are clear of chest wall. (Courtesy of Colqhhoun, M., Handley, A.J. & Evans, T.R. (1995) *ABC of Resuscitation*, 3rd edn. BMJ Publishing Group.)

established that there is no breathing artificial ventilation must be commenced and maintained. If there are no aids to ventilation available then direct mouth-to-mouth ventilation should be used. However this method has two disadvantages. First, it only delivers about 16% oxygen to the patient and, second, there may be risks to the first responder from direct contact with body fluids (Baskett 1993).

Where possible, aids to ventilation should be used. One of the most easily learnt aids is the 'mouth to face mask' method. This is where a valved exhaled air ventilation

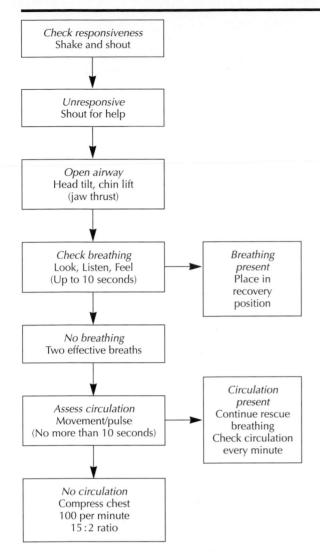

Send or go for assistance as soon as possible according to guidelines.

Figure 8.2 Adult Basic Life Support assessment. (Courtesy of the Resuscitation Council, UK.)

mask with an oxygen attachment valve is used. The mask directs the patient's exhaled air and any fluid away from the responder and the oxygen port allows attachment of oxygen with enrichment up to 60%.

If the operator is skilled in airway management an Ambu bag and mask may be used. When the bag is attached to oxygen, high levels, of up to 90%, can be obtained. However it should be emphasized that to manipulate the head, tilt, and hold on a face mask while squeezing a bag is a procedure that requires practice (Shoemaker *et al.* 1995).

The most effective method of airway management is to use an endotracheal tube, thus enabling the application of

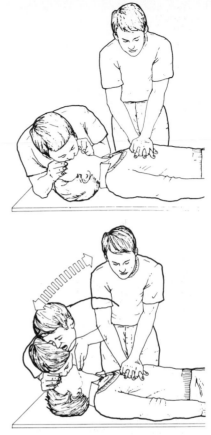

Figure 8.3 Establishing circulation by external cardiac massage. (*Below*) When only one rescuer is present, compression to ventilation ratio is 15:2. (*Above*) When two rescuers are present, compression to ventilation ratio is 5:1. (Courtesy of Colqhhoun, M., Handley, A.J. & Evans, T.R. (1995) *ABC of Resuscitation*, 3rd edn. BMJ Publishing Group.)

100% oxygen (Baskett 1993). This method of airway management is included in the advanced life support section.

Circulation

The rescuer should assess whether the patient has a pulse by palpating a major artery. The carotid, femoral or brachial arteries are most commonly used as the pulse is most easy to palpate. If no pulse is detected after a count of 10 then circulation must be established and maintained by external cardiac massage (Fig. 8.3).

External cardiac massage should be applied at a rate of 100 per minute. It is important that the rescuer positions themselves carefully during this procedure as awkward positioning could result in back injury. The responder should be able to utilize their body mass to provide the strength through their arms. This is best achieved by ensuring a position close to the patient and high enough above them. This may necessitate using a raised platform or kneeling on the bed.

Ratio of breaths to compressions

If there is only one rescuer the ratio is 2 breaths to 15 compressions. If there are two or more rescuers the ratio is 1 breath to 5 compressions (Robertson & Holmberg 1992).

Causes of a cardiorespiratory arrest

A useful way to remember the eight most common causes of a cardiorespiratory arrest is to remember that four start with T and four start with H.

Hypoxia

There are many reasons why a patient may become severely hypoxic (see Chap. 28, Observations and Chap. 35, Respiratory Therapy), the most common being the following:

1 Acute respiratory failure
2 Airway difficulties
3 Acute lung injury
4 Severe anaemia
5 Neuromuscular disorders.

For healthy cell metabolism the body requires a constant supply of oxygen. When this is interrupted for more than 3 minutes in most situations (except when there is severe hypothermia) cell death occurs, followed by lactic acidosis and very rapidly a cardiorespiratory arrest.

Hypovolaemia

Hypovolaemia becomes critical when the patient loses so much of their circulating volume that they have an inability to carry oxygen. This is because the haem molecule in the red blood cell has an affinity for oxygen and if the haemoglobin is reduced below 8 mmol/l there will be an intolerable oxygen deficit at cellular level.

The most common causes of severe blood loss are:

1 Trauma
2 Surgical procedure
3 Gastrointestinal mucosa erosion
4 Oesophageal varices
5 Peripheral vessel erosion (by tumour usually)
6 Clotting abnormality.

Note: blood loss, although usually overt, can be covert such as a gastrointestinal bleed which may only become apparent when the patient collapses.

The treatment for hypovolaemia is to replace the volume with the appropriate fluid – therefore if the patient has lost blood it is imperative that they receive blood. Other colloid fluids, e.g. plasma expanders, can be used while waiting for blood, but only blood can carry oxygen and overtransfusion with other fluids will dilute the red cells further, and result in greater oxygen delivery problems (Von Planta & Chamberlain 1992).

Hypothermia

When the core body temperature falls below approximately 30°C there is a resultant shift in the pH of the blood. This alteration in the pH severely affects cell metabolism and results in a rapid progression to cell death and lactic acidosis. Such severe hypothermia is usually associated with being exposed to severe weather conditions or near drowning. The treatment is to gently warm the patient at a rate of a degree an hour by using warming blankets and the instillation of warmed fluids into the abdomen as well as intravenously via a warming device specially designed for this purpose.

Hypo/hyperkalaemia

Because potassium is so closely linked with muscle and nerve excitation any imbalance will affect both the nervous conduction and the muscular working of the heart. Therefore a severe rise or fall in potassium can cause arrest arrhythmias. The causes of hypokalaemia are:

1 Gastrointestinal fluid losses
2 Urinary fluid loss
3 Drugs that affect cellular potassium, e.g. antifungal agents such as amphotericin.

The immediate treatment for hypokalaemia which has resulted in an arrest is to give concentrated boluses of potassium while carefully monitoring the serial potassium measurements. Most ITU/A&Es and CCUs will have an arterial blood gas analyser that enables the potassium to be measured in 1 minute.

The cause of hyperkalaemia is renal failure. The immediate treatment for hyperkalaemia is to give intravenous calcium. This binds to the potassium and removes it from the cell. However the patient may still require some form of renal replacement therapy post arrest as although the potassium has been removed from the cell it will return to the cell unless it has been removed from the body.

Thromboembolism

Myocardial infarction is the most common cause for cardiac arrest, accounting for approximately 60% of cases (Skinner & Vincent 1997). Pulmonary embolism is less common but is of concern in certain patient groups, for example after major surgery or in patients who have a pelvic malignancy (Skinner & Vincent 1997).

Tension pneumothorax

A tension pneumothorax is the sudden collapse of a lung, usually under pressure, which results in a severe change in intrathoracic pressure and cessation of the heart as a pump. The most common causes are:

1 Trauma
2 Acute lung injury
3 Mechanical ventilation of the newborn.

The immediate treatment is the insertion of an intravenous cannula into the second to third intercostal space on the affected side. As soon as air is heard exiting through the cannula a formal intercostal drain should be inserted in the mid-axillary line on the affected side.

Tamponade

This is where there is an acute effusion of fluid in the pericardial space and as it enlarges, the heart is splinted and finally cannot beat. The fluid is usually blood but can be malignant or infected fluid. The most common cause for a sudden tamponade is trauma. The immediate treatment is to relieve the pericardial compression by aspirating the blood. When the patient has recovered from their cardiac arrest they may then require further cardiac surgery.

Toxicity – drug or metabolic

In this case the heart or its control mechanism (the CNS) has been directly affected by a noxious stimulant. This toxin may be external or endogenous to the body. Examples of external toxins are drugs used with therapeutic intent or recreationally. Internal toxins might be lactic acid, diabetic keto-acidosis or thyrotoxicosis. The treatment is to administer an antidote where possible or to reverse the cause.

Treatment

Treatment of cardiac arrest is carried out in three stages:

1 Restoration of breathing and circulation
2 Correction of acid–base balance
3 Assessment and correction of fluid and electrolyte imbalance.

Drugs

The drugs used in the treatment of cardiac arrest are:

1 Epinephrine (adrenaline) 1 mg (10 ml of a 1 : 10 000 solution) given intravenously. The main purpose of adrenaline is to utilize its inotropic effect to maintain coronary and cerebral perfusion during a prolonged resuscitation attempt.
2 Atropine 3 mg given intravenously once only reduces cardiac vagal tone, increases the rate of discharge of the sinoatrial node and increases the speed of conduction through the atrioventricular node. It is advisable to give atropine for asystole following administration of adrenaline because it blocks all parasympathetic activity (Tinker & Zapol 1991).
3 Calcium chloride (10 ml of 10%) is used for the treatment of electromechanical dissociation when the cause is hyperkalaemia, hypocalcaemia, or when calcium antagonist toxicity is present. Calcium has no proven efficacy in asystolic cardiac arrest (Tinker & Zapol 1991).
4 Sodium bicarbonate 8.4% is only used in prolonged cardiac arrest or according to serial blood gas analyses.

Potential adverse effects of excessive sodium bicarbonate administration include hypokalaemia, exacerbation of respiratory acidosis and increased affinity of haemoglobin for oxygen. The high concentration of sodium can also exacerbate cerebral oedema. Other adverse effects are increased cardiac irritability and impaired myocardial performance. The usual dose of sodium bicarbonate is aliquots of 10–20 mmol, repeated as necessary (Oh 1995).

The Resuscitation Council of the United Kingdom has issued new guidelines for drug administration and defibrillation sequence (ERC Guidelines 1998). Cardiopulmonary resuscitation should not be interrupted for more than 10 seconds, and should be continued for up to 2 minutes after each drug is administered. If an intravenous access cannot be established, then double doses of adrenaline may be given via the endotracheal tube, but drug absorption is unpredictable using this method. When intravenous access is problematic, the intra-osseus route may be utilized. The intra-osseus route is sometimes used in accident and emergency departments when venous access is difficult, especially in children (ERC Guidelines 1998).

Defibrillation

Defibrillation causes a simultaneous depolarization of the myocardium and aims to restore normal rhythm to the heart. This is the immediate treatment for ventricular fibrillation and pulseless ventricular tachycardia.

The carrying out of defibrillation by nurses in special units, i.e. coronary care and intensive care, is becoming an accepted practice, provided nurses have received proper training. This also depends on guidelines laid down in hospital policies.

Please see Fig. 8.4 for the European Resuscitation Council algorithm of electromechanical dissociation, ventricular fibrillation and asystole.

The resuscitation team

Most hospitals now have a designated cardiac arrest team. It is essential that the team works in an efficient and effective manner, with one member acting as coordinator. There are usually four or five team members (Colqhhoun et al. 1995):

1 A duty medical registrar
2 An anaesthetic registrar
3 Senior house officer
4 A porter (and trolley)
5 A nurse skilled in resuscitation or trained in ALS.

The team will require bleeps, with a speech channel so that the operator can give the exact location of the emergency.

Statistics

Sudden cardiac death most frequently occurs in the first 1–2 hours after the onset of symptoms, such as pain (ret-

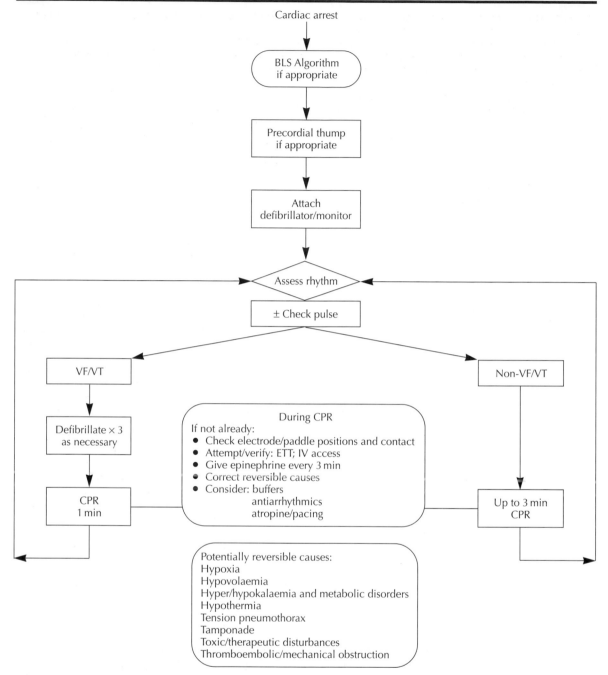

Figure 8.4 ALS Algorithm for management of cardiac arrest in adults. Note that each successive step is based on assumption that the one before has been unsuccessful. (Courtesy of the Resuscitation Council, UK.)

rosternal in origin) and breathlessness, due to fatal arrhythmias, usually ventricular fibrillation (Tinker & Zapol 1991).

Cozart Rosequist (1987) suggests that if cardiopulmonary resuscitation is initiated quickly and promptly by well-trained lay people or emergency medical personnel, then between 40 and 80% of patients with documented ventricular fibrillation can be resuscitated successfully.

In the UK, community resuscitation has been slower to improve. However, with the advent of a nationwide programme of extended training of ambulance staff in resuscitation, and the introduction of a training programme aimed at the general public by a few hospitals (Ferguson 1990), this situation has shown improvements during the 1990s with more hospital staff attending regular ALS updates (Gwinutt 1998).

Of equal importance is the fact that hospital staff often do not possess the necessary skills. Wynn (1987) has shown the poor performance by nursing staff in resuscitation. This indicates an obvious need for more training, and a revision of skills.

Cardiopulmonary resuscitation training requirements

A cardiac arrest is the most acute medical emergency faced by nursing staff. The situation is frequently unexpected and its successful management requires staff who are well trained and rehearsed in basic and advanced life support.

As evidence-based practice and technology in the field of resuscitation has improved, so too has the application of basic and advanced life support. In the last 3 years this has been reflected in an increase in the number of people successfully resuscitated (Handley & Swain 1996). However, if there is a lack of training or refresher courses, cardiopulmonary resuscitation is often poorly performed (Gwinutt 1998).

The Resuscitation Council (UK) started the first UK BLS and ALS courses in 1993, and by the end of 1998 35000 candidates had successfully completed the course. Whether nurses are trained in BLS or ALS will depend on their area of practice and nurses who are regularly part of an arrest team, for example in A&E or coronary care, are required to be trained in ALS. All training programmes should be consistent with the ALS guidelines as produced by the European Resuscitation Council. These guidelines are assessed every year and adjusted in line with current multicentre research findings (Cummins & Chamberlain 1997). It is recommended that those nurses who are part of an arrest team undertake the ALS course every 3 years and those who are not regularly involved in an arrest situation undertake basic life support training every year (Cummins & Chamberlain 1997).

Ethics

The increases in skills, knowledge, technology and pharmacological support have proved very effective in prolonging quality of life. However, the assessment of patients suitable for resuscitation is controversial. There are many important factors which need to be considered in deciding whether or not to resuscitate a patient:

1 The patient's disease and prognosis.
2 Events leading to cardiopulmonary arrest.
3 The patient's wishes and the wishes of the family or friends.
4 The quality of life of the patient and expected quality after discharge.

Decision-making: not for resuscitation

There is a growing corpus of literature and guidelines from professional bodies in recognition that the clinical professions need to consider carefully when resuscitation is advisable and when it is not. In recognition of the needs of their patients/families and clinicians many NHS Hospitals have now accepted responsibility for formulating a policy to deal with situations where to attempt to prolong life would not be in the best interests of the patient (Doyal & Wilsher 1993). It is not proposed that the number of Do Not Resuscitate orders should increase, but rather that the decision-making process should be transparent and that this decision should then be carefully documented in the medical and nursing notes.

The following guidelines are based on those provided by the British Medical Association, the Royal College of Nursing and the European Resuscitation Council. *Note*: where there is any doubt or a decision has not yet been made, routine cardiopulmonary resuscitation (CPR) should be performed without delay.

1 The question of resuscitation should be raised as soon as possible following a patient's admission to hospital.
2 A decision *not* to resuscitate may be made with regard to the patient's wishes and the medical consultant's agreement for the following reasons:
   • A deterioration in the patient's quality of life as judged by the patient and clinical staff.
   • Where the patient's chronic condition has not responded to treatment and where no further treatment is possible.
   • Where there is no available treatment for the alleviation of a life-threatening condition.
3 The patient/family and multi-disciplinary team may initiate and take part in the discussion *but* the final decision can only be made by the medical consultant in charge of the patient's care. The medical consultant may nominate a proxy, for example the relevant specialist registrar (SpR).
4 Once the decision has been made where possible this should be communicated to the patient and where appropriate the family.
5 The decision must then be recorded in the medical notes using the following formula:
   (a) The date
   (b) Do Not Resuscitate (DNR) – written in full (code words are not recommended)
   (c) The rationale for the decision, e.g. 'Progressive disease despite optimum therapy'
   (d) By whom the decision was made – medical consultant or proxy
   (e) Signature and printed name of the medical officer completing the notes – this can be the senior house officer (SHO)
   (f) Whether the decision has been communicated to the patient and/or family and what was said.

Once the decision has been made it is imperative that it is communicated to all the ward staff and recorded in the nursing notes. If the patient is transferred to another ward or care area, his or her resuscitation status must be clearly outlined. Finally, it should be noted that a DNR order applies *only* to CPR and should not reduce the standard of medical or nursing care.

Dangers associated with resuscitation

Diseases such as autoimmune deficiency syndrome (AIDS) and hepatitis B and C have now come into focus with regard to mouth to mouth resuscitation. Research into the human immunodeficiency virus (HIV) being transmitted during resuscitation is still in its infancy, although there is no evidence to date that HIV is transmitted by saliva, and there are airway adjuncts which can be used. Pocket face masks and mouth shields are available commercially, but such devices must not hinder airflow.

References and further reading

Baskett, P.F.J. (1993) Ethics in resuscitation. *Resuscitation*, **25**, 1–8.

Cavanagh, S.J. (1990) Education aspects of cardiopulmonary resuscitation (CPR) training. *Intens Care Nurs*, **6**(1), 38–40.

Chamberlain, D. (1999) Peri-arrest arrhythmias. *Care Crit Ill*, **15**(2), 43–7. Stockton Press, Oxford.

Colqhhoun, M. *et al.* (1995) *ABC of Resuscitation*, 3rd edn. BMJ Publishing Group, London.

Cozart Rosequist, C. (1987) Current standards and guidelines for cardiopulmonary resuscitation and emergency cardiac care. *Heart and Lung Journal of Critical Care (Heart Lung)*, **16**(4), 408–18.

Craig, G.M. (1996) On withholding artificial hydration and nutrition from terminally ill sedated patients. The debate continues. *J Med Ethics*, **22**, 147–53.

Cummins, R.O. & Chamberlain, D. (1997) Recommended guidelines for reviewing, reporting and conducting research on in-hospital resuscitation: the in-hospital 'Utstein style'. *Resuscitation*, **34**, 151–83.

Dando, P. (1992) Medico-legal problems associated with resuscitation. *J Med Defence Union*, **8**.

Dimond, B. (1992) Not for resuscitative treatment. *Br J Nurs*, **1**(2), 93–4.

Doyal, L. & Wilsher, D. (1993) Withholding cardiopulmonary resuscitation: proposals for formal guidelines. *Br Med J*, **306**, June, 1593–6.

Edwards, P. (1995) The issue of resuscitation. *Nurs Times*, **91**(20), 31–3.

ERC Guidelines (1998). Resuscitation Council, London.

Ferguson, A. (1990) Cardiopulmonary resuscitation . . . a teaching guide. *Nurse Educ Today*, **10**(1), 50–53.

Gwinutt, C.L. (1998) *National Audit of In-Hospital Cardiac Arrests*. Resuscitation Council, London.

Handley, A.J. & Swain, A. (eds) (1996) Ethics and legal aspects. In: *Advanced Life Support Manual*. Resuscitation Council, London.

Handley, A.J., Becker, L.B., Allen, M. *et al.* (1997) Single rescuer adult basic life support: an advisory statement by the Basic Life Support Working Group of the International Liaison Committee on Resuscitation. *Resuscitation*, **34**, 101–107.

Hilberman, M., Kutner, J., Parsons, D. & Murphy, D.J. (1997) Marginally effective medical care: ethical analysis of issues in cardiopulmonary resuscitation (CPR). *J Med Ethics*, **23**, 361–7.

Holmberg, S. & Ekstrom, L. (1992) Ethics and practice of resuscitation – a statement for the Advanced Life Support Working Party of the European Resuscitation Council. *Resuscitation*, **24**(3), 239–44.

McPhail, A. *et al.* (1981) One hospital's experience with a 'do not resuscitate' policy. *Can Med Assoc J*, **125**, 830–36.

Neatherlin, J.S. & Brillhart, B. (1988) Glasgow Coma Scores in the patient: post-cardiopulmonary resuscitation. *J Neurosci Nurs*, **20**(2), 104–109.

Oh, T.E. (1995) *Intensive Care Manual*. Butterworths, Sydney.

Page, S. & Meerabeau, L. (1996) Nurses' accounts of cardiopulmonary resuscitation. *J Adv Nurs*, **24**, 317–25.

Quinn, T. (1998) Cardiopulmonary resuscuitation. *Nurs Stand*, **12**(46), 49–56.

RCN and BMA (1993) Cardiopulmonary resuscitation: a statement from the RCN and the BMA. *Issues in Nursing and Health*, 20, Re-order no. 000 244.

Robertson, C. & Holmberg, S. (1992) Compression techniques and blood flow during cardiopulmonary resuscitation. *Resuscitation*, **24**, 123–32.

Shoemaker, W., Ayres, S., Grenvik, A. & Holbrook, P. (1995) *Textbook of Critical Care*. W.B. Saunders, Philadelphia.

Skinner, D.V. & Vincent, R. (1997) *Cardiopulmonary Resuscitation*, pp. 31–43. Oxford University Press, Oxford.

Sowden, G.R., Baskett, P.F.J. & Robins, D.W. (1984) Factors associated with survival and eventual cerebral status following cardiac arrest. *Anaesthetics*, **39**, 1.

Tinker, J. & Zapol, W. (1991) *Care of the Critically Ill Patient*. Springer, London.

Von Planta, M. & Chamberlain, D. (1992) Drug treatment of arrhythmias during cardiopulmonary resuscitation. *Resuscitation*, **24**, 227–32.

Wynn, G. (1987) Inability of trained nurses to perform basic life support. *Br Med J*, **294**(6581), 1198.

GUIDELINES · Cardiopulmonary resuscitation

Equipment

All hospital wards and appropriate departments, i.e. computerized axial tomography (CT) scanning departments, should have a cardiac arrest trolley or box. A list of the items should be drawn up and checked weekly or immediately after use, by ward staff or designated personnel.

1 Airways (different sizes).
2 Mouth to face resuscitation mask.
3 Ambu-bag with valve and mask.
4 Oxygen tubing.
5 Suction apparatus.
6 Oropharyngeal suction catheters.

7 Laryngoscope with spare bulbs and batteries.
8 Magill's forceps.
9 Pre-prepared endotracheal tubes (different sizes according to patient populations), and introducer.
10 Gauze swabs.
11 Lubricating jelly.

12 10 ml syringe for use with endotracheal tube.
13 Artery forceps.
14 Endotracheal suction catheter.
15 Bandage or tracheostomy tape.
16 Scissors.
17 Catheter mount with swivel connector.
18 Emergency cardiac drugs (prefilled syringes).
19 Intravenous infusion administration sets including large bore central venous catheters.

20 Selection of intravenous cannulae – including large bore central venous catheters.
21 Strapping.
22 Syringes and needles (various sizes).
23 70% isopropyl alcohol swabs.
24 Intravenous infusion stand.
25 ECG monitor plus adhesive electrodes.
26 Defibrillator with conductive gel pads for defibrillation.

Procedure

Action	*Rationale*
1 Note time of arrest, if witnessed.	Lack of cerebral perfusion for approximately 3–4 minutes can lead to irreversible brain damage.
2 Give patient pre-cordial thump.	This may restore cardiac rhythm, which will give a cardiac output.
3 Summon help. If a second nurse is available, he/she can call for the cardiac arrest team, bring emergency equipment and screen off the area.	Cardiopulmonary resuscitation is more effective with two rescuers. One is responsible for inflating the lungs, and the other for chest compressions. Continue until medical help arrives.
4 Lie patient flat on firm surface. A King's Fund bed now provides such a surface; failing this, a board may be placed under the mattress, or the patient may be placed on the floor.	Effective external cardiac massage can be performed only on a hard surface.
5 If patient is in bed, remove bed head, and ensure adequate space between back of bed and wall.	To allow easy access to patients' head in order to facilitate intubation.
6 Ensure a clear airway. If cervical spine injury is excluded, extend, not hyperextend, the neck (thus lifting the tongue off the posterior wall of the pharynx). This is best achieved by lifting the chin forwards with the finger and thumb of one hand while pressing the forehead backwards with the heel of the other hand. If this fails to establish on airway, there may be obstruction by a foreign body. Try to remove the obstruction if possible.	To establish and maintain airway, thus facilitating ventilation.
Do not remove well-fitted dentures.	They help to create a mouth seal during ventilation.
7 Insert airway, and place mask over patient's mouth and nose, making sure a seal is created.	To ventilate lungs, and avoid escape of air around face mask. It avoids contact with patient's mouth, thus minimizing risk of disease transmission.
8 Locate the base of the sternum, then place one hand the width of two fingers above this point over the lower third of the sternum, midline. Ensure that only the heel of the dominant hand is touching the sternum.	To ensure accuracy of external cardiac compression.
Place the other hand on top, straighten the elbows and make sure shoulders are directly over the patient's chest.	
The sternum should be depressed sharply by 2–4 cm. The cardiac compressions should be forceful, and sustained at a rate of 60–80 per min.	Pressure on the lower half of the sternum of sufficient weight will compress the sternum and force blood out of the ventricles and improve blood flow (Oh 1995).
9 Compress the Ambu-bag in a rhythmical fashion: the bag should be attached to an oxygen source. In order to deliver 100% oxygen, a reservoir may be attached to the Ambu-bag. If, however, oxygen is not immediately available, the Ambu-bag will deliver ambient air.	To ensure a constant and steady supply of oxygen. The brain and heart have a very low tolerance to hypoxia, and any increase in the blood oxygen content will improve the chances of survival of these organs. Room air contains only 21% oxygen (Oh 1995).

Guidelines • Cardiopulmonary resuscitation (cont'd)

Action	Rationale
10 Maintain cardiac compression and ventilation at a ratio of 15:2 for one-rescuer resuscitation, and 5:1 for two-rescuer resuscitation (Fig. 8.2). This rate can be achieved effectively by counting out loud 'one and two' etc. There should be a slight pause to ensure that the delivered breath is sufficient to cause the patient's chest to rise. This must continue until cardiac output returns and the patient has a palpable blood pressure.	Counting aloud will ensure coordination of ventilation and compression ratio. To maintain circulation and oxygenation, thus reducing risk of damage to vital organs.
11 When the cardiac arrest team arrives, it will assume responsibility for the arrest in liaison with the ward staff.	To ensure an effective expert team coordinates the resuscitation.
12 Attach patient to ECG monitor using three electrodes or defibrillation patches/paddles.	To obtain adequate ECG signal. Accurate recording of cardiac rhythm will determine the appropriate treatment to be initiated.

Intubation

Action	Rationale
13 Continue to ventilate and oxygenate the patient before intubation.	The risks of cardiac arrhythmias due to hypoxia are decreased.
14 Equipment for intubation should be checked before handing to appropriate medical/nursing staff: (a) Suction equipment is operational. (b) The cuff of the endotracheal tube inflates and deflates. (c) The endotracheal tube is well lubricated. (d) That catheter mount with swivel connector is ready for use.	
15 During intubation, the anaesthetist may request cricoid pressure. This involves compressing the oesophagus between the cricoid ring and the sixth cervical vertebra to prevent regurgitation.	Aspiration of stomach contents during intubation can cause a chemical pneumonitis with an increased mortality (Oh 1995).
16 Recommence ventilation and oxygenation once intubation is completed.	Intubation should interrupt resuscitation only for a maximum of 16 sec (Handley *et al.* 1997) to prevent the occurrence of cerebral anoxia.

Intravenous access

Action	Rationale
17 Venous access must be established through a large vein as soon as possible.	To administer emergency cardiac drugs and fluid replacement.
18 Asepsis should be maintained throughout.	To prevent local and/or systemic infection.
19 The correct rate of infusion is required.	To ensure maximum drug and/or solution effectiveness.
20 Accurate recording of the administration of solutions infused and drugs added is essential.	To maintain accurate records, provide a point of reference in the event of queries and prevent any duplication of treatment.

Defibrillation

Used to terminate ventricular fibrillation or ventricular tachycardia.

Post-resuscitation care

Complete recovery from cardiac arrest does not happen immediately. The patient may require between 12 and 24 hours of mechanical ventilation after cardiac arrest.

1 Check the patient by assessing airway, breathing, circulation, blood pressure and urine output.
2 Check arterial blood gases and electrolytes.
3 Monitor patient's cardiac rhythm.
4 Chest X-ray should be taken.
5 Continue respiratory therapy.
6 Assess patient's level of consciousness. This can be done by use of the Glasgow Coma Scale. Although this is intended primarily for head injury, it is clinically relevant. It contains five levels of consciousness:
  (a) Conscious and alert
  (b) Drowsy but responsive to verbal commands
  (c) Unconscious but responsive to minimal painful stimuli
  (d) Unconscious and responsive to deep painful stimuli
  (e) Unconscious and unresponsive.
  See Chap. 26, Neurological Observations.
7 The patient should be made comfortable and nursed in the appropriate position, i.e. upright or in the recovery position. Avoid nursing supine as this physiologically hinders cardiac output and respiration. Careful explanation and reassurance is vital at all times, particularly if the patient is conscious and aware.

The patient should be transferred to a special unit, i.e. coronary care or intensive care.

Continent Urinary Diversions

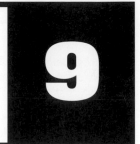

Definition

A urinary diversion is a surgically created system for removing urine from the body when either the bladder or urethra is either non-existent or no longer viable. There are two main types: a urostomy (see Chap. 39, Stoma Care) and continent urinary diversions. *Continent* urinary diversions differ in that a system is created to collect and store urine before it is removed from the body.

Indications for formation of a continent urinary diversion

A continent urinary diversion may be formed to:

1 Store and expel urine from the body if the lower urinary tract is defective or absent
2 Offer patients a choice of urinary diversion
3 Improve or maintain the individual's body image, psychological and social well-being by removing the necessity of wearing external devices, e.g. urostomy pouch, or incontinence pads.

(Randles 1990; Leaver 1997)

Reference material

Principles of a continent urinary diversion

A continent urinary diversion is surgically constructed to replace a defective or non-existent lower urinary tract. It consists of three components:

1 A reservoir to store urine
2 A continence mechanism to retain urine in the reservoir
3 A channel or tunnel to let the urine out

(Leaver 1996, 1997).

The reservoir can be the bladder itself, an augmented bladder or made completely of ileum, colon or a combination of the two. The continence mechanism may be constructed during the operation using the same tissues used to construct the reservoir or an existing valve or sphincter may be utilised (Leaver 1997). Five types of continence systems have been identified;

1 The flutter valve, created by the intussusception of a segment of bowel, usually ileum, e.g. Kock nipple

2 The flap valve, created by tunnelling a narrow tube between the muscle and mucosal layers of the reservoir, e.g. Mitrofanoff valve
3 The ileocaecal valve
4 The urethral sphincter
5 The anal sphincter.

The channel or tunnel component can be formed by utilizing other tube/tunnel-like structures such as the appendix, ureter or fallopian tube. Alternatively, a segment of ileum or colon can be used (Leaver 1996).

There are a number of different types of continent diversions performed today (Table 9.1). These procedures differ in construction, using different structures to form the reservoir and tunnel and different techniques to create the continence mechanism. The outcome for patients and the nursing care involved is essentially similar in most cases. The most commonly performed procedure in the UK is arguably the Mitrofanoff (Leaver 1996) (Figs. 9.1 and 9.2).

Continent urinary diversions are increasingly available as an alternative to the conventional ileal conduit (see Chap. 39, Stoma Care). The aim of these diversions is to mimic, as far as possible, the normal bladder function. The goal is:

1 To create a pouch with the ability to hold an adequate volume of urine at low pressure
2 To preserve and protect the upper tract by preventing reflux
3 To prevent or minimize the absorption of urine, thus avoiding metabolic disturbances
4 To control urine voiding by self-catheterisation

(Razor 1993; Leaver 1996).

The continent urinary diversion involves the patient having two admissions into hospital. The first is to form the continent urinary diversion. Following the operation, a sterile fine-bore tube is left in the continent urinary stoma

Table 9.1 Types of continent urinary diversion with catheterizable stomas

1 Mitrofanoff pouch
2 Kock pouch
3 Benchekroun pouch
4 Mainz pouch
5 Indiana pouch
6 Le bag

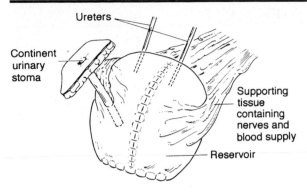

Figure 9.1   Continent urinary diversion.

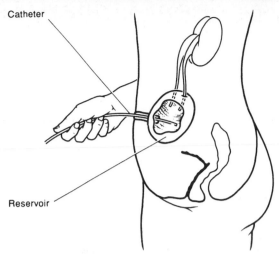

Figure 9.2   Self-catheterization into the continent urinary stoma.

to keep it patent and allow the urine to drain into a catheter bag. After recovering from the operation, patients are taught how to take care of the tubing, leg bags and night drainage systems. Patients are then discharged home to be readmitted 6 weeks after the operation to be taught self-catheterization. This admission lasts between 24 and 48 hours. During this time, patients are taught self-catheterization and encouraged to practise the technique. Nursing staff are available to detect and rectify any problems. This allows patients time to gain confidence in self-catheterization before they return home.

In a continent urinary diversion the urine drains into the urinary reservoir or bladder through the ureters. Patients can self-catheterize into the continent urinary stoma every 4–6 hours to empty the urine reservoir (Fig. 9.2). This is achieved by the patient adjusting any restrictive clothing and inserting a special tube into the continent urinary stoma, pointing the other end into the toilet. When urine has drained out the tube is removed, washed with water and replaced in its container (usually a plastic bag, spectacle case or cosmetic bag).

Before each discharge, patients are given verbal and written advice (Horn 1990), and can contact the hospital 24 hours a day.

The Mitrofanoff pouch was devised in the late 1970s/early 1980s by Paul Mitrofanoff (1980) in France. Initially, it was devised for patients with bladder neck obstruction or incompetence. The bladder was preserved and the appendix was used as the continent urinary stoma. One end of the appendix is buried in a submuscular tunnel in the bladder, forming an obstructing flap valve. The other end is brought to the surface of the abdominal wall to form a continent stoma. As the bladder fills with urine more pressure is put on the valve, causing it to become even more obstructed. A catheter is passed into the stoma along the channel, through the valve and into the bladder when the patient wants to empty their bladder (Leaver 1996).

Mitrofanoff's principle can be adapted to suit each individual patient taking into account their underlying condition and the available body tissues (Duckett & Snyder 1985; Leaver 1994). For example, patients with urinary incontinence may have their bladder preserved and urethra oversown, a tunnel may then be fashioned using

their appendix. Other patients with bladder cancer following cystectomy may have a new 'bladder' constructed from a segment of ileum and, in the absence of an appendix, another segment of ileum may be used to construct the tunnel.

Indications for surgical formation of a continent urinary diversion

The indications for the formation of a continent urinary diversion and an ileal conduit are similar (see Chap. 39, Stoma Care). These include:

1 Congenital abnormalities, e.g. bladder exstrophy
2 Pelvic cancers, e.g. bladder, cervical
3 Neuropathic bladder – a condition where the nerve impulses do not reach the bladder as the result of an underlying disease or injury, e.g. myelomeningocele
4 Trauma
5 Incontinence
6 Interstitial cystitis
7 Radiation fibrosis
8 Irreparable fistula
9 An existing urinary diversion, e.g. ileal conduit

(Horn 1990; Woodhouse 1991; Leaver 1994)

Patient selection

Patients are selected carefully for this type of surgery. They must be physically and psychologically able to undergo lengthy major surgery. Patients need to have an adequate renal function and a healthy bowel, particularly if the bladder is to be replaced with a reservoir constructed from a segment of bowel (Horn 1990; Razor 1993; Leaver 1996). They must also be motivated towards self-catheterization and be dextrous enough to manipulate a nelaton catheter.

Table 9.2 Advantages and disadvantages of an ileal conduit (from Horn 1990)

Advantages	Disadvantages
1 Tried and tested technique, in use since 1950 (Bricker & Eisenman 1950, cited in Boyd & Lieskovsky 1988).	1 Continual urine leakage necessitating the wearing of an appliance.
2 Surgery is not as extensive as with a continent urinary diversion.	2 Potential problem of skin excoriation.
3 The skills to care for an ileal conduit are relatively easy to learn.	3 Potential problem of altered body image to patients and others.
4 Lower incidence of postoperative problems.	4 Fear of maintaining or creating new relationships.

Specific pre-operative preparation

Patients undergo the usual preparation for anaesthesia (see Chap. 30, Peri-Operative Care). Only the specific preparation is discussed here although physical preparation may vary according to the individual surgeon's preference.

Pre-operative counselling

Once patients have been selected as suitable candidates, psychological preparation should begin as soon as possible. Boore (1978), Hayward (1978), Zeimer (1983), Morris *et al.* (1989), Raleigh *et al.* (1990) and Roberts (1991) have illustrated the importance of pre-operative information and explanation in reducing postoperative physical and psychological stress to the individual following the formation of a stoma (ileal conduit or colostomy). Their research is also applicable to patients receiving continent urinary diversion stomas. This is discussed in Chap. 39, Stoma Care.

Patients should receive a full explanation of the operation and its effects. The amount and type of information should be adapted to the individual's requirements. When circumstances permit, patients have the opportunity to choose between an ileal conduit and a continent urinary diversion. This usually takes place in an outpatients clinic, and is reiterated when the patient has been admitted to the ward. The formation of an ileal conduit as well as a continent urinary diversion is discussed with the patient; the advantages and disadvantages of both operations should be fully discussed (Tables 9.2 and 9.3). They should be shown pictures of the continent urinary diversion and ileal conduit stomas, and are encouraged to familiarize themselves with the equipment: pouches, wafers, catheterization tubes and bladder syringes.

Useful aids

Useful aids for teaching patients and helping them to understand the procedure and the implications it may have on their lives include the following:

1 Information booklets
2 Videos
3 Diagrams
4 Samples of equipment

5 Visits from individuals with a continent urinary diversion (ideally of a similar age, sex and background to the patient).

Bowel preparation

Patients are admitted 2–3 days before surgery to commence a regime to evacuate all faecal matter from the intestine. The regime used depends on the surgeon's preference. It is necessary to clear the bowel to:

1 Prevent hard faecal masses from impacting proximal to an anastomosis
2 Prevent faeces spilling from the cut ends of the bowel during the operation
3 Reduce bacterial contamination when the bowel is opened

(Alexander Williams 1980).

Patients undergoing this procedure are at risk of developing hypovolaemia and electrolyte imbalance. Therefore, it is important that the fluid loss is replaced orally or intravenously (Skinner & Lieskovsky 1988; Woodhouse 1989).

Sexual dysfunction

Following the formation of a continent urinary diversion possible sexual impairment for both men and women may occur. This is the same as for other stoma patients and is discussed in Chap. 39, Stoma Care.

Pre- and postoperative counselling is given to each patient and partner. Each person's potential sexual dysfunction should be discussed and treated on an individual basis.

Specific postoperative care

Reconstruction of the lower urinary tract is a lengthy procedure and has a significant complication rate (Leaver 1996). Patients may require a short stay in intensive care or a high dependency unit after surgery. Postoperative care is similar to that for major abdominal surgery, with special attention to urinary output and the patency of the many drainage tubes (Fig. 9.3). Extensive experience has shown that to allow healing of the continent diversion and to reduce the risk of urine leaking into the peritoneum it is

Table 9.3 Advantages and disadvantages of a continent urinary diversion (from Horn 1990; Galister & Woodhouse 1991)

Advantages	Disadvantages
1 No need to wear an appliance.	1 Patient must be enthusiastic and motivated towards self-catheterization.
2 Small stoma, 0.5–1 cm in diameter.	2 There are problems with the operation technique, which is being refined to improve stoma continence.
3 No urine leakage.	3 Operation still involves a laparotomy and drain-site scars, which do fade but may cause an altered body image.
4 Improves or maintains body image by removing the need to wear external devices and by having control over voiding urine.	4 Consider whether patient will have the physical ability to be able to self-catheterize in 5–10 years' time.
5 No skin excoriation.	5 It is a long operation with a high risk of postoperative problems, and requires two hospitalizations.
	6 Lack of familiarity in outside specialist centres.
	7 Long-term problems are unknown.
	8 Surgical and nursing care techniques are modified regularly.
	9 Patients may fear they are being used to test the operation.

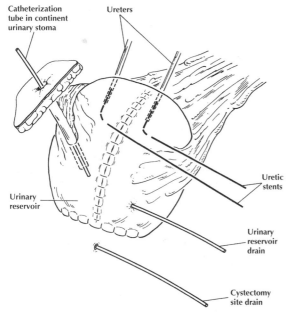

Figure 9.3 Siting of wound drains to reduce risk of haematoma and abscess formation.

important that the reservoir is kept empty for 6–8 weeks. A stoma catheter and a pouch catheter drain the reservoir. If the patient's ureters have had to be re-implanted then there will be one or two ureteric stents (fine bore catheters) in place. These stents will initially drain most of the urine. The catheters draining the reservoir can become blocked by debris or mucus produced by the bowel utilized to form it. Therefore in order to keep the stoma and pouch catheters patent they should be flushed twice daily with

20 ml of sterile 0.9% sodium chloride, commencing day 1 postoperatively. This should be increased to twice daily gentle washouts of the reservoir, using 100 ml of sterile 0.9% sodium chloride on day 4 postoperatively. Once the patient is able they should be taught how to perform this procedure, as it will have to be maintained following their discharge home.

The ureteric stents, if present, are gently pulled on day 7 after the operation to remove them. If resistance is felt the stents should be left in and the procedure repeated on a daily basis, until the stents slide out. Generally the stents are totally removed by day 10. By this time wound drains, the nasogastric tube or gastrostomy tube and all intravenous catheters should also have been removed. After this time the patient may have a cystogram or 'pouchogram' performed to check that the reservoir is intact. If there are no leaks detected on this examination the pouch catheter is removed. The stoma catheter will therefore drain all the urine from the pouch. Patients are discharged home for 4–6 weeks with this catheter in place on 'free drainage' and with instructions to carry out at least twice daily washouts. This is to ensure that the urine drains and that the reservoirs are not stretched at any time. Some patients prefer to be discharged with both the stoma catheter and pouch catheter in place, although only one is usually on free drainage.

Patient education before first discharge

Before discharge, patients should be taught how to flush the continent urinary stoma tubing using tap water (Lapides 1971), secure the tube in place and attach drainage bags. They are taught how to recognize a urinary tract infection and advised to drink at least 2–3 litres of fluid daily to reduce risk of this happening. They are also advised to wear a medical aid bracelet, so that if they are found unconscious at any time a doctor or nurse will know how to empty the urine drainage system.

When patients are well enough to be discharged, they are able to go home for a few weeks before being readmitted to be taught self-catheterization. Patients should be seen by the nurse specialist before discharge and a request for community nurses to continue support at home should be made. An explanatory letter and the relevant literature is supplied. Patients are encouraged to seek advice from the ward staff at any time.

Second admission

Patients are readmitted 6 weeks after the operation to expand the pouch and to be taught intermittent self-catheterization. The stoma catheter is clamped and patients are encouraged to drink fluids. This allows the pouch to fill up with urine and helps the patient establish what sensation is experienced as this happens. Patients have described this sensation as a feeling of fullness, bloated feeling, discomfort or an ache. However, some patients experience no sensations at all when the pouch is full and have to establish a voiding programme to avoid overfilling of the pouch. The stoma catheter is released after 2–3 hours, depending on how the patient tolerates the sensation and on the amount of fluid drunk. This process is repeated 1–2 times more, during the day, to continue expanding the pouch. Experience has shown that at this stage the average pouch capacity is 250–300 ml. The pouches are generally constructed to hold 500 ml and it may take several weeks to reach this target. Patients continue to expand their pouch at their own pace once they are discharged.

Once the pouch has been initially stretched, the catheter is removed and the catheterization procedure is explained and demonstrated. See 'Teaching intermittent self-catheterization', below. Patients should be supervised during the catheterization process until they are competent and confident with the procedure. Generally, patients remain in hospital 1–2 days.

Second discharge advice

Once proficient with intermittent self-catheterization, patients are discharged home with a 2–4 week outpatient clinic appointment to see the surgeon and nurse specialist. Before patients are discharged they should be informed about the following:

1 To empty pouch every 4–6 hours to prevent overdistension and to always empty pouch before participating in strenuous activities to minimize the pressure put on the pouch. If the pouch becomes too full there is a risk of trauma to, or rupture of, the pouch, leakage of urine via the tunnel or, because of increased pressure on the valve, it may make catheterization difficult or impossible (Leaver 1997).

2 To ensure an undisturbed sleep by reducing the amount of fluid the patient drinks 3 hours before going to sleep. The patient should catheterize before going to sleep and on waking.

3 To keep a catheter available at all times (in suit, car, handbag, at work and at home), in case patient needs to empty the urine.

4 A small amount of mucus may leak from the continent urinary stoma and a piece of gauze can be worn to protect clothing.

5 On discharge, patients are given a supply of low friction self-catheterization catheters. These are generally PVC, male-length nelaton-type. This is because the female length catheters are too short to reach into the reservoir to empty all of the urine and for the urine to drain cleanly into the toilet. Various makes of catheter are available on prescription and patients are given information on how to obtain further supplies.

6 Catheters may be re-used for up to 7 days provided they are rinsed out with tap water, patted dry with a tissue and stored in a clean dry receptacle (plastic bag, cosmetic bag, spectacle case) between uses. Patients are advised to ascertain the manufacturer's recommendations for care of their particular appliance.

7 If the patient finds it difficult to insert the catheter into the stoma, he or she is advised to pause and rest for 10 minutes before attempting to insert the catheter again. This is to allow any swelling around the stoma to subside (Horn 1990, 1991). If it is still difficult, then a warm bath sometimes dilates the stoma. The patient should then try again, with a size smaller tube. If it is still difficult, the hospital should be contacted.

8 If there is trauma during catheterization, such as some spotting of blood, the patient should wait 10 minutes and then try again. Trauma may be caused by rough catheterization technique, using the wrong size of catheter or by a problem with the continent urinary stoma which requires further investigation. A doctor should be consulted if the bleeding continues or increases.

9 Patients should be told that it can take a while to become confident with this procedure. However, they can contact the hospital at any time for advice and reassurance.

Long- and short-term problems

A number of complications have been identified; these may be short-term 'teething' problems while the pouch settles down and the patient becomes familiar with it. However, some patients require further surgery or treatment to rectify problems to ensure their pouch function is acceptable. The most common complications are:

1 Infection
2 Stenosis of the stoma
3 Leakage via the stoma
4 Inability to empty pouch
5 Loss of tunnel
6 High-pressure bladder system
7 Stone formation
8 Metabolic acidosis
9 Renal damage
10 Pouch rupture

(Wagstaff *et al.* 1991; McCahill *et al.* 1992; Woodhouse 1994). As the formation of a continent urinary diversion is a relatively new surgical technique the long-term complications (other than those listed above) are unknown. Therefore patients remain on long-term follow-up at those centres where these procedures are performed.

Psychological effects

Several surveys have been undertaken to compare ileal conduits with Mitrofanoff/Kock's continent urinary diversions in terms of social and sexual effects, and to assess the effect on the patient of converting an ileal conduit to a continent urinary diversion (Boyd et al. 1987; Mansson et al. 1988, 1991; Oishi et al. 1993). Each examined the effect of cystectomy and investigated issues such as depression, adjustment to the new skills required for self-catheterization or use of stoma appliances, and changes in social, sports and sexual activity. The evidence suggests that patients are able to learn the manual skills required of them, but that all experience some degree of depression and altered body image. Patients with ileal conduits reported a more negative body image and a higher incidence of depression compared with the other two groups. Patients with a primary continent urinary diversion also exhibited depression and altered body image. Patients whose ileal conduit was converted to a continent urinary diversion experienced less depression and fewer negative changes in body image. It is conjectured that this is because these patients perceive a definite improvement in their situation when the conversion is carried out (Boyd et al. 1987; Mansson et al. 1988, 1991; Oishi et al. 1993).

These studies did not investigate altered body image or psychological morbidity in patients whose ileal conduits or continent urinary diversions were performed for non-malignant disease. Kennedy et al. (1993), however, describe the experiences of four women who had successful pregnancies following continent urinary diversions for non-malignant disease.

The importance of the role of stoma therapists and nursing staff in providing information tailored for the individual and in teaching new skills is recognized by patients, and it is suggested that these functions play a part in adjustment to changes brought about by surgery (Boyd et al. 1987; Mansson et al. 1988, 1991; Oishi et al. 1993).

Useful addresses

The Urostomy Association
Central Office
'Buckland'
Beaumont Park
Danbury
Essex
CM3 4DE
Tel.: 01245 224294

Impotence Information
  Centre
PO Box 1130
London
WC1X 9JN

The Royal Marsden
  Hospital
Fulham Road
London
SW3 6JJ
Tel.: 0207 3528171

Medic-Alert Foundation
17 Bridge Wharf
156 Caledonian Road
London
N1 9UU
Tel.: 0171 833 3034

References and further reading

Alexander Williams, J. (1980) Cleaning the gut for colonic surgery. *World Med*, **15**(10), 18–19.

Arai, Y. *et al.* (1993) Long-term follow-up of the Kock and Indiana pouch procedures. *J Urol*, **150**(1), 51–5.

Boore, J.R.P. (1978) *A Prescription for Recovery: The Effects of Pre-operative Preparation of Surgical Patients on Post-operative Stress, Recovery and Infection*. Royal College of Nursing, London.

Boyd, S.D. & Lieskovsky, D. (1988) Creation of the continent Kock ileal reservoir as an alternative to cutaneous urinary diversion. In: *Diagnosis and Management of Genitourinary Cancer* (eds D. Skinner & D. Lieskovsky), Chap. 46. W.B. Saunders, Philadelphia.

Boyd, S.D. *et al.* (1987) Quality of life survey of urinary diversion patients: comparison of ileal conduits versus continent urinary reservoirs. *J Urol*, **138**, 1386–9.

Brocklehurst, J.C. & Brocklehurst, S. (1978) Management of indwelling catheters. *Br J Urol*, **50**(2), 102–105.

Cummings, J. *et al.* (1987) The choice of suprapubic continent catheterisable urinary stoma. *Br J Urol*, **60**, 227–30.

Delvin, H.B. & Plant, J. (1979) Sexual function – an aspect of stoma care. *Br J Sex Med*, **1**, pp. 2, 6, 22, 26, 33–4, 37.

Diokno, A.C. *et al.* (1983) Fate of patients started on clean intermittent self-catheterisation therapy ten years ago. *J Urol*, **3**(2), 191–3.

Duckett, J.W. & Snyder, H.M. (1985) Use of the Mitrofanoff principle in urinary reconstruction. *World J Urol*, **3**, 191–3.

Duckett, J.W. & Snyder, H.M. (1986) Continent urinary diversion – the Mitrofanoff principle. *J Urol*, **136**, 58–62.

Fillingham, S. & Douglas, J. (1997) *Urological Nursing*, 2nd edn. Baillière Tindall, London.

Galister, J.S. & Woodhouse, C.R. (1991) Role of continent suprapubic diversion in pelvic cancer. *Br J Urol*, **68**(4), 376–9.

Hayward, J. (1978) *Information – A Prescription Against Pain*. Royal College of Nursing, London.

Horn, S.A. (1990) Nursing patients with a continent urinary diversion. *Nurs Stand*, **4**(21), 24–6.

Horn, S.A. (1991) *Continent Urinary Diversions – Your Questions Answered. Patients' Information Booklet*. Royal Marsden Hospital, London.

Jeffrey, L. *et al.* (1988) The Mitrofanoff principle: an alternative form of continent urinary diversion. *J Urol*, **140**, 1529–31.

Jones, M.A. *et al.* (1981) Life with an ileal conduit: results of a questionnaire – surveys of patients and urological surgeons. *Br J Urol*, **52**, 21–5.

Kennedy, W.A. *et al.* (1993) Pregnancy after orthotopic continent urinary diversion. *Surg, Gynaecol Obstet*, **177**(4), 405–409.

Kock, N.G. *et al.* (1987) Appliance-free sphincter controlled bladder substitute. *J Urol*, **138**, 1150–54.

Lapides, S. (1971) Clean intermittent self-catheterization in the treatment of urinary tract disease. *Trans-Am Assoc Genitourin Surg*, **63**, 92.

Lapides, J. *et al.* (1974) Follow-up on unsterile intermittent self-catheterisation. *J Urol*, **11**(1), 184.

Leaver, R.B. (1994) The Mitrofanoff pouch: a continent urinary diversion. *Prof Nurse*, **9**(11), 748–53.

Leaver, R.B. (1996) Continent urinary diversions – the Mitrofanoff principle. In: *Stoma Care Nursing – A Patient-Centred Approach* (C. Myers). Edward Arnold, London.

Leaver, R.B. (1997) Reconstructive surgery for the promotion of continence. In: *Urological Nursing* (S. Fillingham & J. Douglas). Baillière Tindall, London.

Lindenhall, B. *et al.* (1994) Long-term intermittent catheterisation: the experience of teenagers and young adults with myelomeningocele. *J Urol*, **152**(1), 187–9.

Mansson, A. *et al.* (1988) Quality of life after cystectomy. *Br J Urol,* **62**(4), 240–45.

Mansson, A. *et al.* (1991) Psychological adjustment to cystectomy for bladder carcinoma and effects on interpersonal relationships. *Scand J Caring Sci,* **5**(3), 129–34.

McCahill, P.D. *et al.* (1992) Toxic shock syndrome: a complication of continent urinary diversion. *J Urol,* **147**(3), 681–7.

Mitrofanoff, P. (1980) Cystomie continente trans appendiclaire dans le traitment des vessies neurologiques. *Chirurgie Pediatr,* **21**, 297–305.

Morris, J. *et al.* (1989) *The Benefits of Providing Information to Patients.* Centre for Health Economics, University of York.

Oishi, K. *et al.* (1993) Quality of life of patients with a continent urinary reservoir. *Hinyokika-kiyo,* **39**(1), 7–14.

Raleigh, E.H. *et al.* (1990) Significant others benefit from preoperative information. *J Adv Nurs,* **15**(8), 941–5.

Randles, J. (1990) The Mitrofanoff pouch. *Nursing,* **4**(18), 20–22.

Randles, J. (1992) An alternative to urinary conduit. *Nurs Stand,* **6**(42), 33–6.

Razor, B.R. (1993) Continent urinary reservoirs. *Semin Oncol Nurs,* **9**(4), 272–85.

Roberts, S. (1991) Theatre nursing operation reassurance, preoperative visiting. *Nurs Times,* **87**(41), 70–71.

Skinner, D.G. & Boyd, S.D. (1984) Techniques of creation of a continent urinary ileal reservoir (Kock pouch) for urinary diversion. *Urol Clin North Am,* **11**(4), 741–9.

Skinner, D.G. & Lieskovsky, D. (1988) Technique of radical cystectomy. In: *Diagnosis and Management of Genitourinary Cancer* (eds D.G. Skinner & D. Lieskovsky). W.B. Saunders, Philadelphia.

Wagstaff, K.E., Woodhouse, C.R.J., Rose, G.A. *et al.* (1991) Blood and urine analysis in patients with intestinal bladders. *J Urol,* **68**, 311–16.

Whitfield, H.N. & Hendry, W.F. (eds) (1985) *Textbook of Genito-Urinary Surgery.* Chap. 101, Pathophysiology of erection and ejaculation (G.S. Brindley); Chap. 102, Investigations and treatment of impotence (J.P. Pryor); Chap. 121, Bladder surgery (W.F. Hendry & H.N. Whitfield). Churchill Livingstone, Edinburgh.

Woodhouse, C.R.J. (1989) The Mitrofanoff principle for continent urinary diversions. *Br J Urol,* **63**(1), 53–7.

Woodhouse, C.R.J. (1991) *Long-term Paediatric Urology.* Blackwell Scientific, Oxford.

Woodhouse, C.R.J. (1994) *The Infective Metabolic and Histological Consequences of Enterocystoplasty.* European Board of Urology, European Urology Update Series, Vol. 3. Union European des Medecins Specialistes.

Woodhouse, C.R.J. (1994) The Mitrofanoff pouch for urethral failure. *Br J Urol,* **73**(1), 55–60.

Zeimer, M.M. (1983) Effects of information on post-surgical coping. *Nurs Res,* **32**(5), 282–7.

Teaching intermittent self-catheterization of a continent urinary diversion stoma

Definition

Intermittent self-catheterization is when patients insert a self-catheterization catheter into the urinary reservoir via the continent urinary stoma using a clean technique. It is performed to evacuate or instill fluids, after which the tube is removed.

Indications

Intermittent self-catheterization may be carried out for the following reasons:

1 To empty the contents of the urinary reservoir every 4–6 hours. If the reservoir is left too long between emptying it can become overstretched and lose its elasticity.
2 To allow irrigation of the urinary reservoir for the removal of mucus which may occlude the continent urinary stoma.

Reference material

The following research has been gathered from urethral self-catheterization. However, the same principles would apply to a continent urinary stoma.

Intermittent self-catheterization is intended to make life easier and not more complicated. It is associated with a lower incidence of urinary tract infection than long-term indwelling catheters (Lapides 1971, 1974; Diokno *et al.* 1983; Lindenhall *et al.* 1994).

Types of tubing used for intermittent self-catheterization

Catheters used for intermittent self-catheterization should be smooth surfaced and flexible. The nelaton-type of catheter, which is made of soft plastic and has two drainage eyes at one end and a funnel at the other, is most commonly used for patients with continent diversions. The smallest size of catheter which will drain the reservoir at an acceptable speed should be used (Fillingham & Douglas 1996). If the continent stoma and tunnel has been constructed from a fine tube-like structure, such as a ureter or fallopian tube, a small gauge catheter (6–10ch) may be needed. Fine-bore feeding tubes have been used in some instances (Horn 1990; see Chap. 43, Urinary Catheterization).

Teaching self-catheterization

Intermittent self-catheterization should be taught in a place that offers privacy, with a good clear light and a full-length mirror (bathroom, toilet or at the patient's bedside) (Horn 1990). It is a clean and not a sterile procedure. Patients can learn self-catheterization with the aid of a mirror or by touch, and are observed and assisted by a nurse until they are proficient (see Procedure, Guidelines • Self-catheterization, below).

During the day patients are encouraged to drink 2–3 litres of fluid to reduce the risk of any urinary tract infection and to catheterize every 4–6 hours to prevent the reservoir becoming distended and losing its elasticity. However, patients can reduce their fluid intake during the evening so that they need catheterize only before they go to sleep and again when they get up in the morning.

GUIDELINES · Self-catheterization

Equipment

1 Catheters for catheterization depending upon the size of the stoma.
2 Catheter-tipped syringe.
3 Tissues.

4 Clean jug or bowl.
5 Low-linting gauze and non-allergenic skin protective tape to cover stoma if it oozes mucus.

Procedure

Action	Rationale
1 Explain and discuss the procedure with the patient.	To ensure that the patient understands the procedure and gives his/her valid consent.
2 Collect all equipment necessary for the procedure.	To ensure all the equipment required is easily available.
3 Take the equipment to the toilet, bathroom or screened bed area. Ensure there is a good light and a full-length mirror.	To ensure the patient's privacy. To ensure the patient can see the stoma clearly.
4 The equipment should be arranged on a clean surface and within easy reach for the procedure.	To reduce the risk of contamination by surface bacteria. So that equipment is easily available.
5 The patient needs to remove any inhibiting clothing.	To ensure the patient can examine the stoma.
6 The patient should wash their hands with soap and water then dry them.	To ensure the hands are clean.
7 The patient should look at the stoma, if necessary with the aid of a hand or full-length mirror.	To look for mucus and swelling around the stoma.
8 The patient should wipe away any mucus with a tissue soaked in warm water and gently pat dry.	To ensure the opening of the stoma is clear and mucus does not block the catheter during insertion into stoma.
9 Remove the plastic tube from its container. Moisten the tip to be inserted with warm, running water or water-soluble lubricant.	To act as a lubricant to allow the tube to enter the urinary reservoir without causing internal trauma.
10 Ensure the untipped end of the tube is in a receiver, i.e. jug, bowl or toilet.	To ensure the urine goes into a bowl and not onto the patient.
11 The patient can use either a mirror to guide the tube into the opening of the stoma or feel the opening with two fingers slightly apart with the stoma between.	To act as a guide to pass the tube into the continent urinary stoma.
12 Insert the tube gently into the stoma following the pathway inside (usually towards the middle of the abdomen) until urine starts to flow, then insert tube a further 4–6 cm to reduce risk of contamination.	The direction of insertion and the diameter of catheter inserted depends on the type, size and shape of continent urinary stoma. To negotiate continence device.
13 When all the urine has stopped flowing advance the catheter to ensure the bladder is completely empty. Slowly remove the catheter using a rotating action. If urine starts flowing again wait until it stops before removing the catheter any further.	To ensure complete emptying of the urinary reservoir. The rotating acting reduces the suction effect and pain due to friction (Leaver 1996).
14 Remove the tube. Hold one end up then the other end.	To allow complete drainage of the tube.

Guidelines • Self-catheterization (cont'd)

Action	Rationale
15 Rinse tubing through with lukewarm tap water and dry with a tissue.	To rinse out any urine.
16 Replace the tube in its plastic container.	To keep the tubing clean.
17 Cover the stoma with a non-adherent dressing and secure with skin-protective tape.	To prevent mucus staining the patient's clothing.
18 The patient should wash the hands with soap and water, and then dry them.	To remove any urine on the hands.
19 The patient can then dress, collect equipment and dispose of any soiled dressings.	To prevent cross-infection.

Nursing care plan

Problem	Cause	Suggested action
Cannot insert the catheter into the stoma.	Using too large a catheter. Unable to locate opening. Opening occluded, e.g. due to swelling.	Advise the patient to try a smaller sized catheter, and to use a magnifying mirror to find the opening. Advise the patient to rest for 10 minutes to let the stoma relax and then to insert catheter. A warm bath may help to dilate the opening. If still unable to catheterize, then patient should contact the hospital.

Doctor may give subcutaneous injection of steroid to reduce swelling. A needle and syringe may be used to draw off a quantity of urine to take pressure off the valve and thus allow the catheter to be inserted. If the opening remains occluded, a suprapubic catheter may be inserted to allow the swelling to subside and drain the urine from the reservoir. The stoma may need to be dilated by a doctor. |
| Partial insertion only of catheter is possible. | Tubing kinked. Stricture in the stoma. | Remove tubing and try with fresh tubing of the same size. Or try with a size smaller tubing. If unable to catheterize, contact the hospital. |
| Patient has not catheterized for 4 h and feels distended, is easily catheterized but no urine is passed. | Tubing not reaching the reservoir. Tubing kinked. Tube is double backing on itself.

Tube blocked with mucus. | Insert tubing further. Do not use force. If there is resistance then stop. Contact the hospital.

Cough. The increased intra-abdominal pressure may dislodge the plug of mucus. While the tube is inserted, flush it with tap water. Remove tubing, examine for mucus and reinsert once it is clear. Flush the urinary reservoir. |

Stoma leaks urine between catheterizations.	Reservoir not emptied regularly. Mucus plug blocking tubing, preventing complete drainage. Stoma failure.	Catheterize every 3–4 h. If the patient has drunk large amounts, or alcohol (a diuretic), or is taking diuretic medication, it may be necessary to catheterize more frequently. Flush reservoir at least twice a day. If still leaking inform the hospital. Surgical fashioning of the stoma may be necessary.
Staining of blood during catheterization.	Trauma due to rough technique. Using wrong type of self-catheterization catheter.	Lubricate the tube well with water and insert gently into stoma. Use lubricating jelly. If blood staining continues or increases in amount then inform the hospital. Use low friction self-catheterization catheter.

Cytotoxic Drugs: Handling and Administration

Definition

The term cytotoxic literally translated means 'toxic to cells'. Hence these drugs are those which kill cells (malignant or non-malignant).

Reference material

Cytotoxic drug handling by nursing, pharmacy and other health care professionals has been acknowledged as an occupational hazard (Valanis et al. 1993). Cytotoxic drugs have been shown to be mutagenic, teratogenic and carcinogenic when given at therapeutic levels to animals and humans to destroy malignant cells (Bingham 1985; Waksvik et al. 1987; Goodman & Riley 1997). Patients have been shown to develop secondary cancers as a result of treatment with cytotoxic drugs and such risks may be acceptable when patients have a life-threatening illness (Cass et al. 1997). However, these effects are not acceptable to personnel involved in the reconstitution and administration of cytotoxic drugs and the handling of waste and spills. The risk to health associated with exposure is measured by the time, dose and routes of exposure. Cytotoxic drugs can be absorbed through the skin (although with the majority of the compounds there is little or no absorption through intact skin, the exceptions are those which are lipid-soluble). Skin exposure can be by contact with contaminated equipment used in preparing or administering the drugs or during the handling and disposal of waste. In the latter instance this is because drugs and metabolites can be excreted in urine and stools up to 48 hours after administration (Valanis et al. 1993; Cass et al. 1997). Drugs can also be ingested by contaminated food, or be inhaled as a result of aerosolization of powder or liquid during reconstitution. On the basis of the evidence available at present, risks to personnel involved in the reconstitution and administration of cytotoxic drugs fall into two categories – local effects and systemic effects:

1 Local effects are usually caused by direct contact with the skin, eyes and mucous membranes, e.g. dermatitis, inflammation of mucous membranes, excessive lacrimation, pigmentation, blistering (associated with mustine) and other miscellaneous, allergic reactions (Weinstein 1997).

2 The systemic effects of cytotoxic drugs may also have harmful short- or long-term effects if inhaled or ingested during preparation. These effects include lightheadedness, dizziness; nausea; headache; alopecia; coughing; pruritus; general malaise (Valanis 1993; Weinstein, 1997).

A number of experimental studies have suggested that serious long-term effects may result from exposure to cytotoxic drugs. Effects include chromosomal abnormalities (Waksvik et al. 1987) and reproductive function disorders including infertility (Selevan et al. 1985; Valanis et al. 1997). Mutagenic substances have been found in the urine and serum of cytotoxic drug handlers, including nurses (Ames et al. 1975; Falck et al. 1979; Vennit et al. 1984; Kaijser et al. 1990; Newman et al. 1994). It has been shown that although alterations in cell structure have been detected, they appear to be transient and of a low level. It has yet to be demonstrated whether these changes in cell structure are harmful and if this level of mutagenesis can be equated with more serious consequences. There are also many limitations in testing blood and urine due to the range of agents which cannot be detected, low levels of drugs and metabolites and reduced sensitivity of the tests (Cass et al. 1997). This has led to difficulties when offering staff monitoring and surveillance and it is less common to do extensive biological testing as there are no data to support a cause and effect.

The hazards of handling cytotoxic drugs are well recognized along with the requirement to adhere to safety measures recommended in order to protect all staff who prepare, administer and handle cytotoxic drugs or waste products. In 1988 *The Control of Substances Hazardous to Health (COSHH)* regulations were introduced, and updated in 1994. Under these regulations employers are obliged to identify substances which are a hazard to staff, as well as who may be exposed, how the drugs should be handled and what to do in the event of a spill or accident. They also ensure that staff have access to the ideal environment, protective clothing, policies and procedures, a system of monitoring and recording effects, and any necessary equipment such as spill kits (Royal College of Nursing Oncology Nursing Society 1989). This includes consideration of the following:

1 The environment: the most effective means of minimizing the hazard is to arrange for all cytotoxic drugs to be prepared on a named patient basis by trained pharmacy staff in a specially equipped area (Royal College of Nursing Oncology Nursing Society 1989; Cass et al. 1997). Chemotherapy should be reconstituted in a vertical class II laminar flow cabinet or an isolator if drugs are prepared on the ward (Royal College of Nursing Oncology Nursing Society 1989; Doyle 1995; Powell 1996;

Cass *et al.* 1997; Goodman & Riley 1997; Weinstein 1997). Cabinets should be situated in a specified or dedicated area with access restricted to trained or supervised personnel.

2 Protective clothing: protective clothing should always be worn during all types of cytotoxic drug handling. There are minimum requirements for the type and degree of protective clothing which are based on possible exposure and type of environment.

(a) Gloves: gloves should be worn at all times and appear to be the only type of protective clothing which most practitioners consistently wear when handling cytotoxic drugs (Dougherty 1999). No type of glove is completely impermeable to every cytotoxic agent and there is no consensus as to which glove material offers the best protection (Doyle 1995; Cass *et al.* 1997; Goodman & Riley 1997; Weinstein 1997). A number of different protective glove materials, including latex, rubber and PVC, have been recommended (Wright 1993). However the literature recommends that practitioners wear one pair of powder-free latex gloves, which should be changed hourly or when they become punctured, torn or contaminated (Doyle 1995; Cass *et al.* 1997; Goodman & Riley 1997; Weinstein 1997). The key points to consider when selecting gloves are thickness and integrity (Laidlaw *et al.* 1984) as the main factors which affect penetration rates include glove thickness, material composition and molecular weight of the drug (Cass *et al.* 1997). It appears that most authors agree that double gloving is only required in the case of dealing with a spill (Doyle 1995; Cass *et al.* 1997; Goodman & Riley 1997; Weinstein 1997).

(b) Gowns: the literature supports the use of a disposable gown for both reconstitution and administration. It has been suggested that a long-sleeved, non-absorbent gown made of a low-linting, low-permeability material such as tyvek is used (Powell 1996; Cass *et al.* 1997; Weinstein 1997). Armlets and plastic aprons can be substituted for long-sleeved gowns during administration.

(c) Goggles: goggles are used to protect the eyes from splashes and particles and should fully cover the eyes to protect the handler. Goggles should meet BS2092C requirements (Cass *et al.* 1997) and be worn whenever reconstituting or dealing with a spill (Doyle 1995; Powell 1996).

(d) Masks: these should be worn whenever there is a possibility of inhalation or the drug is being prepared in an uncontrolled environment. A suitable dust mask or particulate respirator, such as the 3M 8810, affords the best protection.

There is no doubt that the existence of a formal hospital policy for handling has been shown to have a positive influence in the use of personal protective equipment (Christensen *et al.* 1990; Mahon *et al.* 1994), but it appears that in spite of this there can still be poor compliance of handlers with guidelines and policies (Wiseman *et al.* 1990;

Nieweg *et al.* 1994; Baker & Connor 1996). The move now is towards national evidence based guidelines (Goodman 1998). The aim of any guidelines should be to minimize exposure, provide adequate protective equipment, ensure regular staff monitoring and to provide effective written procedures for dealing with preparation, administration, disposal and dealing with spills and accidents (Dougherty 1999). In order to limit exposure, cytotoxic drugs should only be prepared by skilled, knowledgeable and experienced health care professionals (Mayer 1992; Cass *et al.* 1997).

References and further reading

Allwood, M., Stanley, A. & Wright, P. (eds) (1997) *The Cytotoxic Handbook*, 3rd edn. Radcliffe Medical Press, Oxford.

Ames, B.N. *et al.* (1975) Methods for detecting carcinogens and mutagens with the salmonella/mammalian microsome mutagenicity test. *Mutat Res*, 31, 347–64.

Baker, E.S. & Connor, T.H. (1996) Monitoring occupational exposure to cancer chemotherapy drugs. *Am J Health Sys Pharm*, 53(22), 2713–23.

Bingham, E. (1985) Hazards to health care professionals from antineoplastic drugs. *New Eng J Med*, 313, 1120–22.

Calvert, A.H. (1981) The long-term sequelae of cytotoxic therapy. *Cancer Topics*, 3(7), 77–9.

Cass, Y. *et al.* (1997) Health and safety aspects of cytotoxic services. In: *The Cytotoxic Handbook* (eds M. Allwood, A. Stanley & P. Wright), 3rd edn., pp. 35–54. Radcliffe Medical Press, Oxford.

Chisholm, L.G. *et al.* (1993) Programmed instruction: alternative administrative routes. *Cancer Nurs*, 16(3), 238–43.

Christensen, C.J., Le Masters, G.K. & Wakeman, M.A. (1990) Work practices and policies of pharmacists preparing antineoplastic agents. *J Occup Med*, 32(6), 508–11.

Colls, B.M. (1985) Safety of handling cytotoxic agents: a cause for concern by pharmaceutical companies. *Br Med J*, 291, 318–19.

Cooke, J. *et al.* (1987) Environmental monitoring of personnel who handle cytotoxic drugs. *Pharm J*, 239(6452, Suppl. R2).

Darbyshire, P. (1986) Handle with care. *Nurs Times*, 82(40), 37–8.

Dougherty, L. (1999) Safe administration of intravenous cytotoxic drugs. In: *Intravenous Therapy in Nursing Practice* (eds L. Dougherty & J. Lamb). Churchill Livingstone, Edinburgh.

Doyle, A. (1995) Oncologic therapy. In: *Intravenous Therapy: Clinical Principles and Practices* (eds J. Terry, L. Baranowski, R.A. Lonsway & C. Hedrick), pp. 249–74. W.B. Saunders, Philadelphia.

Elliot, T.S.J. & Tebbs, S.E. (1998) Prevention of central venous catheter related infection. *J Hosp Infect*, 40, 193–201.

Falck, K. *et al.* (1979) Mutagenicity in urine of nurses handling cytotoxic agents. *Lancet*, 1, 1250.

Gibbs, J. (1991) Handling cytotoxic drugs. *Nurs Times*, 87(11), 54–5.

Goodman, I. (1998) Development of national evidence based clinical guidelines for the administration of cytotoxic chemotherapy. *Eur J Oncol Nurs*, 2(1), 43–50.

Goodman, M. & Riley, M.B. (1997) Chemotherapy administration. In: *Cancer Nursing* (eds S.L. Groenwald, M.H. Frogge, M. Goodman & C. Henke Yarbro), 4th edn., pp. 317–404. Jones & Bartlett, Boston.

Harris, J. & Dodds, L. (1985) Handling waste from patients receiving cytotoxic drugs. *Pharm J*, 235(6345), 289–91.

Health and Safety Executive (1983) *Precautions for the Safe Handling of Cytotoxic Drugs. Medical Series*. Stationery Office, London.

Health and Safety Executive (1988) *The Control of Substances Hazardous to Health Regulations*. Stationery Office, London.

Health and Safety Executive (1994) *The Control of Substances Hazardous to Health Regulations*. Stationery Office, London.

Hecker, J. (1988) Improved techniques in IV therapy. *Nurs Times*, **84**(34), 28–33.

Kaijser, G.P. *et al.* (1990) The risks of handling cytotoxic drugs, 1. Methods of testing exposure. *Pharm Weekbi*, **12**(6), 217–27.

Kotilainen, H.R. (1989) Latex and vinyl examination gloves – quality control procedures and implications for health care workers. *Arch Intern Med*, **149**, 2749–53.

Labuhn, K. *et al.* (1998) Nurses' and pharmacists' exposure to antineoplastic drugs: findings from industrial hygiene scans and urine mutagenicity tests. *Cancer Nurs*, **21**(2), 79–89.

Laidlaw, J.L. *et al.* (1984) Permeability of latex and polyvinyl chloride gloves to 20 antineoplastic drugs. *Am J Hosp Pharm*, **41**, 2018–23.

Lee, L. (1993) The risks of handling cytotoxic therapy. *Nurs Stand*, **7**(49), 25–8.

Mahon, S.M. *et al.* (1994) Safe handling practices of cytotoxic drugs: the result of a chapter survey. *Oncol Nurs Forum*, **21**(7), 1157–65.

Mayer, D.K. (1992) Hazards of chemotherapy – implementing safe handling practices. *Cancer*, **70**, 988–92.

Newman, M.A. *et al.* (1994) Urinary biological monitoring markers of anticancer drug exposure in oncology nurses. *Am J Public Health*, **84**(5), 852–5.

Nguyen, T.V. *et al.* (1982) Exposure of pharmacy personnel to mutagenic antineoplastic drugs. *Cancer Res*, **42**, 4792–6.

Nieweg, R.M., De Boer, M., Dubbleman, R.C. *et al.* (1994) Safe handling of antineoplastic drugs: results of a survey. *Cancer Nurs*, **17**(6), 501–511.

Oakley, P. & Reeves, E. (1984) Setting up a reconstitution service. *Pharm J*, **232**(6282), 739–40.

Oldcorne, M.A. *et al.* (1987) Letters to the editor. Handling cytotoxic drugs. *Pharm J*, 18 April, **238**, 488.

Powell, L.L. (ed.) (1996) *Cancer Chemotherapy Guidelines and Recommendations for Practice*. Oncology Nursing Press, Pittsburgh.

Otto, S.E. (1995) Advanced concepts in chemotherapy drug delivery. *Reg Ther J Intraven Nurs*, **18**(4), 170–76.

Priestman, T.J. (1989) *Cancer Chemotherapy: An Introduction*, 3rd edn. Springer, Berlin.

Reymann, P.E. (1993) *Chemotherapy: Principles of Administration in Cancer Nursing* (eds S.L. Groenwald *et al.*), 3rd edn., Chap. 15. Jones & Bartlett, Boston.

Rittenberg, C.N., Gralla, R.J. & Rehmeyer, T.A. (1995) Assessing and managing venous irritation with vinorelbine tartrate. *Oncol Nurs Forum*, **22**(4), 707–710.

Robinson, S. (1993) Principles of chemotherapy. *Eur J Cancer Care*, **2**, 55–65.

Royal College of Nursing Oncology Nursing Society (1989) *Safe Practices with Cytotoxics*. Scutari Projects, Middlesex.

Selevan, S.G. (1986) Letter. *New Engl J Med*, **16**, 1048–51.

Selevan, S.G. *et al.* (1985) A study of occupational exposure to antineoplastic drugs and fetal loss in nurses. *New Engl J Med*, **19**, 1173–8.

Speechley, V. (1984) Administration of cytotoxic drugs. *Nurs Mirror*, **158**(2), 22–5.

Stokes, M. *et al.* (1987) Permeability of latex and polyvinyl chloride gloves to fluorouracil and methotrexate. *Am J Hosp Pharm*, **44**, 1341–6.

Stuart, M. (1981) Sequence of administering vesicant cytotoxic drugs, Part A. *Oncol Nurs Forum*, **9**(1), 53–4.

Taskinen, H.K. (1990) Effects of parental occupational exposures on spontaneous abortion and congenital malformation. *Scan J Work Environ Health*, **16**, 297–314.

Thomas, P.H. & Fenton May, V. (1987) Protection offered by gloves to carmustine exposure. *Pharm J*, **238**, 775–7.

Tsavaris, N.B., Komitsopoulou, P., Karagiaouris, P., *et al.* (1992) Prevention of tissue necrosis due to accidental extravasation of cytostatic drugs by a conservative approach. *Cancer Chemother Pharm*, **30**, 330–33.

Tully, J.L., Friedland, G.H., Baldrini, L.M. *et al.* (1981) Complications of intravenous therapy with steel needles and teflon catheters: a comparative study. *Am J Med*, **70**, March, 702–706.

Valanis, B.G., Vollmer, W.M., Labuhn, K.T. *et al.* (1993) Acute symptoms associated with antineoplastic drug handling among nurses. *Cancer Nurs*, **16**(4), 288–95.

Valanis, B. *et al.* (1997) Occupational exposure to antineoplastic agents and self reported infertility among nurses and pharmacists. *J Occup Environ Med*, **39**(6), 574–80.

Vennit, S. *et al.* (1984) Monitoring exposure of nursing and pharmacy personnel to cytotoxic drugs: urinary mutation assays and urinary platinum as markers of absorption. *Lancet*, **1**, 74–6.

Waksvik, H. *et al.* (1987) Chromosome analysis of nurses handling cytostatic agents. *Cancer Treat Rep*, **65**, 607–610.

Weinstein, S.M. (ed.) (1993) *Principles and Practices of Intravenous Therapy*, 5th edn. J.B. Lippincott, Philadelphia.

Weinstein, S.M. (1997) Antineoplastic therapy. In: *Plumer's Principles and Practice of Intravenous Therapy*, (S.M. Weinstein), 6th edn., pp. 463–530. J.B. Lippincott Philadelphia.

Wiseman, K.C., Wachs, K.C. & Wachs, J.E. (1990) Policies and practices used for the safe handling of antineoplastic drugs. *AAOHN J*, **38**(11), 517–23.

Working Party of the Pharmaceutical Society of Great Britain on the Handling of Cytotoxic Drugs (1983) Guidelines for the handling of cytotoxic drugs. *Pharm J*, **230**(6215), 230–31.

Wright, M.P. (1993) Protective clothing. In: *The Cytotoxic Handbook* (eds M. Allwood & P. Wright), 2nd edn. Radcliffe Medical Press, Oxford.

GUIDELINES · Protection of the environment

The safest method of reconstituting cytotoxic drugs outside a pharmacy department is to use an isolator. There is a variety of systems and each will have specific instructions for its use. The following procedure is for the Envair 'Mini-Iso' isolator. The system creates a negative pressure in the isolator by drawing air out by a fan and passing it through a HEPA filter, which will trap any cytotoxic drug powder or aerosol which may escape from the drug vial during reconstitution.

When used as instructed the isolator will minimize the risk to nurses when reconstituting any dose of cytotoxic drugs, but it will not protect the drug from the risk of microbial contamination so aseptic technique must always be used.

Safe reconstitution using an isolator

Equipment

1 One pair of disposable non-sterile gloves.
2 Syringes, needles.

3 Drug to be reconstituted and appropriate diluent.
4 Appropriate cleaning solution.

Procedure

Action	*Rationale*
1 Prior to commencing reconstitution carefully check the gauntlets, especially the fingers and at the point of attachment to the isolator.	The gauntlets are designed for prolonged use, they need to be changed when torn or punctured.
2 Place hand through slot on right of the top cover of the isolator and press the green button.	To enable the isolator to be switched on.
3 Allow the isolator to run for 3–4 minutes and ensure that the gauge needle is reading over 50 pascals before use.	To ensure that the isolator is prepared and will allow it to be operated safely.
4 Assemble all equipment required.	To avoid interruption of work.
5 Put on a pair of non-sterile gloves which should be worn under the isolator gloves and when passing equipment into or out of the isolator.	To provide extra operator protection in case of tears in the gauntlets while preparing the drug.
6 Open the door on the right side of the isolator by turning the handle anticlockwise through 180°.	To allow equipment to be placed inside the isolator.
7 Place equipment into the isolator and close and lock the door (by turning 180° clockwise).	To ensure that negative pressure can be achieved when doors are securely closed.
8 Place hands into gauntlets.	
9 Reconstitute the dose in the usual way (see Chap. 12, Drug Administration) using aseptic technique.	To minimize the risk of contamination.
10 Move everything to the right prior to removing hands from gauntlets.	To enable easy removal of the prepared drug and waste
11 Leave the isolator fan on.	To ensure any spills/aerosols are contained within the isolator
12 Open the isolator door and remove all equipment.	
13 Dispose of equipment in usual way.	To reduce the risk of contamination and needlestick injury.
14 Moisten a sheet of paper with cleaning spray provided and wipe inside of isolator.	To maintain equipment in good clean working order
15 Turn off isolator by pushing green button.	
16 Complete cytotoxic reconstitution surveillance form and send to occupational health dept.	To ensure follow-up and health surveillance check.

Management of spillage

Equipment

1 Two plastic overshoes.
2 Two disposable armlets.
3 Two clinical waste bags.
4 Two pairs of disposable non-sterile latex gloves.
5 Goggles (non-disposable) – BS 2092C.
6 Particulate respirator mask.

7 Plastic apron.
8 Gown.
9 Paper towels.
10 Plastic bucket.
11 Copy of spillage procedure.

Guidelines • Protection of the environment (cont'd)

Procedure

Action	*Rationale*
1 Act immediately.	Any spillage may become a health hazard.
2 Collect spillage kit.	It contains all necessary equipment.
3 Put on latex gloves, goggles and a gown and then a disposable plastic apron over the gown.	To provide personal protection.
4 If there is visible powder spill, put on a good-quality particulate respirator mask.	To prevent inhalation of powder.
5 If spillage is on the floor, put on overshoes.	For protection and to minimize the spread of contamination.
6 Wipe up powder spillage quickly with well dampened paper towels, starting at the outer edge of the spill area and working in a circular motion towards the middle to contain spill (Cass *et al*. 1997), and dispose of them as 'high-risk' waste.	To prevent dispersal of powder. To prevent spread of contamination to a wider area. To protect others and ensure safe disposal by incineration.
7 Mop up liquids which have been spilled on a hard surface with paper towels, starting at the outer edge of the spill area and working in a circular motion towards the middle to contain spill (Cass *et al*. 1997), and dispose of them as 'high risk' waste.	To prevent spread of contamination to a wider area. To protect others and ensure safe disposal by incineration.
8 Wash hard surfaces at least twice with copious amounts of cold, soapy water and dry with paper towels. The floor should then be given a routine clean as soon afterwards as possible. If spillage has occurred on a carpet it will require cleaning as soon as possible.	To remove residual contamination.
9 If spillage is on clothing, remove it as soon as possible and treat as 'soiled linen'.	To decontaminate clothing without hazard to laundry staff.
10 If spillage has penetrated clothing, wash contaminated skin liberally with soap and cold water.	To decontaminate skin and prevent drug absorption.
11 If spillage is on bed linen put on gloves and an apron, change it immediately and treat as 'soiled linen'.	To protect the patient. To protect the laundry staff.
12 If an accident or spillage involving direct skin contact occurs, the area should be washed thoroughly with soapy water as soon as possible. In the event of a cytotoxic splash to the eye, irrigate thoroughly with 0.9% sodium chloride or tap water for approximately 2 minutes.	To decontaminate the area and minimize the risk of drug absorption and damage.
13 Any accident or spillage involving direct skin contact with a cytotoxic drug by staff must be reported to the occupational health department and manager (see Guideline: Protection of nursing staff when handling cytotoxic drugs, below) and the appropriate documentation completed.	To ensure that details of accidental contact are entered in the nurse's health record, and appropriate follow-up initiated.

Disposal of waste

Action	*Rationale*
1 'Sharps' should be placed in the special container provided.	To ensure incineration and to prevent laceration and/or inoculation during transit and disposal.

2 Dry waste, intravenous administration sets and other contaminated material should be placed in 'high-risk' waste disposal bags.	To ensure careful handling and disposal by incineration.
3 Any part dose of a drug remaining should be placed in a special waste container. However, a small amount (a part dose) of drug solution may be flushed down the main drainage system, using copious amounts of cold water, if no alternative means of safe disposal is available.	Many water authorities prohibit drug waste disposal in the drainage system. This route of disposal must be used *only* if the waste cannot be safely transported elsewhere for disposal.
4 Re-usable trays and other equipment should be washed with copious amounts of water followed by the usual procedure for disinfection.	To reduce the risk of cross-contamination and cross-infection.
5 Unused doses of cytotoxics should be returned, unopened, to the pharmacy.	To enable them to be relabelled and re-issued, stability permitting, or to be destroyed safely.

Disposal of excreta from patients receiving cytotoxic drugs

Few cytotoxic agents are excreted as unchanged drug or active metabolites in urine or faeces. However, in order to comply with safe technique and practice, gloves should now always be worn, thus minimizing risks to all staff.

GUIDELINES · Protection of nursing staff when handling cytotoxic drugs

Nursing staff should not be involved in routine reconstitution of cytotoxic drugs, as this is the function of the pharmacy unit. However, there may be emergency situations when the nurse is requested to prepare chemotherapy and it is essential that this is performed safely. It should only be undertaken by competent, confident staff who have received appropriate training and have previous experience in the procedures required. The following procedure should be used for guidance.

Procedure

Action	*Rationale*
1 Nursing staff should receive instruction in the techniques of reconstitution and the reasons for these recommendations.	To ensure staff are safe to practise and are aware of the risks involved.
2 Reconstitution of cytotoxic drugs should take place in a clinical room or treatment room on the ward. Doors and windows should be closed to prevent draughts.	To prevent any unnecessary airborne exposure from possible powder or droplet aerosol released.
3 While reconstitution is in progress no other activities should be carried out within the area. Movement in and out of that area should be restricted, as far as possible during reconstitution.	As above.
4 The area must contain a sink and running water.	To clean surfaces and/or skin if spillage or contamination occurs.
5 The work surface should be smooth and impermeable.	To enable cleaning of surfaces to be undertaken easily and quickly.
6 Reconstitution should take place in a plastic tray or equivalent.	To enable containment of spillage and ease of cleaning.
7 Direct contact with drug solution can be entirely avoided by use of suitable personal protective clothing	To minimize exposure to handler.

and
(a) Personal protective equipment
  • Cover all cuts and scratches.

To prevent infiltration of the skin if damage to gloves occurs.

Guidelines • Protection of nursing staff when handling cytotoxic drugs (cont'd)

Action	Rationale
• Use protective goggles or glasses.	To prevent contact between drugs and the eyes. If the nurse wears glasses these should provide protection.
• Wash protective goggles with soap and water after use.	To minimize the risk of cross-contamination and/or cross-infection.
• Wear a 3M 8810 particulate respirator mask when reconstituting dry powder, especially if presented in an ampoule, e.g. bleomycin.	To prevent inhalation of any powder released during reconstitution.
• Put on a disposable plastic apron or tabard.	To provide a barrier between the drug and the handler.
• Continue to wear gloves/tabard during administration as the nurse is still handling the drugs and may become contaminated.	To reduce the risk of contamination at a later stage of the procedure.

(b) Good technique

• Hold ampoules away from the face and cover with a sterile gauze swab when breaking them.	To prevent contamination of the gloves and skin. To prevent formation of aerosols or liberation of powder.
• Use luer-locking syringes.	To reduce the incidence of accidental disconnection and spillage of drug.
• Where applicable, use a filtered air venting needle. The alternative 'no airway' technique involves a 'push-pull' use of the syringe to add cyclically small quantities of diluent to, and remove air from, the closed vial. This technique is not recommended (see Chap. 12 Drug Administration, under the heading Guidelines • Administration of injections).	To prevent the development of pressure differentials between syringe and vial. In inexperienced hands, the 'no airway' technique results in the danger of contamination. In extreme circumstances the vial and closure may separate, the syringe/needle junction may leak or the vial may explode.
• Introduce the diluent slowly down the inside wall of the vial or ampoule.	To ensure that the powder is thoroughly wet before agitation, and is not released into the atmosphere.
• Cap needles using one-handed method before the expulsion of air, or the tip should be covered with a sterile swab or the air should be expelled into the vial or ampoule.	To prevent aerosol formation.

Adverse incidents

8 Contamination of the skin, mucous membranes and eyes should be treated promptly. All areas should be washed with copious amounts of tap water or 0.9% sodium chloride for approximately 2 minutes. Eye wash may be available.	To minimize the risk of any local damage to tissue.
9 Accidental infiltration of the skin with a vesicant drug should be treated as an extravasation and the appropriate procedure followed (see Management of extravasation of vesicant drugs, below).	To minimize the risk of any local damage to tissue.
10 If erythema and/or other local reaction occurs in any circumstances, contact the occupational health unit or a member of the medical staff so that appropriate treatment may be advised.	To prevent further damage and/or complications.
11 It is essential after any accident involving direct contact with a cytotoxic drug, or if any local or systemic symptoms occur after handling such a drug, that the occupational health unit should be contacted.	To assist with recording and monitoring of staff exposure.
12 If pregnancy is suspected or intended, the occupational health unit should be contacted.	To discuss future work patterns and any anxiety that may be felt.

Routes of administration

Cytotoxic drugs can be administered via a variety of routes (see Chap. 12, Drug Administration). However, regardless of the route used there are certain pre-administration activities, which should be performed by the nurse, or the nurse should ascertain that the doctor has performed the relevant checks.

1 *Provision of information*: the patient should be fully informed of all the possible side-effects of chemotherapy, how to cope with any effects at home and the types of supportive therapy they may receive, as well as where and how they are to receive the drugs. They should then receive written information, which should be used to reinforce verbal explanation and will enable patients to spend time reading and formulating any questions about treatments.
2 *Gaining the patient's consent*: consent must be obtained before chemotherapy is commenced and every time the patient is changed from one protocol/regimen to another.
3 *Ascertaining whether the patient is fit for treatment*, e.g. full blood count, renal function etc.: certain blood results are required in order to
  (a) Calculate the dose of drug, e.g. in the case of platinum-based drugs ethylenediaminetetra-acetic acid (EDTA) or 24-hour urine collection for creatinine is required
  (b) Ensure that the patient is fit enough to receive the treatment and if any of the blood results are too low, then supportive therapy may be prescribed.
4 *Calculating body surface area*: this is obtained by using the patient's height and weight and should be performed at each visit. The surface area is then determined using a nomogram, and this will then be used to calculate the dose of drug.

Intravenous administration

Definition

This is the administration of cytotoxic drugs via a peripheral or central vein and is the most commonly used route for the administration of cytotoxic drugs.

Indications

Intravenous administration enables:

1 Rapid and reliable delivery of a cytotoxic drug to the tumour site; and
2 Rapid dilution of a drug which reduces local irritation and the risk of tissue damage.

Reference material

Choosing the appropriate device

Cytotoxic drugs may be administered via a winged infusion device, a peripheral cannula or a central venous access device. A winged infusion device is used mainly for bolus injections of non-vesicant drugs, due to the potential risk of infiltration associated with steel needles (Tully *et al.* 1981). A peripheral cannula is used for bolus injections and short or intermittent infusions of both vesicant and non-vesicant drugs (see Table 10.1). This device is associated with phlebitis and requires repeated resiting (Hecker 1988). A central venous catheter is useful for patients with poor venous access, those at high risk of extravasation and for those undergoing long-term, high-dose or continuous infusional chemotherapy (Weinstein 1997; Dougherty 1999). These devices are associated with infection and thrombosis (Elliott & Tebbs 1998).

When the peripheral route is used a winged infusion device or cannula may be used. The insertion site of choice should be the large veins of the forearm (cephalic or basilic) as these are easier to access, reduce the risk of chemical phlebitis and result in less problems if extravasation should occur (Weinstein 1997). The next area of choice would be the dorsum of the hand, then the wrist. The antecubital fossa should only be used as the last resort as it can limit movement and is associated with problems if extravasation occurs in this area (Doyle 1995; Weinstein 1997; Dougherty 1999). The general rule is to start distally and proceed proximally where possible and also to alternate the arms (Weinstein 1997) to ensure that the same veins are not being used and damaged by the chemical and mechanical irritation.

When using the peripheral intravenous route the following should be adhered to:

Table 10.1 Arguments for using either a large- or small-gauge peripheral vascular access device.

Larger	Smaller
1 Enables irritant drugs to reach general circulation quickly, without irritating peripheral veins.	1 Less chance to puncture posterior wall of vein.
2 Administration time is decreased and therefore patient does not need to spend as much time in a stressful environment.	2 Less likely to cause trauma and result in scar formation.
	3 Less pain on needle insertion.
	4 Increased blood flow around small needle increases dilution of drug and reduces risk of chemical phlebitis.

Table 10.2 Controversial issues: use of antecubital fossa

For	Against
1 Larger veins permit rapid infusion of drug.	1 Mobility is restricted.
2 Larger veins allow irritant drugs to reach general circulation more quickly and with less irritation than small veins.	2 Risk of extravasation increased if patient tends to be mobile.
3 Easier to palpate and therefore increases successful insertion of device.	3 Early recognition of extravasation is difficult due to the deep veins. This means there is less chance of observing swelling which could go undetected. The patient may also have a delayed reaction to pain.
	4 Damage can result in loss of structure and function, ulceration and fibrosis.

1 Patency should be checked at the start of administration by withdrawing blood and flushing with 5–10 ml of 0.9% sodium chloride to ensure there is no resistance, swelling or pain. Blood return should then be checked after every 2–5 ml of drug is administered (Doyle 1995; Weinstein 1997; Dougherty 1999).
2 The site should be assessed for signs of phlebitis.
3 The site should be observed when a bolus injection is administered, particularly if a vesicant drug, for signs of infiltration or extravasation.
4 Certain vesicants must not be administered as infusions into a peripheral vein as the risk of extravasation and damage is greater than via the central venous route (Weinstein 1997).

In addition, where possible a new site should be used for vesicants, to ensure the vein is healthy and patent, although this may not be possible. There are some controversial issues related to peripheral intravenous cytotoxic drug administration (see Table 10.2).

Central venous access devices have the advantage of providing a more reliable form of vascular access. This is because the problems associated with peripheral devices such as phlebitis, venous irritation and pain are eliminated as central venous access enables rapid dilution and circulation of the drug. However, extravasation can still occur as a result of a damaged catheter, port needle dislodgement or as a result of fibrin sheath formation along the length of the catheter (Mayo 1998).

Methods

Cytotoxic drugs may be administered as a direct bolus injection, a bolus via the side arm of a rapid infusion of 0.9% sodium chloride or as a continuous infusion. The choice is dependent on:

1 The type of cytotoxic drug, e.g. etoposide is only given as an infusion
2 Pharmacological considerations, e.g. stability, need for dilution
3 Degree of venous irritation, e.g. vinorelbine is a highly irritant drug
4 Whether the drug is a vesicant
5 The type of device in situ (Dougherty 1999).

The advantage of the bolus injection is that the integrity of the vein and any early signs of extravasation can be observed more easily than during an infusion. However, bolus injections can increase the risk of venous irritation due to the constant contact of the drug with the intima of the vein, resulting in venospasm and pain (Dougherty 1999). It could also lead to inappropriate rapid administration of the drug (Weinstein 1997).

Bolus injections administered via the side arm of a rapid infusion of solution ensure greater dilution of potentially irritating drugs and enable rapid removal of the drug from the insertion site and smaller vessels. The disadvantages are that a small vein may not allow rapid flow of the infusate and this may result in the drug backing up the tubing. The practitioner also has to interrupt the flow in order to check blood return (Dougherty 1999).

Adding the drug to an infusion bag allows for greater dilution, thus reducing the possibility of chemical irritation. Some drugs may only be administered as infusions due to the type of side-effects associated with them (e.g. hypotension with etoposide) and long-term continuous infusions, e.g. 5FU, may also be necessary to reduce the risk of side-effects such as diarrhoea. Patency and device position cannot be easily assessed and the longer the infusion, the greater the possibility of device dislodgement, extravasation or infiltration and general complications associated with the device (Doyle 1995).

GUIDELINES • Intravenous administration of cytotoxic drugs

The aim of the procedure for administration of chemotherapy intravenously is to protect both nurse and patient from contamination and also to prevent extravasation of drugs which could result in local tissue damage. The large majority of cytotoxic agents will be delivered to the ward/unit individually packaged for delivery to a named patient, by injection or infusion. If this is not so, specific guidelines should be followed (see Guidelines • Protection of nursing staff when handling cytotoxic drugs, above).

Procedure

Action	Rationale
1 Explain and discuss the procedure with the patient. Evaluate the patient's knowledge of cytotoxic therapy. If this knowledge appears to be faulty or incorrect, offer an explanation of the use, action, dose and potential side-effects of the drug or drugs involved.	To ensure that the patient understands the procedure and gives his/her valid consent. A patient has a right to information.
2 Put on gloves and an apron before commencing the procedure.	To protect the nurse from local contamination of skin or clothing. *Note*: with careful handling technique, this risk is minimal but splashes can occur when changing syringes or infusion containers.
3 Prepare necessary equipment for an aseptic administration procedure, and ensure that this is followed carefully (see Chap. 12, Drug Administration).	To minimize the risk of local and/or systemic infection. Patients are frequently immunosuppressed and at greater risk.
4 Check that all details on the syringe or infusion container are correct when compared with the patient's prescription, before opening the sterile packaging.	To ensure the patient is given the correct drug which has been dispensed for him/her. To prevent wastage.
5 Be aware of the immediate effects of the drug.	To know what to observe during administration. To be prepared to manage any side-effects that occur.
6 Take the medication and the prescription chart to the patient. Check the patient's identity and the dose to be given.	To prevent error.
7 Inspect the device site, and consult the patient about sensation around the device insertion site.	To detect any phenomena, e.g. phlebitis, which would render the vein unusable.
8 Check the patency of the vein using 0.9% sodium chloride.	To determine whether the vein will accommodate the extra fluid flow and irritant drugs and remain patent.
9 Administer drugs in the correct order, i.e. vesicants first.	To ensure that those agents likely to cause tissue damage are given when venous integrity is greatest, i.e. at the beginning. *Note*: because of their irritant nature (approximately pH 3–3.5) antiemetics should be given half an hour before chemotherapy administration or at the end of the sequence.
10 Ensure the correct administration rate.	To prevent 'speed shock'. To prevent extra pressure and irritation within the vein.
11 Observe the vein throughout for signs of infiltration or extravasation, e.g. swelling or leakage at the site of injection. Note the patient's comments about sensation at the site, e.g. pain.	To detect any problems at the earliest moment. To prevent any damage to soft tissue, and to enable the remainder of the drug(s) to be given correctly at another site. To enable prompt treatment to be given, thus minimizing local damage, and possibly preserving venous access for future treatment. (For further information see Management of extravasation of vesicant drugs, below.)
12 Flush the device with 0.9% sodium chloride between drugs and after administration.	To prevent drug interaction. To prevent leakage of drug from the puncture site.
13 Be aware of the patient's comfort throughout the procedure.	To minimize trauma to the patient. To involve the patient in treatment and detect any side-effects and/or problems that may then be avoided at the next treatment.
14 Record details of the administration in the appropriate documents.	To prevent any duplication of treatment and to provide a point of reference in the event of queries.
15 Protect the patient from contact with the drugs by: (a) Ensuring the needle (if used) is inserted or a syringe (if using a needleless injection system) is	To prevent exiting on the other side and contaminating or inoculating the patient.

Guidelines • Intravenous administration of cytotoxic drugs (cont'd)

Action	Rationale
attached carefully into the injection site of the giving set, extension set or cannula injection cap.	
(b) Carefully removing the blind hub and changing needles/syringes, plus care when inserting the administration set into the infusion container or changing bags (which must be done with the bag laying flat on a hard surface).	To avoid leakage or splashes and contamination of the nurse or patient. To prevent mis-spiking the bag and puncturing it.
(c) Securing a good bond between needle and syringe, always use Luer lock syringes.	To prevent leakage or separation, which may occur due to pressure during administration, resulting in spray and contamination.
(d) Checking the injection site or injection cap at the end of the procedure.	To ensure that there is no leakage.
(e) Acting promptly if any contamination is noted and washing the area with cold water or saline.	To prevent any local reaction and absorption on skin, mucous membranes, etc.

Extravasation of vesicant drugs

Definition

Extravasation is the inadvertent administration of vesicant drugs into surrounding tissues which can lead to tissue necrosis, while infiltration is the inadvertent administration of non-vesicant solutions/medications into the surrounding tissues (Weinstein 1997; How & Brown 1998). A vesicant is any drug which has the potential to cause tissue damage, while irritant drugs may cause local tissue inflammation and discomfort but do not result in necrosis and therefore tend to be dealt with more conservatively.

Reference material

Prevention of extravasation

The incidence of extravasation during the administration of vesicant cytotoxic drugs is estimated to be between 0.1 and 6% (McCaffrey Boyle & Engelking 1995). Even when practitioners have many years of experience, extravasation of vesicant agents can occur and is an extremely stressful event. Early detection and treatment are crucial if the consequences of an untreated or poorly managed extravasation are to be avoided. These may include:

1 Pain from necrotic areas
2 Physical defect
3 The cost of hospitalization and plastic surgery
4 Delay in the treatment of disease
5 Psychological distress
6 Litigation – nurses are now being named in malpractice allegations and extravasation injuries are an area for concern (McCaffrey Boyle & Engelking 1995; Weinstein 1997; Camp Sorrell 1998; Schulmeister 1998).

However it is prevention which remains the most effective strategy for managing this hazard to patients. This includes the following strategies:

1 The use of steel needle winged infusion devices is associated with a greater risk of extravasation and should be discouraged, a plastic cannula should be used instead (How & Brown 1998).
2 Siting over joints should be avoided as tissue damage in this area may limit joint movement in the future. It is also recommended that the antecubital fossa should never be used for the administration of vesicants because of the risk of damage to local structures such as nerves and tendons (Rudolph & Larson 1987; Beason 1990; McCaffrey Boyle & Engelking 1995; Allwood *et al.* 1997; Goodman & Riley 1997; Dougherty 1999).
3 Extra caution and observation should be carried out in patients who are at increased risk of extravasation. Those at increased risk include:
   (a) Elderly patients
   (b) Patients with fragile veins
   (c) Patients who are thrombocytopenic
   (d) Paediatric patients
   (e) Unconscious, sedated or confused patients.
4 Vesicants should be given first (see Table 10.3).
5 The longer the cannula is in situ the more chance there is of an extravasation as the vein is not as healthy.
6 Early recognition and prompt action comes from ensuring only skilled and knowledgeable practitioners administer vesicant drugs and/or insert the device (McCaffrey Boyle & Engelking 1995).
7 Adequate information given to patients will ensure early recognition and cooperation as patients are the first to notice pain (McCaffrey Boyle & Engelking 1995; How & Brown 1998).

Drugs capable of causing tissue necrosis

Before administration of vesicant cytotoxic drugs the nurse should know which agents are capable of producing tissue necrosis. The following is a list of those in common use:

Table 10.3 Drug sequencing – rationale for administering vesicant drugs first or last

Vesicants first	Vesicants last
1 Vascular integrity decreases over time.	1 Vesicants are irritating and increase vein fragility.
2 Vein is most stable and least irritated at start of treatment.	2 Venous spasm may occur and mask signs of extravasation.
3 Initial assessment of vein patency is most accurate.	
4 Patient's awareness of changes more acute.	

Group A drugs
Vinca alkaloids
   Vinblastine
   Vindesine
   Vinorelbine

Group B drugs
Amsacrine
Carmustine (concentrated solution)
Dacarbazine (concentrated solution)
Dactinomycin
Daunorubicin
Doxorubicin
Epirubicin
Idarubicin
Mithramycin
Mitomycin C
Mustine
Streptozocin

If in any doubt, the drug data sheet should be consulted or reference made to a research trial protocol. Drugs should not be reconstituted to give solutions which are higher than the manufacturer's recommended concentration, and the method of administration should be checked, e.g. infusion, injection.

A variety of vesicant non-cytotoxic agents in frequent use are also capable of causing severe tissue damage if extravasated. They include:

Group A drugs
Calcium chloride
Calcium gluconate
Phenytoin
Hypertonic solutions of
   sodium bicarbonate
   (greater than 5%)

Group B drugs
Aciclovir
Amphotericin
Cefotaxime
Diazepam
Digoxin
Ganciclovir
Potassium chloride (if greater
   than 40 mmol/l)

This potential hazard should always be remembered. The actions listed in this procedure may not be appropriate in all these instances. Drug data sheets should always be checked and the pharmacy departments should be consulted if the information is insufficient.

Signs and symptoms of extravasation

Extravasation should be suspected if:

1 The patient complains of burning, stinging pain or any other acute change at the injection site. This should be distinguished from a feeling of cold, which may occur with some drugs.
2 Induration, swelling or leakage occurs at the injection site.
3 Erythema of the skin occurs around the injection site; it may not present immediately. It is important that this is distinguished from a 'flare' reaction which is a red streak,

flush or even 'blistering' associated with doxorubicin and other red coloured drugs. This occurs in about 3% of patients and does not cause any pain, although the area may feel itchy. It is caused by a venous inflammatory response to histamine release and is characterised by redness, blotchiness and may result in the formation of small weals, having a similar appearance to a nettle rash. It usually subsides within 30 to 45 minutes with or without treatment, but it responds well within a few minutes to the application of a topical steroid (Beason 1990; Wood & Gullo 1993).

4 No blood return is obtained when the plunger of the syringe is pulled back – this may indicate lack of patency and incorrect position of the device. If no other signs are apparent this should not be regarded as an indication of a non-patent vein, as a vein may not bleed back for a number of reasons and extravasation may occur even in the event of good blood return. Any change in blood flow should be investigated.
5 A resistance is felt on the plunger of the syringe if drugs are given by bolus.
6 There is absence of free flow when administration is by infusion (Reymann 1993).

Note: one or more of the above may be present. If extravasation is suspected or confirmed, action must be taken immediately (Weinstein 1997).

Management of extravasation

The management of the extravasation of chemotherapeutic agents is controversial and there is little documented evidence of efficacy: controlled clinical trials are lacking and it is often difficult to ascertain whether an extravasation has actually occurred (Weinstein 1997). Some studies performed on animals have demonstrated both effective and ineffective treatments, but extrapolation from animals to humans is limited (Powell 1996). In the past, studies have often been small with low numbers of patients (Cox *et al.* 1988) and most have been conducted on anthracyclines with few on the other vesicant drugs (How & Brown 1998).

The management of extravasation involves several stages including:

Stage 1: stopping infusion and withdrawing (aspirating) drug

It appears that most authors are agreed that withdrawing as much of the drug as possible, as soon as extravasation is suspected, is beneficial (Rudolph & Larson 1987; Cox et al. 1988; Doyle 1995; Powell 1996; Weinstein 1997). It may help to reduce the size of the lesion. The likelihood of withdrawing blood (as suggested by Ignoffo & Friedman 1980) is small and the practitioner may waste valuable time attempting this (Dougherty 1999) which could lead to delay in the rest of the management procedure.

Stage 2: removing device

Some clinicians advocate that the vascular access device be left in situ in order to instil the antidote via the device and into the affected tissues (Ignoffo et al. 1980; Cox et al. 1988; Powell 1996; Weinstein 1997). However, others recommend that the device should be removed to prevent any injected solution increasing the size of the affected area (Rudolph & Larson 1987; Doyle 1995). There appears to be no research evidence to support either practice.

Stage 3: applying hot or cold packs

Cold packs are used to cause vasoconstriction which reduces the local destructive effect by reducing local uptake of the drug by the tissues, reducing local oedema and slowing metabolic rates of the cells (Dougherty 1999). The increase in blood supply may also help promote healing (Weinstein 1997). The time suggested for application ranges from 15 minutes four times a day (Rudolph & Larson 1987) to every 20–40 minutes for 24–48 hours (Cox et al. 1988).

Hot packs are recommended specifically for the management of non-DNA binding drugs such as vinca alkaloids. They are used to increase blood supply and increase dispersion and absorption of the neutralizing agent (Dougherty 1999).

Stage 4: use of antidotes

A number of antidotes are available, but again there is a lack of scientific evidence to demonstrate their value. Many are based on personal opinion and attempts to neutralize the drug (Rudolph & Larson 1987). There appear to be two main types, one is used to dilute the drug, e.g. hyaluronidase, and the other to neutralize the drugs and reduce inflammation, e.g. steroids (Allwood et al. 1997; Dougherty 1999). Hyaluronidase is an enzyme which destroys tissue cement and helps to reduce or prevent tissue damage by allowing rapid diffusion of the extravasated fluid and promoting drug absorption. The usual dose is 1500 IU. The evidence is divided regarding the use of steroids, especially for the management of anthracycline extravasations (How & Brown 1998).

Stage 5: elevation of limb

This is recommended as it minimizes swelling (Rudolph & Larson 1987; Powell 1996) and movement should be encouraged to prevent adhesion of damaged areas to underlying tissue (Dougherty 1999).

Stage 6: surgery

Some centres suggest a plastic surgery consultation be performed as part of the management procedure in order to

Suspect an extravasation if:
1 Patient complains of burning or stinging pain or
2 There is evidence of swelling, induration, leakage at the site or
3 There is resistance on plunger of syringe or absence of free flow of infusion or
4 There is no blood return (if found in isolation, this should not be regarded as an indication of a non-patent vein)

Stop the injection/infusion
Withdraw as much of the drug as possible
Remove the cannula
Collect the extravasation pack

Group A drugs
Inject 1500 IU hyaluronidase subcutaneously around site.
Apply warm pack to aid absorption of hyaluronidase.
Warm pack to remain in situ for 2–4 hours

Group B drugs
Apply cold pack to cause vasoconstriction.
Inject dexamethasone 4–8 mg subcutaneously around site.
Replace cold packs regularly for 24 hours.

Elevate the limb

Apply hydrocortisone cream to reduce local inflammation (twice daily)

Inform medical staff

Document in duplicate – one copy in patient's notes and one to IV team

Give patient a patient information sheet

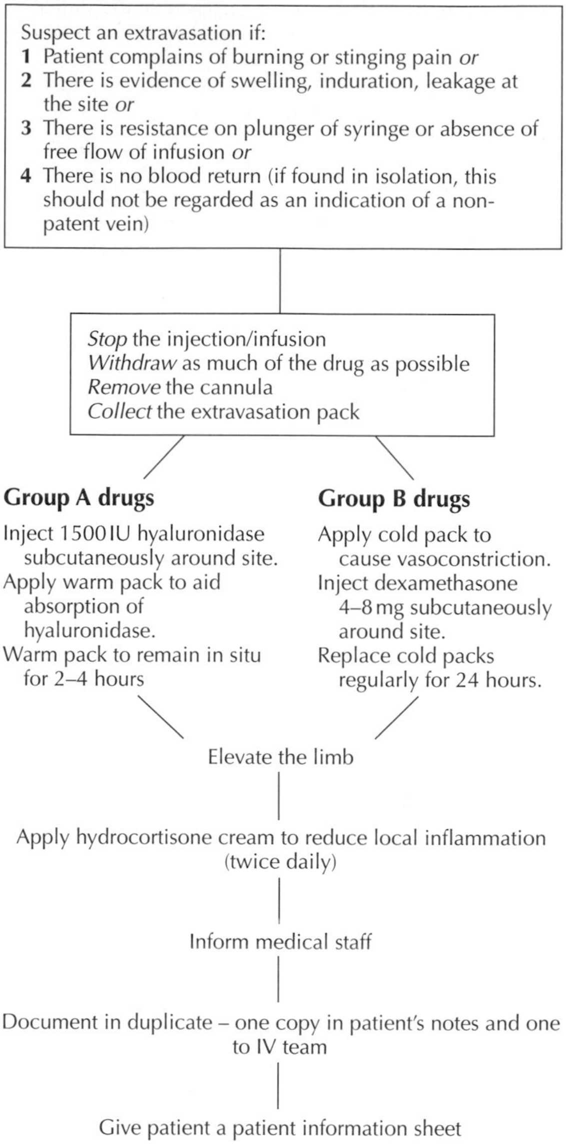

Figure 10.1 Treatment of extravasation.

remove the tissue containing the drug, thereby removing the damaging effects which can continue while the drug remains in situ. Requirement for surgery is usually based upon the size and location of the extravasation as well as the type of drug which has extravasated (Heckler 1989). The use of saline flushing conducted within the first 24 hours has been suggested as a less traumatic and cheaper procedure than surgery (Gault 1993). The saline flushout technique involves four small stab incisions; it facilitates cleansing of any drug from the subcutaneous tissues and is advocated for use with DNA-binding vesicants such as doxorubicin (How & Brown 1998).

The use of extravasation kits has been recommended (Beason 1990). Kits should be assembled according to the particular needs of individual institutions. They should be kept in all areas where staff are regularly administering vesicant drugs, so staff have immediate access to equipment (Dougherty 1999). The kit should be simple to avoid confusion, but comprehensive enough to meet all reasonable needs (Allwood et al. 1997). (See guidelines for minimal content.) Instructions should be clear and easy to follow and the use of a flow chart enables staff to follow the management procedure in easy steps (see Fig. 10.1).

Consideration should be given to the mananagment of mixed vesicant drug extravasation in terms of which drug to treat with which antidote. For example, in the case of VAMP chemotherapy – a mixture of vincristine and doxorubicin – should it be the drug of greatest volume?

An extravasation must be reported and fully documented as it is an accident and the patient will require follow-up care. Information may also be used for statistical purposes, for example collation and analysis using the green card scheme devised by St Chads Hospital, Birmingham. Finally it may be required in case of litigation.

Patients should always be informed when an extravasation has occurred and be given an explanation of what has happened and what management has been carried out (McCaffrey Boyle & Engelking 1995). An information sheet should be given to patients with instructions of what symptoms to look out for and when to contact the hospital during the follow up period (Dougherty 1999).

The procedure detailed here represents the policy of the Royal Marsden Hospital for the management by nursing staff of extravasation injury, drawn up with the assistance of pharmacist and medical colleagues. It relates specifically to the management of extravasation of a drug from a peripheral cannula. CVAD extravasation can occur as a result of a leaking or damaged catheter, fibrin sheath formation (Mayo 1998) or a port needle dislodgement (Schulmeister 1989). The consequences of an extravasation from a central venous access device are more serious and require immediate consultation with the medical team.

References and further reading

Allwood, M., Stanley, A. & Wright, P. (eds) (1997) *The Cytotoxic Handbook*, 3rd edn. Radcliffe Medical Press, Oxford.

Beason, R. (1990) Antineoplastic vesicant extravasation. *J Intraven Nurs*, March/April, 111–14.

Camp Sorrell, D. (1998) Developing extravasation protocols and monitoring outcomes. *J Intraven Nurs*, 21(4), 232–9.

Cox K., Stuart-Harris, R.A., Addini, G. et al. (1988) The management of cytotoxic drug extravasation: guidelines drawn up by a working party for the Clinical Oncological Society of Australia. *Med J Aust*, 148, 185–9.

Dougherty, L. (1999) Safe administration of intravenous cytotoxic drugs. In: *Intravenous Therapy in Nursing Practice* (eds L. Dougherty & J. Lamb). Churchill Livingstone, Edinburgh.

Doyle, A. (1995) Oncologic therapy. In: *Intravenous Therapy: Clinical Principles and Practices* (eds J. Terry, L. Baranowski, R.A. Lonsway, et al.), pp. 249–74. W.B. Saunders, Philadelphia.

Gault, D.T. (1993) Extravasation injuries. *Br J Plast Surg*, 46(2), 91–6.

Goodman, M. & Riley, M.B. (1997) Chemotherapy administration. In: *Cancer Nursing* (eds S.L. Groenwald, M.H. Frogge, M. Goodman & C. Henke Yarbro), 4th edn., pp. 317–404. Jones & Bartlett, Boston.

Hastings-Tolsma, M.T. et al. (1993) Effect of warm and cold applications on the resolution of IV infiltrations. *Res Nurs Health*, 16, 171–8.

Heckler, F.R. (1989) Current thoughts on extravasation injuries. *Clin Plast Surg*, 16(3), 557–63.

How, C. & Brown, J. (1998) Extravasation of cytotoxic chemotherapy from peripheral veins. *Eur J Oncol Nurs*, 2(1), 51–8.

Ignoffo, R.J. & Friedman, M.A. (1980) Therapy of local toxicities caused by extravasation of cancer chemotherapeutic drugs. *Cancer Treat Rev*, 7, 17–27.

Mayo, D.J. (1998) Fibrin sheath formation and chemotherapy extravasation: a case report. *Supp Care Cancer*, 6, 51–6.

McCaffrey Boyle, D. & Engelking, C. (1995) Vesicant extravasation: myths and realities. *Oncol Nurs Forum*, 22(1), 57–65.

Powell, L.L. (ed.) (1996) *Cancer Chemotherapy Guidelines and Recommendations for Practice*. Oncology Nursing Press, Pittsburgh.

Reymann, P.E. (1993) Chemotherapy: principles of administration. In: *Cancer Nursing. Principles and Practice* (eds. S.L. Groenwald, M. Goodman, M.H. Frogge, et al.), 3rd edn. Jones & Bartlett, Boston.

Rudolph, R. & Larson, D.L. (1987) Etiology and treatment of chemotherapeutic agent extravasation injuries: a review. *J Clin Oncol*, 5(7), 1116–26.

Schulmeister, L. (1989) Needle dislodgement from implanted venous access devices – inpatients and outpatient experiences. *J Intraven Nurs*, 12, 90–92.

Schulmeister, L. (1998) A complication of vascular access device insertion. *J Intraven Nurs*, 21(4), 197–202.

Smith, R. (1985a) Extravasation of intravenous fluids. *Br J Parenteral Ther*, 6(2), 30–33, 42.

Smith, R. (1985b) Prevention and treatment of extravasation. *Br J Parenteral Ther*, 6(5), 114–20.

Weinstein, S.M. (1993) *Plumer's Principles and Practice of Intravenous Therapy*, 5th edn. J.B. Lippincott, Philadelphia.

Weinstein, S.M. (1997) Antineoplastic therapy. In: *Plumer's Principles and Practice of Intravenous Therapy* (S.M. Weinstein) 6th edn., pp. 463–530. J.B. Lippincott, Philadelphia.

Wood, L.S. & Gullo, S.M. (1993) IV vesicants: how to avoid extravasation. *Am J Nurs*, April, 42–50.

GUIDELINES • Management of extravasation when using a peripheral cannula

Equipment

To assist the nurse, an extravasation kit should be assembled and should be readily available in each ward/unit. It contains:

1 Instant cold pack × 1/instant hot pack × 1 (or reusable packs which can be frozen or heated as required).

2 Dexamethasone injection 8 mg in 2 ml × 1/hyaluronidase 1500 IU.

Guidelines • Management of extravasation when using a peripheral cannula (cont'd)

3 Hydrocortisone cream 1% 15 g tube × 1.
4 2 ml syringes × 1.
5 25 g needles × 2.
6 Alcohol swabs.

7 Documentation forms.
8 Copy of extravasation management procedure.
9 Patient information leaflet.

Procedure

Action

1 Explain and discuss the procedure with the patient.

2 Stop injection or infusion *immediately*, leaving the cannula in place.

3 Aspirate any residual drug from the device and suspected extravasation site.

4 Remove the cannula.

5 Collect the extravasation pack and take it to the patient.

6 Group A drugs:
Draw up hyaluronidase 1500 IU in 1 ml water for injection and inject volumes of 0.1–0.2 ml subcutaneously at points of the compass around the circumference of the area of extravasation. Apply warm pack.

Group B drugs:
Apply cold pack or ice instantly.

Draw up a dexamethasone injection 4–8 mg and inject 0.1–0.2 ml subcutaneously at each point of the compass around the circumference of the area of extravasation. Ensure the whole area is infiltrated.

7 Where possible elevate the extremity and/or encourage movement.

8 Inform a member of the medical staff at the earliest opportunity.

9 Apply hydrocortisone cream 1% twice daily, and instruct the patient how to do this. Continue as long as erythema persists.

10 Heat pack (Group A drugs) should be reapplied after initial management for 2–4 h. Cold pack (Group B drugs) should be reapplied after initial management for up to 24 h.

11 Provide analgesia as required.

12 Document the following details, in duplicate, on the form provided:
(a) Patient's name/number
(b) Ward/unit

Rationale

To ensure that the patient understands the procedure and gives his/her valid consent.

To minimize local injury. To allow aspiration of the drug to be attempted.

To minimize local injury by removing as much drug as possible. Subsequent damage is related to the volume of the extravasation, in addition to other factors.

To prevent the site from being used as an intravenous route.

It contains all the equipment necessary for managing extravasation.

This is the recommended agent for group A drugs. The warm pack speeds up absorption of the drug by the tissues.

To localize the area of extravasation, slow cell metabolism and decrease the area of tissue destruction. To reduce local pain.
To reduce local inflammation and improve the survival of tissues, especially those marginally injured.

To minimize swelling and to prevent adhesion of damaged area to underlying tissue, which could result in restriction of movement.

To enable actions differing from agreed policy to be taken if considered in the best interests of the patient. To notify the doctor of the need to prescribe drugs.

To reduce local inflammation and promote patient comfort.

To localize the steroid effect in the area of extravasation. To reduce local pain and promote patient comfort.

To promote patient comfort. To encourage movement of the limb as advised.

To provide an immediate full record of all details of the incident, which may be referred to if necessary. To provide a baseline for future observation and monitoring of patient's condition.

(c) Date, time
(d) Signs and symptoms.
(e) Venepuncture site (on diagram).
(f) Drug sequence.
(g) Drug administration technique, i.e. 'bolus' infusion.
(h) Approximate amount of the drug extravasated.
(i) Diameter, length and width of extravasation area.
(j) Appearance of the area.
(k) Nursing management/action taken/medical officer notified.
(l) Patient's complaints, comments, statements
(m) Signature of the nurse,

13 Explain to the patient that the site may remain sore for several days.

To reduce anxiety and ensure continued cooperation.

14 Observe the area regularly for erythema, induration, blistering or necrosis. *Inpatients*: monitor daily.

To detect any changes at the earliest possible moment.

15 All patients should receive written information explaining what has occurred, what management has been carried out and what they need to observe for at the site and when to report any changes. For example, increased discomfort, peeling or blistering of the skin should be reported immediately.

To detect any changes as early as possible, and allow for a review of future management. This may include referral to a plastic surgeon.

16 If blistering or tissue breakdown occurs, begin sterile dressing techniques.

To minimize the risk of a superimposed infection.

17 Consider referral for plastic surgery if no healing occurs and the patient's condition permits.

To prevent further pain or other complications as chemically induced ulcers rarely heal spontaneously.

Oral administration

Definition

The administration of cytotoxic drugs via the oral route.

Indications

The oral route is convenient, economical, non-invasive and sometimes less toxic than the other routes (Powell 1996; Goodman & Riley 1997). Most oral drugs are absorbed well if the gastrointestinal tract is functioning normally. However the oral route can be unreliable for a number of reasons, including:

1 Patients may not comply with therapy (although this is uncommon with chemotherapy), may forget or may feel the side-effects associated are too unpleasant, e.g. nausea and vomiting, hot flushes (Goodman & Riley 1997).
2 Patients may not take medications as instructed.
3 Some patients may experience difficulty taking tablets or capsules, and therefore attempt to crush them which could result in changes to the tablets' disposition and effectiveness.

Reference material

Nurses dispensing tablets or capsules should use a non-touch technique to avoid damage and contamination of the tablets or capsules and contamination of themselves. If tablets have to be counted, this should be done using a triangle, which should be washed and dried after use. Many tablets are coated and this protects the drug in its inner core. There is no risk of contamination if these coatings are not broken. A small number of tablets are compressed powders, but there appears to be no risk of contamination where there is no free powder visible. It is important that these tablets are not crushed because they will then release powder which could be inhaled. Capsules are also not a risk if they have not been opened, broken or have not leaked. They should not be crushed or opened and the powder tipped out. Any visible spillage should be dealt with as previously directed (see Guidelines • Protection of the environment, above).

Intramuscular and subcutaneous injection

Definition

The administration of cytotoxic drugs by injection into the muscle or subcutaneous tissues (Goodman & Riley 1997).

Indications

Intramuscular and subcutaneous injections are a useful route when administering therapy in the community and for patient convenience, and when regular administration is required and journeys to the hospital are impractical, e.g.

younger or elderly patients on maintenance therapy. It is also useful if venous access is limited although only small volumes (up to 3 ml) are recommended using this route (Goodman & Riley 1997).

Only a few cytotoxic drugs can be administered via these routes due to a number of factors:

1 The irritant nature of the drugs and/or tissue damage
2 Incomplete absorption may occur
3 Bleeding as a result of thrombocytopenia
4 Discomfort of regular injections.

Cytotoxic and biological agents administered in this way are:

1 Methotrexate
2 Bleomycin
3 Cytosine arabinoside
4 L-asparaginase
5 Ifosfamide
6 Interferon
7 Colony stimulating factor.

(Allwood *et al.* 1997).

Although the volume of drug and diluent handled is less than for the intravenous route, preparation and reconstitution of the agents should be commensurate with the information listed under Guidelines • Protection of nursing staff when handling cytotoxic drugs, above. The nurse should continue to wear gloves during administration. Spillage and disposal of equipment should be dealt with as previously directed (see Guidelines • Protection of the environment, above) and systems of work modified to ensure these guidelines are followed. Where community nurses are to be responsible for administration, they must be supplied with adequate information when the patient is discharged.

Recommendations about administration should be followed carefully, e.g. deep intramuscular injection using a Z-track technique to prevent leakage onto the skin (Goodman & Riley 1997) and rotation of sites to prevent local irritation developing. The skin should be cleaned with antiseptic prior to injection (Powell 1996) and the smallest needle used, the gauge of which will allow passage of the solution to minimize discomfort and scarring.

Topical application

Definition

Topical application is the application of cream or ointments containing cytotoxic agents.

Indications

Topical application is only suitable for superficial lesions and has been found to be useful in the treatment of cutaneous malignant lesions, e.g. cutaneous T-cell lymphomas, basal cell carcinoma, squamous cell carcinoma and Kaposi's sarcoma (Goodman & Riley 1997).

Topical agents include mustine and 5-fluorouracil (5-FU) (Allwood *et al.* 1997). The most widely used is 5% 5-FU cream, which is usually applied once or twice daily until significant penetration of the damaged or diseased skin can be achieved, and a typical response pattern has been observed. This can take up to 4 weeks when local erythema, blistering and ulceration occurs. Once the affected skin starts sloughing, regranulization of normal tissue will begin to occur (within 8 weeks) (Priestman 1989).

Considerations include safe handling when applying the cream by wearing gloves and using low-linting swabs or non-metal applicators. It is important to protect the normal skin and avoid the eyes and other mucus membranes. The affected area should not be washed vigorously during the treatment (Goodman & Riley 1997). The area should be observed for any adverse reactions such as pain, pruritus and hyperpigmentation, which may result in discontinuation and subsequent dose reduction.

Intrathecal administration

Definition

Intrathecal administration is the administration of cytotoxic drugs into the central nervous system via the cerebrospinal fluid. This is usually achieved using a lumbar puncture (Chisholm *et al.* 1993; Otto 1995; Allwood *et al.* 1997).

Indications

Intrathecal administration has proved to be of benefit in prophylactic treatment in cases of leukaemias and some lymphomas, where the central nervous system (CNS) may provide a sanctuary site for tumour cells not reached during systemic chemotherapy (Allwood *et al.* 1997). It has no place in the treatment of CNS metastases of solid tumours (Allwood *et al.* 1997).

Intrathecal administration is only appropriate for a limited number of drugs:

1 Thiotepa
2 Cytarabine
3 Methotrexate
4 Hydrocortisone
5 Interferon.

The advantage of this route is that it allows the direct access to the CNS of drugs which do not normally cross the blood–brain barrier in sufficient amounts (Allwood *et al.* 1997; Goodman & Riley 1997) and thus ensures constant levels of the drug in this area (Powell 1996). The main disadvantage is that it requires a standard lumbar puncture before the drug can be injected, and this may need to be performed on a daily to weekly basis (Powell 1996; Allwood *et al.* 1997). Although this can be quick and easy to perform it can be distressing for the patient, and could even result in CNS trauma and infection. It may also only reach the epidural or subdural spaces and therefore the concentrations in the ventricles may only be a tenth of that in spinal cord (Priestman 1989). However, central instillation of the drug into the ventricle can be achieved via an Ommaya reservoir which is surgically implanted through the cranium (Goodman & Riley 1997). It carries more risks but provides permanent access and can be inserted under local or general anaesthetic (Goodman & Riley 1997).

The preparation of the drug must be performed using aseptic technique to reduce the risk of infection and the drug should be free from preservatives to reduce neurotoxicity. Cerebrospinal fluid removal and medications should not be more than 2 ml/min (Otto 1995). Expected side-effects of neurotoxicity related to the drugs include headache, nausea and vomiting, drowsiness, fever, stiff neck, ataxia and blurred vision and, rarely, meningitis (Chisholm *et al.* 1993; Powell 1996). Neurologic and vital signs checks should be obtained at least every 1–2 hours initially, and then on a scheduled frequency (Otto 1995). Observations should include signs of infection, headache and signs of increasing intracranial pressure and monitoring the function of the pump or reservoir.

Intrapleural instillation

Definition

Introduction of cytotoxic drugs, or other substances, into the pleural cavity.

Indications

Pleural effusion is a common complication of malignant disease and may pose a considerable management problem. Instillation should occur following drainage of an effusion to prevent or delay a recurrence caused by malignant cells, as after aspiration alone 60% will recur (Chisholm *et al.* 1993).

The most common neoplasms associated with the development of malignant pleural effusions are those of the:

1 Breast
2 Lung
3 Gastrointestinal tract
4 Prostate
5 Ovary.

The incidence of pleural effusions varies, but may be as high as 80% in patients with primary lung or breast carcinoma (Allwood *et al.* 1997). Such effusions can be very distressing to the patient, causing progressive discomfort, dyspnoea and death from respiratory insufficiency.

The alteration in normal anatomy due to the pressure of an effusion is illustrated in Fig. 10.2. In health less than 5 ml of transudate fluid are present between the visceral

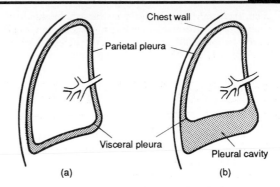

Figure 10.1 Lung anatomy. (a) Normal lung anatomy showing pleura. (b) Lung demonstrating presence of pleural effusion.

and parietal pleurae. This fluid acts as a lubricant and hydraulic seal. (See Chap. 21, Intrapleural drainage.) Infections and malignancies disrupt this mechanism, often repeatedly. Patients may survive for months or years, therefore effective palliation is important in maintaining or improving their quality of life. Administering chemotherapy via this route may alleviate symptoms and also has the potential for delivering the drugs to a site of poor systemic penetration (Allwood *et al.* 1997).

Reference material

Several methods have been used to treat pleural effusions, including:

1 Surgical techniques, such as ablation of the pleural space
2 Radiotherapy
3 Systemic chemotherapy and more recently
4 The insertion of a small bore catheter placement (Parker *et al.* 1989) and the installation of a pleural shunt (Tsang *et al.* 1990) to deliver cytotoxic agents.

In addition, instillation of sclerosing agents into the pleural space has been used for over 30 years and has been reported to have highly variable success rates of 20–88% (Allwood *et al.* 1997). These agents have included talc, radioactive phosphorus, BCG, tetracycline and, more recently, cytotoxic drugs. The drug most frequently instilled is bleomycin (Reymann 1993), but others include mitozantrone, doxorubicin, mustine and thiotepa (Allwood *et al.* 1997).

Cytology may show the presence of tumour cells in effusion fluid, but even when these are absent, instillation of drugs may be effective in preventing recurrence due to the inflammatory reaction which obliterates the pleural space.

Improvements in equipment used, for example flexible cannulae or catheters, and lengthening of both the initial drainage period and that following instillation of the drug have contributed to increased patient comfort and greater effectiveness. The insertion of small-bore percutaneously placed catheters or ports, as well as pleuroperitoneal shunts (Tsang *et al.* 1990) have been found to be useful for recurrent effusions.

The literature recommends that the patient should be turned regularly following instillation of the drug to facilitate its complete distribution over the pleural surfaces (Powell 1996). The recommended timing varies and only one paper (Wood 1981) provides a detailed procedure. The rationale for such turning is based on clinical observation and there is a lack of work comparing patients who were turned with those who were not.

Local pleural pain and inflammation can last for 24–48 hours after instillation. Good symptom management should focus upon emesis control, adequate analgesia and emotional support and chest tube security to ensure patient comfort (Chisholm 1993; Reymann 1993).

References and further reading

Allwood, M., Stanley, A. & Wright, P. (eds) (1997) *The Cytotoxic Handbook*, 3rd edn. Radcliffe Medical Press, Oxford.

Chisholm, L.G. *et al.* (1993) Programmed instruction: alternative administration routes. *Cancer Nurs*, **16**(3), 238–43.

Goodman, M. & Riley, M.B. (1997) Chemotherapy: principles of administration. In: *Cancer Nursing* (eds S.L. Groenwald, M.H. Frogge, M. Goodman *et al.*), 4th edn., pp. 317–404. Jones & Bartlett, Boston.

Otto, S.E. (1995) Advanced concepts of chemotherapy drug delivery. *Reg Ther J Intraven Nurs*, **18**(4), 170–76.

Parker, L.A. *et al.* (1989) Small bore catheter drainage and sclerotherapy for malignant pleural effusions. *Cancer*, **64**, 1218–21.

Powell, L.L. (ed.) (1996) *Cancer Chemotherapy. Guidelines and Recommendations for Practice*. Oncology Nursing Press, Pittsburgh.

Priestman, T.J. (1989) *Cancer Chemotherapy: An Introduction*, 3rd edn. Springer, Berlin.

Reymann, P.E. (1993) Chemotherapy: principles of administration. In: *Cancer Nursing. Principles and Practice* (eds S.L. Groenwald, M. Goodman, M.H. Frogge & C.H. Yarbro), 3rd edn. Jones & Bartlett, Boston.

Taylor, L. (1962) A catheter technique for intrapleural adminstration of alkylating agents: a report of ten cases. *Am J Med Sci*, **244**(6), 706–16.

Tsang, V. *et al.* (1990) Pleuroperitoneal shunt for recurrent malignant pleural effusion. *Thorax*, **45**, 369–72.

Wood, H. (1981) Developments in the support of patients with malignant pleural effusion. In: *Cancer Nursing Update* (ed. R. Tiffany), pp. 69–76. Baillière Tindall, London.

GUIDELINES • Administration of intrapleural drugs

The procedure and nursing care plans related to intrapleural drainage (see Chap. 21) should be consulted for all aspects of thoracic drainage. The following information covers specific points regarding drug instillation.

Procedure

Instillation of drug

Action	Rationale
1 Explain and discuss the procedure with the patient.	To ensure that the patient understands the procedure and gives his/her valid consent.
2 Administer premedication to patients if precribed.	To relax the patient.
3 Prepare the required equipment (see Chap. 12, Drug Administration, Guidelines • Administration of injections) and cytotoxic drug with protective wear as necessary.	To ensure the procedure goes smoothly without interruption.
4 Assist the doctor with the instillation and provide support for the patient.	To increase the efficiency of the procedure and reduce discomfort for the patient.
5 At the end of the procedure clamp the drainage tube and leave for the desired period.	To prevent back-flow of the drug.

Rotation of patient

Action	Rationale
1 Assess the clinical status of the patient and ability to tolerate the desired rotation.	To prevent discomfort the patient may feel and to ensure that the doctor is informed of the patient's inability to comply.

2 Turn the patient in the following rotation:
  (a) Left side
  (b) Supine
  (c) Right side
  (d) Prone
	To ensure that the drug coats and washes the pleural cavity completely.

3 Carry out the rotations as instructed.
  Examples are as follows:
  (a) 5 minutes in each position, repeated once, equals 20 minutes.
  (b) 30 minutes in each position, repeated once, equals 2 h.
  (c) 1 h in each position equals 4 h.
	As above.

4 Observe regularly for patient comfort. Administer analgesic as required.	To keep the patient comfortable and free from pain.
5 Record the patient's respirations and colour at least every15 minutes for 1 h, then every hour until stable, then 4-hourly, or as frequently as the patient's condition dictates. Record temperature at least 4-hourly	To ensure there is no change in respiratory function following the procedure. To observe for pyrexia, a common side-effect that may indicate a developing infection or a reaction to chemotherapy.

Drainage of thoracotomy tube

Action	*Rationale*
1 Ensure the patient is in a comfortable position, and is aware of any limitations about movement.	To prevent discomfort or dislodgement of the drainage tube.
2 Unclamp the chest tube.	To allow drainage of the drug instilled.
3 Maintain the underwater seal until a volume of less than 50 ml is drained during 24 h for 2 consecutive days or for a maximum of 7 days, or in consultation with medical staff.	To allow complete drainage of the drug instilled, and any additional fluid.
4 Record the colour and amount of fluid drained on the appropriate documents.	To monitor the immediate effectiveness of therapy.

Nursing care plan

Problem	*Cause*	*Suggested action*
Local or systemic effects associated with specific cytotoxic drugs, e.g. rigors due to bleomycin.	Absorption of the drug into circulation in sufficient quantities to cause toxicity.	Be aware that this can occur. Initiate preventive action, e.g. obtain a prescription for corticosteroid cover to prevent rigors, or observe for a reaction and treat symptomatically.

Intravesical instillation

Definition

Intravesical instillation is the instillation of cytotoxic drugs directly into the bladder, via a urinary catheter.

Indications

Intravesical instillation has been shown to be effective in the treatment of small, multiple, superficial, well differenti-ated, non-invasive papillomatous carcinomas. It also mini-mizes recurrence in patients with a history of multiple tumours known readily to seed locally (Goodman & Riley 1997).

Reference material

Instillation of cytotoxic agents, and now immunotherapy, into the bladder via a urinary catheter has been used for many years in selected cases and has proven to be an effec-tive and simple method of controlling and treating superficial bladder cancer (Reymann 1993). In measurable disease, average response rates are 60%. Approximately 30% of patients experience a complete response. Cytotoxic drugs found to be effective include:

1 Thiotepa
2 Mitomycin C
3 Doxorubicin
4 Epirubicin
5 Mitoxantrone
6 BCG.

Intravesical instillation allows a high concentration of drug to bathe the endothelium, which enables localized treatment to the tumour and limits the systemic absorption so toxicity is reduced. Systemic toxicity is a problem with thiotepa, but otherwise the main problems are local inflammation, pain, burning on urination, frequency and occasional haematuria. There is also the inconvenience for the patients. In addition a urinary tract infection may develop so the procedure should be performed using an aseptic technique.

Treatment protocols vary. Instillation involves the insertion of a urinary catheter and drainage of the bladder. Instillation of the drug usually takes about 50–60 minutes; it is retained for 1–2 hours with frequent movement to disperse the drug through the bladder (Powell 1996; Goodman & Riley 1997). Therapy may be repeated on alternating days for three doses or weekly for varying lengths of time (4–12 weeks).

Patients should be instructed in good personal hygiene such as washing hands and genitalia thoroughly after voiding and the toilet should be flushed at least twice after voiding. Increased intake during dwell time will increase the dilution of medication required and may reduce side-effects.

References and further reading

Garnick, M.B. et al. (1987) A determination of appropriate end-points in assessing efficacy of intravesical therapies in superficial bladder cancer. *Proceedings of the American Society of Clinical Oncology*, Abstract no. 412.

Goodman, M. & Riley, M.B. (1997) Chemotherapy: principles of administration. In: *Cancer Nursing* (eds S.L. Groenwald, M.H. Frogge, M. Goodman et al.), 4th edn., pp. 317–404. Jones & Bartlett, Boston.

Mulhall, A.B. et al. (1993) Maintenance of closed drainage systems: are practitioners more aware of the dangers? *J Clin Nurs*, **2**, 135–40.

Powell, L.L. (ed.) (1996) *Cancer Chemotherapy Guidelines and Recommendations for Practice*. Oncology Nursing Press, Pittsburgh.

Reymann, P.E. (1993) *Chemotherapy: Principles of Administration in Cancer Nursing. Principles and Practice* (eds S.L. Groenwald, M. Goodman, M.H. Frogge & C.H. Yarbro), 3rd edn, Chapter 15. Jones & Bartlett Publishers, Boston.

Swittes, D.D., Soares, S.E. & White, R.W. (1992) Nursing care of the patient receiving intravesical chemotherapy. *Urol Nurse*, **12**(4), 136–9.

GUIDELINES • Intravesical instillation of cytotoxic drugs

Other relevant procedures are urinary catheterization (see Chap. 43) and bladder lavage and irrigation (see Chap. 5). Details of required procedure and problems which may be encountered are given in these chapters. The following guidelines and care plan deal with specific aspects of chemotherapy administration.

Equipment

1 Urotainer containing prescribed drug in clinically clean tray (delivered from pharmacy reconstitution unit).
2 Sterile, latex gloves.
3 Disposable apron and eye protection.
4 Gate clip or equivalent clamp for catheter.
5 Catheter drainage bag, if catheter is to remain in position.
6 10 or 20 ml sterile syringe.
7 Small dressing pack, containing sterile field.

Procedure

Action	*Rationale*
1 Explain and discuss the procedure with the patient.	To ensure that the patient understands the procedure and gives his/her valid consent.
2 Check the patient's full blood count, as instructed by the medical staff, and inform them of any deficit before administration.	Absorption of the drug through the bladder wall may cause some myelosuppression. However, there are differing opinions as to whether regular checks are necessary.
3 Check all the details on the container of cytotoxic drug against the patient's prescription chart.	To minimize the risk of error and comply with legal requirements.
4 Assemble all necessary equipment, including the cytotoxic drug container, and proceed to the patient.	To ensure that the instillation proceeds smoothly and without interruption.
5 Screen the patient's bed/couch.	To ensure privacy during the procedure.

6	Check that the patient's identity matches the patient's details on the prescription chart.	To ensure that the correct patient has been identified. To reduce the risk of error.
7	If patient does not have a catheter in situ, then pass a catheter (see Chap. 5, Bladder Lavage and Irrigation).	
8	Ensure the bladder is empty of urine.	To prevent dilution of the drug.
9	Put on an apron/eye protection.	To protect the nurse from contact with the cytotoxic drugs. With correct technique the risk of contamination is minimal, but splashes can occur.
10	Using aseptic technique and sterile latex gloves, proceed to place a receiver under the end of the catheter to catch any urine and disconnect the drainage bag.	To protect the patient from infection. To protect the nurse from drug spillage. To gain access to the catheter. To prevent urine from soiling the bed.
11	Remove the cover from the urotainer, connect to the catheter and release the clamp.	To facilitate drug instillation.
12	Allow gravity to instil the cytotoxic drug into the bladder. Gentle squeezing may be needed to assist this process.	Rapid instillation would be uncomfortable for the patient, especially if the bladder is small or scarred from previous treatment or disease.
13	When the correct volume has been instilled, slide urotainer clamp over filling port.	To prevent drainage of drug from the bladder.
14	If the catheter is to be removed, withdraw the water from the catheter balloon using the sterile syringe and remove the catheter using gentle traction. Dispose of equipment into yellow clinical waste bag and seal.	The catheter may not be required for continued urinary drainage, and may have been inserted to facilitate drug administration, particularly in the outpatient department. The risk of infection is greater if the catheter remains in situ.
15	Make the patient comfortable.	
16	Provide outpatients with information about the amount of movement required.	Following outpatient instillation, the journey home is usually sufficient to coat the bladder mucosa.
17	When the drug has been in the bladder for 1 h, request the patient to micturate or slide clamp across filling port and place receiver under connectors. Disconnect urotainer and connect new drainage bag.	One hour is the usual time specified for intravesical drugs to ensure the maximum therapeutic effect with minimum toxicity. To prevent contamination of bed linen.
18	Advise the patient on fluid intake, suggesting ways in which he or she may increase it in the following 24-h period. Patients should be aware that their urine may be cloudy.	To provide a good fluid output, washing out the bladder and reducing the likelihood of local irritation or difficulty in urination due to debris from the tumour. To make patients aware of this side-effect.
19	Instruct the patient to report any discomfort or inability to pass urine immediately to ward staff or general practitioner/district nurse, or to telephone the hospital if anxious.	To detect and resolve any problems at the earliest moment. To reduce anxiety experienced by the patient.

Nursing care plan

Problem	*Cause*	*Suggested action*
No drainage of urine when the catheter is inserted.	Bladder is empty or the catheter is in the wrong place, e.g. in the urethra or in a false track. False tracks may develop after repeated cystoscopy or bladder surgery.	Do not inflate the balloon but tape the catheter to the skin to keep it in position. Check when the patient last micturated. Encourage the patient to drink a few glasses of fluid Do not give the drug until urine flow is seen or correct positioning of the catheter is established. Inform a doctor if no urine has drained during the next 30 minutes.

Problem	Cause	Suggested action
Haematuria.	Trauma of catheterization or loosening of blood clots following cystoscopy by fluid injected into the bladder.	Inform a doctor. Observe the patient for signs of clot retention, shock, haemorrhage or fluid retention. Encourage the patient to drink fluids.
Leakage from around the catheter following administration of the drug.	Catheter slipping out of the bladder or bladder spasm caused by the drug.	Check the position of the catheter. Inform a doctor if leakage persists. Protect the patient's skin by wrapping sterile topical swabs around the catheter. Estimate the volume lost by leakage. Wash contaminated skin thoroughly.
Patient unable to retain the requisite drug volume in the bladder for the time required.	Low bladder capacity; weak sphincter muscles; unstable detrusor muscle causing uncontrolled bladder contractions.	Note actual duration of the drug in the bladder and inform a doctor.
Patient has pain during instillation of the drug or while the drug is in the bladder.	Following resection of mucosa, the bladder can become acutely sensitive to irritants, thus causing painful spasm resulting in possible expelling of the cytotoxic agent.	Allow the drug to drain out and/or stop instillation if the pain is severe. Inform a doctor. Administer Entonox if appropriate (see Chap. 14, Entonox Administration) and have analgesics prescribed for subsequent administration.
Patient unable to pass urine after the drug has been in situ for the required length of time.	Anxiety; poor bladder tone; prostatism.	Reassure the patient. Encourage the patient to drink fluids.
Urine does not drain from the catheter when the clamp is released.	Catheter wrongly placed. Catheter blocked with clots and/or debris.	Check the position of the catheter. Perform bladder lavage.

Intraperitoneal administration

Definition

Intraperitoneal administration is the introduction of cytotoxic drugs into the peritoneal cavity, following drainage of ascites to prevent or delay a recurrence.

Indications

Treatment failures of primary malignant tumours of the colon and rectum as well as ovary occur most frequently as local regional disease. Extensive tumours may be present intra-abdominally without evidence of disease at other sites in the body. In view of this, chemotherapy treatment given intraperitoneally has been shown to have some effect in treating locally recurrent ovarian and colon cancers. This can be either by controlling ascites following aspiration or by control of the tumour (Jenkins *et al.* 1982).

Reference material

The peritoneal space is semi-permeable, which allows high concentrations of the drugs to be achieved at the site of the tumour throughout the peritoneal space, but with lower

concentrations entering the blood stream thus reducing the toxicity (Otto 1995; Young *et al.* 1996). Therefore increased dosages of drug can be delivered to the tumour site than could be delivered systemically.

Large volumes of fluid containing chemotherapy agents should be administered intermittently (Jenkins *et al.* 1982). The chemotherapy agents used include:

1 Cisplatin
2 Carboplatin
3 Etoposide
4 Doxorubicin
5 Bleomycin
6 Paclitaxel
7 Mitoxantrone
8 Cytarabine

(Otto 1995; Allwood *et al.* 1997).

There are three methods of accessing the peritoneal space:

1 Intermittent placement of a temporary indwelling catheter. This is used for a short time such as for symptom relief or palliation.
2 Placement of an external catheter such as a Tenckhoff. This is surgically placed through the anterior abdominal wall and the catheter exits through the skin on the

abdomen. This is the most widely used method and the Tenckhoff catheter has the advantages of allowing a high flow rate (2 litres in 10–15 minutes) and also allows for manipulation to dislodge fibrin deposits (Jenkins *et al.* 1982). Problems include occlusion (Powell 1996), infection, leakage around the catheter and body image problems.

3 Placement of an implantable peritoneal port. The port is internal with no care required when not accessed and therefore has a lower rate of infection and may be more acceptable to the patient. However, ports tend to provide a slower flow rate than a catheter (Otto 1995).

General complications of intraperitoneal chemotherapy include respiratory distress, abdominal pain and distension, discomfort and diarrhoea (which all result in increased abdominal pressure) (Otto 1995; Goodman & Riley 1997). Other problems include mechanical difficulties with the catheter (inflow and outflow obstructions), electrolyte imbalance and peritonitis caused by chemical irritation of the peritoneal space, or by infection or both. In general, intraperitoneal chemotherapy is usually tolerated well by patients and provides a safe and effective treatment in the management of peritoneal disease.

References and further reading

Allwood, M., Stanley, A. & Wright, P. (eds) (1997) *The Cytotoxic Handbook*, 3rd edn. Radcliffe Medical Press, Oxford.

Chisholm, L.G. *et al.* (1993) Programmed instruction: alternative administrative routes. Cancer Nurs, **16**(3), 238–43.

Goodman, M. & Riley, M.B. (1997) Chemotherapy: principles of administration. In: *Cancer Nursing* (eds S.L. Groenwald, M.H. Frogge, M. Goodman, *et al.*), 4th edn., pp. 317–404. Jones & Bartlett, Boston.

Jenkins, J. *et al.* (1982) Technical considerations in the use of intraperitoneal chemotherapy administered by Tenckhoff catheter. *Surgery*, **154**, 858–64.

Powell, L.L. (ed.) (1996) *Cancer Chemotherapy Guidelines and Recommendations for Practice*. Oncology Nursing Press, Pittsburgh.

Otto, S.E. (1995) Advanced concepts in chemotherapy drug delivery. *Reg Ther J Intraven Nurs*, **18**(4), 170–76.

Young, A. *et al.* (1996) Intraperitoneal chemotherapy: a prolonged infusion of 5Fluorouracil using a novel carrier solution. *Br J Nurs*, **5**(9), 539–43.

GUIDELINES • Intraperitoneal instillation of cytotoxic drugs

Details of the procedure for ascitic drainage and problems encountered are given in Chap. 2, Abdominal paracentesis. The following guidelines and care plan deal with specific aspects of chemotherapy administration.

Equipment

1 Syringe or infusion bag containing prescribed drug in clinically clean tray (delivered from pharmacy reconstitution unit).
2 Sterile, latex gloves.
3 Disposable apron and goggles.
4 Gate clip or equivalent clamp for catheter.
5 Catheter drainage bag, if catheter is to remain in position.
6 10 or 20 ml sterile syringe.
7 Small dressing pack, containing sterile field.

Procedure

Action	*Rationale*
1 Explain and discuss the procedure with the patient.	To ensure that the patient understands the procedure and gives his/her valid consent
2 Administer premedication to patient if prescribed.	To ensure the patient is more relaxed during the procedure
3 Check all the details on the container of the cytotoxic drug against the patient's prescription chart.	To minimize the risk of error and comply with legal requirements.
4 Assemble all necessary equipment, including the cytotoxic drug container, and proceed to the patient.	To ensure that the installation proceeds smoothly and without interruption.
5 Prior to instillation, prewarm infusion to body temperature (Powell 1996).	To prevent cramping.
6 Use a Y-tube irrigation set. The catheter is attached by this Y-tube to a bottle of dialysate and a drainage bag.	To ensure minimum intervention in draining peritoneal cavity.
7 Instill fluid at prescribed rate, usually 1–2 litres over 10–15 min, but can be extended to 30–60 min (Otto 1995).	To ensure the correct instillation at the correct rate.

Guidelines • Intraperitoneal instillation of cytotoxic drugs (cont'd)

Action	Rationale
8 Wait prescribed period of time after administration prior to draining off excess fluid. This may be from 1 to 3 h.	To ensure fluid has coated all parts of peritoneal cavity.
9 Observe regularly for patient comfort and intervene as appropriate.	To keep patient comfortable and pain free.
10 Record temperature 4-hourly.	To observe for pyrexia, a common side-effect that may indicate a developing infection or a reaction to chemotherapy.
11 Unclamp drainage tube and, where necessary, flush port or pump using appropriate flushing solution. The catheter may be removed after drainage is complete.	To allow drainage of drug.
Note: if there is leakage around drain site or a drainage bag is attached, nurses must remember that the fluid may still contain cytotoxic drug and should therefore take the same precautions as when handling any cytotoxic waste.	To reduce the risk of contamination to the patient and staff.
12 Record accurate fluid balance.	To assess amount of drug received by patient.

Nursing care plan

Problem	Cause	Suggested action
Local or systemic effects as a complication of dialysis, that is abdominal pain or discomfort.	1 Peritoneal irritation following placement of catheter.	Knowledge of these side-effects.
	2 Incomplete drainage of the dialysate solution.	Observe for a reaction and treat symptomatically.
	3 Failure to warm dialysate solution to body temperature.	
	4 Chemical peritonitis resulting from chemotherapeutic agent.	
	5 Bacterial peritonitis.	
Leakage from around the catheter following administration of the drug.	Peritoneum is not intact or catheter is not entirely within peritoneal cavity.	Strict aseptic technique required. Dressings to be changed frequently. When skin around the catheter has healed, there should be no further leakage.

Intra-arterial administration

Definition

Intra-arterial administration is the delivery of a cytotoxic drug to the tumour site by catheterization of the artery providing the blood supply to the affected organ. This allows a high concentration of drug to be delivered.

Indications

Intra-arterial chemotherapy has been used to treat a variety of malignancies at a number of different sites. These include:

1 Head and neck lesions
2 Liver metastases from colorectal cancer
3 Sarcomas/melanomas of upper and lower limb (including isolated limb perfusion)
4 Carcinoma of the stomach
5 Carcinoma of the breast
6 Carcinoma of the cervix.

The tumour site determines which artery will be used to deliver the chemotherapy since it is the artery supplying the tumour which is cannulated. The commonest route is the hepatic artery (Chisholm *et al.* 1993; Allwood *et al.* 1997).

Reference material

The advantage of the route is that it facilitates the delivery of high concentrations of drug to the primary or secondary tumour mass (Otto 1995). A reduction in systemic circulating levels of drugs has been shown to occur in many circumstances resulting in a corresponding reduction in side-effects to the patient, although this is difficult to predict (Reymann 1993). The cytotoxic drugs used vary with the histology and site of the tumour. All of the following have been administered via the intra-arterial route:

1 Actinomycin D
2 BCNU (carmustine)
3 Bleomycin
4 Cisplatin
5 Doxorubicin
6 5-FU (5-fluorouracil)
7 5-FUDR (floxuridine)
8 Methotrexate
9 Melphalan
10 Mitomycin C
11 Vincristine.

The main disadvantage of this route is that very high levels of drug in a perfused organ may result in excessive tissue damage (Allwood *et al.* 1997). It also requires the insertion of an arterial device. Two main methods are used for infusional chemotherapy; these are termed external or internal arterial infusions.

The external method involves radiographic placement of an arterial catheter and attachment to an external infusion pump for 3–7 days, during which time the patient remains flat (Powell 1996). Temporary catheter placement is used for short-term therapies, i.e. from hours up to 5 days (Otto 1995). Therapy can be given intermittently for several courses. This method is unsuitable for long-term use (6 months or longer) as it is uncomfortable, inconvenient and expensive, although a subcutaneous implanted port increases the patient's comfort and freedom (Goodman & Riley 1997).

Once the catheter is in place and secured, cytotoxic drugs may be administered by:

1 Injection – using a syringe
2 Small volume infusion – using a syringe pump
3 Large volume infusion – using a volumetric pump.

Internal or implantable methods involve the surgical placement of a totally implantable pump and appear to have a lower complication rate than the external method. The catheter is inserted into an appropriate artery and attached to the pump, which is filled with chemotherapy. This approach is more frequently used for colorectal cancer metastases to the liver (Otto 1995).

Confirmation that the artery supplies the desired area can be achieved by instillation of yellow fluorescent dye if the tumour site is visible, or contrast medium if an internal organ such as the liver is the target area.

All delivery systems must provide adequate pressure to combat arterial pressure, i.e. 300 mmHg (Miller 1995; Weinstein 1997). The majority of infusion pumps meet this requirement (Weinstein 1997). Patient education is very important as the patient may have to maintain the implantable pump and be able to recognize any complications or malfunctions.

Principles of nursing care

Insertion is an operative procedure and consent must be obtained. Adequate explanation to the patient is essential, especially what to expect on return to the ward.

The area of insertion should be shaved or otherwise prepared and the period of fasting should be checked with the anaesthetist.

The catheter is inserted in theatre or in the X-ray department and its position checked at that time. The catheter is then secured and an occlusive dressing applied. This should *not* be touched as it is essential that the catheter is *not* displaced.

A three- or one-way tap is connected to the catheter and it is at this point that all manipulations take place. An extension set should be connected to this at the time of insertion or on return to the ward to prevent unnecessary handling near the skin exit site.

The system will consist of: catheter/tap/extension set/administration set and infusion device.

Certain general rules apply:

1 The dressing must not be touched but should be observed regularly for signs of bleeding. This should be reported immediately to the medical staff, including the radiologist.
2 All procedures or manipulations associated with the pathway must use aseptic technique.
3 All connections must be Luer locking to prevent exsanguination, air embolism or disconnection under pressure.
4 The catheter must be clamped securely or switched off using the tap in situ before any equipment changes.
5 A positive pressure greater than arterial pressure must be maintained at all times.
6 When chemotherapy is not being infused, the flushing solution must be used to maintain patency. This should be via a syringe or syringe pump during transfer between wards or departments, or via a syringe pump or infusion pump in the ward. A nurse escort may be necessary for transfers. It should be delivered at the minimum rate sufficient to combat arterial pressure and maintain patency, approximately 3–5 ml per hour or 10 drops per minute, dependent on the device used (Weinstein 1997). If a specialist delivery system is used, then manufacturers' instructions should be followed.
7 The patient must be instructed on the amount of mobility allowed. This may vary depending on the site of the catheter. Assistance may be needed to maintain personal hygiene and relieve pressure in order to prevent the development of pressure ulcers on all points of contact.
8 The position of the catheter may be checked daily by X-ray, which will be performed on the ward. Fluoroscopy and instillation of dye are other methods of confirming position.
9 At the end of treatment, the patency of the arterial line should be maintained using an appropriate flushing solution until a decision has been made about removal. Instructions for this and the amount of heparin to be

used should be prescribed in advance to enable the nurse to initiate the procedure when appropriate.

10 Before removal, the tap may be switched off and the catheter allowed to clot. The catheter should be removed by a doctor and firm pressure applied for at least 5 minutes or until all bleeding has ceased. A dressing should be applied to the site. Pressure dressings are not indicated if bleeding has ceased and can obscure the formation of a haematoma.

Complications associated with intra-arterial chemotherapy

Any problems should be referred to the medical staff (Consertino 1987) or a radiologist as he/she is the expert in catheter placement and management of complications.

1 Arterial occlusion and thrombosis: the literature indicates that thrombosis occurs in over 40% of arteries catheterized for over 48 hours. However, this is dependent on the vessel used. Most catheters used for chemotherapy delivery pose no problem and will remain patent for the treatment period. However, a thrombus may embolize causing vascular insufficiency, distal or central embolism. When occlusion occurs due to thrombus formation or spasm, blood flow is usually maintained by the collateral circulation until the vessel recovers. Presence of a pulse and the colour of the area should be checked daily or a Doppler flow meter may be used. Any abnormality should be reported to the medical staff and radiologist. The catheter should be removed by the doctor using firm, steady traction, in an attempt to prevent dislodging any thrombus present. The condition of the patient and the limb/area should be observed carefully at the time that vital signs are measured.

2 Damage to the artery, arteriovenous fistula, aneurysm formation: the incidence of these is low and the likelihood of problems occurring can be minimized by gentle handling of the catheter and immobilization of the limb/area as soon as appropriate.

3 Chemical hepatitis and biliary sclerosis: the occurrence of these will be evident from elevated liver enzymes.

Therefore, monitoring of liver function tests is important. Any elevation is usually transient.

4 Exsanguination/air embolism: the seriousness of an air embolus depends on the siting of the arterial catheter and whether it is a direct route to the carotid artery and so to the brain. Luer lock connections must be used throughout the pathway. These should be checked at regular intervals, and continuous flow maintained. Care must be taken when changing equipment to prevent blood loss occurring or air entering the catheter, e.g. shut off the tap, firm clamping, if necessary.

References and further reading

Allwood, M., Stanley, A. & Wright, P. (eds) (1997) *The Cytotoxic Handbook*, 3rd edn. Radcliffe Medical Press, Oxford.

Chisholm, L.G. *et al.* (1993) Programmed instruction: alternative administrative routes. *Cancer Nurs*, 16(3), 238–43.

Consertino, F. (1987) Chapter 23. In: *Principles and Practice of Intravenous Therapy* (eds A. Plumer & F. Consertino), 4th edn, pp. 477–504. Little, Brown & Co, Boston.

Goodman, M. & Riley, M.B. (1997) Chemotherapy: principles of administration. In: *Cancer Nursing* (eds S.L. Groenwald, M. Goodman, M.H. Frogge & C.H. Yarbro), 4th edn., pp. 317–404. Jones & Bartlett, Boston.

Miller, T.A. (1995) Haemodynamic monitoring. In: *Intravenous Therapy: Clinical Principles and Practice* (eds J. Terry *et al.*). W.B. Saunders, Philadelphia.

Otto, S.E. (1995) Advanced concepts in chemotherapy drug delivery. *Reg Ther J Intraven Nurs*, 18(4), 170–76.

Powell, L.L. (ed.) (1996) *Cancer Chemotherapy Guidelines and Recommendations for Practice*. Oncology Nursing Press, Pittsburgh.

Reymann, P.E. (1993) Chemotherapy: Principles of Administration. In: *Cancer Nursing* (eds S.L. Groenwald, M. Goodman, M.H. Frogge & C.H. Yarbro), 3rd edn. Jones & Bartlett, Boston.

von Roemeling, R. *et al.* (1986) Chemotherapy via implanted infusion pump. New perspectives for delivery of long-term continuous treatment. *Oncol Nurs Forum*, 13, 17–24.

Taylor, I. (1985) Hepatic arterial infusion of anti-cancer drugs. *Cancer Top*, 5(5), 50–51.

Weinstein, S.M. (1993) *Plumer's Principles and Practice of Intravenous Therapy*, 5th edn. J.B. Lippincott, Philadelphia.

Weinstein, S.M. (1997) *Principles and Practice of Intravenous Therapy*, 6th edn. J.B. Lippincott, Philadelphia.

Nursing care plan

Problem	Cause	Action
Haemorrhage.	Excessive movement.	Observe the dressing at regular intervals. Monitor pulse and blood pressure at least 4 hourly. Instruct the patient on the amount of movement permitted and to report any feeling of faintness, or oozing noted on dressing.
	Insufficient pressure on site following removal of catheter.	After removal of the catheter, vital signs and the dressing should be observed at least every 15 min for 2 h.

		Whether the patient should remain on bedrest for 24 h is dependent on the site where the patient has been catheterized.
		If bleeding occurs, pressure should be applied immediately and a member of the medical staff contacted.
Displacement of the catheter.	Dressing disturbed.	Do not disturb the dressing placed in the X-ray department.
	Excessive movement by patient.	Instruct the patient on amount of movement permitted. Check position daily.
Infection.	Poor aseptic technique.	Strict asepsis must be maintained for all procedures and manipulations of the arterial catheter. Temperature must be taken at least every 4 h and any pyrexia investigated.
Extravasation of drugs/failure of drug to reach target area (both rare).	Incorrect placement of catheter.	If there is any doubt concerning the placement of the catheter the doctor and radiologist should be notified, as extravasation of the drug may lead to ulceration and necrosis.

Discharge Planning

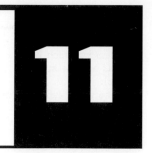

Definition

Discharge planning is the process of developing a plan of care for a patient who is transferred from one environment to another (Jupp & Simms 1986).

Reference material

Discharge from hospital can be a major life event for both patient and carer(s). It also has substantial implications for the use of health and social care resources. Good quality discharge should not be a matter of chance (DoH 1994). Hospital discharge arrangements are based upon legislation and guidance and over the past decade a series of government initiatives has attempted to focus attention and resources away from acute hospital services to primary and preventive care (for example, DoH 1986, 1989a, 1991, 1993, 1998). This places a responsibility on local authorities, health authorities and health providers to work together to assess, plan and meet the needs of people leaving hospital (Henwood & Wistow 1994).

All hospitals should have a discharge policy which is developed, agreed and ideally jointly published with all the relevant local health and social service agencies. Standards should be applicable to the planning and delivery of care at all stages: pre-admission and admission; the period as an inpatient; predischarge; the discharge process and post-discharge (Health Services Accreditation 1996). Patient admission clinics are an ideal opportunity to assess care required on discharge.

The Patient's Charter (DoH 1995c) states that 'before you are discharged from hospital, you can expect a decision to be made about how to meet any needs you may have. Your hospital will agree arrangements with agencies such as community nursing services and local authority social services departments. You, and if you agree, your carers will be involved in making these decisions and will be kept up to date with information at all stages.' Discharge planning, therefore, should be a multidisciplinary process by which needs and resources of patients and carers are assessed and where areas of care/responsibility of health and social services are clearly defined and agreed (Bristow et al. 1986). All patients, whether short- or long-stay, those with few needs or those with complex needs, should receive comprehensive discharge planning. For complex discharges, it is helpful if a key worker or coordinator is appointed to manage the discharge and, where appropriate, for family meetings/case conferences to take place to include the

patient/carer, multi-disciplinary and primary health care team and representatives (Health Services Accreditation 1996; Salter 1996). Good discharge planning prevents unplanned readmission due to breakdown of services at home (Heeks et al. 1991).

Discharge planning is a complex process which cannot be examined in isolation from what has occurred before or separated from the consequences that follow (Armitage 1990). Healthy individuals have sufficient self-care abilities to enable them to meet their needs with assistance from either a nurse or personal carers from social services, or they may be dependent upon someone to meet their needs for them until they are capable of resuming that self-care. In certain circumstances their needs may fluctuate due to their disease process and so self-care may not be a realistic goal. Discharge planning is therefore a vital procedure to assist these individuals who require help to maintain their self-care or to assist them with care needs when they leave one care environment for another (Jackson 1994).

Ineffective discharge planning has been shown to have detrimental effects on a patient's psychological and physical wellbeing and their illness experience (Smith 1996; Nazarko 1998). Planning care, providing adequate information and involving patients, families and health care professionals, keeps disruption to a minimum.

Aims of discharge planning

1 To prepare the patient/family physically and psychologically for transfer home or to an agreed environment.
2 To provide the patient and carers with written and verbal information to meet their needs on discharge.
3 To facilitate a smooth transfer, by ensuring that all necessary health care facilities are prepared to receive the patient.
4 To promote the highest possible level of independence for the patient, partner and family by, where appropriate, encouraging self-care activities.
5 To provide continuity of care between the hospital and the agreed environment by facilitating effective communication.

Principles of good discharge planning

When planning discharge from one care environment to another, certain principles should be followed. These include:

1 Discharge planning should be a multi-disciplinary process by which needs and resources of patients and carers are put in place (Tierney & Closs 1993; Salter 1996).

2 Discharge procedures should be of a consistently high standard for all patients.

3 Patients' needs should always be a priority when discharge is being planned.

4 Patients should be discharged to a safe and adequate environment.

5 Continuity of care between environments should be paramount.

6 Discharge planning should commence on the initial contact with patients.

7 Information about discharge arrangements should be disseminated between professionals and patients/carers, with the latter being provided with written information of ongoing care.

8 Patients' beliefs and culture should be considered when planning discharges.

The discharge planning process and the primary/secondary care interface

The discharge planning process can begin either in the community with the primary health care team (PHCT) or local authority (LA) staff in the patient's own home prior to admission, or in pre-admission clinics for prebooked admissions, or on admission (Health Services Accreditation 1996). Importance is attached to developing a primary care-led NHS, reinforced by the government's white paper, 'The New NHS: Modern, Dependable' and the establish-

ment of primary care groups (PCGs) that came into force in April 1999 (DoH 1998). The focus on quality, patient-centred care and services closer to where people live will be dependent on primary, secondary and tertiary professionals working together (Davis 1998). To this end, the trigger questions shown in Fig. 11.1 are a useful tool for screening patients who may have high social needs.

The discharge planning process takes into account a patient's physical, psychological, social, cultural and economic needs. It involves not only patients but can involve families, friends, carers, the hospital multi-disciplinary team and the community health/social services teams (Nixon *et al.* 1998), with the emphasis on health and social services departments working jointly.

In addition, the frequently used phrase 'quicker and sicker' increasingly describes the process of hospital discharge planning for the 1990s, in that in-patient care is reduced to the minimum (Jackson 1994). The notion of a seamless service may, therefore, be too idealistic because of the time constraints and care needs of such discharges (Smith 1996). Despite well-documented concern about the quality of procedures for the discharge of patients from hospital, shortcomings persist (DoH 1994; Marks 1994; Social Services Inspectorate 1998). In Saville & Bartholomew's (1994) study, less than a third of patients were discharged with the ideal 48 hours' notice being given to the district nurse, while one quarter of all hospital discharges occurred at the weekend (despite this being the least desirable time for discharge as far as community services are concerned). To bridge this gap, information booklets for patients have been used (Vaughan & Taylor 1988) and Neill & Williams (1992) suggest that a 'going home folder' could be utilized, where professionals, as well as patients and carers, can

---

The Royal Marsden Hospital

These trigger questions are designed for use by nursing staff to screen patients with potentially high social care needs whose eligibility for community care services has to be assessed in more detail by a hospital-based social worker. Discussion with the social services team should be initiated regarding appropriate assessment of patient and/or their family's needs.

Patient's name: Hospital no.:   Ward: Estimated data of discharge:

Care needs
1 Significant change in ability to care for self due to the effects of treatment or the debilitating symptoms of progressive disease. ☐
2 Patient has, and is aware of, limited prognosis, requiring a complex package of palliative and community care. ☐
3 Patient appears to have very high social and nursing care needs which suggest a residential or nursing home as a placement option. ☐
4 Patient appears to be in need of NHS-funded continuing care. ☐

Social network
5 High dependency on a carer for all or most aspects of physical care. ☐
6 Carer shows signs of stress, or questions own ability to continue caring. ☐
7 Patient is carer for partner, vulnerable adult dependant and/or children under 18. ☐

Environment
8 Housing unsuitable, access problems or inadequate heating, electricity, water supplies. ☐
9 Patient is homeless or threatened by homelessness. ☐

Signature of referrer: Job title: Date of referral:

Figure 11.1 Trigger questions for social services referrals.

The Royal Marsden Hospital

Definition
A discharge delay is when a patient remains in hospital beyond the date agreed by the multi-disciplinary team and beyond the time when they are medically fit to leave.

Monitoring
For every patient who is 'delayed' the ward nurse will complete a 'delayed discharge' form and return it to the clinical nurse specialist (CNS) community liaison.
The CNS, community liaison will monitor all 'delays' of 7 days or more.

Procedure
Any patient who is 'delayed' for 7 days or more for reasons other than medical need will be discussed at a multi-disciplinary meeting including medical staff, where appropriate. A discharge plan should be formulated and documented in the multidisciplinary care plan.

If there is no resolution at that meeting the CNS, community liaison or social worker will contact the patient services manager. If a long 'delay' is anticipated even when a discharge plan has been agreed, the CNS community liaison or the social worker should inform the patient services manager in writing.

All details of the reasons for the delay and actions taken must be documented in the multidisciplinary care plan.

Source: The Royal Marsden Hospital's Discharge Delay Policy/Procedure (1999).

DISCHARGE DELAY MONITORING FORM
Name of patient:
Hospital number:
Ward:
Expected date of discharge:
Reason for delay:
Signature.

Figure 11.2 Discharge delays.

The Royal Marsden Hospital

Nursing staff responsibility
If a patient wishes to take his/her own discharge the ward sister/coordinator should contact:

1 A member of the medical team
2 The senior nurse manager
3 The clinical nurse specialist (CNS), community liaison.

The CNS, community liaison, will inform social services if appropriate.

Out of hours, following a risk assessment, the senior nurse manager will contact the local social services department if appropriate and inform the hospital social services department the following day.

Medical staff responsibility
The doctor, following consultation with the patient, should complete the appropriate form prior to the patient leaving the hospital. The form must be signed by the patient and the doctor and filed in the medical notes.

The doctor must immediately contact the patient's GP.

Figure 11.3 Patients taking discharge against medical advice. (*Source:* The Royal Marsden Hospital's Discharge Policy/Procedure 1999.)

(The Royal Marsden Hospital Discharge and Policy Procedure 1999). Studies indicate that the greater the level of patient and family involvement in the discharge planning process, the more patients perceive themselves ready for discharge (Jacobs *et al.* 1985; Jupp & Simms 1986). The DoH (1989b) white paper 'Caring for People' explicitly acknowledged that the majority of care is provided by informal carers and that carers need help and support to fulfil that role. A critical time to help carers is during hospital discharge when community care plans are being set up (George 1995). However, in Henwood's (1998) study, 7 out of 10 carers said they did not receive a copy of the discharge plan. Half the carers felt that they had not been informed of the type of care they were expected to give at home and more than a third did not feel their concerns were taken into consideration by the staff planning the discharge. Policy guidance has suggested that carers' needs should be seen as being just as important as those of service users (DoH 1990; Social Services Inspectorate 1998). The *Carer's (Recognition and Services) Act* (DoH 1995b) gives carers a statutory right to request an assessment of their ability to provide care (Henwood 1998). Carers' needs should be acknowledged so that health care professionals adopt a proactive approach to addressing such needs. Voluntary services play a key role in supporting patients and carers at home (Daly 1999).

record facts relevant to discharge (Marks 1994). This meets the need for providing written information for the patient/carer (Robinson & Miller 1996).

Occasionally the discharge process may not proceed as planned. For example, a discharge may be delayed because of a number of reasons and a system should be in place to provide for this (see Fig. 11.2). Patients may take their own discharge against medical advice and this should be documented accordingly (see Fig. 11.3). Some patients receiving news of a poor prognosis may prefer to go home to die and plans would need to be set up at short notice (see Fig. 11.4).

The role of informal carers

Patients and their carers/advocates should be actively involved at all stages of the planning and discharge process

Communication and discharge planning

Inadequate communication networks and a lack of interpersonal cooperation between hospital and community

The Royal Marsden Hospital

This form has been designed to assist with planning an urgent discharge home for terminal care. It should be used as a trigger in conjunction with the discharge policy. Please document all relevant comments in the Multidisciplinary Care Plan.

Emergency Discharge Plan   Date of discharge: ....

(Tick when arranged or cross if not appropriate)
1 Plan agreed and discussed with patient and carers.   ☐
2 Patient and family fully aware of condition and prognosis.   ☐
3 Transport booked   ☐
  Date and time: ....
  Oxygen/suction requested   ☐
  Paramedic crew requested   ☐
  Stretcher   ☐
  Escort (family/nurse)   ☐
4 Oxygen ordered through GP and delivery date organized for ....   ☐
5 Patient/carer given list of contact numbers of community services   ☐
6 Block bed for 24–48 hour period   Yes/No

Nursing issues
1 Contact district nurse (DN) and discuss   ☐
  (a) Patient needs   ☐
  (b) Planned date and time of DN's first visit ....   ☐
  (c) Night nursing service   ☐
      • Starting ....
      • Contact numbers ....
  (d) Marie Curie provision   ☐
      • Starting ....
  (e) Return of RMH syringe driver   ☐
  (f) Delivery of equipment   ☐
      • Hospital bed (adjustable height)   ☐
      • Pressure relieving equipment   ☐
      • Commode/urinal   ☐
      • Hoist   ☐
      • Backrest/mattress variator   ☐
      • Other (please state) ....   ☐
2 Contact hospice home care team   ☐
  Planned date and time of first visit ....
3 Nursing letter for DN and hospice home care team   ☐
4 Medical letter of authorization for drugs to be administered by community nurses   ☐

---

5 List of medication to go with patient   ☐
6 Provide 3–4 days' supply of:
  (a) Dressing and continence aids   ☐
  (b) Syringe driver giving sets   ☐
  (c) Butterfly needle and dressing to secure   ☐
7 Convert syringe driver to a 24-hour pump and aim for it to be changed every morning   ☐

Medical issues
1 Medical team contact GP to discuss:
  (a) Patient needs   ☐
  (b) Drugs prescribed on discharge   ☐
  (c) Need to review patient in community   ☐
2 Prescribe adequate supply of TTOs (include diluent used in syringe driver).   ☐
  (Consider prognosis)
3 Crisis pack for use in the event of an emergency, including diamorphine, midazolam and instructions for use   ☐
4 Medical summary faxed to GP, copy with patient   ☐
5 Medical proforma for ambulance crew stating resuscitation status (signature of consultant/senior registrar)   ☐

If you have any queries please contact the community liaison team or the palliative care team.

Figure 11.4   Emergency Discharge Plan Checklist.

have been identified as contributing to problems with discharge (Tierney & Closs 1993). With the discharge process spanning organizational and professional boundaries, what is required is effective communication and more multidisciplinary and joint approaches to planning. The involvement of patient, carers, community nurses (Guerrero 1990; Worth et al. 1994) and local authority home care managers in the discharge process facilitates closer links between care environments, promotes continuity of care for patients and also ensures that services commence on discharge, with no delays in service contact (McMahon 1988).

To this end, in the 1970s the introduction of liaison nursing posts was seen as a means of improving continuity of care (Gatt et al. 1973) and, although such posts have proliferated, there are differing views as to their effectiveness (Armitage 1990; Evers 1991). The Royal College of Nursing (1992b), Smith (1996) and Nixon et al. (1998) have endorsed the value of liaison nurses in a climate where shorter hospital stays and the early discharge of patients will become the norm (Audit Commission 1992), asserting the belief that the liaison nursing service is essential to the success of discharge planning. The role of the multidisciplinary team in assessing and planning for discharge is vital. Continuous assessment of patients' needs and early liaison with the primary health care team/local authority are essential if appropriate care and a safe environment are to be provided in the community (Tierney 1993).

Interprofessional record keeping

This remains rare in UK hospitals. In most circumstances, nurses, doctors, physiotherapists, occupational therapists, speech and language therapists and care managers keep their own records. This practice has the potential to lead to poor communication and to inhibit team working. The discharge coordinator should operate across professional boundaries and introduce interprofessional working and record keeping to allow effective discharge to take place (Nazarko 1998). Patient-held records (transferable from hospital to community) can improve communication for patients as long as they are used efficiently and do not add to the patient's anxiety (Drury et al. 1996). Computerized patient records will, it is hoped, alleviate many of these problems.

The *NHS and Community Care Act (1990)*

The government's stated key objectives in the *NHS and Community Care Act (1990)* are the promotion of choice and independence for individuals with assessed community care needs. This approach has shifted the balance to take account of the financial consequences of providing care. This Act has had major implications for professionals working in health and social care as well as for patients and their carers. The intention of the Act is to enable elderly, frail, sick and disabled people to live at home for as long as possible. The Act means that hospital discharge policies and procedures must also take full account of the requirements for local authority social services departments to undertake needs-based assessments for community care. It emphasizes the need for continuity of health and social care and promotes choice for consumers. It stresses that patients should not leave hospital until a community care package has been formulated and agreed to meet their needs. The Act also states that resources cannot be committed without prior agreement of the agencies involved. This has implications for health and social carers as it is often not in the financial interests of the local authority to discharge patients early (Marks 1994). Local agreements and contracts are therefore recommended to prevent a clash of interests between those agencies involved.

Residential care

Residential care (whether it be in the form of a residential or nursing home) requires careful thought as for many patients the concept and planning of giving up their own home is one of the most traumatic events that the older person has to consider and that has serious repercussions if a wrong decision is made (Macabee 1994). When a patient is transferred from an inpatient palliative care service to a nursing home, a specific prognosis may not be given, although there is an expectation that death is not imminent, or a nursing home placement, as a longer term facility, should not have been considered. The present government was concerned about the transfer of frail, elderly patients between hospitals and care homes, and such transfers may be stopped or severely restricted if the results of an investigation support the health secretary's impression that too many old people die as a result of being moved (Thorpe 1993). Alternatives such as nurse-led 'hospital at home' schemes (Busby 1995; Jester 1998) or 'immediate response/discharge teams' (usually local authority led) may well enable a person to remain in their own home.

Longer-term health care needs and eligibility criteria

The NHS (1997) survey comments in some detail on the implications of allowing health authorities to set local criteria for eligibility to receive free, NHS funded, long-term care. The NHS argued that these local criteria might create inequity, with individuals in some parts of the country receiving free NHS care, while others in identical circumstances elsewhere contribute towards the cost of care commissioned by local authorities. The NHS called for the national framework to include national eligibility criteria 'to define what the NHS, as a national service . . . always provide' (NHS 1997, para. 8). There will, of course, always have to be a judgement made as to what is the level of care above which domiciliary care packages cease to be realistically affordable, bearing in mind the equally valid needs of other people in the community.

Cost of care

The financial implications of the changes brought by the *NHS and Community Care Act (1990)* have led to a vigorous debate. For the most part this centres on the difference between the continuing care facilities purchased by social services departments, which are means tested, and the continuing care provided within the NHS, which is free at the point of delivery. There is much debate on what constitutes health care (free at the point of delivery) and social care (which is cost-driven) (Roberts *et al.* 1995). It is critically important that the charging system should not contain perverse incentives for local authorities to steer individuals towards residential rather than domiciliary care (Porrock *et al.* 1999).

Audit and the discharge process

It is the responsibility of health authorities, in collaboration with social services departments, to monitor the way in which discharges from hospitals are being undertaken and, if problems occur, to establish the reasons so that any necessary changes are made to address the local needs, for example, monitoring discharge failures (DoH 1989a). Similarly, the United Kingdom Central Council for Nurses, Midwives and Health Visitors (Registrar's letter 18/1995) emphasizes that every ward should have at least a basic system of audit and quality control of discharge practice and procedures. Closs & Tierney (1993) suggest that patient/carer/professional satisfaction surveys appear to be the most useful form of obtaining audit information in this area. Indeed, the National Survey of Hospital Patients (NHS 1994) highlighted implications for discharge practice, for example negotiating the discharge date with the patient/carer. The survey provides a useful basis for local units wishing to audit discharge in their area. Responsibility for the review, monitoring and evaluation of discharge procedures remains with clinical staff and first level management (Handcock & Knight 1992).

Patients with particular care needs

The following categories of patients were identified as having particular care needs. These include patients who:

1 Live alone
2 Are frail and/or elderly
3 Have care needs which place a high demand on carers and carers who find difficulty coping
4 Have a limited prognosis
5 Have serious illnesses, who may be returning to hospital for further treatments
6 Have continuing disability
7 Have learning difficulties
8 Have mental illness or dementia
9 Have dependants
10 Have limited financial resources
11 Are homeless or those living in poor housing
12 Do not have English as their first language
13 Have been in hospital for an 'extended stay'
14 Require aids/equipment at home.

(Adapted from DoH 1989a and NHS 1997.)

Conclusion

From the patient's and carer's perspective, discharge may be one of the most important events of the hospital stay. It is essential, therefore, that discharge planning is considered as an integral part of care.

References and further reading

Armitage, S. (1990) *Liaison and Continuity of Nursing Care. Executive Summary.* Welsh Office, Cardiff.
Audit Commission (1992) *Lying in Wait: The Use of Medical Beds in Acute Hospitals.* HMSO, London.
Baylis, S. (1998) Planning for home – the role of the occupational therapist. *Palliat Care Today,* **VII**(1), 8–9.
Bone, L., Fahey, M. & Klein, L. (1992) Impact of hospital discharge planning on meeting patient needs after returning home. *Health Serv Res,* **27**(1), 155–75.
Bristow, O., Stickney, C. & Thompson, S. (1986) *Discharge Planning for Continuity of Care.* Publication no. 21-1604. National League of Nursing, New York.
Busby, R. (1995) Redefining homesickness. *Nurs Stand,* **9**(24), 22–3.
Butler, P. (1995) The twilight zone. *Health Serv J,* 2 March.
Closs, J. & Tierney, A. (1993) The complexities of using a structure, process and outcome framework: the case of an evaluation of discharge planning for elderly patients. *J Adv Nurs,* **18**(8), 1279–87.
Cooper, J. (1997) *Occupational Therapy in Oncology and Palliative Care.* Whurr, London.
Daly, N. (1999) Campaigning for carers. *Commun Care,* 18–24 February, 1260.
Davis, S. (1998) *Primary secondary care interface.* Proceedings of conference, 25 March. NHS Executive, June, Issue 2.
DoH (1986) *Primary Health Care.* Stationery Office, London.
DoH (1989a) *Discharge of Patients from Hospital.* Health Circular (89) 5. Stationery Office, London.
DoH (1989b) *Caring for People: Community Care in the Next Decade and Beyond.* Stationery Office, London.
DoH (1990) *NHS and Community Care in the Next Decade and Beyond; Policy Guidance.* Stationery Office, London.
DoH (1991) *Integrating Primary and Secondary Care.* Stationery Office, London.
DoH (1992) *The Health of the Nation.* Stationery Office, London.
DoH (1993) *Working Together for Better Health.* Stationery Office, London.
DoH (1994) *The Hospital Discharge Workbook: A Manual on Hospital Discharge Practice.* Stationery Office, London.
DoH (1995a) *Developing and Implementing Eligibility Criteria for Continuing Health Care: A Checklist for Publishers.* Stationery Office, London.
DoH (1995b) *Carer's (Recognition and Services) Act.* Stationery Office, London.
DoH (1995c) *The Patient's Charter.* Stationery Office, London.
DoH (1998) *The New NHS: Modern, Dependable.* Stationery Office, London.
Drury, M., Harcourt, J. & Minon, M. (1996) The acceptability of patients with cancer holding their own shared-care record. *Psycho-Oncol,* **5**, 119–25.

Embling, S. (1997) Reducing risks to patients on discharge: a managerial case study. *Br J Ther Rehab*, **4**(5), 245–63.

Evers, H. (1991) Issues in community care services. (Problems in communication between hospital and community following discharge.) *Nurs Stand*, **5**, 13 Feb, 29–31.

Gatt, R. *et al.* (1973) Team venture in the north-east: A study in co-operation with Aberdeen Royal Infirmary and the domiciliary services. *Nurs Mirror*, **137**, 35–6.

George, M. (1993) Funding the Act. *Nurs Times*, **89**(3), 214–25.

George, M. (1995) Collaborative nursing. *Nurs Stand*, **12**(46), 22–3.

George, M. (1998) Gentle persuasion. *Commun Care*, 1–7 October, 30–31.

Guerrero, D. (1990) Working towards a partnership. *Commun Outlook*, September, 14–18.

Ham, C., Hunter, D. & Robinson, R. (1994) Evidence based policymaking. *Br Med J*, **310**, 14 Jan, 71–2.

Handcock, M. & Knight, D. (1992) Improving discharge planning standards. *Nurs Stand*, **6**(21), 29–31.

Haywood, K. (1998) Patient-held oncology records. *Nurs Stand*, **12**(35), 44–6.

Health Services Accreditation (1996) *Service Standards for Discharge Care*. NHS, E. Sussex.

Heeks, A., Friel, M. & Howard, R. (1991) Return to hospital. *J District Nurs*, August, 8–10.

Henwood, M. (1993) Key task 2, residential and nursing homes. *Commun Care*, 21 January, 17.

Henwood, M. (1994) Hospital discharge. *Health Serv J*, 31 March, 22–4.

Henwood, M. (1998) Helping the helpers. *Commun Care*, 13–19 August, 13–15.

Henwood, M. & Wistow, G. (1994) *Hospital Discharge and Community Care: early Days*. Stationery Office, London.

Jackson, M. (1994) Discharge planning: issues and challenges for gerontological nursing. A critique of the literature. *J Adv Nurs*, **19**, 492–502.

Jacobs, L., Fontana, R. & Albert, D. (1985) Is that geriatric patient really ready to go home? *Reg Nurse*, **48**(11), 40, 43.

Jester, R. (1998) Hospital at home: the Bromsgrove experience. *Nurs Stand* **12**(20), 40–42.

Jupp, M. & Simms, S. (1986) Going home. *Nurs Times*, **83**(33), 40–42.

Kinn, S. *et al.* (1994) *The Nursing Audit Handbook*. University of Glasgow, Glasgow.

Kline, R. (1998) Opportunity knocks. *Nurs Times*, **94**(35), 10.

Macabee, J. (1994) The effect of transfer from a palliative care unit to nursing homes – are patients' and relatives' needs met? *Palliat Med*, **8**, 211–14.

McMahon, R. (1988) Home truths. *Geriat Nurs Home Care*, **8**(9), 16–17.

Marks, L. (1994) *Seamless Care or Patchwork Quilt? Discharging Patients from Acute Hospital Care*. Research Report 17. The King's Fund Institute, London.

National Council for Hospice and Palliative Care Services (1993) *Care in the Community for People Who Are Terminally Ill. Guidelines for Health Authorities and Social Services Departments*. National Council for Hospice and Specialist Palliative Care Services, London.

NHS (1994) *National Survey of Hospital Patients*. Stationery Office, London.

NHS (1997) *Services for Older People: Addressing the Balance. NHS Health Advisory Thematic Review*. Stationery Office, London.

Nazarko, L. (1998) Improving discharge: the role of the discharge co-ordinator. *Nurs Stand*, **12**(49), 35–7.

Neill, J. & Williams, J. (1992) Leaving hospital – elderly people and their discharge to community care. Research Unit, National Institute for Social Work, London. In: *Seamless Care or Patchwork quilt? Discharging Patients from Acute Hospital Care* (L. Marks), Research Report 17. King's Fund Institute, London.

Nixon, A., Whitter, M. & Stitt, P. (1998) Audit in practice: planning for discharge from hospital. *Nurs Stand*, **12**(26), 35–8.

North, M. (1991) Discharge planning: increasing client and nurse satisfaction. *Rehab Nurs*, **16**(6), 327–9.

Patterson, B. (1995) The process of social support: adjusting to life in a nursing home. *J Adv Nurs*, **21**, 682–9.

Porrock, D., Martin, K., Oldham, L., *et al.* (1997) Relocation stress syndrome: the case of palliative care patients. *Palliat Med*, **11**(6), 444–50.

Roberts, C., Crosby, D., Dunn, R. *et al.* (1995) What do we mean by 'care'? *Health Serv J*, 30 March, 21.

Robinson, A. & Miller, M. (1996) Making information accessible: developing plain English discharge instructions. *J Adv Nurs*, **24**, 528–35.

Royal College of Nursing (1992a) *Good Practice in Early Discharge*. RCN, London.

Royal College of Nursing (1992b) *Standards of Care for Liaison Nursing*. RCN, London.

Salter, M. (1996) Nursing the patient in the community. In: *Nursing the Patient with Cancer* (ed. V. Tschudin). Prentice Hall, Hemel Hempstead.

Salter, M. (1998) Future planning of care. In: *Neuro Oncology for Nurses* (ed. D. Guerrero). Whurr, London.

Saville, R. & Bartholomew, J. (1994) Planning better discharges. *J Commun Nurs*, June, 10–14.

The Royal Marsden Hospital Discharge Policy and Procedure (1999) (unpublished).

Smith, S. (1996) Discharge planning: the need for effective communication. *Nurs Stand*, **10**(38), 39–41.

Social Services Inspectorate (1998) A Matter of Chance for Carers? Stationery Office, London.

Thorpe, G. (1998) Enabling more dying people to remain at home. *Br Med J*, **307**(9), 915–18.

Tierney, A.J. (1993) An evaluation of hospital discharge. *Nurs Times*, **89**(47), 11–12.

Tierney, A. & Closs, J. (1993) Discharge planning for elderly patients. *Nurs Stand*, **7**(52), 30–33.

United Kingdom Central Council for Nurses, Midwives and Health Visitors (1995) *Annexe One to Registrar's Letter (18/1995). Discharge of Patients from Hospital*. UKCC, London.

Vaughan, B. & Taylor, K. (1988) Homeward bound. *Nurs Times*, **84**(15), 28–31.

Worth, A., Tierney, A. & Lockerbie, L. (1994) Community nurses and discharge planning. *Nurs Stand*, **8**(21).

Young, L. (1998) Understanding primary care groups. *Prim Health Care*, **8**(3).

GUIDELINES • Discharge planning

Procedure

Action   *Rationale*

Initial assessment (within first 24–48 h of admission)

1 The admitting nurse is responsible for ensuring that an initial assessment is completed when the patient is admitted and is documented in the multidisciplinary care plan. Assessment should be ongoing and regularly reviewed with the multidisciplinary team.

To enable the physical, psychological and social care needs of the patient and carers to be identified at an early stage.

2 An expected date of discharge should be established.

To ensure planning for discharge commences.

3 Clarify whether the patient has dependants, e.g. elderly relatives, children or a disabled partner who is unwell. If so, establish who is looking after them and whether they receive any services.

Arrangements may need to be made for alternative carer or an increase in services. Notification may need to be made to, e.g., school nurse/teacher if patient has children at school.

4 Establish who else is involved in giving care/support and the type of help given, e.g. local support group, voluntary agency, church.

To assess the support that the patient and carers may require at home so that appropriate services can be mobilized. To establish social network in order to coordinate care between voluntary and statutory agencies.

5 Ascertain the type of accommodation the patient is living in, e.g. flat, bungalow (council or privately owned), residential or nursing home, sheltered housing.

To identify early potential housing problems which may entail social work intervention. To identify need for occupational therapy intervention (for equipment to aid independence).

6 Ascertain the names and telephone numbers of sheltered housing wardens or officers in charge of homes.

To enable contact to be made and to establish that an appropriate degree of care and support can continue to be provided, once the patient is discharged from hospital.

7 Ensure that the home address and telephone number of the patient are documented accurately in the care plan. Establish where the patient will be going on discharge and document the discharge address if different from the permanent address.

Personal information may not have been updated on previous nursing or medical records. It is crucial that this information is accurate when making referrals to community services, to ensure appropriate service provision.

8 Ensure that the patient is registered permanently with a general practitioner (GP) and with a GP on a temporary basis if going to a different address on discharge. Check the names, addresses and telephone numbers with the patient.

Community nursing services are unable to accept the patient without medical support. Accurate information is required to establish which district nurse will have responsibility for patient care. It is important for the patient that medical care can be provided at home.

9 Establish whether any statutory community health or social services have been involved before the patient's admission. Include the health visitor when the patient has children under the age of 5 years.

To enable contact for exchange of information. Valuable information can be obtained from community services to assist in assessing potential needs on discharge.

Referrals

10 Assess the patient's ability to carry out activities of daily living at home prior to admission, e.g. was she/he able to climb stairs? Consider patient's current level of functioning and whether this will change as a result of treatment and/or rehabilitation.

To establish at an early stage whether an occupational therapy assessment is required. Home assessment may be required by occupational therapy prior to discharge which may involve complex planning and preparation.

11 Refer to other hospital personnel as soon as potential needs are recognized, e.g. occupational therapist, physiotherapists, dietitian. Referral as soon as possible after admission is essential – do not wait until treatment is completed and discharge is imminent.

To ensure multidisciplinary planning and coordination. Considerable time may be needed to arrange community services and early referral helps to prevent discharge delays.

Guidelines • Discharge planning (cont'd)

Action	Rationale

12 Patients identified as requiring local authority social services support are referred to the social services department. Some hospitals use a 'trigger' form as an aid to assessment, an example of which can be found in Fig. 11.1.

To ensure early and appropriate referral to the social services department for assessment.

13 A discharge planning 'area of care' should be commenced in the care plan; all members of the multidisciplinary team should document in the care plan their assessment, plans and action taken.

To facilitate multidisciplinary planning, coordination and communication.

14 Where there is a designated community liaison nurse/ adviser, she/he can act as a resource offering support and education to the ward team in the preparation of discharge plans, especially for those patients requiring a complex package of care.

To facilitate effective discharge planning and utilize expertise appropriately.

15 Formulate a discharge plan in conjunction with patient and carers and all involved hospital and community personnel and agree a discharge date.

To collate information and coordinate planning.

16 For complex discharges a discharge planning meeting should be held.

To coordinate continuity of care planning.

17 The ward based nurse is responsible for arranging and coordinating community nursing services (including Macmillan/hospice home care nurse) in consultation with the community liaison nurse if applicable.

To facilitate continuity of care between hospital and community.

18 Refer to the community nursing services with a minimum of 48h notice. If a complex package of care is being organized more notice will be required. Invite community nurses to visit the ward where appropriate.

Community nurses may wish to assess the patient's nursing care needs and ensure preparation of the home prior to discharge. They need time to liaise with other agencies to coordinate care and to obtain any equipment required.

19 Ascertain whether district nurses are able to carry out necessary clinical procedures in accordance with their health authority policy, e.g. care of skin-tunnelled catheters. Consider alternative arrangements if necessary. Give written information and instructions

District nurses may not have been trained in certain procedures or may be unfamiliar with particular equipment.

20 Details of patient's MRSA status (or other infections) must be given to community personnel and written in referral details.

To reduce risk of cross-infection. The district nurse requires full knowledge of the patient's history and nursing requirements.

21 Complete the community care referral form or update letter.

The form/letter should be completed and signed and a copy provided for the Macmillan/hospice home care team.

Provide information for community staff to ensure that they have accurate information.

22 Ensure any essential medical/nursing aids or equipment have been obtained before discharge by community services, e.g. oxygen, nebulizers, commode, pressure-relieving mattress, hoist.

Home assessment may be required by occupational therapy prior to discharge.

Some equipment may not be available or may take a long time to obtain. Equipment may be loaned from the community or from hospital and appropriate legislation procedures must be followed for safety reasons.

23 Patients requiring community nursing, physiotherapy, occupational therapy, stoma care, speech therapy and/or dietetic support on discharge will be referred by the appropriate hospita-based health care professional to their equivalent in the community.

To ensure continuity of specialist care.

Leaving hospital

24 Medical staff are responsible for assessing the patient's medical fitness for discharge and for liaising with other members of the multi-disciplinary team regarding arrangements for meeting the patient's care needs in the community.

To ensure that both health and social care needs are taken into consideration when formulating discharge plans.

25 Notify the sheltered housing wardens or officer in charge of the nursing/residential home of discharge date.

To ensure preparation of accommodation.

26 Ensure that patient and, with his/her agreement, carers have full information regarding the patient's medical condition and care required.

To prepare carers and to enable patient and carers to support each other.

27 Teach the patient and carers any necessary skills, allowing sufficient time to practise before discharge. This should include information on the safe use of equipment, e.g. a hoist.

To enable the patient to be as independent as possible and promote an understanding of self-care techniques.

28 Ensure that the patient has a door key and can gain entrance to their residence. Wherever possible, ensure that someone is at home to receive the patient.

The patient may have left their key with a neighbour. It is helpful for someone to be available to welcome the patient and attend to any immediate needs.

29 Book transport if required with 48 hours' notice, using relevant form. Specify if patient needs a stretcher or chair, or requires escort. Ensure that transport is also booked for return clinic appointment if necessary.

The patient may not have private transport facilities and may be too weak to use public transport.

Cancel transport if discharge date or outpatients department appointment is altered.

To prevent a waste of resources.

30 Patients should be given an appropriate supply of medication and, where necessary, a supply of wound management dressings or medical equipment.

To ensure the safe and continuous administration of medication and use of equipment at home. Time is needed to obtain items in the community.

31 Discharge plans should not be altered without consultation with all the hospital personnel who have been involved in the planning, e.g. occupational therapist, social worker, community liaison nurse and also patient/family carers.

If there is no consultation this causes considerable confusion and stress for the patient, family and friends, and all involved services. It may result in the patient being unsupported at home.

32 If discharge is cancelled or postponed, or if the patient dies, ensure that all relevant community services are informed.

To avoid distress to relatives. To avoid wasted visits and promote good community relations.

33 Weekend discharge: patients who require a high level of health services and social services support should not be discharged home on a Friday or Saturday or a public holiday. This applies particularly to patients who were previously unknown to community services.

All community services will be operating at a reduced level and emergency medical back-up may be difficult to obtain.

Note: assessment and planning for weekend leave are as important as for final discharge

Patient information

34 Inform the patient and carers of potential side-effects of treatment and management.

To alleviate anxiety and to promote patient comfort, knowledge and safety.

35 Ensure that patient and carers have information on local support groups or national specialist organizations as appropriate.

Some patients may benefit from the kind of support offered by the organizations.

36 Reinforce any special instructions with written information or by giving an approved education booklet, e.g. one of the Royal Marsden Hospital series.

To promote an understanding of disease and treatment. To confirm arrangements made. To enable the patient to contact the appropriate services.

Guidelines • Discharge planning (cont'd)

Action	*Rationale*
37 Information on community services arranged, including names and telephone numbers and expected date of first visit, should be given to the patient and carers prior to discharge. This information should also be documented in the patient's care plan.	To confirm arrangements made. To enable the patient to contact the appropriate services.
The social worker informs the patient and carers of local authority arrangements upon discharge, provides them with a summary of their care plan and gives contact names, including the care manager or equivalent in the patient's local social services department.	To confirm with patient and carers arrangements made upon discharge.
38 Ensure that arrangements have been made to provide patient with food at home on discharge and that there will be adequate heating.	To supply immediate needs.
39 Ensure that the patient and carers are given verbal and written information on the dosage, route, frequency and side-effects of any medication and how to obtain further supplies.	Lack of information makes it difficult for the GP to provide the medical care required.

After discharge

40 A follow-up phone call should be made to establish how the patient is managing.	To ensure services are in place.

Drug Administration

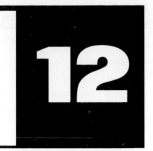

Definition

The giving by a nurse or other authorized person of a drug to a patient (Anderson & Anderson 1995).

Indications

Drugs can be administered for the following purposes:

1 Diagnostic purposes, e.g. assessment of liver function or diagnosis of myasthenia gravis.
2 Prophylaxis, e.g. heparin to prevent thrombosis or antibiotics to prevent infection.
3 Therapeutic purposes, e.g. replacement of fluids or vitamins, supportive purposes (to enable other treatments, such as anaesthesia), palliation of pain and cure (as in the case of antibiotics).

Reference material

The United Kingdom Central Council for Nursing, Midwifery and Health Visiting (UKCC) states that the administration of drugs is not a 'mechanistic task to be performed in strict compliance with the written prescription of a medical practitioner'. It is a process which requires thought and the application of professional judgement, the safety and well being of the patient being of paramount importance (UKCC 1992a). Drug administration involves the medical practitioner, pharmacist and other health care professionals as well as the nurse who usually administers the medication.

While administering medicines the nurse must meet the requirements set out in the document *Standards for the Administration of Medicines* (UKCC 1992a). This document provides guidance regarding the professional responsibility of the nurse involved in the administration of drugs.

Legislation

The manufacture, supply and use of medicines (and the interactive wound dressings) are controlled by two statutes, the *Medicines Act 1968* and the *Misuse of Drugs Act 1971*.

The Medicines Act 1968

This defines 'medicinal products' as substances sold or supplied for administration to humans (or animals) for medic-

inal purposes. Part 3 of the Act, and regulations and orders made under it, control the manufacture and sale or supply of medicines and for this purpose broadly classifies them into three groups:

1 Prescription-only medicines (POM)
2 Pharmacy medicines (P)
3 General sales list medicines (GSL).

Different requirements apply to the sale, supply and labelling of medicines in each group. In NHS hospitals, adherence to the Act usually means that the purchasing and supply of medicines is supervised by a pharmacist, and that supply or administration to a patient is only on a doctor's prescription.

Sections 9, 10, and 11 of the Act exempt doctors, dentists, pharmacists and nurses, respectively, from many restrictions otherwise imposed by the act on the general public, and thus allow them to supply and use drugs in the practice of their respective professions.

The Misuse of Drugs Act 1971

This designates and defines as controlled drugs a number of 'dangerous or otherwise harmful' substances. These substances are all also by definition prescription only medicines under the *Medicines Act 1968*.

The controls imposed by the *Misuse of Drugs Act* are therefore additional to those under the *Medicines Act*.

The purpose of the 1971 Act is to prevent abuse of controlled drugs, most of which are potentially addictive or habit forming, by prohibiting their manufacture, sale or supply except in accordance with regulations made under the Act. Other regulations govern safe storage, destruction and supply to known addicts.

The level of control to be exercised is related to the potential for abuse or misuse of the substances concerned. Under the current (1985) regulations, controlled drugs are classified into five schedules, each representing a different level of control. The requirements of the Act as they apply to nurses working in a hospital with a pharmacy department are described in Table 12.1. Schedule 2 is the most relevant to everyday nursing practice.

Summary

Hospital wards and departments are authorized to hold a stock of controlled drugs. These are obtained by the use of a special duplicate order form signed by the nurse in charge

Table 12.1   Summary of legal requirements for handling of controlled drugs as they apply to nurses in hospitals with a pharmacy

	Schedule 1	Schedule 2	Schedule 3	Schedule 4	Schedule 5
Drugs in schedule	Cannabis + derivatives but excluding nabilone, LSD (lysergic acid diethylamide)	Most opioids in common use including: alfentanyl amphetamines cocaine diamorphine methadone morphine papaveretum fentanyl phenoperidine pethidine codeine dihydrocodeine pentazocine } injections only	Minor stimulants. Barbiturates (but excluding: hexobarbitone thiopentone methohexitone). Diethylpropion. Buprenorphine. Temazepam[7]	Part 1: anabolic steroids. Part 2: benzodiazepines	Some preparations containing very low strengths of: cocaine codeine morphine pholcodine and some other opioids
Ordering	Possession and supply permitted only by special licence from the Secretary of State issued (to a doctor only) for scientific or research purposes	A requisition must be signed in duplicate by the nurse in charge. The requisition must be endorsed to indicate that the drugs have been supplied. Copies should be kept for 2 years	As Schedule 2	No requirement[1]	No requirement[1]
Storage[5]	As Schedule 2	Must be kept in a suitable locked cupboard to which access is restricted	Buprenorphine and diethylpropion: as Schedule 2. All other drugs: no requirement	No requirement[1]	No requirement[1]
Record keeping	As Schedule 2	Controlled drugs[3] register must be used	No requirement	No requirement[1]	No requirement[1]
Prescriptions	As Schedule 2	See below for detail of requirements[4]	As Schedule 2 except for phenobarbitone[2]	No requirement[1]	No requirement[1]
Administration to patients	As Schedule 2. Under special licence only	A doctor or dentist or anyone acting on their instructions may administer these drugs to anyone for whom they have been prescribed	As Schedule 2	No requirement[1]	No requirement[1]

[1] 'No requirement' indicates that the *Misuse of Drugs Act* imposes no legal requirements additional to those imposed by the *Medicines Act 1968*.

[2] All references to phenobarbitone should be taken to include all preparations of phenobarbitone and phenobarbitone sodium. Because of its use as an anti-epileptic, phenobarbitone is exempt from the handwriting requirements only of the full prescription requirements (see 4 below).

[3] *Record keeping.*

There is no legal requirement for the nurse in charge or acting in charge of a ward or department to keep a record of Schedule 1 or 2 controlled drugs obtained or supplied. However, the Aitken Report (1958) recommended that this should be done and in practice a controlled drug register is invariably kept according to the following guidelines:

(a) Each page should be clearly headed to indicate the drug and preparation to which it refers. Records for different classes of drug should be kept on separate pages.

(b) Entries should be made as soon as possible after the relevant transaction has occurred and always within 24 hours.

(c) No cancellations or obliteration of an entry should be made. Corrections should be made by means of a note in the margin or at the foot of the page and this should be signed, dated and cross-referenced to the relevant entry.

(d) All entries should be indelible.

(e) The register should be used for controlled drugs only and for no other purposes.

(f) A completed register should be kept for two years from the date of the last entry.

[4] *Prescription requirements.*

(a) The prescription *must* state:

• The name and address of the patient.

• The drug, the dose, the form of preparation (e.g. tablet).

• The total quantity of drug, or the total number of dosage units to be supplied. This quantity must be stated in *words* and *figures*. All of the above must be written indelibly in the prescriber's own handwriting and he/she must sign the prescription.

• The date of the prescription.

• If the prescription is to be dispensed in instalments, the number of instalments and the intervals between them.

Table 12.1   *Continued*

It is illegal to write or dispense a prescription which does not comply with these requirements.

(b) The full handwriting requirements and statement of quantity to be supplied do not apply to prescriptions for hospital inpatients if the controlled drugs concerned are administered from ward or department stocks. They do, however, apply to prescription for drugs 'to take home' or for outpatients.

[5] *Storage and safe custody.*

(a) All controlled drugs should be stored in a suitably secure (usually metal) cupboard which is kept locked and to which access is restricted. This cupboard (which may be within a second outer cupboard) should be used only for the storage of controlled drugs.

(b) The Aitken Report (1958) recommends that all controlled drug record entries be checked by two nurses. In conjunction with the pharmacy a procedure should be developed to ensure regular checking of records and reconciliation of receipts and issues.

(c) A programme for regular stock checking should be established and adhered to.

[6] *Destruction.*

Unwanted or unused controlled drugs in Schedule 2 should normally be returned to the pharmacy.

[7] Temazepam preparations are exempt from record keeping and prescription requirements, but are subject to storage requirements.

who is then responsible for them. They should be stored in a locked cupboard used exclusively for this purpose. They may be administered only to a patient in that ward or department when prescribed by a doctor. Appropriate records of their use must be maintained. Completed registers and copies of orders should be kept for two years. Unwanted drugs should normally be destroyed in the pharmacy but may, under some circumstances be disposed of on the ward under the supervision of a pharmacist. An appropriate entry should then be made in the ward register.

Types of medicinal preparations of drugs

Preparations for oral administration

Tablets

These come in a great variety of shapes, sizes, colours and types. The formulation may be very simple and result for instance in a plain, white, uncoated tablet, or complex and designed with specific therapeutic aims. Sugar coatings are used to improve appearances and palatability. In cases where the drug is a gastric irritant or is broken down by gastric acid, an enteric coating may be used. This is designed to allow the tablet to remain intact in the stomach and to pass unchanged into the small bowel where the coating dissolves and hence the drug is released and absorbed. Tablets may be formulated specifically to achieve control of the rate of release of drug from the tablet as it passes through the alimentary tract. Terms such as 'sustained-release', 'controlled-release' and 'modified-release' are used by manufacturers to describe these preparations. Tablets may also be formulated specifically to dissolve readily ('soluble' or 'effervescent'), to be chewed or to be held under the tongue ('sublingual') or placed between the gum and inside of the mouth ('buccal'). Unscored or coated tablets should not be crushed or broken, nor should most 'slow-release' or 'sustained action' tablets, since this can alter the rate of release of drug from the tablet.

Capsules

These consist of a gelatin shell in which is contained the drug powder or granules. They offer a useful method of formulating drugs which are difficult to make into a tablet or are particularly unpalatable. Slow-release capsule formulations also exist. Capsules should not normally be broken or opened.

Lozenges and pastilles

These are designed to be sucked for local treatment of the mouth and throat.

Linctuses, elixirs, syrups

These are usually sweet, syrup-like solutions used to treat coughs or where, in children for instance, a tablet or capsule may be inappropriate.

Mixtures

These are flavoured solutions or suspensions of drugs used mainly when patients cannot swallow a tablet or the drug is not available as a tablet. It is particularly important the suspensions are thoroughly mixed by shaking before each dose is measured. This ensures that the measured volume always contains the correct amount of drug.

Rectal and vaginal preparations

Enemas

These are solutions which are instilled into the rectum as laxatives or to obtain other localized therapeutic effects, or for diagnostic purposes.

Suppositories

These are solid wax pellets for rectal administration. They may either melt at body temperature or dissolve or disperse in the mucous secretions of the rectum. They may be used to obtain local effect (e.g. as laxatives) or for systemic therapy. Many drugs, such as the opioids for example, are well absorbed when administered this way. Suppositories sometimes offer a useful alternative to injections for very sick patients unable to take drugs orally.

Pessaries

These are solid pellets for vaginal administration and are usually designed to have a local therapeutic action.

Topical preparations

Creams

These are semisolid emulsions containing a high proportion of water. When applied they are quickly absorbed into the skin leaving little or no greasy residue. They may be used as a 'base' in which a variety of drugs may be applied for local therapy (British National Formulary 1999).

Ointments

These are similar to cream but contain a higher proportion of oil. They are absorbed more slowly into the skin and leave a greasy residue. They have similar uses to creams, and are particularly suitable for dry, scaly lesions (British National Formulary 1999).

Transdermal patches

A number of drugs such as hyoscine to prevent motion sickness, oestrogens for hormone replacement therapy, and fentanyl for pain control are now available in 'transdermal patches'. A very small volume of drug solution is contained in a reservoir which is stuck on the skin. Drug molecules diffuse at a constant rate through a semi-permeable membrane which is in direct contact with the skin when the patch is applied. The drug is absorbed through the skin and into the capillary blood supply from where it enters the systemic circulation. Advantages include a constant rate of drug administration over several days which may reduce the incidence of side-effects and improve patient compliance.

Wound products

See Chap. 47, Wound Management.

Injections

Injections are sterile solutions, emulsions or suspensions. They are prepared by dissolving, emulsifying or suspending the active ingredient and any added substances in water for injections, in a suitable non-aqueous liquid or in a mixture of these vehicles (*European Pharmacopoeia* 1990).

Single-dose preparations

The volume of the injection in a single-dose container is sufficient to permit the withdrawal and administration of the nominal dose using a normal technique.

Multi-dose preparations

Multi-dose aqueous injections contain a suitable antimicrobial preservative at an appropriate concentration except when the preparation itself has adequate antimicrobial properties. When it is necessary to present a preparation for parenteral use in a multidose container, the precautions to be taken for its administration and more particularly for its storage between successive withdrawals are given.

Parenteral infusions

Parenteral infusions are sterile, aqueous solutions or emulsions with water; they are free from pyrogens and are usually made isotonic with blood. They are principally intended for administration in large volume. Parenteral infusions do not contain any added antimicrobial preservative (*European Pharmacopoeia* 1990).

Inhalations

The term 'inhalation' once referred solely to the inhalation of volatile constituents of such preparations as compound tincture of benzoin. In modern therapeutics two techniques – nebulization and aerosolization – permit the inhalation of a range of drugs with the aim of a localized therapeutic effect.

Nebulization involves the passage of air (or sometimes oxygen) through a solution of the drug concerned to create a fine spray. Some antibiotics and bronchodilators may be given in this way.

Aerosolization involves the use of a solution of drug in an inert diluent. Passing a metred volume of this solution through a valve under pressure allows the delivery to the patient of a measured dose of drug in a very fine spray of controlled particle size. Bronchodilators and steroids are administered commonly in this way. Although a very small total dose of drug is administered, the concentration achieved at the site of action is high. Rapid and effective control of symptoms is achieved but without the side-effects commonly associated with an equivalent systemic (oral or parenteral) dose of the drug(s).

There are now available on the market aerosol and non-aerosol inhaler devices. Each device has its own advantages and disadvantages dependent on the particular situation.

GUIDELINES · Storage of drugs

Certain general principles apply to the storage of medicinal preparations (DoH 1988).

Principle	Rationale
1 Security: locked cupboards. When not in use drug trolleys should not only be kept locked but should also be secured to a wall and thus immobilized.	To prevent unauthorized access and deter abuse and/or misuse.

2 *Separate storage*: for medicines and nonmedicines (e.g. syringes, needles).	To prevent confusion and hence danger to patients.
Separate storage: for preparations for oral use and those for topical use.	To prevent errors and therefore danger to the patient.
3 *Stability*: no medicinal preparation should be stored where it may be subject to substantial variations in temperature, e.g. not in direct sunlight or over a radiator.	To maintain efficacy of the medicines.
Stability: some preparations require storage under well-defined conditions, e.g. 'below 10°C' or 'store in a refrigerator'.	To maintain efficacy of the medicines.
4 *Labelling*: the wording of labels is chosen carefully to convey clearly all essential information. Printed labels should always be used.	To ensure that the user has all the necessary information.
5 *Containers*: the type of container used may have been chosen for specific reasons.	The design and material of which the container is made may significantly influence the stability of the contents, e.g. GTN provided in glass containers rather than PVC.
Medicinal preparations should never be transferred (in bulk) from one container to another except in the pharmacy.	As above. Inadequate labelling of repackaged medicines is dangerous.
6 *Stock control*: a system of stock rotation must be operated (e.g. 'first in, first out') to ensure that there is no accumulation of 'old' stocks. Regular stock checks should be carried out, if possible by pharmacy staff.	All medicinal preparations, even when stored correctly retain activity only for a limited period of time.

The label on the pack should in most cases give guidance about storage conditions for individual preparations. The term 'a cool place' is normally interpreted as meaning between 1 and 15°C for which a refrigerator (between 2 and 8°C) will normally suffice. 'Room temperature' allows a range of approximately 15–25°C.

If you are in any doubt about the storage requirements for any preparation you should check with a pharmacist, but the following points are noteworthy:

1 Aerosol containers should not be stored in direct sunlight or over radiators – there is a risk of explosion if they are heated.
2 Creams may deteriorate rapidly if subjected to extremes of temperature.
3 Eye drops and ointments may become contaminated with micro-organisms during use and thus pose a danger to the recipient. Therefore in hospitals, eye preparations should be discarded seven days after they are first opened. For use at home this limit is extended to 28 days.
4 Mixtures may have a relatively short shelf-life. Most antibiotic mixtures require refrigerated storage and even then have a shelf-life of only 7–14 days. Always check the label for details.
5 Tablets and capsules are relatively stable but are susceptible to moisture unless correctly packed. They should be stored only in the containers in which they were supplied by the pharmacy.
6 Vaccines and similar preparations usually require refrigerated storage and may deteriorate rapidly if exposed to heat.

Administration

The effective and safe administration of drugs to patients demands a partnership between the various health professionals concerned, i.e. doctors, pharmacists and nurses. The nurse is responsible for the correct administration of prescribed drugs to patients in his/her care. To achieve this the nurse must have a sound knowledge of the use, action, usual dose and side-effects of the drugs being administered. Various studies have shown that this is not always the case.

Institutional policies and procedures also assist the nurse to administer drugs safely and a sound knowledge of local procedures is essential, since most errors in hospital are the result of procedural error (Malseed 1990). The importance of reporting errors to the appropriate authority can never be underestimated as research suggests that many undeclared medication errors are made by nurses. One survey demonstrated that of every ten medication errors that occurred only one was reported (Kuhn 1989), which may be because of fear of reprisal (Osborne *et al.* 1999). The immediate and honest disclosure that an error has occurred results in the patient receiving the required emergency treatment. Organizational policies therefore need to reflect a culture that encourages disclosure and in which the management of medication errors are viewed as a learning process as opposed to a punitive act (Martin 1994; Gladstone 1995).

It must be recognized, however, that errors in drug administration can have traumatic consequences for the individual nurse involved and that disciplinary procedures invoke fear in most nurses (Arndt 1994). The UKCC, when giving guidance to managers dealing with medication errors, states that there should be a distinction made between errors which result from a serious pressure of work as opposed to those which are a result of reckless practice (UKCC 1992b).

Prescriptions should be written legibly in ink or otherwise as to be indelible. Also, nurses should record in the appropriate documents that the prescribed medication has been administered.

Supply and administration of medicines under group protocols by nurses

In 1989 the *Report of the Advisory Group on Nurse Prescribing* ('Crown One', DoH 1989) recommended that certain nurses holding district nurse or health visitor qualifications and who have completed an approved prescribing course should be allowed to:

1 Prescribe from a limited formulary
2 Supply within a group protocol agreed for a particular clinical service
3 Adjust the timing and dosage of medicines within a patient-specific protocol (DoH 1989).

The necessary legislation to enable nurse prescribing was in place in 1992 and was commenced in 1994. Following a successful pilot scheme where nurse prescribing was assessed (see Luker *et al.* 1998), it was announced in April 1998 that this was to be extended across England (NHSE 1998a; Cresswell 1999). The roll out for district nurses and health visitors is to be completed by March 2001 (NHSE 1998b).

At present nurses – other than those with the district nurse or health visitor qualifications (or equivalent) and who have completed an approved prescribing course – cannot prescribe. However, the *Review of Prescribing, Supply and Administration of Medicines. Final Report* ('Crown Three', DoH 1999) recommends that new groups of professionals (including nurses) should 'be able to apply for authority to prescribe in specific clinical areas, where this would improve patient care and where patient safety could be assured' (p. 3). However, until this time many nurses wishing to provide patient-focused care make use of group protocols in order to supply and/or administer medicines to support their practice.

Group protocols to supply and administer medicines have been used for several years within The Royal Marsden Hospital to support nursing initiatives such as nurse-led clinics (Laverty *et al.* 1997; Mallett *et al.* 1997). A small evaluation indicated that the use of protocols within a nurse-led neuro-oncology clinic reduced the time patients waited for their medications, thereby facilitating early alleviation of symptoms (Mallett *et al.* 1997). Nevertheless, it was not until 1998 that clear guidance was provided for the supply and administration of medicines under group protocols (DoH 1998). This document, *Review of Prescribing, Supply and Administration of Medicines. A Report on the Supply and Administration of Medicines under Group Protocols*, known as 'Crown Two' helped to clarify processes such

as 'supply', 'administration', and 'independent' and 'dependent' prescribing, and as a consequence of this group protocols underwent further rigorous review. The current framework for group protocols utilizes the definition produced by the Crown Review Team whereby a Group Protocol is defined as:

> a specific written instruction for the supply or administration of named medicines in an identified clinical situation. It is drawn up locally by doctors, pharmacists and other appropriate professionals, and approved by the employer, advised by the relevant professional advisory committees. It applies to groups of patients or other service users who may not be individually identified before presentation for treatment

(DoH 1998, p. 5). There are a number of other recommendations within the Crown Two Report which have resulted in the expansion of the protocols to ensure adequate documentation of all aspects associated with this activity (see Fig. 12.1). These include 'Competency of nurse', 'Plan of care', 'Medicine', 'Audit trail' and 'Authorization of protocol'. A protocol, including all of the above, should be completed for each symptom or condition to be managed and this will be agreed by the nominated nurse, the chief nurse, the relevant consultant and the chief pharmacist. The use of algorithms may facilitate completion of the protocols and should be included where appropriate. In addition, systems should be in place and effectively functioning to support and monitor the development of protocols as well as the protocols themselves, for example pharmacovigilance safety systems.

Intravenous administration

The involvement of nursing staff in the administration of intravenous drugs was formally recognized in the mid-1970s following the publication of the Breckenridge Report (DHSS 1976). The report proposed a rational approach to intravenous drug administration, established guidelines for documentation and outlined the responsibilities of health authorities and health professionals. The responsibility of medical staff was to ensure that the drug was administered by the most effective and safest route and that the instructions to facilitate this were clearly written.

An intravenous additive service provided by pharmacists was favoured. In situations where this was not practical, pharmacists were to act as an information source for other personnel. It was accepted that nursing staff could undertake the addition of drugs to intravenous infusion bags and administration of intravenous drugs. The nurse, however, should be qualified (i.e. should be a registered general nurse or an enrolled nurse) and have undergone a period of training and assessment in both the theoretical knowledge and practical procedures involved in such drug administration. Guidance on the scope of professional practice (UKCC 1992b) states that 'the nurse must endeavour always to achieve, maintain and develop knowledge, skill and competence to respond to the needs and interests of the patient or client'.

In all intravenous therapy the nurse's responsibility continues to include the following (RCN 1999):

FRAMEWORK FOR SUPPLY AND ADMINISTRATION OF MEDICINES UNDER GROUP PROTOCOLS		
COMPETENCY OF NURSE		
NURSE SPECIALIST		
DESIGNATION		
COMPETENCY/QUALIFICATIONS	**INDICATORS**	**Assessed**
• **Level of assessment and care provided by nurse sufficient for protocolised nurse administration of medicines** (evidence provided by the nurse, their manager and job description)	Expert level of assessment and care provided assessed by nurse and manager.	
• **Registered nurse and or registered children's nurse**	Appropriateness of qualifications to relevant clinical area assessed by nurse and manager.	
• **UKCC registration**	UKCC Registration checked and assessed by manager.	
• **Oncology certificate or equivalent, relevant other**	Certification checked by manager.	
• **One year's experience in relevant clinical area at senior level** (minimally at 'F' grade)	Appropriateness of experience to relevant clinical area.	
• **Knowledge of key topics of pharmacy** as evidenced by professional qualifications and testing of knowledge and understanding of basic general pharmacology and other relevant details of the drug(s) concerned including: ◇ the names of the drugs/medicines concerned; ◇ the legal status of drugs/medicines concerned (e.g. POM, P or GSL); ◇ dose and/or permissible dose range and the criteria for deciding on the dose to be administered or recommended; ◇ method and route of administration; ◇ if more than one dose is required, the permitted frequency of administration ◇ the permitted total dose and maximum number of doses allowed in a given time ◇ information on any follow-up or concurrent necessary treatment ◇ advice and product information to be given to the patient and/or carer including (side effects, interactions, contraindications, precautions etc., including the use of manufacturer's Product Information Leaflets; identification and management of adverse events or outcomes; the concurrent use of other drugs/medicines) ◇ arrangements for referral to a doctor when desired or necessary ◇ facilities and supplies which should be readily available	Knowledge of key topics of pharmacy assessed by pharmacist (signature) and relevant consultant (signature):	
TRAINING		
◇ Pharmacy course prior to use of protocol ◇ Yearly update training by pharmacy	Successful completion of course as assessed by pharmacist and consultant (signatures)	
REVIEW OF COMPETENCY	One year following last competency assessment as assessed by nurse, their manager, pharmacist and consultant	

Figure 12.1   Framework for Group Protocols developed by the Royal Marsden Hospital to accommodate recommendations in the Crown Two Report (DoH 1998).

MEDICINE	
	Draft example only
MEDICINE	
LEGAL STATUS OF MEDICINE (POM, P or GSL)	
MODE OF ACTION	
INDICATIONS FOR TREATMENT	
CONCURRENT MEDICINES	
DOSE RANGE WITHIN WHICH MEDICINE CAN BE SUPPLIED OR ADMINISTERED (that is, timing and dose – this must be within normal accepted range as stated in the British National Formulary)	
CRITERIA FOR DECIDING DOSE AND CHANGES IN DOSE WITHIN ABOVE RANGE	
FREQUENCY OF ADMINISTRATION AND MAXIMUM NUMBER OF DOSES IF MORE THAN ONE DOSE REQUIRED	
PERIOD OF TIME OVER WHICH THE MEDICINE CAN BE ADMINISTERED	
METHOD OR ROUTE OF ADMINISTRATION OF MEDICINE	
INDICATIONS FOR REVIEW	
RATIONALE FOR REFERRAL TO PHYSICIANS AND ARRANGEMENTS FOR ACHIEVING THIS	
INCOMPATIBLE MEDICINES	
CONTRAINDICATIONS, INTERACTIONS AND SIDE EFFECTS	
REPORTING OF SUSPECTED ADVERSE DRUG REACTIONS	These should be reported immediately to relevant doctor and pharmacist and documented in patient's clinical notes.
ARRANGEMENTS FOR PHARMACOVIGILANCE COMMUNICATIONS AND AMENDMENTS TO PROTOCOLS AS THE RESULT OF NEW SAFETY INFORMATION	This will minimally include reporting of adverse incidents, communication of new safety information, withdrawal of drugs etc between relevant professionals and also to external agencies. (details of system to ensure effective pharmacovigilance be developed jointly)

Figure 12.1 Framework for Group Protocols (*cont'd)*

PLAN OF CARE	
DIAGNOSIS/CONDITION	
(POTENTIAL) SYMPTOM(S)/CLINICAL CRITERIA UNDER WHICH THE PATIENT WILL BE ELIGIBLE FOR INCLUSION IN THE PROTOCOL	
AIMS OF TREATMENT OR CARE	
CRITERIA UNDER WHICH THE PATIENT WILL BE EXCLUDED FROM CARE WITHIN THE PROTOCOL	
ACTIONS TO BE TAKEN FOR PATIENTS WHO ARE EXCLUDED FROM TREATMENT UNDER THE PROTOCOL	
ACTIONS TO BE TAKEN FOR PATIENTS WHO DO NOT WISH TO RECEIVE, OR DO NOT ADHERE TO, CARE UNDER THE PROTOCOL	
METHODS (including patient education and information with regard to medicine and side effects – must include the authorised Patient Information Leaflet if one is available)	
IDENTIFICATION AND MANAGEMENT OF ADVERSE REACTIONS	
FOLLOW-UP TREATMENT WHICH MAY BE REQUIRED	
EVALUATION OF TREATMENT/CARE (see also audit trail)	

AUDIT TRAIL Records required for a documented audit trail	
HEALTH CARE PROFESSIONAL PROVIDING TREATMENT	
PATIENT IDENTIFIERS	
PATIENT (POTENTIAL) SYMPTOMS	
MEDICINE BEING PROVIDED	
ADVERSE DRUG REACTIONS	
EVALUATION OF TREATMENT/CARE	
CLEAR DOCUMENTATION WITHIN CLINICAL NOTES	

Figure 12.1 *Continued*

AUTHORISATION OF PROTOCOL	
SIGNATURE OF CHAIR ON BEHALF OF DRUGS AND THERAPEUTICS COMMITTEE	
SIGNATURE OF CHAIR ON BEHALF OF PATIENT SERVICES COMMITTEE	
SIGNATURE OF CHAIR ON BEHALF OF THE MEDICAL MANAGEMENT COMMITTEE	
SIGNATURE OF NURSE PRESCRIBER (this confirms understanding of the content of the protocol, that necessary education and training has been given to implement the protocol effectively and agreement to work within the protocol)	
SIGNATURE OF PHYSICIAN	
SIGNATURE OF CHIEF NURSE/DIRECTOR OF PATIENT SERVICES	
SIGNATURE OF CHIEF PHARMACIST	
DATE PROTOCOL AGREED	
RATIONALE FOR REVIEW	Initial assessment of protocol
FREQUENCY OF REVIEW	(To be agreed for individual protocols – not less than six monthly)
DATE PROTOCOL TO BE REVIEWED (after which the protocol is no longer valid)	(To be agreed for individual protocols – not less than six monthly)
CLINICAL AREAS IN WHICH A COPY OF PROTOCOL TO BE KEPT	

Figure 12.1   Framework for Group Protocols (cont'd)

1 Identifying the patient and verifying the prescription.
2 Checking the infusion fluid and container for any obvious faults or contamination.
3 Ensuring the administration of the prescribed drug or fluid to the correct patient.
4 Checking that the intravenous device remains patent.
5 Inspecting the site of insertion and reporting abnormalities.
6 Controlling the rate of flow as prescribed.
7 Monitoring the condition of the patient and reporting any changes.
8 Maintaining appropriate records.

In general nurses administer intravenous drugs or fluids via an established vascular access device using the following methods:

1 Continuously, or intermittently, by addition to an intravenous infusion in a bottle, bag or burette. This method may include the use of a variety of equipment, e.g. a small-volume syringe pump or a Y administration set.
2 Intermittently by injection into the injection site or side arm of an intravenous administration set.
3 Intermittently by injection into a vascular access device directly via an injection cap or via other equipment, e.g. an extension set or three-way tap.

Single nurse administration of medicines

Certain nurses may administer drugs by themselves provided it is the policy of the health authority by whom they are employed. Some nurses feel they are able to administer in this way, and others may be opposed and concerned about the dangers (Winson 1991). Some authorities have policies which require that nurses have received specific training, both in theory and practice, and are in possession of a certificate stating their proficiency in the technique.

It is thought that single nurse administration of medicines will result in greater care being given since the nurse will be aware that she/he is solely responsible and accountable.

Those nurses who wish or need to have their administration supervised will retain the right to do so until such time as all parties agree that the requested level of proficiency has been achieved. This is in keeping with the principles of the scope of professional practice (UKCC 1992b).

Self-administration of medicines

Hospital patients approaching discharge, who will continue on a prescribed regimen of medicines at home, benefit significantly from the opportunity to adjust to the responsibility of self-administration while still having access to professional support (UKCC 1992a).

Teaching patients to take their own medication correctly forms part of their programme of rehabilitation, which should begin with the first multidisciplinary assessment on their arrival in hospital (Crome *et al.* 1980). However, repeated studies have shown high levels of non-compliance resulting in inadequate control of symptoms, hoarding of drugs and errors of over- or underdosage and incorrect dosing times. Non-compliance can result in slower recovery from illness, reduced health potential, and poorer quality of life (Williams 1991). However, the advantages of patient participation and independence outweigh these disadvantages (Davis 1991).

Ultimately it is often patients themselves who are responsible for administering prescribed medicines at home. Health professionals can no longer assume that people are passive recipients of care (Kennedy 1981). Bird (1990) suggests that

> for the majority of hospital patients, self-administration of drugs would appear to be a more appropriate method than the conventional system. Self-administration is not merely the process of patients taking their own drugs, it can also help clients retain or regain control over their health.

Patients taught to self-administer their drugs in hospital are encouraged to regain independence and to participate in their own care. Problems which would otherwise only arise after discharge may be identified earlier and addressed before discharge. Although, by definition, self-administration of medicines shifts the balance of responsibility for this part of care firmly towards the patient, it in no way diminishes the fundamental professional duty of care. It is therefore essential that local policies, procedures and records are adequate to ensure that this duty is, and can be shown to be, discharged.

Observation of the patient receiving medication is important. No drug produces a single effect. The combined effect of two or more drugs taken together may be different from the effects when taken separately. The effectiveness of any drug should be noted and any signs of resistance or dependence reported. Side-effects may vary from slight symptoms to severe reaction and any signs must be brought to the attention of the appropriate personnel.

Injections and infusions

Injections can be described as the act of giving medication by use of a syringe and needle, and an infusion is defined as an amount of fluid in excess of 100 ml designated for parenteral infusion because the volume must be administered over a long period of time. However, medications may be given in small volumes (50–100 ml) or over a shorter period 30–60 minutes (Weinstein 1997).

There are a number of routes for injection or infusion. The selection may be predetermined as in intra-arterial, intra-articular, intracardiac, intralesional and intrathecal injections. The choice of the remaining routes will normally depend on the desired therapeutic effect and the patient's safety and comfort.

Intra-arterial

This special technique allows the delivery of a high concentration of drug to the tissues supplied by a particular artery. This route can be used for the administration of chemotherapy, vasodilators and for diagnostic purposes. Injection of drugs into an artery is a rare and hazardous procedure. The introduction of the cannula or catheter must be performed with care as the vessel may go into spasm, causing pain and occlusion. This could result in necrosis of an organ or part of a limb. Injection of irritant chemicals increases the risk of spasm and its sequelae (see Chap. 44, Vascular access devices: insertion and management). In patients with some forms of cancer, however, arterial catheterization is occasionally performed when it is desirable to deliver a high concentration of a drug to a tumour mass (see Chap. 10, Cytotoxic drugs: handling and administration). The most common procedures are catheterization of the hepatic artery and isolated limb perfusion.

Intra-articular

This may be used in the treatment of acute local inflammatory conditions. Corticosteriods are absorbed locally reducing toxicity but using this route can be painful for the patient.

Intrathecal

This may be used when the drug concerned does not penetrate the blood–brain barrier. The intrathecal route can be used for the administration of local anaesthetics, antibiotics, X-ray or contrast media and cytotoxic therapy which necessitates administration into the cerebro spinal fluid (CSF) (Malseed 1990).

Intradermal

The intradermal route provides a local, rather than systemic, effect and is used primarily for diagnostic purposes such as allergy or tuberculin testing. It can also be used for the administration of local anaesthetics (Workman 1999). Observation of an inflammatory reaction is a priority, so the best sites are those that are highly pigmented, thinly keratinized and hairless. Chosen sites are the inner forearms and the scapulae. The injection site most commonly used is the medial forearm area. The injections are best performed using a 25g needle inserted at a 10–15° angle, bevel up, just under the epidermis. Volumes of 0.5 ml or less should be used (Workman 1999).

Subcutaneous

Subcutaneous infusions of fluids (hypodermoclysis)

The administration of fluids by the subcutaneous route is a safe and reliable method of treating dehydration and symptoms of thirst in the elderly and the palliative care patients (Schen & Singer-Edelstein 1981; Constans et al. 1991). It is particularly useful in patients who have difficulty in taking fluids orally, such as those who have dysphagia which results in decreased oral intake and symptom distress (Fainsinger et al. 1994; Ellershaw et al. 1995; Fainsinger et al. 1997). Due to the relative ease in setting up and administering subcutaneous fluids, the procedure can be carried out in the home setting by district nurses, relatives or carers. There is a reduction in the risk of infection when compared with intravenous fluids and it has very few side-effects. However, one study did indicate that prolonged use with large volumes of fluid in a 24 hour period can lead to localized pain and oedema (Schen & Singer-Edelstein 1981). Caution is required in patients who have pre-existing oedema (as swelling at site would not be easily observed) and any clotting disorders (which may predispose the patients to bleeding at cannula sites).

There are three recommended ways to administer fluids via this route. The fluid should be limited to 3 litres in 24 hours and given as a

1 24-hour infusion
2 12-hour infusion
3 Bolus.

It is possible and advisable to use more than one infusion site if the patient requires more than one litre to be infused (Bruera et al. 1996; Ferrand & Campbell 1996). If medications are required it is advisable to administer them via a syringe driver which allows easier control of the rate of delivery.

Hyaluronidase is an enzyme which increases the rate of subcutaneous absorption of fluids. It is usually used if more than one litre is to be infused at one site. It can cause discomfort and local irritation when used for prolonged periods of time (Hypodermoclysis Working Group 1998). A randomized double blind study compared the absorption and side-effect profile of administering subcutaneous fluids with or without hyaluronidase. It found that there was no significant difference in the infusion rate of the fluids or the amount or degree of side-effects caused by its use. However, it did show that on measuring the limb around the site of the infusion, those with hyaluronidase in the

fluid showed a decrease in limb size compared to those without hyaluronidase (Constans et al. 1991).

In the context of single drug infusions, instability is not a clinically significant problem. The drug simply has to be:

1 Available in injectable form
2 Suitable for subcutaneous administration
3 Stable in solution for the duration of the infusion (usually 12–48 hours).

For example, diamorphine hydrochloride is stable in solution for up to 2 weeks (Jones & Hanks 1986).

Problems of drug instability and incompatibility arise when higher drug concentrations and combinations of two or more drugs are used. There is a paucity of pharmaceutical data available regarding compatibility of combining drugs and most information remains anecdotal (David 1992). Where drug compatibility is doubtful or unknown, and more than two drugs are required for adequate control of symptoms, a second syringe driver may be a reasonable option. In addition, exposure of drug solutions to direct light and increased storage temperatures (up to 32°C) also result in drug instability.

Where drug combinations (commonly an analgesic and an anti-emetic) are used, further criteria must be met:

1 The drugs must be compatible with each other.
2 The diluents must be compatible with each other.
3 Each drug must be compatible with the diluent(s) of the other drug(s) in the combination.

Studies by Allwood (1984) and later work by Regnard & Davies (1986) have examined the stability and compatibility of analgesic/antiemetic combinations and as a result were able to make the following recommendations:

1 Protect the syringe from direct light whenever possible.
2 Visual inspection of drug solutions should be made daily, and the syringe discarded if signs of crystallization, precipitation or discoloration occur.
3 Avoid high concentrations of drugs if used in combination.
4 Avoid mixing more than two drugs in one syringe.
5 Do not infuse anti-emetics for more than 24 hours, particularly if part of a combination of drugs, due to problems of precipitation.

Subcutaneous injections

These are given beneath the epidermis into the fat and connective tissue underlying the dermis. Injections are usually given using a 25g needle, at a 45° angle. However, following the introduction of shorter needles the recommendation for insulin injections is at an angle of 90° (Burden 1994). Infusions require the insertion of a 25g winged infusion set or a 24g cannula. These may be inserted at an angle of 45° and secured with a transparent dressing (Springhouse Corporation 1999). The skin should be gently pinched into a fold to elevate the subcutaneous tissue which lifts the adipose tissue away from the underlying muscle (Workman 1999). It is no longer necessary to aspirate after the needle has been inserted, as it has been shown that piercing a blood vessel during a subcutaneous injection is rare (Peragallo-Dittko 1997; Workman 1999). It has also been noted that aspiration of heparin increases the risk of haematoma formation (Springhouse Corporation 1993). The maximum volume tolerable using this route for injection is 2 ml and drugs should be highly soluble to prevent irritation (Workman 1999).

Injection sites

Chosen sites are the lateral aspects of the upper arms and thighs, the abdomen in the umbilical region, the back and lower loins. Absorption from these sites through the capillary network is slower than that of the intramuscular route. Rotation of these sites decreases the likelihood of irritation and ensures improved absorption. Subcutaneous injections given in the upper arm are thought to be less painful since there are fewer large blood vessels and less painful sensations in those areas.

Infusion sites

The best sites to use for continuous infusion of drugs or fluids are the lateral aspects of the upper arms and thighs, the abdomen, the anterior chest below the clavicle and, occasionally, the back (Nicholson 1986). This is because these sites usually have adequate amounts of subcutaneous tissue and will not interfere with the patient's mobility. Areas that should not be used for cannula placement are:

1 Lymphoedematous limbs: the rate of absorption from a skin site would be adversely affected. A cannula breaches skin integrity, thus increasing the risk of infection in a limb that is already susceptible.
2 Sites over bony prominences: the amount of subcutaneous tissue will be diminished, impairing the rate of drug absorption.
3 Previously irradiated skin area: radiotherapy can cause sclerosis of small blood vessels, thus reducing skin perfusion (Tiffany 1988).
4 Sites near a joint: excessive movement may cause cannula displacement and patient discomfort.

Preparation of the skin

The infusion site should be renewed when there is evidence of inflammation (erythema or reddening) or poor absorption (a hard subcutaneous swelling). The time taken for this to occur can vary from hours to over 3 weeks, dependent on the patient and the drug(s) being infused (Regnard & Newbury 1983; Coyle et al. 1986; Nicholson 1986; Brenneis et al. 1987; Bruera et al. 1987). There would appear to be a relationship between the concentration of drug(s) being infused and the duration of a skin site (Nicholson 1986). In one study, the average frequency of needle resiting was 5.1 days for patients receiving 7.5–30 mg of diamorphine per 24 hours, but only 2.4 days for those receiving 1000–2000 mg per 24 hours (Nicholson 1986). Another study noted no statistically significant relationship between duration of skin site and sex and age of patients, type or dose of narcotic, rate of infusion or triceps skinfold measurement (Brenneis et al. 1987). Clearly,

further research into the factors influencing skin site survival is required.

If skin sites break down rapidly, suggestions include:

1 Further dilute the drug infused or change the diluent
2 Change the infusion device
3 Use a different site cleanser
4 Change the site dressing
5 Add 0.5 mg dexamethasone to the pump (this is currently being researched).

Intramuscular

Many drugs may be administered by this route provided they are not irritant to soft tissues and are sufficiently soluble. Absorption is usually rapid and can produce blood levels comparable to those achieved by intravenous bolus injection, relatively large doses, from 1 ml in the deltoid site to 5 ml elsewhere in adults can be given. These values should be halved in children because muscle mass is less (Workman 1999). Intramuscular injections should, where possible, be avoided in thrombocytopenic patients.

Intramuscular injections are given at five sites (see Fig. 12.2 for some examples):

1 *Mid-deltoid:* used for the injection of such drugs as narcotics, sedatives, absorbed tetanus toxoid, vaccines, epinephrine in oil and vitamin B_{12} (Workman 1999). It has the advantage of being easily accessible whether the patient is standing, sitting or lying down. It is also a better site than the gluteal muscles for small-volume (less than 2 ml), rapid onset injections because the deltoid has the greatest blood flow of any muscle routinely used for intramuscular injections. However, as the area is small, it limits the number and size of the injections that can be given at this site.
2 *Gluteus medius:* used for deep intramuscular and Z-track injections. The gluteus muscle has the lowest drug absorption rate. The muscle mass is also likely to have atrophied in elderly, non-ambulant and emaciated patients. This site carries with it the danger of the needle hitting the sciatic nerve and the superior gluteal arteries (Workman 1999). The Z-track method involves pulling the underlying skin downwards or to one side of the injection site, inserting the needle at a right angle to the skin, which moves the cutaneous and subcutaneous tissues by approximately 1–2 cm (Workman 1999). The injection is given and the needle withdrawn, while releasing the retracted skin at the same time. This manoeuvre seals off the puncture tract. Exercising the limb afterwards is believed to assist absorption of the drug by increasing blood flow to the area (Beyea & Nicholl 1995). In the past this method was only used for medications which may cause subcutaneous irritation should they leak and preparations such as iron which may discolour the skin (Malseed 1990), but it is now recommended for use with all IM medications (Beyea & Nicholl 1995).
3 *Ventrogluteal:* used for antibiotics, antiemetics, deep intramuscular and Z-track injections in oil, narcotics and sedatives; typical volume is 1–4 ml. It is best used

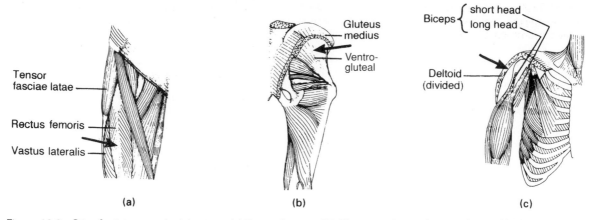

Figure 12.2 Sites for intramuscular injections. (a) Rectus femoris. (b) Gluteus medius and ventrogluteal. (c) Mid-deltoid.

when large-volume intramuscular injections are required and for injections in the elderly, non-ambulant and emaciated patient as it provides the safer option to accessing the gluteus medius muscle. This is because the site is away from major nerves and vascular structures and there have been no reported complications (Beyea & Nicholl 1995; Workman 1999).

4 *Rectus femoris:* used for antiemetics, narcotics, sedatives, injections in oil, deep intramuscular and Z-track injections. It is rarely used in adults but is the preferred site for infants and for self-administration of injections (Springhouse Corporation 1993).

5 *Vastus lateralis:* used for deep intramuscular and Z-track injections. This site is free from major nerves and blood vessels. It is a large muscle and can accommodate repeated injections. This is the site used for children up to 7 months (Beyea & Nicholl 1995) since the muscle mass will be greater in this area but the ventrogluteal site is the optimum choice.

Skin preparation

There are many inconsistencies regarding skin cleansing prior to subcutaneous or IM injections. Previous studies have suggested that cleansing with an alcohol swab is not always necessary, does not result in infections and may predispose the skin to hardening (Dann 1969; Koivistov & Felig 1978; Workman 1999).

Dann (1969) has shown that there is no experimental evidence that skin bacteria are introduced into the deeper tissues by injection, thereby causing infection. Antiseptics in current use cannot act in the time allowed in practice (5 seconds on average) and cannot possibly cause complete sterility. Over a period of 6 years, during which time more than 5000 injections were given to unselected patients via all the injection routes, without using any form of skin preparation, no single case of local and/or systemic infection was reported. Only before injections where strict asepsis is needed, as in intrathecal or intra-articular injections, is skin preparation required. Koivistov & Felig

(1978) carried out a survey into the need for skin preparation before giving an insulin injection and found that skin preparation did reduce skin bacterial count but was not necessary to prevent infection at the injection site. Some Trusts accept that if the patient is physically clean and the nurse maintains a high standard of hand hygiene and asepsis during the procedure, skin disinfection is not necessary (Workman 1999).

However the risk of infection may be increased in immunocompromised patients. Therefore the practice at the Royal Marsden Hospital is to continue to clean the skin prior to injection in order to reduce the risk of contamination from the patient's skin flora. The recommendation is to clean the skin with an alcohol swab for 30 seconds using a circular motion with friction from the centre of the chosen site and progress outwards. The skin should then be allowed to dry for 30 seconds otherwise skin cleansing is ineffective and results in the patient feeling a stinging pain on needle entry (Simmonds 1983).

Needle bevel

Three categories of needle bevel are available:

1 *Regular:* for all intramuscular and subcutaneous injections.
2 *Intradermal:* for diagnostic injections and other injections into the epidermis.
3 *Short:* rarely used.

Intramuscular needle gauge size and length

Needles should be long enough to penetrate the muscle and still allow a quarter of the needle to remain external to the skin (Workman 1999). The most common sizes are 21 or 23 g and 2.5–5 cm long. Lenz (1983) states that when choosing the correct needle length for intramuscular injections it is important to assess the muscle mass of the injection site, the amount of subcutaneous fat and the weight of the patient. Without such an assessment, most injections intended for gluteal muscle are deposited in the gluteal fat. The following are suggested by the author as ways of determining the most suitable size of needle to use.

Deltoid and vastus lateralis muscles

The muscle to be used should be grasped between the thumb and forefinger to determine the depth of the muscle mass or the amount of subcutaneous fat at the injection site.

Gluteal muscles

The layer of fat and skin above the muscle should be gently lifted with the thumb and forefinger for the same reasons as before. Use the patient's weight to calculate the needle length required. Lenz (1983) recommends the following guide:

31.5–40 kg	2.5 cm needle
40.5–90 kg	5–7.5 cm needle
90+ kg	10–15 cm needle

Intramuscular injections and pain

Patients are often afraid of receiving injections because they perceive the injection will be painful (Workman 1999). Torrence (1989) listed a number of factors that cause pain:

1 The needle
2 The chemical composition of the drug/solution
3 The technique
4 The speed of the injection
5 The volume of drug.

Workman (1999) listed a number of techniques that could be utilized to reduce pain and discomfort experienced by the patient such as adequate preparation of the patient, using ice or freezing spray to numb the skin, correct choice of site and technique and positioning of the patient so that the muscle are relaxed. Field (1981) attempts to answer the question of what it is like to give an injection, and goes on to explore the meaning and use of language relating to injections, the feelings involved in preparing and administering injections, and the meaning of the patient's response to the nurse.

Intravenous

Advantages of using the intravenous route

1 An immediate, therapeutic effect is achieved due to rapid delivery of the drug to its target site, which allows a more precise dose calculation and therefore more reliable treatment.
2 Pain and irritation caused by some substances when given intramuscularly or subcutaneously are avoided.
3 The vascular route affords a route of administration for the patient who cannot tolerate fluids or drugs by the gastrointestinal route.
4 Some drugs cannot be absorbed by any other route; the large molecular size of some drugs prevents

absorption by the gastrointestinal route, while other drugs, unstable in the presence of gastric juices, are destroyed.
5 The intravenous route offers the facility for control over the rate of administration of drugs; prolonged action can be provided by administering a dilute infusion intermittently or over a prolonged period of time (Campbell 1996; Weinstein 1997).

Disadvantages of using the intravenous route

1 There is an inability to recall the drug and reverse the action of it. This may lead to increased toxicity or a sensitivity reaction.
2 Insufficient control of administration may lead to speed shock or circulatory overload. This is characterized by a flushed face, headache, congestion, tightness in the chest, etc.
3 Additional complications may occur, such as the following:
  (a) Microbial contamination (extrinsic or intrinsic).
  (b) Vascular irritation, e.g. chemical phlebitis.
  (c) Drug incompatibilities and interactions if multiple additives are prescribed (Campbell 1996; Weinstein 1997).
4 Needle phobia.
5 Altered body image especially with central vascular access devices (Daniels 1995).
6 Time taken for administration (Hockley *et al.* 1995).

Principles to be applied throughout preparation and administration

Asepsis and reducing the risk of infection

Aseptic technique must be adhered to throughout all intravenous procedures (see Chap. 3, Aseptic Technique). The nurse must employ good hand washing and drying techniques using a bactericidal soap or a bactericidal alcohol hand rub. If asepsis is not maintained, local infection, septic phlebitis or septicaemia may result (Nystrom *et al.* 1983; Maki 1992; Springhouse Corporation 1999).

The insertion site should be inspected at least once a day for complications such as infiltration or any indication of infection, e.g. redness at the insertion site of the device or pyrexia (RCN 1999). These problems may necessitate the removal of the device and/or further investigation (Goodinson 1990b; Nichols 1999).

It is desirable that a closed system of infusion is maintained wherever possible, with as few connections as is necessary for its purpose (Speechley 1986). This reduces the risk of bacterial contamination. The use of three-way taps should be kept to a minimum as it has been shown there is an increased risk of contamination associated with these devices. This can be related to the dead space in this equipment, which has been identified as a reservoir for microorganisms which may be released into the circulation (Cheeseborough & Finch 1984). Streamlined adaptors are now available and are preferred (Brismar *et al.* 1984; Cheeseborough & Finch 1984; Weinbaum 1987).

The injection sites on administration sets or bungs

should be cleaned using an alcohol-based antiseptic, allowing time for it to dry. Connections should be cleaned before changing administration sets and manipulations kept to a minimum. Administration sets should be changed according to use (intermittent/continuous therapy), type of device and type of solution and the set must be labelled with the date and time of change (Perucca 1995; RCN 1999):

1 Blood administration sets should be changed at least every 12 hours (HMSO 1996).
2 Sets used for administering parenteral nutrition should be changed every 24 hours (Perucca 1995; Weinstein 1997; Intravenous Nursing Society 1998; RCN 1999; Springhouse Corporation 1999).
3 Research has indicated that routine changing of administration sets (used for infusing solutions) every 48–72 hours instead of every 24 hours is not associated with an increase in infection and could result in considerable savings for hospitals (Band & Maki 1979; Josephson *et al.* 1985; Maki & Ringer 1987; RCN 1999). However if the therapy is being administered intermittently and/or given via a central venous access device then the recommendation is to change the set every 24 hours (Glynn 1997; Weinstein 1997). This is because central venous catheters are associated with a high rate of infection, while intermittent use increases the risk of bacterial contamination because of increased manipulations. Otherwise it is acceptable to change sets every 72 hours (Glynn 1997; RCN 1999; Springhouse Corporation 1999).

Inspection of fluids, drugs, equipment and their packaging must be undertaken to detect any points where contamination may have occurred during manufacture and/or transport. This intrinsic contamination may be detected as cloudiness, discoloration or the presence of particles (Perucca 1995; Weinstein 1997; British National Formulary 1999). Infusion bags should not be left hanging longer than 24 hours. In the case of blood and blood products this is reduced to 5 hours (Perruca 1995; RCN 1999).

Safety

All details of the prescription and all calculations must be checked carefully in accordance with hospital policy in order to ensure safe preparation and administration of the drug(s). The volume required can be calculated using the following calculation:

$$\frac{\text{strength required}}{\text{stock strength}} \times \text{volume of stock solution}$$

$$= \text{volume required}$$

(Pelletier 1995; Weinstein 1997; Hutton 1998; Pickstone 1999). The nurse must also check the compatibility of the drug with the diluent or infusion fluid. The nurse should be aware of the types of incompatibilities, and the factors which could influence them. These include pH, concentration, time, temperature, light and the brand of the drug. If insufficient information is available, a reference book (e.g. *The British National Formulary*) or the product data sheet must be consulted. If the nurse is unsure about any aspect

of the preparation and/or administration of a drug, they should not proceed and should consult with a senior member of staff (UKCC 1992a). Constant monitoring of both the mixture and the patient is important. The preferred method and rate of intravenous administration must be determined.

Drugs should never be added to the following: blood; blood products i.e. plasma or platelet concentrate; mannitol solutions; sodium bicarbonate solution, etc. (Springhouse Corporation 1999). Only specially prepared additives should be used with fat emulsions or amino acid preparations.

Accurate labelling of additives and records of administration are essential.

Any protective clothing which is advised should be worn, and vinyl gloves should be used to reduce the risk of latex allergy (Springhouse Corporation 1999). In addition, needleless injection systems should be utilized to reduce the risk of needlestick injury, along with safe practices such as not resheathing needles and correct disposal of waste (Springhouse Corporation 1999).

Comfort

Both the physical and psychological comfort of the patient must be considered. Comprehensive explanation of the practical aspects of the procedure together with information about the effects of treatment will contribute to reducing anxiety (Wilson-Barnett & Carrigy 1978; Wilson-Barnett & Batehup 1992) and will need to be tailored to each patient's individual needs.

Methods of administering intravenous drugs

There are three methods of administering intravenous drugs: continuous infusion, intermittent infusion and intermittent injection.

Continuous infusion

Continuous infusion may be defined as the intravenous delivery of a medication or fluid at a constant rate over a prescribed time period, ranging from 24 hours to days to achieve a controlled therapeutic response. The greater dilution also helps to reduce venous irritation (Weinstein 1997; Pickstone 1999).

A continuous infusion may be used when:

1 The drugs to be administered must be highly diluted.
2 A maintenance of steady blood levels of the drug is required.

Preprepared infusion fluids with additives such as those containing potassium chloride should be used whenever possible. This reduces the risk of extrinsic contamination, which can occur during the mixing of drugs (Weinstein 1993). Only one addition should be made to each bottle or bag of fluid after the compatibility has been ascertained. More additions can increase the risk of incompatibility occurring, e.g. precipitation (Weinstein 1997; Pickstone 1999; Sani 1999; Trissel 1999). The additive and fluid must be mixed well to prevent a layering effect which can occur with some drugs (Sani 1999). The danger is that a bolus injection of the drug may be delivered. To safeguard against this, any additions should be made to the infusion fluid and the container inverted a number of times to ensure mixing of the drug and prevent a bolus of the drug being infused, before the fluid is hung on the infusion stand. The infusion container should be labelled clearly after the addition has been made. Constant monitoring of the infusion fluid mixture (Weinstein 1997; Sani 1999) for cloudiness or presence of particles should occur, as well as checking the patient condition and IV site for patency, extravasation or infiltration.

Intermittent infusion

Intermittent infusion is the administration of a small-volume infusion, i.e. 50–250 ml, over a period of between 20 minutes and 2 hours. This may be given as a specific dose at one time or at repeated intervals during 24 hours (Pickstone 1999).

An intermittent infusion may be used when:

1 A peak plasma level is required therapeutically.
2 The pharmacology of the drug dictates this specific dilution.
3 The drug will not remain stable for the time required to administer a more dilute volume.
4 The patient is on a restricted intake of fluids.

Delivery of the drug by intermittent infusion may utilize a system such as a 'Y' set, if the primary infusion is of a compatible fluid, or a burette set with a chamber capacity of 100 or 150 ml. This is when the drug can be added to the burette and infused while primary infusion is switched off. A small-volume infusion may also be connected to a cannula specifically to keep the vein open, and maintain patency.

All the points considered when preparing for a continuous infusion should be taken into account here, e.g. pre-prepared fluids, single additions of drugs, adequate mixing, labelling and monitoring.

Direct intermittent injection

Direct intermittent injection is a procedure for the introduction of a drug(s) into a vascular access device or the injection site of the administration set using a needle and syringe. Most must be administered anywhere from 3–5 minutes up to 30 minutes depending on the drug (Weinstein 1997; Pickstone 1999).

A direct injection may be used when:

1 A maximum concentration of the drug is required to vital organs. This is a 'bolus' injection which is given rapidly over seconds, as in an emergency, e.g. adrenaline.
2 The drug cannot be further diluted due to pharmacological or therapeutic reasons or does not require dilution. This is given as a controlled 'push' injection over a few minutes.
3 A peak blood level is required and cannot be achieved by small-volume infusion.

Rapid administration could result in toxic levels and an anaphylactic-type reaction. Manufacturers' recommendations of rates of administration (i.e. millilitres or milligrams per minute) should be adhered to. In the absence of such recommendations, administration should proceed slowly, over 5–10 minutes.

Delivery of the drug by direct injection may be via the cannula through a resealable needleless bung, extension set or via the injection site of an administration set.

1 If a peripheral device is in situ the bandage and dressing must be removed to inspect the insertion of the cannula, unless a transparent dressing is in place.
2 Patency of the vein must be confirmed prior to administration and the vein's ability to accept an extra flow of fluid or irritant chemical must also be checked.

Administration into the injection site of a fast-running drip may be advised if the infusion in progress is compatible in order to dilute the drug further and reduce local chemical irritation. Alternatively, a stop–start procedure may be employed if there is doubt about venous patency. This allows the nurse to constantly check the patency of the vein and detect early signs of extravasation. If the infusion fluid is incompatible with the drug, the administration set may be switched off and a syringe of 0.9% sodium chloride used as a flush.

If a number of drugs are being administered, 0.9% sodium chloride must be used to flush in between each drug to prevent interactions. 0.9% sodium chloride should also be used at the end of the administration to ensure that all of the drug has been delivered. The device should then be flushed to ensure patency is maintained (see Chap. 44, Vascular Access Devices: Insertion and Management).

Summary

The nurse is responsible for administering drugs safely by the methods listed. In order to do this he/she requires a thorough knowledge of the principles and their application, and a responsible attitude which ensures that medications are not given without full knowledge of immediate and late effects, toxicities and nursing implications. The nurse must also be able to justify any actions taken and be prepared to be accountable for the action taken (UKCC 1992).

References and further reading

Adamson, L. (1978) Control of medicines in the UK. *Nurs Times*, **74**, 973–5.

Allwood, M.C. (1984) Diamorphine mixed with antiemetic drugs in plastic syringes. *Br J Pharm Pract*, **6**, 88–90.

Arndt, M. (1994) Research and practice: how drug mistakes affect self-esteem. *Nurs Times*, **90**(15), 27–31.

Band, J. & Maki, D. (1979) Safety of changing intravenous delivery systems at longer than 24-hour intervals. *Ann Intern Med*, **90**, 173–8.

Baranowski, L. (1993) Central venous access devices, current technologies, uses and management strategies. *J Intraven Nurs*, **16**(3), 167–94.

Barrett, P. & Lester, R. (1990) Heparin versus saline flushing solutions in a small community hospital. *Hosp Pharm*, **25**, 115–18.

Bayliss, P.F.C. (1980) *Law on Poisons, Medicines and Related Substances*, 3rd edn. Ravenswood, London.

Beyea, S.C. & Nicholl, L.H. (1995) Administration of medications via the intramuscular route: an integrative review of the literature and research based protocol for the procedure. *Appl Nurs Res*, **5**(1), 23–33.

Bird, C. (1990) A prescription for self-care. *Nurs Times*, **86**(43), 52–5.

Brenneis, C. *et al.* (1987) Local toxicity during subcutaneous infusion of narcotics. *Cancer Nurs*, **10**(4), 172–6.

Brismar, B. *et al.* (1984) Bacterial contamination of intravenous cannula injection ports and stopcocks. *Clin Nutr*, **3**, 23–6.

British Medical Association/Pharmaceutical Society of Great Britain (1988) *British National Formulary*. BMA, London.

British National Formulary (1995) *British Medical Association and Royal Pharmaceutical Society of Great Britain*. No. 30, September, Appendix **6**, 584–94.

British National Formulary (1999) *British Medical Association and Royal Pharmaceutical Society of Great Britain*. No. 38, September, Appendix 6, pp. 642–54.

Brock, A.M. (1979) Self-administration of drugs in the elderly. *Nurs Forum*, **18**(4), 340–57.

Bruera, E., Legis, M.A. & Kuehn, N. (1990) Hypodermoclysis for the administration of fluids and narcotic analgesics in patients with advanced cancer. *J Pain Sympt Manage*, **5**(4), 218–20.

Burden, M. (1994) A practical guide to insulin injections. *Nurs Stand*, **8**(29), 25–9.

Campbell, J. (1996) Intravenous drug therapy. *Prof Nurses*, **11**(7), 437–42.

Central Health Services Council (1958) *Report of Joint Sub-Committee on the Control of Dangerous Drugs and Poisons in Hospitals* (Chairman J.K. Aitken). Stationery Office; London.

Cheeseborough, J.S. & Finch, R. (1984) Side ports – an infection hazard? *Br J Parenteral Ther*, July, 155–7.

Clarkson, D. (1995) The future of infusion. *Hosp Equip Supplies*, June, 17.

Constans, T. *et al.* (1991) Hypodermoclysis in dehydrated elderly patients – local effects with and without hyaluronidase. *J Palliat Care*, **7**(2), 10–12.

Cresswell, J. (1999) *Nurse Prescribing Handbook*. Association of Nurse Prescribing and Community Nurse, UK.

Crome, P. *et al.* (1980) Drug compliance of elderly hospital in patients. *Practitioner*, **224**, 728.

Cyganski, J. *et al.* (1987) The case for the heparin flush. *Am J Nurs*, **87**, 796–7.

Dale, J.R. & Appelbe, G.E. (1983) *Pharmacy, Law and Ethics*, 3rd edn. Pharmaceutical Press, London.

Daniels, L.E. (1995) The physical and psychosocial implications of central venous access devices in cancer patients: a review of the literature. *J Cancer Care*, **4**, 141–5.

Dann, T.C. (1969) Routine skin preparation before injection: an unnecessary procedure. *Lancet*, **2**, 96–7.

David, J. (1992) A survey of the use of syringe drivers in Marie Curie Centers *Eur J Cancer Care*, **1**(4), 23–8.

David, J.A. (1983) *Drug Round Companion*, Chapters 3, 7 and 8. Blackwell Science, Oxford.

Davis, S. (1991) Self administration of medicine. *Nurs Stand*, **5**(15), 29–31.

DHSS (1973) *Medicines Commission Report on Prevention of Microbial Contamination of Medicinal Products*. Stationery Office, London.

DHSS (1976) *Health Services Development, Addition of Drugs to Intravenous Fluids*, HC(76)9 (Breckenridge Report). Stationery Office, London.

DoH (1988) *Guidelines for the Safe and Secure Handling of Medicines* (The Duthie Report). Stationery Office, London.

DoH (1989) *Report of the Advisory Group on Nurse Prescribing*. Crown One. Stationery Office, London.

DoH (1998) *Review of Prescribing, Supply and Administration of Medicines. A Report on the Supply and Administration of Medicines under Group Protocols*. Crown Two. Stationery Office, London.

DoH (1999) *Review of Prescribing, Supply and Administration of Medicines. Final Report*. Crown Three. Stationery Office, London.

Dorr, T. & Von Hoff, D. (1993) *Cancer Chemotherapy Handbook*, 2nd edn. Appleton & Lange, Hemel Hempstead.

Dougherty, L. (1997) Reducing risks of complications in IV therapy. *Nurs Stand*, **12**(5), 40–42.

Downie, G. *et al.* (1987) *Drug Management for Nurses*. Churchill Livingstone, Edinburgh.

Drugs and Therapeutics Bulletin (1977) Storage and shelf life of drugs: when is it important? *Drugs Therap Bull*, **15**(21), 81–3.

Dunn, D. & Lenihan, S. (1987) The case for the saline flush. *Am J Nurs*, **87**(6), 798–9.

Ellershaw, J. *et al.* (1995) Dehydration and the dying patient. *J Pain Sympt Manage*, **10**(3), 192–7.

Epperson, E.L. (1984) Efficacy of 0.9% sodium chloride injection with and without heparin for maintaining indwelling intermittent injection sites. *Clin Pharm*, **3**, 626–9.

European Pharmacopoeia (1990) 2nd edn, Monograph 520. Maisonneuve sa. Council of Europe, Strasbourg.

Fainsinger, R. & Bruera, E. (1997) When to treat dehydration in a terminally ill patients. *Support Care Cancer*, **5**, 205–11.

Fainsinger, R. *et al.* (1994) The use of hypodermoclysis for rehydration of terminally ill cancer patients. *J Pain Symp Manage*, **9**, 298–302.

Falconer, M. (1971) Self administered medication. *Hosp Admin Can*, **13**(5), 28–30.

Ferrand, S. & Campbell, A. (1996) Safe, simple subcutaneous fluid administration. *Br J Hosp Med*, **55**(11), 690–92.

Field, P.A. (1981) A phenomenological look at giving an injection. *J Adv Nurs*, **6**(4), 291–6.

Fink, J.L. (1983) Preventing lawsuits. *Nurs Life*, **3**(2), 27–9.

Francis, G. (1980) Nurses' medication errors: a new perspective. *Supervisor Nurse*, **11**(8), 11–13.

Gatford, J. & Anderson, R. (1998) *Nursing Calculations*, 5th edn. Churchill Livingstone, Edinburgh.

Gladstone, J. (1995) Drug administration errors: a study into the factors underlying the occurrence and reporting of drug errors in a district general hospital. *J Adv Nurs*, **22**(4), 628–37.

Glynn, A. *et al.* (1997) *Hospital Acquired Infection – Surveillance Policies and Practice*. Central Public Health Laboratory, London.

Goode, C.J. *et al.* (1991) A meta analysis of effects of heparin flush and saline flush – quality and cost implications. *Nurs Res*, **40**(6), 324–30.

Goodinson, S.M. (1990a) The risks of IV therapy. *Prof Nurse*, February, 235.

Goodinson, S.M. (1990b) Keeping the flora out. *Prof Nurse*, August, 572.

Goodinson, S.M. (1990c) Good practice insures minimum risk factors. *Prof Nurse*, December, 175.

Goodinson, S. *et al.* (1988) A survey of intravenous catheters and other inserts. *Proceedings of 2nd International Conference on Infection Control*, pp. 13–80.

Hamilton, R.A. *et al.* (1988) Heparin sodium versus 0.9% sodium chloride injection for maintaining patency of indwelling intermittent infusion devices. *Clin Pharm*, **7**, 439–43.

Haynes, S. (1989) Infusion phlebitis and extravasation. *Prof Nurse*, December, 160–61.

Hecker, J. (1988) Improved technique in IV therapy. *Nurs Times*, **84**(34), 28–33.

HMSO (1996) *Handbook of Transfusion Medicine*, 2nd edn. Stationery Office, London.

Hockley, J. *et al.* (1995) Audit to pinpoint IV drug administration pitfalls. *Nurs Times*, **91**(51), 33–4.

Hoffman, K.K. *et al.* (1992) Transparent polyurethane film as an intravenous catheter dressing – a meta analysis of the infection risks. *J Am Med Assoc*, **267**(15), 2072–6.

Hook, M. (1990) Heparin vs 0.9% sodium chloride. Letters to the Editor. *J Intraven Nurs*, **13**(3), 150–51.

Hopkins, S.J. (1987) *Drugs and Pharmacology for Nurses*, 9th edn. Churchill Livingstone, Edinburgh.

Hudek, K. (1986) Compliance in intravenous therapy. *J Can Intraven Nurs Assoc*, **2**(3), 7–8.

Hutton, M. (1998) Numeracy skills for IV calculations. *Nurs Stand*, **12**(43), 49–56.

Hypodermoclysis Working Group (1998) Hypodermoclysis – Guidelines on the Technique. CP Pharmaceuticals, Wrexham.

Intravenous Nursing Society (1998) Revised intravenous nursing standards of practice. *J Intraven Nurs*, **21**(15), Suppl. 1S.

Jones, V.A. & Hanks, G.W. (1986) New portable infusion pump for prolonged administration of opioid analgesics in patients with advanced cancer. *Br Med J*, **292**, 1496.

Josephson, A. *et al.* (1985) The relationship between intravenous fluid contamination and the frequency of tubing replacement. *Infect Control*, **9**, 367–70.

Keenleyside, D. (1993) Avoiding an unnecessary outcome. *Prof Nurse*, February, 288–91.

Kennedy, B. (1981) Self-medication. *Cancer Nurs*, **77**, 336–7.

Koivistov, V.A. & Felig, P. (1978) Is skin preparation necessary before insulin injection? *Lancet*, **1**, 1072–3.

Kuhn, M.M. (1989) *Pharmacotherapeutics. A Nursing Process Approach*, 2nd edn. F.A. Davis, Philadelphia.

Lamb, J. (1999) Local and systemic complications of intravenous therapy. In: *Intravenous Therapy in Nursing Practice*. (eds L. Dougherty & J. Lamb). Churchill Livingstone, Edinburgh.

Laverty, D., Mallett, J. & Mulholland, J. (1997) Protocols and guidelines for managing wounds. *Prof Nurse*, **13**(2), 79–80.

Lenz, C.L. (1983) Make your needle selection right to the point. *Nursing (US)*, **13**(2), 50–51.

Loebl, S. *et al.* (1980) *The Nurse's Drug Handbook*, 2nd edn., pp. 10–22. John Wiley, Chichester.

Luker, K.A., Austin, L., Hogg, C. *et al.* (1998) Nurse–patient relationships: the context of nurse prescribing. *J Adv Nurs*, **28**, 235–42.

Lydiate, P.W.H. (1977) *The Law Relating to the Misuse of Drugs*. Butterworth, London.

Maki, D. (1977) A semi-quantative culture method for identifying intravenous catheter-related infections. *New Engl J Med*, **296**, 1305–6.

Maki, D.G. (1991) *Proceedings of International Congress and Symposium*. 9 March, London. Royal Society of Medicine (Series 179).

Maki, D.G. (1992) Infections due to infusion therapy. In: *Hospital Infections* (eds J.V. Bennett & P.S. Bradman), 3rd edn. Little, Brown & Co, Boston.

Maki, D.G. & Ringer, M. (1987) Evaluation of dressing regimens for prevention of infection with peripheral intravenous catheters. *J Am Med Assoc*, **256**(17), 2396–403.

Maki, D. *et al.* (1987) Prospective study replacing administration sets for intravenous therapy, at 48 to 72 hour intervals. *J Am Med Assoc*, **258**(13), 1777–81.

Mallett, J., Faithfull, S., Guerrero, D. *et al.* (1997) Nurse prescribing by protocol. *Nursing Times*, **93**(8), 50–52.

Malseed, R.T. (1990) *Pharmacology. Drug Therapy and Nursing Considerations*, 3rd edn. J.B. Lippincott, Philadelphia.

Markowitz, J.S. *et al.* (1981) Nurses, physicians, and pharmacists: their knowledge of hazards of medication. *Nurs Res*, **30**(6), 366–70.

Martin, P.J. (1994) Professional updating through open learning as a method of reducing errors in the administration of medicines. *J Nurs Manage*, **2**(5), 209–12.

National Health Service Executive (1998a) *Nurse Prescribing. A Guide for Implementation*. Stationery Office, London.

National Health Service Executive (1998b) *Nurse Prescribing. Implementing the Scheme Across England*. HSC 1998/232. Stationery Office, London.

Nichols, M. (1999) Safe administration of IV therapy. In: *Intravenous Therapy in Nursing Practice* (eds L. Dougherty & J. Lamb). Churchill Livingstone, Edinburgh.

Nicolson, H. (1986) The success of the syringe driver. *Nurs Times*, **82**, 49–51.

Nystrom, B. *et al.* (1983) Bacteraemia in surgical patients with intravenous devices: a European multicentre incidence study. *J Hosp Infect*, **4**, 338–49.

Oldman, P. (1991) A sticky situation? *Prof Nurse*, **6**(5), 265–9.

Osbourne, J., Blais, K. & Hayes, J.S. (1999) Nurses' perceptions: when is it a medication error? *J Nurs Admin*, **29**(4), 33–8.

Ostrow, L.S. (1981) Air embolism and central venous lines. *Am J Nurs*, **81**(11), 2036–9.

Parish, P. (1982) Benefits to risks of IV therapies. *Br J Intraven Ther*, **3**(6), 10–19.

Pearson, R.M. & Nestor, P. (1977) Drug interactions. *Nurs Mirror*, **145**, Suppl. XI.

Pelletier, G. (1995) Intravenous therapy calculations. In: *Intravenous Therapy: Clinical Principles and Practices* (eds J. Terry, L. Baranowski, R.A. Lonsway, *et al.*), pp. 366–78. W.B. Saunders, Philadelphia.

Peragallo-Dittko, V. (1997) Rethinking subcutaneous injection technique. *Am J Nurs*, **97**(5), 71–2.

Perdue, L. (1995) Intravenous complications. In: *Intravenous Therapy: Clinical Principles and Practices* (eds J. Terry, L. Baranowski, R.A. Lonsway, *et al.*), pp. 419–46. W.B. Saunders Philadelphia.

Perucca, R. (1995) Obtaining vascular access. In: *Intravenous Therapy: Clinical Principles and Practices* (eds J. Terry, L. Baranowski, R.A. Lonsway, *et al.*), pp. 377–91. W.B. Saunders, Philadelphia.

Peters, J. *et al.* (1984) Peripheral venous cannulation: reducing the risks. *Br J Parent Ther*, **5**(2), 56–88.

Pickstone, M. (1999) A Pocketbook for Safer IV Therapy. Medical Technology and Risk Series, Scitech.

Powys Health Authority (1984) *All Wales Working Party of Review of the Administration of Drugs by Nurses*. Powys Health Authority, Bronllys.

Plumer, A.L. (1987) *Principles and Practice of Intravenous Therapy*, 4th edn. Little, Brown & Co., Boston.

RCN (1999) *Guidance for Nurses Giving intravenous Therapy*. Royal College of Nursing, London.

Regnard, C.F. & Davies, A. (1986) *A Guide to Symptom Relief in Advanced Cancer*. Haigh and Hochland, Manchester.

Reville, B. & Almadrones, L. (1989) Continuous infusion chemotherapy in the ambulatory setting: the nurse's role in patient selection and education. *Oncol Nurs Forum*, **16**, 529–35.

Roberts, R. (1978) Self medication trial for the elderly. *Nurs Times*, **74**(23), 976–7.

Sager, D. & Bomar, S. (1980) *Intravenous Medications*. J.B. Lippincott, Philadelphia.

Sager, D. & Bomar, S. (1983) *Quick Reference to Intravenous Drugs*. J.B. Lippincott, Philadelphia.

Sani, M. (1999) Pharmacological aspects of IV therapy. In: *Intravenous Therapy in Nursing Practice* (eds L. Dougherty & J. Lamb). Churchill Livingstone, Edinburgh.

Scales, K. (1996) Legal and professional aspects of intravenous therapy. *Nurs Stand*, **11**(3), 41–8.

Schen, R. & Singer-Edelstein, M. (1981) Subcutaneous infusions in the elderly. *J Am German Soc*, **29**, 583–5.

Simmonds, B.P. (1983) CDC guidelines for the prevention and control of nosocomial infections: guidelines for prevention of intravascular infections. *Am J Infect Control*, **11**(5), 183–9.

Smith, R. (1985a) Extravasation of intravenous fluids. *Br J Parent Ther*, **6**(2), 30–35.

Smith, R. (1985b) Prevention and treatment of extravasation. *Br J Parent Ther*, **6**(5), 114–19.

Smolders, C. (1988) Infusion phlebitis. *Can Intraven Nurs Assoc*, **4**(2), 20–22.

Speechley, V. (1986) The nurse's role in intravenous management. *Nurs Times*, 2 May, 31–2.

Speechley, V. & Toovey, J. (1987) Factsheets: problems in IV therapy 1, 2, 3. *Prof Nurse*, **2**(8), 240–42; **2**(12), 413; **3**(3), 90–91.

Springhouse Corporation (1993) *Medication, Administration and IV Therapy Manual*, 2nd edn. Springhouse, Pennsylvania.

Springhouse Corporation (1999) *Handbook of Infusion Therapy*. Springhouse, Pennsylvania.

Steiner, N. & Bruera, E. (1998) Methods of hydration in palliative care patients. *J Palliat Care*, **14**(2), 6–13.

Thomas, S. (1979) Practical nursing – medicines: care and administration. *Nurs Mirror*, **148**, 28–30.

Torrence, C. (1989) Intramuscular injection, part 1 and 2. *Surg Nurses*, **2**(5), 6–10; **2**(6), 24–7.

Trissel, L.A. (1999) *Handbook on Injectable Drugs*, 10th edn. American Society of Health System Pharmacists, Bethesda.

United Kingdom Central Council for Nursing, Midwifery and Health Visiting (1992a) *Standards for the Administration of Medicines*. UKCC, London.

United Kingdom Central Council for Nursing, Midwifery and Health Visiting (1992b) *The Scope of Professional Practice*. UKCC, London.

Weinbaum, D.L. (1987) Nosocomial bacterias. In: *Infection Control in Intensive Care* (ed. B.F. Faser), pp. 39–58. Churchill Livingstone, New York.

Weinstein, S.M. (ed.) (1993) *Plumer's Principles and Practices of Intravenous Therapy*, 5th edn. J.B. Lippincott, Philadelphia.

Weinstein, S.M. (1997) *Plumer's Principles and Practice of Intravenous Therapy*, 6th edn. J.B. Lippincott, Philadelphia.

Williams, A. (1984) Medicine management. *Nurs Mirror*, **159**(12), Suppl. 1, i–viii.

Williams, B. (1991) Medication education. *Nurs Times*, **87**(29), 50–52.

Wilson-Barnett, J. & Batehup, L. (1992) *Patients' Problems: A Research Base for Nursing Care*, Chapter 3. Scutari Press, London.

Wilson-Barnett, J. & Carrigy, A. (1978) Factors influencing patients' emotional reactions to hospitalization. *J Adv Nurs*, **3**, 221–9.

Winson, G. (1991) A survey of nurses' attitudes towards single administration of medicines. *Nurse Practitioner*, **4**(3), 20–23.

Workman, B. (1999) Safe injection techniques. *Nurs Stand*, **13**(39), 47–52.

Wright, A. *et al.* (1985) Use of transdermal glyceryl trinitrate to reduce failure of intravenous infusion due to phlebitis and extravasation. *Lancet*, **11**, 1148–50.

GUIDELINES · Self-administration of drugs

Procedure

Action	Rationale
1 Take a drug history from the patient on admission.	To ensure an accurate record of: all medicines being taken (prescribed or otherwise); dietary supplements, e.g. multivitamins, herbal remedies, complementary therapies; allergies or hypersensitivities; understanding of current medicines; possible problems with self-administration.
2 Review proposed (inpatient) prescription in liaison with pharmacist and compare with details given by patient and medicines in their possession.	If frequent changes of drug or dose are expected, immediate self-administration may be undesirable and/or impractical. Appropriate medicines already in the patient's possession may be used, subject to local policy and agreement with the pharmacist.
3 Consider whether there are any constraints on self-administration, and if so, how they might be overcome. Discuss this with appropriate members of the multidisciplinary team.	To promote successful and safe self-administration and ensure that medicines are dispensed and labelled appropriately for the patient's needs. Constraints such as physical or visual handicap must be addressed. Changes in performance status may result from the underlying condition or its treatment, and must be allowed for. If a compliance aid such as a 'dosette' box is to be used, responsibility for filling and labelling the aid, especially whilst used on the ward, must be agreed and documented in local policies.

4 Discuss self-administration with the patient and prepare a jointly agreed plan for: teaching; secure storage of drugs; monitoring and recording progress.

Teach any special skills required, e.g. correct use of aerosol inhalers.

To promote the informed commitment and involvement of patients in their own care, where appropriate. To ensure that treatment is received as intended.

5 Check that drugs are taken as intended, and that the necessary records are kept.

To discharge the nurse's overall responsibility for patient care and well-being. To maintain a record of responsibilities undertaken.

Particular care with record keeping is needed in the period of gradual transition from nurse administration to self-administration. Any problems encountered must be addressed.

The detail and format of the record may vary according to: the patient's needs and performance status; the complexity of treatment; and local circumstances and policy.

6 Monitor changes in the patient's prescription.

To ensure that: changes are put into effect promptly; drugs are properly relabelled or redispensed; any discontinued drugs are retrieved from the patient.

7 Check when drug supplies are expected to run out and make arrangements for re-supply. Order TTOs (drugs 'to take out') as far in advance as possible.

To ensure that drugs are represcribed and dispensed in time to allow uninterrupted treatment and to facilitate planned discharge.

8 Evaluate the effectiveness of the self-administration teaching programme and record any difficulties encountered and interventions made.

To identify further learning and teaching needs and modify care plan accordingly.

GUIDELINES · Oral drug administration

Procedure

Action

1 Wash hands with bactericidal soap and water or bactericidal alcohol hand rub.

Rationale

To minimize the risk of cross-infection.

2 Before administering any prescribed drug, check that it is due and has not been given already. Check that the information contained in the prescription chart is complete, correct and legible.

To protect the patient from harm.

3 Before administering any prescribed drug, consult the patient's prescription sheet and ascertain the following:
(a) Drug
(b) Dose
(c) Date and time of administration
(d) Route and method of administration
(e) Diluent as appropriate
(f) Validity of prescription
(g) Signature of doctor
(h) The prescription is legible.

To ensure that the patient is given the correct drug in the prescribed dose using the appropriate diluent and by the correct route.
To protect the patient from harm.
To comply with UKCC (1992a) standards for administration of medicines.

4 Select the required medication and check the expiry date.

Treatment with medication that is outside the expiry date is dangerous. Drugs deteriorate with storage. The expiry date indicates when a particular drug is no longer pharmacologically efficacious.

5 Empty the required dose into a medicine container. Avoid touching the preparation.

To minimize the risk of cross-infection. To minimize the risk of harm to the nurse.

Guidelines • Oral drug administration (cont'd)

Action	Rationale
6 Take the medication and the prescription chart to the patient. Check the patient's identity by asking the patient to state their full name and date of birth and check the dose to be given.	To prevent error.
7 Evaluate the patient's knowledge of the medication being offered. If this knowledge appears to be faulty or incorrect, offer an explanation of the use, action, dose and potential side-effects of the drug or drugs involved.	A patient has a right to information about treatment.
8 Administer the drug as prescribed.	
9 Offer a glass of water, if allowed.	To facilitate swallowing the medication.
10 Record the dose given in the prescription chart and in any other place made necessary by legal requirement or hospital policy.	To meet legal requirements and hospital policy.
11 Administer irritant drugs with meals or snacks.	To minimise their effect on the gastric mucosa.
12 Administer drugs that interact with foods, or drugs destroyed in significant proportions by digestive enzymes, between meals or on an empty stomach.	To prevent interference with the absorption of the drug.
13 Do not break a tablet unless it is scored. Break scored tablets with a file or a tablet cutter. Wash after use.	Breaking may cause incorrect dosage, gastrointestinal irritation or destruction of a drug in an incompatible pH. To reduce risk of contamination between tablets.
14 Do not interfere with time-release capsules and enteric coated tablets. Ask patients to swallow these whole and not to chew them.	The absorption rate of the drug will be altered.
15 Sublingual tablets must be placed under the tongue and buccal tablets between gum and cheek.	To allow for correct absorption.
16 When administering liquids to babies and young children, or when an accurately measured dose in multiples of 1 ml is needed for an adult, an oral syringe should be used in preference to a medicine spoon or measure.	A syringe is much more accurate than a measure or a 5 ml spoon. Use of a syringe makes administration of the correct dose much easier in an uncooperative child. Special syringes are available for this purpose, and usually available from pharmacy. (a) They are washable and re-usable; the graduations do not readily rub off. (b) They have a non-luer fitting to which it is impossible to attach a needle in error.
17 In babies and children especially, correct use of the syringe is very important. The tip should be gently pushed into and towards the side of the mouth. The contents are then *slowly* discharged towards the inside of the cheek, pausing if necessary to allow the liquid to be swallowed. In difficult children it may help to place the end of the barrel between the teeth!	To prevent injury to the mouth and eliminate the danger of choking the patient. To get the dose in and to prevent the patient spitting it out.

Controlled drugs

Action	Rationale
1 Consult the patient's prescription sheet, and ascertain the following: (a) Drug	To ensure that the patient is given the correct drug in the prescribed dose using the appropriate diluent and by the correct route.

(b) Dose

(c) Date and time of administration

(d) Route and method of administration

(e) Diluent as appropriate

(f) Validity of prescription

(g) Signature of doctor.

2 Select the correct drug from the controlled drug cupboard.

3 Check the stock against the last entry in the ward record book. (At The Royal Marsden Hospital, a second person is required to check the stock level.)

To comply with hospital policy.

4 Check the appropriate dose against the prescription sheet.

5 Return the remaining stock to the cupboard and lock the cupboard.

6 Enter the date, dose and the patient's name in the ward record book.

7 Take the prepared dose to the patient, whose identity is checked.

To prevent error and confirm patient's identity.

8 Administer the drug after checking the prescription chart again. Once the drug has been administered, the prescription chart is signed by the nurse responsible for administering the medication.

9 Record the administration on appropriate sheets.

To maintain accurate records, provide a point of reference in the event of any queries and prevent any duplication of treatment.

GUIDELINES · Administration of injections

Equipment

1 Clean tray or receiver in which to place drug and equipment.

2 21 g needle(s) to ease reconstitution and drawing up, 23 g if from a glass ampoule.

3 21, 23 or 25 g needle, size dependent on route of administration.

4 Syringe(s) of appropriate size for amount of drug to be given.

5 Swabs saturated with isopropyl alcohol 70%.

6 Sterile topical swab, if drug is presented in ampoule form.

7 Drug(s) to be administered.

8 Patient's prescription chart, to check dose, route, etc.

9 Recording sheet or book as required by law or hospital policy.

10 Any protective clothing required by hospital policy for specified drugs, such as antibiotics or cytotoxic drugs (see Chap. 10, Cytototoxic Drugs: Handling and Administration).

Procedure

Action

1 Collect and check all equipment.

2 Check that the packaging of all equipment is intact.

3 Wash hands with bactericidal soap and water or bactericidal alcohol hand rub.

4 Prepare needle(s), syringe(s), etc. on a tray or receiver.

Rationale

To prevent delays and enable full concentration on the procedure.

To ensure sterility. If the seal is damaged, discard.

To prevent contamination of medication and equipment.

Guidelines • Administration of injections (cont'd)

Action	*Rationale*
5 Inspect all equipment.	To check that none is damaged; if so, discard.
6 Consult the patient's prescription sheet, and ascertain the following: (a) Drug (b) Dose (c) Date and time of administration (d) Route and method of administration (e) Diluent as appropriate (f) Validity of prescription (g) Signature of doctor.	To ensure that the patient is given the correct drug in the prescribed dose using the appropriate diluent and by the correct route.
7 Check all details with another nurse if required by hospital policy.	To minimize any risk of error.
8 Select the drug in the appropriate volume, dilution or dosage and check the expiry date.	To reduce wastage. Treatment with medication that is outside the expiry date is dangerous. Drugs deteriorate with storage. The expiry date indicates when a particular drug is no longer pharmacologically efficacious.
9 Proceed with the preparation of the drug, using protective clothing if advisable.	
10 Evaluate the patient's knowledge of the medication being offered. If this knowledge appears to be faulty or incorrect, offer an explanation of the use, action, dose and potential side-effects of the drug or drugs involved.	A patient has a right to information about treatment.
11 Administer the drug as prescribed.	
12 Record the administration on appropriate sheets.	To maintain accurate records, provide a point of reference in the event of any queries and prevent any duplication of treatment.

Single-dose ampoule: solution

Action	*Rationale*
1 Inspect the solution for cloudiness or particulate matter. If this is present, discard and follow hospital guidelines on what action to take, e.g. return drug to pharmacy.	To prevent the patient from receiving an unstable or contaminated drug.
2 Tap the neck of the ampoule gently.	To ensure that all the solution is in the bottom of the ampoule.
3 Cover the neck of the ampoule with a sterile topical swab and snap it open. If there is any difficulty a file may be required.	To aid asepsis. To prevent aerosol formation or contact with the drug which could lead to a sensitivity reaction. To reduce the risk of injury to the nurse.
4 Inspect the solution for glass fragments; if present, discard.	To minimize the risk of injection of foreign matter into the patient.
5 Withdraw the required amount of solution, tilting the ampoule if necessary.	To avoid drawing in any air.
6 Replace the sheath on the needle and tap the syringe to dislodge any air bubbles. Expel air.	To prevent aerosol formation. To ensure that the correct amount of drug is in the syringe.

Note: replacing the sheath should **not** be confused with resheathing used needles.

An alternative to expelling the air with the needle sheath in place would be to use the ampoule or vial to receive any air and/or drug.

7	Change the needle, and discard used needle into appropriate sharps container.	To reduce the risk of infection. To avoid tracking medications through superficial tissues. To ensure that the correct size of needle is used for the injection. To reduce the risk of injury to the nurse.

Single-dose ampoule: powder

Action

1 Tap the neck of the ampoule gently.

2 Cover the neck of the ampoule with a sterile topical swab and snap it open. If there is any difficulty a file may be required.

3 Add the correct diluent carefully down the wall of the ampoule.

4 Agitate the ampoule.

5 Inspect the contents.

6 When the solution is clear withdraw the prescribed amount, tilting the ampoule if necessary.

7 Replace the sheath on the needle and tap the syringe to dislodge any air bubbles. Expel air.

8 Change the needle, and discard used needle into appropriate sharps container.

Rationale

To ensure that any powder lodged here falls to the bottom of the ampoule.

To aid asepsis. To prevent contact with the drug which could cause a sensitivity reaction. To prevent injury to the nurse.

To ensure that the powder is thoroughly wet before agitation and is not released into the atmosphere.

To dissolve the drug.

To detect any glass fragments or any other particulate matter. If present, continue agitation or discard as appropriate.

To ensure the powder is dissolved and has formed a solution with the diluent. To avoid drawing in air.

To prevent aerosol formation. To ensure that the correct amount of drug is in the syringe.

To reduce the risk of infection. To avoid tracking medications though superficial tissues. To ensure that the correct size of needle is used for the injection. To reduce the risk of injury to the nurse.

Multi-dose vial: powder

Action

1 Clean the rubber cap with the chosen antiseptic and let it dry.

2 Insert a 21 g needle into the cap to vent the bottle (Fig. 12.3a).

3 Add the correct diluent carefully down the wall of the vial.

4 Remove the needle and the syringe.

5 Place a sterile topical swab over the venting needle (Fig. 12.3b) and shake to dissolve the powder.

Rationale

To prevent bacterial contamination of the drug.

To prevent pressure differentials, which can cause separation of needle and syringe.

To ensure that the powder is thoroughly wet before it is shaken and is not released into the atmosphere.

To prevent contamination of the drug or the atmosphere. To mix the diluent with the powder and dissolve the drug.

Note: the nurse may encounter other presentations of drugs for injection, e.g. vials with a transfer needle, and should follow the manufacturer's instructions in these instances.

6 Inspect the solution for cloudiness or particulate matter. If this is present, discard. Follow hospital guidelines on what action to take, e.g. return drug to pharmacy.

7 Clean the rubber cap with an appropriate antiseptic and let it dry.

8 Withdraw the prescribed amount of solution, and inspect for pieces of rubber which may have 'cored out' of the cap (Fig. 12.3c).

To prevent patient from receiving an unstable or contaminated drug.

To prevent bacterial contamination of the drug.

To prevent the injection of foreign matter into the patient.

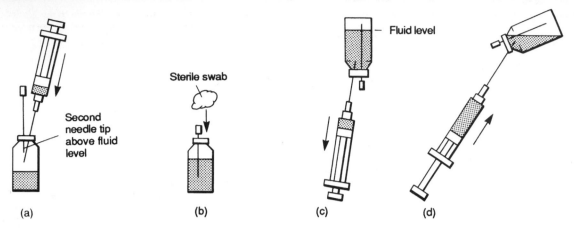

Figure 12.3 Suggested method of vial reconstitution to avoid environmental exposure. (a) When reconstituting vial, insert a second needle to allow air to escape when adding diluent for injection. (b) When shaking the vial to dissolve the powder, push in second needle up to Luer connection and cover with a sterile swab. (c) To remove reconstituted solution, insert syringe needle and then invert vial. Ensuring that tip of second needle is above fluid, withdraw the solution. (d) Remove air from syringe without spraying into the atmosphere by injecting air back into vial.

Guidelines • Administration of injections (cont'd)

Action	Rationale
Note: coring can be minimized by inserting the needle into the cap, bevel up, at an angle of 45° to 60°. Before complete insertion of the needle tip, lift the needle to 90° and proceed (Fig. 12.4).	
9 Remove air from syringe without spraying into the atmosphere by injecting air back into the vial (see Fig. 12.3d) or replace the sheath on the needle and tap the syringe to dislodge any air bubbles. Expel air.	To reduce risk of contamination of practitioner. To prevent aerosol formation. To ensure that the correct amount of drug is in the syringe.
10 Change the needle.	To reduce the risk of infection. To avoid possible trauma to the patient if the needle has barbed. To avoid tracking medications through superficial tissues. To ensure that the correct size of needle is used for the injection.

Subcutaneous injections

Action	Rationale
1 Explain and discuss the procedure with the patient.	To ensure that the patient understands the procedure and gives his/her valid consent.
2 Consult the patient's prescription sheet, and ascertain the following: (a) Drug (b) Dose (c) Date and time of administration (d) Route and method of administration (e) Diluent as appropriate (f) Validity of prescription (g) Signature of doctor.	To ensure that the patient is given the correct drug in the prescribed dose using the appropriate diluent and by the correct route.
3 Assist the patient into the required position.	To allow access to the chosen site.

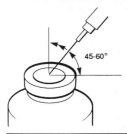

45-60°

Figure 12.4   Method to minimize coring.

4	Remove appropriate garments to expose the chosen site.	To gain access for injection.
5	Choose the correct needle size.	To minimize the risk of missing the subcutaneous tissue and any ensuing pain.
6	Clean the chosen site with a swab saturated with isopropyl alcohol 70%.	To reduce the number of pathogens introduced into the skin by the needle at the time of insertion. (For further information on this action see 'Skin preparation', above.)
7	Gently pinch the skin up into a fold.	To elevate the subcutaneous tissue, and lift the adipose tissue away from the underlying muscle (Workman 1999).
8	Insert the needle into the skin at angle of 45° and release the grasped skin (unless administering insulin when an angle of 90° should be used). Inject the drug slowly.	Injecting medication into compressed tissue irritates nerve fibres and causes the patient discomfort (Malseed 1990). The introduction of shorter insulin needles makes 90° the more appropriate angle (Burden 1994).
9	Withdraw the needle rapidly. Apply pressure to any bleeding point.	To prevent haematoma formation.
10	Record the administration on appropriate sheets.	To maintain accurate records, provide a point of reference in the event of any queries and prevent any duplication of treatment.
11	Ensure that all sharps and non-sharp waste are disposed of safely and in accordance with locally approved procedures. For example, sharps into sharps bin and syringes into yellow clinical waste bag.	To ensure safe disposal and to avoid laceration or other injury to staff.

Intramuscular injections

Action   *Rationale*

1	Explain and discuss the procedure with the patient.	To ensure that the patient understands the procedure and gives his/her valid consent.
2	Consult the patient's prescription sheet, and ascertain the following: (a) Drug (b) Dose (c) Date and time of administration (d) Route and method of administration (e) Diluent as appropriate (f) Validity of prescription (g) Signature of doctor.	To ensure that the patient is given the correct drug in the prescribed dose using the appropriate diluent and by the correct route.
3	Assist the patient into the required position.	To allow access to the chosen site and to ensure the designated muscle group is flexed and therefore relaxed.
4	Remove the appropriate garment to expose the chosen site.	To gain access for injection.

Guidelines • Administration of injections (cont'd)

Action	Rationale
5 Clean the chosen site with a swab saturated with isopropyl alcohol 70% for 30 seconds and allow to dry for 30 seconds (Workman 1999).	To reduce the number of pathogens introduced into the skin by the needle at the time of insertion, to prevent stinging sensation if alcohol is taken into the tissues upon needle entry. (For further information on this action see 'Skin preparation'.)
6 Stretch the skin around the chosen site.	To facilitate the insertion of the needle and to displace the underlying subcutaneous tissue.
7 Holding the needle at an angle of 90°, quickly plunge it into the skin.	To ensure that the needle penetrates the muscle.
Leave a third of the shaft of the needle exposed.	To facilitate removal of the needle should it break.
8 Pull back the plunger. If no blood is aspirated, depress the plunger at approximately 1 ml every 10 seconds and inject the drug slowly. If blood appears, withdraw the needle completely, replace it and begin again. Explain to the patient what has occurred.	To confirm that the needle is in the correct position. This allows time for the muscle fibres to expand and absorb the solution (Workman 1999). To prevent pain and ensure even distribution of the drug.
9 Wait 10 seconds before withdrawing the needle.	To allow the medication to diffuse into the tissue.
10 Withdraw the needle rapidly. Apply pressure to any bleeding point.	To prevent haematoma formation.
11 Record the administration on appropriate sheets.	To maintain accurate records, provide a point of reference in the event of any queries and prevent any duplication of treatment.
12 Ensure that all sharps and non-sharp waste are disposed of safely and in accordance with locally approved procedures, e.g. put sharps into sharps bin and syringes into yellow clinical waste bag.	To ensure safe disposal and to avoid laceration or other injury to staff.

GUIDELINES • Administration of rectal and vaginal preparations

Equipment

1 Disposable gloves.
2 Topical swabs.

3 Lubricating jelly.
4 Prescription chart.

Procedure

Rectal preparations

For further information about the administration of rectal medication see the relevant sections in Chap. 6, Bowel care.

Vaginal pessaries

Action	Rationale
1 Explain and discuss the procedure with the patient.	To ensure that the patient understands the procedure and gives his/her valid consent.
2 Consult the patient's prescription sheet, and ascertain the following: (a) Drug (b) Dose (c) Date and time of administration (d) Route and method of administration	To ensure that the patient is given the correct drug in the prescribed dose using the appropriate diluent and by the correct route.

(e) Diluent as appropriate
(f) Validity of prescription
(g) Signature of doctor.

3 Select the appropriate pessary and check it with the prescription chart.

To ensure that the correct medication is given to the correct patient at the appropriate time.

4 Assist the patient into the appropriate position, either left lateral with buttocks to the edge of the bed or supine with the knees drawn up and legs parted.

To facilitate the correct insertion of the pessary.

5 Wash hands with bactericidal soap and water or bactericidal alcohol hand rub, and put on gloves.

To minimize the risk of cross-infection.

6 Apply lubricating jelly to a topical swab and from the swab on to the pessary.

To facilitate insertion of the pessary and ensure the patient's comfort.

7 Insert the pessary along the posterior vaginal wall and into the top of the vagina.
Note: This procedure is best performed late in the evening when the patient is unlikely to get out of bed.

To ensure that the pessary is retained and that the medication can reach its maximum efficiency.

8 Wipe away any excess lubricating jelly from the patient's vulval and/or perineal area with a topical swab.

To promote patient comfort.

9 Make the patient comfortable and apply a clean sanitary pad.

To absorb any excess discharge.

10 Record the administration on appropriate sheets.

To maintain accurate records, provide a point of reference in the event of any queries and prevent any duplication of treatment.

GUIDELINES • Topical applications of drugs

Equipment

1 Clean non-sterile gloves.
2 Sterile topical swabs.
3 Applicators.

Procedure

Action

Rationale

1 Explain and discuss the procedure with the patient.

To ensure that the patient understands the procedure and gives his/her valid consent.

2 Check the patient's prescription chart.

To ensure that the patient is given the correct drug and dose.

3 Use aseptic technique if the skin is broken.

To prevent local or systemic infection.

4 Remove semisolid or stiff preparations from their containers with a gloved hand.

To minimize the risk of cross-infection from one part of the wound to another.

5 If the medication is to be rubbed into the skin, the preparation should be placed on a sterile topical swab. The wearing of gloves may be necessary.

To minimize the risk of cross-infection. To protect the nurse.

6 If the preparation causes staining, advise the patient of this.

To ensure that adequate precautions are taken beforehand and to prevent unwanted stains.

7 Record the administration on appropriate sheets.

To maintain accurate records, provide a point of reference in the event of any queries and prevent any duplication of treatment.

GUIDELINES • Administration of drugs in other forms

Procedure

Inhalations

Action	Rationale
1 Explain and discuss the procedure with the patient.	To ensure that the patient understands the procedure and gives his/her valid consent.
2 Seat the patient in an upright position if possible.	To permit full expansion of the diaphragm.
3 Consult the patient's prescription sheet, and ascertain the following: (a) Drug (b) Dose (c) Date and time of administration (d) Route and method of administration (e) Diluent as appropriate (f) Validity of prescription (g) Signature of doctor.	To ensure that the patient is given the correct drug in the prescribed dose using the appropriate diluent and by the correct route.
4 Administer only one drug at a time unless specifically instructed to the contrary.	Several drugs used together may cause undesirable reactions or they may inactivate each other.
5 Measure any liquid medication with a syringe.	To ensure the correct dose.
6 Clean any equipment used after use, and discard all disposable equipment in appropriate containers.	To minimize the risk of infection.
7 Correct use of inhalers is essential (see manufacturer's information leaflet) and will be achieved only if this is carefully explained and demonstrated to the patient. If further advice is required, contact the hospital pharmacist.	Incorrect use may result in most of the dose remaining in the mouth and/or being expelled almost immediately. This renders treatment ineffective.
8 Record the administration on appropriate sheets.	To maintain accurate records, provide a point of reference in the event of any queries and prevent any duplication of treatment.

Gargles

Action	Rationale
1 Throat irrigations should not be warmer than body temperature.	Any liquid warmer may cause discomfort or damage tissue.

Nasal drops

Action	Rationale
1 Explain and discuss the procedure with the patient.	To ensure that the patient understands the procedure and gives his/her valid consent.
2 Consult the patient's prescription sheet, and ascertain the following: (a) Drug (b) Dose (c) Date and time of administration (d) Route and method of administration (e) Diluent as appropriate (f) Validity of prescription (g) Signature of doctor.	To ensure that the patient is given the correct drug in the prescribed dose using the appropriate diluent and by the correct route.

3 Have paper tissues available.	To wipe away secretions and/or medication.
4 Clean the patient's nasal passages, with tissues or damp cotton bud.	To ensure maximum penetration for the medication.
5 Hyperextend the patient's neck.	To obtain the best position for insertion of the medication.
6 Avoid touching the external nares with the dropper.	To prevent the patient from sneezing.
7 Request the patient to maintain his/her position for 1 or 2 minutes.	To ensure full absorption of the medication.
8 Each patient should have his/her own medication and dropper.	To minimize the risk of cross-infection.
9 Record the administration on appropriate sheets.	To maintain accurate records, provide a point of reference in the event of any queries and prevent any duplication of treatment.

Eye medications

For information on eye care see Chap. 17.

Ear drops

Action	*Rationale*
1 Explain and discuss the procedure with the patient.	To ensure that the patient understands the procedure and gives his/her valid consent.
2 Consult the patient's prescription sheet, and ascertain the following: (a) Drug (b) Dose (c) Date and time of administration (d) Route and method of administration (e) Diluent as appropriate (f) Validity of prescription (g) Signature of doctor.	To ensure that the patient is given the correct drug in the prescribed dose using the appropriate diluent and by the correct route.
3 Ask the patient to lie on his/her side with the ear to be treated uppermost.	To ensure the best position for insertion of the drops.
4 Warm the drops to body temperature if allowed.	To prevent trauma to the patient.
5 Pull the cartilaginous part of the pinna backwards and upwards.	To prepare the auditory meatus for instillation of the drops.
6 Allow the drop(s) to fall in direction of the external canal.	To ensure that the medication reaches the area requiring therapy.
7 Request the patient to remain in this position for 1 or 2 minutes.	To allow the medication to reach the eardrum and be absorbed.
8 Record the administration on appropriate sheets.	To maintain accurate records, provide a point of reference in the event of any queries and prevent any duplication of treatment.

GUIDELINES • Administration of intravenous drugs by continuous infusion

This procedure may be carried out by the infusion of drugs from a bag, bottle or burette.

Guideline • Administration of intravenous drugs by continuous infusion (cont'd)

Equipment

1 Clinically clean receiver or tray containing the prepared drug to be administered.
2 Patient's prescription chart.
3 Recording sheet or book as required by law or hospital policy.

4 Protective clothing as required by hospital policy for specific drugs.
5 Container of appropriate intravenous infusion fluid.
6 Swab saturated with isopropyl alcohol 70%.
7 Drug additive label.

Procedure

Action	*Rationale*
1 Explain and discuss the procedure with the patient.	To ensure that the patient understands the procedure and gives his/her valid consent.
2 Inspect the infusion in progress.	To check it is the correct infusion being administered at the correct rate and that the contents are due to be delivered on time in order for the next prepared infusion bag to be connected. To check if the patient is experiencing any discomfort at the site of insertion, which might indicate the peripheral device needs to be resited.
3 Before administering any prescribed drug check that it is due and has not been given already.	To protect the patient from harm.
4 Before administering any prescribed drug, consult the patient's prescription sheet and ascertain the following: (a) Drug (b) Dose (c) Date and time of administration (d) Route and method of administration (e) Diluent as appropriate (f) Validity of prescription (g) Signature of doctor (h) The prescription is legible.	To ensure that the patient is given the correct drug in the prescribed dose using the appropriate diluent and by the correct route. To protect the patient from harm. To comply with UKCC standards for administration of medicines.
5 Wash hands with bactericidal soap and water or bactericidal alcohol hand rub, and assemble the necessary equipment.	
6 Prepare the drug for injection described in the procedure Guidelines • Administration of injections.	
7 Check the name, strength and volume of intravenous fluid against the prescription chart.	To ensure that the correct type and quantity of fluid are administered.
8 Check the expiry date of the fluid.	To prevent an ineffective or toxic compound being administered to the patient.
9 Check that the packaging is intact and inspect the container and contents in a good light for cracks, punctures, air bubbles.	To check that no contamination of the infusion container has occurred.
10 Inspect the fluid for discoloration, haziness and crystalline or particulate matter.	To prevent any toxic or foreign matter being infused into the patient.
11 Check the identity and amount of drug to be added. Consider: (a) Compatibility of fluid and additive (b) Stability of mixture over the prescription time (c) Any special directions for dilution, e.g. pH, optimum concentration, etc. (d) Sensitivity to external factors such as light (e) Any anticipated allergic reaction.	To minimize any risk of error. To ensure safe and effective administration of the drug. To enable anticipation of toxicities and the nursing implications of these.

If any doubts exist about the listed points, consult the pharmacist or appropriate reference works.

12	Any additions must be made immediately before use.	To prevent any possible microbial growth or degradation.
13	Wash hands thoroughly using bactericidal soap and water or bactericidal alcohol hand rub.	To minimize the risk of cross-infection.
14	Place infusion bag on flat surface.	To prevent puncturing the side of the infusion bag when making additions.
15	Remove any seal present.	To expose the injection site on the container.
16	Clean the site with the swab and allow it to dry.	To reduce the risk of contamination.
17	Inject the drug using a new sterile needle into the bag, bottle or burette. A 23 or 25 g needle should be used.	To minimize the risk of contamination. To enable resealing of the latex or rubber injection site.
18	If the addition is made into a burette at the bedside:	
	(a) Avoid contamination of the needle and inlet port.	To minimize the risk of contamination.
	(b) Check that the correct quantity of fluid is in the chamber.	To ensure the correct dilution.
	(c) Switch the infusion off briefly.	To ensure a bolus injection is not given.
	(d) Add the drug.	
19	Invert the container a number of times, especially if adding to a flexible infusion bag.	To ensure adequate mixing of the drug.
20	Check again for haziness, discoloration and particles. This can occur even if the mixture is theoretically compatible, thus making vigilance essential.	To detect any incompatibility or degradation.
21	Complete the drug additive label and fix it on the bag, bottle or burette.	To identify which drug has been added, when and by whom.
22	Place the container in a clean receptacle. Wash hands and proceed to the patient.	To minimize the risk of contamination.
23	Check the identity of the patient with the prescription chart and infusion bag.	To minimize the risk of error and ensure the correct infusion is administered to the correct patient.
24	Check that the contents of the previous container have been delivered.	To ensure that the preceding prescription has been administered.
25	Switch off the infusion. Place the new infusion bag on a flat surface and then disconnect empty infusion bag.	To ensure that the administration set spike will not puncture side wall of infusion bag.
26	Push the spike in fully without touching the spike and hang the new infusion bag on the infusion stand.	To reduce the risk of contamination.
27	Restart the infusion and adjust the rate of flow as prescribed.	To ensure that the infusion will be delivered at the correct rate over the correct period of time.
28	If the addition is made into a burette, the infusion can be restarted immediately following mixing and recording and the infusion rate adjusted accordingly.	
29	Ask the patient if any abnormal sensations, etc. are experienced.	To ascertain whether there are any problems that may require nursing care and refer to medical staff where appropriate.
30	Discard waste, making sure that it is placed in the correct containers, e.g. 'sharps' into a designated receptacle.	To ensure safe disposal and avoid injury to staff. To prevent reuse of equipment.
31	Complete the patient's recording chart and other hospital and/or legally required documents.	To maintain accurate records. To provide a point of reference in the event of any queries. To prevent any duplication of treatment.

GUIDELINES • Administration of drugs by intermittent infusion

Equipment

Equipment for this procedure is as described for the previous procedure (i.e. items 1–7), together with the following:

8 Intravenous administration set.
9 Intravenous infusion stand.
10 Clean dressing trolley.
11 Clinically clean receiver or tray.
12 Sterile needles and syringes.
13 0.9% sodium chloride, 20 ml for injection.

14 Heparin, in accordance with hospital policy, plus sterile bung.
15 Alcohol-based lotion for cleaning injection site, e.g. chlorhexidine in 70% alcohol.
16 Alcohol-based hand wash solution or rub.
17 Sterile dressing pack.
18 Hypoallergenic tape.

Procedure

Action	*Rationale*
1 Explain and discuss the procedure with the patient.	To ensure that the patient understands the procedure and gives his/her valid consent.
2 Before administering any prescribed drug, check that it is due and has not been given already. Check that the information contained in the prescription chart is complete, correct and legible.	To protect the patient from harm.
3 Before administering any prescribed drug, consult the patient's prescription sheet and ascertain the following: (a) Drug (b) Dose (c) Date and time of administration (d) Route and method of administration (e) Diluent as appropriate (f) Validity of prescription (g) Signature of doctor (h) The prescription is legible.	To ensure that the patient is given the correct drug in the prescribed dose using the appropriate diluent and by the correct route. To protect the patient from harm. To comply with UKCC standards for administration of medicines.
4 Prepare the intravenous infusion and additive as described for the previous procedure (i.e. items 2–13) .	
5 Prime the intravenous administration set with infusion fluid mixture and hang it on the infusion stand.	To ensure removal of air from set and check that tubing is patent. To prepare for administration.
6 Draw up 10 ml of 0.9% sodium chloride for injection in two separate syringes, using an aseptic technique.	To ensure sufficient flushing solution is available.
7 Draw up flushing solution, as required by hospital policy.	To prepare for administration.
8 Place the syringes in a clinically clean receiver or tray on the bottom shelf of the dressing trolley.	To ensure top shelf is used for sterile dressing pack in order to minimize the risk of contamination.
9 Collect the other equipment and place it on the bottom shelf of the dressing trolley.	To ensure all equipment is available to commence procedure.
10 Place a sterile dressing pack on the top of the trolley.	To minimize risk of contamination.
11 Check that all necessary equipment is present.	To prevent delays and interruption of the procedure.
12 Wash hands thoroughly using bactericidal soap and water or bactericidal alcohol hand rub before leaving the clinical room.	To minimize the risk of cross-infection.

13 Proceed to the patient. Check patient's identity with prescription chart and prepared drugs.	To minimize the risk of error and ensure the correct drug is given to the correct patient.
14 Open the sterile dressing pack.	To minimize the risk of cross-infection.
15 Add lotion for cleaning the skin to the gallipot in order to wet the low-linting swabs.	To ensure the swabs can be used for cleaning when sufficient alcohol-based lotion is applied.
16 Wash hands with bactericidal soap and water or with a bactericidal alcohol hand rub.	To minimize the risk of cross-infection.
17 If peripheral device is in situ remove the patient's bandage and dressing.	To observe the insertion site.
18 Inspect the insertion site of the device.	To detect any signs of inflammation, infiltration, etc. If present, take appropriate action.
19 Wash hands as above (see item 16).	To minimize the risk of contamination.
20 Put on gloves, if appropriate.	To protect against contamination with hazardous substances, e.g. cytotoxic drugs.
21 Place a sterile towel under the patient's arm.	To create a sterile area on which to work.
22 (a) If using a needleless injection system, clean the cap with alcohol-soaked swabs.	To minimize the risk of contamination and maintain a closed sytem.
(b) If using an injectable cap, then clean the connection between the cap and the device/ extension set then remove the cap while applying digital pressure at the point in the vein where the cannula tip rests.	To minimize the risk of contamination and to prevent blood spillage.
23 Inject gently 10 ml of 0.9% sodium chloride for injection.	To confirm the patency of the device.
24 Check that no resistance is met, no pain or discomfort is felt by the patient, no swelling is evident, no leakage occurs around the device and there is a good back-flow of blood on aspiration.	To ensure the device is patent.
25 Connect the infusion to the device.	To commence treatment.
26 Open the roller clamp.	To check the infusion is flowing freely.
27 Check the insertion site and ask the patient if he/she is comfortable.	To confirm that the vein can accommodate the extra fluid flow and that the patient experiences no pain, etc.
28 Adjust the flow rate as prescribed.	To ensure that the correct speed of administration is established.
29 Tape the administration set in a way that places no strain on the device, which could in turn damage the vein.	To reduce the risk of mechanical phlebitis or infiltration.
30 If peripheral device is in situ cover it with a sterile topical swab and tape it in place.	To maintain asepsis.
31 Remove gloves, if used.	
32 If the infusion is to be completed within 40 minutes, bandaging is unnecessary and the patient may be instructed to keep the arm resting on the sterile towel.	
33 If the infusion is to be in progress for longer than 40 minutes a bandage should be applied to the peripheral device site and the equipment must be cleared away and new equipment prepared for discontinuing the infusion.	To reduce the risk of dislodging the device. To ensure that the equipment used is sterile prior to use.

Guidelines • Administration of drugs by intermittent infusion (cont'd)

Action	Rationale
34 Monitor flow rate and device site frequently.	To ensure the flow rate is correct, the patient is comfortable and for signs of infiltration.
35 When the infusion is complete, wash hands using bactericidal soap and water or bactericidal alcohol hand rub, and recheck that all the equipment required is present.	To maintain asepsis and ensure that the procedure runs smoothly.
36 Stop the infusion when all the fluid has been delivered.	To ensure that all of the prescribed mixture has been delivered and prevent air infusing into the patient.
37 Wash hands with bactericidal soap and water or bactericidal alcohol hand rub.	To maintain asepsis.
38 Put on non-sterile gloves, if appropriate.	To protect against contamination with hazardous substances.
39 Disconnect the infusion set and flush the device with 10 ml of 0.9% sodium chloride for injection. (A 'minibag' may be used to flush the drug through the tubing but the cost implications of this as well as the risk to patients on restricted intake should be considered before this is adopted routinely.)	To flush any remaining irritating solution away from the cannula.
40 Attach a new sterile injection cap if necessary.	To maintain a closed system.
41 Flushing must follow.	To maintain the patency of the device.
42 Clean the injection site of the bung with a swab saturated with chlorhexidine in 70% alcohol.	To minimize the risk of contamination.
43 Administer flushing solution (using a 23 or 25 g needle if necessary) using the push pause technique and ending with positive pressure technique.	To maintain the patency of the device and if needle used enable reseal of the latex injection site.
44 If a peripheral device is in situ cover the insertion site and cannula with a new sterile low-linting swab. Tape it in place. Apply a bandage.	To minimize the risk of contamination of the insertion site. To reduce the risk of dislodging the cannula.
45 Ensure that the patient is comfortable.	
46 Record the administration on appropriate sheets.	To maintain accurate records, provide a point of reference in the event of any queries and prevent any duplication of treatment.
47 Discard waste, placing it in the correct containers, e.g. 'sharps' into a designated container.	To ensure safe disposal and avoid injury to staff. To prevent re-use of equipment.
48 Remove gloves, if used.	

GUIDELINES • Administration of drugs by direct injection, bolus or push

This procedure may be carried out via any one of the following:

1 The injection site of an intravenous administration set.
2 An injection cap attached to any vascular access device.

3 An extension set, multiple adaptor or stopcock (one-, two- or three-way).

Equipment

1 Clinically clean receiver or tray containing the prepared drug(s) to be administered.
2 Patient's prescription chart.

3 Recording sheet or book as required by law or hospital policy.

4 Protective clothing as required by hospital policy or specific drugs.
5 Clean dressing trolley.
6 Clinically clean receiver or tray.
7 Sterile needles and syringes.
8 0.9% sodium chloride, 20 ml for injection.

9 Flushing solution, in accordance with hospital policy.
10 Alcohol-based solution for cleaning injection site, e.g. chlorhexidine in 70% alcohol.
11 Sterile dressing pack.
12 Hypoallergenic tape.
13 Sharps container.

Procedure

Action	Rationale
1 Explain and discuss the procedure with the patient.	To ensure that the patient understands the procedure and gives his/her valid consent. To protect the patient from harm.
2 Before administering any prescribed drug, check that it is due and has not been given already. Check that the information contained in the prescription chart is complete, correct and legible.	
3 Before administering any prescribed drug, consult the patient's prescription sheet and ascertain the following: (a) Drug (b) Dose (c) Date and time of administration (d) Route and method of administration (e) Diluent as appropriate (f) Validity of prescription (g) Signature of doctor (h) The prescription is legible.	To ensure that the patient is given the correct drug in the prescribed dose using the appropriate diluent and by the correct route. To protect the patient from harm. To comply with UKCC standards for administration of medicines.
4 Select the required medication and check the expiry date.	Treatment with medication that is outside the expiry date is dangerous. Drugs deteriorate with storage. The expiry date indicates when a particular drug is no longer pharmacologically efficacious.
5 Wash hands with bactericidal soap and water or bactericidal alcohol hand rub, and assemble necessary equipment.	To minimize the risk of infection.
6 Prepare the drug for injection as per procedure described earlier.	
7 Prepare a 20-ml syringe of 0.9% sodium chloride for injection, as described, using aseptic technique	To use for flushing between each drug.
8 Draw up flushing solution, as required by hospital policy.	To prepare for administration.
9 Place syringes in a clinically clean receptacle on the bottom shelf of the dressing trolley, along with the receptacle containing any drug(s) to be administered.	To ensure top shelf is used for sterile dressing pack in order to minimize the risk of contamination.
10 Collect the other equipment and place it on the bottom of the trolley.	To ensure all equipment is available to commence procedure.
11 Place a sterile dressing pack on top of the trolley.	To minimize the risk of contamination.
12 Check that all necessary equipment is present.	To prevent delays and interruption of the procedure.
13 Wash hands thoroughly.	To minimize the risk of infection.
14 Proceed to the patient and check identity with prescription chart and prepared drug.	To minimize the risk of error and ensure the correct patient.
15 Open the sterile dressing pack. Add lotion to wet the low-linting swab.	

Guidelines • Administration of drugs by direct injection, bolus or push (cont'd)

Action	Rationale
16 Wash hands with bactericidal soap and water or with bactericidal alcohol hand rub.	To reduce the risk of infection.
17 If a peripheral device is in situ, remove the bandage and dressing.	To observe the insertion site.
18 Inspect the insertion site of the device.	To detect any signs of inflammation, infiltration, etc. If present, take appropriate action (see Nursing Care Plan).
19 Observe the infusion, if in progress.	To confirm that it is infusing as desired.
20 Check if the infusion fluid and the drugs are compatible. If not change the infusion fluid to 0.9% sodium chloride to flush between the drugs.	To prevent drug interaction. Some manufacturers may recommend that the drug is given into the injection site of a rapidly running infusion.
21 Wash hands or clean them with an alcohol hand rub.	To minimize the risk of infection.
22 Place a sterile towel under the patient's arm.	To create a sterile field.
23 Clean the injection site with a swab saturated with chlorhexidine in 70% alcohol and allow to dry.	To reduce the number of pathogens introduced by the needle at the time of the insertion. To ensure complete disinfection has occurred.
24 Switch off the infusion or close the fluid path of a tap or stopcock	To prevent excessive pressure within the vein. To prevent contact with an incompatible infusion fluid. To allow the nurse to concentrate on the site of insertion and injection.
25 If a peripheral device is in situ use a sterile 23 or 25 g needle if the injection is made through a resealable latex site and gently inject 0.9% sodium chloride. This may not be necessary if the patient has a 0.9% sodium chloride infusion in progress.	To enable resealing of the site at the end of the injection. To confirm patency of the vein. To prevent contact with an incompatible infusion solution.
26 Open the roller clamp of the administration set fully. Inject the drug at a speed sufficient to slow but not stop the infusion and inject the drug smoothly in the direction of flow at the specified rate.	To prevent a back-flow of drug up the tubing. To prevent excessive pressure within the vein. To prevent speed shock.
27 Ensure used needles and syringes are disposed of immediately into appropriate sharps container (or are returned to tray). Do not leave any sharps on opened sterile pack.	To reduce the risk of needlestick injury and to prevent contamination of pack.
28 Observe the insertion site of the device throughout.	To detect any complications at an early stage, e.g. extravasation or local allergic reaction.
29 Blood return and/or 'flashback' must be checked frequently throughout the injection.	To confirm that the device is correctly placed and that the vein remains patent.
30 Consult the patient during the injection about any discomfort, etc.	To detect any complications at an early stage, and ensure patient comfort.
31 If more than one drug is to be administered, flush with 0.9% sodium chloride between administrations by restarting the infusion or changing syringes.	To prevent drug interactions.
32 At the end of the injection, flush with 0.9% sodium chloride by restarting the infusion or attaching a syringe containing 0.9% sodium chloride.	To flush any remaining irritant solution away from the device site.
33 Observe the insertion site of the cannula carefully.	To detect any complications at an early stage. Extra pressure within the vein caused by both fluid flow and injection of the drug may cause rupture.

34 After the final flush of 0.9% sodium chloride adjust the infusion rate as prescribed or open the fluid path of the tap/stopcock or use flushing solution.

To continue delivery of therapy.
To maintain the patency of the cannula.

35 If a peripheral device is in situ cover the insertion site with new sterile low linting swab and tape it in place.

To minimize the risk of contamination of the insertion site.

36 Apply a bandage.

To reduce the risk of dislodging the cannula.

37 Make sure that the patient is comfortable.

38 Record the administration on appropriate sheets.

To maintain accurate records, provide a point of reference in the event of any queries and prevent any duplication of treatment.

39 Dispose of used syringes with needles, unsheathed, directly into a sharps container during procedure or place back on to plastic tray and then dispose of in a sharps container as soon as possible. *Do not* disconnect needle from syringe prior to disposal. Other waste should be placed into the appropriate plastic bags.

To avoid needlestick injury.

Nursing care plan

The problems associated with injection and infusion of intravenous fluids and drugs fall into two categories:

1 Local venous complications associated with the cannula insertion site.
2 Systemic problems which affect the whole patient, exerting effects on vital organs and their functions.

The nurse must observe regularly the insertion site, the infusion and the patient to detect any complications at the earliest possible moment and to prevent progression to more serious conditions. Early detection is aided by paying attention to the patient's comments of discomfort or pain. The patient's symptoms and physical signs both constitute reasons for a resiting of the peripheral device or discontinuation of the infusion. Signs and symptoms are used as problem headings.

Problem	Possible causes	Preventive nursing measures	Suggested action
Infusion slows or stops.	Change in position of the following:		
	(a) Patient.	Check the height of the fluid container if the patient is active and receiving an infusion using gravity flow.	Adjust the height of the container accordingly. But the infusion should not hang higher than 1 m (above the patient) as the increased height will result in increased pressure and possible rupture of the vessel/device.
	(b) Limb.	Prevent by avoiding use of joints when inserting peripheral devices. Instruct the patient on the amount of movement permitted. Continued movement could result in mechanical phlebitis.	Move the arm or hand until infusion starts again. Retape, bandage or splint the limb again carefully in the desired position. Take care not to cause damage to the limb.
	(c) Administration set.	Tape the administration set so that it cannot become kinked or occluded.	Check for kinks and/or compression if the patient is active or restless and correct accordingly.

Problem	Possible causes	Preventive nursing measures	Suggested action
	(d) Cannula.	Tape the cannula firmly to prevent movement. It may come into contact with the vein wall or a valve. Infusions sited in small veins are prone to this problem.	Remove the bandage and dressing and manoeuvre the peripheral device without pulling it out of the vein gently until the infusion starts again. Retape carefully.
	Technical problems:		
	(a) Negative pressure prevents flow of fluid.	Ensure that the container is vented using an air inlet.	Vent if necessary, using venting needle.
	(b) Empty container.	Check fluid levels regularly.	Replace the fluid container before it runs dry.
	(c) Venous spasm due to chemical irritation or cold fluids/drugs.	Dilute drugs as recommended. Remove solutions from the refrigerator a short time before use.	Apply a warm compress to soothe and dilate the vein, increase blood flow and dilute the infusion mixture.
	(d) Injury to the vein.	Detect any injury early as it is likely to progress and cause more serious conditions (see below).	Stop the infusion and request a resiting of the cannula.
	(e) Occlusion of the device due to fibrin formation.	Maintain a continuous, regular fluid flow or ensure that patency is maintained by flushing or by placement of a stylet. Instruct the patient to keep arm below the level of the heart if ambulant.	Remove extension set/injection cap and attempt to flush the cannula gently using a 10 ml syringe of 0.9% sodium chloride. If resistance is met, stop and request a resiting of the device.
	(f) The cannula has become displaced either completely or partially, i.e. it has 'tissued'.	Tape the cannula and the administration set so that no stress is placed on them. Instruct the patient on the amount of movement permitted.	Confirm that infiltration of drugs has/has not occurred by: (i) inspecting the site for leakage, swelling, etc.; (ii) testing the temperature of the skin – it will be cooler if infiltration has occurred; (iii) comparing the size of the limb with the opposite limb; (iv) lowering the infusion below the height of the limb. If the vein is patent, blood will flow back into the administration set. Once infiltration has been confirmed, stop the infusion and request a resiting of the device. If the infusion is allowed to progress, discomfort and tissue damage will result. Apply cold or warm

			compresses to provide symptomatic relief, whichever provides the most comfort for the patient. Reassure the patient by explaining what is happening.
Erythoma (inflammation) around the insertion site, and/or pain and swelling	Phlebitis due to:		Failure to detect and act when phlebitis is at an early stage, for whatever reason, will result in painful and incapacitating thrombophlebitis. Dislodgement of a thrombus could cause a pulmonary embolus (Weinstein 1997; Lamb 1999).
	(a) Sepsis.	Adhere to aseptic techniques when performing all intravenous procedures (RCN 1999)	Stop the infusion, remove the device and request a resiting of the cannula. Follow hospital policy about sending equipment for bacterial analysis. Clean the area and apply a sterile dressing. Check regularly.
	(b) Chemical irritation.	Dilute drugs according to instructions. Check compatibilities carefully to reduce the risk of particulate formation. Administer the drugs as an infusion instead of a bolus injection. Be aware of the factors involved, e.g. pH (Wright *et al.* 1985; Smolders 1988; Haynes 1989). Apply local heat above the cannula site (Lamb 1999). Apply a glycerol trinitrate (GTN) patch to aid vasodilatation (Wright *et al.* 1985; Hecker 1988).	Stop the infusion and request a resiting of the device. If the infusion is allowed to progress, tissue damage and severe pain will result. Apply cold or warm compresses to provide symptomatic relief. Encourage movement of the limb. Reassure the patient by explaining what is happening.
	(c) Mechanical irritation.	Tape, bandage or splint the limb if the infusion is sited at a point of flexion. Use an extension set to minimize direct handling if cannula sited in awkward position. Instruct the patient on the amount of movement permitted (Hecker 1988; Goodison 1990a).	Stop the infusion and remove the device and request a resiting of the device. Although inflammation of this type progresses more slowly, it will cause discomfort. Provide symptomatic relief as above. Encourage movement and reassure the patient by explaining what is happening.

Problem	Possible causes	Preventive nursing measures	Suggested action
	Infection with or without discharge.	Adhere to aseptic techniques when performing all intravenous procedures. Observe all recommendations for equipment changes, etc.	Stop the infusion and request a resiting of the device. Follow hospital policy about sending equipment for bacterial analysis. Clean the area and apply a sterile dresing. Check regularly. Observe the patient for signs of systemic infection.
	Cellulitis due to: (a) Sepsis. (b) Non-specific sterile inflammation.	As above.	As above. Due to the nature of the connective tissue any infection or inflammation spreads quickly, especially if the limb is oedematous.
	Local allergic reaction, e.g. flare reaction which occurs with doxorubicin.	Ask if the patient has any allergies before administration of any drugs or fluids, including sensitivities to topical solutions, which may cause erythema at the site. Check whether the particular medication is commonly associated with local or venous flushing.	Observe the patient for systemic reaction. Treat the local area symptomatically. Reassure the patient. Inform medical staff.
Local oedema.	During infusion or injection: (a) Infiltration. (b) Phlebitis. (Haynes 1989) (c) Extravasation of medication (see Chap. 10, Cytotoxic Drugs: Handling and Administration).	Tape the device and administration set so that no stress is placed on the cannula. Use an extension set. Instruct the patient on the amount of movement permitted. Check regularly for swelling, e.g. tightness of bandages or any rings. Observe the patient carefully throughout drug administration.	Stop the infusion and request a resiting of the cannula before proceeding. Apply warm compresses to provide symptomatic relief. Reassure the patient by explaining what is happening. Stop the injection immediately extravasation is suspected. Act in accordance with hospital policy. Some drugs may cause inflammation and supportive, symptomatic relief will be required. Others may have the potential to cause necrosis of tissue and further action may be necessary.
Oedema of the limb.	Infiltration.	Tape the device and administration set so that no stress is placed on the device, which in turn can lead to damage of the vein. Use an extension set. Instruct the patient on the	Stop the infusion and request a resiting of the device. Provide symptomatic relief and support. Reassure the patient.

		amount of movement permitted. Check regularly for swelling, as above.	
	Circulatory overload.	Administer infusion fluids at the prescribed rate and do not make sudden alterations of flow. Use infusion equipment wherever possible and administration set with anti free flow systems. Be aware of the patient's renal and cardiac status. Monitor intake and output routinely (Weinstein 1997; Lamb 1999).	Slow the infusion. Monitor vital signs for increase in blood pressure and respirations. Place the patient in an upright position and keep him/her warm to promote peripheral circulation and relieve stress on the central veins. Reassure the patient. Notify a doctor immediately.
Pain at the insertion site.	All of the previous listed conditions may be accompanied by soreness or pain.	As previously listed.	Provide local symptomatic relief, e.g. warmth, as required. Administer systemic analgesia, as prescribed, if necessary.
Pyrexia, rigors, tachycardia.	Septicaemia.	Adhere to aseptic techniques when performing all intravenous procedures. Inspect all equipment, infusion fluids, etc., before use. Observe recommendations for additives, equipment changes and general management. Avoid the use of equipment that can increase the risk of contamination, e.g. stopcocks (Cheeseborough & Finch 1984; Lamb 1999).	Notify a doctor immediately. Follow hospital policy about sending equipment for bacterial analysis.
Decrease in blood pressure, tachycardia, cyanosis, unconsciousness.	Embolism: (a) Air.	Check the containers and change before they run through, especially bottles. Clear all air from tubing before commencing infusion. Check all connections regularly and make sure they are secure. Use infusion equipment with air in line detectors.	Turn the patient onto left side and lower the head of the bed to prevent air from entering the pulmonary artery. Notify a doctor immediately. Administer oxygen (Ostrow 1981; Weinstein 1997; Lamb 1999; RCN 1999). Reassure the patient.
	(b) Particle.	Check all infusion fluids before and after any additions have been made. Check drug compatibility and stability. Observe the solution throughout the infusion for precipitate formation (Trissel 1999).	As above, but also change the container and administration set. Replace with new equipment and 0.9% sodium chloride infusion from a different batch. Follow hospital policy about sending

Problem	Possible causes	Preventive nursing measures	Suggested action
			contaminated fluid and equipment for bacterial analysis.
Itching, rash, shortness of breath.	Allergic reaction due to sensitivity to an intravenous fluid, additive or drug.	Ask the patient if he/she has any allergies *before* administration of any drugs or fluids. Check whether the particular medication is commonly associated with any allergic reactions and observe the patient during treatment.	Stop drug infusion or injection and maintain the patency of the VAD using 0.9% sodium chloride. Notify a doctor immediately. Reassure the patient. Ensure that hydrocortisone and adrenaline are available.
Flushed face, headache, congestion of the chest, possibly progressing to loss of consciousness.	Speed shock due to too rapid administration of drugs. May be a small volume (Perdue 1995; Lamb 1999)	Administer drugs and infusion at the correct rate. Check the flow rate frequently. Use infusion equipment with anti free flow administration sets if the delivery rate is crucial.	As above.

Ear Syringing

13

Definition

Ear syringing is the irrigation of the external auditory canal of the ear with water at body temperature using an ear syringe or electronic pulsed water unit. It is usually carried out by practice nurses to remove ear wax (cerumen) and, in some circumstances, foreign bodies. Irrigation of the ear should only be prescribed by a medical practitioner and only undertaken by an appropriately qualified practitioner.

Reference material

Anatomy of the ear

The ear can be divided into three parts: the external ear, the middle ear and the inner ear. Syringing is directed only at the external ear. The pinna (or auricle), the external auditory meatus and the tympanic membrane (ear drum) make up the external ear (Fig. 13.1).

The *pinna* is the prominent, visible part of the external ear which sits over the temporal bone of the skull. It consists of cartilage covered by perichondrium and skin. The *external auditory meatus* is an S-shaped canal which leads down from the pinna to the tympanic membrane. It is lined with epithelium continuous with that on the tympanic membrane. The meatus is 24–25 mm long in the adult with the outer third made of cartilage and the inner two-thirds made of bone (Corbridge 1998). Hair and sebaceous glands cover the cartilaginous part. Cerumen is produced in this area by modified sweat glands or apocrine glands (known as ceruminous glands). The *tympanic membrane* (or ear drum) forms the inner end of the external auditory canal. It is normally shiny and described as transparent, opaque or pearly grey (Ignatavicius *et al.* 1995). As part of the normal ageing process, the ear drum becomes whiter and duller (Webber-Jones 1992). Some structures of the middle ear are faintly visible through the normal tympanic membrane.

Foreign bodies

Foreign bodies are sometimes inserted into the external canal and may become lodged. Alternatively, insects or debris may be blown into the ear (Beare & Myers 1998). If the foreign body is composed of vegetable matter, irrigation and the use of liquids (e.g. mineral oil) are contraindicated because vegetable matter (e.g. peas, beans) is absorbent and swells up on contact with the liquid. Once swollen, the foreign body becomes more firmly lodged and therefore more difficult to remove.

Insects may be removed by instilling mineral oil, vegetable oil or diluted alcohol into the ear. The insect is usually killed and floats to the entrance of the auditory canal where it can be retrieved with Tilley's or other grasping forceps. Foreign bodies should only be removed by specialized medical staff. Referral to an ENT department must be made if the attempt is unsuccessful, there is suspected trauma to the ear drum or there is a risk of damaging the eardrum during removal (Corbridge 1998). To extract a solid foreign body a hook or Jobson horn probe is passed beyond the foreign body and gently pulled out (Corbridge 1998). Attempting this procedure without the necessary skills may result in the foreign body being forced into the bony portion of the canal, the skin in the canal being damaged, or the eardrum being perforated (Brunner & Suddarth 1989). Occasionally (for example if the patient is very young) general anaesthesia is required to remove foreign bodies.

Impaction of cerumen

Cerumen is continuously produced by ceruminous glands. The secretions mix with keratin debris produced by the migration of epithelial cells, in the external meatus (Rodgers 1997a). Cerumen protects and waterproofs the meatal skin and is slightly acidic, thereby providing antibacterial and antifungal properties (Rodgers 1997a). It is gradually moved towards the entrance of the auditory canal by the action of muscles used in chewing and talking and by surface migration. Hooper (1991) points out that 'people seem to be unaware that wax is necessary to protect the external auditory meatus and view its presence as a sign of poor personal hygiene'. Such public misconception contributes considerably to the amount of syringing performed (Sharp *et al.* 1990). Cotton-tipped swabs ('cotton buds') are used in an attempt to remove ear wax; however, this frequently pushes wax further into the canal and causes it to become impacted (Webber-Jones 1992).

If cerumen production is excessive, or if an obstruction prevents it moving towards the entrance to the auditory canal, the canal may become blocked with wax which hardens over time. People with large amounts of hair in their ears, or who work in dusty or dirty atmospheres, are

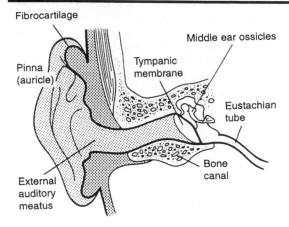

Figure 13.1 External auditory canal. The external one-third is formed of fibrocartilage; the inner two-thirds are bony.

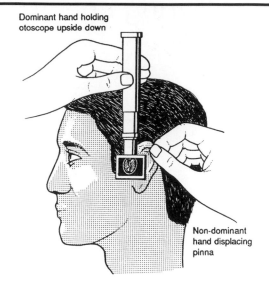

Figure 13.2 Technique for otoscopic examination.

more likely to experience excessive build-up of ear wax (Beare & Myers 1998).

Routine cleaning of the ear

In normal circumstances ear hygiene can be maintained by washing the pinna and external auditory meatus with soap and water and a face cloth. Patients should be advised not to insert anything into the ear further than the part that can be seen from the outside (Beare & Myers 1998). Cotton buds, match sticks and hairpins can damage the wall of the canal, cause wax to become impacted, increase the likelihood of otitis externa or perforate the tympanic membrane.

Examining the outer ear

The external auditory meatus and tympanic membrane must be examined with an otoscope by a qualified practitioner before the decision to irrigate the ear can be made. This has an ear piece (speculum), illumination to visualize the eardrum and magnification for accurate assessment (Phipps 1993).

A full history must be obtained from the patient of any relevant problems, particularly any previous perforations (Price 1997). It is also important to allow patients to describe their symptoms in detail. If pressure or movement of the pinna is painful, the patient may have an infection of the outer ear (otitis externa). Otitis externa is also associated with redness, scaling, itching, swelling, watery discharge and crusting of the external ear (Phipps 1993). Pain, hearing loss, tinnitus and otorrhoea (ear discharge) may indicate an infection of the middle ear, known as otitis media (Corbridge 1998). Otitis media may also be associated with headache, loss of appetite and nausea and vomiting (Brunner & Suddarth 1992). If an infection of the outer or middle ear is suspected, advice from a specialized medical practitioner should be sought. Blockage of the ear with impacted cerumen may cause a feeling of pressure or

fullness, muffled hearing, whistling, squeaking and crackling noises and discomfort (rarely pain).

Otoscopic examination using an appropriately sized speculum is carried out by first pulling the pinna upwards and backwards, which stretches the cartilaginous part of the external meatus (Fig. 13.2). The otoscope is held in the dominant hand while the pinna is gently pulled up and back by the non-dominant hand. The external auditory canal can be inspected as the speculum is carefully inserted into the ear. The walls of the canal are very sensitive and fragile. Rough contact with the end of the speculum is painful, and should be avoided. Holding the otoscope so that the ulnar surface of the hand is stabilized on the patient's temple (when the otoscope is reversed) or the patient's jaw or occiput (when the otoscope is upright) prevents scratching of the auditory canal with the speculum if the patient moves (Webber-Jones 1992).

In infants and young children the pinna is pulled down and back. The cartilaginous part of the external auditory meatus is proportionately smaller, and only a small, narrow speculum can be used. Otoscopic examination is therefore difficult. It is important that young patients have their head held gently and firmly by a skilled practitioner or trusted carer (Fig. 13.3) as sudden movement may damage the external canal or tympanic membrane (Ignatavicius et al. 1995).

The appearance of the tympanic membrane should be assessed (Fig. 13.4). In normal circumstances the tympanic membrane is intact (without perforations). The long and short processes of the malleus (a small bone in the middle ear) are visible through the membrane as white markings, and the umbo, where the malleus is connected with the tympanic membrane, appears as a white spot.

Light from the otoscope is reflected off the normal tympanic membrane from a triangle formed by the annulus and the umbo (the 'light reflex'). If the light is reflected in

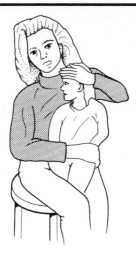

Figure 13.3 Holding a small child for examination of the ear.

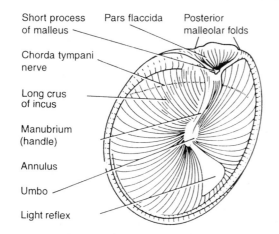

Short process of malleus
Pars flaccida
Posterior malleolar folds
Chorda tympani nerve
Long crus of incus
Manubrium (handle)
Annulus
Umbo
Light reflex

Figure 13.4 Right tympanic membrane.

an uneven way, the light reflex is said to be diffuse, and is abnormal.

Changes in the colour of the tympanic membrane, which is normally shiny, translucent and pearly grey, and the shape, which is normally slightly concave, may indicate an infection of the middle ear. Otitis media may make the tympanic membrane red; serous otitis may cause it to be dull or retracted. A bulging tympanic membrane indicates the presence of exudate in the middle ear.

Normally, the surface of the tympanic membrane is smooth and unmarked. Scarring is caused by previous infections and/or perforations. Ear syringing is contraindicated if the patient has a history of the following:

- Previous perforation of the tympanic membrane or surgery, e.g. mastoid, as syringing may result in unsterile water being forced into the middle ear or the mastoid cavity (Cook 1998).

- Recent or current middle ear infections, e.g. otitis media, as the tympanic membrane may be under pressure from mucus or pus and syringing would cause pain as well as the risk of perforating the membrane (Cook 1998).

Microsuction is used for patients with chronic ear disease, e.g. chronic otitis externa or media, and is performed by an ENT surgeon (Zeitoun *et al.* 1997). For this procedure the ear is examined using a speculum and a light microscope, an aural sucker is then used to identify and remove debris (Zeitoun *et al.* 1997).

Any abnormality identified in the external ear should be brought to the attention of appropriate medical staff, and advice on further action sought.

Irrigation of the external auditory canal

Irrigation is carried out with tap water at body temperature (37°C) using an ear syringe. Water that is too cold or too hot is uncomfortable, may damage tissues and can cause nausea, vomiting and dizziness by triggering the vestibular reflex. Approximately 300 ml are used in total, although no more than 50–70 ml are instilled at one time (Ignatavicius *et al.* 1995).

Electronic pulsed water units (e.g. the *Propulse* syringe) are available. These incorporate variable pressure settings, and are operated either by foot or hand controls. Detailed guidelines for the *Propulse* syringe are available from the Primary Ear Care Centre, Rotherham Health Authorities, which was set up in 1990. The Medical Devices Agency recommends that electric irrigators are connected to an isolated mains power supply to reduce the risk of electric shock, which may occur if water leaks inside the unit (Cook 1998).

A cerumenolytic product or baby oil, mineral oil or olive oil may be prescribed to soften ear wax that is too thick or dry to be removed immediately. These can be instilled 2–3 days prior to the procedure (Thurgood & Thurgood 1995). In certain circumstances softening agents may be used for up to 7 days (Sharp *et al.* 1990). Ear wax solvents can significantly reduce the need for syringing by breaking up the wax and allowing natural expulsion in 50% of patients with impacted ears (Keane *et al.* 1995). Ignatavicius *et al.* (1995) point out that removal of wax is a slow process, and may not be completed in one session.

Patients should be seated where there is a good source of light. Having assembled and prepared the equipment (see Guidelines, below) the tap water is warmed to body temperature. It is important to ensure that the ear syringe nozzle is firmly secured. An otoscopic examination of the external meatus is carried out to check the position of the ear wax and to confirm that the tympanic membrane is intact and there are no signs of external ear or middle ear infection. A waterproof covering is placed around the patient's neck and shoulder, and a receiver or Noots tank placed or held (by an assistant or the patient) under the ear. A Noots tank is a conical metal container shaped on one side of the rim to fit under the ear, and on the other to allow the syringe to be angled upwards.

The syringe is filled with 50–70 ml water. With the patient's head in an upright position, the ear is gently pulled upwards and backwards (downwards and backwards in children) and the tip of the syringe placed at an angle so that a low-pressure stream of water is directed upwards and backwards, rather than directly at the tympanic membrane (Bull 1996; Cook 1998) (Fig. 13.5). Directing a jet of water at the ear drum can cause a temporary perforation (Price 1997). The tip of the syringe should not occlude the meatus. The returning fluid should be examined for traces of the cerumen plug. Irrigation should be repeated with a further 50–70 ml of water. The ear should be examined intermittently throughout the procedure (Kaufman 1998), using the otoscope to ascertain the position of the wax plug and the condition of the external meatus. Irrigation may cause the tympanic membrane to appear pink. If the patient becomes nauseous or dizzy at any point during the procedure irrigation should be discontinued. If the cerumen has not been removed, irrigate with a further 50–70 ml. If it cannot be dislodged, medical advice about a suitable softening agent should be sought. An ENT surgeon may alternatively use microsuction to remove the wax (Corbridge 1998). In children ear drops are prescribed initially, then wax is removed by either a medical practitioner or an ENT surgeon. If the wax is hard, the child is very young or non-compliant or the attempt fails, the wax can be removed under a short acting anaesthetic (Birrell 1986).

Following the irrigation procedure, the canal should be examined to assess the effect of the irrigation and then dried. The head should be tilted to allow water and remaining debris to drain out. Where necessary a piece of cotton wool can be placed in the V formed by the tragus and antitragus to catch remaining irrigating solution (Webber-Jones 1992) (Fig. 13.5).

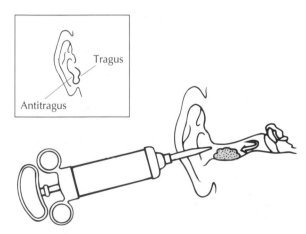

Figure 13.5 Irrigation of the ear with an ear syringe. A low-pressure stream of water is directed upwards and backwards towards the roof of the canal (Bull 1996; Cook 1998).

Follow-up and prevention

Lewis-Cullinan & Janken (1990) suggest that impacted cerumen is a common condition in the hospitalized elderly. Of a random sample of 226 patients, 35% were found to have either bilateral or unilateral cerumen impaction. Improved hearing was demonstrated in 75% of ears after cerumen had been removed. On the basis of this study the researchers suggest that the hearing health of the elderly can be promoted by routine otoscopic examinations by nurses in acute care of the elderly settings, followed by ear canal irrigation when impacted cerumen is found.

A patient with recurring buildup and plugging of excess cerumen may be taught to use a prescribed non-irritant softener regularly. Through education, patients will develop an understanding of how to prevent ear problems, recognizing the first signs of recurrence, and will therefore seek treatment sooner (Rodgers 1997b).

References and further reading

Beare, P.G. & Myers, J.L. (eds) (1998) *Principles and Practice of Adult Health Nursing*, 3rd edn., pp. 1160–84. Mosby, St Louis.

Birrell, J.F. (1986) *Paediatric Otolaryngology*, 2nd edn., Chapter 18. Wright, Bristol.

Booth, L. (1998) Ear syringing. *Practice Nurse*, **16**(9), 580–81.

Brunner, L.S. & Suddarth, D.S. (1989) *The Lippincott Manual of Medical–Surgical Nursing*, 2nd edn., pp. 867–83. Harper & Row, London.

Brunner, L.S. & Suddarth, D.S. (1992) *The Textbook of Adult Nursing*, pp. 950–70. Chapman & Hall, London.

Bull, P.D. (1996) *Lecture Notes on Diseases of the Ear, Nose and Throat*, 8th edn., pp. 30–37. Blackwell Science, Oxford.

Cook, R. (1998) Ear syringing. *Nurs Stand*, **13**(13–15), 56–61.

Corbridge, R.J. (1998) *Essential ENT Practice. A Clinical Text*, pp. 90–120, 156–62. Edward Arnold, London.

Hampson, G.D. (1994) *Bolden & Takle's Practice Nurse Handbook*, 3rd edn. Blackwell Scientific, Oxford.

Hooper, M. (1991) Aural hygiene and the use of cotton swabs. *Nurs Times*, **6**(12), 38–9.

Ignatavicius, D.D. *et al.* (eds) (1995) *Medical–Surgical Nursing: A Nursing Process Approach*, Vol. 2, pp. 1351–90. W.B. Saunders, Philadelphia.

Kaufman, G. (1998) Ear problems: care and prevention. *Practice Nurse*, **15**(6), 338, 340, 342.

Keane, E.M., Wilson, H., McGrane, D. *et al.* (1995) Use of solvents to disperse ear wax. *Br J Clin Pract*, **49**, 71–2.

Lewis-Cullinan, C. & Janken, J.K. (1990) Effect of cerumen removal on the hearing ability of geriatric patients. *J Adv Nurs*, **15**, 594–600.

Phipps, W.J. (1993) The patient with ear problems. In: *Medical–Surgical Nursing. A Nursing Process Approach*, 3rd edn. (eds B. Long, W. Phipps & V. Cassmeyer), pp. 1327–51. Mosby, St Louis.

Price, J. (1997) Problems of ear syringing. *Practice Nurse*, **14**(2), 126, 128.

Rodgers, R. (1997a) How safe is your syringing? *Commun Nurse*, **3**(5), 28, 29.

Rodgers, R. (1997b) Letters. Ear care advice should be updated. *Practice Nurse*, **14**(3), 214.

Sharp, J.F., Wilson, J.A., Ross, L. *et al.* (1990) Ear wax removal: a survey of current practice. *Br Med J*, **301**, 1251–3.

Thurgood, K. & Thurgood, G. (1995) Ear syringing: a clinical skill. *Br J Nurs*, **4**(12), 682–7.

Webber-Jones, J. (1992) Doomed to deafness? *Am J Nurs*, November, 37–9.

Zeitoun, H., Demajumdar, R., Hemmings, C. *et al.* (1997) Developing a nurse-led aural clinic. *Nurs Times*, **93**(45), 46, 47.

GUIDELINES • Irrigating the external auditory canal

Irrigation of the external auditory canal to remove impacted cerumen is normally carried out by nursing staff, particularly practice nurses. Only suitably qualified nurses should perform this procedure.

Equipment

1 Lamp.
2 Tray.
3 Otoscope and range of specula.
4 200–300 ml tap water in suitable container.
5 Lotion thermometer.
6 Waterproof covering.
7 Ear syringe/pulsed water unit.
8 Receiver/Noots tank.
9 Cotton swabs.
10 Yellow clinical waste bag.

Procedure

Action	Rationale
1 Explain and discuss the procedure with the patient.	To ensure that the patient understands the procedure and gives his/her valid consent.
2 Position the patient's chair and direct the lamp.	To allow the nurse to move freely and to illuminate the ear clearly.
3 Examine the ear with the otoscope.	To confirm position of the cerumen and that there are no contraindications to irrigation (e.g. perforations in ear drum; infection; vegetable matter foreign body; grommets).
4 Ask the patient to sit with head in upright position.	To facilitate drainage of irrigation fluid.
5 Arrange waterproof covering over patient's neck and shoulder.	To protect clothing from irrigation fluid and debris.
6 Ask assistant or patient to hold the receiver or Noots tank below the ear, close to the head.	To catch irrigation fluid and debris.
7 Check temperature of water with lotion thermometer.	Irrigation fluid should be at body temperature to avoid triggering vestibular reflex.
8 Draw up water into the ear syringe and holding the nozzle upwards, expel any air.	To ensure an even flow of water without air bubbles.
Or, run water through tubing of the pulsed water unit.	To expel any air or cold water remaining in the tubing.
9 Make sure the syringe nozzle or tip of the pulsed water unit is firmly secured.	The auditory canal may be damaged or the ear drum perforated if the nozzle or tip flies off under pressure from the water.
10 Pull ear gently upwards and backwards (adults); downwards and backwards (children).	To stretch and straighten external auditory canal; to hold the ear steady to prevent injury.
11 Place tip of ear syringe at entrance to meatus but do not occlude it; direct low-pressure stream of water (50–70 ml) upwards and backwards towards the roof of the canal (Bull 1996; Cook 1998).	Water should flow behind the cerumen plug and back along the canal to wash it out; too forceful a stream of water may force the plug back along the canal or rupture the tympanic membrane.
12 If the patient experiences dizziness or nausea, discontinue the irrigation.	To prevent further triggering of the vestibular reflex.
13 Observe solution in receiver/Noots tank for traces of dislodged ear wax.	To evaluate effect of irrigation.

Guidelines • Irrigating the external auditory canal (cont'd)

Action	Rationale
14 Examine external auditory meatus with otoscope.	To determine position and size of cerumen plug and monitor condition of ear.
15 Irrigate ear with 50–70 ml water once or twice more if necessary.	To remove remaining ear wax.
16 Ask patient to tilt head to allow water to drain, and place cotton swab below meatus.	To dry ear without irritating or damaging canal.
17 Carry out final examination of ear with otoscope.	To confirm removal of cerumen, and monitor condition of external meatus and tympanic membrane.
18 If any abnormality is observed, refer patient to medical practitioner.	Medical advice is required if cerumen plug has not been removed, or further treatment is necessary.
19 Remove waterproof covering and ensure patient is comfortable.	
20 Wash the aural speculum and syringe nozzle in hot soapy water, and dry.	To maintain hygiene.
21 To disinfect equipment, wash in hot soapy water, dry and then immerse in 70% ethanol. Dry equipment after immersion.	To reduce the risk of cross-infection. 70% ethanol does not penetrate organic matter.
22 If equipment can be autoclaved, it may be sterilized by this method.	Autoclaving is the most effective sterilization method.
23 Wipe over the syringe plunger with instrument lubricating oil.	To ensure free movement when the plunger is depressed.

Entonox Administration

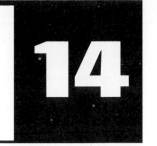

14

Definition

Entonox is a gaseous mixture of 50% oxygen and 50% nitrous oxide which acts as an analgesic agent when inhaled. The mixture of oxygen and nitrous oxide remains stable at temperatures of above –6°C.

Indications

Nitrous oxide is a powerful analgesic in sub-anaesthetic concentrations. It has the advantage of providing very rapid onset of analgesia (BOC 1998a). It is extensively used in obstetrics and the ambulance service. It has also proved highly effective in controlling the pain of myocardial infarctions and various uncomfortable interventions during intensive care. The duration of its analgesic effect is limited by its effect upon bone marrow (BOC 1998a).

Entonox is used exclusively for the relief of pain. The use of Entonox is indicated before and during a number of painful procedures because it has several advantages:

1 It has a rapid onset of analgesic effect.
2 It has a very short half-life and thus can wear off within 2–5 minutes (BOC 1998a).
3 The gas has no depressive effects on respiratory or cardiovascular functions. It can, therefore, be considered for short-term relief for procedures inevitably involving pain, such as:
   (a) Wound and burn dressing, wound debridement and suturing.
   (b) Normal labour.
   (c) Changing or removing of packs and drains.
   (d) Removal of sutures from sensitive areas, e.g. the vulva.
   (e) Invasive procedures such as catheterization and sigmoidoscopy.
   (f) Removal of radioactive intracavity gynaecological applicators.
   (g) Altering the position of a patient who experiences incident pain.
   (h) Manual evacuation of the bowel in severe constipation.
   (i) Acute trauma, e.g. applying orthopaedic traction following pathological fracture.
   (j) Physiotherapy procedures, particularly postoperatively.

Contraindications

Entonox should not be used with any of the following conditions:

1 Maxilofacial injuries – as the patient may not be able to hold the mask tightly to the face or use the mouthpiece adequately. There is a risk of causing further damage to facial wounds and there may also be a significant risk of blood inhalation.
2 Head injuries with impairment of consciousness.
3 Heavily sedated patients – as they would be unable to breathe in the Entonox on demand and to potentiate sedation further may be hazardous.
4 Intoxicated patients – as drowsiness and aspiration would be a hazard in the event of vomiting.
5 Pneumothorax, bowel obstruction or abdominal distension (BOC 1998a). The nitrous oxide constituent of Entonox passes into all gas-containing spaces in the body faster than nitrogen passes out. Therefore, Entonox must not be used where air is entrapped within a body and where its expansion might be dangerous.
6 Decompression illness or a recent dive (the 'bends') – as nitrous oxide escapes into the blood stream and increases the size of the nitrogen bubbles in the tissues.
7 Laryngectomy patients – as they will be unable to use the apparatus.
8 Temperatures of below –6°C as separation of the gases occurs.

Caution

The very young and very old may require additional care in the administration of Entonox due to possible mask fitting difficulties or inability to understand instructions for use. Consideration should be given to the patient's ability to use the Entonox, for example very dyspnoeic patients or those with reduced lung capacity may not be able to tolerate deep inhalation of the gas.

Reference material

Despite increasing awareness of pain control by health professionals and the availability of a wide variety of analgesic agents, the area of pain control for patients undergoing painful procedures is often inadequate. There are many reasons for this including inadequate assessment, prior to a procedure, underestimation of a patient's pain and difficulty of judging at the outset how painful a procedure will prove to be. The specific goal of clinical pain assessment should be to expand our knowledge of the existing types of pain and to develop assessment techniques for treatment, which have a valid, scientific basis (Foley 1997) (see also

Chap. 29, Pain assessment and management). Hollinworth (1995) describes poor assessment and management of pain control at wound dressing changes and discusses the difficulties clinicians may have in assessing pain, which during a dressing change may be brief but intense (Entonox is recommended in this situation). This is often true for many other procedures, and Entonox provides an effective analgesia which can be self-administered to provide immediate pain relief.

Nurses, midwives and physiotherapists may be able to administer Entonox (according to local policy) without a written prescription from a doctor. Entonox also provides patients with some control over their pain during painful procedures with minimal side-effects.

To wait for a doctor to prescribe analgesia or to wait for a prescribed analgesic to take effect is sometimes difficult or unacceptable. In these situations an analgesic which could be prescribed and administered by other qualified health care professionals, which would take immediate effect and be rapidly excreted from the body with few side-effects is the ideal (Diggory 1979). Entonox fulfils these criteria but is underutilized. Hollinworth (1995) advocates wider availability of Entonox and staff training through workshops to improve its use and heighten awareness of health professionals to its potential.

Equipment

The Entonox cylinder is coloured blue and has a white band on the shoulder (Fig. 14.1). The apparatus needed for administration consists of the cylinder, the Bodok seal, inhalation tubing and the handpiece. Either a mask or a mouthpiece may be used.

Principle of administration

Entonox is designed for self-administration by the patient. The apparatus works as a demand unit, i.e. gas can be obtained only by the patient inhaling from the mouthpiece or mask and producing a negative pressure (Fig. 14.2). The gas flow stops when the patient removes the mouthpiece or mask from their face. Therefore, the patient must hold the mask firmly over the face or mouthpiece to the lips to produce an airtight fit and breathe in before the gas will flow. Expired gases escape by the expiratory valve on the handpiece. It is essential to adhere to this method of self-administration as it is then impossible for patients to overdose themselves because if they become drowsy they will relax their grip on the handset and the gas flow will cease when no negative pressure is applied. Doses may be self-

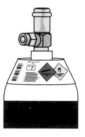

Figure 14.1 Collar-type cylinder label. [Reproduced with kind permission of BOC Group plc (1999). BOC and BOC GASES are trademarks of the BOC Group plc.]

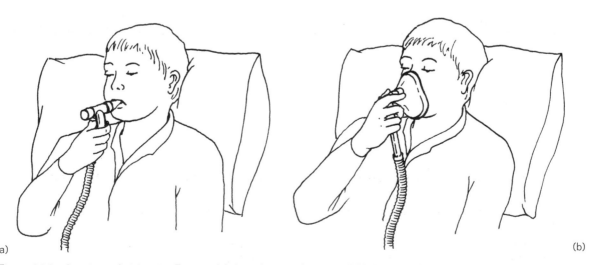

(a)

(b)

Figure 14.2 A patient administering Entonox (a) through a mouthpiece and (b) through a face mask. (Courtesy of BOC Medical Gases.)

regulated, but additionally may be administered by attendant medical personnel trained in its use, e.g. within obstetric/accident and emergency units, and accident ambulances. Since pain is usually relieved with a concentration of 25% nitrous oxide (BOC 1998a), continued inhalation does not usually occur. However, should inhalation continue, light anaesthesia supervenes and the mask drops away as the patient relaxes.

Entonox has an oxygen content two-and-a-half times that of air and is, therefore, a good way of giving extra oxygen as well as providing analgesia.

Use during pregnancy and lactation

It has been suggested that prolonged exposure to high levels of nitrous oxide may affect a woman's ability to become pregnant (BOC 1998a). Mild skeletal teratogenic changes have been observed in pregnant rat embryos when the dam (pregnant mother) has been exposed to high levels of nitrous oxide during the period of organogenesis. However, no increased incidence of fetal malformation has been discovered in eight epidemiological studies and case reports in human-beings (Matheson Gas Products 1971; Compressed Gas Association 1990). No published material shows that nitrous oxide is toxic to the human fetus. Therefore, there is no absolute contraindication to its use in the first 15 weeks of pregnancy.

Complications

Inappropriate inhalation of Entonox will ultimately result in unconsciousness, passing through stages of increasing lightheadedness and intoxication. The treatment is removal to fresh air, mouth to mouth resuscitation and, if necessary, the use of an oxygen resuscitator (BOC 1998a).

References and further reading

BOC (1994) *Gas Safe – In the Hospital* (video). BOC Gases, Manchester.

BOC (1995) *Entonox in Midwifery* (video). BOC Gases, Manchester.

BOC (1997) *Gas Safe – With Medical Gases. A Guide to the Safe Use of Medical Gas Cylinders.* BOC Gases, Manchester.

BOC (1998a) *BOC Gases Data Sheet.* BOC Gases, Manchester.

BOC (1998b) *Safe Under Pressure.* BOC Gases, Manchester.

BOC (1999) *Inhalation Pain Control* (video). BOC Gases, Manchester.

Compressed Gas Association (1990) *Handbook of Compressed Gases.* Van Nostrand Reinhold, New York.

Diggory, G. (1979) Entonox and its role in nursing care. *Nursing,* April, 28–31.

Doyle, D., Hanks, G.W.C. & MacDonald, N. (eds) (1994) *Oxford Textook of Palliative Medicine.* Oxford Medical Publications, Oxford.

Foley, K.M. (1997) The treatment of cancer pain. *New Engl J Med,* **1085**(3131), 84–95.

Hollinworth, H. (1995) Nurses' assessment and management of pain at wound dressing changes. *J Wound Care,* 4(2), 77–83.

Matheson Gas Products (1971) *Gas Data Book.* Matheson Gas Products, Wisconsin.

Msi, J. (1981) The use of Entonox for the relief of pain experienced by cancer patients. In: *Cancer Nursing Update* (ed. R. Tiffany). Baillière Tindall, London.

Reynolds, J.E.F. (ed. Martindale) (1993) *The Extra Pharmacopoeia,* 13th edn. Pharmaceutical Press, London.

Toulson, S. (1990) More than a lot of hot air. *Nursing,* 4(2), 23–6.

GUIDELINES · Entonox administration

Equipment

1 Entonox cylinder and head.
2 Face mask and/or mouthpiece.

Procedure

Action	*Rationale*
1 Explain and discuss the procedure with the patient.	To ensure that the patient understands the procedure and gives his/her valid consent.
2 Turn the tap on the Entonox cylinder in an anticlockwise direction.	To ascertain if there is any Entonox in the cylinder.
3 Examine the gauge to determine how much gas is in the cylinder.	To ensure an adequate supply of gas throughout the procedure.
4 Ensure that the patient is in as comfortable a position as possible.	

Guidelines • Entonox administration (cont'd)

Action	Rationale
5 Demonstrate how to use the apparatus by holding the mask tightly to your face. Explain to the patient that when the patient breathes in and out regularly and deeply a hissing sound will be heard, indicating that the gas is being inhaled.	To ensure that the patient understands what to do and what to expect before any painful procedure commences.
6 Allow the patient to practise using the apparatus.	To enable the patient to adopt the correct technique and for the nurse to observe the analgesic effect of the gas before the procedure commences.
7 Encourage the patient to breathe gas in and out for at least 2 min before commencing any painful procedure.	To allow sufficient time for an adequate circulatory level of nitrous oxide to provide analgesia. (When the patient inhales, gas enters first the lungs then the pulmonary and systemic circulations. It takes 1–2 min to build up reasonable concentrations of nitrous oxide in the brain.)
8 During the procedure encourage the patient to breathe in and out regularly and deeply.	To maintain adequate circulatory levels, thus providing adequate analgesia.
9 At the end of the procedure observe the patient until the effects of the gas have worn off.	Some patients may feel a transient drowsiness or giddiness and should be discouraged from getting out of bed until these effects have worn off. It is rare for the patient to experience transient amnesia (BOC 1999).
10 Evaluate the effectiveness of Entonox with the patient throughout, and following procedures, by verbal questioning and encouraging the patient to self-assess the analgesic effect.	To establish whether the Entonox has been a useful analgesic for the procedure. This should then be documented to assist any subsequent procedures, e.g. dressing changes.
11 Turn off Entonox supply from the cylinder by turning the tap in a clockwise direction. The gauge should read 'Empty'.	To avoid potential seepage of gas from the apparatus.
12 Depress the diaphragm under the valve.	To remove residual gas from tubing.
13 Wash the face mask, expiratory valve and handpiece in hot soapy water.	To reduce the risk of cross-infection.
Note: if the patient is known or suspected to be infected, e.g. hepatitis B or MRSA, then the equipment must be sent to the Sterile Services Department for disinfection.	
14 Record the administration on appropriate documentation.	To promote continuity of care, maintain accurate records and provide a point of reference in the event of any queries.

Nursing care plan

Problem	Cause	Suggested action
Patient not experiencing adequate analgesic effect.	Entonox cylinder empty. Apparatus not properly connected.	Check before procedure commences.
	Patient not inhaling deeply enough.	Encourage the patient to breathe in until a hissing noise can be heard from the cylinder. Reassess suitability of patient for Entonox use. The patient may not be strong enough or have reduced lung capacity to inhale deeply.

	Patient inhaling pure oxygen, i.e. cylinder has been stored below −6°C and nitrous oxide has liquified and settled at the bottom of the cylinder. (All cylinders should be stored horizontally at a temperature of 10°C or above for 24h before use.)	Initially safe, but later the patient may inhale pure nitrous oxide and be asphyxiated. Discontinue the procedure. Ensure adequate warming of the cylinder and inversion of the cylinder to remix the gases adequately.
	Not enough time has been allowed for nitrous oxide to exert its analgesic effect.	Allow at least 2min of Entonox use before commencing the procedure.
Patient experiences generalized muscle rigidity.	Hyperventilation during inhalation.	Discontinue Entonox and allow the patient to recover. Explain the procedure again, stressing deep and regular inspiration. Use a mouthpiece in place of a mask.
Patient unable to tolerate a mask.	Smell of rubber, feeling of claustrophobia.	Use a mouthpiece in place of a mask.
Patient feels nauseated, drowsy or giddy.	Effect of nitrous oxide accumulation.	Discontinue Entonox administration – the effect will then rapidly disappear.
Patient afraid to use Entonox.	Associates gases with previous hospital procedures, e.g. anaesthesia before surgery.	Reassure patient and reiterate instructions for use and short-term effects.

Epidural Analgesia

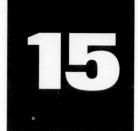

Definition

Epidural analgesia is the administration of analgesics and anti-inflammatory drugs into the epidural space. Analgesic drugs may be divided into two categories:

1 Local anaesthetics, which provide a conduction block for sensory stimuli.
2 Opiates which act within the central nervous system by attaching to specific opiate receptors in the substantia gelatinosa and the thalamus (Marieb 1996).

Both groups of drugs provide excellent analgesia and each has its own specific side-effects:

1 Local anaesthetics. The main side-effects are related to sympathetic and motor neuronal blockade. Sympathetic blockade may result in hypotension, due to vascular dilatation, requiring treatment with volume expanders and/or vasoconstrictors such as Ephedrine. Motor blockade will result in temporary paralysis of muscle groups supplied by the affected nerve segments.
2 Opiates. The main side-effect is that of respiratory depression, which may require treatment with intravenous naloxone and respiratory therapy. A further minor, though significant, side-effect can be pruritis, requiring treatment with antihistamine and calamine (McNair 1990).

A side-effect common to both classes of analgesics is urinary retention which may require catheterization.

Indications

1 Provision of analgesia during labour.
2 As an alternative to general anaesthesia, e.g. in severe respiratory disease or for patients with malignant hyperthermia.
3 As a supplement to general anaesthesia.
4 Provision of postoperative analgesia.
5 Provision of analgesia for pain resulting from trauma, e.g. fractured ribs, which may result in respiratory failure due to pain on breathing.
6 Management of chronic intractable pain, e.g. from bone metastases.
7 To relieve muscle spasm and pain resulting from lumbar cord pressure due to disc protrusion or local oedema and inflammation.

Contraindications

These may be absolute or relative.

Absolute:

1 Patients with coagulation defects, which may result in epidural haematoma formation and spinal cord compression, e.g. iatrogenic (anticoagulated patient) or congenital (haemophiliacs), or thrombocytopenia due to disease or as the result of anticancer treatment (Horlocker & Wedel 1998).
2 Local sepsis at the site of proposed epidural injection; the result might be meningitis or epidural abscess formation.
3 Proven allergy to the intended drug.
4 Unstable spinal fracture.
5 Patient refusal to consent to the procedure.

Relative:

1 Unstable cardiovascular system.
2 Spinal deformity.
3 Raised intracranial pressure (a risk of herniation if a dural tap occurs).
4 Certain neurological conditions, e.g. multiple sclerosis (Morgan 1989).

Reference material

Anatomy of the epidural space

The epidural space lies between the spinal dura and ligamentum flavum. Its average diameter is 0.5 cm and it is widest in the midline posteriorly in the lumbar region. The contents of the epidural space include a rich venous plexus, spinal arterioles, lymphatics and extradural fat (Fig. 15.1).

Spinal nerves traverse the epidural space laterally. There are 31 pairs of spinal nerves of varying size. The two main groups of nerve fibres are:

1 Myelinated – myelin is a thin, fatty sheath which insulates the fibres, preventing impulses being transmitted to adjacent fibres. Myelin also protects fibres and speeds of impulses.
2 Unmyelinated – delicate fibres, more susceptible to hypoxia and toxins than myelinated fibres.

The spinal nerves are composed of a posterior and anterior root, which join to form a spinal nerve:

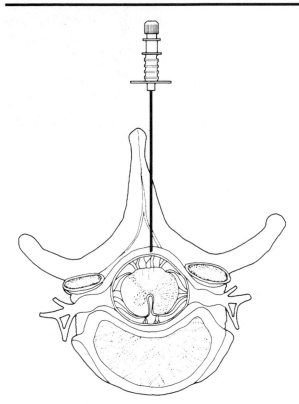

Figure 15.1 Positioning of Tuohy needle. [Courtesy of Crul, B. & Delhaas, E. (1991) Technical complications during long-term subarachnoid or epidural administration of morphine in terminally ill cancer patients. *Regional Anaesthesia*, **16**, 209–13.]

1 Posterior root – transmits ascending sensory impulses from the periphery to the spinal cord.
2 Anterior root – transmits descending motor impulses from the spinal cord to the periphery by means of its corresponding spinal nerve.

Common solutions used

1 Local anaesthetics – either plain or with adrenaline 1 : 200 000: A solution containing adrenaline is used primarily during surgery to minimize blood loss. Adrenaline achieves this by causing constriction of blood vessels.
   (a) Bupivacaine: slower onset of action, but longer duration (2–8 hours).
   (b) Lignocaine 0.5–2%: rapid onset, short duration (1–2 hours).
2 Opiates: diamorphine, morphine and fentanyl are the most commonly used opiates.

Spread of local anaesthetic solutions

Spread of local anaesthetic solutions is influenced by the following:

1 Volume injected.
2 Integrity of central nervous system.
3 Force of injection.
4 Level of catheter.
5 Drug concentration.

Mode of injection

1 Bolus injections
2 Continuous infusions
3 Combined infusion/bolus method, i.e. background infusion with boluses as required if analgesia inadequate.

Methods of administration: acute pain management

1 Continuous infusions
   An increasing number of units are using a combination of one or more drugs as a continuous infusion. Drugs used vary according to the clinical situation. A variety of opiates may be used, e.g. diamorphine, fentanyl. In most cases, a 30 or 60 ml syringe containing the selected drug is run at a rate prescribed by the anaesthetic team. The rate can be increased or decreased as necessary. The syringe pump should be monitored to ensure that the correct dose is given and that the pump is working accurately.
   The most important, and potentially fatal, complication of spinal opiates is respiratory depression, which may be delayed up to 12 hours after the continuous infusion is commenced. *All* patients must be observed constantly and the rate of their respiration, depth and pattern recorded. The use of pulse oximeters to continually display oxygen saturation is now employed in most units. Blood gases may need to be taken and oxygen therapy administered if appropriate (McNair 1990).
   After 24 hours if there have been no complications and the pain control is judged to be acceptable by the patient/nursing staff, the patient may be transferred to a general ward area. However, hourly observation of respiratory rate and oxygen saturation levels must be maintained (Royal College of Anaesthetists 1991).
2 Bolus administered by nurse or doctor, when required.
3 Patient-controlled administration using a microprocessor-controlled infusion device (see Chap. 20, Infusion Devices).

Complications of epidural analgesia

1 Headache or backache or lack of mobilization.
2 Backache has been produced occasionally from local irritation caused by the needle or catheter.
3 Intraocular haemorrhage has been reported after rapid injection of 30 ml of fluid. This is thought to raise cerebrospinal fluid pressure, with resultant intraocular bleeding.
4 Extradural abscess may take up to 16 days to develop. Extradural abscess or haematoma should be drained on diagnosis, otherwise paraplegia may result (Mackenzie *et al.* 1998).

Epidural analgesia for patients with cancer and chronic pain

Epidural analgesia may be chosen for cancer patients with intractable pain. When the epidural route is chosen for this indication, there are several issues that are only relevant in the chronic setting. The next section will apply to the special considerations required in the chronic setting. It is also important to remember the clinical guidelines that are followed, i.e. stringent postoperative observations in acute care of epidural pain management, essential following general anaesthetic, may not be appropriate in the chronic pain setting.

Analgesia given as an infusion via the epidural route has been used since the late 1970s to relieve the chronic pain experienced by patients with cancer (Wang *et al.* 1979). The rationale for selecting the epidural route is based on the premise that lower doses of opioids are required to effect pain control and that the patient should therefore experience fewer side-effects (De Conno *et al.* 1995).

It has been demonstrated that there are many logistical and technical complications associated with an indwelling spinal catheter and the use of a pump (Ben *et al.* 1991). It is therefore expected that only those patients whose pain is refractory to oral or parenteral therapy, or who have intolerable side-effects from standard analgesia, will be selected for a trial of epidural analgesia.

Indications

If the patient is to stay in the hospital or hospice setting but all other routes for pain management have failed.

Contraindications

Absolute contraindications:

1 Evidence of severe systemic infection
2 Grossly abnormal clotting
3 Platelet count below 50×10^9/litre.

Social contraindications:

1 The patient/family or their primary care team may not be able to fulfil the recommendations described above.

Discharge planning

To ensure that patients have previously received optimum systemic therapy they should have been assessed by the palliative care team. Before any decision is made to use the epidural route it is imperative to assess the individual patient's suitability and this assessment should be completed before any discharge date is discussed with the patient/family.

The patient should be assessed for the following:

1 Physical and mental ability to comply
2 Availability of personnel trained in the delivery of epidural analgesia
3 Availability of a suitable electronic pump.

If the patient wishes to go home it is essential that certain issues have been addressed. First, that the general practitioner and the district nursing team are willing to be involved and be trained in the care. Second, that the patient is geographically located near a centre that regularly uses epidural analgesia. It is also important that there is a family or social network that can support the patient if there are problems with the catheter or pump. Finally, reconstitution of the syringes/bags needs to be provided as well as organization of transport to the home.

Once the decision has been made that the patient can receive treatment at home, it should be explained that they will need a period of time in hospital, following insertion of the catheter, to allow for dose adjustment and ensure that optimum pain management is achieved. During this time coordination of community services to manage the care of the epidural can be arranged. A discussion must also take place with the patient and family before consent is obtained to insert the catheter to ensure that they are aware of likely side-effects, particularly altered sensation in their legs and possible alterations in mobility.

Dose calculations

In order to ensure that the patient will receive the optimum opioid dose, the palliative care team will review the patient's previous opioid prescription and convert the dose to the equivalent epidural dose as described below:

1 *Conversion of oral to epidural:* the epidural opiate dose is one tenth of the oral dose, for example 180 mg morphine sulphate twice a day converts to 36 mg of opiate via the epidural route in 24 hours.
2 *Conversion of subcutaneous to epidural:* the epidural dose is one third of the subcutaneous dose, for example 90 mg diamorphine subcutaneously over 24 hours is the same as 30 mg of epidural diamorphine over 24 hours.
3 *Local anaesthetic drugs:* the drug of choice is bupivacaine due to its long duration of action and predominant action on sensory rather than motor fibres. Bupivacaine is normally commenced in a concentration of 0.125%, but concentrations up to 0.5% are often required to block resistant pain. However, concentrations above 0.25% are associated with motor block (weakness) and autonomic block (urinary retention requiring catheterization).

References and further reading

Adam, S. (1985) Epidural anaesthesia. *Nurs Mirror*, **160**(10), 38–41.

Allcock, N. (1996) The use of different research methodologies to evaluate the effectiveness of programmes to improve the care of patients in postoperative pain. *J Adv Nurs*, **23**, 32–8.

Atkinson, R. & Murray, P. (1995) Opioids and non-steroidal anti-inflammatory drugs in chronic pain. *Curr Opin Anaesth*, **8**, 342–6.

Ben, J.P., Crul, M.D. & Delhaas, E.M. (1991) Technical complications during long-term subarachnoid or epidural administration of morphine in terminally ill cancer patients: a review of 140 cases. *Reg Anesth*, **16**, 209–13.

Bibbings, J. (1984) Epidural analgesia. *Nurs Times*, **80**(35), 53–5.

Brown, E. (1990) Narcotics via the epidural route (Part 1). *Nurs Stand*, **4**(38), 24–39; Part II, *Nurs Stand*, **4**(39), 37–9.

Crul, B. & Delhaas, E. (1991) Technical complications during long-term subarachnoid or epidural administration of morphine in terminally ill cancer patients. *Reg Anesth*, **16**, 209–13.

de Boek, R. *et al.* (1990) *Patient-Controlled Analgesia*. The Royal Marsden Hospital (Patient Information Series) (unpublished), London.

De Conno, F., Ripamonte, C. & Ticozzi, C. (1995) Intraspinal opioids and local anaesthetics for cancer pain. *Eur J Palliat Care*, **1**(4), 162–8.

De Jong, P.C. & Kansen, P.J. (1994) A comparison of epidural catheters with or without subcutaneous injection ports for treatment of cancer pain. *Reg Anesth Pain Manage*, **78**, 94–100.

De Leon-Casasola, O.A., Myers, D.P., Donaparthi, S. *et al.* (1993) A comparison of post-operative epidural analgesia between patients with chronic cancer taking high doses of oral opioids versus opioid-naïve patients. *Anesth Analg*, **76**, 302–307.

Du Pen, S.L., Kharasch, E.D., Williams, A. *et al.* (1992) Chronic epidural bupivacaine – opioid infusion in intractable cancer pain. *Pain*, **49**, 293–300.

Du Pen, S.L. & Williams, A.R. (1994) The dilemma of conversion from systemic to epidural morphine: a proposed conversion tool for treatment of cancer pain. *Pain*, **56**, 113–18.

Greenland, S. (1995) A review of the uses of epidural analgesia. *Nurs Stand*, **9**(32), 33–5.

Hancock, H. (1996) Implementing change in the management of postoperative pain. *Intens Crit Care Nurs*, **12**, 359–62.

Hansberry, J.L., Bannick, K.H. & Durkan, M.J. (1990) Managing chronic pain with a permanent epidural catheter. *Nursing*, October, 53–4.

Hicks, F., Simpson, K.H. & Tosh, G.C. (1994) Management of spinal infusions in palliative care. *Palliat Med*, **8**, 325–32.

Hogan, Q., Haddox, J., Abram, S. *et al.* (1991) Epidural opiates and local anesthetics for the management of the cancer pain. *Pain*, **46**, 271–9.

Horlucker, T. & Wedel, D. (1998) Spinal and epidural blockade and perioperative low molecular weight heparin: smooth sailing on the Titanic. *Anaesth Analg*, **8**, 1153–6.

MacConnacline, A.M. (1996) Low molecular weight heparins. *Intens Crit Care Nurs*, **12**, 309–10.

Mackenzie AR. *et al.* (1998) Spinal epidural abscess: the importance of early diagnosis and treatment. *J Neurosurg Psychiatry*, **65**(2), 209–12.

MacLellan, K. (1997) A chart audit reviewing the prescription and administration trends of analgesia and documentation of pain, after surgery. *J Adv Nurs*, **26**, 345–50.

Marieb, E.N. (1996) *Human Anatomy and Physiology*. Benjamin/ Cummings, Wokingham.

Mallett, J. & Bailey, C. (1996) *The Royal Marsden NHS Trust Manual of Clinical Nursing Procedures*, 4th edn. Blackwell Science, Oxford.

McNair, N.D. (1990) Epidural narcotics for post-operative pain – nursing implications. *J Neurosci Nurs*, **22**(5), 275–9.

Mercadante, S. (1994) Intrathecal morphine and bupivacaine in advanced cancer pain patients implanted at home. *J Pain Sympt Manage*, **9**(3), 201–207.

Morgan, M. (1989) The rational use of intrathecal and extradural opioids. *Br J Anaesth*, **63**, 165–8.

Olsson, G.L., Leddo, C.C. & Wild, L. (1989) Nursing management of patients receiving epidural narcotics. *Heart Lung*, **18**(2), 130–38.

Owen, H. *et al.* (1988) The development and clinical use of patient-controlled analgesia. *Anaesth Intens Care*, **16**, 437–47.

Royal College of Surgeons of England and College of Anaesthetists (1990) *Report of the Working Party on Pain After Surgery*, pp. 15–17.

Stephenson, N.L. (1994) A comparison of nurse and patient perceptions of postsurgical pain. *J Intraven Nurs*, **17**(5), 235–9.

Tanelian, D.L. & Cousins, M.J. (1989) Failure of epidural opioid to control cancer pain in a patient previously treated with massive doses of intravenous opioid. *Pain*, **36**, 359–62.

Wang, J.K., Nauss, N.A. & Thomas, J.E. (1979) Pain relief by intrathecally applied morphine in man. *Anesthesiology*, **50**, 149–51.

Yap K.B. (1994) Epidural infection associated with epidural catheterization in a cancer patient with back pain: case report. *Palliat Med*, **8**, 251–3.

Yarde, A. (1989) Epidural analgesia. *Prof Nurse*, **4**, Part 12, 608–13.

GUIDELINES · Insertion of an epidural catheter

Note: patients undergoing epidural analgesia should always have venous access or an intravenous infusion in situ before the procedure as reaction to the opiate or local anaesthetic can rarely cause emergencies necessitating immediate IV access such as respiratory depression or sympathetic blockade.

Equipment

1 Chlorhexidine in 70% alcohol.
2 Local anaesthetic.
3 Selection of needles and syringes.
4 Sterile dressing pack.
5 Face mask.
6 Tuohy needle or assorted gauge lumbar puncture needles.
7 Epidural catheter.
8 Bacterial filter.
9 Waterproof dressing and plastic adhesive dressing to tape catheter securely.

Procedure

Action

1 Explain and discuss the procedure with the patient.
   If the intention is to provide postoperative analgesia then explanation and consent should have been discussed the day before surgery.

Rationale

To ensure that the patient understands the procedure and gives his/her valid consent and to ensure patient has time to assess information and ask questions.

Guidelines • Insertion of an epidural catheter (cont'd)

Action	Rationale
2 Assist the patient into the required position: (a) Lying: 　Position pillow under patient's head. 　Firm surface. 　On side with knee drawn up to the abdomen and clasped by the hands. 　Support the patient in this position.	To ensure maximum widening of the intervertebral spaces, providing easier access to the epidural space. To prevent the catheter being dislodged and sudden movement which could result in accidental malplacement of the epidural needle.
(b) Sitting: 　Patient sits on firm surface with arms resting on a table, and with the head resting on the arms.	Allows proper identification of the spinal processes and therefore invertebral spaces.
3 Support, encourage and observe the patient throughout the procedure.	As procedure takes place behind the patient, reassurance is very important.
4 Assist the doctor as required. The doctor will proceed as follows:	
(a) Clean the skin with alcohol-based solution (e.g. chorhexidine in 70% isopropyl alcohol).	To maintain asepsis.
(b) Identify the area to be punctured and inject the skin and subcutaneous layers with local anaesthetic.	
(c) Introduce Tuohy or spinal needles usually between third and fourth lumbar vertebrae.	
(d) Ensure epidural space has been entered.	To prevent anaesthesia being given directly into spinal cord or intravenously by means of the dural veins.
(e) Inject test dose of drug (may be performed).	To ensure the position of the needle.
(f) Thread epidural catheter through barrel of Tuohy needle.	To facilitate intermittent topping-up of anaesthesia and to allow greater control.
(g) Attach the bacterial filter.	To prevent injection of contaminants into epidural space.
(h) Apply transparent occlusive dressing and tape to the catheter insertion site.	To prevent the catheter being dislodged and to aid visibility of the site.
(i) Inject solution into epidural space via catheter.	To provide anaesthesia.
5 Position the patient according to the doctor's instructions, tilting if appropriate.	To ensure spread of solution to provide optimum effect.
6 Take vital signs observations: blood pressure and respirations at least every 6 minutes for 30 minutes, and then 15 minutes for next 90 minutes. Take pulse every 15 minutes for 2 hours, or more frequently if the patient's condition dictates.	To monitor for signs of hypotension and respiratory depression.
7 Make the patient comfortable. Usually the patient is nursed flat for the first 3–6 hours, then slowly elevated into a sitting position. Bedclothes should not constrict the feet.	To ensure that any CNS leak is minimized and to prevent the patient developing a headache. To prevent the development of footdrop.
8 Assess pain regularly using a visual analogue scale or pain chart if appropriate. Observe the patient's movements and facial expressions. Discuss insufficient or ineffective analgesia with the anaesthetist.	To ensure optimal pain management and that the patient is involved in his or her pain management.

Nursing care plan • Emergencies

Problem	Cause	Suggested action
Rapid fall in blood pressure.	Sympathetic blockade producing hypotension.	Turn off infusion pump if in progress. If systolic blood pressure falls below 70–80 mmHg:

1 Summon duty anaesthetist or doctor.
2 Tilt the patient's head down unless contraindicated.
3 Give oxygen 4 litres per minute via a mask.

To prevent hypoxia caused by reduction in cardiac output:

1 Increase intravenous infusion (unless contraindicated, i.e. congestive cardiac failure).
2 Prepare 15–30 mg ephedrine for intravenous injection which may be requested urgently by medical staff. Ephedrine increases heart rate and therefore cardiac output.

Respiratory depression.	Opiate analgesia.	Call for medical assistance. Turn off infusion pump or patient-controlled analgesia (PCA) pump if in progress. Prepare naloxone 0.4 mg intravenously. If prescribed, give dose according to criteria, i.e. respiratory rate less than 8 per minute. Dosage counteracts respiratory depression and might also reverse the analgesic effect. If no improvement, administer second dose. A further 0.4 mg naloxone intravenously can be given 5–10 minutes after first. Prepare emergency equipment to support respiration.
		The patient's respiratory rate, pattern and depth should be observed at all times. Maintain continuous monitoring of tissue oxygen saturation, e.g. with pulse oximeter. Access to blood gas machines should be available. Observe pupil constriction.
Total spinal anaesthesia.		Prepare emergency equipment to support respiration. Call for medical assistance. Turn patient into the supine position. Ventilate the lungs. Elevate the legs. Prepare emergency drugs. Connect intravenous infusion of crystalloid fluid and administer at a high rate unless contraindicated. Prepare equipment for intubation.
Total central neurological blockade: 1 Marked hypotension. 2 Apnoea. 3 Dilated pupils. 4 Loss of consciousness.		Call for medical assistance and initiate emergency procedures.
Toxicity due to injected drug:		Call for medical assistance and initiate emergency procedures.

Problem	Cause	Suggested action
1 Disorientation. **2** Twitching. **3** Convulsions. **4** Apnoea.		
Nausea or vomiting.	Side-effect of opiates. Due to stimulation of the vomiting centre in the brain stem and stimulation of the chemoreceptor zone in the fourth ventricle of the brain.	Administer antiemetics as prescribed. Inform an anaesthetist. Continue to monitor and change antiemetics as necessary.
Headache.	May be caused by accidental dural puncture.	Administer systemic analgesia. Lie patient flat. Oral and intravenous fluids may be increased to encourage cerebrospinal fluid formation.
Pruritis, especially of the face and/or neck.	Histamine release following administration of opiates.	Inform anaesthetist. Administer antihistamine as prescribed. Keep patient cool. Use calamine lotion. If there is no improvement, the opiate may have to be discontinued and local anaesthetic used alone.
Urinary retention.	Due to parasympathetic block at the sacral level of the spinal cord.	Inform anaesthetist. Insert urinary catheter as required. The majority of patients on an intensive therapy unit or high dependency unit are catheterized.
Infection.		Check temperature at least 4-hourly. Check catheter entry site for inflammation or exudate. Remove epidural cannula if appropriate and send complete catheter to microbiology.

GUIDELINES • Topping up epidural analgesia

Usually performed by the doctor. Local anaesthetic agents *or* opioids may be given by nursing staff as part of an extended role, according to local policy. This should follow an agreed period of education and supervised practice, which must be documented.

Equipment

1 Antiseptic cleaning agent.
2 Syringes and needles.
3 Drug as prescribed.
4 Water or 0.9% sodium chloride for injection as necessary.
5 Patient's prescription chart.
6 Sterile hub/bung.

Procedure

Action	Rationale
1 Wash hands with bactericidal soap and water or bactericidal alcohol hand rub.	To reduce risk of cross-infection.
2 Check the drug to be administered and diluents, according to policy.	To ensure the correct drug, amount and concentration is administered to the correct patient.

3 Draw up the drug.

4 Check patient's nameband against prescription.　　To ensure correct patient receives correct drug.

5 Clean the access portal of the bacterial filter.　　To prevent the introduction of contaminants and micro-organisms into the epidural space.

6 Inject drug as prescribed.

7 Make the patient comfortable.

8 Monitor vital signs, blood pressure and respirations at least every 5 minutes for 30 minutes, then every 15 minutes for 60 minutes. Take pulse if the patient's condition dictates.　　To monitor signs of hypotension and respiratory depression.

9 Dispose of the equipment appropriately.

10 Maintain pain control assessment.　　To ensure optimum pain control and ensure that the patient feels involved in their pain management programme.

GUIDELINES • Removal of an epidural catheter

Note: before an epidural catheter is removed it is essential to consider the clotting status of the patient's blood. If the patient is fully anticoagulated a clotting profile must be performed and advice sought from the medical staff as to when the catheter can be removed. If the patient is receiving prophylactic anticoagulant, the catheter should be removed 6 hours before the next dose (Horlucker & Wedel 1998). This is to minimize the risk of an epidural haematoma.

Equipment

1 Dressing pack.
2 Skin cleansing agent, i.e. 0.9% sodium chloride.
3 Occlusive dressing.

Procedure

Action

1 Explain and discuss the procedure with the patient.

2 Wash hands with bactericidal soap and water or bactericidal alcohol hand rub.

3 Open dressing pack.

4 Wash hands and remove tape and dressing from catheter insertion site.

5 Gently, in one swift movement, remove catheter. Check that it is removed intact by observing marks along the catheter.

6 Apply an occlusive dressing and leave *in situ* for 24 hours.

The epidural tip may be sent for culture and sensitivity if infection is suspected, or according to local policy.

Rationale

To ensure the patient understands the procedure and gives his/her valid consent.

To minimize cross-infection.

To minimize risk of cross-infection.

To ensure the catheter is removed intact with the minimum of discomfort to the patient.

To prevent inadvertent access of micro-organisms along the tract.

GUIDELINES • Pre-insertion management of an epidural for chronic pain

If the patient is taking a slow release preparation of morphine, e.g. MST or MXL, they should be converted to immediate release morphine, either orally, intravenously or as a subcutaneous infusion for 24 hours before the insertion of the catheter. This is in order to minimize the risk of opioid overdose and the risk of respiratory depression. Once it has been decided that the patient is to have an epidural, a decision will need to be made regarding its fixation. As the catheter may need to stay in situ for several weeks/months it will either be tunnelled subcutaneously or anchored in place with medical glue and sutures.

Equipment

1 Chlorhexidine in 70% alcohol.
2 Syringes and needles.
3 Analgesia as prescribed.
4 0.9% sodium chloride for injection.
5 Patient's prescription chart.
6 Dressing pack.
7 IV administration set.
8 Epidural catheter set.
9 Suture material.
10 Transparent dressing.

Procedure

Action	Rationale
1 Explain and discuss the procedure with the patient and relatives/carers, obtain written consent.	To ensure that the patient understands the procedure and gives his/her valid consent.
2 Blood analysis for full blood count (FBC) and clotting.	To assess the risk of haemorrhage and/or epidural haematoma.
3 Assess and document patient's current pain: its location, duration, type and intensity of impact.	To obtain baseline information to guide the epidural therapy.
4 Assess and document motor and sensory function.	To obtain baseline information to guide the epidural therapy.
5 Discuss with the patient about the choices they would like to make and their individual goals – expectations of tolerable pain scores and expectations of motor or sensory deficit.	In the chronic pain setting – it may sometimes be necessary to accept reduced independence (motor function) to achieve reasonable pain control.
6 Ensure adequate community support/expertise.	Essential if the patient is to be discharged from hospital.

GUIDELINES • Changing the dressing over the epidural insertion site

The dressing over the epidural site needs to fulfil the following three functions:

1 To help anchor the epidural catheter.
2 To maintain asepsis and minimize the risk of infection.
3 To allow observation of the site without disturbing the dressing.

The frequency of dressing changes will be dictated by the type of dressing chosen – most polymeric/transparent occlusive dressings will be ideal for this purpose. To reduce the risk of microbial contamination and the possibility of disturbing the position of the catheter an occlusive dressing should be selected which can maintain a barrier for a minimum of 7 days. There is little agreement in the literature and in clinical practice about how often the administration set should be changed. Until good evidence exists, clinical practice needs to be guided by the manufacturer's instructions and individual hospital policy. There is also no clear evidence for the use of, or frequency of, filter changes and this will therefore be guided by the manufacturer's instructions and hospital policy (Hicks *et al.* 1994).

Changing the dressing when the epidural is anchored by the use of medical glue and sutures

If the catheter is not skin tunnelled, the medical adhesive glue will need to be reapplied once a week.

Equipment

1 Sterile dressing pack containing a gallipot, low-linting gauze, sterile field, disposable bag.

2 Sterile 0.9% sodium chloride for cleaning.

3 Can of medical adhesive glue.

4 Occlusive dressing.

Procedure

Action

1 Explain and discuss the procedure with the patient.

2 Clean trolley (or plastic tray in the community) with chlorhexidine in 70% alcohol with a paper towel.

3 Position the patient comfortably on their side or sitting forward so that the site is easily accessible without undue exposure of the patient.

4 Prepare trolley or tray with sterile field and cleaning solution.

5 Remove old dressing and place in disposable bag.

6 Wash hands with bactericidal hand rub

7 Observe site for any signs of infection such as redness, swelling or purulent discharge.

8 Clean site with sodium chloride 0.9%.

9 Using the medical adhesive spray the area around the site where the catheter is coiled on the skin (around the exit site) and ensure the catheter is well stuck down on to the skin.

10 Apply transparent occlusive dressing over the whole area.

11 Ensure that the patient is comfortable.

12 Dispose of all material in the clinical waste bag.

13 Wash hands with bactericidal soap and water.

Rationale

To ensure that the patient understands the procedure and gives his/her valid consent.

To provide a clean working surface.

To maintain the patient's dignity and comfort. This is especially important when carers are attending to an area that is not visible to the patient.

To minimize risk of infection and ensure equipment available.

To minimize the risk of infection.

To minimize the risk of microbial contamination.

To ensure careful monitoring of site to minimize the chance of any infection.

To minimize the risk of infection.

To ensure that the catheter is maintained in position.

Retention of catheter, to minimize the risk of microbial contamination and to allow frequent observation.

To prevent environmental contamination. Yellow is the recognized colour for clinical waste.

To reduce the risk of cross-infection.

GUIDELINES · Postinsertion monitoring of respiratory and cardiac function in chronic pain management

It should be noted that the monitoring required in this patient group is different to that required in the postoperative setting. In the chronic setting, patients have already been taking opioids and have not received a general anaesthetic and are therefore less likely to suffer respiratory depression or alterations to their blood pressure (De Leon-Casasaola *et al.* 1993).

Procedure

Action

1 Monitor the patient's respiratory and cardiovascular function whilst in a recovery or high dependency area for 1 hour postinsertion.

Rationale

To monitor for signs of respiratory depression and hypotension and to allow for immediate intervention where indicated.

Guidelines • Postinsertion monitoring of respiratory and cardiac function in chronic pain management (cont'd)

Action	Rationale
2 On return to the ward for a minimum of 4h perform hourly assessment of: respiratory rate and SaO$_2$, blood pressure and pulse for 2 hours.	To monitor for signs of respiratory depression and hypotension and to allow for intervention if indicated.
3 If patient stable, 4-hourly observations of the above for 24 hours.	To monitor patient safety whilst minimising invasive procedures in patients with chronic problems.

After 24 hours if patient is stable, monitoring should only be reintroduced if deemed necessary by the Multidisciplinary Team.

Pain assessment

Action	Rationale
1 Assess the patient for their comfort/freedom from pain at rest and on movement, utilizing the same tool as used pre-insertion.	This allows the clinician and the patient to make a valid comparison.
2 Pain assessment should be performed by the clinician and patient/family together.	To gain the patient's trust and to give the patient some control over their quality of life.
3 Pain assessment should be performed initially at least hourly and then a minimum of 4 hourly until the patient and clinician feel that an optimum target has been achieved.	To aid patient comfort and the adjustment of drug dosages.
4 Document pain assessment.	To provide the patient/family with a visual record of achievement and to allow continuity of information for different clinicians.
5 Assess sensory and mobility quality.	Monitor for any loss of sensation, bladder function and motor function.

GUIDELINES • Setting up the epidural infusion (utilizing a syringe pump or driver)

Equipment

1 Chlorhexidine in 70% alcohol.
2 Syringes and needles.
3 Analgesia as prescribed.
4 0.9% sodium chloride for injection.

5 Patient's prescription chart.
6 Dressing pack.
7 IV administration set.

Procedure

Action	Rationale
1 Explain and discuss the procedure with the patient	To ensure that the patient understands the procedure and gives his/her valid consent.
2 Wash hands with bactericidal soap and water or bactericidal alcohol hand rub.	To reduce risk of cross-infection.
3 Check the drugs to be administered and diluents according to policy.	To ensure the correct drugs, amount and concentration are administered to the correct patient.
4 Draw up the drugs and diluent into the syringe, affix drug identification label and attach the administration set.	To ensure safe checking for different clinicians.

5 Draw up 10 ml of 0.9% sodium chloride in a syringe as a flush.

To ensure patency of the catheter.

6 Clean the access portal of the bacterial filter with the chlorhexidine in 70% isopropyl alcohol.

To prevent the introduction of contaminants and micro-organisms into the epidural space.

7 Inject 0.9% sodium chloride – the catheter has a very narrow gauge so expect some resistance.

To ensure patency of the catheter before commencing the infusion.

8 Commence the infusion at the prescribed rate.

9 Check regularly that the light indicator is flashing and that the infusion is being delivered and the syringe is emptying.

To ensure that the patient is receiving their analgesia.

10 Document date, time and dosage at commencement of infusion.

To ensure optimum management of pain and to establish a baseline.

11 Dispose of the equipment appropriately.

To prevent a sharps injury and reduce the risk of infection.

12 Maintain pain control assessment.

To ensure optimum pain control.

GUIDELINES • Setting up of epidural infusion (utilizing an ambulatory pump)

As above except:

Procedure

Action

Rationale

1 Instil prescribed drugs and diluent into appropriate infusion bag and attach relevant administration set; apply drug information label.

To ensure infusion is ready to connect.

2 Check patency of epidural catheter as above.

3 Insert administration set into ambulatory pump, ensuring that manufacturer's instructions are followed.

To ensure optimal functioning of the device.

4 Before attaching to the patient, prime the administration set following the manufacturer's guidelines.

To ensure set is free from air when the infusion is commenced, thus minimizing the risk of air entering the catheter.

5 Clean as above (see Guidelines for changing the dressing, points 6–9).

6 Attach administration set to epidural catheter and start pump; ensure that indicator light is flashing (as above).

To ensure that pump is working and the drugs are being delivered.

7 Place pump and infusion bag into 'carry bag/pouch', ensuring that the tubing is not kinked.

To ensure comfort for the patient and to avoid obstruction to the infusion.

GUIDELINES • Discharge planning

An epidural infusion should not be seen as a barrier to the patient leaving hospital. Patients can be safely managed in the community provided the following areas are addressed.

Guidelines • Discharge planning

Procedure

Action

1 Convert patient's infusion to one that requires the minimum of changing, i.e. an infusion bag and ambulatory pump rather than a 20 ml syringe and driver.

2 Ensure that the patient will not be alone at home.

3 Arrange preparation of epidural drug infusion bags, usually in batches to provide enough delivery for one week. This can be arranged at the cancer centre or the referring hospital if they have the appropriate pharmaceutical arrangements.

4 Discuss how the infusion bags will be collected each week; they cannot be posted because they contain drugs that are categorized as controlled drugs.

5 The patient/family should be provided with the following equipment to take home:
(a) Spare battery.
(b) Bottle of bactericidal hand rub.
(c) Bottle of chlorhexidine in 70% alcohol.
(d) Sterile gauze.
(e) Syringes and needles.
(f) Sodium chloride for injection.
(g) ×1 Spare bacterial filter.
(h) ×1 Week's supply of reconstituted epidural infusion bags.
(i) Written advice re contact numbers/troubleshooting and prescription.

6 Patient/family and district nurse/GP should be taught and trained in the following areas:
(a) Setting up the infusion.
(b) The functions of the ambulatory device, including alarms and visual displays.
(c) Loading the administration set into the pump and priming the line.
(d) Observation of the epidural for signs of infection – redness, swelling, leakage of pus.
(e) The prescribed therapy for breakthrough pain.
(f) Troubleshooting (as described below).
(g) The procedure for obtaining medical/nursing help locally or at the cancer centre 24 hourly and every day of the week.
(h) Dressing of the epidural site.

Rationale

This will reduce the workload of the patient/family or district nurse and also minimizes the number of interruptions to the patient circuit, thus minimizing the chance of microbial contamination.

Epidural catheters can obstruct, become dislodged and the battery can fail on the device – most patients need immediate reassurance and practical help in these situations.

Pharmacy reconstitution ensures aseptic preparation, thus minimizing the chance of microbial contamination, and reduces the workload and anxiety for family/district nurse. It should also be noted that epidural infusions may contain a combination of drugs and pharmacy reconstitution may help to reduce preparation error.

The method of collection needs to be discussed at an early stage with the family/district nurse to ensure continuity of epidural delivery and avoid any anxiety or delay to discharge.

To ensure that the first week of therapy continues smoothly. To reduce anxiety and increase patient comfort and trust.

Nursing care plan • Troubleshooting: the following can be used for nursing staff and then adapted for use by the patient/family

Problem	Cause	Suggested action
1 Ambulatory pump auditory alarm.	(a) Battery failure is most likely (batteries usually last 3 weeks).	(a) Stop pump, remove old and replace with new battery; ensure battery is fitted up snugly to connections. Turn on pump and ensure light indicator is flashing.
	(b) Catheter occlusion.	(b) Stop pump, draw up 0.9% sodium chloride and flush catheter, if catheter clears reattatch pump, press start and ensure light indicator is flashing. If catheter is still obstructed and will not flush, phone cancer centre/GP.
2 Sudden acute pain.	Catheter obstruction; catheter movement; change in pathology.	Take prescribed breakthrough analgesia, e.g. a dose of Oromorph/Sevredol; document date and time taken; flush catheter as indicated above; inform cancer centre/GP/district nurses. If possible, once breakthrough analgesia taken, try to see if another position for the patient might help.
3 Leakage of clear coloured fluid from around the epidural site.	Disconnection of catheter; movement of catheter; kinking of catheter.	If the patient is experiencing any pain take breakthrough drug as prescribed. Observe and check the patient administration set and pump for any loose connections. Try to estimate the degree of fluid leak, i.e. a 50 p coin size, etc., contact district nursing team/GP and describe the leak.
4 Disconnection of epidural catheter from filter.	Patient movement – typically turning in bed at night.	Stop pump. Call district nursing team. Clean the end of the line with chlorhexidine, allow to dry. Reinsert the end of the catheter furthest away from the patient into the replacement filter screw into connection firmly. Restart pump.
5 Redness, swelling or leakage of discoloured fluid from site.	Infection *or* local irritation at site from skin interaction with the plastic catheter.	Take oral temperature. Contact cancer centre/district nurses/GP. **Ensure** that a clinician does see the area as soon as possible – it may be necessary to remove the catheter/administer prescribed systemic antibiotics.

External Compression and Support in the Management of Lymphoedema

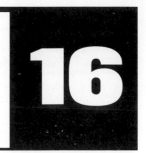

Definition

'Support may be defined as the retention and control of tissue without the application of compression . . . Compression implies the deliberate application of pressure' (Thomas 1991a). The application of both support and compression results in pressure; the differences between the two techniques are, firstly, that the resulting pressure arises from different mechanisms and, secondly, that the relationship between resting pressures and active pressures is different (Thomas 1991b).

In the case of support, pressure arises from the body tissues pushing outwards against the stocking or bandage. The pressure from compression results from the forces in the stocking or bandage exerting pressure on the tissues beneath. Thus it is the type of material from which stockings or bandages are made that determines whether support or compression is being applied. Short-stretch or extensible bandages and the more rigid types of hosiery will result in support, as the tissues push out against the firm rigid casing provided by the stocking/bandage. Elastic hosiery or bandages will result in compression, as the elastic properties of the material pull in against the tissues (Thomas 1991b).

Under support the resting pressure is relatively low and the active pressure relatively high, resulting in a massaging effect on the tissues beneath. Under compression the difference between the resting and active pressure is less pronounced and the massaging effect diminished (Thomas 1991b).

Indications

External graduated pressure in the form of support or compression is the mainstay of conservative management for lymphoedema. It is important for several reasons:

1 It ensures that fluid in the limb travels towards the root of the limb.
2 It limits the formation of fluid in the tissues.
3 It contains the tissues of the swollen limb and helps to maintain a normal shape to the limb.
4 It helps to maximize the effect of the muscle pump (Gaylarde et al. 1993).

Elastic compression is primarily indicated when the lymphoedema is mild and uncomplicated (Badger 1996). It is also used to maintain the reduced size of a swollen limb after the use of bandaging. Support, provided by low stretch bandages or the more rigid types of hosiery, is indicated when the lymphoedema is moderate to severe and the limb has swollen out of shape. It is also effective when fibrosis of the subcutaneous tissues is present, due to the massaging effect on the tissues of the low resting pressures and high working pressures.

Contraindications for external graduated pressure

1 Arterial disease in the arm or leg
2 Acute stages of deep vein thrombosis in the leg
3 Acute infections of the limb, e.g. cellulitis
4 Cardiac oedema

(Callam et al. 1997).

Reference material

There are many reasons why a limb may swell and the appearance of oedema represents an increase in extracellular fluid volume (Mortimer 1995). Dependency or gravitational oedema is commonly seen in the immobile patient when the immobility results in minimal lymph drainage. Swelling can also occur in chronic venous disease of the lower limbs as a result of lymph drainage failure and increased capillary filtration (Mortimer 1996).

Lymphoedema occurs because the lymphatics are reduced in number, obstructed, obliterated or simply fail to function. Tissue swelling then appears due to the failure of lymph drainage (Mortimer 1996). Lymphoedema is most commonly seen in cancer patients as a result of damage to lymph nodes following surgery and/or radiotherapy, but it can also occur as a result of local tumour obstruction in lymph node areas. A survey of 1200 breast cancer patients on the south coast of England reported the prevalence of chronic arm oedema as 28%. The prevalence increased with time following treatment in patients who had received postoperative radiotherapy (Mortimer et al. 1996). There is no research to indicate the incidence of leg oedema following treatment for abdominal and pelvic tumours, soft tissue sarcomas and melanomas, although lymphoedema is known to occur following treatment for these tumours (Logan 1995).

Lymphoedema can affect any part of the body including the face and head, but it most commonly affects a limb (Mortimer 1995). The swelling can have physical, psychological and psychosocial implications for the patient and is associated with a number of complications arising from its development. Limb heaviness may lead to impaired function, reduced mobility and musculoskeletal problems. Skin and tissue changes develop with increased lymph stasis in the oedematous limb and give rise to the characteristic deepened skin folds, distorted limb shape and hyperkeratosis associated with long-standing lymphoedema. There is an increased risk of local and systemic infection as a result of poor lymph drainage and recurrent acute inflammatory episodes are common (Mortimer 1996).

The experience of living with lymphoedema as a long-term chronic condition is a unique experience for each patient and can have an impact on many areas of the individual's life. Studies of breast cancer patients with arm swelling have highlighted the degree of psychological and psychosocial distress that can be experienced when lymphoedema develops (Tobin *et al.* 1993; Woods 1993; Woods *et al.* 1995). The physical and psychological effects of lymphoedema are not short-lived and enormous motivation and perseverance coupled with adaptation is demanded in order to achieve control or reduction of the swelling.

Assessment of the patient with lymphoedema

Definition

Assessment has been defined as an expert activity (Benner 1984) which can have a dramatic effect on outcome for the individual patient (Derdiarian 1990). As lymphoedema is a unique experience for each patient, accurate assessment is essential if an individualized approach is to be achieved and the most appropriate treatment chosen.

Indications

When the use of external compression and support is being considered, a full and careful assessment will highlight the patient's main problems and any co-existing complications. This information is then used to set realistic treatment goals and to determine the approach to treatment. A number of treatments are used in combination during the management of lymphoedema and their choice and usefulness can be determined by the therapist and patient at the time of assessment.

A full assessment should include the following elements:

1 *Physical assessment:* to determine the cause of the swelling and any symptoms or complicating factors, i.e. the cause and extent of the oedema, assessment of skin condition and limb shape, disease status.
2 *Psychological assessment:* to determine the effect of the swelling on the patient, i.e. effect on relationships, personal concerns and fears.
3 *Psychosocial assessment:* to determine the influence of the swelling upon the patient's life, i.e. influence upon limb function and mobility, employment, hobbies, activities, personal roles.

In order to evaluate the outcome of a plan of treatment, suitable outcome indicators are required (Sitzia *et al.* 1997). The measurement of limb volume using surface measurement is the most frequently used means of assessing response to treatment in lymphoedema management (Sitzia *et al.* 1997). The effect of treatment on the patient's psychological and psychosocial wellbeing should, however, also be monitored and this is frequently achieved in a more subjective manner where the patient's views are sought.

Measurement of limb volume

Definition

The measurement of limb volume is calculated from a series of circumference measurements taken along the length of the limb and applied to the formula for the volume of a cylinder (Sitzia 1995).

Indications

As part of the initial assessment of the patient, limb volume measurements can be calculated in order to:

1 Determine the total excess volume of the swollen limb compared to the patient's contralateral normal limb.
2 Establish the distribution of the swelling along the limb.
3 Provide information to assist in the choice of external pressure.

Measurements can also be used to provide an objective method of determining response to treatment by indicating:

1 Changes in the size and shape of the limb over time.
2 Changes in the excess volume.
3 The distribution of any volume loss or gain in the limb.

Reference material

A reliable method of assessing response to treatment is the measurement of limb volume. A variety of methods to measure volume have been used, including:

1 Volume measured by water displacement (Kettle *et al.* 1958; Engler & Sweat 1962)
2 Volume measured using an optoelectronic device (Stanton *et al.* 1997)
3 Volume calculated from surface measurements (Sitzia 1995).

Each of these methods has advantages and disadvantages. The calculation of limb volume from surface measurements, however, is uncomplicated and inexpensive. Reproducibility is accurate if care is taken with the procedure and a standard format for the recording of the measurements is used (Woods 1994; Badger 1997).

The following points should be considered when using surface measurements in order to calculate limb volume:

1 Ensure that the same position is used for the same patient each time the limb is measured. The position of the limb will affect the measurements taken because the degree to which muscles are flexed or relaxed will influence the shape and size of the limb.

The formula for calculating the volume of a cylinder is $\dfrac{circumference^2}{\pi}$. The formula must be applied to each circumference measurement ($circ_1$, $circ_2$, ... $circ_n$) in order to calculate the volume of each segment; the volumes are totalled to give the total limb volume.

$$So\left(\frac{circ_1 \times circ_1}{3.1415}\right) + \left(\frac{circ_2 \times circ_2}{3.1415}\right) + \left(\frac{circ_3 \times circ_3}{3.1415}\right) + \dots \text{etc.}$$

Use of a programmable calculator will speed up the process of calculation.

Figure 16.1 Procedure for calculating volume from circumferences.

2 The limb should be marked afresh on each measuring occasion with a washable ink, even when measuring on consecutive days. Any increase or decrease in limb volume will influence the position of the marks on the limb.

3 Tension should not be exerted on the tape measure during measuring. If tension is applied it will vary between measurers and recordings will not be consistent.

4 The tape measure should be positioned so that it is horizontal around the limb, taking care to ensure that it is not pulled tightly.

5 The same number of measurements should be taken on both limbs each time measurements are taken. Although the normal limb would not be expected to change significantly in volume except following vigorous exercise or where there has been weight loss or gain, the normal limb acts as a control in patients with unilateral swelling.

6 The starting point for the taking of measurements should be clearly identified by measuring and clearly recording the distance from the tip of the middle finger to the wrist. This starting point on the wrist should be used each time.

7 A standard format for the recording of measurements should be adopted to ensure that key points can be referred to.

Once measurement of the limb has been completed, a number of formulae may be used to calculate the limb volume (Sitzia 1995; Badger 1997). The formula for the volume of a cylinder (Fig. 16.1) considers the limb as a series of cylinders, each with a height of 4 cm, and limb volume is calculated by totalling the volume of each section.

Phases of treatment: introduction

Treatment of lymphoedema can be approached in two phases: the maintenance phase and the reduction phase (Todd 1998). The difference between the phases is primarily focused upon the choice of external graduated pressure applied to the swollen limb. In the maintenance phase of treatment, elastic hosiery is used to provide compression and in the reduction phase, external support is provided with short stretch extensible bandages.

Not all patients will follow both phases of treatment and many may only need to follow the maintenance phase.

Maintenance phase of treatment

Indications

Elastic compression hosiery is used during the maintenance phase of lymphoedema management in order to control limb swelling or to maintain a reduction in limb size following bandaging. It is usually combined with other elements of treatment including:

1 A skin-care regimen to minimize the risks of infection.
2 Exercise to promote lymph drainage.
3 Massage to stimulate lymph drainage.

Elastic compression hosiery is most effective when patients have mild, uncomplicated swelling. It can also be used to control swelling and to provide support in the palliative treatment of oedema.

Contraindications

Elastic hosiery should not be used where there is:

1 Arterial disease; blood supply may be further compromised.
2 Distortion of limb shape; the garment will not fit.
3 Skin folds; the garment will cause ridges and a torniquet effect to the limb.
4 Open wounds; the garment will become soiled and pose an infection risk.
5 Fragile skin; application and removal of the garment may cause further damage to the skin.
6 Lymphorrhoea; the garment will become wet and may cause skin excoriation.

Choosing compression hosiery

The choice and fitting of a compression garment should follow a detailed assessment of the patient (Armstrong 1997) and should only be attempted by a health care professional with knowledge and appropriate skills to ensure patient safety.

A wide range of garments are available in different styles, materials and compression classes. Garments can be 'off the shelf' or 'made to measure'. Consideration of the patient's ability must be taken into account when choosing a garment as a high degree of dexterity and strength may be required during its application and removal and this may be impractical for the patient.

Compression stockings are available in two compression standards, British and continental, which differ in the amount of compression applied to the limb. The highest compression provided by a stocking when fitted can be found at the ankle. The compression is then graduated along the length of the limb to encourage movement of fluid out of the limb. British standard compression garments achieve lower compression at the ankle and are available on prescription, whilst the continental standard compression garments achieve higher compression at the ankle and are only available from specialist orthotics suppliers (Table 16.1).

All areas influenced by swelling must be contained within the compression garment or further swelling will develop. Once fitted, the garment should feel comfortable and supportive, not tight and restrictive. The patient should be instructed concerning the application, removal and care of the garment to ensure that maximum effectiveness is achieved through its use.

Reduction phase of treatment

The reduction or intensive phase of treatment should always be carried out by a skilled therapist with the necessary skills and experience to apply bandages to the swollen limb, ensuring that pressure is graduated towards the root of the limb and evenly applied (Badger 1996). Damage to the skin and tissues can occur if the bandages are incorrectly or inappropriately applied (Thomas 1990a,b).

Indications

The reduction phase of treatment is usually carried out for a short specified period of 2–3 weeks, necessitating daily bandaging of the swollen limb. Indications for this phase of treatment include:

1 Large limbs: containment hosiery used on large swollen limbs may be ineffective due to the difficulties of applying sufficient tension to compress the limb (Stillwell 1973).
2 Misshapen limbs: containment hosiery will promote the development of deep skin folds when the limb is awkwardly shaped. Foam or soft padding under bandages will smooth out the folds and restore normal shape to the limb.
3 Severe lymphoedema: large limbs with long-standing oedema require high pressures to break down tissue fibrosis. Bandages provide a low resting and high active pressure which enables hardened tissues to soften.

4 Lymphorrhoea: the leakage of lymph fluid from the skin responds readily to external pressure provided by bandages.
5 Damaged or fragile skin: containment hosiery can cause damage to fragile skin. Bandages should be used until the skin condition improves (Mortimer et al. 1993).

Palliative care

Bandaging can be versatile and extremely useful in the palliative care setting when volume reduction may be unrealistic or not indicated. Support and comfort can be provided to a limb using a low level of pressure with a modified technique of bandaging designed around the patient's needs. The bandages can be left in place for 2–3 days and should not prevent the patient from maintaining full movement in their bandaged limb (Mortimer et al. 1993).

Principles to be followed in multi-layer bandaging

Low-stretch bandages should always be used. These provide a low resting pressure to the swollen limb when the muscle is inactive and a high working pressure during activity when the muscle is pumping against the resistance created by the bandage (Staudinger 1993). The bandages should provide an even pressure around the circumference of the limb (Thomas 1990). In awkwardly shaped limbs this can be achieved with the use of soft foam or padding to smooth out skin folds and promote a suitable profile. The pressure from the bandages should be graduated towards the root of the limb with the greatest pressure over the hand or foot, gradually reducing as the limb is bandaged upwards. This is achieved by controlling the amount of bandage tension and overlap used. Moderate tension only should be maintained on the bandages. The bandages should never be stretched to their maximum length.

The bandages should be left in place day and night and removed once every 24 hours. This enables skin hygiene to be attended to and the condition of the skin to be checked. Reapplication of the bandages then ensures that effective compression is maintained on the changing limb shape (Staudinger 1993).

The bandages should be comfortable for the patient and removed at any time if they cause any pain, numbness or discoloration (blueness) in the fingers or toes. This may indicate a variety of causes including too great a compression on the limb. A satisfactory outcome of treatment should be achieved within 2–3 weeks. The patient may then begin the maintenance phase of treatment where containment hosiery is fitted.

Evaluation of the bandaging procedure

Evaluation of each stage of the bandaging procedure is essential to ensure that the bandage and padding have been used appropriately and correctly.

The process of evaluation must be thorough and exhaustive and should include:

Table 16.1 British and continental standard compression rates (in mm Hg) measured at the ankle

Compression class	British standard	Continental standard
1	14–17	18.4–21.1
2	18–24	25.2–32.3
3	25–35	36.5–46.6

1 Continuous attention to the colour of the digits. Too much pressure will result in compromised circulation.
2 Continuous attention to the sensations experienced in the bandaged limb. The bandages should not cause pain, numbness or tingling.
3 The shape of the limb. A cylindrical contour should be achieved with the use of soft foam and padding.
4 The overlap of the bandages. This should be even and consistent with no gaps in the bandages.
5 The pressure achieved. This should feel even to the patient and there should be no creases in the bandages. Layers should be used appropriately.

Patient evaluation

The patient should feel comfortable and able to move their limb. Information should be given concerning when and how to remove the bandages if necessary.

References and further reading

Armstrong, A. (1997) Compression hosiery. *Prof Nurse*, **12**(7), Suppl. 49–54.

Badger, C. (1996) Treating lymphoedema. *Nurs Times*, **92**(11), 84–8.

Badger, C. (1997) A study of the efficacy of multi-layer bandaging and elastic hosiery in the treatment of lymphoedema and their effects on the swollen limb. PhD thesis, Institute of Cancer Research.

Benner, P. (1984) *From Novice to Expert*. Addison-Wesley, California.

Callam, M.J., Ruckley, C.V., Dale, J.J. *et al.* (1997) Hazards of compression treatment of the leg: an estimate from Scottish surgeons. *Br Med J*, **295**, 1382.

Derdiarian, A. (1990) Effects of using systematic assessment instruments on patient and nurse satisfaction with nursing care. *Oncol Nurs Forum*, **17**(1), 95–101.

Engler, H. & Sweat, R. (1962) Volumetric arm measurements: techniques and results. *Am Surg*, **28**, 465–8.

Gaylarde, P., Sarkany, I. & Dodd, H. (1993) The effect of compression on venous stasis. *Br J Dermatol*, **128**, 255–8.

Kettle, J., Rundle, F. & Oddie, T. (1958) Measurement of upper limb volumes: a clinical method. *Aust N Z J Surg*, **27**, 263–70.

Logan, V. (1995) Incidence and prevalence of lymphoedema: a literature review. *J Clin Nurs*, **4**, 213–19.

Mortimer, P. (1995) Managing lymphoedema. *Clin Exp Dermatol*, **20**, 98–106.

Mortimer, P. (1996) Lymphoedema. *Vasc Surg*, 73–7.

Mortimer, P., Badger, C. & Hall, J.G. (1993) Lymphoedema. In: *Oxford Textbook of Palliative Medicine* (eds D. Doyle, G. Hanks & N. McDonald). Oxford Medical Publications, Oxford.

Mortimer, P., Bates, D., Brassington, H. *et al.* (1996) The prevalence of arm oedema following treatment for breast cancer. *Q J Med*, **89**, 377–80.

Sitzia, J. (1995) Volume measurement in lymphoedema treatment: examination of the formulae. *Eur J Cancer Care*, **4**, 11–16.

Sitzia, J., Stanton, A. & Badger, C. (1997) A review of outcome indicators in the treatment of chronic limb oedema. *Clin Rehab*, **11**, 181–91.

Stanton, A., Northfield, J., Holroyd, B. *et al.* (1997) Validation of an optoelectronic limb volumeter (Perometer). *Lymphology*, **30**, 77–97.

Staudinger, P. (1993) Compression bandaging for lymphoedema. *Nat Lymphoedema Network Newsl USA*, **5**(3), 5–6.

Stillwell, G. (1973) The Law of Laplace: some clinical applications. *Mayo Clinic Proc*, **48**, 863–9.

Thomas, S. (1990a) Bandages and bandaging: the science behind the art. *CARE Sci Pract*, **8**(2), 56–60.

Thomas, S. (1990b) Bandages and bandaging. *Nurs Stand*, **4**(39), Suppl. 8, 4–6.

Tobin, M., Mortimer, P., Meyer, L. *et al.* (1993) The psychological morbidity of breast cancer related arm swelling. *Cancer*, **72**(11), 3348–52.

Todd, J. (1998) Lymphoedema – a challenge for all health care professionals. *Int J Palliat Nurs*, **4**(5), 230–39.

Woods, M. (1993) Patients' perceptions of breast-cancer related lymphoedema. *Eur J Cancer Care*, **2**, 125–8.

Woods, M. (1994) An audit of swollen limb measurements. *Nurs Stand*, **9**(5), 24–6.

Woods, M., Tobin, M. & Mortimer, P. (1995) The psychological morbidity of breast cancer patients with lymphoedema. *Cancer Nurs*, **18**(6), 467–71.

GUIDELINES · Calculation of limb volume

Equipment

1 Ruler, preferably 30 cm or longer.
2 Tape measure; avoid those made from fabric which tends to stretch.

3 Felt-tip pen for marking the limb.
4 Record chart and pen.

Procedure for measuring lower limbs

Action	Rationale
1 Place the patient in a sitting position with the legs outstretched horizontally, preferably on a firm couch with adjustable height.	The lower limbs are relaxed and supported and the adjustable height means that the measurer can work without straining the back.
2 Standing on the outside of the leg, ask the patient to flex the foot to a right angle. Measure the distance	This establishes a reproducible fixed starting point for all subsequent measurements.

from the base of the heel to the ankle, along the inside of the leg; mark the ankle, allowing at least 2 cm of leg to lie below the mark, and record the distance on the chart.

3 Ask the patient to relax the foot. From the starting point mark the inside of the leg at 4 cm intervals along the length of the leg up to the groin; use the ruler for this.

4 Place the tape measure around the limb and measure the circumference at each marked point, recording each measurement on the chart. Make sure that the tape lies smoothly around the relaxed limb and that it does not lie at an angle. Decide at the outset whether the tape is to be placed above, below or on the mark and keep to the same position every time.

5 Repeat the process on the other leg, whether or not it is swollen.

6 If desired, a circumference measurement may be taken of the foot but this is *not* included in the calculation of volume.

Note: the marks represent a point midway through each cylinder segment, they do not represent the base of the cylinder, therefore at least half the segment (i.e. 2 cm) must lie below the mark.

Reducing the limb to 4 cm segments improves the accuracy of measurement since these segments resemble a cylinder more closely than does the whole limb. The formula used here assumes that the measurements are 4 cm apart.

Ensuring that there are no gaps between the limb and the tape and ensuring that the procedure is the same each time reduces error.

If only one limb is affected the normal limb acts as the patient's own control.

The foot cannot be considered to be a cylinder and it is therefore inappropriate to include it in the calculation of volume.

Procedure for measuring upper limbs

Action

1 Sit the patient in a chair with the arms extended in front and resting on the back of a chair. The arms should be as close to an angle of 90° to the body as possible.

2 Measure the distance from the tip of the middle finger to the wrist. Mark the wrist, allowing at least 2 cm from where the hand joins the arm, and note down the distance.

3 From the starting point mark along the length of the arm at 4 cm intervals up to the axilla; use the ruler for this.

4 Place the tape measure around the limb and measure the circumference at each marked point, recording each measurement on the chart. Make sure that the tape lies smoothly around the relaxed limb and that it does not lie at an angle. Decide at the outset whether the tape is to be placed above, below or on the mark and keep to the same position every time.

5 Repeat the process on the other arm whether or not it is swollen.

6 If desired, a circumference measurement may be taken of the hand but this is *not* included in the calculation of volume.

Rationale

The arms are supported and accessible at a standard height. Changing the angle of the arms to the body will result in changes in the measurements.

This establishes a reproducible fixed starting point for all subsequent measurements. *Note*: The marks represent a point midway through each cylinder segment, they do not represent the base of the cylinder, therefore at least half the segment (i.e. 2 cm) must lie below the mark.

Reducing the limb to 4 cm segments improves the accuracy of measurement since these segments resemble a cylinder more closely than does the whole limb.

Ensuring that there are no gaps between the limb and the tape and ensuring that the procedure is the same each time reduces error.

If only one limb is affected the normal limb acts as the patient's own control.

The hand cannot be considered to be a cylinder and it is therefore inappropriate to include it in the calculation.

GUIDELINES · The application of elastic hosiery

The application of hosiery can be greatly eased by the wearing of household rubber gloves during application which facilitate control of the garment. Any moisturizing creams should be applied at night-time rather than in the morning before putting the garment on. A very fine layer of talcum powder applied to hot sticky skin can ease application. If this is the first time that the patient has worn compression hosiery, the therapist should explain to the patient that the feeling of pressure may feel strange for the first few hours, but that it should not cause pain in the limb or numbness in the digits or toes.

Procedure for applying hosiery to the leg

Action	*Rationale*
1 Explain and discuss the procedure with the patient.	To ensure that the patient understands the procedure and gives his/her valid consent.
2 If possible, position the patient seated upright on a bed or couch and raise the height to a comfortable level.	To ensure the comfort of both the patient and nurse.
3 Turn the stocking inside-out to the heel.	This makes it easier to ease the stocking up.
4 Pull the foot of the stocking over the patient's foot.	
5 Turn the rest of the stocking back over the foot and up the leg.	
6 Ask the patient to keep the leg straight and if possible to push against the nurse.	
7 Starting at the foot, gradually ease the stocking into place over the heel and up the leg a bit at a time, until it is in its final position.	Since it is the material of the stocking that provides the pressure, it must be distributed evenly to ensure an even distribution of pressure.
8 Do not pull from the top.	This will cause the stocking top to become overstretched and will lead to an uneven distribution of the stocking material.
9 Once the stocking is in place, check that there are no creases or wrinkles, particularly around the joints.	Wrinkles cause chafing of the skin and constricting bands of pressure.
10 Check that the patient finds the stocking comfortable and ask that any feelings of pain, tingling or numbness be reported.	Pain, tingling or numbness indicate that the stocking has been either inappropriately applied or fitted.
11 To remove the stocking, peel the stocking off the limb from the top downwards. Do not roll it down.	Rolling the stocking can result in tight bands of material forming, which are difficult to move.

Procedure for applying hosiery to the arm

Action	*Rationale*
1 Explain and discuss the procedure with the patient.	To ensure that the patient understands the procedure and gives his/her valid consent.
2 The patient may be seated or standing.	
3 Turn the sleeve inside-out to the wrist. Pull over the patient's hand. *Note*: if the handpiece is separate from the sleeve, always put the handpiece on before the sleeve.	To avoid increasing swelling in the hand.
4 Turn the rest of the sleeve back over the hand and up the arm.	
5 Ask the patient to grip something stable, such as a towel rail or the back of a chair.	This steadies the arm and gives the patient something to pull against.

6 Working from the hand or wrist, gradually ease the sleeve up the arm.

7 Do not pull up from the top.

8 Once the sleeve is in place, check that there are no creases or wrinkles, particularly around the joints.

9 Check that the patient finds the sleeve comfortable and ask that any signs of pain, tingling or numbness be reported.

10 To remove the sleeve peel the sleeve off the limb from the top. Do not roll it down.

Since it is the material that provides the pressure, it must be evenly distributed to ensure an even distribution of pressure.

This will cause the top to become overstretched and will result in an uneven distribution of pressure.

Wrinkles and creases cause chafing of the skin and constricting bands of pressure.

Pain, tingling or numbness indicate that the sleeve has been either inappropriately applied or fitted.

Rolling the sleeve down can lead to tight bands of material forming which are difficult to move.

GUIDELINES • Standard multi-layer compression bandaging

This procedure should not be attempted by anyone who has not had specialist education in this area. The swollen limb should be clean and well moisturized with a bland cream (e.g. E45) before being bandaged. Pressure must be applied in a graduated profile, i.e. highest over the hand or foot, and gradually reducing as the limb is bandaged upwards, to ensure that fluid is encouraged to drain towards the root of the limb. The degree of pressure is influenced by:

1 The circumference of the limb − pressure will be highest over a small circumference and lowest over a large circumference [Laplace's law (Stillwell 1973)].
2 The amount of tension placed on the bandage.
3 The amount of bandage overlap.
4 The number of bandage layers (Thomas 1990).

Thus, on a normally shaped limb, maintaining the same amount of bandage tension and the same amount of bandage overlap all the way up the limb will result in a natural graduation of pressure due to the gradual increase in the size of the limb from ankle to groin, or wrist to axilla. In cases where swelling has distorted the shape of the limb, additional padding is used to create a suitable profile on which to bandage, and adjustments may be needed in bandage tension and bandage overlap. Very large limbs may also require extra layers of bandage to be used in order to ensure that sufficient pressure is applied.

Equipment for bandaging an arm

1 Stockinette.
2 Light retention bandages, 6 and 10 cm to bandage digits and to hold foam padding in place.
3 Padding, 6 cm roll.

4 Foam.
5 Low-stretch compression bandages, 6 and 8 cm.
6 Tape.
7 Scissors.

Procedure

Action

1 Explain and discuss the procedure with the patient.

2 If possible, the patient should be seated in a chair. The nurse should be positioned in front of the patient.

3 Cut a length of stockinette long enough to fit the patient's arm. Cut a small hole for the thumb and slip over the patient's arm.

4 The fingers must be bandaged (Fig. 16.2). Using a narrow light retention bandage anchor the bandage loosely at the wrist and bring across the back of the hand to the thumb. Bandage around the thumb from the tip downwards (start at the level of the nail bed). Do not pull the bandage tight but go gently and firmly. Take the bandage under the wrist and back over the back of the hand to the index finger (Fig. 16.3). Again, bandage from the nail bed

Rationale

To ensure that the patient understands the procedure and gives his/her valid consent.

To ensure the comfort of both the patient and nurse.

To protect the skin from chafing.

To reduce or prevent swelling.

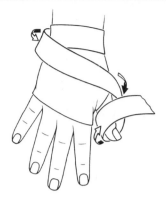

Figure 16.2 Bandaging swollen fingers.

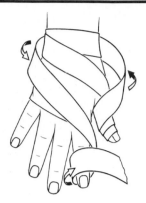

Figure 16.3 Bandage is taken under wrist, back over hand, to index finger.

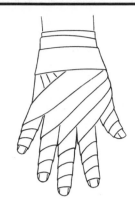

Figure 16.4 Finished bandage.

Guidelines • Standard multi-layer compression bandaging (cont'd)

Action	Rationale
down to the webs of the finger. Repeat the same procedure for all fingers. Finish by tucking in the end of the bandage (Fig. 16.4).	
5 Check the colour and temperature of the tips of the fingers.	To ensure that the blood supply is not compromised.
6 Check that the patient can move the fingers and make a fist.	To check that the bandage is not too tight.
7 Using the roll of padding, cover the hand in a figure of eight, padding out the palm and back of the hand (Fig. 16.5).	Padding out the hand ensures even pressure distribution and protects the bony areas of the hand.

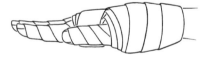

Figure 16.5 Palm and back of hand are padded out.

Action	Rationale
8 Using foam and padding, even out any exaggerated contours of the limb.	To create a smooth profile on which to apply the bandage.
9 Cut foam to fit the length of the arm from the wrist to axilla. Ensure that the width is sufficient to encircle the arm with a small overlap.	To protect the elbow joint and provide a smooth, even profile on which to bandage.
10 Wrap the foam around the arm, securing with a light retention bandage. Finish by tucking in the end of the bandage (Fig. 16.6).	
11 Take a 6 cm compression bandage and start by anchoring it loosely at the wrist. Bandage the hand firmly in a figure of eight until all of the hand is covered (Fig. 16.7). Continue the rest of the bandage up the forearm in a spiral, covering half of the bandage with each turn. Keep the bandage as smooth as possible.	To avoid constriction at the wrist.

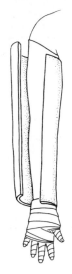

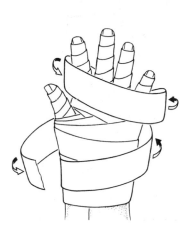

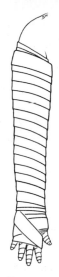

Figure 16.6 Foam is wrapped around arm, secured with a light retention bandage.

Figure 16.7 Hand is bandaged firmly in a figure of eight using a 6 cm compression bandage.

Figure 16.8 Starting at wrist, an 8 or 10 cm bandage is used to cover to top of arm, in a spiral fashion.

12 Take an 8 or 10 cm bandage and, starting at the wrist, bandage in a spiral, still covering half of the bandage with each turn, up to the top of the arm (Fig. 16.8).

Two layers are used on the forearm to ensure that pressure is highest distally.

13 Secure the end of the bandage with tape.

14 Once again, check the colour and sensations of the finger tips and check that the patient can move all joints.

To check that the blood flow is not compromised.

15 Remind the patient to use the limb as normally as possible and to report any feelings of discomfort, tingling or numbness.

To ensure good lymph flow.

Equipment for bandaging a leg

1 Stockinette.
2 Light retention bandages, 6 and 10 or 12 cm.
3 Padding, 10 and 20 cm.
4 Foam.

5 Low-stretch compression bandages, 8, 10 and 12 cm.
6 Tape.
7 Scissors.

Procedure for bandaging a leg and the toes

Action

Rationale

1 Explain and discuss the procedure with the patient.

To ensure that the patient understands the procedure and gives his/her valid consent.

2 If possible, the patient should be seated upright on a bed or treatment couch. Raise the bed or couch to a comfortable height.

To ensure the comfort of both the patient and nurse.

3 Cut a length of stockinette long enough to fit the patient's leg. Slip over the leg.

To protect the skin from chafing.

4 If the toes are swollen or have a tendency to swell they must be bandaged. The little toe can be omitted.

To reduce or prevent swelling.
To prevent friction to and around the little toe.

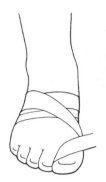

Figure 16.9

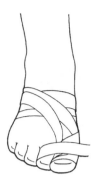

Figure 16.10

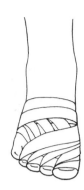

Figure 16.11

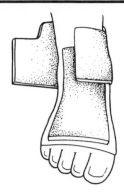

Figure 16.12 Foam is used to cover dorsum of foot and around ankle.

Guidelines • Standard multi-layer compression bandaging (cont'd)

Action	Rationale
Using a narrow light retention bandage anchor the bandage around the foot and bring across the top of the foot to the big toe (Fig. 16.9). Bandage around the toe from the tip downwards (start at the level of the nail bed). Do not pull the bandage tight but gently and firmly. Take the bandage under the foot and back over the top of the foot to the next toe (Fig. 16.10). Repeat the same procedure for each toe that needs to be bandaged. Finish by tucking in the end of the bandage (Fig. 16.11).	
5 Cut the foam into pads to fit over the dorsum of the foot, around the ankle (Fig. 16.12) and behind the knee (Fig. 16.13).	To protect bony prominences and joint flexures.
6 Secure the pads firmly in place with light retention bandages.	
7 Using foam and padding even out any exaggerated contours of the limb.	To create a smooth profile on which to apply the bandages.
8 Using a 10 cm roll of padding, apply firmly in a spiral up the leg, starting around the foot. Use the 20 cm padding over the thigh (Fig. 16.14).	To protect the skin and create a smooth profile on which to bandage.
9 Take an 8 cm compression bandage and start by anchoring it loosely at the ankle. Bandage the foot, starting as close as possible to the toes (Fig. 16.15). Use a spiral over the instep, covering half of the bandage with each turn, and use a figure of eight over the heel and ankle. Bandage firmly and do not leave any gaps.	To avoid constriction at the ankle.
	Fluid will accumulate in any unbandaged areas.
10 Using a 10 cm bandage, continue from where the first bandage finished, using a spiral up the leg and covering half of the bandage with each turn. Remember to bandage firmly. Use the widest bandage over the thigh. Secure the end of the last bandage with tape.	
11 Apply a second layer of bandage, from ankle to thigh, using a figure of eight. Secure the end with tape (Fig. 16.16).	

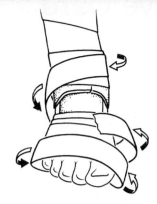

Figure 16.15 Bandaging foot using an 8 cm compression bandage and starting close to toes.

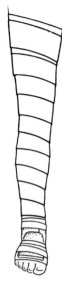

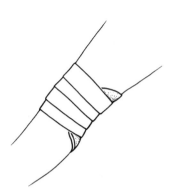

Figure 16.13 A foam pad is bandaged into position behind knee.

Figure 16.14 Rolls of padding are applied firmly in a spiral up leg, starting around foot.

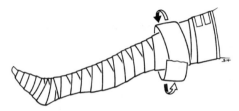

Figure 16.16 Applying a second layer of bandage, from ankle to thigh.

12 Check the colour and temperature of the patient's toes. It may be difficult for the patient to flex the knee at first but this should get easier as the bandages loosen slightly.	To check that the blood flow is not compromised.
13 Remind the patient to use the limb as normally as possible and to report any feelings of discomfort, tingling or numbness.	To ensure good lymph flow.

Eye Care

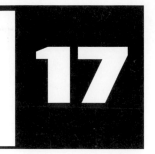

17

Definition

Eye care is the practice of assessing, cleansing or irrigating the eye and/or the instillation of prescribed ocular preparations.

Indications

Eye care may be necessary under the following circumstances:

1 To relieve pain and discomfort.
2 To prevent or treat infection.
3 To prevent further injury to the eye.
4 To detect disease at an early stage.
5 To detect drug-induced toxicity at an early stage.
6 To prevent damage to the cornea in sedated or unconscious patients.

(Cloutier 1992; Ashurst 1997; Cunningham & Gould 1998.)

Reference material

If able, and after appropriate instruction, patients should be encouraged to carry out many of the procedures involved in eye care themselves. However, in the case of postoperative, very ill or unconscious patients, it is often the nurse who is responsible for eye care. A poor eye care technique may lead to the transmission of infection from one eye to the other or the development of irreversible damage to the eye (Ashurst 1997; Cunningham & Gould 1998). In some cases this can lead to loss of sight.

Anatomy and physiology

The eye consists of three main areas: the orbit, the globe (eyeball) and the extrinsic structures. The orbit, or socket, is formed by seven bones of the skull and is lined with fat; it supports and protects the globe and its accessory structures and provides attachments for the ocular muscles. The globe itself can be divided into three layers (Fig. 17.1):

1 The outer layer or fibrous tunic, composed of the cornea and sclera.
2 The middle layer or vascular tunic, composed of the choroid, ciliary body and iris.
3 The inner layer or nervous tunic, composed of the retina.

The function of the outer layer is protective and gives shape to the eyeball. The middle layer contains the globe's

vascular supply and is darkly pigmented. The inner layer contains the light sensitive cells know as the rods and cones and is also the site of the macula lutea (yellow spot) and central fovea (area of highest visual acuity). Extrinsic structures of the eye include the eyelids, eyelashes, eyebrows and lacrimal (tear) apparatus. These structures protect the globe from external injury (SoftKey Multimedia 1995; Tortora & Grabowski 1996). The blood vessels inside the eye may be readily viewed with an ophthalmoscope and examined for changes due to systemic diseases, such as diabetes or hypertension, or local disease processes, such as senile macular degeneration (Tortora & Grabowski 1996).

The optic nerve (cranial nerve II) exits the eye to the side of the macula lutea at an area called the optic disc or blind spot. The optic nerve passes from the orbit, through the optic foramen and into the brain. The two separate optic nerves meet at the optic chiasma and in this area some optic nerve fibres cross over to the opposite side of the brain. The nerves then continue along the optic tracts and terminate in the thalamus. From there projections extend to the visual areas in the occipital lobe of the cerebral cortex (Tortora & Grabowski 1996) (Fig. 17.2). An additional blind spot, or scotoma, may be indicative of a brain tumour. For example, in pituitary gland tumours it is common to develop bilateral defects in the field of vision due to invasion of the optic chiasma (Wickham & Rohan 1997).

The inside of the globe is divided into two chambers by the lens: the anterior cavity, anterior to the lens, and the vitreous chamber, posterior to the lens. The anterior cavity is divided into the anterior chamber and the posterior chamber by the iris. It contains a clear, watery fluid called the aqueous humour. The vitreous chamber is filled with a jelly-like substance called the vitreous body or vitreous humour. Together these two fluid-filled cavities help maintain the shape of the eyeball and the intra-ocular pressure (Marieb 1989; Tortora & Grabowski 1996) (Fig. 17.3).

The aqueous humour is continuously secreted by the choroid plexus of the ciliary process (a part of the ciliary body) located behind the iris. This fluid then permeates the posterior chamber, passing between the lens and the iris, and flows through the pupil into the anterior chamber. From the anterior chamber the aqueous humour drains into the scleral venous sinus (canal of Schlemm) (see Fig. 17.5) and is absorbed back into the blood stream. The aqueous humour is the principal source of nutrients and waste removal for the lens and cornea, as these structures have no direct blood supply. If the outflow of aqueous humour is blocked, excessive intra-ocular pressure may

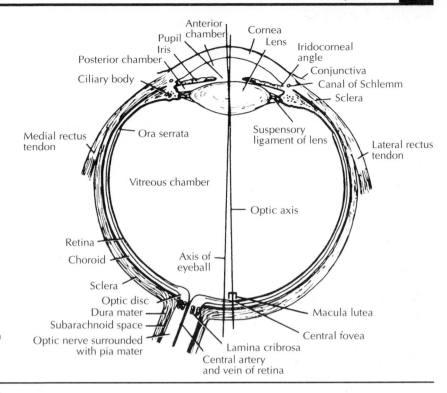

Figure 17.1 Horizontal section through eyeball at level of optic nerve. Optic axis and axis of eyeball are included.

develop, leading to the disease process known as glaucoma. This excess pressure can cause degeneration of the retina and blindness. The vitreous humour, unlike the aqueous humour, is produced during foetal development and is never replaced (Marieb 1989; Tortora & Grabowski 1996).

Tears are produced in the lacrimal glands located at the upper, outer edge of the eye (Fig. 17.4). They are excreted onto the upper surface of the globe and washed over the globe by the action of blinking. The function of tears is to cleanse, moisten and lubricate the globe and eyelids. Tears also provide antisepsis as they contain an enzyme called lysozome that is able to rupture the cell membranes of some bacteria leading to their lysis and death (Tortora & Grabowski 1996).

The tears collect in the nasal canthus (inner, medial aspect of the eye) where they drain into the upper and lower lacrimal puncti. The puncti are small openings leading to the lacrimal canaliculi (or canals), these in turn drain into the lacrimal sac. From here the tears pass into the naso-lacrimal duct and empty into the nasal cavity (Marieb 1996; Tortora & Grabowski 1996; SoftKey Multimedia 1995).

General principles of eye care

Aseptic technique is necessary only in certain circumstances, for example, when the eye is damaged or following ophthalmic surgery.

Position of patient

The patient should be sitting or lying with his or her head tilted backwards and chin pointing upwards. This allows for easy access to the eyes and is usually a good position for patient comfort and compliance.

Position of light source

A good light source is necessary prior to commencing eye care procedures to enable careful assessment of the eyes and to avoid damage to their delicate structures. The light source should be positioned above and behind the nurse. It should never be allowed to shine directly into the patient's eyes, as this will be extremely uncomfortable for the patient.

Instillation of drops

Most types of drops are instilled into the upper rim of the inferior fornix (i.e. just inside the lower eyelid) as the conjuctiva in this area is less sensitive than that overlying the cornea. Also, the drops will run into the pocket of the inferior fornix preventing immediate loss of the drops into the naso-lacrimal drainage system. Exceptions to this instillation technique are as follows:

1 *Drugs used to lubricate the cornea*: oil-based drops produce less corneal reaction than aqueous ones as they do not

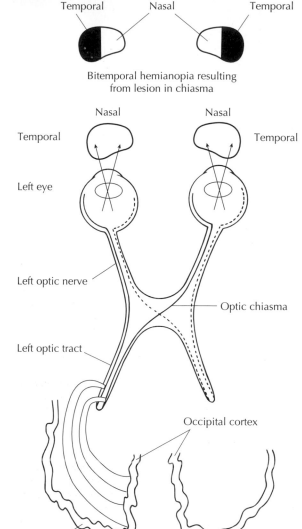

Bitemporal hemianopia resulting
from lesion in chiasma

Temporal

Nasal

Left eye

Left optic nerve

Left optic tract

Optic chiasma

Occipital cortex

Left cerebral hemisphere

Figure 17.2 Visual pathways and visual fields.

1 *Oil-based solutions*: these are used for lubricating the eyeball. Usually one drop is instilled and repeated as required.
2 *Anaesthetic drops*: it is usual to instil two or three drops at a time. This is repeated until the drop cannot be felt on the eye.

The dropper should be held as close to the eye as possible without touching either the lids or the cornea. This will avoid corneal damage and reduce the risk of cross-infection. If the drop falls from too great a height it is difficult to control and will also be uncomfortable for the patient.

A variety of droppers and bottles are available for the instillation of eye preparations. These include pipettes, bottles incorporating pipettes, plastic bottles with a dropper attachment and single dose packs. Pipettes are easy to use but need to be dried and sterilized between doses. Plastic bottles can be squeezed and so avoid the need for a pipette and they are also cheaper than glass bottles with a dropper. Each patient should have their own, individual eye drop container and single dose containers should be used for all patients in eye clinics or in accident and emergency departments (British National Formulary 1999).

Instillation of ointments

Ointments are also applied to the upper rim of the inferior fornix using a similar technique to eye drops. A 2 cm line of ointment should be applied from the nasal canthus outwards. Similarly to the instillation of eye drops, the nozzle should be held approximately 2.5 cm above the eye to avoid contact with the cornea and eyelids.

Contact lenses and eye preparations

Contact lenses may affect the distribution and absorption of eye preparations. Some drugs and preservatives in eye preparations may accumulate in soft hydrogel lenses and induce a toxic reaction. For these reasons contact lenses should be removed prior to instillation of eye drops or ointments and not worn for the period of treatment (British National Formulary 1999).

Eye irrigation

The most common use of eye irrigation is for the removal of caustic substances from the eye, e.g. domestic cleaning agents or medications, particularly cytotoxic material. This should be done as soon as possible to minimize damage. The procedure is also used as a pre-operative preparation or to remove infected material. The fluids most commonly used are sterile 0.9% sodium chloride, 'for irrigation', or sterile water, 'for irrigation'. In an emergency tap water may be used (McConnell 1991). The volume used will vary depending on the degree of contamination; copious amounts are needed for corrosive chemicals and smaller volumes for removal of eye secretions.

feel as cold to the cornea when administered. They may therefore be instilled directly into the inferior fornix.
2 *Anaesthetic drops*: the first drop should be instilled into the inferior fornix for absorption and then directly onto the cornea one drop at a time until the patient is no longer able to feel the drops.
3 *Drops used to treat the nasal passages*: these should be instilled at the nasal canthus end of the eye.

The number of drops instilled depends on the type of solution used and its purpose. Usually, one drop only is ordered and will be sufficient if it is instilled in the correct manner. The exceptions to the 'one drop' rule are:

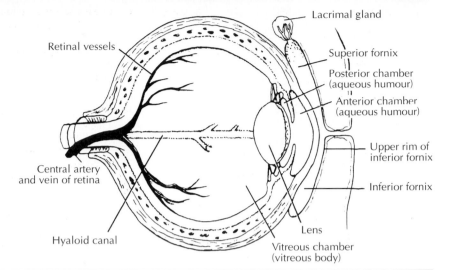

Figure 17.3 Anterior cavity in front of lens is incompletely divided into anterior chamber (anterior to iris) and posterior chamber (behind iris), which are continuous through pupil. Aqueous humour, which fills the cavity, is formed by ciliary processes and reabsorbed into venous blood by the canal of Schlemm.

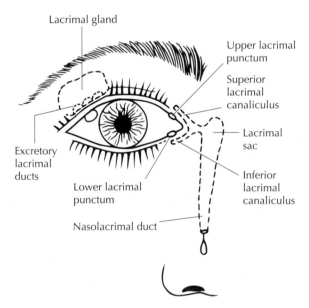

Figure 17.4 Lacrimal apparatus.

Care of the insensitive eye

If the eye-blink reflex is absent the eye's surface will dry out, causing irreversible corneal damage. The cornea may become ulcerated or infected, leading to scarring and possibly loss of vision. This is a particular problem in the sedated, ventilated or unconscious patient. When the patient has lost this protective reflex, the nurse must institute measures to maintain eye moisture and corneal integrity. The surface of the eye and surrounding structures should be keep clean and moist by gentle cleansing with sterile 0.9% sodium chloride and, when necessary, the instillation of lubricating preparations. If there is no eye-blink reflex the eyelids should be kept closed by the use of hypoallergenic tape or by the application of hydrogel sheet preparations, e.g. Geliperm. If the eyes become infected the relevant medication should be prescribed and administered (Ashurst 1997).

With each of these measures care must be taken not to spread infection between the eyes. Any alteration to the appearance of the eye must be reported to the doctor.

Eye medications

Drugs may be given either systemically or topically to exert an effect on the eye. However, if given systemically the prescribing doctor needs to take account of the physiological barrier and the blood–aqueous barrier which exists within the eye and which is selective in allowing drugs to pass into the intraocular fluids. Permeability of this barrier may be altered in inflammatory conditions and following paracentesis (removal of excess fluid with a needle or cannula).

Medications applied locally meet some resistance at the barrier presented by the lacrimal system (tear film barrier). A further barrier is that of the cornea which is selectively permeable and only allows the passage of water and not drugs. However, the corneal resistance may alter if there is damage to the corneal epithelium. Many drugs will produce a similar effect on both the healthy and diseased eye. Drugs for use in the eye are usually classified according to their action.

Mydriatics and cycloplegics

These drugs produce their effects by paralysing the ciliary muscle, by stimulating the dilator muscle of the pupil or by a combination of both (Fig. 17.5). They are used mainly for diagnostic purposes and most have an anticholinergic action. The most commonly used preparations are

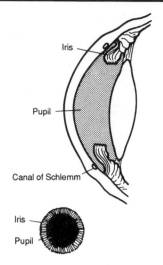

Figure 17.5 Effect of mydriatics.

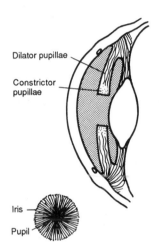

Figure 17.6 Effect of miotics.

cyclopentolate hydrochloride and tropicamide (British National Formulary 1999).

Miotics

These drugs produce their effects by constricting the pupil and contracting the ciliary muscle (Fig. 17.6). Miotics help in the drainage of aqueous humour and are used primarily in the treatment of glaucoma. Examples are pilocarpine and carbachol (British National Formulary 1999).

Local anaesthetics

These render the eye and the inner surfaces of the lids insensitive. They are used before minor surgery, removal of

foreign bodies and tonometry (measurement of intra-ocular pressure). The most widely used eye anaesthetics are oxybuprocaine and amethocaine. Cocaine is no longer used as an eye anaesthetic due to corneal toxicity and the possibility of patients developing an idiosyncrasy to it and suddenly collapsing (British National Formulary 1999).

Anti-inflammatories

Anti-inflammatory drugs include steroids, antihistamines, lodoxamide and sodium cromoglycate. The most commonly used steroid preparations are dexamethasone, prednisolone and betamethasone (British National Formulary 1999).

Corticosteroid eye drops should be used with caution as they can cause a gradual rise in intraocular pressure in a small percentage of people (especially if they have a history of glaucoma).

Antibacterials/antivirals

Antibacterials and antivirals can be used for the active treatment of infections or as prophylactic treatment for eye surgery, after removal of a foreign body or following an eye injury. Antibiotic preparations in common use are chloramphenicol, neomycin and framycetin. Aciclovir is the only antiviral available as an eye preparation (British National Formulary 1999).

Artificial tears

Artificial tears are used when there is a deficiency in natural tear production. This can be due to a disease process, postradiotherapy treatment, as a side-effect of certain drugs and when the eye-blink reflex is absent. These artificial lubricants commonly contain hypromellose or hydroxyethylcellulose (British National Formulary 1999).

Toxic effects of common systemic drugs on the eye

As the eye may be the first place to show signs of systemic disease, so some systemic drugs may show their toxic effects in the eye. These effects range from pruritis, irritation, redness, epiphora (excess tear production with overflow), photophobia and blepharoconjunctivitis (inflammation of the eyelids and conjunctiva), to disturbance of vision (Cloutier 1992). Particular effects of specific drugs are listed below:

1 *Methotrexate and related antimetabolites:* these drugs can affect the meibomian glands (specialized sebaceous glands in the eyelids), causing blepharoconjunctivitis. They may also induce photophobia, epiphora, periorbital oedema and conjunctival hyperaemia.
2 *5-Fluorouracil (5-FU):* 5-FU can cause canalicular fibrosis and oculomotor disturbances (probably secondary to a local neurotoxicity affecting the brainstem).

3 *Antihistamines:* these drugs decrease tear production and may lead to 'dry eye', especially in patients with Sjögren's syndrome (a wasting disease of the salivary glands), ocular pemphigus (rare, autoimmune disease of the skin), those who wear contact lenses and in the elderly.

4 *Tamoxifen:* this drug can cause subepithelial whirl-like deposits in the corne, and retinal lesions.

5 *Indomethacin:* this can cause corneal deposits and retinal pigmentary toxicity.

6 *Oral contraceptives:* these can stimulate corneal steeping and intolerance to contact lenses.

7 *Atropine, scopalamine and belladonna-like substances:* such drugs cause mydriasis (widening of the pupil) and cycloplegia (paralysis of the ciliary muscle that moves the iris) (Martin 1996).

8 *Corticosteroids:* prolonged use of corticosteroids produces posterior subcapsular cataracts.

9 *Chloramphenicol:* chloramphenicol treatment can lead to optic neuritis.

10 *Ethambutol:* this drug can cause damage to the optic nerve.

11 *Rifampicin:* stains soft contact lenses.

12 *Digoxin:* in overdose results in blurred vision and yellow/green vision.

13 *Oxygen:* in neonates, high concentrations for a long period can cause retrolental fibroplasia (abnormal proliferation of fibrous tissue behind the lens causing blindness) (Martin 1996).

Tumours of the eye

There are a number of tumours associated with the eye and they may involve the orbit, globe or extrinsic structures. To appreciate the spread of disease and clinical features associated with eye tumours, it is important to be aware of the relationship between the eye and other local structures. The anterior cranial fossa lies superiorly, the nasal cavity and ethmoid labyrinth medially, the maxillary antrum inferiorly and the infratemporal and middle cranial fossa laterally to the eye (Lund 1987; Tortora & Grabowski 1996).

Tumours of the orbit

While orbital tumours are rare, primary and metastatic lesions do occur. However, metastases are more likely to arise in the globe than in the orbit. The most common primary tumours of the orbit are rhabdomyosarcoma in children and lymphoma in adults. Occurring less often are meningiomas, soft tissue sarcomas and nerve sheath tumours (including optic nerve gliomas) (Henderson 1980; Char 1993; Souhami & Tobias 1998). Development of metastases in the orbit is indicative of a primary tumour elsewhere in the body. Metastases may vary from a rapidly developing mass, often invading local soft tissues and bone, to slow scarring of the soft tissues of the eye. The primary tumours most likely to develop orbital metastases arise in the thyroid, bronchus, breast, prostate, kidney and skin (Tijl *et al.* 1992; Souhami & Tobias 1998).

Signs and symptoms

Most orbital tumours push the eye away from its normal visual axis in a sagittal or vertical plane. In almost all cases the direction of displacement is opposite to the growing tumour (Moeloek 1993). Lack of room for growth due to the rigid bony cavity causes the eye to protrude (proptosis), often to a large degree. The average volume of the orbital cavity is 24 ml and an increase in volume of only 4 ml will produce 6 mm of proptosis. Therefore proptosis, with signs of diplopia (double vision), is the main clinical feature of orbital tumours and this can be a very disfiguring and distressing symptom for the patient (Tijl *et al.* 1992; Char 1993; Moeloek 1993; Souhami & Tobias 1998). It should be noted that bilateral proptosis is most commonly related to hyperthyroidism (Leitman 1988).

If the tumour involves the muscles of the eye it may cause ophthalmoplegia (paralysis of the eye muscles); this may also occur if cranial nerve III is involved. Chemosis (swelling of the conjuctiva) may occur and, in conjunction with an infection, may be misdiagnosed as cellulitis. In addition, panophthalmitis (inflammation of the interior of the eye) can develop and may lead to perforation of the globe and unilateral blindness. This is common with advanced tumours (Souhami & Tobias 1998).

Visual changes can occur with tumours that involve the optic nerve or its sheath, or that press against its surface externally. Diplopia, excess tear production, a visible mass, ptosis (drooping of the upper eyelid), epiphora and pain are other clinical features of orbital tumours (Lund 1987; Tijl *et al.* 1992; Char 1993; Moeloek 1993; Souhami & Tobias 1998).

Tumours of the globe

Retinoblastoma (malignant tumour of the retina) and malignant melanoma are the most common tumours occurring in the globe. Melanoma occurs most often in adults and retinoblostoma is generally a disease of childhood, with most cases presenting before the age of 5. Forty percent of retinoblastomas are hereditary and 60% are spontaneous (non-hereditary). Retinoblastoma has a good prognosis, with a 5-year disease-free period in 80–90% of childhood cases. The most common site for melanoma of the globe is in the vascular tunic (choroid, ciliary body and iris). There are about six cases per million a year and the majority (85%) occur in the choroid. Because this layer of the eye is very vascular, metastases are common and suggest a poor prognosis. Melanomas of the iris and ciliary body are usually diagnosed earlier as they are more visible, whereas choroidal tumours may remain undiagnosed for some time unless they cause a disturbance in the visual field, for example if they are in the macula lutea or cause retinal detachment. As the choroid is a common site of secondary deposits from cutaneous melanoma, the possibility of the tumour being metastatic and not a primary must be ruled out (Souhami & Tobias 1998; National Cancer Institute 1999a,b).

Melanoma and squamous cell carcinoma (SCC) are occasionally found in the conjunctiva. Conjunctival melanoma has a good overall prognosis with about 75% of patients surviving for over 5 years; however for patients presenting with large lesions the risk of disseminated disease is high. A precancerous lesion known as ocular melanosis can occur in the conjunctiva and this must be differentiated from a true melanoma. These lesions should be managed by careful observation, as a malignant change can develop but may take many years to do so. The early diagnosis of conjunctival SCC is important and with the correct treatment there is generally a good prognosis (Souhami & Tobias 1998).

Tumours of the extrinsic structures

Basal cell carcinoma (BCC) and SCC are fairly common tumours of the eyelid, particularly in the elderly. The lower eyelid and inner canthus are the areas most commonly affected (Henk 1976; Souhami & Tobias 1998). BCC grows slowly and rarely metastasizes; however, it can spread by direct growth into adjacent structures such as the orbit and, ultimately, even the brain. SCC has a similar epidemiology to BCC but it grows more rapidly and may metastasize to regional lymph nodes, particularly in the neck. Metastatic SCC carries a poor prognosis (National Cancer Institute 1999d).

Investigations

Comprehensive clinical examination by a specialist consultant is imperative. Additional investigations include:

1 Histology
2 Computerized tomography
3 Magnetic resonance imaging
4 Orbital venography
5 Carotid angiography
6 Ultrasound.

The last three techniques have become less popular with the advent of computerized tomography and magnetic resonance imaging (Lund 1987). Histological confirmation of the tumour type should be performed if possible, by either biopsy or cytology. Care needs to be taken during these procedures as tumour spillage, haemorrhage and blindness are potential risks with either method of sampling. If the tumour is encapsulated it is suggested that it be excised in entirety (Souhami & Tobias 1998).

Treatment

The treatment of any eye malignancy is always based on the principle of curing the disease and preserving sight. In the instance of large or invasive tumours this is not always possible so the aim then is to maintain a suitable cosmetic appearance. Clinicians should be reminded that any decision on preservation of the orbital contents must be based on a clear and unemotional decision that will not compromise the overall prognosis (Lund 1987). It should also be remembered that the final decision on treatment

must be made by the patient. In order to make this decision the patient must be fully informed and aware of all treatment or non-treatment options available to them, and the likely outcome of each option.

Rhabdomyosarcomas are usually treated with radiotherapy and adjuvant chemotherapy with good results (National Cancer Institute 1999c). The standard treatment for orbital lymphoma is radiotherapy alone (Souhami & Tobias 1998). Orbital metastases are treated according to the type of primary tumour. With metastatic breast cancer, radiotherapy is given in the first instance with chemotherapy and hormonal therapy also used if proven effective. Prostate cancer is generally radiosensitive, therefore radiotherapy is used to treat orbital deposits. Radiotherapy is again used for thyroid secondaries and may be an external beam or in the form of radioactive iodine (Tijl *et al.* 1992). These are usually palliative measures and are only appropriate if the patient is well enough to tolerate them. They can help to preserve vision, reduce pain and, consequently, improve quality of life.

Treatment of retinoblastoma will depend on the size of the tumour. Small tumours may be controlled with ablative therapies (cryotherapy or photocoagulation, for example), brachytherapy ('short distance' therapy, see Chap. 33, Radioactive Source Therapy: Sealed Sources) or external beam radiotherapy. If the tumour is large, radiotherapy is often combined with adjuvant chemotherapy, giving a 5-year survival rate of about 75%. When the tumour is very extensive and/or the eye is beyond the point of useful recovery then enucleation (removal of the globe) is considered the treatment of choice (Souhami & Tobias 1998; National Cancer Institute 1999b). The management of ocular melanoma has recently changed from the use of extensive surgery, usually enucleation, to a more conservative approach of close observation and intervention only if symptoms develop. This approach is commonly taken in elderly patients. When treatment is needed, the choice again depends on the size of the tumour. The approach is the same as for retinoblastoma, with surgical excision, ablative therapies and local irradiation being the mainstays of treatment for small tumours. For larger tumours enucleation is usual, possibly in conjunction with preoperative external beam radiotherapy (Souhami & Tobias 1998; National Cancer Institute 1999a).

The most common treatments for squamous cell and basal cell carcinomas of the external eye are surgery or ablative therapies and radiotherapy, either alone or in combination. Early diagnosis of conjuctival melanoma and SCC is essential as small lesions may be effectively treated by radiotherapy, conserving the eye and preserving vision. Surgical excision followed by brachytherapy is also a common treatment for these lesions (Souhami & Tobias 1998; National Cancer Institute 1999d).

Any tumour of the eye may necessitate enucleation if it is very large or has local extension, if the optic nerve is involved or retinal detachment has occurred. It may also be necessary for the control of pain or if secondary glaucoma has developed. However, minimally invasive tumours of the orbit that do not involve the ocular muscles may be resected without enucleation and any defect to the periosteum reconstructed using the temporalis facia. This procedure is usually followed by postoperative radiotherapy (Goldberg & Cantore 1997).

Summary

Like most disfigurements of the head and neck, orbital tumours are also difficult to camouflage. Commonly patients will wear tinted glasses, or wear an eye pad/protector so that it looks more like protection from an eye injury rather than camouflage of a tumour. Eye patches are occasionally worn, but most patients feel that this is indicative of eye loss.

Patients with orbital disease need skilled emotional support. This is particularly true if the disease is inoperable and/or end stage. The tumour may be exophytic, proptosed or causing splaying of the nasal and ethmoid bones. Such disfiguring complications may lead to social isolation, avoidance and despair. These patients not only live with disfigurement and dysfunction, but also the threat to their survival from the disease process. It is suggested that eye tumours, for example childhood retinoblastoma (National Cancer Institute 1999b) and choroidal melanoma (Foss *et al.* 1999), be treated at specialist centres for the optimal prognostic outcome. Nursing and medical staff in these centres are more likely to have the experience and knowledge required in dealing with these relatively rare and demanding disease processes and their consequences. In addition, they may be more aware of community support networks and can ensure that, when necessary, patients are referred to an appropriate specialist prosthetic department.

Primarily, the nurse will be involved in helping the patient cope with the diagnosis and treatment of their disease, care of the eye (or cavity if enucleation has been performed) and any prostheses the patient has had fitted. Reintegration into the community and workplace must be followed up closely through outpatient clinics or via telephone contact to help reduce any feelings of isolation and abandonment once discharged from hospital. Further nursing interventions include observation and early detection of any eye irregularities and clinical management of symptoms. This will involve assessment and management of pain (see Chap. 29, Pain Assessment and Management), maintaining the eye in a clean and comfortable state and administering eye preparations as prescribed. The eye may need to be covered for protection, patient comfort or as a means of camouflage.

References and further reading

Ashurst, S. (1997) Nursing care of the mechanically ventilated patient in ITU: 1. *Br J Nurs*, **6**(8), 447–54.

Belden, C.J. & Zinreich, S.J. (1997) Orbital imaging techniques. *Semin Ultrasound CT MRI*, **18**(6), 413–22.

British National Formulary (1999) *Number 37 (March)*. British Medical Association/Royal Pharmaceutical Society of Great Britain, London.

Bryant, W.M. (1981) Common toxic effects of systemic drugs on the eye. *Occup Health Nurs*, **29**, 15–17.

Char, D.H. (1993) Management of orbital tumours. *Mayo Clin Pract*, **68**, 1081–96.

Chilman, A.M. & Thomas, M. (1987) *Understanding Nursing Care*, 3rd edn. Churchill Livingstone, Edinburgh.

Cloutier, A.O. (1992) Ocular side effects of chemotherapy: nursing management. *Oncol Nurs Forum*, **8**(19), 1251–9.

Cunningham, C. & Gould, D. (1998) Eyecare for the sedated patient undergoing mechanical ventilation: the use of evidence-based care. *Int J Nurs Stud*, **35**, 32–40.

Darling, V.H. & Thorpe, M.R. (1981) *Ophthalmic Nursing*, 2nd edn. Baillière Tindall, London.

Foss, A.J.E., Cree, I.A., Dolin, P.J. et al. (1999) Modelling uveal melanoma. *Br J Ophthalmol*, **83**, 588–94.

Goldberg, S.H. & Cantore, W.A. (1997) Tumours of the orbit. *Curr Opin Ophthalmol*, **815**, 51–6.

Gorman, C.A. (1978) The presentation and management of endocrine ophthalmopathy. *Clin Endocrinol Metab*, **7**, 67–96.

Henderson, J.W. (1980) Metastatic carcinoma. In: *Orbital Tumours* (ed. J.W. Henderson), 2nd edn, pp. 451–71. Decker, New York.

Henk, J.M. (1976) Neoplasms of the head and neck. In: *Radiotherapy in Modern Clinical Practice* (ed. H.F. Hope-Stone), pp. 108–42. Crosby Lockwood Staples, London.

Leitman, M.W. (1988) *Manual for Eye Examination and Diagnosis*, 3rd edn. Medical Economics Body, New Jersey.

Lund, V.J. (1987) The orbit. In: *Otolaryngology* (ed. A.G. Kerr), 5th edn. Butterworth, London.

McConnell, E.A. (1991) How to irrigate the eye. *Nursing*, **91**, March, 28.

Marieb, E.N. (1987) *Human Anatomy and Physiology Laboratory Manual*. Benjamin Cummings, California.

Marieb, E.N. (1996) *Human Anatomy and Physiology*. Benjamin Cummings, California.

Marshall, E.C. (1993) Epidemiology of tumours affecting the visual system. *Optomet Clin*, **3**(3), 1–16.

Martin, E.A. (1996) *Concise Colour Medical Dictionary*. Oxford University Press, Oxford.

Moeloek, N.F. (1993) Updates in orbital tumours. *Eye Sci*, **9**(1), 40–44.

National Cancer Institute (1999a) Intraocular melanoma. http://cancernet.nci.nih.gov/clinpdq/soa/intraocular_melanoma physician.html

National Cancer Institute (1999b) Retinoblastoma. http://cancernet.nci.nih.gov/clinpdq/soa/retinoblastoma_physician.html

National Cancer Institute (1999c) Childhood rhabdomyosarcoma. http://cancernet.nci.nih.gov/clinpdq/soa/childhood_rhabdomyosarcoma_physician.html

National Cancer Institute (1999d) Skin cancer. http://cancernet.nci.nih.gov/clinpdq/soa/skin_cancer_physician.html

Phillips, M. (1982) Ophthalmic preparations. *Nurs Mirror*, **155**, 69–71.

Rooke, E.C.E. et al. (1980) *Ophthalmic Nursing – Its Practice and Management*. Churchill Livingstone, Edinburgh.

Smith, J. & Nachazel, D.P. (1980) *Ophthalmologic Nursing*. Little, Brown, Boston.

SoftKey Multimedia (1995) *BodyWorks 5.0 for Windows* CD-ROM. SoftKey International, Cambridge, Massachusetts.

Souhami, R. & Tobias, J. (1998) *Cancer and its Management*. Blackwell Science, Oxford.

Tijl, J. et al. (1992) Metastatic tumours to the orbit – management and prognosis. *Graefe's Arch Clin Exp Ophthalmol (Amsterdam)*, **230**, 527–30.

Tortora, G.J. & Grabowski, S.R. (1996) *Principles of Anatomy and Physiology*, 8th edn. Harper Collins, Menlo Park, California.

Wickham, R. & Rohan, K. (1997) Endocrine malignancies. In: *Cancer Nursing: Principles and Practice* (eds S.L. Groenwald, M. Hansen Frogge, M. Goodman, et al.), 4th edn., pp. 1055–81. Jones and Bartlett, Sudbury, Massachusetts.

Zhao, D., Dhields, C.L., Shields, J.A. et al. (1998) New developments in the management of retinoblastoma. *J Ophthal Nurs Tech*, **17**(1), 13–18.

GUIDELINES · Eye swabbing

Equipment

1 Sterile dressing pack.
2 Sterile 0.9% sodium chloride for irrigation or sterile water for irrigation.

Procedure

Action	*Rationale*
1 Explain and discuss the procedure with the patient.	To ensure that the patient understands the procedure and gives his/her valid consent.
2 Assist the patient into the correct position: (a) Head well supported and tilted back. (b) Preferably the patient should be in bed or lying on a couch.	The patient needs to be discouraged from flinching or making unexpected movements and so should be in the most comfortable position possible at the start of the procedure.
3 Ensure an adequate light source, taking care not to dazzle the patient.	To enable maximum observation of the eyes without causing the patient harm or discomfort.
4 Wash hands thoroughly using bactericidal soap and water or bactericidal alcohol hand rub, then dry hands.	To reduce the risk of cross-infection.
5 Always treat the uninfected or uninflamed eye first.	To reduce the risk of cross-infection.
6 Always bathe lids with the eyes closed first.	To reduce the risk of damaging the cornea.
7 Using a slightly moistened low-linting swab, ask the patient to look up and gently swab the lower lid from the nasal corner outwards. Use an aseptic technique for the damaged or postoperative eye.	If the swab is too wet the solution will run down the patient's cheek. This increases the risk of cross-infection and causes the patient discomfort. Swabbing from the nasal corner outwards avoids the risk of swabbing discharge into the lacrymal punctum, or even across the bridge of the nose into other eye. Aseptic technique reduces the risk of cross-infection.
8 Ensure that the edge of the swab is not above the lid margin.	To avoid touching the sensitive cornea.
9 Using a new swab each time, repeat the procedure until all the discharge has been removed.	To reduce risk of infection.
10 Gently swab the upper lid by slightly everting the lid margin and asking the patient to look down. Swab from the nasal corner outwards and use a new swab each time until all discharge has been removed.	To effectively remove any foreign material from eye. To reduce the risk of cross-infection.
11 Once both eyelids have been cleansed and dried, make the patient comfortable.	
12 Remove and dispose of equipment.	
13 Wash hands.	To reduce the risk of cross-infection.
14 Record the procedure in the appropriate documents.	To monitor trends and fluctuations.

Note: for information about obtaining an eye swab for pathological investigations, see the appropriate section in Chap. 37, Specimen Collection.

GUIDELINES • Instillation of eye drops

Equipment

1 Sterile dressing pack.
2 Sterile 0.9% sodium chloride for irrigation or sterile water for irrigation.
3 Appropriate eye drops. (Any preparation must be checked against the doctor's prescription.)
4 Low-linting swab.

Procedure

Action	*Rationale*
1 Explain and discuss the procedure with the patient.	To ensure that the patient understands the procedure and gives his/her valid consent.
2 If there is any discharge, proceed as for eye swabbing.	To remove any infected material and thus ensure adequate absorption of the drops.
3 Consult the patient's prescription sheet, and ascertain the following: (a) Drug. (b) Dose. (c) Date and time of administration. (d) Route and method of administration, including which eye the drops are prescribed for. (e) Expiry date on bottle. (f) Validity of prescription. (g) Signature of doctor.	To ensure that the patient is given the correct drug in the prescribed dose in the correct eye, and that the drug has not expired.
4 Assist the patient into the correct position, i.e. head well supported and tilted back.	To ensure that drops are instilled into the pocket of the inferior fornix and to avoid excess solution running down the patient's cheek.
5 Wash hands thoroughly using bactericidal soap and water or bactericidal alcohol hand rub, and dry them.	Asepsis is essential, particularly when the patient has a damaged eye or has just had an operation on the eye. Infection can lead to loss of an eye.
6 Place a wet low-linting swab on the lower lid against the lid margin and gently pull down to evert the lower eyelid.	To absorb any excess solution which may be irritating to the surrounding skin and open the inferior fornix.
7 Ask the patient to look up immediately before instilling the drop.	This opens the eye and allows the drop to be instilled into the upper rim of the ïnferior fornix. If done too soon the patient may blink as the drop is instilled.
8 Ask the patient to close the eye. Keep the wet low-linting swab on the lower lid.	To ensure absorption of the fluid and to avoid excess running down the cheek.
9 Make the patient comfortable.	
10 Remove and dispose of equipment.	
11 Wash hands with bactericidal soap and water.	To reduce the risk of cross-infection.
12 Complete the patient's recording chart and other hospital and/or legally required documents.	To maintain accurate records. To provide a point of reference in the event of any queries. To prevent any duplication of treatment.

GUIDELINES • Instillation of eye ointment

Equipment

1 Sterile dressing pack.
2 Sterile 0.9% sodium chloride for irrigation or sterile water for irrigation.

3 Appropriate eye ointment. (Any preparation must be checked against the doctor's prescription.)
4 Low-linting swab.

Procedure

Action

1 Explain and discuss the procedure with the patient.

2 If there is any discharge, and to remove any previous application of ointment, proceed as for eye swabbing.

3 Consult the patient's prescription sheet, and ascertain the following:
(a) Drug.
(b) Dose.
(c) Date and time of administration.
(d) Route and method of administration, including which eye the ointment is prescribed for.
(e) Expiry date on bottle.
(f) Validity of prescription.
(g) Signature of doctor.

4 Wash hands thoroughly using bactericidal soap and water or bactericidal alcohol hand rub.

5 Place a wet low-linting swab on the lower lid against the lid margin.

6 Slightly evert the lower lid by pulling on the low-linting swab. Ask the patient to look up immediately before applying the cream.

7 Apply the ointment by gently squeezing the tube and, with the nozzle 2.5 cm above the eye, drawing a line along the inner edge of the lower lid from the nasal corner outward.

8 Ask the patient to close the eye and remove excess ointment with a new wet low-linting swab.

9 Warn the patient that, when the eye is opened, vision will be a little blurred for a few minutes.

10 Make the patient comfortable.

11 Remove and dispose of equipment.

12 Wash hands with bactericidal soap and water.

13 Complete the patient's recording chart and other hospital and/or legally required documents.

Rationale

To ensure that the patient understands the procedure and gives his/her valid consent.

To remove any infected material and previous ointment to allow for absorption of ointment.

To ensure that the patient is given the correct drug in the prescribed dose in the correct eye, and that the drug has not expired.

To reduce the risk of cross-infection.

To absorb excess ointment which may be irritating to the surrounding skin.

To allow the application to be made inside the lower lid into the lower fornix.

To reduce the risk of cross-infection, contamination of the tube and trauma to the eye.

To avoid excess ointment irritating the surrounding skin.

To prepare patient and to avoid anxiety.

To reduce the risk of cross-infection.

To maintain accurate records. To provide a point of reference in the event of any queries. To prevent any duplication of treatment.

GUIDELINES • Eye irrigation

Equipment

1 Sterile dressing pack.
2 Sterile 0.9% sodium chloride for irrigation or sterile water for irrigation (in an emergency tap water may be used).
3 Receiver.
4 Towel.

5 Plastic cape.
6 Irrigating flask.
7 Warm water in a bowl to heat irrigating fluid to tepid temperature.
8 Anaesthetic drops.

Procedure

Action	*Rationale*
1 Explain and discuss the procedure with the patient.	To ensure that the patient understands the procedure and gives his/her valid consent.
2 Instil anaesthetic drops if required (proceed as for instillation of eye drops).	To avoid any discomfort.
3 Prepare the irrigation fluid to the appropriate temperature.	Tepid fluid will be more comfortable for the patient. The solution should be poured across the inner aspect of the nurse's wrist to test the temperature.
4 Assist the patient into the appropriate position: (a) Head comfortably supported with chin almost horizontal. (b) Head inclined to the side of the eye to be treated.	To avoid the solution running either over the cheek into the other eye or out of the affected eye and down the side of the nose.
5 Wash hands using bactericidal soap and water or bactericidal alcohol hand rub, and dry.	To reduce risk of infection.
6 If there is any discharge proceed as for eye swabbing.	To prevent washing the discharge down the lacrimal duct or across the cheek.
7 Ask the patient to hold the receiver against the cheek below the eye being irrigated.	To collect irrigation fluid as it runs away from the eye.
8 Position the towel and plastic cape.	To protect the patient's clothing.
9 Hold the patient's eyelids apart, using your first and second fingers, against the orbital ridge.	The patient will be unable to hold the eye open once irrigation commences.
10 Do not press on the eyeball.	To avoid causing the patient discomfort or pain.
11 Warn the patient that the flow of solution is going to start and pour a little onto the cheek first.	To allow time for adjustment of feeling of water flow.
12 Direct the flow of the fluid from the nasal corner outwards.	To wash away from the lacrimal punctum and prevent contaminating other eye.
13 Ask the patient to look up, down and to either side while irrigating.	To ensure that the whole area is washed.
14 Evert lids while irrigating.	To ensure complete removal of any foreign body.
15 Keep the flow of irrigation fluid constant.	To ensure swift removal of any foreign body.
16 When the eye has been thoroughly irrigated, ask the patient to close the eyes and use a new swab to dry the lids.	For patient comfort.
17 Take the receiver from the patient and dry the cheek.	To prevent spillage of receiver contents and promote patient comfort.

Guidelines • Eye irrigation (cont'd)

Action	Rationale
18 Make the patient comfortable.	
19 Remove and dispose of equipment.	
20 Wash hands with bactericidal soap and water.	To reduce the risk of cross-infection.
21 Complete the patient's recording chart and other hospital and/or legally required documents.	To maintain accurate records. To provide a point of reference in the event of any queries. To prevent any duplication of treatment.

Gene Therapy for the Management of Cancer

18

Definition

Gene therapy is the insertion, augmentation or substitution of a functioning gene into a cell to provide the cell with a new function, which will correct a genetic disorder or correct a malformation to achieve a therapeutic effect (Palu *et al.* 1999).

Reference material

Normal cells contain the mechanisms to repair damage to the genetic material. Cancer can occur when such mechanisms are absent or fail to protect against genetic error through cell division. This failure allows multiplication of abnormal cells, invasion of local tissue and ultimately distant metastases (Trahan Rieger 1997). The overall goal of gene therapy is to improve health by correcting the gene alteration in affected cells (Lea 1997).

The process by which genes are inserted, augmented or substituted into a cell is termed genetic modification. Genetic modification in relation to an organism means the altering of the genetic material by a method which does not occur naturally, e.g. by mating and/or natural recombination (HSE 1996). This can take the form of *ex vivo* (outside body) or *in vivo* (inside body) therapy. *Ex vivo* gene therapy is achieved by introducing the gene into the patients cells and reinfusing them into the patient. *In vivo* describes the direct administration of the genetic material into the patient using an appropriate delivery system such as a virus, by methods such as injections or infusion (Sandhu *et al.* 1997).

Genetic modification involves the manipulation of nucleic acid and, in particular, DNA. Molecules of DNA contain information for cellular structure and function. Every cell in an organism contains a complete set of genes, 'the genome', which are found on chromosomes. Gene therapy involves ascertaining which gene controls which inherited feature, and then introducing, deleting or enhancing a particular trait in an organism, by altering its genetic composition. In most cases this involves extracting DNA from one organism, manipulating or restructuring it and then transferring it into another organism. Transfer usually takes place by attaching the gene of interest to another DNA carrier (vector). The most commonly used vectors are plasmids and viruses (Jenkins *et al.* 1994).

For example, one of the best viruses in terms of its potential ability to deliver therapeutic genes to cancer cells is the adenovirus. The adenovirus contains DNA and can, therefore, be manipulated to transport a genetically modified gene into any cell it invades. The virus will do no harm as long as genes conferring virulence are removed when the new genes are inserted. Genetic modification of the virus means its virulence is reduced and it can no longer replicate, which ensures viral infection cannot occur. The manipulated virus is called an 'attenuated' adenovirus. Viruses are useful as vectors as they are capable of invading living cells and replicating themselves only within the target cell. For example, an adenovirus can be genetically altered in such a way that it assumes command of tumour cells but not healthy ones. The virus replicates in the tumour causing cell death, however healthy non-tumour cells remain unaffected (Trahan Rieger 1997)

There are four potential uses for gene therapy:

1 Enhancement gene transfer, which involves transferring a gene that would enhance or improve a specific desirable trait.
2 Eugenics, which is genetic engineering of society to favour certain desirable human traits.
3 Somatic cell gene transfer, which places a gene in a body cell other than an egg or sperm cell. Somatic cells are all of the body's non-reproductive cells. They are targets for gene therapy, as they cannot pass on the new trait to the patient's offspring.
4 Germline gene transfer, which makes inheritable alterations to egg or sperm cells, which can be passed on to future humans (Halsey Lea 1997).

Gene therapy has the potential to be used to treat disorders caused by a defect in a single gene. This may be inherited diseases such as cystic fibrosis, or diseases such as cancer (Bank 1996). Gene therapy is experimental and much is unknown about the immediate and later safety and toxicity effects. The only form of gene therapy currently being used is somatic cell therapy for human clinical trials in patients with incurable diseases.

Gene therapy has the potential to enhance useful properties or reduce unwanted properties of the genes being used. There are many different approaches to the choice of the genes. Examples include:

1 Tumour suppressor genes: if the tumour suppressor genes that prevent or control abnormal cell growth become mutated, the cells may grow uncontrollably and become malignant.
2 Tumour susceptibility genes: the tumour susceptibility genes are a class of genes which include oncogenes, tumour suppressor genes and DNA repair genes, that predispose an organism to the development of tumours (Jenkins 1992).

The goal of traditional cancer treatments is to eliminate cancer cells, however during this process many normal cells may also be eliminated. Gene therapy is a novel therapeutic approach that targets disease directly at the molecular and cellular levels and is expected to be less toxic than traditional treatments such as chemotherapy and radiotherapy. Gene therapy should therefore improve the quality of life for the patient with cancer. However, gene therapy research is still in its infancy and it is, therefore, too early to identify benefits (De Cruz *et al.* 1996).

Regulatory controls for gene therapy

All work with genetically modified organisms (GMO), including gene therapy, is controlled by the following regulations, the majority of which focus on safety. For example:

1 *The Genetically Modified Organisms (Contained Use) (Amendment) Regulations 1996.* These regulations implement the requirements of the EC Directive 90/129 EEC on the contained use of genetically modified organisms. The regulations have been made under the powers of the *Health and Safety at Work etc. Act (1974)* and the *European Communities Act (1972)*. The regulations are concerned with protecting both human health and the environment and are designed to ensure the safe use and handling of genetically modified organisms under containment. 'Contained use' means any operation in which organisms are genetically modified or in which such genetically modified organisms are cultured, stored, used, transported, destroyed or disposed of and for which physical barriers, or a combination of physical barriers with chemical or biological barriers or both, are used to limit their contact with the general population and the environment (HSE 1996).

2 *The Control of Substances Hazardous to Health Regulations (1996).* These regulations require formal risk assessments and appropriate control measures to be provided in order to reduce potential health risks to those working with the genetically modified micro-organisms. Information on the classification of genetically modified biological agents is provided within the Health and Safety Commission Advisory Committee on Genetic Modification (ACGM) Compendium of Guidance (HSE 1996).

3 *The Management of Health and Safety at Work Regulations (1992)* requires a suitable and sufficient assessment of the risk to the health and safety of employees to which they are exposed at work, and of the risk to others arising out of their work activities.

4 *The Genetically Modified Organisms (Deliberate Release) Regulations (1995)* deal with the deliberate release into the environment of genetically modified organisms to ensure adverse effects to the environment do not occur.

5 The use of viral vectors for gene therapy requires rigorous control of production and safety testing methods. Approval from the Medicines Control Agency and the Gene Therapy Advisory Committee (GTAC) should be obtained before any gene therapy research is attempted on humans.

6 Other legislation that has a bearing on work with genetically modified organisms include the *Medicine Acts 1985, 1971 and 1968*; *European Council Regulations No (EEC) 2309/93* and *The Personal Protection Equipment Regulations 1992*.

Regulation requirements

The main requirements of the Genetically Modified Organisms (Contained Use) (Amendment) Regulations (1996) are for each organization wishing to undertake gene therapy to

1 Establish a local Genetic Modification Safety Committee. All risk assessments for work with genetically modified organisms must to be formally discussed and approved by the local Genetic Modification Committee. It should be noted that research treatments such as gene therapy also need to be formally agreed by the health care organization's own local ethics committee and by the Department of Health's Gene Therapy Advisory Committee (GTAC).

2 Carry out risk assessments to assess the risks to human health and to the environment.

3 Record the risk assessments and identify appropriate categorization of the work.

4 Submit advanced notification to the Health and Safety Executive (HSE) of an intention to use premises for genetic modification purposes and in certain circumstances receive HSE consent before work can start. Consideration of the recipient, the nature, activity and function of the vector, the insert sequence, and the overall combination of host, vector and insert will need to be made before categorization can be decided.

5 Notify the HSE of individual activities and, for some activities, await consent before proceeding.

The Genetically Modified Organisms (Contained Use) (Amendment) Regulations (1996) and the Control of Substances Hazardous to Health Regulations (1996) are enforced by the HSE. Failure to comply can lead to enforcement action and/or prosecution.

Classification

The Genetically Modified Organisms (Contained Use) (Amendment) Regulations (1996) define two hazard groups for genetically modified organisms: group I and group II. Classification is made by considering the recipient organism, the nature, activity and function of the vector, insert sequences and the overall combination of the host, vector and insert.

To be classified as group 1 the following three criteria must be met:

1 The recipient or parental micro-organism is unlikely to cause disease to humans, animals or plants. Disease might be infection, toxic, mutagenic, tumorigenic, allogenic or the overexpression of hormones or cytokines.

2 Whether what has been modified in the organism will result in a harmful phenotype.

3 The genetically modified organism (GMO) is unlikely to cause disease to humans, animals or plants and is unlikely to cause adverse effects on the environment.

Those which do not meet the above safety criteria are classified as group II genetically modified organisms.

HSE notification procedures currently relate to these two classifications, but may change in the future when proposed new regulations are adopted.

Risk assessments

One of the most important features of the Genetically Modified Organisms (Contained Use) (Amendment) Regulations (1996) is that a risk assessment must be made before any genetic modification work is undertaken. The risk assessment process must involve the classification of the genetically modified organism involved and decisions about the appropriate level of containment required for safety.

Each individual risk assessment will, therefore, vary. However, each risk assessment should identify:

1 The hazards of the activity.
2 The likelihood that the activity will give rise to harm (i.e. an accident, injury, ill-health or infection).
3 The safety control measures and procedures needed to reduce risk.

The assessment should consider any hazards associated with the vector's pathogenicity, the inserted gene product, the area of use and the survivability of the organism in the environment. In addition, with respect to gene therapy, the risk assessment should also consider possible risks to the patients receiving the treatment, other patients and visitors in the treatment area and to health care workers and others likely to come in contact with the genetically modified organism and/or the gene therapy patient. The assessment should identify the appropriate hazard rating for each part of the work activity and the relevant containment classifications and controls.

Once the written risk assessment has been completed (usually by the principal investigator for the study) a copy must be reviewed and approved by the local Genetic Modification Safety Committee.

Standard operating procedures

Safety procedures must be prepared for all areas and staff involved in the gene therapy study. This would include areas involved in preparing and administering the therapy, those involved in diagnostic investigation following the administration of the therapy and those involved in the general care of the patient. Safety procedures for staff involved in ancillary tasks such as cleaning and waste disposal tasks should also be completed under the risk assessment requirements of the Genetically Modified Organisms (Contained Use) (Amendment) Regulations (1996). The safety procedure documentation must reflect the safe practices necessary for the specified gene therapy protocol and identify responsibilities for compliance in each of the work areas identified.

The structure of the safety documentation should essentially include:

1 A preamble, which describes the protocol and the genetically modified organism involved and the level of risk to those potentially affected by the work activity.
2 Storage and preparation procedures.
3 Administration precautions for pharmacy staff.
4 Safety procedures for staff involved in the care of the patient.
5 Safety procedures for transportation, analysis, packaging, storage and disposal of all biological samples and specimens taken during the gene therapy treatment period.
6 Waste disposal procedures.
7 Action to be taken for decontamination of spills of the genetically modified organisms.
8 Action to be followed for accidental exposure of staff to genetically modified organisms.
9 Arrangements for staff training (HSE 1996).

Nursing care

Potential safety issues include the immediate and long-term complications of gene therapy to the health care worker, patient, visitors and other patients. There is no current information related to the risk of health care workers to genetically modified organisms and no severe toxicity has been seen related to gene therapy (Halsey Lea 1997). However, studies are limited at this stage and, therefore, strict safety precautions must be observed at all times.

Current standards of safe practice are as follows:

1 The patient receiving gene therapy must be admitted into a single room with en-suite facilities. This room will have previously been agreed by the local Genetic Modification Safety Committee as suitable, when the protocol and risk assessment documentation was undertaken. Consideration may need to be given to the appropriateness of the ward to be used depending on the patient population and potential health issues associated with the vector used.
2 Negative pressure air conditioning is an advantage in eliminating any airborne contamination, but is not essential.
3 Only those persons who are providing direct patient care should enter the room during the treatment period.
4 Nursing staff should observe barrier nursing principles and ensure appropriate protective clothing is worn, i.e. water-repellent tabard or gown, gloves, respiratory face mask, safety goggles or spectacles, plus overshoes if contamination has occurred (see Chap. 4, Barrier Nursing).
5 Hand washing procedures should be observed before and after entering the patient's room (see Chap. 3, Aseptic Technique).
6 In some cases the gene therapy can be administered to patients in the outpatient setting. The therapy should be administered in a room in outpatients or the day care department which has been approved previously as suit-

able. Although these patients are receiving their therapy on an outpatient basis, the restrictions and segregation that are adopted for inpatients are used in the outpatient setting. The patient should be instructed to go directly to the designated room upon arriving at the hospital. In some cases a respiratory face mask may need to be worn by the patient on entering the hospital and removed on leaving the site. This requirement highlights the need to protect vulnerable patients within the hospital setting.

7 While genetic modification of the vector ensures that the virulence of the vector is reduced, microbiological monitoring of blood and body fluids is required to ensure that the patient is no longer excreting the vector, before barrier nursing restrictions can be reduced (Young 1997).

There is a need for nurses to appreciate the importance that gene therapy may play in cancer prevention and control in the future (Peters 1997). Nurses must be familiar with the gene therapy protocol to be able to provide help, support, education and advice to the patients and their families and at the same time good direct clinical care (Lea 1997). Anxiety and fatigue may result from being included in a treatment trial. Patients may also experience reduced levels of concentration and therefore the nurse may need to repeat instructions and provide encouragement during the treatment period (Jenkins *et al.* 1994). Continuing observations are essential to identify toxicities as soon as possible.

In a survey carried out by Jenkins *et al.* (1994), which investigated the public's perception of gene therapy, it was found that the potential benefits were thought to be cure, prevention of genetic disease, disease control, medical advance and overall benefit to humanity worldwide. However, this survey group also expressed concerns related to the risk of genetic manipulation, including the danger of human misuse.

One concern about the use of viral vectors is that changes in the virus's genetic material could occur which would cause them to revert back to replication competent viruses, which could multiply after administration to the patient and cause a viral infection. Alternatively, retroviruses could insert themselves into the DNA of the patient to cause inactivation of a tumour suppressor gene, or activation of an oncogene, resulting in a malignancy. In addition, an immunological reaction to the viral vector protein may occur. For instance, the immune system may attack and neutralize the virus before it reaches its target.

To date, no serious adverse effects have been reported. Strict health and safety and infection control principles must be maintained at all times to reduce the risk of any adverse effect to a level as low as practically possible.

Consent

Patients must be fully informed of the experimental nature of gene therapy treatments (Robinson *et al.* 1996). As much information as is available should be given to the patient in order for them to make an informed decision as to whether they wish to be included in the study or not.

The patient must sign a consent form (Young 1997) (see Chap. 1, Care in Context: Assessment, Communication and Consent).

Gene therapy options in the future

Ardern–Jones (1999) discusses how cancer due to inherited genetic factors represents 5–10% of the total cases of cancer. The identification of inherited cancer susceptibility genes and advances in gene therapy technology may, in the future, lead to modification of these genes by gene therapy (Flygenring 1999) to treat or prevent cancer.

References and further reading

Alexandroff, A.B. *et al.* (1998) Sicky and smelly issues: lessons on tumour cell and leucocyte trafficking, gene and immunotherapy of cancer. *Br J Cancer*, **77**(11), 1806–11.

Ardern-Jones, A. (1999) Developing roles of nursing in cancer prevention: the clinical nurse specialist in cancer genetics. *Oncol Nurs Today*, **4**(2), 11–13.

Bank, A. (1996) Human somatic cell gene therapy. *Bioassays*, **18**(12), 999–1007.

Clayman, G.L. (1995) Gene therapy for head and neck cancer. *Head Neck*, **17**(6), 535–41.

Gore, M.E. *et al.* (1994) Gene therapy for cancer. *Eur J Cancer*, **30**A(8), 1047–9.

De Cruz, E.E. *et al.* (1996) The basis for somatic therapy of cancer. *J Exp Ther Oncol*, **1**(2), 73–83.

Flygenring, B.G. (1999) Comments from Iceland. *Oncol Nurs Today*, **4**(2), 13–14.

Kinnon, C. *et al.* (1990) Gene therapy for cancer. *Eur J Cancer*, **26**(5), 638–40.

Komiya, T., Hirashima T., & Kawasw, I. (1999) Clinical significance of p53 in non-small-cell lung cancer. *Oncol Rep*, **6**(1), 19–28.

Halsey Lea, D. (1997) Gene therapy: current and future implications for oncology nursing practice. *Semin Oncol Nurs*, **13**(2), 115–22.

HSE (1996) *A guide to The Genetically Modified Organisms (Contain Use) Regulations 1992, amended 1996.* Health and Safety Executive, London.

Jenkins, J. (1992) Biology of cancer: current issues and future prospects. *Semin Oncol Nurs*, **8**(1), 63–9.

Jenkins J., Wheeler, V. & Albright, L. (1994) Gene therapy for cancer. *Cancer Nurs*, **17**(6), 447–56.

Lea, D.H. (1997) Gene therapy: current and future implications for oncology nursing practice. *Semin Oncol Nurs*, **13**(2), 115–22.

Palu, G., Bonaguro, R. & Marcello, A. (1999) In pursuit of new developments for gene therapy of human diseases. *J Biotechnol*, **68**(1), 1–13.

Peters, K.F. & Hadley, D.W. (1997) The human genome project. *Cancer Nurs*, **20**(1), 62–71. Quiz 72–75.

Peters, J.A (1997) Applications of genetic technologies to cancer screening, prevention, diagnosis, prognosis and treatment. *Semin Oncol Nurs*, **13**(2), 74–81.

Peters, J., Dimond, E. & Jenkins, J. (1997) Clinical applications of genetic technologies to cancer care. *Cancer Nursing*, **20**(5), 359–77.

Robinson, K.D., Abernathy, E. & Conrad, K.J. (1996) Gene therapy of cancer. *Semin Oncol Nurs*, **12**(2), 142–51.

Romano, G., Pacilio, C. & Giordano, A. (1999) Gene transfer technology in therapy: current applications and future goals. *Stem Cells*, **17**(4), 191–202.

Roth, J.A. *et al.* (1998) Gene therapy for non-small cell lung cancer: a preliminary report of a phase 1 trial of adenoviral p53 gene replacement. *Semin Oncol*, **25**(3), Suppl. **8**, 33–7.

The Control of Substances Hazardous to Health Regulations 1994 (COSHH) SI 1994/3246. Stationery Office, London.

The Health and Safety at Work Etc Act 1974. Stationery Office, London.

The Management of Health and Safety at Work Regulations (1992) SI 1992/2051. Stationery Office, London.

Sandhu, J.S., Keating, A. & Hozumi, N. (1997) Human gene therapy. *Crit Rev Biotechnol*, **17**(4), 307–26.

Sikora, K. (1994) First five years of gene therapy for cancer. *Lancet*, **344**(8937), 1109–1110.

Tomizawa, Y. *et al.* (1999) Correlation between the status of the p53 gene and survival in patients with stage 1 non-small cell lung carcinoma. *Oncogene*, **18**(4), 1007–1014.

Trahan Rieger, P. (1997) Emerging strategies in the management of cancer. *Oncol Nurs Forum*, **24**(4), 728–37.

Weber, C.E. (1998) Cytokine-modified tumour vaccines: an anti-tumor strategy revisited in the age of molecular medicine. *Cancer Nurs*, **21**(3), 167–77.

Young, A. (1997) Gene therapy for oncology patients. *Nurs Times*, **93**(37).

Environmental Protection Act 1990. Stationery Office, London.

European Community Act 1972. Stationery Office, London.

HSE (1995) *The Genetically Modified Organisms (Deliberate Release) Regulations 1995.* Health and Safety Executive, London.

Medicine Act 1985 and 1971. Stationery Office, London.

European Council Regulations No. (EEC) 2309/93. Stationery Office, London.

The Personal Protection Equipment Regulations 1992. Stationery Office, London.

GUIDELINES • Care of patients receiving gene therapy

Preparation of patient

Action	Rationale
1 Explain and discuss the procedure with the patient	To ensure that the patient understands the procedure and gives his/her valid consent.
2 Ensure the patient is aware of the barrier nursing restrictions, and the need to remain in the room during the treatment period.	Patients who understand the need for restrictions are more likely to comply and be satisfied with their care.
3 Ensure the relatives and visitors are aware of the reasons why barrier nursing restrictions are required.	In order for relatives to be able to encourage and support the patient during the barrier nursing care.
4 Encourage patients to bring books and entertainment items into the room.	To prevent a feeling of loneliness and boredom.
5 Ensure that all personal items are washable.	In the event of contamination with genetically modified material personal items will need to be cleaned before removal from the room.

Preparation of room

Action	Rationale
1 Room should include a television and video.	To prevent the patient being bored and leaving the single room.
2 Room should be stocked with all necessary equipment. This will include observation equipment.	Equipment used regularly by the patient should be left within the barrier nursing area to prevent possible spread of infection.
3 Place a clinical waste bag on a bag holder in the room.	To contain all waste, including used protective clothing.
4 Place a special waste bin with a biohazard label and a sharps disposal bin in the room.	To ensure immediate and safe disposal of special waste and sharps.
5 Place a specimen carrying box in room.	To store and transport specimens.
6 Put water-repellent tabard or gowns, disposable gloves, respiratory face mask with filtering face piece protection level 3 (FFP3), safety goggles or spectacles and overshoes outside the room.	To reduce the risk of contamination to clothing, skin, eyes, nose and mouth, and to reduce the risk of inhalation or ingestion of GMO. Staff and visitors are more likely to use the protective clothing if it is readily available.

Guidelines • Care of patients receiving gene therapy (cont'd)

Action	Rationale

7 Ensure hand wash basin is stocked with bactericidal detergent, paper towels and bactericidal alcoholic hand rub.

To ensure hand washing is undertaken before and after patient contact.

Entering the room

1 Ensure staff and visitors aware of restrictions related to entering the room.

To ensure compliance with restrictions and ensure non-essential persons do not enter the patients room.

2 Visitors and staff should be restricted to essential persons only.

To restrict entry to the room to those who are aware of the need to comply to the restrictions.

3 Pregnant persons should seek advice from occupational health staff before they enter the room.

There is no information to suggest there is a risk to the foetus, but as research is limited occupational health should undertake a risk assessment.

4 Young children and babies must not enter the room.

Young persons are unlikely to understand or be able to comply with restrictions.

5 Wash hands with bactericidal detergent or alcoholic rub.

To reduce the risk of cross-infection.

6 Put on appropriate protective clothing before entering the room. This will include:
(a) Water-repellent tabard or gown.
(b) Disposable gloves.
(c) Respiratory face mask (FFP3).
(d) Safety goggles or spectacles.
(e) Overshoes (if contamination of the floor has occurred).

To protect staff and visitors from contamination.

7 Enter the room closing the door behind you.

To reduce the risk of airborne contamination leaving the room.

Attending to patient

1 Serve meals using normal crockery and cutlery.

Nicely prepared and served food will encourage the patient to eat their food.

2 Dispose of any uneaten food in the clinical waste bag in the room.

Food may be contaminated by saliva.

3 Wash used crockery and cutlery immediately in the ward's dishwasher.

Mechanical washing and heat will remove or kill all micro-organisms.

4 Place waste in yellow clinical waste bag, seal the bag with an identification tie and send for incineration when half full.

Yellow is the national colour for clinical waste and must be incinerated. To prevent contamination of the environment.

5 Label specimens with a biohazard warning label, double bag in biohazard specimen carrying bag (also labelled by a biohazard warning label) and take to the appropriate laboratory in a sealable box.

To warn laboratory workers of the possible risk. The box and double bag will contain spillages, if the specimen container becomes damaged.

Administration of gene therapy

1 Ensure only identified 'designated' staff should be involved in the administration of the gene therapy treatment.

To minimize the number of persons who could become contaminated if an accident occurs during administration of the gene therapy vaccine.

2 Staff who directly administer the gene therapy vaccine should attend the occupational health department and, if appropriate, provide a sample of blood which will be stored in a freezer for 40 years.

Occupational health will ensure staff are fit to undertake this task and maintain appropriate health surveillance as required by the COSHH Regulations (1996).

3 Administer the treatment using an aseptic technique. For example, intravenously, subcutaneously, directly into the tumour or via an intraperitoneal catheter (see Chap. 12, Drug Administration).

To minimize risk of cross-infection. As far as possible the administration procedures should minimize the potential risk of airborne exposure and/or inoculation.

4 Identify all equipment used to administer gene therapy as clinical waste and autoclave before incineration.

To comply with statutory waste disposal procedures.

Accidental inoculation or spillage of gene therapy

1 In the event of an inoculation accident or contamination occurring during the administration of gene therapy, immediate action should be:
(a) Make the inoculation area bleed.
(b) Wash the area thoroughly.
(c) Inform the occupational health department.
(d) Inform the infection control officer.
(e) Complete an accident report form.

To ensure appropriate care is provided. An accident occurring at the time of treatment has increased significance due to the concentrated nature of the gene therapy.

2 Implement the follow-up care for inoculation and contamination accidents at the time of administration, which will be included in the risk assessment documentation.

To ensure that staff are aware of appropriate emergency procedures.

3 In the event of a sharps accident occurring after administration of gene therapy, handle as for routine sharps accidents.

Sharps accidents that occur which are not involved with the administration of gene therapy are not as significant as those that occur when gene therapy is involved, due to the diluted nature of the gene therapy following administration.

4 Clear up spillages using a standard spillage kit containing chlorine releasing tablets.

To contain and remove the contamination.

Readmission following gene therapy

1 Barrier nursing restrictions to be reinstated, if patient is readmitted within one week of discharge, until the clinician can reassess the condition of the patient.

The time during which excretion of the gene therapy occurs is unknown, therefore precautions are necessary until a risk assessment shows that barrier nursing is not necessary, i.e. the patient is no longer shedding.

Domestic staff

1 Thoroughly prepare and clean patient's room prior to the start of the gene therapy treatment.

To provide a pleasant and safe environment for the patient.

2 The room should only be cleaned while the patient is being barrier nursed following the administration of the gene therapy, if stated in the risk assessment document.

If contamination of the environment is likely, the domestic staff should not enter the room.

3 In the event that the risk assessment states the domestic staff may enter the room, cleaning should be undertaken as for guidelines for barrier nursing (see Chap. 4, Barrier Nursing).

Employing barrier nursing principles will reduce risk of contamination of staff and the environment.

4 In the event that the risk assessment states the domestic may not enter the room, the patient should be informed of this before admission and asked to undertake minor cleaning tasks. This may include flushing the toilet with disinfectant after use.

Patients expect their hospital accommodation to be kept clean by the domestic department. Prior warning that this will not occur may help prevent patient dissatisfaction and complaint. To ensure disinfection of the toilet.

5 Following discharge of the patient the room and bathroom should be thoroughly cleaned using a detergent/bleach solution.

To ensure any contamination is removed. Bleach is particularly useful in destroying viruses.

6 Once cleaning is completed, the room can be used as normal.

Cleaning will remove any contamination, making it safe for other patients to be admitted into this area.

Guidelines • Care of patients receiving gene therapy (cont'd)

Action	Rationale

Linen

1 Place used linen in a red alginate bag, then in an outer red bag.

Red is the recognized colour for foul or infected linen. The laundry will process this type of laundry in a hot barrier wash.

Discontinuing restrictions

1 Discontinue restrictions when microbiological sampling shows that the patient is not excreting the micro-organism.

For some gene therapy trials it is possible to test the patient to see if they are infected. Early notification can result in a reduction in stringent barrier nursing procedures.

Discharge home

1 The patient will be discharged home when the clinician is satisfied that it is safe to do so.

Generally, restrictions are less once the patient is discharged into the community.

Haematological Procedures: Specialist, Diagnostic and Therapeutic

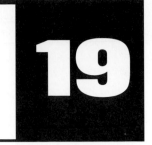

Definition

Haematological procedures include bone marrow procedures and apheresis procedures (donor and therapeutic).

Bone marrow procedures

Bone marrow procedures involve the removal of haemopoietic tissue from the iliac crest, sternum and spinal processes using a special needle. In children aged less than 2 years the upper end of the tibia may be used (Dacie & Lewis 1994). Bone marrow procedures include the following:

1 *Aspiration:* withdrawal of the bone marrow fluid. Tests performed on this sample include observation of haemopoiesis, cytology of cells and infiltrates, assessment of iron stores, cytochemistry and immunotyping (MIMS 1994).
2 *Trephine biopsy:* removal of a core of the bone including marrow. Tests performed on this sample include histological examination and assessment of marrow cellularity, classification of marrow infiltrates, diagnostic information where the aspirate is unsatisfactory and imprint preparations for cytology (MIMS 1994).
3 *Harvest:* withdrawal of bone marrow including haemopoietic stem cells.

Indications

The study of bone marrow in haematological diseases was first introduced by Arinkin in 1929. Tests on the bone marrow are performed for haematological conditions where there is a decrease or increase in a blood element, e.g. anaemia, leukaemia and for diagnosis of diseases not primarily affecting the blood system, e.g. malignancies, infections and hereditary conditions (Monteil 1996). Bone marrow is harvested for autologous or allogeneic transplantation or cryopreservation for both malignant and non-malignant conditions.

Apheresis procedures (donor or therapeutic)

Apheresis is the separation and collection of one or more blood components. It may be performed using either a single arm or two arm technique via a peripheral cannula. It can be performed by a continuous or intermittent flow depending on the apheresis machine used (Burgstaler &

Pineda 1994). The procedure for performing apheresis is complex and beyond the scope of this chapter and should only be performed by specially trained operators. Further information can be gained from the individual apheresis operator's manual. Apheresis procedures include the following:

1 *Platelet depletion:* removal of circulating platelets, either from a donor or in order to reduce dangerously high levels such as in essential thrombocythaemia to prevent thrombosis.
2 *Therapeutic plasma exchange:* removal of part of the plasma pool and replacing it with disease free plasma. Used in diseases such as multiple myeloma, autoimmune disorders and idiopathic thrombotic thrombocytopenic purpura.
3 *Red cell exchange:* used on patients with haematological disorders such as sickle cell anaemia, thalassaemia, polycythaemia and haemochromatosis. In sickle cell anaemia exchange transfusion may be needed if there is neurological damage, visceral sequestration or repeated painful crisis (Hoffbrand & Pettit 1993).
4 *Rapid red cell transfusion:* for outpatient transfusion (to minimize length of time in hospital) and prevention of fluid overload in volume sensitive patients (McLeod *et al.* 1994).
5 *White blood cell (mononuclear cell or polymorphonuclear cell) procedures:* used to remove excess white blood cells in patients with leukaemia, collecting donor T lymphocytes for immunotherapy or collecting donor granulocytes for treatment of acute sepsis (Hoffbrand & Pettit 1993).
6 *Peripheral blood stem cell procedures:* used to harvest haemopoietic stem cells for autologous or allogeneic transplantation or cryopreservation for both malignant and non-malignant conditions.

Reference material

Anatomy and physiology

In early gestation the yolk sac is the primary area for haemopoiesis. From 6 to 7 months of fetal life through to adulthood the bone marrow then becomes the only source of haemopoiesis (Monteil 1996). The bone marrow is specialized soft tissue filling the spaces in cancellous bone in the epiphyses (Mosby 1997). It is one of the largest organs in the body, representing 3.4–4.6% of the total body weight (Monteil 1996).

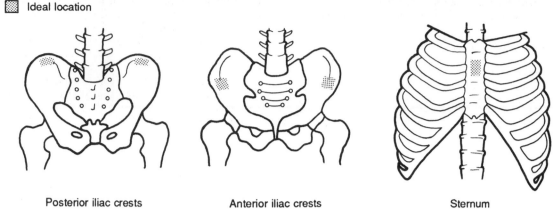

▨ Ideal location

Posterior iliac crests   Anterior iliac crests   Sternum

Figure 19.1   Common sites for bone marrow examination, arranged in order of preference. Normally, only aspirations and not biopsies are done on the sternum because of its small size and proximity to vital organs.

Haemopoietic stem cells give rise to all haemopoietic cell lines. Stromal cells, fat cells and a microvascular network provide a suitable network for stem cell growth and development (Hoffbrand & Pettit 1993). There are two types of bone marrow:

1 Red bone marrow: this is responsible for haemopoeisis. It is found in the proximal epiphyses of the humerus and femur and in the sternum, ribs and vertebral bodies of adults (Mosby 1997).
2 Yellow bone marrow: this consists of fat cells, blood vessels, reticulum cells and fibres. Some of the fatty bone marrow is capable of reversion to haemopoeisis (Hoffbrand & Pettit 1993).

Blood cells

Blood cell growth and development is regulated by haemopoietic growth factors. Some growth factors are found naturally in the plasma but others are only detectable following an inflammatory or other stimulus (Hoffbrand & Pettit 1993). Growth factors include GM-CSF (granulocyte macrophage colony stimulating factor), G-CSF (granulocyte colony stimulating factor) and IL-6 (interleukin 6). All mature blood cells are derived from a common pluripotent haemopoietic stem cell. These cells mature and differentiate to provide the three types of blood cells:

1 Red blood cells (erythrocytes): the main function is to carry oxygen to the tissues and to return carbon dioxide to the lungs. This gaseous exchange is facilitated by the protein haemoglobin contained in the erythrocyte (Hoffbrand & Pettit 1993). The normal values of haemoglobin and erythrocytes vary according to gender (see Table 19.1).
2 White blood cells (leucocytes): the main function is to protect the body from infection. Leucocytes are divided into neutrophils, eosinophils and basophils (granulocytes); monocytes; and lymphocytes (T and B).
3 Platelets: the main function is the formation of mechanical plugs during the normal haemostatic response to vascular injury (Hoffbrand & Pettit 1993).

The most common sites for obtaining bone marrow tissue are the posterior iliac crest, sternum, anterior superior iliac crest and spinal processes (Monteil 1996) (Fig. 19.1). Peripheral blood haemopoietic stem cells can be harvested via apheresis following mobilization of immature cells into the peripheral circulation by haemopoietic growth factors and/or chemotherapy such as cyclophosphamide. Haemopoietic stem cells can also be harvested from foetal tissue and umbilical cord blood (Amos & Gordon 1995).

Aspiration and trephine biopsy

Patients may be anxious about the procedure and a mild sedative may be indicated. The procedure is performed under local anaesthetic, although due to the nature of the pain (often described as a dragging sensation) the actual aspiration procedure may still remain painful even when the site is numb. The iliac crests are often used for patients requiring frequent marrow procedures as the use of the right and left crests can be alternated, both anterior and posterior surfaces may be used and there are no vital organs nearby that may be punctured by the procedure. The posterior iliac crest is often preferred as the procedure can

Table 19.1   Normal values (Hoffbrand & Pettit 1993)

	Males	Females	Males and females
Haemoglobin (g/dl)	13.5–17.5	11.5–15.5	
Erythrocytes ($\times 10^{12}$/l)	4.5–6.5	3.9–5.6	
Leucocytes ($\times 10^{9}$/l)			4.0–11.0
Platelets ($\times 10^{9}$/l)			150–400

then be performed outside the patient's field of vision. The procedure normally takes between 15 and 30 minutes.

Contraindications

Bone marrow aspirate and trephine biopsy are contraindicated in those patients who are unable to cooperate or have a coagulation defect such as increased clotting time, unless this is correctable, as excessive bleeding or bruising may occur. Patients in extreme pain may not be able to adopt the lateral position for posterior iliac crest sampling. In this case the anterior iliac crest or, if biopsy is not needed, the sternum can be used (MIMS 1994).

Bone marrow harvest

Bone marrow harvests are performed under a general anaesthetic. This is done because:

1 The procedure may last approximately 1 hour compared with the 5–15 minutes for an aspiration and biopsy.
2 Multiple puncture sites are used and the patient may be approached from both sides (i.e. from both the pelvis and the sternum).
3 The procedure can be very painful.

A volume of 1 litre or more (dependent on the harvest cell count in relation to the recipient's body weight) is aspirated from multiple puncture sites. If large volumes of marrow are harvested the patient may require a blood transfusion. The marrow may be harvested for immediate use or may be cryopreserved for the future.

Complications of bone marrow procedures

Complications of bone marrow procedures are extremely rare but include the following:

1 Cardiac tamponade: this is compression of the heart produced by the accumulation of blood or fluid in the pericardial sac. It can be due to rupture of a blood vessel in the myocardium caused by the aspirate or trephine needle. The actual risks associated with a sternal puncture are extremely small (Dacie & Lewis 1994), especially with the use of a guarded needle which prevents too deep an insertion.
2 Haemorrhage: this occurs almost exclusively in those patients with thrombocytopenia. It may be avoided by applying pressure to the puncture site for a few minutes following the procedure and by the administration of platelet transfusions where indicated.
3 Infection, particularly in the neutropenic patient.
4 Bone fractures, particularly in small children due to the pressure exerted.

Complications of apheresis procedures

Complications of apheresis procedures are usually mild and transient. They include the following:

1 Hypocalcaemia (with use of citrate phosphate dextrose as anticoagulant): the relationship between plasma phosphorous and ionized calcium is reciprocal (Horne *et al.* 1997). Therefore if plasma phosphorous is increased plasma calcium will decrease. Oral calcium supplements may be required.
2 Venous access difficulties: large-bore cannulae are predominantly used in the antecubital fossa, therefore good venous access is required.
3 Arm discomfort: due to keeping arms straight during procedure.
4 Miscellaneous symptoms: anxiety, headache, lightheadedness, fever, chills, haematoma, hyperventilation, nausea and vomiting, syncope, urticaria, hypotension and allergic reactions (COBE Spectra 1996).
5 Transfusion reaction (with red cell exchange procedures) (see Chap. 41, Transfusion of Blood and Blood Products).

References and further reading

Abrahams, P. & Webb, P. (1975) *Clinical Anatomy of Practical Procedures*. Pitman Medical, London.

Amos, T.A. & Gordon, M.Y. (1995) Sources of human hemopoietic stem cells for transplantation – a review. *Cell Transpl*, **4**(6), 547–69.

Arinkin, M.J. (1929) Intravitale Untersuchungsmethodik der Knochenmarks. *Folia Haematol (Leipz)*, **38**, 233.

Ayliffe, G., Lowbury, E., Geddes, A. *et al.* (1996) *Control of Hospital Infection: A Practical Handbook*, 3rd edn. Chapman & Hall, London.

Bevan, J. (1994) *A Pictorial Handbook of Anatomy and Physiology*. Mitchell Beazley, London.

Booth, J.A. (1983) *Handbook of Investigations*. Harper & Row, London.

Brunner, L.S. & Suddarth, D.S. (1996) *The Lippincott Manual of Medical–Surgical Nursing*, Vol. 2. Harper & Row, London.

Burgstaler, E.A. & Pineda, A.A. (1994) Therapeutic cytapheresis: continuous flow versus intermittent flow apheresis systems. *J Clin Apheresis*, **9**(4), 205–209.

COBE Spectra Apheresis System Operators' Manual (for use with versions 4.7, 5.1 and 6.0 software programs) 1996/10.

Dacie, J. & Lewis, S.M. (1994) *Practical Haematology*, 8th edn. Churchill Livingstone, Edinburgh.

Frazer, I. & Gough, K.R. (1968) Bone marrow biopsy. In: *Biopsy Procedures in Clinical Medicine* (ed. A.E. Read). John Wright, Bristol.

Henke, Y.C. (1990) Physiology of normal bone marrow. *Semin Oncol Nurs Adult Leuk*, **6**(1), 3–8.

Horne, M., Heitz, U. & Swearingen, P. (1997) *Pocket Guide to Fluid, Electrolyte, and Acid-Base Balance Unit II* (Mosby's Pocket Guide Series), 3rd edn., p. 107. Mosby, London.

Hoffbrand, A. & Pettit, J. (1993) *Essential Haematology*, 3rd edn., pp. 36–52, 299–317, 392–405. Blackwell Scientific Publications, Oxford.

Keele, C., Neil, E. & Joels, N. (1983) *Samson Wrights Applied Physiology*, 13th edn., Part I, pp. 22–6. Oxford University Press, Oxford.

Markus, S. (1981) Taking the fear out of bone marrow examinations. *Nursing* (US), **11**(4), 64–7.

McLeod, B.C., Reed, S., Viernes, A. *et al.* (1994) Rapid red cell transfusion by apheresis. *J Clin Apheresis*, **9**(2), 142–6.

MIMS (1994) *Handbook of Haematology*, Part 4, pp. 43–55. Haymarket, London.

Monteil, M.M. (1996) Bone marrow. In: *Clinical Hematology and Fundamentals of Hemostasis* (eds D. Harmening Pittiglio & R.A. Sacher), 3rd edn. F.A. Davies, Philadelphia.

Mosby (1997) *Mosby's Medical, Nursing and Allied Health Dictionary*, 5th edn. Mosby, London.

Navarett, D. (1981) Assisting with bone marrow aspiration. In: *Mosby's Manual of Clinical Nursing Procedures* (eds J. Hirsch & J. Hancock). Mosby, St Louis.

Pagnana, K.D. & Pagnana, T.J. (1994) *Diagnostic Testing and Nursing Implications*, 4th edn. Mosby, St Louis.

Skydell, B. & Crowder, A. (1975) *Diagnostic Procedures – A Reference for Health Practitioners and a Guide for Patient Counseling*. Little, Brown, Boston.

GUIDELINES · Bone marrow aspiration and trephine biopsy

Equipment

1 Antiseptic skin cleansing agent (chlorhexidine in alcohol 70%).
2 Sterile dressing pack.
3 Selection of syringes and needles for administration of local anaesthetic.
4 Local anaesthetic.
5 Marrow aspiration needle and guard, e.g. Salah needle.
6 Microscope slides and coverslips.
7 Specimen bottles (plain and with heparin).
8 Polyurethane semipermeable dressing.

Procedure

Action	*Rationale*
1 Explain and discuss the procedure with the patient.	To ensure that the patient understands the procedure and gives his/her valid consent.
2 Give medication, such as sedation, as ordered, allowing sufficient time for it to have effect.	Usually this is only necessary for very anxious patients.
3 Help the patient into the correct position: (a) Supine. (b) Prone or on side.	To enable access for sternal puncture or for anterior or posterior iliac crest puncture.
4 Continue to observe the patient throughout the procedure. Assist the doctor as required. Reassure the conscious patient. Follow the appropriate procedure if the patient is anaesthetized.	To detect signs of discomfort or pain and to minimize anxiety.
5 Procedure is performed by a doctor: (a) Skin is cleansed with antiseptic solution.	To maintain asepsis throughout the procedure and thus minimize the risk of infection.
(b) Local anaesthetic is injected intradermally and through the various layers until the periosteum is infiltrated.	To minimize pain during the procedure. Transitory pain will be felt both as the periosteum is punctured and when the marrow is aspirated.
(c) Once the local anaesthetic has taken effect the doctor inserts the marrow needle with the guard on, into the anaesthetized area.	The needle guard ensures the correct positioning of the needle in the marrow cavity and diminishes the risk, particularly in the sternal puncture, of inadvertently puncturing vital organs.
(d) If the patient has not been anaesthetized, the doctor warns the patient he/she will feel a brief episode of sharp pain as the marrow is withdrawn. The needle is advanced into the bone marrow and the required amount of marrow is withdrawn.	To allay anxiety and to ensure the patient's maximum cooperation.
(e) The needle is removed from the puncture site.	
6 Once the doctor has removed the needle, apply pressure over the puncture site using a sterile topical swab until the bleeding stops.	To minimize bruising and to prevent haematoma formation. Prolonged pressure, 5–10 min, is required if the patient has a low platelet count (thrombocytopenia).
7 Once the bleeding stops, cover the site with polyurethane semipermeable dressing. Ask the patient not to bathe or wash the area for 24 h.	To provide an airtight seal over the puncture site and to prevent the entry of bacteria.

8 Make the patient comfortable. He/she may be mobile, as desired, depending on the level of sedation.

Some patients will have this procedure performed in the outpatient department and will be asked to wait in the clinic for a further 30 min to ensure that no further bleeding occurs.

9 Ensure equipment is removed and disposed of safely. Some types of needles are disposable, others can be reused following sterilization.

To reduce the risk of infection and needlestick injury.

10 Record necessary information in the appropriate documents and ensure that specimens are sent to the appropriate laboratory department, correctly labelled and with the necessary forms.

To maintain accurate records.
To ensure that the specimens from the right patient are delivered to the laboratory.

Nursing care plan

Problem	Cause	Suggested action
Pain experienced over the puncture site for 1–2 days following the procedure.	Bruising of the tissues at the time of puncture or haematoma formation due to inadequate pressure on the puncture site following the procedure.	Administer a mild analgesic as prescribed by the doctor.
Haemorrhage from the puncture site following the procedure.	Low platelet count or inadequate pressure on the puncture site following the procedure.	Ensure that pressure is applied for a minimum of 5 min on the puncture site. Report excessive or uncontrollable bleeding to the appropriate personnel.
Haematoma formation over the puncture site.	Haemorrhage following the procedure.	Administer analgesics as prescribed. If the haematoma is severe, report this to the doctor as aspiration may be required.

GUIDELINES • Bone marrow harvest

Equipment

1 Sterile syringes: 1 × 2 ml, 1 × 5 ml.
2 Transfer pack 600 ml – collect from the haematology department.
3 Small sterile dressing.
4 Full blood count haematology forms.
5 Sterile sampling coupling spike, usually obtained from haematology department.
6 Sterile gown pack.
7 Sterile gloves.
8 Swab saturated with 70% isopropyl alcohol.
9 64 ml of CPD (citrate phosphate dextrose) per transfer pack if marrow to be infused fresh, usually obtained from haematology department.

10 Chlorhexidine 0.5% in 70% alcohol.
11 500 ml bag of 0.9% sodium chloride.
12 5 ml ampoules of heparin, 1000 units per ml (preservative free).
13 Aspiration needles (short sternal needles) of appropriate size.
14 Bone marrow needles (e.g. Islam) of appropriate size.
15 Sterile pack containing 5-inch bowl, Gallipot, gauze swabs, two sponge holders, five towel clips, drapes.

Procedure

Follow pre-, intra- and postoperative guidelines for general care during bone marrow harvest procedure.

Action

1 Prepare the area (iliac crests or sternum) cleaning with 0.5% chlorhexidine in 70% alcohol.

Rationale

To reduce risk of wound contamination (Ayliffe *et al*. 1996).

Guidelines • Bone marrow harvest (cont'd)

Action	Rationale
2 Drape the area with sterile towels. Secure the towels with towel clips.	To provide and maintain a sterile field around the operation site.
3 Place two swabs on the towels.	To be available to remove blood exudate from the puncture site.
4 Flush syringe and aspiration needles with heparinized saline solution prepared on sterile trolley.	To reduce risk of clotting in the aspiration needle and syringe.
5 Using the appropriate size aspiration needle make a small hole in the skin over the posterior iliac crest.	To facilitate smooth introduction of the bone marrow needle.
6 Introduce the bone marrow aspiration needle into the bone with firm controlled pressure. Initially it should enter the bone to a depth of approximately 1 cm.	The posterior iliac crest is 5–7 cm thick and there are no structures in the surrounding area which can be damaged by the introduction of a needle.
7 Firmly site the bone marrow needle.	To prevent slippage.
8 Remove the trocar.	To enable aspiration of the bone marrow.
9 Place a 20 ml syringe which has been flushed with the heparinized solution on the end of the aspiration needle, taking a volume of 10–25 ml.	To draw marrow into syringe for collection.
10 Pass the syringe containing marrow to a nurse who injects the bone marrow into the heparinized transfer pack.	To maintain the sterility of the operating personnel. The transfer pack is not sterile on the outer surface.
11 After two aspirations from the same site, replace trocar and move the position of the bone marrow needle to another place in the bone approximately 2 cm from the first entry site.	To reduce risk of wound infection and excessive cell depletion. No further skin puncture is necessary due to the elasticity of the skin. If more than two aspirates are taken from one site the cells become depleted.
12 Move the bone marrow needle around over an area 2.5–5 cm from the entry site in the skin and introduce the needle every 2 cm until 400–500 ml of marrow have been removed in total.	The required amount of bone marrow can be harvested using the original hole in skin. It is normally possible to obtain sufficient bone marrow from the patient's iliac crests. If any more is required the sternum is used.
13 Place bone marrow in the transfer pack.	The number of cells required for re-engraftment is calculated using the recipient's body weight. Generally, 2×10^8/kg body weight of cells are required, although more can be obtained if desired.
14 Take sample of aspirate from transfer pack and place in full blood count specimen container and send to the laboratory.	To establish the white cell count of the bone marrow aspirate and the number of stem cells present in each pack.
15 Seal the transfer pack with sterile plug.	To maintain sterility and prevent spillage.
16 Record amount in millilitres of bone marrow aspirate on outside of the transfer bag.	To establish total amount of bone marrow in each bag.
17 If the bone marrow is to be used fresh add 64 ml CPD to the bone marrow in the transfer pack.	To prolong the life of the bone marrow and maintain its liquid form for up to 24 h.
18 Withdraw needle and place gauze swab over site; apply digital pressure for 5 min, or longer if required.	To stop leakage and formation of haematoma.
19 Inspect puncture site for bleeding. Apply small sterile dressing.	To reduce risk of wound infection.
20 Take fresh bone marrow to designated fridge in haematology laboratories.	To ensure constant temperature and viability of stem cells.

Infusion Devices

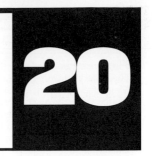

20

Definition

An infusion device is designed to deliver measured amounts of drug or fluid (either intravenously or subcutaneously) over a period of time. This is set at an appropriate rate to achieve the desired therapeutic response and prevent complications.

Indications

The nurse has a responsibility to determine the correct rate in individual circumstances and to maintain that rate throughout the infusion. The nurse can achieve this by mechanical means such as gravity flow or by the use of an electronic infusion device. The following factors should be considered when selecting an appropriate infusion delivery system:

1 Risk to the patient of:
   (a) Overinfusion
   (b) Underinfusion
   (c) Uneven flow
   (d) High delivery pressure
   (e) Inadvertent bolus
   (f) Extravascular infusion
2 Delivery parameters:
   (a) Infusion rate and volume required
   (b) Accuracy required (over a long or short period of time)
   (c) Alarms required
   (d) Ability to infuse into site chosen (venous, arterial, subcutaneous)
   (e) Suitability of device for infusing drug (e.g. ability to infuse viscous drugs)
3 Environmental features:
   (a) Ease of operation
   (b) Frequency of observation and adjustment
   (c) Type of patient (neonate, child, very sick)
   (d) Mobility of patient

(Wittig & Semmler-Bertanzi 1983; Medical Devices Agency 1995).

Reference material

The aim of using an infusion device is to ensure the delivery of a drug or fluid to a patient at a constant rate over a set period of time with no adjustment to 'catch up'. This is not only to ensure a therapeutic response but also to avoid complications of over- and underinfusion (Table 20.1)

The nurse must have knowledge of the solutions, their effects and the factors which affect their flow, as well as the complications which could occur when flow is not controlled. The nurse should have an understanding of which groups require accurate flow control in order to prevent complications (Table 20.2) and how to select the most appropriate device for accuracy of delivery to best meet the patient's flow control needs (according to age, condition, setting and prescribed therapy).

The use of infusion devices both mechanical and electronic has increased the level of safety in IV therapy. However, the equipment is only as good as the person who is selecting and setting it up. A locally agreed policy is essential for the selection and purchase of infusion devices and should form part of an overall policy for medical device management (Medical Devices Agency 1995; Morling & Ford 1997).

The Medical Devices Agency regulations (1995) provide guidance on the selection and purchase of infusion devices and recommendations include:

1 That the number of different models in use within a unit should be minimized as far as possible; and
2 Systems should be evaluated on site wherever possible.

Criteria for selection of an infusion device include clinical requirement, education, compatibility with other equipment, disposables, product support, costs, service and maintenance and regulatory issues, e.g. compliance with European Community directives (Morling & Ford 1997). Strategies need to be developed for replacement of old, obsolete or inappropriate devices (Morling & Ford 1997) as well as planned service and maintenance programmes.

As infusion devices become increasingly more sophisticated there is an increase in the necessity for user training (Clarkson 1992). As the main users of infusion devices in direct patient care, nurses must be competent with both simple and complex devices (Wilkinson 1993; McConnell 1996). Education can be problematic, often inadequate, and its nature and quality vary greatly (McConnell 1995). The most frequently identified methods of training for staff are reading the user/instruction manual, trial and error (self taught) and consulting policy and procedure manuals (McConnell 1995; McConnell et al. 1996). 'Hands on' training is a major constituent of learning to use the equipment and teaching may be carried out by another member of staff or as part of in-service training. During education and training nurses should be competent at simple 'trouble shooting' and be aware of the limitations of their abilities (Leggett 1990b; UKCC 1992; Morling & Ford 1997). They

Table 20.1 Complications of inadequate flow control

Complications associated with overinfusion:
1 Fluid overload with accompanying electrolyte imbalance.
2 Metabolic disturbances during parenteral nutrition, mainly related to serum glucose levels.
3 Toxic concentrations of medications, which may result in a shock-like syndrome ('speed shock').
4 Air embolism, due to containers running dry before expected.
5 An increase in venous complications, e.g. chemical phlebitis, caused by reduced dilution of irritant substances (Weinstein 1993).

Complications associated with underinfusion:
1 Dehydration.
2 Metabolic disturbances.
3 A delayed response to medications or below therapeutic dose.
4 Occlusion of a cannula/catheter due to slow cessation of flow.

Table 20.2 Groups at risk of complications associated with flow control

1 Infants and young children.
2 The elderly.
3 Patients with compromised cardiovascular status.
4 Patients with impairment or failure of organs, e.g. kidneys.
5 Patients with major sepsis.
6 Patients suffering from shock, whatever the cause.
7 Postoperative or post-trauma patients.
8 Stressed patients, whose endocrine homeostatic controls may be affected.
9 Patients receiving multiple medications, whose clinical status may change rapidly (Weinstein 1993).

should also be made aware of the mechanism for reporting faults with devices and procedures for adverse incident reporting both within their trust and to the Medical Devices Agency (Richardson 1995; Medical Devices Agency 1997).

Constant beeping noises, being unsure how to use a device, setting up the equipment in a hurry and fear of harming the patients have been found in studies (McConnell 1996) to be reasons for causing nurses stress during the setting up and using of infusion devices. This in turn can result in user error, which is the more common reason for inappropriate delivery of drugs than pump/device error (Wilkinson 1993; Richardson 1995). Seventy per cent of errors with equipment occur with the syringe pump (Richardson 1995). Common problems often occur when pumps are not regularly serviced and cleaned, and may include:

1 Free flow of infusate when sets are being removed from, or attached to, infusion bags and the roller clamp is not closed.
2 Patient or relative interference (Wilkinson 1993; Richardson 1995).

Factors influencing flow rates

The following factors may increase or decrease IV flow rates, particularly with mechanical devices using gravity flow.

Type of fluid and container

The composition, viscosity and concentration of the fluid affect flow (Sager & Bomar 1980; Weinstein 1997). For example, an infusion of cold blood (which is viscous when cold, Macklin 1999) will result in venospasm and impede the flow rate. Intravenous fluids run by gravity and so any changes in the height of the container will alter the flow

rate (Weinstein 1997). The optimum height of the container above the patient is 1 m and it will usually provide 70 mmHg of pressure, which is adequate to overcome venous pressure (normal range in an adult is 25–80 mmHg) (Macklin 1999; Pickstone 1999; Springhouse Corporation 1999). Therefore any alterations in the patient's position may alter the flow rate and necessitate a change in the speed of the infusion to maintain the appropriate rate of flow (Auty 1989; Weinstein 1997; Dolan 1999).

Type of administration set

The flow rate of the infusion may be affected in several ways:

1 The roller clamps on administration sets, which are used to control fluid flow, may slip, loosen or distort the tubing causing a phenomenon known as 'cold flow'. Any marked tension or stretching of the tubing, due to movement by the patient, can render the clamp ineffective (Sager & Bomar 1980; Luken & Middleton 1990).
2 The diameter/inner lumen size of the tubing will also affect flow. Microbore sets have a narrow lumen and flow is restricted to some degree. However, these sets may be used as a safeguard against 'runaway' or bolus infusions (Jensen 1995).
3 Inclusion of other in-line devices may also affect the flow rate, e.g. filters (Weinstein 1993).

Type of vascular access device

The flow rate may be affected by any of the following:

1 The condition and size of the vein, e.g. phlebitis can reduce the lumen size and decrease flow (Weinstein 1997).
2 The gauge of the cannula/catheter.
3 The position of the device within the vein, i.e. if it is up against the vein wall.
4 The site of the vascular access device, e.g. the flow may be affected by the change in position of a limb – such as a decrease in flow when a patient bends their arm if a cannula is sited over the elbow joint.

5 Kinking, pinching or compression of the cannula/ catheter or tubing of the administration set may cause variation in the set rate.
6 Occlusion of the device due to clot formation, which may result from a BP cuff on the infusion arm, with the patient lying on the side of the infusion (Weinstein 1997).

The patient

Patients occasionally adjust the control clamp or other parts of the delivery system, for example changing the height of the infusion container, thereby making flow unreliable. Some pumps now have tamper-proof features (Jensen 1995). Positioning of the patient will affect flow and patients should be instructed to keep the arm lower than the infusion if on a gravity device (Dolan 1999).

Complications associated with lack of flow control

Fluid/electrolyte imbalance

Circulatory overload

The most common disorder of fluid and electrolyte balance is circulatory overload, which is *isotonic fluid expansion*. It is caused by infusion of fluids of the same tonicity as plasma into the vascular circulation, for example 0.9% sodium chloride. As isotonic solutions do not affect osmolarity, water does not flow from the extracellular to the intracellular compartment. The result is that the extracellular compartment expands in proportion to the fluid infused (Weinstein 1997). Because of the electrolyte concentration, no extra water is available to enable the kidneys selectively to excrete and restore the balance. In children, where the heart and circulation are smaller, and in renal and cardiac patients, overload can occur more rapidly (Perdue 1995; Weinstein 1997). Elderly patients must also be carefully monitored because they have a lower tolerance to fluids and electrolytes.

Early manifestations include:

1 Weight gain.
2 A relative increase in fluid intake compared to output.
3 A high bounding pulse pressure, indicating a high cardiac output.
4 Raised central venous pressure measurements.
5 Peripheral hand vein emptying time longer than normal. (Peripheral veins will usually empty in 3–5 seconds when the hand is elevated and will fill in the same length of time when the hand is lowered to a dependent position; Weinstein 1997.)
6 Peripheral oedema.

Progression of circulatory overload will lead to dyspnoea and cyanosis due to pulmonary oedema and neck vein engorgement (Weinstein 1997). Early detection results in simple treatment and consists of withholding all fluids until excess water and electrolytes have been eliminated by the body and/or administration of diuretics to promote rapid

diuresis (Perdue 1995). However, careful monitoring should continue to prevent isotonic contraction occurring (where there is loss of fluid and electrolytes isotonic to the extracellular fluid such as blood and large volumes of fluid from diarrhoea and vomiting; Weinstein 1997).

If a patient is receiving large quantities of electrolyte-free water, such as glucose 5% in water to replace losses from gastric suction, vomit, diarrhoea, diuresis or insensible loss, *hypotonic expansion* may develop. This involves both extracellular and intracellular compartments (Weinstein 1993).

Hypertonic expansion occurs when the volume of body water is increased by infusion of hypertonic saline, whilst *hypertonic contraction* (dehydration) occurs when water is lost without a corresponding loss of salts (Weinstein 1997).

Dehydration

This occurs when water is lost without corresponding loss of salts and occurs in patients unable to take sufficient fluids (elderly, unconscious or incontinent patients) or who have excess insensible water loss via skin and lungs or as a result of certain drugs in excess. Manifestations include:

1 Thirst (although this may be absent in the elderly)
2 Weight loss
3 Negative fluid balance
4 Irritability and restlessness
5 Skin turgor diminishes
6 Dry mouth and furrowed tongue.

Hypotonic contraction occurs when fluids containing more salt than water are lost and this results in a decrease in osmolarity of the extracellular compartment. Infants are at greatest risk, especially if they have diarrhoea (Wheeler & Frey 1995; Weinstein 1997). It may also result from the loss of salt from various sources – excess diuresis, fistula drainage, burns, vomiting or sweating. Manifestations include:

1 Weight loss
2 Negative fluid balance
3 Weak, thready, rapid pulse rate
4 Increased 'hand filling time'
5 Increased skin turgor.

Treatment of dehydration is replacement of fluids and electrolytes.

Metabolic disturbances

Metabolic disturbances are related to parenteral nutrition and most commonly to glucose intolerance. This may result in either a hyper- or hypoglycaemic state in the patient. Signs of hypoglycaemia include weakness, headache, thirst and a cold clammy skin. Hyperglycaemia will lead rapidly to coma (Weinstein 1997).

Accurate control of flow rates of all feeding solutions is essential and the rates should never be adjusted by more than 10% as too rapid a rate can result in hyperglycaemic reactions (Weinstein 1997).

Speed shock

This should not be confused with pulmonary oedema, which relates to the volume of fluid infused into the patient. Speed shock is related to the rapidity with which medication is administered and can occur even with small volumes (Perdue 1995). Rapid, uncontrolled administration of drugs will result in toxic concentrations reaching vital organs. Toxicity may be manifested by an exaggeration of the usual pharmacological actions of the drug or by signs and symptoms specific for that drug or class of drugs. The most extreme toxic response which can occur if a drug is given at a dose or rate exceeding that recommended is the lethal response.

Signs of speed shock may include:

1 Flushed face
2 Headache and dizziness
3 Congestion of the chest
4 Tachycardia and fall in blood pressure
5 Syncope
6 Shock
7 Cardiovascular collapse (Weinstein 1997).

Prevention of speed shock is achieved by reducing the drop size, for example by the use of paediatric burette sets or infusion devices. When commencing an infusion using gravity flow, check that the solution is flowing freely before adjusting the rate. Movement of the patient or the device within the vessel can cause the infusion to flow more or less freely after a few minutes of setting the rate (Weinstein 1997). Always close the roller clamp prior to removing the set from the pump. Although most pumps have an anti-free-flow mechanism, it is still recommended to switch off the clamp (Pickstone 1999). Administration must be slowed down or discontinued and the medical staff notified. If speed shock occurs it may be necessary to administer antidotes and diuretics (see Nursing care plan).

Air embolism

Medical opinion is divided about the volume of air which can cause complications (Auty 1995). Even a small air bubble (100 µl) could constitute a hazard and might induce a stroke in certain circumstances (Auty 1995), therefore, most infusion equipment has an air-in-line detector as a feature. An air-in-line detector is usually located where the administration set exits from the device and can be designed to detect only visible bubbles or microscopic 'champagne' sized bubbles (Jensen 1995). Air can enter the IV system if not cleared from an administration set prior to use, if bags are left hanging once all the solution has infused or during disconnection of a set. Therefore it is important that care is taken during manipulations to minimize this risk.

Venous complications

Increased contact time with the intima of the vein by irritant drugs can lead to vasoconstriction, phlebitis and possible infiltration. In the long term this may result in reduced venous access and difficulty with fluid replacement. It may be necessary either to select the central venous route or to infuse fluids subcutaneously, known as hypodermoclysis (Weinstein 1997), which does not require the use of veins (see Chap. 12, Drug Administration).

Paediatric considerations

In a child, especially a clinically compromised one, even the smallest error can cause serious problems (Sager & Bomar 1980). Therefore paediatrics is an area where extra care is required with flow control. Maintenance of flow at a constant rate can be achieved by the use of special sets such as burettes or by electronic infusion devices. Observation of intake and output are vital (Table 20.3) as well as weight, general condition, vital signs and behaviour, e.g. tachycardia, raised blood pressure and respirations, oedema, headache, abdominal cramps. Assessment of fluid needs is often based on body surface area, and weight and medications are calculated to an accuracy of 0.1 mg or ml (Wheeler & Frey 1995).

Principles of equipment selection and application

The Medical Devices Agency (1995) has made recommendations on the safety and performance of infusion devices in order to enable users to make the appropriate choice of equipment to suit most applications. The Medical Devices Agency (1995) has developed a classification system for infusion devices according to the perceived risk of, and suitability for, particular applications. Infusion devices are classified into one of three risk categories, which are:

1 Neonatal: this is the highest risk category. Consistency of flow, availability of very low flow rates with 0.1 ml increments, high accuracy (both short- and long-term), comprehensive alarm features with very short alarm

---

Table 20.3 Measuring fluid balance in the paediatric patient

Intake
1 An hourly record of the amount and type of fluid.
2 A running total of the amount administered.
3 Regular checks of the infusion device and the rate of flow.
4 Recording the volume of diluent used in drug reconstitution.
5 Checking the electrolyte content of drug presentations, especially sodium and potassium.
6 Consideration of additional water needs due to a faster metabolic rate and a greater loss in urine due to immature renal function.

Output
1 Careful recording of all output, including weighing nappies.
2 Recording any other drainage, e.g. from a wound site.
3 Adjustments to allow for insensible loss via a greater surface area.

delays, very low bolus of drug/solution on release of an occlusion and automatic changeover to battery operation on mains failure are essential.

2 High risk: these are typically the infusion of drugs where consistency of flow, high accuracy (both short- and long-term), comprehensive alarm features with short alarm delays, very low bolus of drug/solution on release of an occlusion and automatic changeover to battery operation on mains failure are essential.

3 Lower risk: these include infusion of simple electrolytes, antibiotics and total parenteral nutrition (TPN) where it may not be required to deliver a given volume in a precise time and where the constant rate of delivery is not so important. A simpler alarm system is also acceptable.

The Medical Devices Agency (1995) has also classified devices which are designed for specific applications, including:

1 Ambulatory infusion pumps (pumps usually carried around by the patient whether in hospital or at home)
2 Patient controlled analgesia (PCA) pumps
3 IV anaesthesia pumps.

It may not be easy for nursing staff to identify which pump should be used in which setting as the Department of Health has issued no universal classification of drugs for IV infusions, although some trusts have devised their own systems (Pickstone 1995). Pumps have been found to be inappropriately selected at ward level, and mismatching can be potentially hazardous if use of a 'lower risk' category of pump is used to administer a drug to a neonate (Pickstone *et al.* 1994, 1995). Systems must be in place to ensure that staff can easily select the most appropriate device for the application (Petty *et al.* 1996).

Requirements of devices

Accuracy of delivery

In order to meet requirements for high risk and neonatal infusions, pumps must be accurate to within ±5% of the set rate when measured over a 60-minute period (Pickstone *et al.* 1994; Jensen 1995). They also have to satisfy short-term, minute to minute accuracy requirements which determine smoothness and consistency of output (Pickstone *et al.* 1994).

Occlusion response and pressure

Flow will occur if the pressure at the tip of an intravascular device is just fractionally above the pressure in the vein; the pressure does not need to be excessive. In an adult peripheral vein pressure is approximately 25 mmHg, while in a neonate it measures 5 mmHg (Auty 1995). Most pumps have a variable pressure setting which allows the user to use their own judgement about the pressure needed to deliver therapy safely. It can be set as low as 100–250 mmHg (2–5 psi) for infusions of vesicants or a maximum of 10 psi in positional central venous catheters. The common

Table 20.4 Performance requirements for infusion devices (DHSS 1990)

	Neonatal	High risk infusion
Occlusion alarm pressure at 1 ml/hour (mmHg)	<300	<500
Bolus following release of occlusion at all flow rates (ml)	<0.3	<0.6
Time to alarm following occlusion at 1 ml/hour (min)	<30	<45

setting is 200–400 mmHg (4–8 psi) (Jensen 1995; Macklin 1999). Flow is dependent upon pressure divided by resistance. If very long extension sets of small internal bore are used the resistance to flow can increase dramatically (Auty 1995). If any set is occluded this increases resistance and infusate will not flow into the vein. The longer the occlusion occurs, the greater the pressure and the pump will continue to pump until an occlusion alarm is activated. There are two types of occlusions defined – upstream, between the pump and the container, and downstream, which is between the pump and the patient (Jensen 1995).

Pumps alarm at a pressure termed 'occlusion alarm pressure' and many pumps allow the user to set the pressure within a range (Auty 1995). Therefore the time it takes to alarm depends on the rate of flow – high rates alarm more quickly. When the alarm is activated, a certain amount of stored bolus will be present and it is important that a large bolus is not released into the vein as this could lead to rupture of the vein or constitute overinfusion (Auty 1995).

The DHSS (1990) has set performance requirements in terms of pressure, occlusion alarm delay time and the size of bolus released (Table 20.4) (Pickstone *et al.* 1994).

Infusion devices

Gravity infusion devices

Gravity flow

Gravity infusion devices depend entirely on gravity to drive the infusion. The system consists of an administration set containing a drip chamber and utilizing a roller clamp to control the flow, which is usually measured by counting drops (Auty 1995). The indications for use are:

1 Delivery of fluids without drug additives.
2 Administration of drugs or fluids where adverse effects are not anticipated if the infusion rate varies slightly.
3 Where the patient's condition does not give cause for concern and no complication is predicted.

Gravity infusions are ideal for infusing fluids which do not need to be infused with absolute precision. The pressure is dependent on the height of the container above the infusion site as well as the other factors mentioned previously. Roller clamps used to adjust and to maintain rates of flow on gravity infusions vary considerably in their efficiency and accuracy (Clarkson 1995). Flow rate is calculated using a formula which requires the following information: the volume to be infused, the number of hours the infusion is running over and the drop rate of the administration set (which will differ depending on type of set). The number of drops per millilitre is dependent on the type of administration set used and the viscosity of the infusion fluid. Increased viscosity causes the size of the drop to increase. For example, crystalloid fluid administered via a solution set is delivered at the rate of 20 drops/ml; the rate of packed red cells given via a blood set will be calculated at 15 drops/ml.

The rate of administration of a continuous or intermittent infusion may be calculated from the following equation (Gatford 1998):

$$\frac{\text{Volume to be infused}}{\text{Time in hours}} \times \frac{\text{Drop rate}}{60\,\text{minutes}} = \text{Drops per minute}$$

In this equation, 60 is a factor for the conversion of the number of hours to the number of minutes.

Advantages and disadvantages

The advantages of the gravity flow system are that it is usually familiar to most staff and is simple to set up. It is low cost and the infusion of air is less likely than with electronic devices. However, the system does require frequent observation and adjustment due to:

1 The tubing changing shape over time.
2 Creep or distortion of tubing made of PVC.
3 Fluctuations of venous pressure which can affect the flow of the solution.
4 The roller clamp can be unreliable, leading to inconsistent flow rates.

There can also be variability of drop size and if the roller clamp is inadvertently left open free flow will occur. Infusion rates with viscous fluids can be reduced (particularly if administered via small cannulae) and there is a limitation on the type of infusion as it is not suitable for arterial infusions – this is because viscosity and arterial flow offer a high resistance to flow which cannot be overcome by gravity flow (Auty 1995; Medical Devices Agency 1995; Dolan 1999).

Gravity controllers

A controller is a mechanical device that operates by gravity; there is no pumping action. It controls the flow of the infusion at the desired rate by constricting the infusion set (Auty 1989; Luken & Middleton 1990; Medical Devices Agency 1995). There are two types:

Drip-rate controllers

These devices control gravity by placing a detector on the drip chamber to count drops and an automatic clamping mechanism to control flow (Auty 1995). The desired flow is set in drops per minute. They are suitable for the majority of lower risk infusions in which volumetric accuracy is of lesser importance.

Advantages and disadvantages

Although they can maintain a drip rate within 1%, volumetric accuracy is not guaranteed and many of the disadvantages associated with gravity flow still remain. The main advantages are they are relatively inexpensive and can usually use standard gravity sets. They also incorporate some audible and visual alarm systems (Auty 1995).

Volumetric controllers

These are calibrated in millilitres per hour and accuracy of flow is dependent mainly on the size of the drop formed. However, drop size is affected by a number of factors including temperature, pressure, the physical nature and condition of the drop-forming orifice, rate of drop formation and type of fluid being infused, fluid viscosity and surface tension (Auty 1995). They are suitable for the majority of lower risk infusions in which volumetric accuracy is required.

Advantages and disadvantages

These devices are fairly easy to operate due to the simplicity of the set and controls. The alarms are very sensitive, they have a low infusion pressure and the infusion of air is unlikely. However, they are more expensive to purchase than drip-rate controllers and a dedicated set is usually required. They cannot be used for arterial infusions and infusion rates may be limited, especially with viscous fluids and small-gauge vascular access devices.

Infusion pumps

Common to all pumps is the ability to overcome resistance to flow by increased delivery pressure. Pumps do not rely on gravity and can therefore be placed in almost any reasonable position relative to the infusion site. If a catheter becomes occluded or displaced, delivery pressures can rise to high values to overcome resistance, leading to the risk of extravascular infusion. However, the default pressure is usually limited and some pumps include a facility for setting very low occlusion alarm pressures (Medical Devices Agency 1995). The performance of these pumps is predictable, but these devices are associated with a number of risks. There are two types:

Drip rate pumps

These were the first infusion pumps which controlled the rate of drop formation using standard gravity sets. They had few alarms and delivered at high pressures. These have become obsolete and are not recommended by the Medical Devices Agency for use in the clinical setting (Auty 1995;

Medical Devices Agency 1995). Today all large volume infusions are administered using a volumetric pump.

Volumetric pumps

A volumetric pump works by calculating the volume delivered. This is achieved when the pump measures the volume displaced in a 'reservoir'. The reservoir is an integral component of the administration set. The pump calculates that every fill and empty cycle of the reservoir delivers a given amount of solution (Weinstein 1997). The mechanism of action may be piston generated or linear peristaltic – where fingers in the pump move in a wave-like manner pushing the fluid out of the chamber (Jensen 1995; Pickstone 1999). The indications for use are all large volume infusions, both venous and arterial.

Most volumetric pumps have a linear peristaltic pumping mechanism, although some use cassettes. All are mains and battery powered, with the rate selected in ml per hour. The accuracy of flow is usually within 5% when measured over a period of time, which is more than adequate for most clinical applications (Auty 1995).

Advantages and disadvantages

These pumps are able to overcome resistance to flow by increased delivery pressure and do not rely on gravity. This generally makes the performance of pumps predictable and capable of accurate delivery over a wider range of flow rates (Medical Devices Agency 1995).

The pumps also incorporate a wide range of features including air-in-line detectors, variable pressure settings and comprehensive alarms such as end of infusion, KVO (keep vein open, where the pump switches to a low flow rate, e.g. 5 ml/hour, in order to continue flow to prevent occlusion of the device) and low battery. Many have a secondary infusion facility, which is to allow for intermittent therapy, e.g. antibiotics. The pump is programmed to switch to a secondary set and, when completed, it reverts back to the primary infusion at the previously set rate.

The disadvantages are that these are usually relatively expensive and often dedicated administration sets are required. The use of the wrong set could result in error even if the pump appears to work. Some are complicated to set up which can also lead to errors (Medical Devices Agency 1995).

Syringe pumps

Syringe pumps are low-volume, high-accuracy devices designed to infuse at low flow rates and the rate is controlled by the drive speed of the piston attached to the syringe plunger (Auty 1995; Jensen 1995).

Syringe pumps are useful in intensive care situations where small volumes of highly concentrated drugs need to be infused.

The volume for infusion is limited to the size of the syringe used in the device which is usually a 60 ml syringe, but most pumps will accept different sizes and brands of syringe. These devices are calibrated for delivery in millilitres per hour.

Advantages and disadvantages

Syringe pumps are mains and/or battery powered, are usually easy to operate and tend to cost less than volumetric pumps. The alarm systems are becoming more comprehensive but include low battery, end of infusion and syringe clamp open alarm. Most of the problems associated with the older models, for example free flow, mechanical backlash (slackness which causes start-up and alarm delays) and incorrect fitting of the syringe, have been eliminated in the newer models (Medical Devices Agency 1995; Pickstone 1999).

Specialist pumps

Patient controlled analgesia (PCA) pumps

PCA devices are typically syringe pumps (although some are based on volumetric designs) (Auty 1995; Medical Devices Agency 1995). The syringe pump forces down on the syringe piston, collapsing the syringe at a preset rate, but the distinguishing feature is the ability of the pump to deliver doses on demand, which occurs when the patient pushes a button (Jensen 1995). Whether or not the dose is delivered is determined by preset parameters in the pump. That is, if the maximum amount of drug over a given period of time has already been delivered, a further dose cannot be delivered.

PCA pumps are useful for patients who require analgesia. PCA pumps are used more in the acute setting, but are also useful in ambulatory situations.

Infusion options of a PCA pump are usually categorized into three types:

1 Basal: a 'baseline' rate can be accompanied by intermittent doses requested by patients. This aims to achieve pain relief with minimal medication, but not necessarily to achieve a pain-free state (Jensen 1995).
2 Continuous: designed for the patient who needs maximum pain relief without the option of demand dosing, e.g. epidural.
3 Demand: drug delivered by intermittent infusion when button is pushed and can be used alone or supplemented by the basal rate. Doses can be limited by a designated maximum amount (Jensen 1995).

The PCA pump can dispense a bolus dose, with an initial bolus dose being called a loading dose. This may benefit patients as the one time dose is significantly higher than a demand dose in order to achieve immediate pain relief.

Advantages and disadvantages

These devices offer a 'lock-out' feature (when a key or a combination of numbers is necessary to gain access to pump controls) which is designed for patient safety. These pumps have an extensive memory capability which can be accessed through the display via a printer or computer. This facility is critical for the pump's effective use in pain relief (Jensen 1995), as it enables the clinician to determine when and how often demand is made by a patient and what total volume has been infused (Auty 1995; Medical Devices Agency 1995). It has also been shown that they increase patient satisfaction, patients require less sedation, anxiety is reduced and so is nursing time and time in hospital (Ripamonti & Bruera 1997).

Anaesthesia pumps

These are syringe pumps designed for delivery of anaesthesia or sedation and must only ever be used for that purpose. They should be restricted to operating or high dependency areas and should be clearly labelled. They infuse at a very high flow rate and have a high rate bolus facility in order to deliver the induction dose of anaesthesia quickly (Medical Devices Agency 1995).

Ambulatory infusion devices

Ambulatory devices are small devices which were developed to allow patients more freedom and enable the patient to continue with normal activities or to move unencumbered by a large infusion device (Jensen 1995; Medical Devices Agency 1995). They are used for small volumes of a variety of drugs and are mainly designed for patients to wear and use when ambulant.

Ambulatory devices range in size and weight from small enough to fit into a pocket to large enough to require a rucksack. The solution containers are often more cumbersome than the actual pump itself. Due to their size the available capacity may be low and alarms provided may be limited. Considerations for selection of an ambulatory device include the following:

1 Type of therapy
2 Patient's ability to understand
3 Drug stability
4 Frequency of doses
5 Reservoir volumes required
6 Control of flow/flow rates
7 Type of access
8 Cost effectiveness
9 Portability
10 Convenience

(Shoernike & Brown 1990; Schelis & Tice 1996). Ambulatory pumps fall into two categories: mechanical and battery-operated infusion devices.

Mechanical infusion devices

These are simple and compact but may not necessarily be cost effective as they are usually disposable. The mechanism for delivery is either by balloon, simple spring or gas-powered.

Elastomeric balloons

These are made of a soft rubberized material capable of being inflated to a predetermined volume and the drug is

then administered over a very specific infusion time. The balloon is encapsulated inside a rigid transparent container which may be round or cylindrical. The rate of infusion is not controlled by the balloon but by the diameter of the restricting outlet located in the preattached tubing. It is designed for single use that supplies the patient's need for a single dose infusion of drugs, e.g. intermittent small volume parenteral therapies such as delivery of antibiotics. Its small size causes little disruption to the patient's daily activities and it tends to be well tolerated (Auty 1995; Jensen 1995; Hamid 1996; Allwood *et al.* 1997; Springhouse Corporation 1999).

Spring mechanism

Spring coil piston syringes have a spring which powers the plunger of a syringe in the absence of manual pressure. The volume is restricted by the size of the syringe, which is usually prefilled. The spring coil container tends to be a multi-dose, small-volume administration device and is a combination of a spring coil in a collapsible flattened disk. Its shape can accommodate many therapies and volumes (Jensen 1995; Medical Devices Agency 1997).

Gas-powered

These devices are activated using hydrogen or carbon dioxide gases, produced by a chemical reaction (Medical Devices Agency 1997). The user activates the chemical reaction, which facilitates a controlled release of gas, in order to start the infusion. The single-use cartridge then pressurizes the syringe plunger or reservoir to deliver the fluid (Medical Devices Agency 1997).

Battery-operated infusion devices

Battery-operated pumps are small and light enough to be carried around by the patient without interfering with most everyday activities (Boutin & Hagar 1992; Koeppen & Caspers 1994). They are operated using rechargeable or alkaline batteries but, due to their size, the available battery capacity tends to be low. The length of time the battery lasts is often dependent on the rate the pump is set at. Most give an output in the form of a small bolus delivered every few minutes. Most devices have an integral case or pouch which allows the pump and the reservoir/syringe to be worn with discretion by the patient. There are two types: ambulatory volumetric infusion pumps and syringe drivers.

Ambulatory volumetric infusion pumps

An ambulatory volumetric infusion pump is an infusion device which pumps in the same way as a large volumetric pump, but by nature of its size it is portable and useful in the ambulatory setting.

This pump is suitable for patients who have been prescribed continuous infusional treatment for a period of time, for example from 4 days to 6 months, and enables the patients, where appropriate, to receive treatment at home, because it is small and portable.

The use of ambulatory devices for the delivery of continuous infusional chemotherapy has dramatically altered cancer treatment (Jones *et al.* 1994), particularly in cancers such as breast, gastrointestinal, myeloma and teratoma. Drugs with relatively short half lives such as doxorubicin and bleomycin are more effective when given by continuous infusion because an effective drug concentration can be present in malignant cells when they replicate (Forgeson *et al.* 1988). Certain cytotoxic drugs have been found to induce prolonged plasma concentrations when given by continuous infusion. The aim of continuous therapy is to achieve the maximum effects while reducing the severity and frequency of side-effects; 5 FU is one such drug (Frail *et al.* 1980; Carlson 1996; Meta Analysis Group in Cancer 1998). Ambulatory chemotherapy which enables patients to receive treatment at home enhances patients' well-being and quality of life by increasing their independence and sense of control (Dougherty *et al.* 1998).

The advantages of the ambulatory pump are that it:

1 Is able to deliver drugs continuously or intermittently.
2 Delivers drugs accurately over a set period of time.
3 Improves potential outcomes of treatment by delivering treatment continuously.
4 Heightens patients' independence and control by allowing them to be at home and participate in their own care.
5 Is compact, light and easy to use.
6 Has audible alarm systems.

The disadvantages are that:

1 It may require the insertion of a central venous access device, which has associated complications and problems.
2 It could malfunction at home, which could be distressing and dangerous for the patient.
3 In spite of its ease of use, some patients may not be able to cope with it at home.
4 Patients may have to adapt their lifestyle to cope with living with a pump continuously.

Syringe drivers

A syringe driver is a portable battery-operated infusion pump. It is used to deliver drugs at a predetermined rate via the appropriate parenteral route. Typical applications include its use in pain control, cytotoxic chemotherapy, coronary care and neonatal care. It may also be used for the administration of heparin and insulin, and treatment of thalassaemia. The syringe driver should be used for patients who are unable to tolerate oral medication for whatever reason, for example, in nausea and vomiting, dysphagia, intestinal obstruction, local disease or sometimes in intractable pain which is unrelieved by oral medications and where rapid dose titration is required. In addition, patients who are weak, agitated or unconscious may benefit from subcutaneous infusions. It is mainly used for administration of drugs via the subcutaneous route, but may be used intravenously too.

The syringe driver was developed in 1979 by Martin Wright for use in treating thalassaemia with infusions of desferrioxamine (Wright & Callam 1979), followed closely by their use in the terminal care setting (Russell 1979).

The use of a portable, battery-operated syringe driver for subcutaneous medications is now a well-established technique in palliative care. This type of device is used to administer analgesics and antiemetics, anxiolytic sedatives and dexamethasone (Coyle *et al.* 1986; Dover 1987; Oliver 1988; Bottomley & Hanks 1990, as cited in Doyle *et al.* 1998) and more recently ketorolac (Blackwell *et al.* 1993; Myers & Trotman 1994) and octreotide (Mercadante 1992; Riley & Fallon 1994).

The Graseby Medical MS16A and Graseby MS26 syringe drivers are typical examples of the drivers in use; however, other types are available and nurses should follow the manufacturer's instruction manual for details of their use. The first models of Graseby Medical MS16A and MS26 were very similar in appearance, however the rate settings were different. The MS16A allows drug administration on an hourly rate (Fig. 20.1). This pump is now clearly marked with a pink '1HR' in the bottom right-hand corner of the driver. The MS26 delivers drugs on a 24-hourly rate. It is important that users are aware that the MS16A syringe driver is calibrated in millimetres per hour, and the MS26 is calibrated in millimetres per day. The MS26 model is now marked with '24 HR' in the bottom right-hand corner to avoid error. The MS series of syringe drivers may be used with most sizes and brands of plastic syringes, although it is preferable to use those with luer lock facility to avoid leakage or accidental disconnection.

The advantages of the syringe driver are:

1 It avoids the necessity of intermittent injections.
2 Mixtures of drugs may be administered.
3 Infusion timing is accurate, which is particularly advantageous in the community where the ability to constantly monitor the rate is not feasible.
4 The device is lightweight and compact, allowing mobility and independence (it usually weighs approximately 175 g including the battery and measures about $165 \times 53 \times 23$ mm).
5 Rate can be increased (see additional notes at end of chapter).
6 Simple calculations of dosage are required over a 12- or 24-hour period.
7 It allows patients to spend more time at home with their symptoms managed effectively.

The disadvantages are:

1 The patient may become psychologically dependent on the device.
2 Inflammation or infection may occur at the site of the cannula insertion.
3 The rate calculation can be confusing for the novice because there are two different types of pumps, particularly if the patient's dose requirements alter (see 'Additional Notes' at end of Guidelines).
4 The alarm system of some syringe drivers, e.g. the Graseby, operates only if the plunger is obstructed. It does not alert the nurse if the flow is too rapid or if the skin site has perished.

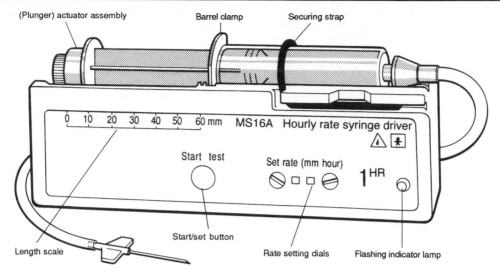

Figure 20.1 Graseby Medical MS16A hourly rate syringe driver.

Summary

Careful calculation and control of flow rates are essential as delivery of fluids and medications may be critical due to any of the factors mentioned above. There are many infusion control devices available to assist the nurse in this task, ranging from the simple to the complex. A knowledge of these systems and of their application is necessary to ensure appropriate choices are made (Manley 1992). Although these devices provide a valuable aid to patient care they do not replace the need for good nursing assessment and intervention (Leggett 1990).

References and further reading

Allwood, M., Stanley, A. & Wright, P. (eds) (1997) *The Cytotoxic Handbook*, 3rd edn, Chap. 5. Radcliffe Medical Press, Oxford.

Auty, B. (1989) Choice of instrumentation for controlled IV infusion. *Intens Ther Clin Monitor*, **10**(4), 117–22.

Auty, B. (1995) Types of infusion pump and their risks. *Br J Intens Care*, Feb, Suppl., 11–16.

Auty, B. & Protheroe, D.T. (1986) Syringe pumps: a review. *Br J Parent Ther*, **7**, 72–7.

Blackwell, N. *et al.* (1993) Subcutaneous ketorolac – a new development in pain control. *Palliat Med*, **7**, 63–5.

Boutin, J. & Hagar, E. (1992) Patients' preference regarding portable pumps. *J Intraven Nurs*, **15**(4), 230–32.

British National Formulary (1987) *Number 14*. British Medical Association/Pharmaceutical Society of Great Britain, London.

British National Formulary (1999) *Number 38, (Sept), Appendix*. British Medical Association/Royal Pharmaceutical Society of Great Britain, London.

Carlson, R. (1996) Continuous intravenous infusion chemotherapy. In: *The Chemotherapy Source Book* (ed. M.C. Perry), pp. 225–51. William & Wilkers, Baltimore.

Clarkson, D. (1992) Internal delivery. *Nurs Times*, **88**(20), 53–8.

Clarkson, D. (1995) The future of infusion. *Hosp Equip Supplies*, June, 17.

Coyle, N. *et al.* (1986) Continuous subcutaneous infusions of opiates in cancer patients with pain. *Oncol Nurs Forum*, **13**(4), 53–7.

DHSS (1990) *Health Equipment Information Evaluation Issue No. 198*. Stationery Office, London.

Dolan, S. (1999) Intravenous flow control and infusion devices. In: *Intravenous Therapy in Nursing Practice* (eds L. Dougherty & J. Lamb), pp. 195–222. Churchill Livingstone, Edinburgh.

Dougherty, L., Viner, C. & Young, J. (1998) Establishing ambulatory chemotherapy at home. *Prof Nurse*, **13**(6), 356–60.

Dover, S.B. (1987) Syringe driver in terminal care. *Br Med J*, **294**, 553–5.

Doyle, D. *et al.* (1998) *Oxford Textbook of Palliative Medicine*, 2nd edn. Oxford University Press, Oxford.

Forgeson, G.V. *et al.* (1988) Vincristine and adriamycin with high dose methyl prednisolone in advanced treated multiple myeloma patients. *Br J Cancer*, **58**, 469–73.

Frail, R.J. *et al.* (1980) Pharmacokinetics of 5FU administered orally by rapid infusion and by slow infusion. *Cancer Res*, **40**, 2323–8.

Gatford, J.D. (1998) *Nursing Calculations*, 5th edn. Churchill Livingstone, Edinburgh.

Hamid, S.K. (1996) A novel device for patient controlled sedation. *Anaesthesia*, **51**(2), 145–50.

Hawkett, S. & Nicholson, R. (1987) Syringe drivers (drug administration for the terminally ill in the community). *J District Nurs*, **5**(8), 4–6.

Hudek, K. (1986) Compliance in intravenous therapy. *J Can Intraven Nurses Assoc*, **2**(3), 7–8.

Jensen, B.L. (1995) Types of intravenous equipment. In: *Intravenous Therapy: Clinical Principles and Practices* (eds J. Terry, L. Baranowski, R.A. Lonsway, *et al.*), pp. 303–338. W.B. Saunders, Philadelphia.

Jones, A.L. *et al.* (1994) Phase 2 study of a continuous infusion 5FU with epirubicin and cisplatin in patients with metastatic and locally advanced breast cancer: an active regimen. *J Clin Oncol*, **12**(6), 1259–65.

Koeppen, M.A. & Caspers, S.M. (1994) Problems identified with home infusion pumps. *Intraven Nurs*, **17**(3), 151–6.

Latham, J. (1987) Syringe drivers in pain control. *Prof Nurse*, **2**(7), 207–209.

Ledger, T. (1986) Administering heparin with syringe pumps. *Prof Nurse*, **1**(7), 176–7.

Leggett, A. (1990a) Intravenous infusion pumps. *Nurs Stand*, **4**(28), 24–6.

Leggett, A. (1990b) Looking at infusion devices. *Nurs Stand*, **4**(30), 29–31.

Luken, J. & Middleton, J. (1990) Intravenous infusion controllers. *Nurs Stand*, **4**(29), 30–32.

Macklin, D. (1999) What's physics got to do with it? – a review of the physical principles of fluid administration. *J Vasc Access Networks*, Summer, 7–11.

Manley, K. (1992) Flow control in intravenous therapy. *Surg Nurse*, 12–15.

McConnell, E.A. (1995) How and what staff nurses learn about the medical devices they use in direct patient care. *Res Nurs Health*, **18**, 165–72.

McConnell, E.A. *et al.* (1996) Australian registered nurse medical device education: a comparison of simple vs complex devices. *J Advanced Nurs*, **23**, 322–8.

Medical Devices Agency (1995) Infusion systems. *Device Bull, MDA DB 9503*, May.

Medical Devices Agency (1997) Selection and use of infusion devices for ambulatory applications. *Device Bull, MDA DB 9703*, March.

Mercadante, S. (1992) Treatment of diarrhoea due to enterocolic fistula with octreotide in a terminal cancer patient. *Palliat Med*, **65**, 257–9.

Meta Analysis Group in Cancer (1998) Efficacy in intravenous continuous infusion of fluorouracil compared with bolus administration in advanced colorectal cancer. *J Clin Oncol*, **16**(1), 301–308.

Miller, J. (1989) Intravenous therapy in fluid and electrolyte imbalance. *Prof Nurse*, Feb, 237.

Morling, S. & Ford, L. (1997) IV therapy: selection, use and management of infusion pumps. *Br J Nurs*, **6**(19), 1094–102.

Myers, K. & Trotman, I. (1994) Use of ketorolac by continuous subcutaneous infusion for the control of cancer related pain. *Postgrad Med J*, **70**, 359–62.

Nicholson, H. (1986) The success of the syringe driver. *Nurs Times*, **82**(9), 49–51.

Oliver, D.J. (1988) Syringe drivers in palliative care: a review. *Palliat Med*, **2**, 21–6.

Perdue, L. (1995) Intravenous complications. In: *Intravenous Therapy: Clinical Principles and Practices* (eds J. Terry, L.

Baranowski, R.A. Lonsway, *et al.*), pp. 419–46. W.B. Saunders Philadelphia.

Petty, D.R. *et al.* (1996) A measure of infusion risk. *Br J Intens Care*, Jan, 33–4.

Pickstone, M. (1999) *A Pocketbook for Safer IV Therapy*. Medical Technology and Risk Series. Scitech, Kent.

Pickstone, M. *et al.* (1994) Intravenous infusion of drugs. *Br J Intens Care*, Nov/Dec, 338–43.

Pickstone, M. *et al.* (1995) Intravenous infusion of drugs, Part 2. *Br J Intens Care*, Jan, 17–24.

Richardson, N. (1995) A review of drug infusion incidents. *Br J Intens Care*, Feb, Suppl., 8–10.

Riley, J. & Fallon, M.T. (1994) Octreotide in terminal malignant obstruction of the GI tract. *Eur J Palliat Care*, **1**, 23–5.

Ripamonti, C. & Bruera, E. (1997) Current status of patient controlled analgesia in cancer patients. *Oncology*, **11**(3), 373–80.

Russell, P.S.B. (1979) Analgesia in terminal malignant disease. *Br Med J*, **1**(6177), 1561.

Sager, D. & Bomar, S. (1980) *Intravenous Medications*. J.B. Lippincott, Philadelphia.

Schoenike, S. & Brown, S. (1990) Ambulatory infusion devices. *CINA*, **6**(4), 7–9.

Schelis, T.G. & Tice, A.D. (1996) Selecting infusion devices for use in ambulatory care. *Am J Health Syst Pharm*, **53**(8), 868–77.

Sepion, B. (1990) Intravenous care for children. *Paed Nurs*, April, 14–16.

Springhouse Corporation (1999) *Handbook of Infusion Therapy*. Springhouse, Pennsylvania.

UKCC (1992) *Code of Professional Conduct*. UKCC, London.

Weinstein, S.M. (ed.) (1993) *Principles and Practices of Intravenous Therapy*, 5th edn. J.B. Lippincott, Philadelphia.

Weinstein, S.M. (1997) *Plumer's Principles and Practice of Intravenous Therapy*, 6th edn. J.B. Lippincott, Philadelphia.

Weston, A. (1989) Graseby syringe driver (brief research project). *Nurs Times Nurs Mirror*, **85**, 60–61.

Wheeler, C. & Frey, A.M. (1995) IV therapy in children. In: *Intravenous Therapy: Clinical Principles and Practices* (eds J. Terry, L. Baranowski, R.A. Lonsway, *et al.*), pp. 467–94. W.B. Saunders, Philadelphia.

Wilkinson, R. (1993) IV therapy – risks, responsibilities and practice. *Nurs Stand* (Poster).

Wilkinson, R. (1996) Nurses' concerns about IV therapy and devices. *Nurs Stand*, **10**(35), 35–7.

Wittig, P. & Semmler-Bertanzi, D.J. (1983) Pumps and controllers: a nurse's assessment guide. *Am J Nurs*, **7**, 1023–5.

Woollons, S. (1996) Infusion devices for ambulatory use. *Prof Nurse*, **11**(10), 689–95.

Wright, B.M. & Callam, K. (1979) Slow drug infusions using a portable syringe driver. *Br Med J*, **2**, 582.

GUIDELINES · Subcutaneous administration of drugs using a syringe driver (e.g. Graseby Medical MS16A)

Equipment

1 Syringe driver MS16A.
2 Battery (PP3 size, 9 volt alkaline).
3 Winged infusion set (e.g. Vygon microflex PVC infusion set tube 100 cm, 0.5 mm G25).
4 Luer lock syringe of suitable size (5 ml or larger).
5 Swab saturated with isopropyl alcohol 70%.
6 Transparent adhesive dressing.
7 Drugs and diluent.
8 Needle (to draw up drug).
9 Drug additive label.
10 Patient's prescription.

Guidelines • Subcutaneous administration of drugs using a syringe driver (e.g. Graseby Medical MS16A) (cont'd)

Calculating the rate setting for administration of drugs using a syringe driver (e.g. Graseby Medical MS16A) over a 12-hour period

1 Measure stroke length in mm. The stroke length is the *length* of fluid to be infused, i.e. the distance the plunger has to travel (irrespective of the number of ml) (Fig. 20.2).

2 Check the delivery time (previously prescribed) in hours.

3 Calculate:

$$\frac{\text{Stroke length (mm)}}{\text{Delivery time (h)}} \times \text{Rate setting}$$

Example:
  Stroke length = 24 mm
  Delivery time = 12 h
  Rate setting = 2 mm/h
Set rate using screwdriver provided.
If the set rate is a single figure, e.g. 2, this must be preceded by 0 (Fig. 20.3).
See instruction booklets provided with individual syringe pumps.

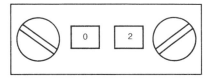

Figure 20.3 Setting the rate.

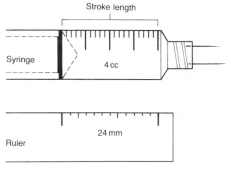

Figure 20.2 Measuring stroke length.

GUIDELINES • Preparation of the syringe for 12-hour drug administration using Graseby Medical MS16A syringe driver

Action

1 Calculate dosage of drugs and minimum volume of diluent required over 12 h (use at least 1 ml diluent per 250 mg diamorphine hydrochloride injection).

2 Draw up drugs with diluent, withdrawing the plunger until the stroke length corresponds with a number divisible by 12, e.g. 24, 36 or 48 mm.

3 Establish the rate setting of the pump and check (or where appropriate educate the patient to check) the rate 4- to 6-hourly.

Rationale

This is more comfortable for the patient. Smaller volumes reduce the risk of inflammation at infusion site.

To ensure accuracy as the infusion rate can only be set in whole numbers.

To monitor rate and ensure the drug is given over the prescribed time period.

GUIDELINES • Priming the infusion set

Action

1 Using previously prepared syringe, connect a 100 cm winged infusion set.

2 Gently depress the plunger until the infusion tubing is filled up to the needle end.

3 Having previously calculated the rate setting, allow time for speedier first infusion rate.

Rationale

This length of tubing allows patient greater freedom of movement.

This removes extraneous air from the system. Adding further diluent to syringe reduces the potency and therefore the effect of drug to be infused.

Ensures patient receives drugs immediately and accurately. (Usually priming the line reduces delivery time by approximately half an hour.) Do not alter previously calculated rate setting despite volume reduction in barrel of syringe.

GUIDELINES • Inserting the winged infusion set

Action	*Rationale*
1 Explain and discuss the procedure with the patient.	To ensure that the patient understands the procedure and gives his/her valid consent.
2 Assist the patient into a comfortable position.	
3 Expose the chosen site for infusion (see subcutaneous infusion sites in Chap. 12, Drug Administration).	
4 Clean the chosen site with a swab saturated with 70% isopropyl alcohol. Wait until the alcohol evaporates.	To reduce the risk of infection.
5 Grasp the skin firmly.	To elevate the subcutaneous tissue.
6 Insert the infusion needle into the skin at an angle of 45° and release the grasped skin.	Positioning shallower than 45° may shorten the life of the infusion site.
7 Tape the infusion wings firmly to the skin using transparent adhesive dressing (see preparation of skin in Chap. 12, Drug Administration).	Transparent dressing allows observation of the infusion site and maintains the correct position of the needle.
8 Connect the syringe to the syringe driver (see instructions below).	To ensure the syringe is connected correctly to the syringe driver.
9 Record, in the appropriate documents, that the infusion has been commenced.	To comply with local drug administration policies and ensure the safe administration and monitoring of the infused drug.

Connecting syringe to syringe driver

1 Place the syringe on the syringe driver along the grooved lines, with barrel clamp firmly in position.	To ensure the syringe is in the correct position.
2 Secure in place with rubber strap.	To ensure the syringe is securely clamped to the barrel.
3 Slide the actuator assembly along the lead screw by pressing white release button as shown in Fig. 20.4, until it rests against the end of the plunger.	To enable the pump mechanism to operate correctly.
4 Secure plunger with additional safety clamp (Fig. 20.5).	To ensure extra security and minimize the risk of errors in infusional rates.
5 Press start/test button to commence infusion. The indicator light should flash to indicate functioning syringe pump.	To check the infusion device is operating correctly.

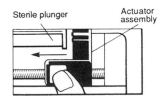

Figure 20.4   Connecting syringe to syringe driver.

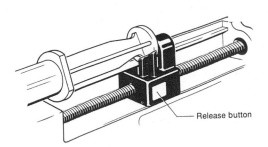

Figure 20.5   Securing the plunger.

Guidelines • Inserting the winged infusion set (cont'd)

Additional notes

1 Different manufacturers of syringes have different barrel sizes, i.e. 4 ml in a 10 ml syringe made by one company may yield a different stroke length to 4 ml in a 10 ml syringe made by another.

2 If more than one drug is to be administered, for example analgesic and antiemetic, it is important not to increase the rate of the syringe driver to yield more pain relief, as this will increase the antiemetic dose.

3 If 'breakthrough' analgesia is required, it is preferable to administer the equivalent of a 4-hourly dose as a separate extra statim subcutaneous injection. Bolus pushes using the boost button are not recommended, for the following reasons:

(a) Those outlined in point 2 above.

(b) A 'boost' push yields only 0.2 mm of extra analgesia.

(c) Pain assessment is more difficult and evaluation of pain control is hindered.

(d) Inaccuracies of infusion time may occur as a result.

4 Accurate documentation of the site, rate, flow, start time and drugs used is imperative in order to avoid confusion and errors among staff.

5 Appropriate education/teaching material is required for both the patients and staff, especially for use in the community where staff may have little or no experience with syringe drivers

Problem solving

Problem	Possible causes	Preventive nursing measures	Suggested action
Pump alarming (a) Air	Air bubbles in administration set.	Ensure all air is removed from all equipment prior to use.	Remove all air from administration set and restart infusion.
	Wrongly loaded set.	Ensure set is loaded correctly.	Check that set is loaded correctly and reload if necessary.
(b) Occlusion	Occlusion in device or administration set.	Ensure the device and administration set is flushed. Do not allow infusion bag to run dry.	Check the device for patency and locate the occlusion, remove if possible.
	Kinking of tubing.	Ensure that tubing is taped to prevent kinking. Reposition tubing whenever set is removed from a pump to prevent crushing.	If tubing kinked, reposition and tape.
	Phlebitis/infiltration or extravasation.	Observe site regularly for signs of swelling, pain and erythema.	Remove device immediately and resite.
Pump malfunctioning (electrical/mechanical)	Not charging at mains. Low battery. Batteries keep requiring replacement.	Ensure that the device is kept plugged in where appropriate. Check lead is pushed in adequately. Do not use small rechargeable batteries in ambulatory pumps	Change device and remove pump from use until fully charged. Send to works department to check plug.
	Technical fault.	Ensure all pumps are serviced regularly.	Remove pump from use and contact clinical

			nurse specialist IV services/company.
	Device soiled inside mechanism.	Maintain equipment and keep clean and free from contamination.	Remove administration set, wipe pump, reload. Do not use alcohol-based solutions on internal mechanisms
Unstable pump	Mounted on old, poorly maintained stands.	Ensure that stands are maintained and kept clean. Replace old stands.	Remove device from stand. Remove stand and send to works department for repair.
	Mounted on incorrect stands.	Ensure the correct stands are used.	Check the stand and change to appropriate stand.
	Equipment not balanced on stand.	Ensure that all equipment is balanced around the stand.	Remove devices and attach to two stands if necessary. Balance equipment.
Under/overinfusion	Technical fault with equipment.	Ensure regular servicing of devices.	Remove device from use immediately and label to prevent further use. Report incident to medical staff and nursing staff. Report to appropriate person, e.g. nurse specialist or an electro-biomedical engineer for checking. Complete an incident form. Inform MDA.
	Incorrect rate setting.	Ensure that the rate is calculated prior to commencing infusion. Check infusion rate regularly within the first hour and at start of each shift to ensure correct rate is set	Check patient's condition. Inform medical staff and senior member of nursing staff.

Intrapleural Drainage

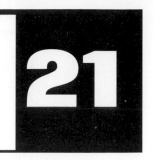

21

Definitions

Intrapleural drainage is a method used to remove a collection of air, fluid, pus or blood from the pleural space in order to restore normal lung expansion and function (Walsh 1989; McMahon-Parkes 1997).

An intrapleural drain is a length of tubing, made of clear, fairly rigid yet pliable plastic which may have a radiopaque strip incorporated into it, which enables X-ray detection. It has a proximal and distal end. The proximal end is inserted into the pleura and has a number of holes at the insertion end which facilitate drainage. The distal end is connected to the drainage system (Carroll 1991; Tomlinson & Treasure 1997).

Indications

1 To allow re-inflation of the lung after injury or surgery (Carroll 1991; Campbell 1993; McManus 1996; Kumar & Clarke 1998).
2 To facilitate removal of air, fluid, blood or pus from the pleural space (Graham 1996; Tomlinson & Treasure 1997).

Reference material

Anatomy and physiology of the pleura

Each lung is surrounded by a double membrane called the pleura. The outer membrane is the parietal pleura; this is attached to the thoracic (chest) wall and contains nerve receptors which detect pain. The inner membrane is the visceral pleura and this adheres to the lung covering the lung fissures, hilar bronchi and vessels (Fig. 21.1). The pleura are thin, serous and porous, which allows for movement of interstitial fluid across these membranes (West 1995; Guyton & Hall 1996).

Pleural space

A space exists between the parietal and visceral pleura commonly known as the pleural space, cavity or potential space. Approximately 10 ml of serous fluid produced by the pleura fills this space, lubricating the pleural surfaces to facilitate smooth and easy movement of the pleura over each other during respiration. In addition, the serous fluid enables the membranes to be held closely together by surface tension forces. A careful balance is required to control the amount of fluid present in the pleural space. This balance is maintained by the oncotic pressure across the pleura and lymphatic drainage.

The natural recoil tendency of the lungs during respiration causes them to try and collapse, but a negative pressure is required on the outside of the lungs to keep them expanded. This is provided by the pleura. This negative pressure also provides suction which holds the two membranes close together and near to the chest wall. During respiration the intrapleural pressure will vary. Before inspiration the pressure within the pleural space is equal to -5 cm H_2O. During inspiration there is a decrease in the intrapleural pressure due to the diaphragm being drawn down and outward with expansion of the chest. The pressure falls to -7.5 cm H_2O and this results in air being drawn in for gaseous exchange. During expiration the lung returns to its pre-inspiratory state by elastic recoil, with collapse of the chest wall and diaphragm and the exhalation of gas, resulting in a subsequent rise in the intrapleural pressure to -4 cm H_2O (West 1995; Guyton 1996). Any injury to the parietal or visceral pleura can effect the intrapleural pressure with a loss of negative pressure which can result in partial or total lung collapse. This can then lead to a reduction in the capacity of the lung available for effective gaseous exchange (West 1995; Guyton 1996).

Conditions that require intrapleural drainage

Pneumothorax

This can be defined as air in the pleural cavity (Kumar & Clarke 1998). It occurs as a result of communication made between the pleural space and the atmosphere when air enters the pleural cavity, resulting in collapse of the lung. It may occur spontaneously or develop as a tension pneumothorax.

Spontaneous pneumothorax is the most common type and it occurs due to a small bleb (blister) on the surface of the lung (West 1995). It can occur in healthy young people due to mechanical stresses on the surface of the lung, and then air enters the pleural space causing partial or total lung collapse (West 1995). Spontaneous pneumothorax can also occur as a result of trauma, surgery, central venous catheter insertion, during positive pressure ventilation, and in those individuals with lung conditions, e.g. asthma, chronic bronchitis, TB, pneumonia or carcinoma of the lung due to the mechanical and physiological processes of

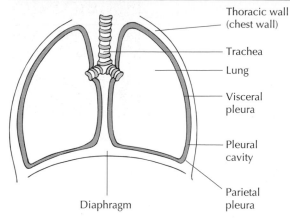

Figure 21.1 Relationship between pleural membranes, chest wall and lungs.

these conditions. If left untreated a spontaneous pneumothorax can become a tension pneumothorax. A tension pneumothorax results when air enters the pleural space during inspiration but cannot escape during expiration. Air continues to enter the pleural space as a one-way valve exists which prevents the exit of air and as a consequence there is collapse of the lung (West 1995). A tension pneumothorax is an emergency and needs immediate intervention. In the case of a tension pneumothorax the increased intrapleural pressure can cause complete collapse of the lung and severe cardiac disarrythmias, which if untreated can lead to cardiac arrest.

Pleural effusion

This is defined as an excessive amount of fluid in the pleural space (Kumar & Clarke 1998). The fluid can be composed of malignant cells, or result from an accumulation of lymph in the pleural space (chylothorax). An effusion occurs as a result of trauma, carcinoma, heart failure, hypoproteinaemia or pneumonia.

Haemothorax

This is defined as blood in the pleural space and usually occurs as a result of chest injury, trauma to the heart, lungs or major vessels or in a patient who has bled on anticoagulant therapy (Yeam & Sassoon 1997).

Haemopneumothorax

This is defined as blood and air in the pleural space, as a combination of factors already mentioned (Yeam & Sassoon 1997).

Empyema

This is defined as pus in the pleural space. Its main causes include rupture of an abscess of the lung, following pneu-

monia, pulmonary TB, or an infection following thoracic surgery (Kumar & Clarke 1998).

Collective signs and symptoms

The following signs and symptoms can occur in the conditions previously mentioned, individually or together depending on the patient's condition:

1 Pallor
2 Cyanosis
3 Dyspnoea
4 Increasing respiratory rate
5 Reduced breath sounds on affected side
6 Dullness of air entry, on listening to the chest with stethoscope
7 Reduced chest movement on affected side
8 Decrease in peripheral tissue oxygen saturations
9 Pleuritic chest pain
10 Cardiovascular change, i.e. increasing heart rate, decreasing blood pressure due to compression of the mediastinum and in turn the heart and surrounding vessels (Kumar & Clarke 1998).

Drain insertion site

Intrapleural drains are usually inserted in what is known as the 'triangle of safety'. This is bound by the anterior axillary line, mid-axillary line and a horizontal line at the level of the nipples which is furthest away from the abdominal contents and major vessels (Graham 1996). The positioning of the drain depends on whether it is being inserted to remove air or fluid.

1 *In the case of air*: the drain would be placed in the second, third or fourth intercostal space in the mid-clavicular line, which is in the anterior and apical part of the chest. This position is chosen as it is high and air will rise (Carroll 1995; Graham 1996).
2 *In the case of fluid*: the drain would be placed in the fifth or sixth intercostal space in the mid-axillary line which is in the posterior and basal part of the chest. Fluid and blood are heavier and use the principle of gravity for drainage (Carroll 1995; Graham 1996).

Drain size

The size of tube used is dependent on the reason for drainage: to remove air, use a size 16–24 Fr gauge catheter; to remove fluid, blood or pus, use a 28–40 Fr gauge catheter (a larger size is required due to the thicker consistency of fluid, blood or pus).

Stripping/milking of intrapleural drains

Intrapleural drains should not be routinely stripped or milked (Carroll 1995). The procedure of stripping involves the temporary occlusion of the drain which creates a momentary subatmospheric negative pressure and when released allows the tubing to open fully and release the obstruction. In doing so it causes a suction effect in the pleural space, which can cause tissue damage and suction of portions of the pleural lung tissue into the chest drain bottle. It is performed by anchoring the tube with one hand and vigorously squeezing with the other hand. Pressures of between −100 and −400 cm H_2O have been recorded; normal pressures would be in the range of −15 to −25 cm H_2O (Duncan & Erickson 1982).

Milking of the drain is a less stressful procedure and therefore causes less trauma to the pleura. Milking is performed by gently squeezing the tubing between the fingers throughout the length of the tubing, or by using specific tube rollers.

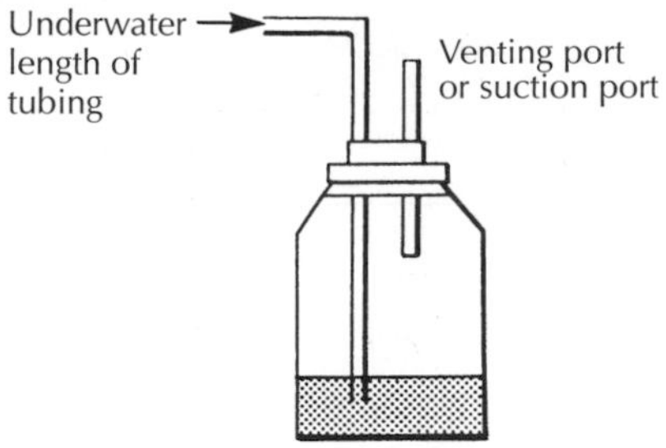

Clamping of intrapleural drains

Drains should only be clamped in the case of tube disconnection or bottle/system breakage and then the clamp should be in place for the least time possible. The reason for not clamping drains is the build-up of pressure that can occur and lead to a tension pneumothorax (Pierce 1995). This would apply when the patient is being moved in bed, to sit in a chair or during transfer to another department.

In the case of disconnection or breakage of the drain or drainage system, the drain would need to be clamped to prevent the occurrence or recurrence of a pneumothorax, but again for the least time possible (Miller & Harvey 1993; Tomlinson & Treasure 1997).

Drainage systems

Four types of drainage system exist: one-, two- and three-bottle glass systems and multi-chamber drainage systems composed of plastic, which are gradually replacing the glass system units. These systems are much lighter and easier to manage and aid patient mobility.

A one-bottle glass system is usually suitable for the drainage of an uncomplicated pneumothorax, haemothorax or a pleural effusion. The bottle has a screw top with two ports. One port has the underwater length of tubing attached. The second port has a shorter length of tubing attached which acts as the venting end and is exposed to air or could be attached to a suction unit. Venting prevents the build-up of pressure in the chest drainage system which could prevent evacuation of air or fluid (Fig. 21.2).

When the drainage bottle is set up, 500 ml of sterile water is placed in the bottle. The distal end of the intrapleural drain is then attached to the underwater seal port of the chest drain bottle and immersed 2.5 cm below the level of the water. Incoming air bubbles through the water which acts as a one-way valve and prevents the backflow of air into the intrapleural space (McMahon-Parkes 1997).

Traditionally, a drainage unit consisted of three glass bottles connected by tubing. The first bottle would act as the collection chamber, the second as the underwater seal

Figure 21.2 One-bottle system.

and the third as the vacuum or suction control, with a venting port. This type of system is bulky and restricts patient mobility, and although still in clinical use, is used less frequently.

The plastic multi-chamber system incorporates the above glass bottle system into one unit. There are three chambers: the first is for drainage, the second chamber is the underwater seal and the third chamber is the vacuum or suction control. When this system is set up, water is placed in the water seal chamber to the indicated mark, and also placed in the suction control chamber to the required level. This system is a great improvement on the previous systems and aids patient mobility (Fig. 21.3).

When the drain is attached to the drainage bottle bubbling or swinging should be observed; this indicates that air is being evacuated from the pleural space. As the lung re-inflates, the bubbling should decrease (Carroll 1991). If bubbling continues, a leak may be present in the patient's lung (Carroll 1991). A careful assessment is then required to check where the leak is and to look at the whole system thoroughly and to ensure that there are no loose connections through the tubing or circuit. This would be done by working from the chest drain bottle back to the drain and drain insertion site, checking the tubing and all connections. The drain needs to be examined to establish whether the leak is within the lung. If the leak continues and when the drain is clamped at the entry site the leak stops, this indicates that the leak is within the lung. Great care needs to be taken when checking the drain, to prevent more trauma and because of the risk of high pressure, due to the clamping process. If no bubbling occurs there should be swinging (tidalling), indicating communication between the pleural cavity and drainage system (Campbell 1993). Swinging (tidalling) reflects a change of pressure in the pleural cavity which occurs as a result of respiratory effort. There would be a rise on inspiration and a fall on expiration. The amount of swinging (tidalling) should reduce, but continue as the lung re-inflates (Campbell 1993). If swinging (tidalling) stops it may indicate that there is a blockage or kinking of the tubing in the drainage system or of the actual drain.

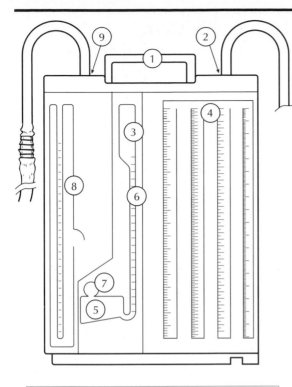

1 Carrying handle
2 High negativity relief valve
3 High negativity float valve and relief chamber
4 Collection chamber
5 Patient air leak meter (only on A-7000)
6 Calibrated water seal
7 Self-sealing diaphragm in water seal chamber
   and suction control chamber
8 Suction control chamber
9 Positive pressure relief valve

Figure 21.3 Multi-chamber drainage system. (Modified from Pierce (1995) *Guide to Mechanical Ventilation and Intensive Respiratory Care*, W.B. Saunders, originally reproduced Courtesy of Deknatel, Inc., Fall River, Mass.)

Suction and its use

If there is a persistent air leak or large collection of fluid etc., suction may be required to remove the air or fluid and restore a negative pressure in the intrapleural space (McMahon-Parkes 1997). Suction can be applied through some of the drainage units or through an independent suction pump. Suction used should be of low pressure. The range of suction normally used is 10–25 cm H_2O (McManus 1996). High levels of suction should be avoided as this can lead to damage of the lung tissue or to too rapid inflation of the lung.

Wet and dry suction units exist. In a wet unit the amount of suction is regulated by the height of water in the suction control unit. The amount of water must be kept at the correct level, which is indicated on the chamber of the drainage bottle. Water in this chamber should bubble gently. In the dry unit the amount of suction is regulated by a spring mechanism or screw valve mechanism attached to an external suction unit. When the dial is set, a pull is applied to the diaphragm controlling a negative pressure in the intrapleural space to allow for re-expansion of the lung (Pierce 1995).

Note: a chest drain connected to a suction unit which is turned off can be considered to be a clamped drain and could potentiate a tension pneumothorax. If suction is turned off then the drain must be disconnected from the suction pump (Tomlinson & Treasure 1997).

References and further reading

Adam, S.K. & Osborne, S. (1997) Respiratory problems. In: *Critical Care Nursing*, pp. 72–5. Oxford Medical Publications, Oxford.

Baumann, M.H. & Strange, C. (1997) The clinician's perspective on pneumothorax management. *Chest*, **112**/(3), 822–8.

Calhorn Thomson, S., Wells, S. & Maxwell, M. (1997) Chest tube removal after cardiac surgery. *Crit Care Nurse*, **17**(1), 34–8.

Campbell, J. (1993) Making sense of underwater sealed drainage. *Nurs Times*, **89**(9), 34–6.

Carroll, P. (1991) What's new in chest tube management. *Reg Nurse*, **54**(5), 35–40.

Carroll, P. (1995) Chest tubes made easily. *Reg Nurse*, **58**(12), 46–55.

Carson, M. (1995) Minimizing pain when removing a chest tube. *Reg Nurse*, **58**(2), 19.

Carson, M.M., Barton, D.M., Morrison, C.G., *et al.* (1994) Managing pain during mediastinal chest tube removal. *Heart Lung*, **23**(6), 500–505.

Couzza, C. (1995) Dislodged chest tube. *Nursing*, **25**(9), 33.

Duncan, C. & Erickson, R. (1982) Pressure associated with chest tube stripping. *Heart Lung*, **11**(4), 166–71.

Ekstrowicz, N. (1997) Managing pain during chest tube insertion. *Nursing*, **27**(11), 28.

Foss, M. (1987) Intercostal drains. *Prof Nurse*, **4**(2), 290–91.

Godden, J. (1998) Managing the patient with a chest drain: a review. *Nurs Stand*, **12**(32), 35–9.

Graham, H. (1996) Chest drain insertion. 'How to' guide series. *Care Crit Ill*, **12**(5).

Grodzin, C.J. & Baik, R.A. (1997) Indwelling small pleural catheter needle thoracentesis in the management of large pleural effusions. *Chest*, **111**(4), 981–8.

Guyton, A.C. & Hall, J.E. (1996) *Textbook of Medical Physiology*, 9th edn., Chaps. 37, 38, pp. 497–8. W.B. Saunders, London.

Kumar, P. & Clarke, M. (1998) *Clinical Medicine*, 4th edn. W.B. Saunders, London.

Lazzara, D. (1996) Why is the Hemlich chest drain valve making a comeback? *Nursing*, **26**(12), 50–53.

McConnell, E. (1995) Clinical do's and don'ts. *Nursing*, **25**(8), 18.

McMahon-Parkes, K. (1997) Management of pleural drains. *Nurs Times*, **93**(52), 48–52.

McManus, K. (1998) Chest drainage systems. 'How to' guide series. *Care Crit Ill*, **14**(4).

Miller, A.C. & Harvey, J.E. (1993) Guide lines for the management of spontaneous pneumothorax. *Br Med J*, **307**, 114–16.

Patz, E.F. (1998) Malignant pleural effusions: recent advances and ambulatory sclerotherapy. *Chest*, **113**(1), Suppl. 1, 74S–77S.

Pettinicchi, T.A. (1998) Trouble shooting chest tubes. *Nursing*, **28**(3), 58–9.

Pierce, L.N.B. (1995) *Guide to Mechanical Ventilation and Intensive Respiratory Care*, Appendix 111, pp. 356–63. W.B. Saunders, London.

Smith, R.D., Fallentine, J. & Kessel, S. (1995) Underwater chest drainage bringing the facts to the surface. *Nursing*, **25**(2), 60–63.

Thomson, S.C., Wells, S. & Maxwell, M. (1997) Chest tube removal after cardiac surgery. *Crit Care Nurse*, **17**(1), 34–8.

Tomlinson, M.A. & Treasure, T. (1997) Insertion of a chest drain: how to do it. *Br J Hosp Med*, **58**(6), 248–52.

Walsh, M. (1989) Making sense of chest drainage. *Nurs Times*, **85**(24), 40–41.

West, J.B. (1995) The essentials. In: *Pulmonary Pathophysiology*, 5th edn., Waverly Europe, London.

Yeam, I. & Sassoon, C. (1997) Haemothorax and chylothorax. *Curr Opin Pulmon Med*, **3**(4), 310–14.

GUIDELINES · Chest drain insertion

Equipment

1 Sterile chest drain pack containing, gallipot, disposable towel, forceps, scalpel holder, scalpel blade and sterile gauze.
2 Suture material.
3 Cleaning solution, chlorhexidine in 70% alcohol.
4 Sterile gloves.
5 Local anaesthetic, lignocaine 1%.
6 Syringes.
7 Needles.

8 Chest drain French gauge cannulae.
9 Sterile dressing.
10 Tape.
11 Chest drain tubing.
12 Chest drain bottle.
13 Sterile water.
14 Chest drain clamps ×2.
15 Suction pump if required.

Intrapleural drain insertion procedure

Action

1 Explain and discuss the procedure with the patient

Note: the procedure might have to be performed under emergency conditions.

2 Administer analgesia prior to procedure after discussion with the doctor, about the type and route of administration. The analgesia should be given at least half an hour before the procedure.

3 Administer sedation on doctor's instruction, if considered appropriate, e.g. for an anxious patient

4 Wash hands with bactericidal soap and water.

5 Prepare trolley, placing equipment on bottom shelf. Take to patient's bedside

6 Assist doctor in setting up sterile procedure pack.

7 Check the correct side of chest for drain insertion.

8 Position patient in preparation for the procedure. The patient may be positioned flat on the bed with the arm on the affected side placed behind his/her head away from the chest wall or abducted to 90°. If patient is able to sit upright, he/she can be positioned resting over a table supported by a pillow.

Rationale

To ensure the patient understands why and how the procedure is to be performed and gives his/her valid consent.
A patient may have become acutely unwell, and so the procedure would prevent respiratory and cardiovascular collapse.

To minimize any pain during the procedure and to ensure the patient is pain-free and able to cooperate.

To relieve anxiety and allow the patient to relax and cooperate and to enable the procedure to go ahead.

To minimize the risk of infection.

To aid with procedure.

To minimize risk of infection and to have equipment ready.

To ensure safety of the patient by checking the chest X-ray.

To facilitate insertion of the intrapleural drain.
To aid patient comfort.

9 Observe the patient throughout procedure, with attention to respiratory status including colour, respiratory rate, respiratory pattern, equal movement of chest and peripheral tissue oxygen saturations. Observe patient for any change to the cardiovascular system by alterations in heart rate or blood pressure.

To look for any change in the patient's condition and report to the doctor, to ensure appropriate intervention, e.g. oxygen therapy.

To look for any change in the patient's condition and report to the doctor to ensure appropriate intervention.

10 Communicate with the patient during the procedure and explain what is happening at each stage.

To keep the patient fully informed and to enable the patient to feel involved and reassured.

11 Assist doctor in procedure as below:

(a) The doctor will wash his hands and apply sterile gloves.

To minimize risk of infection.

(b) The area for planned insertion of the drain will be cleaned with chlorhexidine in alcohol.

To minimize risk of infection.

(c) Local anaesthetic will be injected into the skin and deeper tissue (intercostal muscle and parietal pleura) along proposed insertion site.

To minimize the feeling of pain on drain insertion.

(d) Wait 2–3 min for local anaesthetic to take.

To ensure local anaesthetic has been effective.

(e) A tract is then created down through to the parietal pleura by blunt dissection with the forceps.

To aid and ease the movement of the drain into the correct position.

(f) A finger may then be manoeuvred through to the parietal pleura to guide the drain into place, between the parietal and visceral pleura in the pleural space (Miller & Harvey 1993; Graham 1996).

To aid the drain into the correct position.

(g) The drain is then clamped using two clamps until connected to the drainage system.

To prevent further lung collapse and entry of air.

(h) Connect the distal end of the drain to the drainage system and ensure that it is well supported and secured.

To allow for inflation of the lung or drainage of fluid, to ensure there is no movement of drain and that it remains in the correct position.

(i) The proximal end of the drain is secured and sutured in place. The drain will require (i) an anchor suture to secure it at the wound site and (ii) a suture to aid with removal, e.g. a purse string suture. This type of suture is threaded around and through the wound edges in a U-shape (Thomson *et al*. 1997; Fig. 21.4).

(i) To secure drain in position.
(ii) To aid wound closure when drain is removed.

12 Clean the site and apply a keyhole dressing of gauze, then an occlusive dressing over the gauze.

To ensure site is well covered and sealed.
To reduce risk of infection.

13 Send patient for chest X-ray.

To ensure the correct position of the drain and to ensure that the lung has re-inflated.

14 Check the drain is well secured.

To prevent movement of drain or loss of drain.

15 Ensure that there is bubbling/swinging of water in the bottle/tubing or drainage fluid and check there are no leaks around the site or that any loose connections exist within the drainage system.

To ensure there is no occlusion or leak which will prevent re-expansion of the lung or drainage of the fluid.

16 Ensure patient comfort following the procedure. Return the patient to an elevated position sitting in bed, well supported by pillows and give further analgesia if required.

To ensure patient comfort in order to aid recovery and breathing.

17 Dispose of waste appropriately.

To reduce risk of cross-infection and sharps injury.

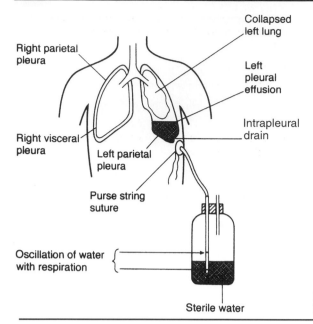

Collapsed left lung

Right parietal pleura

Left pleural effusion

Intrapleural drain

Right visceral pleura

Left parietal pleura

Purse string suture

Oscillation of water with respiration

Sterile water

Figure 21.4 An intrapleural drain and underwater seal bottle are used to drain a left pleural effusion.

Guidelines • Chest drain insertion (cont'd)

Post drain procedure

Action

1 Observe patient for any change in respiratory status:
(a) Colour.
(b) Respiratory rate and pattern.
(c) Unequal chest movement.
(d) Peripheral tissue oxygen saturations.
(e) Blood gases.
Observe patient for any change in cardiovascular status:
(a) Heart rate.
(b) Blood pressure.

2 Ensure the drain remains well secured with suture and dressing.

3 Ensure the drain is well positioned with no loops or kinks.

4 Ensure drain tubing is well supported at the side of the bed using tape and clamps.

5 Ensure drain tubing and connections are secure and attached to the drainage unit.

6 Ensure a pair of clamps is available beside the patient in case of accidental disconnection.

7 Do not clamp drains other than in the case of accidental disconnection.

8 Ensure chest drain remains at a level below the chest at all times.

Rationale

These symptoms may indicate a change of chest drain position, occlusion of the drain or recurrence of pneumothorax or collection of fluid.

May indicate pressure on the cardiovascular system.

To prevent movement of drain and ensure safety of patient.

To prevent occlusion of drain.

To prevent drain pulling and dragging, causing trauma to the patient or movement of or the risk of the drain falling out.

To ensure a sealed unit exists to prevent air entry into the pleura which could lead to further lung collapse.

To clamp drain and prevent further lung collapse.

To prevent a high positive pressure which can be created when the drain is clamped and which can result in a tension pneumothorax.

This prevents backflow of fluid into the pleural space.

9 Do not milk or strip tubing other than in an emergency such as removal of an obstruction after discussion with doctor.

Milking or stripping can cause an increase in negative pressure which could result in damage to lung tissue.

10 Observe drainage by placing adhesive tape vertically along length of bottle in order to measure drainage. Observe volume and type of drainage; is it clear/bloodstained, etc? Record on a fluid chart and in the nursing notes.

To ensure monitoring of type and volume of fluid loss.

11 Position patient comfortably in bed, sitting upright, well supported by pillows.

To aid patient comfort. To aid breathing and allow for full expansion of the lungs.

12 Change the position of the patient while in bed.

To reduce risk of breakdown in skin integrity.

13 Encourage mobilization of the patient, e.g. to sit in chair and also to walk aided by physiotherapist or nurse.

To encourage patient independence and prevent complications, e.g. pulmonary embolus, deep vein thrombosis, breakdown in skin integrity.

14 Ensure patient maintains mobility of arm on side of drain.

To prevent complications and reduce risk of immobility of arm.

15 Ensure patient remains pain-free.

To relieve pain and aid recovery.

16 Maintain patient hygiene and mouth care. Assist patient in washing/mouth care because of restriction of movement due to drain.

To aid patient comfort and reduce the risk of infection.

17 Maintain normal oral and dietary intake.

To aid healing process. To reduce risk of dehydration and malnutrition. To reduce risk of infection.

18 Maintain a normal sleep pattern.

To allow patient to rest and aid recovery.

19 Ensure patient is kept occupied, e.g. reading, watching TV, listening to the radio.

To relieve boredom and aid recovery.

GUIDELINES • Removal of a chest drain

Equipment

1 Sterile dressing pack containing gallipot, gauze, sterile towel.
2 Cleaning solution, e.g. 0.9% sodium chloride.
3 Sterile gloves.

4 Stitch cutter.
5 Sterile dressing.
6 Tape.
7 Chest drain clamps ×2.

Two nurses/assistants are required to facilitate safe removal of a chest drain. One is required to tie the suture and seal the site, and the other to remove the drain.

Procedure

Action

1 Prepare patient for removal of the drain. Explain and discuss each step of the procedure with the patient.

2 Encourage patient to practise breathing exercises, as these are required to help with the procedure. The patient should be instructed to take three deep breaths in and out and on fourth breath to hold the breath in. It is on this breath that the drain will be removed.

Rationale

To ensure the patient is well prepared, and to ensure their cooperation and consent.

To prepare the patient and encourage cooperation. To allow the patient to practise the breathing exercises. To prevent the entry of air which can occur due to a negative intrathoracic pressure (Tomlinson & Treasure 1997).

Guidelines • Removal of a chest drain (cont'd)

Action	Rationale
Note: another procedure which can be used during the removal is the Valsalva manoeuvre. Instead of holding the fourth breath as above, the patient bears down on exhalation of the fourth breath.	
3 Administer analgesia prior to procedure after discussion with doctor about the type and route of administration. The analgesia should be given at least half an hour before the procedure.	To minimize any pain during the procedure and to ensure the patient is pain-free and able to cooperate.
4 Administer sedation on doctor's instruction, if considered appropriate, e.g. for an anxious patient.	To relieve anxiety and allow the patient to relax and cooperate and to enable the procedure to go ahead.
5 Discontinue suction if in use.	To prevent a tension pneumothorax.
6 Prepare trolley for procedure.	To aid the procedure.
7 Assist or set up the sterile procedure pack.	To minimize risk of infection and to have equipment ready.
8 Position patient comfortably.	To aid patient comfort.
9 Place protective pad underneath the patient and drain.	To absorb any ooze from the drain. To reduce risk of contamination of the patient and bed clothing.
10 Wash hands with bactericidal soap and water before touching the drain or dressing.	To reduce risk of infection.
11 Remove dressing from around drain site, examine sutures present: (a) tube retaining suture (anchor suture) and (b) purse string suture; expose the ends of these sutures.	To prepare for drain removal and check what type of suture is present so that the suture can be used to form an airtight seal when the drain is removed.
12 Both assistants for the procedure must wash their hands and apply sterile gloves.	To reduce risk of infection.
13 First nurse/assistant prepares purse string suture and loosens ends ready to tie the suture when the drain is removed.	To prepare for drain removal.
14 Second nurse/assistant prepares and cuts the anchor suture and ensures the drain is mobile and ready to remove.	To prepare for drain removal.
15 Second nurse/assistant asks the patient to start deep breathing exercises: to take three deep breaths then hold his/her breath on the fourth one while the drain is pulled out steadily and smoothly.	To aid in drain removal. Deep breathing exercises can help to prevent a tension pneumothorax. If a drain is removed too quickly or without due care a pneumothorax can occur due to rupture of the pleura.
16 First nurse/assistant will tie the purse string suture securely to the skin.	To form an airtight seal and prevent air entry and formation of a pneumothorax.
17 Clean around site with 0.9% sodium chloride and apply an occlusive dressing.	To clean site, form an airtight seal, prevent air entry and reduce risk of infection.
18 Ensure that the patient is comfortable on completion of procedure by sitting the patient upright, and support with pillows.	To ensure patient comfort.
19 Dispose of waste appropriately.	To ensure safety and reduce risk of infection.
20 Observe and measure amount of drainage. Document on fluid chart and in nursing notes.	To maintain an accurate record of a legal document and to provide a point of reference for any queries.

Nursing care plan

Problem	Cause	Suggested action
Patient shows signs of respiratory distress, increased respiratory rate, uneven chest movement, decreasing peripheral tissue oxygen saturations.	Pneumothorax or tension pneumothorax.	Observe patient continually for change in vital signs. Inform doctor and administer oxygen. Prepare for re-insertion of chest drain.
Lack of drainage.	Kinking, looping or pressure on the tubing may cause reflux of fluid into the intrapleural space or may impede drainage, causing blocking of the intrapleural drain.	Check the system and straighten tubing as required. Secure the tubing to prevent a recurrence of the problem.
Drain not swinging.	Drain occluded due to position or occlusion.	Check no loops or kinks present in tubing. Lift drain, not higher than the patient's chest, to see if the obstruction will clear. Seek medical advice as the drain may need replacing.
Drain not bubbling.	Drain occluded or not correctly positioned.	Check no loops or kinks in the tubing. Lift tubing to see if it will clear. Gently squeeze between two fingers to see if it bubbles. If no bubbling inform the doctor as the drain may need to be repositioned.
Continual bubbling in chest drain bottle.	Air leak in system.	Check system for loose connections in tubing or around drainage unit. If no leak present in the drainage tubing the leak may be present in the lung. If the drain is clamped and the leak stops the problem is in the lung. The drain may need re-inserting. Inform doctor. Prepare chest drain insertion pack.
Leakage from drain site.	Bleeding or infection.	Remove the dressing and observe the site. Inform doctor, take swab. Clean and redress site.
Drainage from around drain site.	As a result of the insertion procedure. Incomplete closure with sutures. Infected insertion site.	Observe drain site, amount and type of drainage. Inform doctor. Take swab from site. Prepare suture pack to be available if required.
Accidental disconnection of the drainage tubing from the intrapleural drain.	Connections not secure.	Apply a clamp to the drain immediately in order to avoid air entering the pleural space. Re-establish the connection as soon as possible in order to re-establish drainage. If necessary, use a clean, sterile drainage tube; tubing may have been contaminated when it became disconnected. Report to the doctor, who may wish to X-ray. Record the incident in the relevant records. The patient may have been upset by the incident and will need reassurance.

Problem	Cause	Suggested action
Intrapleural drain falls out.	Drain not secure.	Pull the purse-string suture immediately to close the wound. Cover the wound with an occlusive sterile dressing. Check the patient's vital signs. Inform a doctor. The objective is to minimize the amount of air entering the pleural space. The drain will probably need reinserting. Prepare chest drain insertion pack. Reassure the patient with appropriate explanations.
Poor arm movement.	Restriction of arm movement due to position of drain.	Encourage movement of limb to keep mobile. Adjust analgesia as required.
Pain.	At the drain insertion site.	Try repositioning tubing, so that it is not dragging or irritating skin. Give analgesia as prescribed.
Restricted mobility of patient.	Due to position of drain and attachment to the drainage unit.	Explore with the patient the movement that is possible and aid them where help is required. Encourage mobility, aid patient to sit in chair. Work in liaison with physiotherapist. Encourage patient to move in bed and change position.

Last Offices

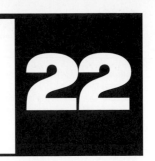

Definition

Last offices is the care given to a deceased patient which is focused on fulfilling religious and cultural beliefs as well as health and safety and legal requirements.

Reference material

The United Kingdom today is a multicultural, multiracial and multireligious society. This offers a great challenge to all areas of health care, but none more so than nursing. It is incumbent upon nurses to be aware of the different religious and cultural rituals which accompany the death of a patient. There are considerable cultural variations between people of different faiths, ethnic backgrounds and national origins in their approach to death and dying. However, those who have settled in a society where there is a dominant faith or culture other than their own increasingly adopt that dominant culture in many ways, but retain, almost deliberately to emphasize differences, their different practices at times of birth, marriage or death (Neuberger 1997). Approaches to death and dying reveal much of the attitude of society as a whole to the individuals it comprises. Funeral rites can be dated back 50 000 years, and from this time show how early men laid down their dead in grief and in some hope of a continued existence (Eiseley 1961). Nurses are also required to possess the information pertinent to the legal requirements for the care of the dead.

It is essential then that the correct procedures are followed during last offices, and that every effort is made to accommodate the wishes of patients' relatives (Speck 1978; Olivant 1986; Neuberger 1987; Hospital Chaplaincies Council 1992). This is central to the concept of holistic care for the patient, and if we disregard such procedures for our patients, we also disregard both patients' and families' dignity (Wald 1986; Spector 1991). For nursing staff, administering last offices can be a rewarding experience as it is the final demonstration of respectful, sensitive care given to a patient. The details of the practices relating to last offices can vary depending on the patient's cultural background and religious practices (Nearney 1998). The following sections provide a guide to cultural and religious variations in attitudes to death, and how individuals may wish to be treated. Two key issues should be considered in the application of this information to practice:

1 Few of us are whole hearted in our acceptance of the ways of our own religious or cultural group.

2 Our motivation to categorize individuals into groups with clearly defined norms can lead to depersonalization of patients and their families (Sampson 1982).

It is imperative that health care professionals establish individual preferences, and encourage patients to talk about the different patterns of observance within their own religious/cultural group.

The bibliography set out below is by no means exhaustive, but may be used by nurses to deepen their understanding of issues surrounding death, and broaden their knowledge of and respect for other cultures and faiths.

References and further reading

General

Ainsworth-Smith, I. & Speck, P. (1982) *Letting Go: Caring for the Dying and the Bereaved*. SPCK, London.

Bishop, P. & Danton, M. (1987) *The Encyclopaedia of World Religions*. Macmillan-Orbis, London.

Black, J. (1987) Broaden your mind about death and bereavement in certain ethnic groups in Britain. *Br Med J*, **295**, 536–67.

Bowker, J. (1993) *The Meaning of Death*. Canto (CUP), Cambridge.

Crowther, C.E. (1991) *AIDS – A Christian Handbook*. Epworth, London.

DoH (1992) *Health Service Guidelines. Meeting the Spiritual Needs of Patients and Staff* HSG (92) 2. Stationery Office, London.

DSS (1990) *What to Do After Death*. Stationery Office, London.

Eisely, L. (1961) *The Firmament of Time*, p. 113. Gollancz, London.

Gentles, I. (1982) *Care of the Dying and the Bereaved*, pp. 121–32. Anglican Book Centre, Toronto.

Green, J. & Green, M. (1992) *Dealing with Death: Practices and Procedures*. Chapman & Hall, London.

Hayes, H. (OSF) & van der Poel, C.J. (CSSp) (eds) (1990) *Health Care Ministry: A Handbook for Chaplains*. Paullist Press, Mawah.

Helman, C.J. (1990) *Culture, Health and Illness*, 2nd edn. Wright, London.

Hospital Chaplaincies Council (1992) *Our Ministry and Other Faiths*. HCC, London.

Housely, J. (ed.) (1992) *Death Customs*. Wayland, Hove.

Hughes, S. & Henley, A. (1990) *Dealing with Death in Hospitals: Procedures for Managers and Staff*. King Edwards Hospital Fund for London, London.

Jewett, C. (1984) *Helping Children Cope with Separation and Loss*. Batsford, London.

Jones, K., Johnston, M. & Speck, P.W. (1989) Despair felt by the patient and the professional carer: a case study of the use of cognitive behavioural methods. *Palliat Med*, **3**, 39–46.

Karmi, G. & McKeigue, P. (eds) (1993) *Ethnic Health Bibliography*. NE and NW Thames RHA, London.

Kübler-Ross, E. (1990) *Living with Dying and Death*. Souvenir, London.

Lundin, T. (1984) Morbidity following sudden unexpected bereavement. *Br J Psychiatry*, **144**, 84–8.

National Council for Hospice and Specialist Palliative Care Services (1995) *Opening Doors: Improving Access to Hospital and Specialist Care Services by People in Black and Ethnic Communities*. Occasional papers series no. 7. National Council for Hospice and Specialist Palliative Care Services, London.

Nearney, L. (1998) Practical procedures for nurses. Last offices. *Nurs Times*, **94**(26).

Neuberger, J. (1987) *Caring for Dying People of Different Faiths*. Lisa Sainsbury Foundation Series, London.

Neuberger, J. (1997) Cultural issues in palliative care. In: *Oxford Textbook of Palliative Medicine* (eds D. Doyle, G.W.C. Hanks & N. MacDonald). Oxford University Press, Oxford.

Olivant, P. (1986) Coping with death: last offices . . . steps nurses should take to help bereaved relatives. *Nurs Times*, **82**(12), 32–3.

Parkes, C.M. (1990) Risk factors in bereavement: implications for the prevention and treatment of pathological grief. *Psychiatric Ann*, **20**, 308–13.

Parkes, C.M., Laungani, P. & Young, B. (1997) *Death and Bereavement Across Cultures*. Routledge, London.

Racial Equality Council (1992) *Religions and Cultures*. Lothian, Edinburgh.

Rankin, J. *et al.* (1993) *Ethics and Religions*. Longman, London.

Rinpoche, S. (1992) *Tibetan Book of the Living and Dying*. Rider, London.

Robbins, J. (ed.) (1989) *Caring for the Dying Patient and the Family*. Harper & Row, London.

Sambi, S.P. & Cole, W.O. (1990) Caring for Sikh patients. *Palliat Med*, **4**, 229–33.

Sampson, C. (1982) *The Neglected Ethic: Religious and Cultural Factors in the Care of Patients*. McGraw-Hill, Maidenhead.

Sharma, D.L. (1990) Hindu attitudes towards suffering, dying and death. *Palliat Med*, **4**, 235–8.

Speck, P. (1978) *Loss and Grief in Medicine*. Ballière-Tindall, London.

Spector, R. (1991) *Cultural Diversity in Health and Illness*, 3rd edn. Appleton & Lange, Connecticut.

Storr, E. (1986) The cost of dying: practical details the relatives have to face. *Geriatric Med*, **16**(16), 40–44.

Wald, F.S. (ed.) (1986) *In Quest of the Spiritual Component of Care for the Terminally Ill*. Yale University Press, New Haven.

Weller, P. (ed.) (1997) *Religions in the UK; A Mutli-Faith Directory*. University of Derby, Derby.

Weymont, G. (1982) The Howie Report. *Nurs Times*, **78**(35), J Infect Control Nurs, Suppl. 16.

Which? (1987) *What to Do When Someone Dies*. Hodder, London.

Zaehner, R.C. (ed.) (1979) *The Concise Encyclopaedia of Living Faiths*. Hutchinson, London.

Specific

Bahai

Compilation from the Sacred Bahai Writings (1983) *The Pattern of Bahai Life*. Bahai Publishing Trust, Oakham, Rutland.

Buddhism

Humphreys, C. (1976) *Buddhism*. Penguin, London.

Shelling, J. (1987) *The Buddhist Handbook. A Complete Guide to Buddhist Teaching and Practice*. Rider, London.

Sibley, D. (1997) Caring for dying Buddhists. *Int J Palliat Nurs*, **3**(1), 26–30.

Williams, P. (1989) *Mahayana Buddhism*. Routledge, London.

Christianity

Cross, F.L. (ed.) (1988) *The Oxford Dictionary of the Christian Church*. Oxford University Press, Oxford.

Feiner, J. & Fisher, L. (1975) *The Common Catechism*. Search Press, London.

Keely, R. (ed.) (1982) *The Lion Handbook of Christian Belief*. London Publishing, Tring.

Searle, M. (1989) *Christening, the Making of Christians*. Kevin Mayhew, Leigh on Sea.

Hinduism

Flood, G. (1996) *An Introduction to Hinduism*. Cambridge University Press, Cambridge.

Henley, A. (1983) *Caring for Hindus and Their families: Religious Aspects of Care*. Asians in Britain Series. National Extension College/DHSS/Kings Fund Centre. National Extension College, Cambridge.

Jackson, R. & Killingley, D. (1988) *Approaches to Hinduism*. John Murray, London.

Karmi, G. (1995) *Traditional Asian Medicine in Britain*. MENAS Press, London.

McAvoy, B.R. & Donaldson, L.J. (1990) *Health Care for Asians*. Oxford University Press, Oxford.

Jainism

Dundas, P. (1992) *The Jains*. Routledge, London.

Oldfield, K. (1989) *Jainism, the Path of Purity and Peace*. CEM, Derby.

Jehovah's Witnesses

Hoekma, A.A. (1979) *Jehovah's Witnesses*. Paternoster, Exeter.

Judaism

Close, B.F. (1993) *Judaism*. Hodder & Stoughton, London.

Lancaster, B. (1993) *The Elements of Judaism*. Element, London.

Samson Katz, J. (1996) Caring for dying Jewish People in a multi-cultural/religious society. *Int J Palliat Nurs*, **2**(1), 43–7.

Mormons

Hoekma, A.A. (1977) *Mormonism*. Paternoster, Exeter.

Muslim (Islam)

Chippendale, P. & Horrie, C. (1990) *What Is Islam?* Virgin, London.

Dawood, N.J. (1990) *The Koran*. Penguin, London.

Guillaume, A. (1990) *Islam*. Penguin, London.

Henley, A. (1982) *Caring for Muslims and Their families: Religious Aspects of Care*. Asians in Britain Series. National Extension College/DHSS/Kings Fund Centre. National Extension College, Cambridge.

Lewis, P. (1994) *Islamic Britain*. I.B. Tauris, London.

Nasr, S. (1986) *The Ideals and Realities of Islam*. George Allen, London.

Rastafarianism

Barrett, L. (1979) *The Rastafarians*. Sangster, Kingston.

Sikhism

Avora, R. (1986) *Sikhism*. Wayland, Hove.

Henley, A. (1983) *Caring for Sikhs and Their Families: Religious Aspects of Care*. Asians in Britain Series. National Extension College/DHSS/Kings Fund Centre. National Extension College, Cambridge.

McAroy, B.R. & Donaldson, L.J. (1990) *Health Care for Asians*. Oxford University Press, Oxford.

McCormack, M. (1987) *Brief Outline of the Sikh Faith*. Sikh Cultural Society of Great Britain, London.

Zoroastrianism

Hinnels, J.R. (1981) *Zoroastrians and the Parsees*. Ward Lock, London.

Paganism

Harvey, G. & Hardman, C. (eds) (1996) *Paganism Today*. Thorsons, London.

GUIDELINES • Last offices

Equipment

1 Bowl, soap, towel, two face cloths.
2 Razor (electric or disposable), comb, nail scissors.
3 Equipment for oral toilet including equipment for cleaning dentures.
4 Identification labels.
5 Documents required by law or hospital policy, e.g. notification of death cards.
6 Shroud or patient's personal clothing: night-dress, pyjamas, clothes previously requested by patient, or clothes which comply with family/cultural wishes.
7 Body bag if required (i.e. in event of actual or potential leakage of bodily fluids and/or infectious disease), and labels for the body defining the nature of the infection/disease.
8 Tape.
9 Dressing pack, tape and bandages if wounds present.
10 Valuables or property book.
11 Plastic bag for waste.

Procedure

Action

1 Inform medical staff. Confirmation of death must be given. This is usually done by medical staff. If an expected death occurs during the night, the senior nurse on duty sometimes confirms death if an agreed policy has been implemented.

An unexpected death must be confirmed by the attending medical officer.

Confirmation of death must be recorded in a patient's medical and nursing notes.

2 Inform the appropriate senior nurse.

3 Inform and offer support to relatives and/or next of kin. Offer support of the Hospital Chaplain or other appropriate religious leader.

4 Inform other patients.

5 Put on gloves and apron.

Rationale

A registered medical practitioner who has attended the deceased person during the last illness is required to give a medical certificate of the cause of death. The certificate requires the doctor to state the last date on which he/she saw the deceased alive and whether or not he/she has seen the body after death.

To maintain continuity of care, and to allow preparations for care of relatives/friends to continue.

To ensure relevant individuals are aware of patient's death. To provide sensitive care.

Other patients are often aware that a death is expected or has occurred. It is important to inform them when someone dies so that they can be offered support and reassurance, and to answer any questions sensitively, so as to allay misconceptions and fears.

To reduce risk of contamination with body fluids, and to reduce risk of cross-infection. Protective clothing, for example gloves and an apron, must be worn for carrying out last offices.

Guidelines • Last offices (cont'd)

Action	Rationale
6 Lay the patient on his/her back. Remove all but one pillow. Support the jaw by placing a pillow or rolled-up towel on the chest underneath the jaw. Remove any mechanical aids such as syringe drivers, heel pads, etc. Straighten the limbs.	To maintain the patient's dignity, as rigor mortis occurs 4–6 h after death.
7 Close the patient's eyes by applying light pressure to the eyelids for 30 sec.	To maintain the patient's dignity, as rigor mortis occurs within 4–6 hours after death.
8 Drain the bladder by pressing on the lower abdomen.	Because the body can continue to excrete fluids after death.
9 Pack orifices if fluid secretion continues or may be anticipated.	Leaking orifices pose a health hazard to staff coming into contact with the body.
10 Exuding wounds should be covered with a clean absorbent dressing and secured with an occlusive dressing (e.g. Tegaderm).	The dressing will absorb any leakage from the wound site. Open wounds pose a health hazard to staff coming into contact with the body. If a post mortem is required existing dressings should be left in situ and covered.
11 Remove drainage tubes, etc., unless otherwise stated. Open drainage sites may need to be sealed with an occlusive dressing (e.g. Tegaderm).	Open drainage sites pose a health hazard to staff coming into contact with the body. If a post mortem is required drainage tubes, etc., should be left in situ.
12 Wash the patient, unless requested not to do so for religious/cultural reasons (please refer to section on individual faiths in this chapter.) If necessary, shave a male patient.	For hygienic and aesthetic reasons.
It may be important to family and carers to assist with washing, to continue to provide the care given in the period before the death.	It is an expression of respect and affection, part of the process of adjusting to loss and expressing grief.
13 Clean the patient's mouth using a foam stick to remove any debris and secretions. Clean dentures and replace them in the mouth if possible.	For hygienic and aesthetic reasons.
14 Remove all jewellery, in the presence of another nurse, unless requested by the patient's family to do otherwise. Jewellery remaining on the patient should be documented on the 'notification of death' form. Record the jewellery and other valuables in the patient's property book and store the items according to local policy.	To meet with legal requirements and relatives' wishes.
15 Dress the patient in personal clothing or shroud, depending on hospital policy or relatives' wishes.	For religious or cultural reasons and to meet family's or carers' wishes.
16 Label one wrist and one ankle with an identification label. Complete any documents such as notification of death cards. Copies of such cards are usually required (refer to hospital policy for details). Tape one securely to shroud.	To ensure correct and easy identification of the body in the mortuary.
17 Wrap the body in a mortuary sheet, ensuring that the face and feet are covered and that all limbs are held securely in position.	To avoid possible damage to the body during transfer and to prevent distress to colleagues, e.g. portering staff.
18 Secure the sheet with tape.	Pins must not be used as they are a health hazard to staff.
19 Place the body in a body bag if leakage of body fluid is a problem or if the patient has certain infectious diseases. Consult local policy for advice.	Actual or potential leakage of fluid, whether infection is present or not, poses a health hazard to all those who come into contact with the deceased patient. The sheet will absorb excess fluid.
20 Tape the second notification of death card to the outside of the sheet (or body bag).	For ease of identification of the body in the mortuary.

21	Request the portering staff to remove the body.	Decomposition occurs rapidly, particularly in hot weather and in overheated rooms, and may create a bacterial hazard for those handling the body. Autolysis and growth of bacteria are delayed if the body is cooled.
22	Screen off the appropriate area.	Avoid causing unnecessary distress to other patients and relatives.
23	Remove gloves and apron. Dispose of equipment according to local policy, and wash hands.	To minimize risk of cross-infection and contamination.
24	Amend appropriate nursing documentation.	To record the time of death, names of those present, and names of those informed.
25	Transfer property, patient records etc. to the appropriate administrative department.	The administrative department cannot begin to process the formalities such as the death certificate or the collection of property by the next-of-kin until the required documents are in its possession.

Nursing care plan

Problem	Suggested action
Death occurring within 24 hours of an operation.	All tubes and/or drains must be left in position. Spigot any cannulae or catheters. Treat stomas as open wounds. Leave any endotracheal or tracheostomy tubes in place. Post-mortem examination will be required to establish the cause of death. Any tubes, drains, etc., may have been a major contributing factor to the death.
Unexpected death.	As above. Post-mortem examination of the body will be required to establish the cause of death.
Unknown cause of death.	As above.
Patient brought in dead.	As above, unless patient seen by a medical practitioner within 14 days before death. In this instance the attending medical officer may complete the death certificate if he/she is clear as to the cause of death.
Patient with leaking wounds/orifices with or without infection present.	Follow procedures outlined in section on hepatitis B (Chap. 4, Barrier Nursing).
Patient with hepatitis B or who is HIV positive.	For further information see the procedures in the sections on hepatitis B and AIDS (Chap. 4).
Patient who dies after receiving systemic radioactive iodine.	For further information, see the procedure on iodine-131 (Chap. 34).
Patient who dies after insertion of gold grains, colloidal radioactive solution, caesium needles, caesium applicators, irridium wires or irridium hair pins.	Inform the physics department as well as appropriate medical staff. Once a doctor has verified death, the sources are removed and placed in a lead container. A Geiger counter is used to check that all sources have been removed. This reduces the radiation risk when completing the last offices procedures. Record the time and date of removal of the sources.
Relatives not present at the time of the patient's death.	Inform the relatives as soon as possible of the death. Consider also that they may want to view the body before last offices are completed.
Relatives or next-of-kin not contactable by telephone or by the general practitioner.	If within UK, local police will go to next-of-kin's house. If abroad, the British Embassy will assist.

Problem	*Suggested action*
Relatives want to see the body after removal from the ward.	Inform the mortuary staff in order to allow time for them to prepare the body. The body will normally be placed in the hospital's chapel of rest. Ask relatives if they wish for a chaplain or other religious leader to accompany them. As required, religious artefacts should be removed from or placed in the non-denominational chapel of rest. The nurse should check that all is ready before accompanying the relatives into the chapel. The relatives may want to be alone with the deceased but the nurse should wait outside the chapel in order that support may be provided should the relatives become distressed. After the relatives have left, the nurse should contact the portering service who will return the body to the mortuary.
Relatives want the body to be placed in the hospital's chapel of rest.	The environment of the mortuary may cause great distress to the relatives. A sympathetic and understanding attitude to grief may help to alleviate some anxieties and if they wish to view the body (see above).

GUIDELINES • Requirements for people of different religious faiths

The following are only guidelines: individual requirements may vary even among members of the same faith. Varying degrees of adherence and orthodoxy exist within all the world's major faiths. The given religion of a patient may occasionally be offered to indicate an association with particular cultural and national roots, rather than to indicate a significant degree of adherence to the tenets of a particular faith. If in doubt, consult the family members concerned.

Bahai

1 Bahai relatives may wish to say prayers for the deceased person, but normal last offices performed by nursing staff are quite acceptable.
2 Bahai adherents may not be cremated or embalmed, nor may they be buried more than an hour's journey from the place of death. A special ring will be placed on the finger of the patient and should not be removed.
3 Bahais have no objection to post-mortem examination and may leave their bodies to scientific research or donate organs if they wish.
4 Further information can be obtained from the nearest Assembly of the Bahais (see telephone directory). Alternatively, contact:

> National Spiritual Assembly of the Bahais of the United Kingdom
> 27 Rutland Gate, London SW7 1PD.
> Tel: 020 7584 2566.

Buddhism

1 There is no prescribed ritual for the handling of the corpse of a Buddhist person, so customary laying out is appropriate. However, a request may be made for a Buddhist monk or nun to be present.
2 There are a number of different schools of Buddhism. It is important to confirm which school the patient belongs to, as ritual requirements differ.
3 When the patient dies, inform the monk or nun if required (the patient's relatives often take this step). The body should not be moved for at least one hour if prayers are to be said.
4 There are unlikely to be objections to post-mortem examination and organ donation, although some Far Eastern Buddhists may object to this.
5 The patient's body should be wrapped in an unmarked sheet.
6 For further information contact:

> The Buddhist Society
> 58 Ecclestone Square, London SW1V 1PH.
> Tel: 020 7834 5858.

Christianity

1 There are many denominations and degrees of adherence within the Christian faith. In most cases customary last offices are acceptable.

2 Relatives may wish staff to call the hospital chaplain, or minister or priest from their own church to either perform last rites or say prayers.

3 Some Roman Catholic families may wish to place a rosary in the deceased patient's hands and/or a crucifix at the patient's head.

4 Some orthodox families may wish to place an ikon (holy picture) at either side of the patient's head.

5 For further information consult the hospital chaplain or consult the telephone directory for the local denominational minister or priest. Alternatively, contact:

Hospital Chaplaincies Council
Church House, Dean's Yard, Westminster, London SW1.
Tel: 020 7898 1000.
or Apostolate of the Sick (Roman Catholic)
Tel: 020 7898 1000.
or Eastern (oriental) and Orthodox Christians:
Fellowship of St Alban and St Sergius
52 Ladbroke Grove, London W10.
Tel: 020 7727 7713.

Hinduism

1 If required by relatives, inform the Hindu priest (Brahmin). If unavailable, relatives may wish to read from the *Bhagavad Gita* or make a request that staff read extracts during the last offices (see Chapters 2, 8 and 15 in *Bhagavad Gita*, edited by Jean Mascaro, Penguin, London, 1962).

2 The family may wish to stay with the patient during last offices. If possible, the eldest son should be present. A Hindu would like to have leaves of the sacred Tulsi plant and Ganges water placed in his/her mouth by relatives before death. It is therefore imperative that relatives are warned that the patient's death is imminent. Relatives of the same sex as the patient may wish to wash his or her body, preferably in water mixed with water from the River Ganges, but some prefer nursing staff to do this. Do not remove sacred threads or jewellery.

3 The patient's family may request that the patient be placed on the floor, and they may wish to burn incense.

4 Post-mortems are viewed as disrespectful to the deceased person, so are only carried out when strictly necessary. Consult the wishes of the family before touching the body.

5 For further information contact the nearest Hindu temple (see telephone directory).

Jainism

1 The relatives of a Jainist patient may wish to contact their Brahman (priest) to recite prayers with the patient and family.

2 The family may wish to be present during the last offices, and also to assist with washing. Not all families will want to perform this task, however.

3 The family may ask for the patient to be clothed in a plain white gown or shroud with no pattern or ornament and then wrapped in a plain white sheet. They may provide the gown themselves.

4 Post-mortems may be seen as disrespectful, depending on the degree of orthodoxy of the patient.

5 Cremation is arranged whenever possible within 24 hours of death.

6 Orthodox Jains may have chosen the path of *Sallekhana*, that is, death by ritual fasting. This unusual approach to death is permitted by the Jainist faith after permission has been granted by family and priests. This act is seen as the supreme path for fulfilling religious obligations.

7 For further information contact:

The Institute of Jainiology
81 Crundale Avenue, Kingsbury, London NW9 9BJ.

Jehovah's Witness

1 Relatives may wish to be present during last offices, either to pray or to read from the Bible. The family will inform staff should there be any special requirements, which may vary according to the patient's country of origin.

2 Further information can be obtained from the nearest Kingdom Hall (see telephone directory).

Judaism

1 The family will contact their own community leader if they have one. If not, the hospital chaplaincy will advise. Prayers are recited by those present.
2 Eight minutes are required to elapse before the body is moved.
3 Usually close relatives will straighten the body, but nursing staff are permitted to perform any procedure for preserving dignity and honour. Nurses may:
   (a) Close the eyes.
   (b) Tie up the jaw.
   (c) Put the arms parallel and close to the sides of the body leaving the hands open. Straighten the patient's legs.
   (d) Remove tubes and instruments (unless contraindicated).
   Patients must not be washed, but may be dressed in a plain shroud. The body will be washed by a nominated group, the Holy Assembly, which performs a ritual purification.
4 Watchers stay with the body until burial (normally completed within 24 hours of death). In the period before burial a separate non-denominational room is appreciated, where the body can be laid on the floor with its feet towards the door.
5 It is not possible for funerals to take place on the Sabbath (between sunset on Friday and sunset on Saturday). If death occurs during the Sabbath, the body should be left. Advice should be sought from the relatives.
6 Post-mortems are permitted only if required by law.
7 If no relative or other suitable person is available to make the funeral arrangements contact:

The Burial Society of the United Synagogue
Tel: 020 8343 3456.

Reformed:
Tel: 020 7723 4404.

Liberal:
Tel: 020 7580 1663.

8 For further information, contact:

Orthodox:
The Office of the Chief Rabbi
Alder House, Tavistock Square, London WC1.
Tel: 020 7387 1966.

Reformed:
Reform Synagogues of Great Britain
80 East End Road, London N3 2SY.
Tel: 020 8349 4731.

Liberal and Progressive:
Union of Liberal and Progressive Synagogues
109 Whitefield Street, London W1.
Tel: 020 7580 1663.

Hassidic Community:
Union of Jewish Congregations
40 Queen Elizabeth's Walk, London N16 OHH.
Tel: 020 8802 6226.

Mormon (Church of Jesus Christ of the Latter Day Saints)

1 There are no special requirements, but relatives may wish to be present during the last offices. Relatives will advise staff if the patient wears a one or two piece sacred undergarment. If this is the case, relatives will dress the patient in these items.
2 For further information contact the nearest Church of Jesus Christ of the Latter Day Saints (see telephone directory).

Muslim (Islam)

1 Family members will probably wish to stay with the dying patient and perform the last rites. If possible the patient's head (never the feet) should point towards Mecca, which in the UK is south east.
2 Ideally the body should be untouched by non-Muslims, but if it must be touched, gloves should be worn. If no family are present, close the patient's eyes and straighten the body. The head should be turned to the right shoulder, and the body covered with a plain white sheet. The body and hair should *not* be washed, nor the nails cut.
3 Where possible, the patient's bed should be turned so that their body (head first) is facing Mecca. If the patient's bed cannot be moved, then the patient can be turned onto their *right* side so that the deceased's face is facing towards Mecca.
4 The patient's body is normally either taken home or taken to a mosque as soon as possible to be washed by another Muslim of the same sex. A wife may wash her husband, but the reverse is not permitted.

5 Burial, never cremation, is preferred within 24 hours of death.
6 Post-mortems are only allowed if required by law, and organ donation is not encouraged.
7 For further information about Islamic groups, contact:

Ahmaddya:
London Mosque
16 Gressen Hall Road, Putney, London SW18.
Tel: 020 8870 8518.

Ismaili:
Institute of Ismaili Studies
19 Portland Place, London W1N 3AF.
Tel: 020 7436 1736.

Shi'ite:
Iranian Embassy
16 Prince's Gate, London SW7.
Tel: 020 7584 8101.

Sunni:
London Central Mosque
146 Park Road, London NW8.
Tel: 020 7742 3362.

Rastafarian

1 Customary last offices are appropriate, although the patient's family may wish to be present during the preparation of the body to say prayers.

2 For further information contact:

The Rastafarian Society
290–296 Tottenham High Road, London N15 4AJ.
Tel: 020 8808 2185.

Afro-Caribbean Community Association.
Tel: 020 8985 0067.

Sikhism

1 Family members (especially the eldest son) and friends will be present if they are able.
2 Usually the family takes responsibility for the last offices, but nursing staff may be asked to close the patient's eyes, straighten the body and wrap it in a plain white sheet.
3 Do not remove the '5 Ks', which are personal objects sacred to the Sikhs:
Kesh: do not cut hair, beard or remove turban.
Kanga: do not remove the semi-circular comb, which fixes the uncut hair.
Kdra: do not remove bracelet worn on the wrist.
Kaccha: do not remove the special shorts worn as underwear.
Kirpan: do not remove the sword: usually a miniature sword is worn.

4 The family will wash and dress the deceased person's body.
5 Post-mortems are only permitted if required by law.
6 Organ donation for transplant is not permitted.
7 For further information contact the nearest Sikh temple or Gurdwara (see telephone directory). Alternatively, contact:

Sikh Council for Inter Faith Relations
43 Dorset Road, Merton Park, London SW19 3EZ.
Tel: 020 8540 4148.

Sikh Missionary Resource Centre
346 Green Lane, Small Heath, Birmingham B9 5DR.
Tel: 0121 772 5365.

Zoroastrian (Parsee)

1 Customary last offices are often acceptable to Zoroastrian patients.
2 The family may wish to be present during, or participate in, the preparation of the body.
3 Orthodox Parsees require a priest to be present, if possible.

4 After washing, the two sacred garments are required: the *Sadra* is placed next to the skin under the sheet, and the *Kusti* is replaced.
5 Relatives may cover the patient's head with a white cap or scarf.
6 It is important that the funeral takes place as soon as possible after death.

7 Post-mortems are forbidden unless required by law.

8 Organ donation is forbidden by religious law.

9 For further information contact:

The Zoroastrian Information Centre
88 Compayne Gardens, London NW6 3RV.
Tel: 020 7328 6018.

In addition to the addresses given above, further information is available from:

The Shap Working Party on World Religions in Education
The National Society's RE Centre
23 Kensington Square, London W8 5HN.
Tel: 020 7937 7229.

Lumbar Puncture

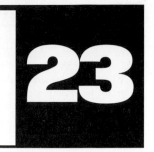

Definition

Lumbar puncture is a medical procedure which involves withdrawing cerebrospinal fluid by the insertion of a hollow spinal needle with a stylet into the lumbar subarachnoid space (Hickey 1997).

Indications

A lumbar puncture and withdrawal of cerebrospinal fluid (CSF), with or without the introduction therapeutic agents, is performed for the following purposes:

1 *Diagnosis:* CSF is normally a crystal clear, colourless and sterile liquid which resembles water. Analysis of the CSF for cells not normally present may be made to determine the presence of a pathological process (Bassett 1997). In addition, CSF pressure can be measured but is contraindicated in patients where raised intracranial pressure (RIP) is suspected or present due to the risk of 'brain herniation'.
2 *Introduction of therapeutic agents:* For example, antibiotics or cytotoxic intrathecal chemotherapy in the presence of malignant cytology (Hickey 1997).
3 *Introduction of spinal anaesthesia for surgery* (Hickey 1997).

Contraindications

The procedure should not be undertaken in the following circumstances:

1 In patients with papilloedema or deteriorating neurological symptoms, where raised intracranial pressure or an intracranial mass is suspected. In this situation, neuro-imaging (CT or MRI scan) should be undertaken prior to LP in order to avoid resultant potentially fatal brainstem compression, herniation or coning.
2 In the presence of infection. Local skin infection may result in meningitis by passage of the bacteria from the skin to the CSF during the procedure (Richards 1992). The presence of frontal sinusitis, middle ear discharge, congenital heart disease or prosthetic heart valves may all give rise to cerebral abscesses and, therefore, careful thought should be given when meningitis is suspected in these cases.
3 In patients who are unable to cooperate or who are too drowsy to give a history. Patient cooperation is essential to minimize the potential risk associated with this procedure.

4 In patients who have severe degenerative spinal joint disease. In such cases difficulty will be experienced both in positioning the patient and in accessing between the vertebrae (Hickey 1997).
5 In those patients undergoing anti-coagulant therapy or who have coagulopathies or thrombocytopenia (less than 50×10^9/litre). These patients are at increased risk of bleeding, therefore careful consideration should be taken and blood product support employed prior to undertaking lumbar puncture.

Reference material

Anatomy and physiology

The spinal cord lies within the spinal column, beginning at the foramen magnum and terminating about the level of the first lumbar vertebra (Fig. 23.1). Like the brain, the

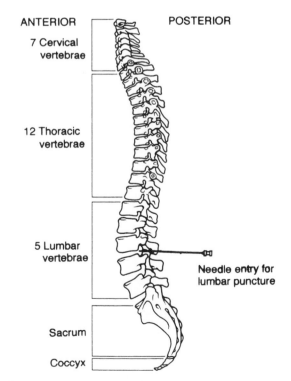

ANTERIOR   POSTERIOR

7 Cervical vertebrae

12 Thoracic vertebrae

5 Lumbar vertebrae

Needle entry for lumbar puncture

Sacrum

Coccyx

Figure 23.1   Lateral view of spinal column and vertebrae, showing needle entry site for lumbar puncture.

spinal cord is enclosed and protected by the meninges, that is, the dura mater, arachnoid mater and pia mater. The dura and arachnoid mater are separated by a potential space known as the subdural space. The arachnoid and pia mater are separated by the subarachnoid space which contains the CSF. Below the first lumbar vertebra the subarachnoid space contains CSF, the filum terminale and the cauda equina (the anterior and posterior roots of the lumbar and sacral nerves) (Weldon 1998). So as to avoid damage to the spinal cord, it is imperative that lumbar puncture is performed below the first lumbar vertebra where the cord terminates (Fig. 23.2).

The cord serves as the main pathway for the ascending and descending fibre tracts that connect the peripheral and spinal nerves with the brain (Weldon 1998). The peripheral nerves are attached to the spinal cord by 31 pairs of spinal nerves.

Cerebrospinal fluid (CSF)

CSF is formed primarily by filtration and secretion from networks of capillaries, called choroid plexuses, located in the ventricles of the brain. Eventually, absorption takes place through the arachnoid villi, which are finger-like projections of the arachnoid mater that push into the dural venous sinuses. CSF is clear, colourless and slightly alkaline with a specific gravity of 1005 (Draper 1989). In an adult, approximately 500 ml of CSF are produced and reabsorbed each day (Weldon 1998), with 120–150 ml present at one time. CSF constituents include:

1 Water
2 Mineral salts
3 Glucose
4 Protein (20–30 mg per 100 ml) (Keele *et al.* 1983)
5 Urea and creatinine.

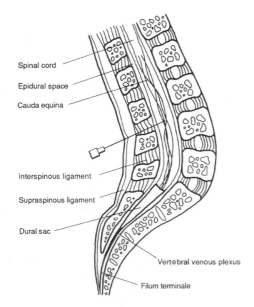

Figure 23.2 Lumbar puncture. Sagittal section through lumbosacral spine. The most common site for lumbar puncture is between L3 and L4 and between L4 and L5 as the spinal cord terminates at L1.

The functions of CSF include:

1 To act as a shock absorber
2 To carry nutrients to the brain
3 To remove metabolites from the brain
4 To support and protect the brain and spinal cord
5 To keep the brain and spinal cord moist (Hickey 1997).

Sampling and CSF pressure

The amount of CSF withdrawn for sampling depends on the investigation required. In practice, approximately 5–10 ml of CSF are usually withdrawn, although investigations for cell count and Gram stain can be performed using 1 ml. The pressure of CSF can be measured at the time of lumbar puncture using a manometer. Normal CSF pressure falls between a range of 60–180 mm H_2O (Hickey 1997). Spinal pressure may be raised in the presence of cerbrovascular accident (Long & Phipps 1989).

Queckenstedt's test

Historically, Queckenstedt's test was performed to check for obstruction in the spinal canal. This was undertaken by compressing, alternately, the jugular veins on either side of the neck, the CSF pressure was then measured by a manometer. Normal response is a sharp rise in pressure followed by a sharp fall as pressure to the jugular vein is removed. Should the rise and fall in pressure be sluggish or absent, it would indicate a blockage of the spinal canal. However, the relative impression of the Queckenstedt's test which gives too many false negative results to be reliable, has meant that it has largely been discarded in clinical practice (Walton 1989). Nowadays, with modern neuroimaging, this test is largely obsolete.

Abnormalities of CSF

1 Reddening of the CSF is indicative of the presence of blood, which is an abnormal finding. If the presence of blood is caused by a traumatic spinal tap, the blood will usually clot and the fluid clear as the procedure continues. If the presence of blood is due to subarachnoid haemorrhage, no clotting will occur (Lindsay *et al.* 1997).
2 Turbidity, cloudy CSF, is indicative of the presence of a large number of white cells and is an abnormal finding. The causes of such turbidity include infection or the secondary infiltration of the meninges with malignant disease, e.g. leukaemia or lymphoma.
3 Presence of different types of blood cells in the CSF can be diagnostic of a variety of neurological disorders, e.g.
   (a) Erythrocytes are indicative of haemorrhage.
   (b) Polymorphonuclear leucocytes are indicative of meningitis or cerebral abcess.
   (c) Monocytes are indicative of a viral or tubercular meningitis or encephalitis.
   (d) Lymphocytes present in larger numbers are indicative of viral meningitis or infiltration of the meninges by malignant disease (Hickey 1997).

(e) The presence of leukaemic blast cells is indicative of infiltration of the meninges by leukaemia.

(f) Viral, bacterial or fungal cultures from the CSF sample are indicative of infection.

Investigations

A number of tests can be performed on cerebrospinal fluid to aid diagnosis (Lindsay *et al.* 1997):

1 *Culture and sensitivity.* Identifying the presence of micro-organisms would confirm the diagnosis of bacterial/fungal meningitis or a cerebral abscess. The isolation of the causative organism would enable the initiation of appropriate antibiotic or antifungal therapy.

2 *Virology screening.* Isolation of a causative virus would enable appropriate therapy to be initiated promptly.

3 *Serology for syphilis.* Tests include: Wasserman test (WR), venereal disease research lab (VDRL) and *Treponema pallidum* immobilization test (TPI).

4 *Protein.* The total amount of protein in cerebrospinal fluid should be 15.45 mg/dl (=154.5 µg/ml). Proteins are large molecules which do not readily cross the blood–brain barrier. There is normally more albumin (80%) than globulin in cerebrospinal fluid as albumins are smaller molecules (Fischbach 1984). Raised globulin levels are indicative of multiple sclerosis, neurosyphilis, degenerative cord or brain disease. However, raised levels of total protein can be indicative of meningitis, encephalitis, myelitis or the presence of a tumour.

5 *Cytology.* Central nervous system tumours or secondary meningeal disease tend to shed cells into the CSF, where they float freely. Examination of these cells morphologically after lumbar puncture will determine whether the tumour is malignant or benign (Fischbach 1984).

Instillation of chemotherapy

A number of drugs do not cross the blood–brain barrier. Lumbar puncture is a method of introducing drugs into the central nervous system. Antibiotics can be instilled to treat specific infections such as bacterial meningitis; some cytotoxic drugs, e.g. methotrexate or cytosine arabinoside, can be instilled to treat malignant diseases such as leukaemia and can also be used prophylactically to prevent recurrence (Weinstein 1993).

Complications associated with lumbar puncture

1 Infection (inadvertently introduced during procedure – there is a greater risk in the presence of neutropenia).

2 Haemorrhage/localized bruising (may be caused by a traumatic procedure or in the presence of thrombocytopenia or a coagulopathy).

3 Transtentorial or tonsillar herniation (if Queckenstedt's test is carried out in the presence of raised intracranial pressure).

4 Headache.

5 Backache.

6 Leakage from puncture site (Hickey 1997).

7 Arachnoiditis (reported when administering intrathecal methylprednisolone) (Latham *et al.* 1997).

References and further reading

Bassett, C. (1997) Medical investigations: principles and nursing management. Lumbar puncture. *Br J Nurs*, **6**(7).

Fischbach, F.T. (1984) *A Manual of Laboratory Diagnostic Tests*, 2nd edn. J.B. Lippincott, Philadelphia.

Guerrero, D., Sardell, S. & Hines, F. (1998) Chemotherapy, pp. 179–200. In: *Neuro-Oncology for Nurses* (ed. D. Guerrero). Whurr, London.

Hickey, J. (1997) *The Clinical Practice of Neurological and Neurosurgical Nursing*, 4th edn. J.B. Lippincott, Philadelphia.

Keele, C.A. *et al.* (1983) *Samson Wright's Applied Physiology.* Oxford Medical Publications, Oxford.

Latham, J.M., Fraser, R.D., Moore, R.J. *et al.* (1997) The pathological effects of intrathecal betamethasone. *Spine*, **22**(14), 1558–62.

Lindsay, K. *et al.* (1997) *Neurology and Neurosurgery Illustrated*, 3rd edn. Churchill Livingstone, Edinburgh.

Long, B. & Phipps, W. (1989) *Medical – Surgical Nursing: A Nursing Process Approach*, 2nd edn. Mosby, London.

Richards, P. (1992) Monitoring of cerebral function. *Br J Hosp Med*, **48**(7), 390–92.

Walton, L. (1989) *Essentials of Neurology*, 6th edn, Chap 3. Churchill Livingstone, Edinburgh.

Weinstein, S. (1993) *Principles and Practice of Intravenous Therapy*, 5th edn. J.B. Lippincott, Philadelphia.

Weldon, K. (1998) Anatomy and physiology of the nervous system, pp. 1–28. In: *Neuro-Oncology for Nurses* (ed. D. Guerrero). Whurr, London.

GUIDELINES • Lumbar puncture

Equipment

1 Antiseptic skin-cleansing agents, e.g. chlorhexidine 70%, isopropyl alcohol or povidine iodine.

2 Selection of needles and syringes.

3 Local anaesthetic, e.g. lignocaine 1%.

4 Sterile gloves.

5 Sterile dressing pack.

6 Lumbar puncture needles of assorted sizes.

7 Disposable manometer.

8 Three sterile specimen bottles. (These should be labelled 1, 2 and 3. The first specimen, which may be bloodstained due to needle trauma, should go into bottle 1. This will assist the laboratory to differentiate between blood due to procedure trauma and that due to subarachnoid haemorrhage.)

9 Plaster dressing or plastic dressing spray.

Guidelines • Lumbar puncture (cont'd)

Procedure

Action

1 Explain and discuss the procedure with the patient.

2 Assist patient into required position on a firm surface:

(a) Lying (Fig. 23.3):
- One pillow under the patient's head.
- On side with knees drawn up to the abdomen and clasped by the hands.
- Support patient in this position by holding him/her behind the knees and neck.

(b) Sitting:
- Patient straddles a straight-backed chair so that his/her back is facing the doctor.
- Patient folds arms on the back of the chair and rests head on them.

3 Continue to support, encourage and observe the patient throughout the procedure.

4 Assist doctor as required. Doctor will proceed to:

(a) Clean the skin with the antiseptic cleansing agents.
(b) Identify the area to be punctured and infiltrate the skin and subcutaneous layers with local anaesthetic.
(c) Introduce a spinal puncture needle between the second and third lumbar vertebrae and into the subarachnoid space.
(d) Ensure that the subarachnoid space has been entered and attach the manometer to the spinal needle, if required.
(e) Decide whether Queckenstedt's manoeuvre may be performed.

(f) Obtain the appropriate specimens of CSF (about 10 ml in total) for analysis. (Cell count and Gram stain can be performed using 1 ml of fluid.)
(g) Withdraw the spinal needle once specimens have been obtained, appropriate pressure measurements taken and intrathecal medication administered if required.

5 When the needle is withdrawn, apply pressure over the lumbar puncture site using a sterile topical swab.

6 When all leakage from the puncture site has ceased, apply a plaster dressing or plastic dressing spray.

Rationale

To ensure that the patient understands the procedure and gives his/her valid consent.

To ensure maximum widening of the intervertebral spaces and thus easier access to the subarachnoid space.

To avoid sudden movement by the patient which would produce trauma.

This position may be used for those patients unable to maintain the lying position. It allows more accurate identification of the spinous processes and thus the intervertebral spaces.

To facilitate psychological and physical well-being.
To monitor any physical or psychological changes.

To maintain asepsis throughout the procedure.
To minimize discomfort from the procedure.

This is below the level of the spinal cord but still within the subarachnoid space.

To obtain a CSF pressure reading (normal pressure is 60–180 mm H_2O).

To check for obstruction to CSF flow in the spinal column. (Obstructon may be caused by a spinal cord tumour or herniated intervertebral disc.)
To establish diagnosis.

To minimize the risks of the procedure.

To maintain asepsis and to stop blood and cerebrospinal fluid flow.

To prevent secondary infection.

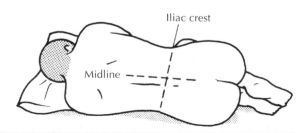

Figure 23.3 Position for lumbar puncture. Head is flexed onto chest and knees are drawn up.

7 Make the patient comfortable. He/she should lie flat or the head should be tilted slightly downwards. Time to lie flat varies from hospital to hospital, but is usually around 4 hours if there is no headache.

To avoid headache and decrease the possibility of brainstem herniation (coning) due to a reduction in cerebrospinal fluid pressure.

8 Observe patient for the next 24 hours for the following:
   (a) Leakage from the puncture site.

There may be a small amount of bloodstained oozing. The presence of clear fluid should be reported immediately to the doctor, especially if accompanied by fluctuation of other observations, as it may be a cerebrospinal fluid leak.

   (b) Headache.

Not unusual following lumbar puncture. Usually relieved by lying flat and, if ordered by the doctor, a mild analgesic.

   (c) Backache.

As above.

   (d) Neurological observations/vital signs.

These may indicate signs of a change in intracranial pressure. (For further information on neurological observations and vital signs, see Chap. 26.)

9 Encourage a fluid intake of 2–3 litres in 24 hours.

To replace lost fluid and assist the patient to micturate, which may be difficult due to the supine position.

10 Remove equipment and dispose of as appropriate.

To prevent the spread of infection.

11 Record the procedure in the appropriate documents.

To promote continuity of care and provide an accurate record for future reference.

12 Ensure that specimens are labelled appropriately and sent with the correct forms to the laboratory.

To ensure that the results are returned to the appropriate patient's notes.

Nursing care plan

Problem	*Cause*	*Suggested action*
Pain down one leg during the procedure.	A dorsal nerve root may have been touched by the spinal needle.	Inform doctor, who will probably move the needle. Reassure patient.
Headache following procedure (may persist for up to a week).	Removal of the sample of cerebrospinal fluid.	Reassure patient that it is a transient symptom. Ensure that he/she lies flat for specified period of time. Encourage a high fluid intake to replace fluid lost during procedure. Administer analgesics as ordered. If headache is severe and increasing, inform a a doctor – there is a possibility of rising intracranial pressure.
Backache following procedure.	(a) Removal of the sample of cerebrospinal fluid. (b) Position required for puncture.	Reassure patient that it is usually a transient symptom. Ensure that he/she lies flat for appropriate period of time. Administer analgesic as ordered.
Fluctuation of neurological observations, i.e. level of consciousness, pulse, respirations, blood pressure or pupillary reaction.	Herniation (coning) of the brainstem due to the decrease of intracranial pressure. (Raised intracranial pressure is a contraindication to lumbar puncture.)	Observe patient constantly for signs of alteration in intracranial pressure. The frequency may be decreased as patient's condition allows. Report any fluctuations in these observations to a a doctor immediately.
Leakage from the puncture site.	(a) Resolution of bleeding. (b) Leakage of cerebrospinal fluid.	(a) No further action required. (b) Report immediately to a doctor, especially if accompanied by fluctuation in neurological observations (see Chap. 26).

Mouth Care

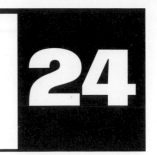

Definition

Mouth care (oral hygiene) is defined as the scientific care of the teeth and mouth (Thomas 1997). The aims of oral care are to:

1 Keep the mucosa clean, soft, moist and intact and to prevent infection
2 Keep the lips clean, soft, moist and intact
3 Remove food debris as well as dental plaque without damaging the gingiva
4 Alleviate pain and discomfort and enhance oral intake
5 Prevent halitosis and freshen the mouth

(Daeffler 1980).

Reference material

Anatomy and physiology

The mouth is the oval cavity at the anterior end of the digestive tract (Mosby 1997). It consists of the mouth cavity (cavum oris proprium) and the vestibule (vestibulum oris), which is bounded by the lips and cheeks, and the gums and teeth. The oral cavity is lined with moist stratified epithelium consisting of 15–20 layers of cells (Hinchliffe & Montague 1988). It is an area of rapid replication designed to meet the constant demands of activities such as chewing and talking (Porter 1994). The tongue forms the greater part of the floor of the oral cavity.

The mouth has three main functions: (1) ingestion of food and water; (2) communication; (3) breathing (with the nasal cavity) (Lippold & Winton 1972).

The mouth is lubricated by secretions from the salivary glands: parotid, submandibular and sublingual. Approximately 1.5 litres of saliva are produced each day (Torrance 1990). The functions of saliva are both protective and digestive in nature.

Predisposing factors to poor oral health are:

1 Inability to take adequate fluids leading to dehydration and dryness of mucosa
2 Poor nutritional status leading to poor cellular repair and vitamin deficiencies
3 Insufficient saliva production leading to infection and dryness of the mucosa
4 Major intervention altering oral status – surgery, radiotherapy or chemotherapy causing structural changes
5 Lack of knowledge or motivation towards maintaining oral hygiene (Trenter & Creason 1986).

Oral complications

Oral complications manifest as pain, ulcers, infection, bone and dentition changes, bleeding and functional disorders affecting verbal and non-verbal communication, chewing and swallowing, taste and respiration (Porter 1994). Stomatitis (inflammation of the oral cavity) results from damage to the mucous membrane (Holmes 1990). It may be induced by trauma, infection or by factors that decrease the proliferation rate of the cells (e.g. chemotherapy and radiotherapy). Xerostomia is an alteration in the production of saliva. Salivary function can be reduced or even destroyed by radiation (Cherry & Glucksmann 1959) as the salivary glands are highly sensitive to radiation (Carl 1983). Radiotherapy may also cause damage to the bone and dentition. Long-term damage may result in severe osteoradionecrosis (Yusef & Bakri 1993).

The oral cavity harbours many varieties of bacteria which do not normally pose any problems (Clarke 1993). However, immunosuppression and systemic treatments such as cytotoxic therapy and antifungal therapy may increase the pathogenicity of these organisms leading to local infection. Common organisms include *Pseudomonas*, *Klebsiella* and *Escherichia coli* (Goepfert & Toth 1979) and *Candida* species (Martin *et al.* 1981). Local infection may lead to systemic or secondary infection such as septicaemia or pneumonia.

Mouth care

Mouth care involves oral assessment, appropriate frequency of care and the use of oral care tools and agents.

Oral assessment

Oral assessment is required in planning effective care (Eilers *et al.* 1988). Thorough assessment of the oral cavity is required to: (1) provide baseline data; (2) monitor response to therapy; and (3) identify new problems as they arise (Holmes & Mountain 1993).

A number of oral assessment tools have been developed. Holmes & Mountain (1993) evaluated three oral assessment guides for reliability, validity and clinical usefulness. In their conclusion they showed a preference for that developed by Eilers *et al.* (1988), but stressed that further work is required to develop a tool that is entirely satisfactory for use in clinical practice and future research.

Frequency of care

Ginsberg (1961) concluded that the incidence of oral complications was reduced by the frequency of care rather than the agents employed. However, since then there has been little research to indicate the most effective frequency. Studies have reported various suggested time intervals including 2 hourly, 4 hourly and after meals (Ginsberg 1961; Howarth 1977; Beck 1979; Dudjak 1987) and there is clearly a need for further research.

Oral care tools

A number of different oral care tools have been reported in the literature including toothbrush, foamstick, dental floss and gauze. The most appropriate tool should be determined by its efficacy together with its potential to damage the gingiva. The use of the toothbrush is well supported by the literature (Howarth 1977; Carl 1983; Trenter & Creason 1986), however the foamstick has been cited as preferable when oral care is administered by the nurse as it may cause less trauma (Dewalt 1975). The foamstick, however, is much less effective than the toothbrush at removing debris from the teeth and gums. Borowski *et al.* (1994) showed that intensive oral hygiene such as dental treatment, gingival and tooth brushing, during aplasia, does not increase the percentage of documented septicaemia. It has been found that this is superior to limited oral care, which excluded gingival and tooth brushing during periods of aplasia. Care must be taken to ensure that the toothbrush is kept free from infection as toothbrushes have been shown to harbour organisms such as Group A beta-haemolytic streptococci, staphylococci, *Candida* and *Pseudomonas*. These have been found to contribute to persistent oropharynx infections (Taji & Rogers 1998; Brook & Gober 1998).

Oral care agents

The choice of an oral care agent is dependent on the aim of care. The agent may be used to remove debris and plaque, prevent superimposed infection, alleviate pain, stop bleeding, provide lubrication or to treat specific problems (Porter 1994). A wide variety of agents are available and should be determined by the individual needs of the patient together with a detailed nursing assessment. The agents described below comprise those included in *The Royal Marsden Hospital Trust Prescribing Guidelines for Mouth Care* (1999).

Chlorhexidine gluconate

Chlorhexidine is a compound with broad-spectrum antimicrobial activity that results in binding to and sustained release from mucosal surfaces (Ferretti *et al.* 1987). It has been shown to protect the patient from infection and to aid resolution of existing infections (Ferretti *et al.* 1987) and causes a reduction in soft tissue disease and oral microbial burden. It is effective against both anaerobes and aerobes as well as *Candida* (Mandel 1988; Walker 1988) and its effi-

cacy is dose-related (Addy & Moran 1991). Efficacy has been shown in doses of 0.01–0.2%. However, Foote *et al.* (1994) identified that patients receiving chlorhexidine mouthwash while undergoing radiation therapy showed a trend to develop more mucositis than a placebo arm, leading to the hypothesis that chlorhexidine may be detrimental in this clinical setting. However, more research needs to done within this area.

Fluconazole

Fluconazole is an orally absorbed antifungal azole which is soluble in water. It has been demonstrated to be effective in the treatment of candidosis of the oropharynx, oesophagus, urinary tract and a variety of deep tissue sites (Brammer 1990).

Sucralfate

Barker *et al.* (1991) showed that consistent daily oral hygiene and use of a mouth-coating agent such as sucralfate in patients receiving radiotherapy results in less pain and may reduce weight loss and interruption of radiation therapy because of severe mucositis. Reduction in pain and increase in oral intake have also been shown in patients with chemotherapy-induced ulcerating or erythematous mucositis taking oral sucralfate (Adams *et al.* 1986).

Nystatin

Nystatin is the best known and most commonly used antifungal agent (Campbell 1995). It is an antifungal antibiotic that is used as an oral suspension (Daeffler 1980). Barkvoll *et al.* (1989) showed in their in vitro study that combinations of nystatin and chlorhexidine gluconate were not effective against *Candida albicans* and recommended that the most efficient treatment plan must be restricted to the use of one of these drugs alone. Bristol-Myers Squibb Pharmaceuticals Ltd (personal communication 1993) has suggested that it is logical to leave a time interval of 15–30 minutes between administration of each agent.

Fluoride

Fluoride helps to prevent and arrest tooth decay, especially radiation caries, demineralization and decalcification. Following its use no food or fluids should be taken for at least 30 min in order for it to work (Myers & Mitchell 1988).

Artificial saliva

Saliva substitutes duplicate the properties of normal saliva (Kusler & Rambur 1992). They buffer the acidity of the mouth and lubricate the mucous membranes (Heals 1993).

Maintaining good oral hygiene

1 Clean teeth with toothpaste and toothbrush after meals.
2 Chlorhexidine gluconate 0.2% 5 ml, four times a day

diluted in 100 ml of water which should be retained in the mouth for at least 1 minute before discarding.

Problems

Oral candidiasis

Prophylaxis

Nystatin mouthwash 1 ml used four times a day. This should be rinsed around the mouth and retained for at least 1 minute before swallowing. A time interval of 15–30 minutes should be allowed between administration of chlorhexidine and nystatin to ensure efficacy.

Treatment

Surgical patients
    First-line: Nystatin 5 ml four times a day
    Second-line: Fluconazole 50 mg tablet, daily for 7 days
Radiotherapy/chemotherapy patients
    First-line: Fluconazole 50 mg orally, daily for 7 days. Use 100 mg IV daily if patients cannot tolerate oral therapy
    Second-line: Fluconazole 200–400 mg IV, daily until able to tolerate oral therapy

Painful mouth

First-line

Aspirin mouthwash four times a day (1–2 × 300 mg soluble tablets) used as mouthwash for oral cavity or a gargle for the oropharynx, mixed with lemon mucilage to aid adherence of aspirin to the mucosa when treating the hypopharynx. Paracetamol is an alternative if aspirin is contraindicated (e.g. in clotting disorders).

Second-line

Lignocaine 2% gel applied four times a day for pain relief of mucositis or ulceration. For extensive mucositis use lignocaine spray. Sucralfate suspension 5 ml, four times a day rinsed around the mouth and swallowed.

Third-line

Low dose opiates by oral, subcutaneous or intravenous route.

Reduced salivary flow

Sodium fluoride (e.g. Fluorigard) mouthwash used after breakfast and subsequent cleaning of teeth and use of chlorhexidine mouthwash. No other mouthwash should be used for at least 1 hour after use as its action may be affected. Fluoride gel (e.g. Gel-Kam) should be brushed on the teeth last thing at night.

Treatment of dry mouth

Artificial saliva (e.g. Glandosane or Luborant), two or three sprays up to four times daily or as often as necessary.

Advances in mouth care

The last few years have seen advances in the management of oral complications. Much of the research has arisen from the dental literature and may need to be researched in the cancer arena.

Local delivery of antimicrobials

Periodontitis is a bacterial infection which often appears in local areas within the oral cavity. Local antimicrobial delivery systems such as tetracycline fibre, doxycycline polymer, chlorhexidine chip, minocycline ointment and metronidazole gel are now available and aim to deliver high concentrations of antimicrobials directly to the site of the infection (Killoy 1998). These systems are currently used predominantly in the treatment of chronic inflammatory periodontal diseases.

Autologous saliva

Sreebny et al. (1995) investigated the use of autologous saliva in patients undergoing radiation for head and neck cancer. Their study showed that it was feasible to collect saliva from patients prior to receiving radiation, sterilize it and ensure that it retained its protective properties. Saliva could then be stored in a saliva bank for use in post-radiation xerostomia.

Growth factors

Studies have been carried out to determine the efficacy of colony stimulating factors such as G-CSF and GM-CSF on the incidence of oral mucositis. Nicolatou et al. (1998) showed that the local administration of GM-CSF significantly reduced and almost healed radiation-induced mucositis in 14 out of 17 patients during radiotherapy. This supports the findings of Kannaan et al. (1997) who also suggest that further study in randomized double-blind trials is warranted. Rovirosa et al. (1998) also showed that GM-CSF was effective in the control of pain, oral intake and weight loss. It has been shown that by giving TGF-beta 3, a potent negative regulator of epithelial and haemopoietic stem cell growth, it is possible to temporarily arrest oral mucosal basal cell proliferation and provide a safe and effective intervention for patients who undergo aggressive regimens of cancer therapy (Spijkervet & Sonis 1998).

Chlorhexidine chewing gum

Smith et al. (1996) showed that the use of a chlorhexidine chewing gum was as effective to oral hygiene and gingival health as a 0.2% chlorhexidine mouthwash. Teeth staining, a common side-effect of chlorhexidine mouthwash, was less with the gum than with the mouthwash, although this was not statistically significant.

Pilocarpine

This has been shown to improve saliva production and relieve symptoms of xerostomia after radiation of head and neck cancer. As a cholinergic drug the minor side-effects associated with its use were limited to sweating (Johnson *et al.* 1993).

Cryotherapy

Dose (1992) found that using ice chips within the oral cavity decreased the incidence of 5-fluorouracil (5-FU) induced stomatitis. 5-FU has a relatively short half life so by reducing the blood supply to the oral mucosa by application of cold before, during and after systemic bolus administration of the drug, the amount of 5-FU taken up by the cells can be reduced, thereby reducing cellular damage.

Tumours of the oral cavity

Clinical presentation

Tumours of the oral cavity include a spectrum of benign, pre-malignant and malignant lesions which usually present as exophytic swellings, mucosal thickenings or painful ulcerative tumours. Benign tumours such as fibromas, granulomas and adenomas of the tongue and buccal mucosa are slow growing, rarely ulcerate except if they are situated on the lateral border of the tongue when they may be traumatized by the teeth, and are easily excised. Pre-malignant lesions include leukoplakia, erythroplakia and chronic hyperplastic candidiasis, but there are other oral conditions such as lichen planus and submucous fibrosis which may be associated with a higher incidence of oral cancer.

Malignant tumours of the mouth are most commonly squamous cell carcinomas arising from the mucosal surface. The most frequent sites are the lateral border of the tongue and the anterior floor of the mouth which, because of their position, often present early. More posterior lesions on the tongue and tonsil produce rather vague symptoms of throat discomfort and may not be diagnosed until they are more advanced, although earlier detection may be predicted by astute investigation of a suspicious lump in the upper neck which is a common presentation of a metastatic cervical lymph node from this site.

The most common aetiological factor in squamous carcinoma of the oral cavity is tobacco which may be taken in several different forms, often associated with excessive alcohol intake. In Western countries where cigarette smoking is the most frequent causative factor, cancers of the upper aerodigestive tract account for about 10% of all cancers, but in the Asian subcontinent where chewing of tobacco and betel nut is common, the incidence is in the region of 40%. Alcohol is a synergistic factor which increases the mucosal absorption of carcinogens which are more soluble in alcohol than in normal aqueous mucus or saliva.

Management

The only curative treatments for squamous carcinoma of the oral cavity are surgery and radiotherapy. These modalities may be combined with postoperative radiotherapy in more advanced tumours depending on the histology and its potential for invasion and spread to the neck. Alternatively brachiotherapy with iridium wire implants may be used for early lesions confined to the tongue, although this technique is not recommended for lesions that encroach near the alveolus because of risk of radionecrosis.

Surgery

Early tumours of the tongue and oral cavity may cause only minimal ulceration or discomfort to the patient, but as they become more advanced they will cause major symptoms due to fungation, trismus, bleeding, foul odour due to secondary infection, loss of eating ability and cosmetic deformity. Temporary limited control of these symptoms may be achieved by basic oral hygiene with the use of oral douches and systemic metronidazole which is an excellent deodoriser for these tumours. The use of tranexamic acid often minimizes the risk of bleeding in haemorrhagic tumours (Sindet-Pedersen & Steubjerg 1986; Waly 1995).

Surgical resection of the tumour, however, provides the most reliable way of removal of the disease, together with any local lymph node metastases. This may be achieved in the small tumour with laser excision and primary closure or leaving the wound open to allow secondary healing. Regular douching of the open wound will help to prevent secondary infection. Alternatively, reconstruction of the remaining tongue with a free radial forearm flap can be achieved with good success and functional rehabilitation.

Malignant tumours of the upper jaw may require partial or total maxillectomy and this operation results in a defect in the palate and maxilla which usually is filled with a complex upper denture prosthesis. This needs to be taken out daily for regular douching and cleaning of the cavity to prevent secondary infection.

Radiotherapy

Treatment with radiotherapy involves implantation of the tumour with iridium afterloading wires and/or external beam irradiation. Local mucositis and ulceration of the mucosa and skin occur frequently towards the end of treatment and are managed by local mouthcare treatment to keep the mouth clean, comfortable and free of candida infection. Radionecrosis of the mandible may occur after irradiation which results in exposure of an area of bone in the floor of mouth. This must be kept clean with regular douching, preferably with a pulsating 'water-pick'. Often this will eventually heal after sequestration of the devascularized piece of bone.

Chemotherapy

Chemotherapy is not a curative treatment for squamous carcinoma of the oral cavity and pharynx. However, it may be used as adjuvant therapy to help eliminate microscopic disease or as neo-adjuvant treatment prior to radiotherapy or surgery (Jones *et al.* 1995). More commonly chemotherapy is used in palliative treatment of recurrent inoperable disease or metastases. This often successfully palliates disease-related symptoms and affords the patient some quality of life.

Summary

It is essential that consideration is given to those patients at risk of potential isolation, social ostracism and prejudice if lesions are visible and if halitosis is evident. Good oral hygiene will help to minimize complications related to infection, foul odour, bleeding and pain. This in turn will facilitate patient comfort especially where oral prostheses are worn. A comfortable mouth will not only assist with appetite and food intake but will help the patient feel more sociable and confident. Sexual relationships can also be disrupted in this group of patients as the mouth plays an important role in oral stimulation and sexual expression. To achieve optimum oral status for each individual patient, it is vital that the nurse uses all resources available and involves members of the multidisciplinary team (clinical nurse specialist, dentist, dental hygienist, maxillofacial prosthodontist, pharmacist, pain control team, speech and language therapist, and dietitian). Any oral regimen must be evaluated frequently for efficacy and the patients should know how to access members of the team for advice and support especially on discharge for continuity of care given.

References and further reading

Adams, S.C. *et al.* (1986) Evaluation of sucralfate as a compound oral suspension for the treatment of mucositis. *Proc Annu Meeting Am Soc Clin Oncol*, **5**, 257.

Addy, M. & Moran, J. (1991) The effect of some chlorhexidine containing mouth rinses on salivary bacterial counts. *J Clin Periodontol*, **18**, 90–93.

Barker, G. *et al.* (1991) The effects of sucralfate suspension and diphenhydramine syrup plus kaolin-pectin on radiotherapy-induced mucositis. *Oral Surg Oral Med Oral Pathol*, **71**(3), 288–93.

Barkvoll, P. *et al.* (1989) Effect of nystatin and chlorhexidine digluconate on *Candida albicans*. *Oral Surg Oral Med Oral Pathol*, **67**, 279–81.

Beck, S. (1979) Impact of a systemic oral protocol on stomatitis after chemotherapy. *Cancer Nurs*, **2**(5), 185–99.

Borowski, B., Benhamou, E., Pico, J.L. *et al.* (1994) Prevention of oral mucositis in patients treated with high dose chemotherapy and bone marrow transplantation: a randomised controlled trial comparing two protocols of dental care. *Eur J Cancer Oral Oncol*, **30B**(2), 93–7.

Brammer, K.W. (1990) Management of fungal infection in neutropenic patients. *Haematol Blood Transf*, **33**, 546–50.

Brook, I. & Gober, A.E. (1998) Persistence of group A beta-hemolytic streptococci in toothbrushes and removable orthodontic appliances following treatment of pharyngotonsillitis. *Arch Otolaryngol Head Neck Surg Sep*, **124**(9), 993–5.

Campbell, S. (1995) Treating oral candidiasis. *Nurse Prescriber*, June, 12–13.

Carl, W. (1983) Oral complications in cancer patients. *Am Fam Physician*, **27**, 161–70.

Cherry, C.P. & Glucksmann, A. (1959) Injury and repair following irradiation of salivary glands in male rats. *Br J Radiol*, **32**, 596–608.

Clarke, G. (1993) Mouth care in the hospitalized patient. *Br J Nurs*, **2**(4), 221–7.

Daeffler, P. (1990) Oral hygiene measures for patients with cancer. I. *Cancer Nurs*, **3**(5), 347–56.

Daeffler, R. (1980) Oral hygiene measures for patients with cancer. II. *Cancer Nurs*, Dec, 427–31.

Dewalt, E.M. (1975) Effect of timed hygienic measures on oral mucosa in a group of elderly subjects. *Nurs Res*, **24**, 104–108.

Dose, A.M. (1992) *Cryotherapy for prevention of 5 fluorouracil induced mucositis. Cancer nursing, changing frontiers*. Proc 7th Int Conf Cancer Nursing, August.

Dudjak, L. (1987) Mouth care for mucositis due to radiation therapy. *Cancer Nurs*, **10**, 131–40.

Eilers, J. *et al.* (1988) Development, testing and application of the oral assessment guide. *Oncol Nurs Forum*, **15**(3), 325–30.

Ferretti, G. *et al.* (1987) Chlorhexidine for prophylaxis against oral infections and associated complications in patients receiving bone marrow transplants. *J Am Dental Assoc*, **114**(4), 461–7.

Foote, R.L., Loprinzi, C.L., Frank, A.R. *et al.* (1994) Randomized trial of a chlorhexidine mouthwash for alleviation of radiation-induced mucositis. *J Clin Oncol*, **12**(12), 2630–33.

Ginsberg, M. (1961) A study of oral hygiene nursing care. *Am J Nurs*, **61**, 67–9.

Goepfert, H. & Toth, B.B. (1979) Head and neck complications of cancer chemotherapy. *Laryngoscope*, **89**, 315–19.

Heals, D. (1993) A key to wellbeing: oral hygiene in patients with advanced cancer. *Prof Nurse*, March, 391–8.

Hinchliffe, S. & Montague, S. (1988) *Physiology for Nursing Practice*. Ballière Tindall, London.

Holmes, S. (1990) *Cancer Chemotherapy*. Lisa Sainsbury Foundation, pp. 180–81. Austen Cornish, London.

Holmes, S. & Mountain, E. (1993) Assessment of oral status: evaluation of three oral assessment guides. *J Clin Nurs*, **2**, 35–40.

Howarth, H. (1977) Mouth care procedures for the very ill. *Nurs Times*, **73**, 354–5.

Johnson, J.T., Feretti, G.A., Nethery, W.J. *et al.* (1993) Oral pilocarpine for post irradiation xerostomia in patients with head and neck cancer. *New Engl J Med*, **329**(6), 390–95.

Jones, A.L. & Gore, M.E. (1995) Medical treatment of malignant tumours of the mouth, jaw and salivary glands. In: Langdon, J.D. & Henk, J.M. *Malignant Tumours of the Mouth, Jaws and Salivary Glands*, 2nd edn., pp. 123–35. Edward Arnold, London.

Kannan, V., Bapsy, P.P., Anantha, N. *et al.* (1997) Efficacy and safety of granulocyte macrophage-colony stimulating factor (GM-CSF) on the frequency and severity of radiation mucositis in patients with head and neck carcinoma. *Int J Radiat Oncol Biol Phys*, **37**(5), 1005–10.

Killoy, W.J. (1998) Chemical treatment of periodontitis: local delivery of antimicrobials. *Int Dent J*, 3 Suppl., 305–15.

Kusler, D.L. & Rambur, B.A. (1992) Treatment for radiation-induced xerostomia: an innovative remedy. *Cancer Nurs*, **15**(3), 191–5.

Langdan, J.D. & Henk, J.M. (1995) *Malignant Tumours of the Mouth, Jaws and Salivary Glands*, 2nd edn. Edward Arnold, London.

Lippold, A.J.C. & Winton, F.R. (1972) *Hearing and Speech Human Physiology*, pp. 443–64. Churchill Livingstone, Edinburgh.

Mandel, I. (1988) Chemotherapeutic agents for controlling plaque and gingivitis. *J Clin Periodontol*, **15**, 488–98.

Martin, U.V. *et al.* (1981) Yeast flora of the mouth and skin during and after irradiation for oral and laryngeal cancer. *J Med Microbiol*, **14**, 457–67.

Mosby (1997) *Mosby's Medical, Nursing and Allied Health Dictionary*, 5th edn. Mosby, London.

Myers, R.E. & Mitchell, L.D. (1988) Fluoride for the head and neck radiation patient. *Military Med*, **153**(8), 411.

Nicolatou, O. *et al.* (1998) A pilot study of the effect of granulocyte-macrophage colony-stimulating factor on oral mucositis in head and neck cancer patients during X-radiation therapy. *Int J Radiat Oncol Biol Phys*, **42**(3), 551–6.

Partridge, J. (1990) *Changing Faces – The Challenge of Facial Disfigurement*. Penguin, Harmondsworth.

Porter, H.J. (1994) Mouth care in cancer. *Nurs Times*, **90**(14), 27–9.

Rhys Evans, F. (1996) Tumours of the head and neck. In: Tshudin, V. (ed.) *Nursing the Patient with Cancer*.

Rovirosa, A., Ferre, J. & Biete, A. (1998) Granulocyte macrophage-colony stimulating factor mouthwashes heal oral ulcers during head and neck radiotherapy. *Int J Radiat Oncol Biol Phys*, **41**(4), 747–54.

Royal Marsden Hospital (1999) *The Royal Marsden Hospital Prescribing Guidelines for Mouth Care*. Drugs and Therapeutic Advisory Committee, September. The Royal Marsden Hospital, London.

Shklar, G. (1984) Oral Cancer. *The Diagnosis, Therapy Management and Rehabilitation of the Oral Cancer Patient*. W.B. Saunders, London.

Sindet-Pederson, S. & Steubjerg, S. (1986) Effect of local antifibrinolytic treatment with tranexamic acid in hemophiliacs undergoing oral surgery. *J Oral-Maxillofacial Surg*, **44**(9), 903–909.

Smith, A.J., Moran, J., Dangler, L.V. *et al.* (1996) The efficacy of an anti-gingivitis chewing gum. *J Clin Periodontol*, **23**(1), 19–23.

Spijkervet, F.K. & Sonis, S.T. (1998) New frontiers in the management of chemotherapy-induced mucositis. *Curr Opin Oncol*, **10**(Suppl. 1), S23–7.

Sreebny, L.M., Zhu, W.X. & Meek, A.G. (1995) The preparation of an autologous saliva for use with patients undergoing therapeutic radiation for head and neck cancer. *J Oral Maxillofacial Surg*, **53**(2), 131–9.

Taji, S.S. & Rogers, A.H. (1998) ADRF Trebitsch Scholarship. The microbial contamination of toothbrushes. A pilot study. *Aust Dent J*, **43**(2), 128–30.

Thomas, C.L. (1997) *Taber's Cyclopedic Medical Dictionary*, 18th edn. F.A. Davis, Philadelphia.

Torrance, C. (1990) Oral hygiene. *Surg Nurse*, **15**, 16–20.

Trenter, P. & Creason, N.S. (1986) Nurse administered oral hygiene: is there a scientific basis? *J Adv Nurs*, **11**, 323–31.

Walker, C. (1988) Microbial effects of mouth rinses containing antimicrobials. *J Clin Periodont*, **15**, 499–505.

Waly, N.G. (1995) Local antifibrinolytic treatment with tranexamic acid in hemophiliac children undergoing dental extractions. *Egypt Dental J*, **41**(1), 961–8.

Yusef, Z.W. & Bakri, M.M. (1993) Severe progressive periodontal destruction due to radiation tissue injury. *J Periodontol*, **64**(12), 1253–8.

GUIDELINES · Mouth care

Equipment

1 Clean tray.
2 Plastic cups.
3 Mouthwash or clean solutions.
4 Appropriate equipment for cleaning.
5 Clean receiver or bowl.
6 Paper tissues.
7 Wooden spatula.
8 Small-headed, soft toothbrush.
9 Toothpaste.
10 Disposable gloves.
11 Denture pot.
12 Small torch.

Items 1–11 may be left in the patient's locker when appropriate, and should be cleaned, renewed or replenished daily.

Procedure

Action	*Rationale*
1 Explain and discuss the procedure with the patient.	To ensure that the patient understands the procedure and gives his/her valid consent.
2 Wash hands with bactericidal soap and water/ bactericidal alcohol hand rub and dry with paper towel.	To reduce the risk of cross-infection.
3 Prepare solutions required.	Solutions must always be prepared immediately before use to maximize their efficacy and minimize the risk of microbial contamination.
4 Remove the patient's dentures if necessary, using paper tissues or topical swabs, and place them in a denture pot.	Removal of dentures is necessary for cleaning of underlying tissues. A tissue or topical swab provides a firmer grip of the dentures and prevents contact with patient's saliva.
5 Inspect the patient's mouth with the aid of a torch and spatula.	The mouth is examined for changes in condition with respect to moisture, cleanliness, infected or bleeding areas, ulcers, etc.

Guidelines • Mouth care (cont'd)

Action	Rationale
6 Using a soft, small toothbrush and toothpaste (or foamstick if the gingiva is damaged) brush the patient's natural teeth, gums and tongue.	To remove adherent materials from the teeth, tongue and gum surfaces. Brushing stimulates gingival tissues to maintain tone and prevent circulatory stasis.
7 Brush the inner and outer aspects of the teeth with firm, individual strokes directed outwards from the gums.	Brushing loosens and removes debris trapped on and between the teeth and gums. This reduces the growth medium for pathogenic organisms and minimizes the risk of plaque formation and dental caries. Foam sticks are ineffective for this.
8 Give a beaker of water or mouthwash to the patient. Encourage patient to rinse the mouth vigorously then void contents into a receiver. Paper tissues should be to hand. If the patient is immunosuppressed do not allow to rinse directly into a sink.	Rinsing removes loosened debris and toothpaste and makes the mouth taste fresher. The glycerine content of toothpaste will have a drying effect if left in the mouth. Reservoirs of stagnant water may harbour *Pseudomonas* bacteria.
9 If the patient is unable to rinse and void, use a rinsed toothbrush to clean the teeth and moistened foam sticks to wipe the gums and oral mucosa. Foam sticks should be used with a rotating action so that most of the surface is utilized.	To remove debris as effectively as possible.
10 Apply artificial saliva to the tongue if appropriate and/or suitable lubricant to dry lips.	To increase the patient's feeling of comfort and well-being and prevent further tissue damage.
11 Clean the patient's dentures on all surfaces with a denture brush or toothbrush. Rinse them well and return them to the patient.	Cleaning dentures removes accumulated food debris which could be broken down by salivary enzymes to products which irritate and cause inflammation of the adjacent mucosal tissue. Some commercial denture cleaners may have an abrasive effect on the denture surface. This then attracts plaque and encourages bacterial growth.
12 Dentures should be soaked in chlorhexidine for 10 minutes if oral *Candida* species are present.	Soaking in chlorhexidine reduces the risk of reinfecting the mouth with infected dentures.
13 Discard remaining mouthwash solutions.	To prevent the risk of contamination.
14 Clean and thoroughly dry the toothbrush	
15 Wash hands with soap and water or alcohol hand rub and dry with paper towel.	To reduce the risk of cross-infection.

Nursing care plan

Problem	Cause	Suggested action
Dry mouth.	Inadequate hydration.	Monitor fluid balance and increase fluid intake where necessary.
	Impaired production of saliva, e.g. as a consequence of radiotherapy or chemotherapy.	Apply artificial saliva to the oral cavity as required. Give the patient ice cubes to suck.
	Presence of specific stressors, e.g. mouth breathing, oxygen therapy, no oral intake, intermittent oral suction.	Inspect the mouth frequently, e.g. half-hourly. Swab mucosa with water.
Dry lips.	As above.	Smear a thin layer of appropriate lubricant.

Thick mucus.	Postoperative closure of a tracheostomy. Radiotherapy. Poor swallowing mechanism.	Use sodium bicarbonate solution in the mouth care procedure. Rinse the mouth afterwards with water or 0.9% sodium chloride.
Patient unable to tolerate toothbrush.	Pain, e.g. postoperatively; stomatitis.	Use foam sticks to clean the patient's gums and mucosa. 0.9% sodium chloride is advisable as a cleansing agent. For severe pain use an anaesthetic mouth spray or mouthwash before giving mouth care.
Toothbrush inappropriate or ineffective.	Infected stomatitis. Accumulation of dried mucus, new lesions, blood or debris.	As above and take a swab of any for culture before giving mouth care.

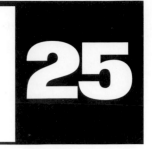

Definition

Manual handling operations are defined as:

> any transporting or supporting of a load (including the lifting, putting down, pushing, pulling, carrying or moving thereof) by hand or bodily force
>
> (HSE 1998)

This chapter is primarily concerned with the manual handling of patients (commonly termed the moving and handling of patients).

Indications

When a patient cannot move independently nurses are involved in the moving and handling of patients (following individual patient assessment).

Reference material

Nurses are involved in the moving and handling of patients as well as inanimate loads such as medical equipment, and in many procedures with the potential to cause postural strain. This is due to the constraints of a poor environment as well as a lack of equipment. In such a demanding and stressful job, nurses are subject to cumulative strain and at risk of musculo-skeletal problems – in particular back problems (Pheasant 1998).

For any manual handling operation to be considered successful it must meet two prime objectives. The handler needs to employ minimal effort, while the patient experiences minimal discomfort. These objectives can be achieved and the risk of injury reduced by undertaking a comprehensive assessment of the task's requirements. Risk assessments must be undertaken when manual handling cannot be avoided and there is a risk of injury. Where relevant, suitable equipment such as hoists, small handling aids and electronic profiling beds should be provided, as well as ongoing supervision in their use. The aim is to have fewer nurses injured and to increase comfort and safety for patients.

The Royal College of Nursing in their 1996 Safer Patient Handling Campaign, recommended that all health care organizations implement a safer patient handling policy (RCN 1996a, 1996b, 1996c). A safer patient handling policy involves far more than simply training nurses in the latest handling techniques. Without management commitment to occupational health and safety, in consultation with employees, the risk to nurses will not be reduced (Fig.

25.1). The patient's perspective also needs to be taken into account – the experience of being moved physically by others can be unpleasant and frightening, especially if no prior explanation of the manoeuvre has been given. It can also be physically damaging to patients (Holmes 1998).

Epidemiology

It is well known that nursing is one of the occupational groups most likely to suffer from back pain. Stubbs and colleagues (1983, 1984) provided a comprehensive account of this, and demonstrated that there is a significant incidence of back problems among nurses, which is a big factor in nurse wastage (Stubbs *et al.* 1986). It is many years since this seminal research yet the picture has not greatly changed. The Confederation of Health Service Employees estimated that each year 3650 nurses leave the profession permanently as a result of back injury, and one in four nurses experience back pain in the course of a working day (COHSE 1992). The National Back Pain Association 'Back Facts' statistics for 1996/97 state that 80000 nurses hurt their back each year and 3600 nurses are invalided out each year. The toll of back injuries is not only counted in terms of the suffering of individual nurses. Training one nurse costs over £30000, not to mention such additional costs involved in litigation, covering sickness absence, recruiting new staff and possible effects on insurance premiums. Over 15000 manual handling accidents in the health care sector were reported to the Health and Safety Executive (HSE) between 1994 and 1997 and more than 60% of them involved patient handling (Health and Safety Commission 1998). Statistics on injuries at work are partly obtained as a result of the Reporting of Injuries, Diseases and Dangerous Occurrences Regulations (RIDDOR) 1995, which require employers to report certain incidents to the HSE. (Reportable incidents include those where an accident at work results in an absence from work of 3 days or more.)

Legal background, ergonomics and risk assessment

The Manual Handling Operations Regulations 1992 came into effect on 1 January 1993 under the terms of the *Health and Safety at Work Act 1974*, thereby implementing European Directive 90/269/EEC. As a result, employers and employees acquired greater responsibilities for the design, development and maintenance of safe systems of practice. The regulations state that all hazardous manual

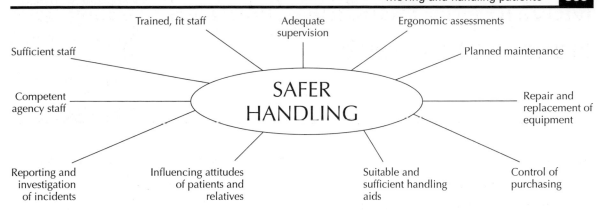

Figure 25.1   Factors that contribute to safer handling. (From *Manual Handling in the Health Services 1998*. Health and Safety Commission, 1998. Crown copyright material is reproduced with the permission of the Controller of Her Majesty's Stationery Office.)

handling tasks must, if reasonably practical, be eliminated. If this is not possible then a 'suitable and sufficient' written assessment of the risk must be undertaken by the employer (or someone designated by the employer). In order for assessments to be considered as suitable and sufficient they must consider the task, the load, the working environment and individual capability. Employers are required to provide suitable mechanical handling aids if the handling operation cannot be avoided, and training for employees in the use of equipment to maintain a safe working environment.

Employees must make use of safe systems of work implemented by their employers, and report to an appropriate person any hazards identified, as well as changes in their own ability to undertake manual handling tasks safely (e.g. pregnancy, back injury or deterioration in health status). In addition, employees are obliged:

> generally to make use of appropriate equipment provided for them in accordance with their training and the instructions, this would include machinery and other aids provided for the safe handling of loads
>
> (HSE 1998)

This law is based on the ergonomic approach of adapting the workplace to suit the needs of the people working there (rather than the other way around). As with much health and safety law, the approach involves risk assessment by competent people.

Manual handling procedures involve both hazards and risks, factors which exist to a greater or lesser extent in any operation which involves the manual handling of a load. A hazard can be defined as something which has the potential to cause harm, while risk is an expression of probability of injury, in relation to the severity of the hazard. Hazards and risks are present for both nurses and patients involved in manual handling, particularly if an unsuitable system or method is employed.

There are many regulations in addition to The Manual Handling Operations Regulations (1992) that are relevant to manual handling, some of which are illustrated in Fig. 25.2.

In the context of legal requirements, the RCN, through the Advisory Panel on Back Pain in Nurses, has published a Code of Practice for the Handling of Patients (RCN 1996b). The Code advocates that no nurse should be expected to move a patient where he/she bears most or all of the patient's weight and a hoist, sliding or other appropriate handling aid should always be used as appropriate, along with the required and associated education and training.

Manual handling assessments must be documented. Individual patient handling assessment involves ascertaining how much the patient can do (for example their ability to stand), and then assessing at what stage help will be required if a patient cannot move independently. This must be documented in detail and should include, for example, the type of hoist to be used for a manoeuvre (such as a stretcher hoist) or if a hoist sling is to be used the size of the sling. Since risk assessment factors (for example a patient's condition) may change, reassessment is crucial and this too must be documented and communicated to all concerned (see Fig. 25.3 for a sample individual patient handling assessment form). More detailed advice on assessments of tasks and patients (including generic patient handling assessments) is given in the RCN's *Manual Handling Assessments in Hospital and the Community* (RCN 1996c).

The risk of injury to both handler and patient can be reduced by fully assessing the task and identifying the best system for completing the procedure. However, assessment of the task and training are not sufficient on their own to minimize the risk or the incidence of back pain (Pheasant & Stubbs 1991). It is important that nurses understand how ergonomic principles contribute to providing and maintaining a safer environment for the handling of patients, and they must develop the ability to change their practices.

Biomechanics of load management

Biomechanics has been defined in the *Oxford Concise Dictionary* as 'the study of the mechanical laws relating to the

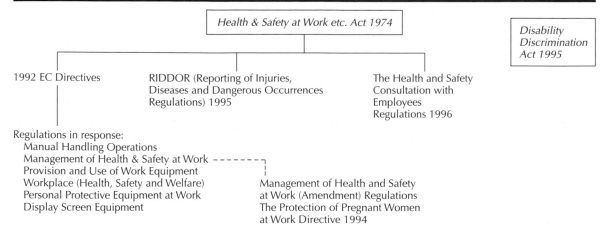

Figure 25.2 Nurses and manual handling: the legal context. In addition to criminal law, duties exist in civil law. These arise either from statutory provisions or from the common law, which is derived from the results of past cases.

movement or structure of living organisms' (Thompson 1995). Leggett (1998) explains in simple terms the biomechanics of human movement covering both mechanically and neurophysiologically based principles. She states that 'efficient movement of the human body involves the application of principles rather than the learning of techniques'.

When a person stands erect, most of the forces applied to the spine are the result of gravity acting upon the head and trunk. These forces are applied directly down through the spinal column, and very little muscular activity is required to maintain a stable upright position. However, when the trunk begins to move forward, away from the erect position, the nature and direction of the forces being applied to the spinal structure can change according to the lever principle. In the erect and near erect position the forces upon the spine are compressive, while in the stooped position forces can acquire harmful, sheering characteristics (Pheasant 1991). So the further a person moves away from an upright position, the more strain is put on the spine.

Due to its gentle 'S' shape the spine is able to withstand considerable compressive forces being applied to it. This can be ten times more than it could withstand if it were a straight structure. Despite this, it can become easily damaged if those forces become torsional, twisting or shearing, affecting the surface of intervertebral discs.

Compression forces are caused by the greater effort exerted by the erector spinae muscles to maintain a counterbalance to the forward weight of the trunk and to the weight of any load being moved. They increase in direct proportion to the distance the load is held away from the operator's body (Pheasant 1991). Rotational or jerking movements can increase shearing forces by up to 400% (Nachemson 1981). It is always safer to move any load with the natural curves of the spine maintained and the object or patient as close to the body as possible with the weight of the load symmetrically spread through both arms. This makes use of the large, strong muscles of the hip and thigh to provide the momentum for the movement of the load, reducing the shearing forces produced in the back. This is

not only safer but is also more mechanically efficient. Mechanical efficiency is further improved by the use of low friction devices and mechanical lifting aids.

It is also important to try to have a wide, stable base when manual handling so that the body is balanced with the line of gravity falling within that base. These basic principles of good manual handling are the cornerstone of back care training programmes. The aim is to encourage people to remember these principles and apply them (Fig. 25.4). Mechanical efficiency is further improved by using manual handling equipment, thus eliminating the need to lift patients physically.

Policy

Health care organizations must have a manual handling policy. The policy should be produced following consultation with all concerned and agreed by a multidisciplinary team. Periodic audit should be undertaken to review progress in ensuring good standards as a part of developing safe systems of work (Fazel 1998); a sample audit form is shown in Fig. 25.5. The RCN recommend the introduction and implementation of a safer patient handling policy within all health care organizations. They suggest that such a policy might state:

> the manual handling of patients is eliminated in all but exceptional or life-threatening situations . . . patients are encouraged to assist in their own transfers and handling aids must be used whenever they can help to reduce risk, if this is not contrary to a patient's needs
> (RCN 1996a)

The policy must be agreed, written down and communicated to all concerned. The roles, duties and responsibilities of managers, employees and occupational health and safety staff should be clear and guidance given on such aspects as assessment, reporting accidents and incidents, training content and requirements and equipment. A useful appendix to such a policy should include samples of assessment paperwork.

SECTION 1. LOAD

AFFIX PATIENT
LABEL

PATIENT'S COMPREHENSION (Tick appropriate box)

GOOD	DEAFNESS	LANGUAGE BARRIER	NO COMPREHENSION	DISORIENTED

DISABILITY/WEAKNESS/DEFORMITY

HANDLING CONSTRAINTS (e.g. pain)

BEHAVIOUR AFFECTING HANDLING

NONE	
LOSS OF CONFIDENCE	
UNPREDICTABILITY	
POOR MOTIVATION	
HISTORY OF FALLS	

PROBLEMS AND CAPABILITIES

PROBLEMS STANDING	
PROBLEMS WALKING	
TRANSFER TO AND FROM BED	
MOVEMENT IN BED	
PROBLEMS TOILETING	

AIDS NORMALLY USED BY THE PATIENT

WEIGHT AND HEIGHT

| kg | |
| cm | |

SECTION 2. ENVIRONMENT

	YES	NO	ACTION TO BE TAKEN
ADEQUATE FLOOR SPACE?			
IS FLOOR SLIP FREE?			
BRAKES IN WORKING ORDER?			
APPROPRIATE BED			

SECTION 3. TASKS

TASK	INDEPENDENT	1 NURSE ASSISTANT	2 NURSE ASSISTANT	TYPE OF MANOEUVRE (SPECIFY)	TYPE OF AID (SPECIFY)	PATIENT EXPECTED TO DO
TURNING						
SITTING UP						
MOVE UP BED						
TOILET IN BED						
TRANSFERS						
BED TO CHAIR						
BED TO WHEELCHAIR						
BED TO TROLLEY						
CHAIR TO CHAIR						
TOILETING						
BATHING						
WALKING						

OTHER PROBLEMS

| REFER TO MANUAL HANDLING COORDINATOR? | YES | NO |
| REFER TO BACK CARE ADVISOR? | YES | NO |

| SIGNATURE | GRADE | DATE |
| PRINT NAME | | |

Figure 25.3 Sample individual patient manual handling assessment form. It is important to constantly review and reassess the situation, completing a new, updated form as necessary.

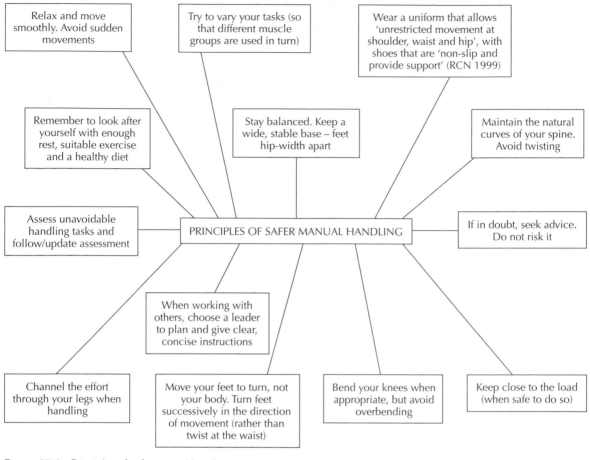

Figure 25.4 Principles of safer manual handling.

Equipment

Wherever patients requiring assisted mobility are cared for, appropriate equipment, for example hoists and sliding aids, and relevant training and supervision should be provided. Employers who do not make this kind of provision are in conflict with the law, as are nurses who choose not to use such equipment and systems of practice which have been implemented for their own safety and protection (DoH 1993). The reason for the use of equipment must be explained to patients and relatives.

Equipment must be appropriate, in good working order, well maintained and serviced, and used and cleaned in accordance with local infection control policy.

Awareness of the existence of and training in the use of manual handling aids is increasing and manufacturers are responding to feedback and continually developing new products. Hoist manufacturers, such as Arjo Ltd, provide follow-up servicing and training. There are many different hoists and small handling aids available to assist with the moving and handling of patients (Disabled Living Foundation 1994). Hoists have now been designed which

have the facility to lift patients from the ground on a stretcher, or hammock, sling attachment. Other hoists help physiotherapists when assisting patients to walk in rehabilitation. Sliding devices (for example Phil-E-Slide roller sheets) may be an effective way to help move someone up or down a bed. The traditional poles and canvas method of transferring a patient from bed to bed or bed to trolley can be replaced by more effective lateral transfer aids such as the Patslide. This information should be ascertained during the assessment. Patients may be able to use small aids such as 'monkey poles', rope ladders or patient hand blocks, which may allow them to be independent of the nurse while moving in bed. These are just a few examples of the hundreds of manual handling aids on the market.

The selection of use of an aid is based on individual patient assessment – one piece of equipment may be ideal for one patient but unhelpful to another. The key is taking account of the principles of safe handling, knowing what equipment is available and whom to contact for help or advice concerning other useful equipment which could be purchased or rented. An example of this is where a patient exceeds the safe working load of the hoist available on a ward

THE ROYAL MARSDEN HOSPITAL
MANUAL HANDLING AUDIT

The department manager should complete the audit form and return to Occupational Health.

SITE	
DEPARTMENT	

POLICY

		Yes	No
1	Have you read the Manual Handling Policy?		
2	Are you aware of your responsibilities under the Policy?		
3	Are staff within your department aware of their responsibilities under the Policy?		
4	Are departmental procedures in place to ensure that all manual handling accidents are reported?		
5	Are procedures in place to ensure that all manual handling equipment faults are reported?		

RISK ASSESSMENT

		Yes	No
1	Are written manual handling assessments prepared for all non-patient handling tasks undertaken within your area of responsibility?		
2	Where completed, have any action points been identified?		
3	Where identified, have action points been implemented? *If NO, please specify reason why:*		
4	Are assessments made available to staff (full time, part time, agency, etc.) as part of team meetings, within departmental procedures, on induction, etc.? *Please specify:*		
5	Are arrangements in place to ensure that assessments are routinely reviewed and revised as appropriate?		

RISK ASSESSMENT – PATIENT HANDLING (Complete as applicable)

		Yes	No
6	Are written patient handling risk assessments completed as part of the patient care plan when appropriate? *If YES, please indicate who completes the assessment and how often it is reviewed:* **Please provide a copy of a recent completed example (name omitted) with the returned form.**		
7	Are generic patient handling assessments completed for the department when appropriate? *If YES, please give examples of generic activities covered:* **Please provide a copy of a recent completed example (name omitted) with the returned form.**		

EQUIPMENT

		Yes	No
1	Is any manual handling equipment provided for staff use within the department within the department/ward, e.g. hoists, step ladders, slings, etc.? *Please complete Appendix A, as appropriate:*		
2	Where provided, is there an equipment inventory for the department?		
3	Where equipment is provided, are there routine maintenance procedures in place?		
4	Are records of equipment maintenance or testing maintained and held by the department?		
5	Are there any additional manual handling equipment needs for the department? *If YES, please specify:*		

TRAINING

1	How many of your staff are involved in undertaking manual handling tasks?		
	Patient handling	Non-patient handling	Both

2	How many staff involved in manual handling tasks have attended RMH manual handling training?	
	Patient handling	Non-patient handling

		Yes	No
3	Have staff received specific training in the use of manual handling equipment provided for use within the department?		
4	Have you attended managers' risk assessment training?		
5	Have you attended practical manual handling training?		

COMPLETED BY

DESIGNATION

DATE

APPENDIX A
PATIENT HANDLING EQUIPMENT INVENTORY

Please identify the following manual handling equipment items available for use within your department:

Item	Number	Manufacturer and serial number(s)	Date of last service
Patient hoist			
Slings for use with hoist (specify type and size)			
Sliding sheets			
Pat slide			
Monkey pole/trapeze			
Wheeled Sanichair			
Height-adjustable bed/trolley or couch			
Electronic profiling bed			
Other (please list) For example: Rope ladder One-way glide Patient handling belt Sliding board Patient hand block			

DETAILS

COMPLETED BY

DESIGNATION

DATE

Figure 25.5   The Royal Marsden Hospital Manual Handling Audit form.

– there should be a procedure already documented stating the action required in this situation. This may involve accessing equipment from elsewhere in the hospital or renting suitable heavy duty equipment. As with all manual handling issues the multidisciplinary approach is best.

Valuable sources of information outside the individual workplaces include the National Back Exchange (an association with a muldisciplinary membership which promotes the exchange and dissemination of information and ideas on back care) and the Disabled Living Foundation.

As the skills of the handler develop, their techniques in the use of these aids become more effective, although it must be recognized that even with the use of mechanical hoists there is still an element of manual handling to be done. Overhead tracking hoists remove the strain of pushing and pulling a mobile hoist, although there is still some effort involved in positioning the sling. Nurses must recognize their own capabilities and seek advice as required. Even when using aids, prior assessment is essential to make the operation as safe as possible.

It must always be remembered that the use of any equipment must be commensurate with the manufacturer's guidelines and instructions, and that the use of such equipment is kept under review for new information and developments in its use.

Training

Training is only one aspect of a comprehensive manual handling programme (Fig. 25.1). Training is crucial, however, and a legal requirement for any staff who are at risk of injury from manual handling. Training for such staff and their managers must include a theoretical component (covering epidemiology, law, anatomy and physiology, biomechanics and ergonomics, 24-hour back care, back pain and risk assessment) as well as the latest practical manual handling techniques. Training must be undertaken by competent trainers (Oakley 1997) and should be in accordance with national guidelines (for example, National Back Exchange 1995, Health and Safety Commission 1998, Lloyd 1998). Such national guidelines are often quoted as examples of good practice in legal cases. Basic core training is to be followed up by refresher training:

> professional trainers have found that three to five days is needed to train healthcare staff who have had no previous relevant training or experience in manual handling. But training is an ongoing process and review or refresher courses need to be planned and implemented.
> (Health and Safety Commission 1998)

Refresher training frequency should be based on risk assessment. Signed training records must be kept by employers as well as details of the content of the training.

As well as a rolling programme of formal theoretical and practical classroom-based training there must be ongoing department-based training and supervision as part of a safe system of work. Managers must ensure that they and their staff understand, and are familiar with, the handling aids in their area and promote good manual handling practice. Training and supervision in the use of equipment is essen-

tial. However, it should be noted that new equipment also brings new hazards (as shown by the Medical Devices Agency hazard and safety notices).

Summary

A team approach to manual handling policy, procedures, equipment selection and problem solving involves physiotherapists, occupational therapists and nurses sharing knowledge and working together for the benefit of the patient. Many patients may be able, with guidance and encouragement, to move themselves or assist nurses while being moved, and should be encouraged to help in ways that are compatible with their capabilities or health status. Manual handling assessments must be documented, implemented and updated. Nurses must be fully and regularly trained in manual handling by competent trainers and must always keep in mind the ergonomic principles of safer manual handling and back care.

References and further reading

COHSE (1992) *Back Breaking Work*. Confederation of Health Service Employees, Banstead.

Disability Discrimination Act 1995. Stationery Office, London.

Disabled Living Foundation (1994) Handling People: Equipment, Advice and Information. Disabled Living Foundation, London.

DoH (1993) *Risk Management in the NHS*. Stationery Office, London.

Fazel, E. (1998) The pain of moving. *Occup Health J*, **50**(8), 22–3.

Health and Safety at Work Etc. Act 1974. Stationery Office, London.

Health and Safety Commission (1994) *The Management of Health and Safety at Work (Amendment) Regulations (1992). The Protection of Pregnant Women at Work Directive*. HSC, London.

Health and Safety Commission (1998) *News release 19th March*. HSC, London.

Health Services Advisory Committee (1998) *Manual Handling in the Health Services*. HSE, Sudbury.

Holmes, D. (1998) Risk assessment: the practice. In: *Guide to the Handling of Patients*, (ed. P. Lloyd), revised 4th edn. National Back Pain Association/RCN, London.

HSE (1992a) *Workplace (Health, Safety and Welfare) Regulations. Approved Code of Practice*. HSE, Sudbury.

HSE (1992b) *Management of Health and Safety at Work Regulations. Approved Code of Practice*. HSE, Sudbury.

HSE (1992c) *Work Equipment. Provision and Use of Work Equipment Regulations. Guidance on Regulations*. HSE, Sudbury.

HSE (1992d) *Personal Protective Equipment at Work Regulations. Guidance on Regulations*. HSE, Sudbury.

HSE (1995) *Reporting of Injuries, Diseases and Dangerous Occurrences Regulations*. HSE, Sudbury.

HSE (1996) *The Health and Safety Consultation with Employees Regulations. Guidance on the Regulations*. HSE, Sudbury.

HSE (1998) *Manual Handling Operations Regulations 1992. Guidance on the Regulations*, 2nd edn. HSE, Sudbury.

Leggett, P. (1998) The Biomechanics of Human Movement. In: *Guide to the Handling of Patients* (ed. P. Lloyd), revised 4th edn. National Back Pain Association/RCN, London.

Lloyd, P. (ed.) (1998) *Guide to the Handling of Patients*, revised 4th edn. National Back Pain Association/RCN, London.

Nachemson, A. (1981) Disc pressure measurement. *Spine*, **6**(1), 93–7.

National Back Exchange (1995) *The Interprofessional Curriculum. A Case for Back Care Advisors.* Scutari Press, Glasgow.

National Back Pain Association (1997) *Back Facts.* Information Sheet. NBPA, London.

Oakley, K. (ed.) (1997) *Occupational Health and Safety.* In: *Occupational Health Nursing,* pp. 108–109. Whurr, London.

Pheasant, S. (1991) *Ergonomics: Work and Health.* Macmillan, Basingstoke.

Pheasant, S. (1998) Back injury in nurses – ergonomics and epidemiology. In: *Guide to the Handling of Patients* (ed. P. Lloyd), revised 4th edn., pp. 30–38. National Back Pain Association/ RCN, London.

Pheasant, S. & Stubbs, D. (1991) Lifting and Handling – An Ergonomic Approach. National Back Pain Association/Thorn EMI UK Rental, London.

RCN (1996a) *Introducing a Safer Patient Handling Policy.* Royal College of Nursing, London.

RCN (1996b) *Code of Practice for Patient Handling.* Royal College of Nursing, London.

RCN (1996c) *Manual Handling Assessments in Hospitals and the Community.* Royal College of Nursing, London.

RCN (1999) *Working Well Initiative. Uniform Leaflet.* Royal College of Nursing, London.

Stubbs, D. & Buckle, P. (1994) The epidemiology of back pain in nursing. *Nursing,* **2**(32), 935–7.

Stubbs, D. *et al.* (1983) Back pain in the nursing profession. Epidemiology and pilot methodology. *Ergonomics,* **26**(4), 755–65.

Stubbs, D. *et al.* (1986) Backing out: nurse wastage associated with back pain. *Int J Nurs Stud,* **23**(4), 325–36.

Thompson, D. (1995) *Oxford Concise Dictionary,* 9th edn. Clarendon Press, Oxford.

GUIDELINES • Moving and handling of patients

Procedure

Action	*Rationale*
1 Assess the needs of the patient, the environment and necessity for the procedure.	To ensure that action is in the patient's best interests. To ascertain whether there is sufficient space and appropriate equipment to perform procedure.
2 Inform all participating staff of the results of the assessment and confirm that details have been understood.	All staff participating in the procedure understand the plan of action in order to coordinate their actions correctly.
3 Prepare area by moving away any unwanted furnishings or equipment	To provide an ergonomic workspace with sufficient space to manoeuvre and perform the required task.
4 Select appropriate equipment as specified in the hospital training programme and the assessments.	To ensure the patient is moved with the minimum of effort, safely, and experiences as little discomfort as is possible.
5 Assist the patient into the desired position, with one handler acting as leader and coordinator for the procedure.	To ensure that effort is exerted at the appropriate time by the handlers to prevent strain on the handlers.
6 Check that the patient is comfortable following the manoeuvre and store equipment correctly and in line with safe practice. Document any significant information.	To evaluate the methods used and maintain a safe working environment.

Neurological Observations

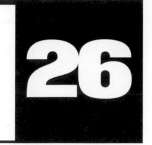

Definition

Neurological observation relates to the evaluation of the integrity of an individual's nervous system.

Indications

Neurological observations are required to monitor and evaluate changes in the nervous system by indicating trends, thus aiding diagnosis and treatment, which in turn may affect prognosis and rehabilitation (Abelson 1982; Jennett & Teasdale 1984).

Reference material

Changes in neurological status can be rapid and dramatic or subtle, developing over minutes, hours, days, weeks or even months depending on the insult (Aucken & Crawford 1998). Therefore the frequency of neurological observations will depend upon the patient's condition and the rapidity with which changes are occurring or expected to occur.

Neurological function is assessed by observing five critical areas:

1 Level of consciousness
2 Pupillary activity
3 Motor function
4 Sensory function
5 Vital signs

Level of consciousness

Alterations in level of consciousness can vary from slight to severe changes, indicating the degree of brain dysfunction (Aucken & Crawford 1998). Consciousness ranges on a continuum, from alert wakefulness to deep coma with no apparent responsiveness. Therefore, nurses must ensure that families and friends are involved at initial history taking and throughout care so as to chronicle accurately any change in neurological symptoms.

Categories of consciousness include the following:

1 *Full consciousness*: the patient is aware of self and environment and this is reflected in the ability of the patient to be aroused, perceive internal or external stimuli and respond appropriately on a cognitive (ability to assess, process, organize and use knowledge effectively) or motor level. Responses may be altered by focal, sensory and/or motor deficits.

2 *Lethargy/drowsiness*: the patient is inactive and indifferent, responds slowly or unpurposefully to stimuli and many not respond verbally.
3 *Coma*: the patient has total absence of awareness of self and environment. Response to arousal from a painful stimulus may be absent (see Chap. 42, The Unconscious Patient).

Coma itself is not a disease process; instead, it reflects some underlying process resulting from a primary central nervous system insult or metabolic or systemic disorder (Aucken & Crawford 1998). The reticular activating system (RAS) is a system of nerves in the brain stem concerned with levels of consciousness, from sleep to full alertness (Martin 1996). Processes that disturb its function will lead to altered consciousness (Fuller 1993) (see Chap. 42, The Unconscious Patient). Therefore, specific diseases and injuries can impair the level of consciousness since they may depress or destroy the RAS (Fig. 26.1).

Arousability

This depends on the integrity of the RAS. This core of nuclei extends from the brainstem to the thalamic nuclei in the cerebral hemispheres. Thus cognitive ability depends on the ability of the cerebral cortex to permit reciprocal stimulation and conscious behaviour.

Awareness

This requires an intact cerebral cortex to interpret sensory input and respond accordingly. This is the content of the consciousness (Nikas 1982; Scherer 1986).

Levels of consciousness may vary and are dependent on the location and extent of any neurological damage (Aucken & Crawford 1998). Previous and/or co-existing problems should be heeded when noting levels of consciousness, for example, deafness, hemiparesis/plegia.

Assessment of level of consciousness

Assessment involves three phases:

1 Eye opening
2 Evaluation of verbal response
3 Evaluation of motor response

Level of consciousness is often measured using the Glasgow Coma Scale (GCS) which was developed in 1974 at the University of Glasgow by Jennett and Teasdale (Fig. 26.2

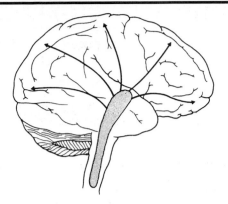

Figure 26.1   Reticular activating system.

and Table 26.1). It was designed as a system to grade the severity of impaired consciousness in patients with traumatic head injuries or intracranial surgery (Aucken & Crawford 1998). It is used worldwide, as it provides a reliable and easy to use measure of conscious level. It also provides an instant graphic representation of the conscious state which can facilitate consistent information of the patient's neurological status.

Evaluation of eye opening

Eye opening indicates that the arousal mechanism in the brain is active. Eye opening may be: spontaneous; to speech, e.g. spoken name; to painful stimulus or none at all. Arousal (eye opening) is always the first measurement undertaken when performing the GCS, as without arousal, cognition cannot occur (Aucken & Crawford 1998). It must, however, be remembered that swollen or perma-

nently closed eyes (e.g. after tarsorrhaphy surgery in which the upper and lower eyelids are partially or wholly joined to protect the cornea (Martin 1996)) will not open and do not necessarily indicate a falling conscious level.

Evaluation of verbal response

Verbal response may be:

1 *Orientated:* the patient is aware of self and environment.
2 *Confused:* the patient's responses to questions are incorrect and patient is unaware of self or environment.
3 *Incomprehensible:* the patient may moan and groan without recognizable words.
4 *None:* the patient does not speak or make sounds at all.

The absence of speech may not always indicate a falling level of consciousness. The patient may not speak English (though he/she can still speak), may have a tracheostomy or may be dysphasic. The nurse should also bear in mind that some patients may need a lot of stimulation to maintain their concentration to answer questions, even though they can answer them correctly. It is, therefore, important to note the amount of stimulation that the patient required as part of the baseline assessment (Aucken & Crawford 1998).

Evaluation of motor response

To obtain an accurate picture of brain function, motor response is tested by using the upper limbs since responses in the lower limbs may reflect spinal function (Aucken & Crawford 1998). The patient should be asked to obey commands; for example the patient should be asked to squeeze the examiner's hands (both sides) with the best motor response recorded. The nurse should note power in the hands and the patient's ability to release the grip. This is

Table 26.1   Scoring activities of the Glasgow Coma Scale (from Aucken & Crawford 1998). Scores are added, with the highest score 15 indicating full consciousness

Eye opening		*Scored 1–4*
Spontaneously	4	Eyes open without need of stimulus
To speech	3	Eyes open to verbal stimulation (normal, raised or repeated)
To pain	2	Eyes open to central pain (tactile) only
None	1	No eye opening to verbal or painful stimuli
Verbal response		*Scored 1–5*
Orientated	5	Able to describe accurately details of time, person and place
Sentence	4	Can speak in sentences but does not answer orientation questions correctly
Words	3	Speaking incomprehensible, inappropriate words only
Sounds	2	Incomprehensible sounds following both verbal and painful stimuli
None	1	No verbal response following verbal and painful stimuli
Motor response		*Scored 1–6*
Obeys command	6	Follows and acts out commands, e.g. lift up right arm
Localizes	5	Purposeful movement to remove noxious stimulus
Normal flexion	4	Flexes arm at elbow without wrist rotation in response to central painful stimulus
Abnormal flexion	3	Flexes arm at elbow with accompanying rotation of the wrist into spastic posturing in response to central pain
Extension	2	Extends arm at elbow with some inward rotation in response to central pain
None	1	No response to central painful stimulus

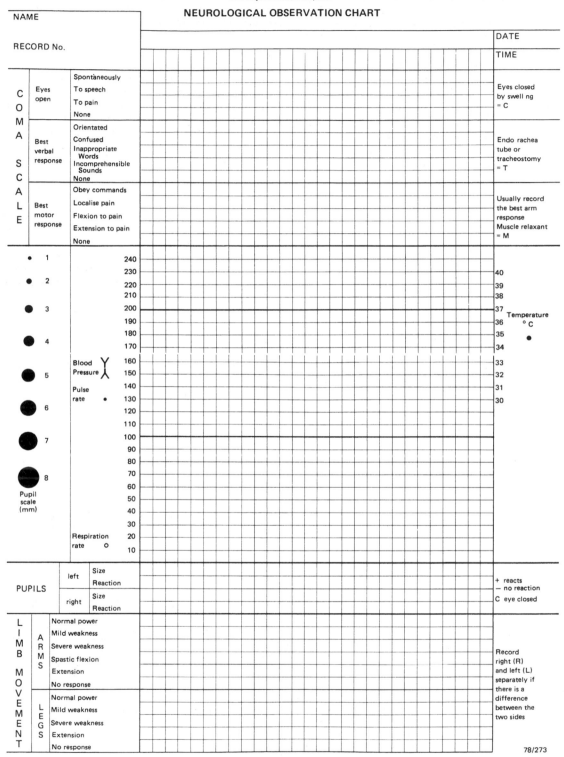

Figure 26.2 Glasgow Coma Scale.

because some patients with cerebral dysfunction, for example those with diffuse brain disease, may show an involuntary grasp reflex where stimulation of the palm of their hand causes them to grip (Aucken & Crawford 1998). If movement is spontaneous, the nurse should note which limbs move, and how, for example whether the movement is purposeful.

Response to painful stimulus may be:

1 Localized; the patient moves the other hand to the site of the stimulus.
2 Flexor; the patient's limb flexes away from pain.
3 Extensor; the patient's limb extends from pain.
4 Flaccid; no motor response at all.

Evaluation of painful stimuli

Painful stimuli should be employed only if the patient does not respond to firm and clear commands. It is always important that the least amount of pressure to elicit a response is applied so as to avoid bruising the patient. As such, it should only be undertaken by experienced professionals (for suggested methods see below.)

As the ability to localize pain is lost, various responses may be observed when painful stimuli are applied (Hudak et al. 1982). It is important to note, when applying a painful stimulus, that the brain responds to central stimulation and the spine responds first to peripheral stimulation (Aucken & Crawford 1998).

Central stimulation can be applied in the following ways (Lindsay et al. 1997; Aucken & Crawford 1998):

1 *Trapezium squeeze*: using the thumb and two fingers, hold 2 inches of the trapezius muscle where the neck meets the shoulder and twist the muscle.
2 *Supraorbital pressure*: running a finger along the supraorbital margin, a notch is felt. Applying pressure to the notch causes an ipsilateral (on that side) sinus headache. This method is not to be used if the facial bones are unstable, facial fractures are suspected or the assessor has sharp fingernails.
3 *Sternal rub*: using the knuckles of a clenched fist to grind on the centre of the sternum. When applied adequately, marks are left on the skin as sternal tissue is tender and bruises easily. Please note that because of the danger of bruising, this method should not be used for repeated assessment.

Peripheral stimuli can be applied in the following way:

1 Place the patient's finger between assessor's thumb and a pencil or pen.
2 Pressure is gradually increased over a few seconds until the slightest response is seen.

Any finger can be used, although the third and fourth fingers are often most sensitive (Frawley 1990). Please note, that because of the risk of bruising, pressure should not be applied to the nail bed. It must be remembered that nail bed pressure is a peripheral stimulus and should only be used to assess limbs that have not moved in response to a central stimulus (Aucken & Crawford 1998).

It cannot be overemphasized that the above methods of patient assessment should only be undertaken by appropriate qualified and trained nurses.

Evaluation of pupillary activity

Careful examination of the reactions of the pupils to light is an important part of neurological assessment (Table 26.2). The size, shape, equality, reaction to light (both direct and consensual responses, that is, the response from the eye that is not directly exposed to light) and position of the eyes should be noted. Are the eyes deviated upwards or downwards? Are both eyes conjugate (moving together) or dysconjugate (not moving together)? Impaired pupillary accommodation signifies that the midbrain itself may be suffering from pressure exerted by a swelling mass in the brain. Pupillary constriction and dilation are controlled by cranial nerve III (oculomotor) and any changes may indicate pressure on this nerve or brain stem damage (Fig. 26.3).

It should be noted that 'normal' visual function depends on a full and conjugate range of eye movements (cranial nerves III, IV, VI) in addition to normally functioning optic and oculomotor nerves and an intact visual centre in the occipital cortex (Aucken & Crawford 1998).

Evaluation of motor function

Damage to any part of the motor nervous system can affect the ability to move. Motor function assessment involves an evaluation of the following:

1 Muscle strength
2 Muscle tone
3 Muscle coordination
4 Reflexes
5 Abnormal movements

Muscle strength

This involves testing the patient's muscle strength against one's own muscle resistance and then against the pull of gravity.

Muscle tone

This involves flexing and extending the patient's limbs on both sides and noting how well such movements are

Table 26.2 Examination of pupils (from Fuller 1993)

What you find	Pupil size	Pupil reactiveness	Indication
Pupils equal	Pinpoint		Opiates or pontine lesion
	Small	Reactive	Metabolic encephalopathy
	Mid-sized	Fixed	Midbrain lesion
		Reactive	Metabolic lesion
Pupils unequal	Dilated	Unreactive	IIIrd nerve palsy
	Small	Reactive	Horner's syndrome

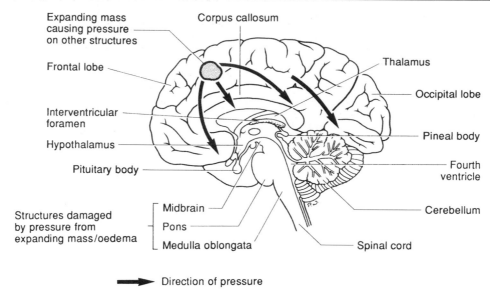

Figure 26.3 Diagrammatic representation of pressure from expanding mass and/or cerebral oedema.

resisted. Increased resistance would denote increased muscle tone and vice versa.

Muscle coordination

Any disease or injury that involves the cerebellum or basal ganglia will affect coordination. Assessment of hand and leg coordination can be achieved by testing the rapidity and rhythm of alternating movements and of point-to-point movements.

Reflexes

Among the most important reflexes are: blink, gag and swallow, oculocephalic and plantar.

1 *Blink:* this is a protective reflex and can be affected by damage to the Vth cranial nerve (trigeminal) and the VIIth cranial nerve (facial). Absence of the corneal reflex (Vth cranial nerve) may result in corneal damage. Facial weakness (VIIth cranial nerve) will affect eye closure.
2 *Gag and swallow:* damage to the IXth cranial nerve (glossopharyngeal) and Xth cranial nerve (vagus) may impair protective reflexes. These two cranial nerves are always assessed together as their functions overlap. Muscle innervation of the palate is from the vagus, while sensation is supplied by the glossopharyngeal nerves (Aucken & Crawford 1998).
3 *Oculocephalic:* this reflex is an eye movement that occurs only in patients with a severely decreased level of consciousness. In conscious patients this reflex is not present. When the reflex is present, the patient's eyes will move in the opposite direction from the side to

which the head is turned. However, in patients with absent brain stem reflexes, the eyes will appear to remain stationary in the centre.
4 *Plantar:* this reflex will help to locate the anatomical site of the lesion. Upgoing plantar (extension) reflex is termed 'positive Babinski' and indicates an upper motor neurone lesion. It should be noted that in babies under 1 year of age upgoing plantar is normal (Aucken & Crawford 1998).

Abnormal movements

When carrying out neurological observations, any abnormal movements such as seizures, tics and tremors must be noted.

Sensory functions

Constant sensory input enables an individual to alter responses and behaviour to suit the environment. When disease or injury damages the sensory pathways, the sensory responses are always affected. Any assessment of sensory function should include an evaluation of the following:

1 Central and peripheral vision.
2 Hearing and ability to understand verbal communication.
3 Superficial sensations (light touch, pain) and deep sensations (muscle and joint pain, muscle and joint position) (Hudak *et al.* 1982; Fuller 1993).

Vital signs

It is recommended that assessments of vital signs should be made in the following order:

Table 26.3 Abnormal respiratory patterns

Type	Pattern	Significance
Cheyne–Stokes	Rhythmic waxing and waning of both rate and depth of respirations, alternating regularly with briefer periods of apnoea	May indicate deep cerebral or cerebellar lesions, usually bilateral; may occur with upper brain stem involvement
Central neurogenic hyperventilation	Sustained, regular, rapid respirations, with forced inspiration and expiration	May indicate a lesion of the low midbrain or upper pons areas of the brain stem
Apnoeustic	Prolonged inspiration with a pause at full inspiration; there may also be expiratory pauses	May indicate a lesion of the lower pons or upper medulla, or hypoglycaemia, or drug-induced respiratory depression
Cluster breathing	Clusters of irregular respirations alternating with longer periods of apnoea	May indicate a lesion of lower pons or upper medulla
Ataxic breathing	A completely irregular pattern with random deep and shallow respirations; irregular pauses may also appear	May indicate a lesion of the medulla

1 Respirations
2 Temperature
3 Blood pressure
4 Pulse

(See also Chap. 28, Observations.)

Respirations

Of these four vital signs, respiratory patterns give the clearest indication of how the brain is functioning since respirations are controlled by different areas of the brain. Any disease or injury that affects these areas may produce respiratory changes. The rate, character and pattern of a patient's respiration must be noted. Abnormal respiratory patterns are listed in Table 26.3.

Temperature

Damage to the hypothalamus, the temperature-regulating centre, may result in grossly fluctuating temperatures (Nikas 1982).

Blood pressure, pulse and respirations

Observations of blood pressure, pulse and respirations will provide evidence of increased intracranial pressure. When intracranial pressure is greater than 33 mm Hg for even a short time cerebral blood flow is significantly reduced. The resulting ischaemia stimulates the vasomotor centre, causing systemic blood pressure to rise. The patient becomes bradycardic and the respiratory rate falls. Abnormalities of blood pressure and pulse usually occur late, after the patient's level of consciousness has begun to deteriorate. This change in the blood pressure was first described by Cushing and is known as the Cushing reflex (Nikas 1982).

Table 26.4 Visual pathways (from Fuller 1993)

Defect	Implication
Monocular field defects	Lesion anterior to optic chiasm
Bitemporal field defects	Lesion at the optic chiasm
Homonymous field defects	Lesion behind the optic chiasm
Congruous homonymous field defects	Lesion behind lateral geniculate bodies

General points

The initial assessment of a patient should include a history (taken from relatives or friends if appropriate) including noting changes in: mood, intellect, memory and personality, since these may be indicators of a longstanding problem, e.g. brain tumour (Barker 1990).

Visual acuity

May be tested using Snellen's chart or newspaper prints, with and without glasses if worn.

Visual fields

Lesions at different points in the visual pathways affect vision (Table 26.4). It should be noted that loss of vision is always described with reference to the visual fields rather than the retinal fields (Weldon 1998).

References and further reading

Abelson, N.M. (1982) Observation of the neurosurgical patient. *Curiatonis*, **5**(3), 32–7.
Allen, D. (1984) Glasgow Coma Scale. *Nurs Mirror*, **158**(2), 32.

Aucken, & Crawford, (1998) Neurological observations, pp. 29–65. In: *Neuro-Oncology for Nurses* (ed. D. Guerrero). Whurr, Edinburgh.

Barker, E. (1990) Brain tumour: frightening diagnosis, nursing challenge. *Registered Nurse*, **53**(9), 46–56.

Frawley, P. (1990) Neurological observations. *Nurs Times*, **86**(35), 29–34.

Fuller, G. (1993) *Neurological Examinations Made Easy*. Churchill Livingstone, Edinburgh.

Hickey, J.V. (1997) *The Clinical Practice of Neurological and Neurosurgical Nursing*, 4th edn. Lippincott-Raven, Philadelphia.

Hudak, C.M. *et al.* (1982) Nervous system (B. Fuller), pp. 321–34; Pathophysiology of CNS, pp. 335–48; Management modalities, pp. 349–78; Assessment skills, pp. 379–89. In: *Critical Care Nursing*, 3rd edn. Lippincott, New Jersey.

Jennett, B. & Teasdale (1984) *An Introduction to Neurosurgery*, 4th edn., pp. 23–9. William Heinemann Medical Books, London.

Lindsay, K.W., Bone, I. & Callander, R. (1997) *Neurology and Neurosurgery Illustrated*, 3rd edn. Churchill Livingstone, Edinburgh.

Martin, E.A. (1996) *Oxford Concise Colour Medical Dictionary*. Oxford University Press, Oxford.

Netter, F.H. (1975) *IHL Printing of CIBA Collection of Medical Illustrations, Volume 1, Nervous System*, pp. 58–9. CIBA, Summit, New Jersey.

Nikas, D. (ed.) (1982) *The Critically Ill Neurosurgical Patient*, pp. 1–27, 77–80, 100–103. Churchill Livingstone, New York.

Scherer, P. (1986) The logic of coma. *Am J Nurs*, 542–9.

Tortora, G.J & Grabowski, S.R. (1996). *Principles of Anatomy and Physiology*, 8th edn. Harper Collins, London.

Vernberg, K. *et al.* (1983) The Glasgow Coma Scale: How do you rate? *Nurse Educator*, **8**(3), 33–7.

Weldon, K. (1998) Neurological observations, pp. 1–28. In: *Neuro-Oncology for Nurses* (ed. D. Guerrero). Whurr, London.

GUIDELINES • Neurological observations and assessment

Note: the following describes a full neurological assessment. It may be inappropriate, unnecessary or impossible for the nurse to carry out all of the procedures every time the patient is observed.

Equipment

1 Pencil torch.
2 Thermometer.
3 Sphygmomanometer.
4 Tongue depressor.
5 Low linting swabs.
6 Patella hammer.
7 Neurotip (disposable).
8 Two test tubes.

Procedure

Action	Rationale
1 Inform the patient, whether conscious or not, and explain and discuss the observations	Sense of hearing is frequently unimpaired even in unconscious patients. To ensure, as far as is possible, that the patient understands the procedure and gives his/her valid consent.
2 Talk to the patient. Note whether he/she is alert and is giving full attention or whether he/she is restless or lethargic and drowsy. Ask the patient who he/she is, the correct day, month and year, where he/she is, and to give details about family.	To establish whether the patient's level of consciousness is deteriorating. If the patient is becoming disorientated, changes will occur in this order: (a) Disorientation as to time. (b) Disorientation as to place. (c) Disorientation as to person.
3 Ask the patient to squeeze and release your fingers (include both sides of the body) and then to stick out the tongue.	To evaluate motor responses.
4 If the patient does not respond, apply painful stimuli. Suggested methods have been discussed earlier.	Responses grow less purposeful as the patient's level of consciousness deteriorates. As the condition worsens, the patient may no longer localize pain and respond to it in a purposeful way (Vernberg *et al.* 1983).
5 Record, precisely, the findings. Write exactly what stimulus was used, where it was applied, how much pressure was needed to elicit a response, and how the patient responded.	Vague terms can be easily misinterpreted. Record the patient's best response (Allen 1984).
6 Hold the eyelids open and note the size, shape and equality of the pupils.	To assess the size, shape and equality of the pupils as an indication of brain damage. Normal pupils are spherical, usually at mid-position and have a diameter ranging from 1.5 to 6 mm (Nikas 1982).

7 Darken the room, if necessary, or shield the patient's eyes with your hands.	To enable a better view of the eye.
8 Hold each eyelid open in turn. Move torch towards the patient from the side. Shine it directly into the eye. This should cause the pupil to constrict promptly.	To assess the reaction of the pupils to light. A normal reaction indicates no lesions in the area of the brainstem regulating pupil constriction.
9 Hold both eyelids open but shine the light into one eye only. The pupil into which the light is not shone should also constrict.	To assess consensual light reflex. Prompt constriction indicates intact connections between the brainstem areas regulating pupil constriction (Scherer 1986)
10 Record unusual eye movements.	To assess cranial nerve damage.
11 Extend your hands and ask the patient to squeeze your fingers as hard as possible. Compare grip and strength.	To test grip and ascertain strength.
12 Ask the patient to close the eyes and hold the arms straight out in front, with palms upwards, for 20–30 sec. The weaker limb will 'fall away'.	To show weakness in limbs.
13 Stand in front of the patient and extend your hands. Ask the patient to push and pull against your hands. Ask the patient to lie on his/her back in bed. Place the patient's leg with knee flexed and foot resting on the bed. Instruct the patient to keep the foot down as you attempt to extend the leg. Flex the knee and place your hand in the flexion. Instruct the patient to straighten the leg while you offer resistance. *Note:* if a patient cannot follow the instruction due to a language barrier or unconsciousness, observe spontaneous movements and note how strong they appear. Then, if necessary, apply painful stimuli.	To test arm strength. If one arm drifts downwards or turns inwards, it may indicate hemiparesis. To test flexion and extension strength in the patient's extremities by having patient push and pull against your resistance.
14 Flex and extend all the patient's limbs. Note how well the movements are resisted.	To test muscle tone.
15 Ask the patient to pat the thigh as fast as possible. Note whether the movements seem slow or clumsy. Ask the patient to turn the hand over and back several times in succession. Evaluate coordination. Ask the patient to touch the back of the fingers with the thumb in sequence rapidly.	To assess hand and arm coordination. The dominant hand should perform better.
16 Extend one of your hands towards the patient. Ask the patient to touch your index finger, then his/her nose, several times in succession. Repeat the test with the patient's eyes closed.	To assess hand and arm coordination.
17 Ask the patient to place a heel on the opposite knee and slide it down the shin to the foot. Check each leg separately.	To assess leg coordination.
18 Ask the patient to look up or hold the eyelid open. With your hand, approach the eye unexpectedly or touch the eyelashes.	To test the blink reflex.
19 Ask the patient to open the mouth, and hold down the tongue with a tongue depressor. Touch the back of the pharynx, on each side, with a low linting swab.	To test the gag reflex.
20 Ask the patient to lie on his/her back in bed. Place your hand under the knee, raise and flex it. Tap the patellar tendon. Note whether the leg responds.	To assess the deep tendon reflex.
21 Stroke the lateral aspect of the sole of the patient's foot. If the response is abnormal (Babinski's response), the big toe will dorsiflex and the remaining toes will fan out.	To assess for upper motor neurone lesion.

Guidelines • Neurological observations and assessment (cont'd)

Action	Rationale
22 Ask the patient to read something aloud. Check each eye separately. If vision is so poor that the patient is unable to read, ask the patient to count your upraised fingers or distinguish light from dark.	To test the visual acuity.
23 Occlude the ear with a cotton wool swab. Stand a short way from the patient. Whisper numbers into the open ear. Ask for feedback. Repeat for both ears.	To test hearing and comprehension.
24 Ask the patient to close the eyes. Using the point of a sterile needle, stroke the skin. Use the blunt end occasionally. Ask patient to tell you what is felt. See if the patient can distinguish between sharp and dull sensations.	To test superficial sensations to pain.
25 Ask the patient to close the eyes. Fill two test tubes with water: one warm, one cold. Touch the patient's skin with each test tube and ask patient to distinguish between them.	To test superficial sensations to temperature.
26 Stroke a low linting swab lightly over the patient's skin. Ask the patient to say what he/she feels.	To test superficial sensations to touch.
27 Ask the patient to close the eyes. Hold the tip of one of the patient's fingers between your thumb and index finger. Move it up and down and ask the patient to say in which direction it is moving. Repeat with the other hand. For the legs, hold the big toe.	To test proprioception (Netter 1975; Tortora & Grabowski 1996). *Definition of proprioception:* the receipt of information from muscles and tendons to the labyrinth that enables the brain to determine movements and the position of the body.
28 Note the rate, character and pattern of the patient's respirations.	Respirations are controlled by different areas of the brain. When disease or injury affects these areas, respiratory changes may occur.
29 Take and record the patient's temperature at specified intervals.	Damage to the hypothalamus, the temperature-regulating centre in the brain, will be reflected in grossly abnormal temperatures.
30 Take and record the patient's blood pressure and pulse at specified intervals.	To monitor signs of increased intracranial pressure. Hypertension and bradycardia usually occur late, after the patient's level of consciousness has begun to deteriorate. Call for medical assistance as soon as it is evident that there is a deterioration in the patient's level of consciousness (Scherer 1986; Tortora & Grabowski 1996).

Nursing care plan

Category	Frequency	Rationale
All patients diagnosed as suffering from neurological or neurosurgical conditions.	At least 4-hourly, affected by the patient's condition.	To monitor the condition of the patient so that any necessary action can be instigated.
Unconscious patients (including ventilated and anaesthetized patients).	Frequency indicated by patient's condition.	To monitor the condition closely and to detect trends so that appropriate action may be taken.

Nutritional Support

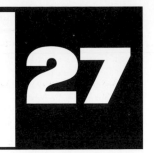

Definition

Nutritional support refers to any method of giving nutrients which encourages an optimal nutritional status. It includes modifying the types of foods eaten, dietary supplementation, enteral tube feeding and parenteral nutrition.

Indications

Nutritional support should be considered for anybody unable to maintain their nutritional status by taking their usual diet.

1 Patients unable to eat their usual diet (e.g. because of anorexia, mucositis, taste changes or dysphagia, see Nursing care plan) should be given advice on modifying their diet.
2 Patients unable to meet their nutritional requirements, despite dietary modifications, should take dietary supplements.
3 Patients unable to take sufficient food and dietary supplements to meet their nutritional requirements should be considered for an enteral tube feed.
4 Patients unable to eat at all should have an enteral tube feed. Reasons for complete inability to eat include carcinoma of the head and neck area or oesophagus, surgery to the head or oesophagus, radiotherapy treatment to the head or neck, fistulae of the oral cavity or oesophagus.
5 Parenteral nutrition (PN) may be indicated in patients with a non-functioning or inaccessible gastrointestinal (GI) tract who are likely to be 'nil by mouth' for 5 days or longer. Reasons for a non-functioning or inaccessible GI tract include bowel obstruction, short bowel syndrome, gut toxicity following bone marrow transplantation or chemotherapy, major abdominal surgery, uncontrolled vomiting or enterocutaneous fistulae.

Patients in any group may have an increased requirement for nutrients due to an increased metabolic rate, as found in patients with burns, major sepsis, trauma or cancer cachexia (Thomas 1994, pp. 80–92; Kinney 1995).

Reference material

Assessment of nutritional status

Before the initiation of nutritional support the patient must be assessed. The purpose of assessment is to identify whether a patient is undernourished, the reasons why this may have occurred and to provide baseline data for planning and evaluating nutritional support (Pichard & Jeejeebhoy 1993). It is useful to use more than one method of assessing nutritional status. For example, a dietary history may be used to assess the adequacy of a person's diet but does not reflect actual nutritional status, whereas percentage weight loss does give an indication of nutritional status. However, percentage weight loss taken in isolation gives no idea of dietary intake and likelihood of improvement or deterioration in nutritional status (Sitges-Serra & Franch-Arcas 1995).

Nutrient intake

Nutrient intake can be assessed by a diet history (Ralph 1993). A 24-hour recall may be used to assess recent nutrient intake and a food chart may be used to monitor current dietary intake. A diet history may also be used to provide information on food frequency, food habits, preferences, meal pattern, portion sizes, the presence of any eating difficulty and changes in food intake (Reilly 1996). A food chart where all current food and fluid taken is recorded is a useful method for monitoring nutritional intake, especially in the hospital setting or when dietary recall is not reliable.

Body weight and weight loss

Body mass index or comparison of a patient's weight with a chart of ideal body weight gives a measure of whether the patient has a normal weight, is overweight or underweight, and may be calculated from weight and height using the following equation:

$$\text{Body mass index (BMI)} = \frac{\text{Weight (kg)}}{\text{Height (m}^2)}$$

These comparisons, however, are not a good indicator of whether the patient is at risk nutritionally, as an apparently normal weight can mask severe muscle wasting. Of greater use is the comparison of current weight with the patient's usual weight. Percentage weight loss is a useful measure of the risk of malnutrition:

$$\% \text{ weight loss} = \frac{\text{usual weight} - \text{actual weight}}{\text{usual weight}} \times 100$$

An unintentional weight loss over 6 months of 10% represents malnutrition and a loss of 20%, severe malnutrition (Jensen et al. 1983; Wyszynski et al. 1998). Obesity and oedema may make interpretation of body weight difficult;

both may mask loss of lean body mass and potential malnutrition (Bistrain 1981; Pennington 1997). Accurate weighing scales are necessary for measurement of body weight. Patients who are unable to stand may require sitting scales for weight to be measured.

It is often not appropriate to weigh palliative care patients who may experience inevitable weight loss as disease progresses. Measures of nutritional status such as clinical examination and food intake may be used to assess patients.

Skinfold thickness

Skinfold thickness measurements can be used to assess stores of body fat. They are rarely used in routine nutritional assessment due to the insensitivity of the technique and the variation between measurements made by different observers. They are more appropriate for long-term assessments or research purposes. Calipers are used to measure the thickness of subcutaneous fat at four sites: the triceps, biceps, subscapular and supra-iliac. The measurements can be used to determine the percentage of body fat of a person (Durnin & Wolmersley 1974). Percentage charts for skinfold thickness measurements may be used to assess nutritional status (Thomas 1994, Appendix 3).

Bioelectrical impedance

Bioelectrical impedance analysis (BIA) is a simple technique which measures total body water and requires little patient cooperation (Walden & Klein 1992). The procedure involves the patient lying on a bed for a period of 5–10 minutes while electrodes are connected to the hand and foot. A small electrical current passes through the body which is undetectable by the patient. The principle of BIA relies on the difference in the electrical conductivity of the fat-free mass and fat mass of the body. Water is a good conductor of electricity and most water in the body is contained within fat-free mass. The small device with electrodes measures the impedance through the body of a small electrical current and calculates the body composition of the patient. It may be used for research studies or for monitoring nutritional status over a period of time (Heitman 1994).

Clinical examination

General nutritional depletion may be seen on clinical examination (Golder 1993). Specific nutritional deficiencies may be identifiable in some patients by a trained observer or clinician; such deficiencies may include polyneuropathy, cardiac enlargement and oedema in thiamin deficiency, or swollen, bleeding gums and poor wound healing in vitamin C (ascorbic acid) deficiency (Thomas 1994, pp. 52–7).

Subjective global assessment

Subjective global assessment is a clinical score, which can be obtained by a trained observer using a standardized questionnaire along with a physical examination, focused on nutritional status. The questionnaire includes questions about food intake, physical symptoms and weight loss and therefore encompasses a number of methods of assessing nutritional status (Naber et al. 1997).

Biochemical investigations

Biochemical tests carried out on blood may give information on the patient's nutritional status. The most commonly used are:

1 Plasma proteins. Changes in plasma albumin may arise due to physical stress, changes in circulating volume, hepatic and renal function, shock conditions and septicaemia. Plasma albumin and changes in plasma albumin are not a direct reflection of nutritional intake and nutritional status as it has been shown that these may remain unchanged despite changes in body composition (Sitges-Serra & Franch-Arcas 1995). It may be useful to review serum albumin concentrations in conjunction with C-reactive protein (CRP) which is an acute phase protein produced by the body in response to injury or trauma. CRP greater than 10 mg/litre and serum albumin less than 30 g/litre suggests 'illness'. CRP less than 10 mg/litre and serum albumin less than 30 g/litre suggests protein depletion (Thomas 1994, pp. 52–7).

2 Haemoglobin. This is often below haematological reference values in malnourished patients (men: 13.5–17.5 g/dl; women: 11.5–15.5 g/dl). This can be due to a number of reasons, such as loss of blood from circulation, increased destruction of red blood cells or reduced production of erythrocytes and haemoglobin, e.g. due to dietary deficiency of iron or folate (Chanarin 1993).

3 Serum vitamin and mineral levels. Clinical examination of the patient may suggest a vitamin or mineral deficiency. For example, gingivitis may be due to a deficiency of vitamin C, vitamin A, niacin or riboflavin. Goitre is associated with iodine deficiency, and tremors, convulsions and behavioural disturbances may be caused by magnesium deficiency (Shenkin 1995). Serum vitamin and mineral levels are rarely measured routinely, as they are expensive and often cannot be performed by hospital laboratories.

4 Immunological competence. Total lymphocyte count may reflect nutritional status although levels may also be depleted with malignancy, chemotherapy, zinc deficiency, age and non-specific stress (Rapin 1995).

If a patient is considered to be malnourished by one or more of the above methods of assessment then a referral to a dietitian should be made immediately (Burnham 1995).

Calculation of nutritional requirements

Energy requirements may be calculated using equations such as those derived by Schofield (1985), which take into account height, weight, age, sex and injury. However, an easier method is to use body weight and allowances based on the patient's clinical condition (Table 27.1).

Table 27.1   Guidelines for estimation of patient's daily protein and energy requirements (per kg body weight)

	Normal	Intermediate (moderate infection, postoperative patients, most cancer patients)	Severely hypermetabolic (multiple injuries, severe infection, severe burns)
Energy (kcal)	30	35–40	40–60
Nitrogen (g)	0.16	0.2–0.3	0.3–0.5
Protein (g)	1	1.3–1.9	1.9–3.1
Fluid (ml)	30–35	30–35	30–35 plus 500–700 ml additional fluid for every 1°C rise in temperature in pyrexial patients

Fluid and nitrogen (or protein) requirements can be calculated in a similar way. If additional nitrogen is being given in situations where losses are increased, for example due to trauma, gastrointestinal losses or major sepsis, then additional energy intake is required to assist in promoting a positive nitrogen balance. Additional fluid of 500–750 ml is necessary for every 1°C rise in temperature in pyrexial patients (Elwyn 1980).

Vitamin and mineral requirements calculated as detailed in the Committee on Medical Aspects of Food Policy (COMA) Report 41 on dietary reference values (DoH 1991) apply to groups of healthy people and are not necessarily appropriate for those who are ill. Some conditions may improve with the use of additional vitamins and minerals, for example a malnourished patient with poor wound healing may benefit from an increased intake of vitamin C and zinc, although the evidence is controversial (Hallböök & Lanner 1972; Taylor et al. 1974; Thomas 1997).

Planning nutritional support

Factors which may influence future food intake (e.g. surgery, chemotherapy or radiotherapy) also need to be considered when planning nutritional support, as clinical experience shows these may exert a deleterious effect on appetite and the ability to maintain an adequate nutritional intake (Feitkau 1991; Newman et al. 1998).

Modification of diet

Timing and frequency of food and drink

Patients unable to eat their usual portions, e.g. patients who have undergone gastrectomy or who have ascites or anorexia, may benefit from small frequent snacks.

Altering food consistency

Patients may benefit from very soft foods or even liquids alone if they have a sore mouth or throat, find it difficult to chew or have dysphagia.

Altering food choice

A sore mouth or throat may be exacerbated by certain flavours or foods, such as salt, spices, vinegar, citrus fruits.

Foods and drinks containing these items should be avoided.

Taste changes may mean foods previously liked are disliked and those previously disliked now enjoyed. Taste blindness may result in the patient feeling that food and drinks are lacking in taste.

Nausea and vomiting may be exacerbated by the smell of hot food and drinks, by fatty and spicy foods and by large quantities of food on a plate. Cold food and drinks, fizzy drinks and small frequent snacks high in carbohydrates (e.g. biscuits and toast) may help reduce nausea and vomiting.

Fortifying food

Food may be fortified with energy and protein for those patients unable to eat and drink sufficient amounts.

Practical information on modification of diet can be found in The Royal Marsden Hospital Patient Information Series No 9, *Overcoming Eating Difficulties*, 1997 (Thomas 1994, pp. 590–93). See also Table 27.2.

Dietary supplements

These may be used to improve an inadequate diet or may be used as a sole source of nutrition if taken in sufficient quantity.

Sip feeds

These come in a range of flavours, both sweet and savoury, and are presented as a powder in a packet or ready prepared in a can or Tetrapak. Sip feeds contain whole protein, hydrolysed fat and carbohydrates. Most are called 'complete feeds' since they provide all protein, vitamins, minerals and trace elements to meet requirements if a prescribed volume is taken. (Thomas 1994, pp. 65–75; Pennington 1997).

Energy supplements

Carbohydrates

Glucose polymers in powder or liquid form contain approximately 350 kcal per 100 g and 187–299 kcal per 100 ml respectively. Powdered glucose polymer is virtually tasteless

Table 27.2 Suggestions for modification of diet

Eating difficulty	Dietary modification
Anorexia	Serve small frequent meals and snacks Make food look attractive with garnish Fortify foods with butter, cream, cheese to increase the energy content of the meal Use alcohol, steroids, megestrol acetate or medroxyprogesterone acetate as an appetite stimulant Encourage food that the patient prefers Offer nourishing drinks between meals
Sore mouth	Offer foods that are soft and easy to eat Avoid dry foods that require chewing Avoid citrus fruits and drinks Avoid salt and spicy foods Allow hot food to cool before eating
Dysphagia	Offer foods that are soft and serve with additional sauce or gravy Some food may need to be blended – make sure that this food is served attractively Supplement the diet with nourishing drinks between meals
Nausea and vomiting	Have cold foods in preference to hot as these emit less odour Keep away from cooking smells Sip fizzy, glucose containing drinks Eat small frequent meals Try ginger drinks and ginger biscuits
Early satiety	Eat small frequent meals Avoid high fat foods which delay gastric emptying Avoid drinking large quantities while eating Use prokinetics, e.g. metoclopramide or cisapride, to encourage gastric emptying

and may be added to anything in which it will dissolve, e.g. milk and other drinks, soup, cereals and milk pudding; liquid glucose polymers may be fruit flavoured or neutral (Thomas 1994, pp. 696–709). Such supplements would be used to increase the energy content of the diet.

Fat

Fat may be in the form of long chain triglycerides (LCT) or medium chain triglycerides (MCT) and comes as a liquid which can be added to food and drinks. These oils provide 416–772 kcal per 100 ml – the oils with a lower energy value are presented in the form of an emulsion and those with a higher energy value are presented as pure oil (Thomas 1994, pp. 696–709).

Mixed fat and glucose polymer solutions and powders are available and provide 150 kcal per 100 ml or 486 kcal per 100 g, depending on the relative proportion of fat and carbohydrates in the product.

Products containing MCT are used in preference to those containing LCT where a patient suffers from gastrointestinal impairment causing malabsorption.

Always check with the manufacturer for the exact energy content of products.

Note: products containing a glucose polymer are unsuitable for patients with diabetes mellitus.

Protein supplements

These come in the form of a powder and provide 55–90 g protein per 100 g. Protein supplement powders may be added to any food or drink in which they will dissolve, e.g. milk, fruit juice, soup, milk pudding.

Energy and protein supplements are not used in isolation as these would not provide an adequate nutritional intake. They are used in conjunction with sip feeds and a modified diet. The detailed nutritional compositions of dietary supplements are available from the manufacturers (Silk 1995).

Vitamin and mineral supplements

When dietary intake is poor a vitamin and mineral supplement may be required. This can often be given as a one-a-day tablet supplement that provides 100% of the dietary reference values.

Enteral tube feeding

While the majority of patients will be able to meet their nutritional requirements orally, there is a group of individuals who will require enteral tube feeding either in the short term or on a more permanent basis. Several different feeding tubes are available.

Types of enteral feed tubes

Nasogastric/nasoduodenal

Nasogastric feeding is the most commonly used enteral tube feed and is suitable for short-term use such as postoperatively or during radiotherapy. Fine-bore feeding tubes should be used whenever possible as these are more comfortable for the patient than wide-bore tubes. They are less likely to interfere with swallowing or cause oesophageal irritation (Payne-James 1995). Polyurethane or silicone tubes are preferable to polyvinyl chloride (PVC) as they withstand gastric acid and can stay in position longer than the 10–14 day lifespan of the PVC tube.

Nasogastric tubes may either have a tungsten-weighted tip or be unweighted. A wire introducer is provided with many of the tubes to aid intubation if necessary. The weighted tip of a tube may facilitate the passage of the tube towards the soft palate and pharynx after insertion into the nasal passage. Weighted tubes may also be used to facilitate duodenal or jejunal intubation in postpyloric feeding for patients with abnormal gastric function where there is risk of aspiration (Thomas 1994, pp. 65–75). However, these tubes may be placed more successfully with an endoscope (Patrick *et al.* 1997).

Gastrostomy

A gastrostomy may be more appropriate than a nasogastric tube where long-term feeding is anticipated. It avoids delays in feeding and discomfort associated with tube displacement and for some patients is cosmetically more acceptable. A gastrostomy tube is also indicated in upper gastrointestinal obstruction where the passage of a nasogastric tube is restricted (Moran 1994). Percutaneous endoscopically guided gastrostomy (PEG) tubes are the gastrostomy tube of choice. They are made from polyurethane or silicone and are therefore suitable for short- or long-term feeding. A flange, flexible dome or inflated balloon holds the tube in position. The use of conventional balloon urinary catheters is now outdated, particularly as these are at risk of allowing gastric acid to leak at the tube entry site. However, gastrostomy tubes held in place with an inflatable balloon have the benefit over urinary catheters of being less likely to leak and are also made from polyurethane or silicone rather than from PVC. Clinical trials have shown that complications with PEG tubes, such as leakage, are rare (Ruppin & Lux 1986). For long-term feeding, (i.e. longer than 1 month), a gastrostomy tube may be replaced with a button which is made from silicone. The entry site for feeding is flush with the skin, making it neat and less obvious than a gastrostomy tube. The button is held in place by a balloon or dome inside the stomach (Griffiths 1996).

PEG tubes may be placed while the patient is sedated, thereby avoiding the risks associated with general anaesthesia. If a patient cannot be endoscoped for insertion of a PEG tube, then a surgically placed gastrostomy may be a more suitable feeding route. Alternatively, a radiologically placed gastrostomy can be used (Righi *et al.* 1998). (See Guidelines for care of the gastrostomy tube site.)

Jejunostomy

A jejunostomy is preferable to a gastrostomy if a patient has undergone upper gastrointestinal surgery or has severe delayed gastric emptying; in some cases it can be used to feed a patient with pyloric obstruction (Thomas 1994, pp. 65–75). Fine-bore feeding jejunostomy tubes may be inserted with the use of a jejunostomy kit, which consists of a needle-fine catheter. The use of needles and an introducer wire allows a fine-bore polyurethane catheter to be inserted into a loop of jejunum. Alternatively, some gastrostomy tubes allow the passage of a fine-bore tube into the jejunum.

Enteral feeding equipment

The administration of enteral feeds may be as a bolus, intermittent or continuous infusion, via gravity drip or pump-assisted (see Table 27.3). There are many enteral feeding pumps available which vary in their range of flow rate from 1 ml to 300 ml per hour. The following systems may be used for feeding via a pump or gravity-drip:

1 Plastic bottles into which the feed is decanted before connection to a giving set. This system may cut down wastage compared with a system which delivers a set amount of feed.
2 A PVC bag into which the feed is decanted. The giving set may be an integral part of the bag and some bags may have a rigid neck to assist filling.
3 A glass or plastic bottle containing feed which is attached directly to the giving set. This gives less flexibility in choice of feed or additional liquids than the plastic bottle or bag, but is quick and easy for the patient on a standard feed (Payne-James 1995). The feed container and administration set should be labelled with date and time of administration. The feed giving set should be changed every 24 hours. 'Ready to hang' sealed containers are also available which may help to reduce the risk of microbial contamination (Silverman *et al.* 1990).

Enteral feeds

Commercially prepared feeds should be used for nasogastric, gastrostomy or jejunostomy feeding. Available in liquid or powder form, they have the advantage of being of known composition and are sterile when packaged.

1 Whole protein/polymeric feeds contain protein, hydrolysed fat and carbohydrate and so require digestion. These may provide 1 kcal/ml or 1.5 kcal/ml (see manufacturer's specifications). As the energy density of the feed increases so does the osmolarity. Hyperosmolar feeds tend to draw water into the lumen of the gut and can contribute to diarrhoea if given too rapidly. The majority of feeds are low residue, although some contain dietary fibre. The fibre may help to reduce the incidence of diarrhoea by stimulating gut function (Silk 1995).
2 Feeds containing medium-chain triglycerides (MCT). In some whole protein feeds a proportion of the fat or long-chain triglycerides may be replaced with medium-chain triglycerides. The feed often has a lower osmolarity, and is therefore less likely to draw fluid from the plasma into the gut lumen. MCT is transported via the portal vein

Table 27.3 Methods of administering enteral feeds

Feeding regimen	Advantages	Disadvantages
Continuous feeding via a pump	Easily controlled rate Reduction of gastrointestinal complications	Patient connected to the feed for majority of the day May limit patient's mobility
Intermittent feeding via gravity or a pump	Periods of time free of feeding Flexible feeding routine May be easier than managing a pump for some patients	May have an increased risk of gastrointestinal symptoms, e.g. early satiety Difficult if outside carers are involved with the feed
Bolus feeding	May reduce time connected to feed Very easy Minimum equipment required	May have an increased risk of gastrointestinal symptoms Can be time consuming

rather than the lymphatic system. These feeds are suitable for patients with mildly impaired gastrointestinal function (Thomas 1994).

3 Chemically defined/elemental feeds. These contain free amino acids, short-chain peptides or a combination of both as the nitrogen source. They are often low in fat or may contain some fat as MCT. Glucose polymers provide the main energy source. These feeds require little or no digestion and are suitable for those patients with impaired gastrointestinal function (O'Morain *et al.* 1984). They are hyperosmolar and low in residue.

4 Special application feeds. Low protein and mineral feeds may be used for patients with liver or renal failure.

High fat, low carbohydrate feeds may be used for ventilated patients because less carbon dioxide is produced per calorie intake compared with a low fat, high carbohydrate feed.

Very high energy and protein feeds may be used where nutritional requirements are exceptionally high, e.g. burns, severe sepsis. These feeds contain approximately double the amount of energy and protein compared to standard whole protein feeds.

5 The value of glutamine, arginine, omega-3 fatty acid enriched feeds to promote immune function has yet to be demonstrated.

Up-to-date information on the exact composition of dietary supplements and enteral feeds can be obtained from the manufacturers (Pichard & Jeejeebhoy 1993; Silk 1995).

Monitoring enteral tube feeding

In order to avoid complications and ensure optimal nutritional status, it is important to monitor the following in patients on enteral tube feeds:

1 Oral dietary intake
2 Body weight
3 Fluid balance
4 Basic biochemical, e.g. urea and electrolytes, and haematological parameters, e.g. haemoglobin, measured at the commencement of enteral feeding and thereafter weekly

Complications of enteral tube feeding

The type and frequency of complications related to tube feeding depend on the access route, underlying disease state, the feeding regimen and the patient's metabolic state (Heberer & Marx 1995) (Table 27.4).

Home enteral feeding

Patients who are unable to take sufficient food and fluids orally may be taught to manage enteral tube feeding at home. Home circumstances and the ability of the patient to manage the feed must be considered before the patient is discharged. Adequate time should be allowed in the hospital setting for patients to become fully accustomed to the techniques of feed administration and care of the feeding tube, prior to discharge home. Support in the form of the general practitioner, community nurse and community dietetic services should be established before discharge. If possible, a multidisciplinary discharge meeting may be of benefit to both the patient and the professionals involved. Many of the commercial feed companies organize for the patient's feed and equipment to be delivered to the patient's home, after consultation with the local community services (BAPEN 1994a).

Termination of enteral tube feeding

It is important to ensure that an individual is able to meet their nutritional requirements orally prior to termination of the feed. Ideally, the feeds should be reduced gradually, according to the dietary intake (BAPEN 1999). It may be useful to maintain an overnight feed while the patient is establishing oral intake.

Parenteral nutrition

Parenteral nutrition (PN) is the direct infusion into a vein, of solutions containing the essential nutrients in quantities to meet all the daily needs of the patient. While enteral feeding is the preferred route of nutritional support in terms of cost and mechanical, septic and metabolic complications

Table 27.4 Complications of enteral feeding

Complication	Cause	Solution
Aspiration	Regurgitation of feed due to poor gastric emptying Incorrect placement of tube	Medication to improve gastric emptying, e.g. metaclopramide, cisapride Check tube placement Ensure patient has head at 45° during feeding
Nausea and vomiting	Related to disease/treatment Poor gastric emptying Rapid infusion of feed	Antiemetics Reduce infusion rate Change from bolus to intermittent feeding
Diarrhoea	Medication such as antibiotics, chemotherapy, laxatives Radiotherapy Disease-related, e.g. pancreatic insufficiency Gut infection	Antidiarrhoeal agent If possible discontinue antibiotics, avoid microbiological contamination of feed or equipment Send stool sample to check for gut infection
Constipation	Inadequate fluid intake Immobility Use of opiates or other medication causing gut stasis Bowel obstruction	Check fluid balance Administer laxatives/bulking agents If possible encourage mobility If in bowel obstruction, discontinue feed
Abdominal distension	Poor gastric emptying Rapid infusion of feed Constipation or diarrhoea	Reduce rate of infusion Gastric motility agents If possible encourage mobility Treat constipation or diarrhoea
Blocked tube	Inadequate flushing or failure to flush feeding tube Administration of medication via the tube	Prevent by flushing with 30–50 ml water before and after feeds or medication Use liquid or finely crushed medications If blocked, try soda water, sodium bicarbonate, fizzy soft drink, pancreatic enzymes

(Mercadante 1998; Reilly 1998), parenteral nutrition may be indicated for patients with a prolonged ileus, uncontrolled vomiting or diarrhoea, severe radiation enteritis, short bowel syndrome or gastrointestinal obstruction.

Route of administration

The traditional method of access is a central venous catheter, usually into the subclavian vein. The major hazard associated with the delivery of PN via a central venous catheter is infection. Therefore catheter insertion should take place in theatre where possible, using aseptic technique (Elliott *et al.* 1994). A skin-tunnelled catheter is the catheter of choice for long-term nutrition. The number of lumens will depend on the patient's peripheral venous access. If veins are considered inadequate then a double or triple lumen catheter should be inserted. This is because PN solutions are hyperosmolar and there is a risk of thrombophlebitis associated with feeding into peripheral veins. However, it has been shown that with care and attention, peripheral veins can be used to provide short-term PN (Mercadante 1998). This would be via a midline or a peripherally inserted central catheter (PICC). (See Chap. 44, Vascular Access Devices: Insertion and Management.)

PN solution

The basic components of a PN regime are provided by solutions of:

1 Amino acids (nitrogen source). Commercially available solutions provide both essential amino acids, usually in proportions to meet requirements, and non-essential amino acids, such as alanine and glycine.
2 Glucose (carbohydrate energy source). Glucose is the carbohydrate source of choice. It provides 3.75 kcal/g.
3 Fat emulsion (fat energy source). Fat generates 9 kcal/g and its inclusion in PN is necessary to provide essential fatty acids. Fat usually provides 30–50% of non-nitrogen energy. Nitrogen:non-nitrogen energy is usually provided in the ratio of 1:150–200. An insufficient energy supply from carbohydrate and fat will encourage the use of nitrogen for energy.
4 Electrolytes, e.g. sodium, potassium.
5 Vitamins: both water-soluble and fat-soluble are required.
6 Trace elements, e.g. zinc, copper, chromium, selenium.

(Thomas 1994, pp. 80–92.)

Choice of a PN regimen

PN is usually administered from a single infusion container in which all the requirements for a 24-hour feed are premixed. Such infusions are prepared either by the hospital pharmacy or are purchased.

The regime for a particular patient may be formulated according to the patient's needs for energy and nitrogen (see calculation of nutritional requirements, Table 27.1).

The majority of commercial vitamin and mineral preparations aim to meet both short- and long-term requirements.

Standard PN regimes may be suitable for some patients who require short-term nutritional support and do not appear to have excessively altered nutritional requirements.

The choice of such regimes depends on the patient's body weight. To allow for the possible need to vary the constituents of the infusion in response to changes in the patient's electrolyte or nutritional requirements, PN solutions should be ordered daily. Once compounded, most PN preparations last up to 7 days and need to be stored in a refrigerator. However, some triple chamber PN bags can be stored at ambient temperatures and require mixing prior to administration.

Delivery of parenteral nutrition and recommendations for IV management

Administration sets should always be changed every 24 hours (Burnham 1999) using an aseptic technique. Existing injection sites on the administration set should never be used for the giving of additional medications as PN is incompatible with numerous medications. If any additional medications, blood products or CVP readings are required then they should be given via a separate lumen or via a peripheral device.

A volumetric infusion pump should be used to ensure accurate delivery of PN. No bag should be used for longer than 24 hours. No adjustment greater than four drops per minute every 15 minutes should be made to the infusion rate. Never attempt to 'catch up' rapidly if the infusion is running too slowly (Weinstein 1997).

If the infusion must be discontinued the catheter should be flushed and patency maintained. Partly used PN bags should not be re-used but must be discarded and a new one requested from the pharmacy.

Monitoring of PN

During intravenous feeding monitoring is necessary to detect and minimize complications (see Table 27.5). Once feeding is established and the patient is biochemically stable then the frequency of monitoring may be reduced if the clinical condition of the patient permits. Additional patient monitoring such as 24-hour urine collection for urinary urea, nitrogen, serum zinc may be carried out where indicated, e.g. in severe malnutrition, poor wound healing.

Metabolic complications of PN

Metabolic complications should be detected by appropriate monitoring. Some more common complications are:

1 *Fluid overload.* This may occur when other blood products and fluids are given concurrently. It may be possible to reduce the volume of a 24-hour bag of PN while maintaining the nutritional content. Pharmacy can advise on the feasibility of making such regimes.

2 *Hyperglycaemia.* This may occur due to stress-induced insulin resistance or carbohydrate overload. A simultaneous sliding scale insulin infusion may be required. Failure to recognize hyperglycaemia may result in osmotic diuresis.

3 *Hypoglycaemia.* Abrupt cessation of PN may result in a rebound hypoglycaemia. A reduction in infusion rate to half the rate prior to stopping the infusion may help prevent this occurring.

4 *Azotaemia.* Raised plasma urea may indicate renal dysfunction or dehydration. Alterations in the non-protein energy content of the PN may be required or an increase in fluid input (Nordenström 1995).

5 *Hypophosphataemia.* This is associated with excessive glucose infusion and the refeeding syndrome in malnourished patients (Nordenström 1995). It is necessary to correct phosphate levels by providing additional phosphate prior to feeding. Phosphate levels should be monitored daily at the start of feeding. Introducing PN gradually in malnourished patients may help to prevent the refeeding syndrome.

Other complications such as metabolic acidosis, electrolyte disturbances, hyperammonaemia, hypernatraemia and hypokalaemia may require a review of the PN solution, rate of administration, additional fluids, blood products and drugs.

Table 27.5 Monitoring of PN (BAPEN 1996)

Parameter	Frequency of monitoring
TPR and blood pressure	Daily
Body weight	Daily
Fluid balance	Daily
Serum urea, creatinine and electrolytes	Initially and at least three times weekly
Blood glucose	Daily for the first week, if normal, twice weekly thereafter
Full blood count	Initially and at least three times weekly
Serum phosphate	48 hours after initiation of feeding, thereafter twice weekly
Serum magnesium	At least twice weekly (may be measured more often if the patient is on magnesium-depleting drugs, e.g. cyclosporin and cisplatin)
Alkaline phosphatase, alanine transaminase, bilirubin	Initially and at least twice weekly
Zinc	At least monthly

Termination of PN

Parenteral nutrition should not be terminated until oral or enteral tube feeding is well established. The patient needs to be taking a minimum of 50% of their nutritional requirements via the enteral route. It is important that all members of the multidisciplinary team are involved in the decision to terminate PN.

The final unit of PN can be given as two halves, each one being administered over 24 hours. This may provide the opportunity for enteral intake to be established whilst continuing to provide nutritional support.

Elective removal of catheter

See Chap. 44, Vascular Access Devices: Insertion and Management.

Home PN

There are few indications for home PN. It may be necessary in patients who have complete intestinal failure, e.g. short bowel syndrome due to Crohn's disease or radiation enteritis. The cost of home parenteral feeding is high and requires first class training with an efficient and comprehensive back-up service. It is recommended that only hospitals which have the appropriate facilities to train patients and provide the necessary care in case of an emergency should be involved in home PN (Lennard-Jones 1992; BAPEN 1994a).

Multidisciplinary team

It is important that all members of the multidisciplinary team, including dietitian, nurse, doctor, pharmacist, catering department and community services, are involved in the patient's nutritional care to ensure a thorough and coordinated approach to nutritional management (BAPEN 1994b).

References and further reading

Appleton, J. & Machin, J. (1998) *Working with Oral Cancer*, 2nd edn. Winslow, Bicester.

BAPEN (1994a) *Enteral and Parenteral Nutrition in the Community* (ed. M. Elia). British Association for Parenteral and Enteral Nutrition, Maidenhead.

BAPEN (1994b) *Organisation of Nutritional Support in Hospitals* (ed. D.B.A. Silk). British Association for Parenteral and Enteral Nutrition, Maidenhead.

BAPEN (1996) *Current Perspectives on Parenteral Nutrition in Adults* (ed. C.R. Pennington). British Association for Parenteral and Enteral Nutrition, Maidenhead.

BAPEN (1999) *Current Perspectives on Enteral Nutrition in Adults* (ed. C.A. McAtear). British Association for Parenteral and Enteral Nutrition, Maidenhead.

Bistrain, B. (1981) Assessment of protein energy malnutrition in surgical patients. In: *Nutrition and the Surgical Patient* (ed. C.L. Hill), pp. 39–57. Churchill Livingstone, Edinburgh.

Burnham, W.R. (1995) The role of a nutrition support team. In: *Artificial Nutrition Support in Clinical Practice* (eds J. Payne-James, G. Grimble & D. Silk), pp. 175–86. Edward Arnold, London.

Burnham, P. (1999) Parenteral nutrition. In: *Intravenous Therapy in Nursing Practice* (eds L. Dougherty & J. Lamb), pp. 377–400. Churchill Livingstone, Edinburgh.

Burns, S.M., Martin, M., Robbins, V. *et al.* (1995) Comparison of nasogastric tube securing methods and tube types in medical intensive care patients. *Am J Crit Care*, **4**(3), 198–203.

Chanarin, I. (1993) Nutritional management of diseases of the blood. In: *Human Nutrition and Dietetics* (eds J.S. Garrow & W.P.T. James), 9th edn., pp. 584–96. Churchill Livingstone, Edinburgh.

DoH (1991) *Dietary Reference Values for Food Energy and Nutrients for the United Kingdom*. COMA Report 41. Stationary Office, London.

Durnin, J.B. & Wolmersley, J. (1974) Body fat assessed from total body density and its estimation from skinfold thickness: measurements on 481 men and women aged from 16 to 72 years. *Br J Nutr*, **32**, 77–9.

Elliot, T.S.J. *et al.* (1994) Guidelines for good practice in central venous catheterisation. *J Hosp Infect*, **28**, 163–76.

Elwyn, D.H. (1980) Nutritional requirements of adult surgical patients. *Crit Care Med*, **8**, 9–20.

Feitkau, R. (1991) Percutaneous endoscopically guided gastrostomy in patients with head and neck cancer. *Recent Results Cancer Res*, **121**, 268–82.

Golder, B.E. (1993) Primary protein – energy malnutrition. In: *Human Nutrition and Dietetics* (eds J.S. Garrow & W.P.T. James), 9th edn., pp. 440–55. Churchill Livingstone, Edinburgh.

Grant, A. & Todd, E. (1987) *Enteral and Parenteral Nutrition*. Blackwell Scientific Publications, Oxford.

Griffiths, M. (1996) Single-stage percutaneous gastrostomy button insertion: a leap forward. *J Parenteral Enteral Nutr*, **20**(3), 237–9.

Groher, M. (1997) *Dysphagia: Diagnosis and Management*, 2nd edn. Butterworth & Heinemann, Boston.

Hallböök, T. & Lanner, E. (1972) Serum zinc and healing of venous leg ulcers. *Lancet*, **14**, 780–82.

Heberer, M. & Marx, A. (1995) Complications of enteral nutrition. In: *Artificial Nutrition Support in Clinical Practice* (eds J. Payre-James, G. Grimble & D. Silk), pp. 247–56. Edward Arnold, London.

Heitman, B. (1994) Impedance: a valid method in assessment of body composition? *Eur J Clin Nutr*, **48**, 228–40.

Jensen, T.G. *et al.* (1983) *Nutritional Assessment – A Manual for Practitioners*. Prentice-Hall, London.

Jones, E. (1998) Surgical excision of a pharyngeal pouch. *Prof Nurse*, **13**(6), 378–81.

Kinney, J.M. (1995) Metabolic response to starvation, injury and sepsis. In: *Artificial Nutrition Support in Clinical Practice* (eds J. Payne-James, G. Grimble & D. Silk), pp. 1–11. Edward Arnold, London.

Lennard-Jones, J.E. (1992) *A Positive Approach to Nutrition as Treatment*. King's Fund Centre, London.

Logemann, J. (1998) *The Evaluation and Treatment of Swallowing Disorders*, 2nd edn. College Hill Press, San Diego.

Mercadante, S. (1998) Parenteral versus enteral nutrition in cancer patients: indications and practice. *Support Cancer Care*, **6**, 85–93.

Metheny, N., Reed, L., Wiersema, L. *et al.* (1993) Effectiveness of pH measurements in predicting tube placement: an update. *Nurs Res*, **42**(6), 324–31.

Moran, B.J. (1994) Access methods in nutritional support. *Proc Nutr Soc*, **53**, 465–71.

Naber, T.H.J., Schermer, T., de Bree, A. et al. (1997) Prevalence of malnutrition in nonsurgical hospitalised patients and its association with disease complications. Am J Clin Nutr, 66, 1232–9.

Naysmith, M.R. & Nicholson, J. (1998) Nasogastric drug administration. Prof Nurse, 13(7), 424–7.

Newman, L.A., Vieira, F., Schwiezer, V. et al. (1998) Eating and weight changes following chemoradiation therapy for advanced head and neck cancer. Arch Otolaryngol Head Neck Surg, 124, 589–92.

Nordenström, J. (1995) Metabolic complications of parenteral nutrition. In: Artificial Nutrition Support in Clinical Practice (eds J. Payne-James, G. Grimble & D. Silk), pp. 333–42. Edward Arnold, London.

Nutricia Clinical Care (1996) The Flocare Gastrostomy Range: A Guide to Professional Care. Nutricia Clinical Care, Cow & Gate Nutricia, Trowbridge.

O'Morain, C. et al. (1984) Elemental diet as a primary treatment of acute Crohn's disease: a controlled trial. Br Med J, 288, 1859–62.

Passwood, R. & Eastwood, M.A. (eds) (1986) Special feeding methods. In: Human Nutrition and Dietetics, pp. 490–501. Churchill Livingstone, Edinburgh.

Patrick, P.G., Marulendra, S., Kirby, D.F. et al. (1997) Endoscopic nasogastric-jejunal feeding tube placement in critically ill patients. Gastrointest Endosc, 45(1), 72–6.

Payne-James, J. (1995) Enteral nutrition: tubes and techniques of delivery. In: Artificial Nutrition Support in Clinical Practice (eds J. Payne-James, G. Grimble & D. Silk), pp. 197–213. Edward Arnold, London.

Pennington, C.R. (1997) Disease and malnutrition in British hospitals. Proc Nutr Soc, 56, 393–407.

Pichard, C. & Jeejeebhoy, K.N. (1993) Nutritional management of clinical undernutrition. In: Human Nutrition and Dietetics (eds J.S. Garrow & W.P.T. James), 9th edn., pp. 421–39. Churchill Livingstone, Edinburgh.

Ralph, A. (1993) Methods for dietary assessment. In: Human Nutrition and Dietetics (eds J.S. Garrow & W.P.T. James), 9th edn., pp. 777–81. Churchill Livingstone, Edinburgh.

Rapin, C.H. (1995) Nutrition support and the elderly. In: Artificial Nutrition Support in Clinical Practice (eds J. Payne-James, G. Grimble & D. Silk), pp. 535–44. Edward Arnold, London.

Reilly, H. (1996) Nutrition in clinical management: malnutrition in our midst. Proc Nutr Soc, 55, 841–53.

Reilly, H. (1998) Parenteral nutrition: an overview of current practice. Br J Nurs, 7(8), 461–7.

Righi, P.D., Reddy, D.K., Weisberger, E.C. et al. (1998) Radiologic percutaneous gastrostomy: results in 56 patients with head and neck cancer. Laryngoscope, 108, 1020–24.

Rollins, H. (1997) A nose for trouble. Nurs Times, 93(49), 66–7.

Ruppin, H. & Lux, G. (1986) Percutaneous endoscopic gastrotomy in patients with head and neck cancer. Endoscopy, 18, 149–52.

Schofield, W.N. (1985) Predicting basal metabolic rate. New standards and review of previous work. Human Nutr Clin Nutr, 39C, Suppl. 15, 41.

Shenkin, A. (1995) Adult micronutrient requirements. In: Artificial Nutrition Support in Clinical Practice (eds J. Payne-James, G. Grimble & D. Silk), pp. 151–66. Edward Arnold, London.

Silk, D.B.A. (1995) Enteral diet choices and formulations. In: Artificial Nutrition Support in Clinical Practice (eds J. Payne-James, G. Grimble & D. Silk), pp. 215–45. Edward Arnold, London.

Silverman, D.W., Campbell, S.M. & Renk, C. (1990) Comparison of two handling techniques on microbiological quality of pre-filled enteral feedings. J Am Diet Assoc, 90, A134.

Sitges-Serra, A. & Franch-Arcas, G. (1995) Nutrition assessment. In: Artificial Nutrition Support in Clinical Practice (eds J. Payne-James, G. Grimble & D. Silk), pp. 125–36. Edward Arnold, London.

Taylor, S.J. (1988) A guide to NG feeding equipment. Prof Nurse, Nov, 91–4.

Taylor, T.V. et al. (1974) Ascorbic acid supplementation in the treatment of pressure sores. Lancet, 7, 544–6.

The Royal Marsden NHS Trust (1994) Patient Information Series No. 9. Overcoming Eating Difficulties. Haigh & Hochland, London.

Thomas, B. (1994) Manual of Dietetic Practice, 2nd edn. Blackwell Science, Oxford.

Thomas, D.R. (1997) Specific nutritional factors in wound healing. Advances Wound Care, 10(4), 40–43.

Todorovic, V.E. & Micklewright, A. (1997) A Pocket Guide to Clinical Nutrition, 2nd edn. British Dietetic Association, Birmingham.

Walden, D. & Klein, S. (1992) Nutritional assessment. Curr Opin Gastroenterology, 8, 286–9.

Weinstein, S.M. (1997) Plumer's Principles and Practice of Intravenous Therapy, 6th edn. J.B. Lippincott, Philadelphia.

Wyszynski, D.F., Crivelli, A., Ezquerro, S. et al. (1998) Assessment of nutritional status in a population of recently hospitalised patients. Mecinina, 58, 51–7.

GUIDELINES · Nasogastric intubation with tubes using an introducer

Equipment

1 Clinically clean tray.
2 Fine-bore nasogastric tube.
3 Introducer for tube.
4 Sterile receiver.
5 Sterile water.
6 10 ml syringe.
7 Hypoallergenic tape.
8 Adhesive patch if available.
9 Glass of water.
10 Lubricating jelly.
11 Indicator strips, e.g. pH Fix, 0–6, Fisher Scientific.

Prior to performing this procedure the patient's medical and nursing notes should be consulted to check for potential complications. For example, anatomical alterations due to surgery, such as a flap repair or the presence of a cancerous tumour, can prevent a clear passage for the nasogastric tube, resulting in pain and discomfort for the patient and further complications.

Procedure

Action	Rationale

Action

Rationale

1 Explain and discuss the procedure with the patient.

To ensure that the patient understands the procedure and gives his/her valid consent.

2 Arrange a signal by which the patient can communicate if he/she wants the nurse to stop, e.g. by raising his/her hand.

The patient is often less frightened if he/she feels able to have some control over the procedure.

3 Assist the patient to sit in a semi-upright position in the bed or chair. Support the patient's head with pillows *Note*: The head should not be tilted backwards or forwards (Rollins 1997).

To allow for easy passage of the tube. This position enables easy swallowing and ensures that the epiglottis is not obstructing the oesophagus.

4 Select the appropriate distance mark on the tube by measuring the distance on the tube from the patient's ear lobe to the bridge of the nose plus the distance from the bridge of the nose to the bottom of the xiphisternum.

To ensure that the appropriate length of tube is passed into the stomach.

5 Wash hands with bactericidal soap and water or bactericidal alcohol hand rub, and assemble the equipment required.

To minimize cross-infection.

6 Inject 10 ml sterile water down the tube before inserting introducer. Lubricate proximal end of tube with jelly.

Contact with water activates coating inside tube and on the tip. This lubricates the tube assisting its passage through the nasopharynx and allowing easy withdrawal of the introducer.

7 Check that the nostrils are patent by asking the patient to sniff with one nostril closed. Repeat with the other nostril.

To identify any obstructions liable to prevent intubation.

8 Insert the rounded end of the tube into the clearest nostril and slide it backwards and inwards along the floor of the nose to the nasopharynx. If any obstruction is felt, withdraw the tube and try again in a slightly different direction or use the other nostril.

To facilitate the passage of the tube by following the natural anatomy of the nose.

9 As the tube passes down into the nasopharynx, ask the patient to start swallowing and sipping water.

To focus the patient's attention on something other than the tube. A swallowing action closes the glottis, enabling the tube to pass into the oesophagus.

10 Advance the tube through the pharynx, as the patient swallows until the predetermined mark has been reached. If the patient shows signs of distress, e.g. gasping or cyanosis, remove the tube immediately.

The tube may have accidentally been passed down the trachea instead of the pharynx. Distress may indicate that the tube is in the bronchus.

11 Remove the introducer by using gentle traction. If it is difficult to remove, then remove the tube as well.

If the introducer sticks in the tube, it may be indicative that the tube is in the bronchus.

12 Check the position of the tube to confirm that it is in the stomach by using one of the following three mathods:

(a) Taking an X-ray of chest and upper abdomen;

To confirm placement of radio-opaque NG tube. X-ray of radio-opaque tubes is the most accurate confirmation of position and is the method of choice in patients with altered anatomy, those who are aspirating or are unconscious with no gag reflex.

(b) Aspirating 2 ml of stomach contents and testing this with pH indicator strips (Rollins 1997). When aspirating fluid for pH testing, wait at least one hour after a feed or medication has been administered (either orally or via the tube). Before aspirating, flush the tube with 20 ml of air to clear other substances (Metheny *et al*. 1993). pH

Indicator strips can distinguish between gastric acid (pH < 3) and bronchial secretions (pH > 6) (Rollins 1997). Wait at least 1 hour before aspirating to enable the feed or medication to be absorbed, otherwise an inaccurate test result will be obtained.

Guidelines • Nasogastric intubation with tubes using an introducer (cont'd)

Action	Rationale
indicator strips should not be used on patients who are receiving acid-inhibiting agents (defined as H2 receptor antagonists). With these patients the pH value of aspirate from the stomach will range from 0 through to 6.0 (Metheny *et al.*, 1993). Certain types of fine-bore feeding tubes cannot be aspirated, therefore it is necessary to use one of the other methods for checking the position of the tube.	
(c) Introducing 5 ml of air into the stomach via the tube and checking for a bubbling sound using a stethoscope placed over the epigastrium (Jones 1998).	Air can be detected by a bubbling sound when entering the stomach.
13 Secure the tube to the nostril with adherent dressing tape, e.g. elastoplast (Burns *et al.* 1995). If contraindicated, a hypoallergenic tape should be used. An adhesive patch (if available) will secure the tube to the cheek.	To hold the tube in place. To ensure patient comfort. Feeding via the tube must not begin until the correct position of the tube has been confirmed.

GUIDELINES • Nasogastric intubation with tubes without using an introducer, e.g. a Ryle's tube

Equipment

1 Clinically clean tray.
2 Nasogastric tube that has been stored in a deep freeze for at least half an hour before the procedure is to begin, to ensure a rigid tube that will allow for easy passage.
3 Topical gauze.
4 Lubricating jelly.
5 Hypoallergenic tape.

6 20 ml syringe.
7 Indicator strips, e.g. pH Fix, 0–6, Fisher Scientific.
8 Receiver.
9 Spigot.
10 Glass of water.
11 Stethoscope.

Procedure

Action	Rationale
1 Explain and discuss the procedure with the patient.	To ensure that the patient understands the procedure and gives his/her valid consent.
2 Arrange a signal by which the patient can communicate if he/she wants the nurse to stop, e.g. by raising his/her hand.	The patient is often less frightened if he/she feels able to have some control over the procedure.
3 Assist the patient to sit in a semi-upright position in the bed or chair. Support the patient's head with pillows.	To allow for easy passage of the tube. This position enables easy swallowing and ensures that the epiglottis is not obstructing the oesophagus.
4 Mark the distance which the tube is to be passed by measuring the distance on the tube from the patient's ear lobe to the bridge of the nose plus the distance from the bridge of the nose to the bottom of the xiphisternum.	To indicate the length of tube required for entry into the stomach.
5 Wash hands with bactericidal soap and water or bactericidal alcohol hand rub, and assemble the equipment required.	To minimize cross-infection.
6 Check the patient's nostrils are patent by asking him/her to sniff with one nostril closed. Repeat with the other nostril.	To identify any obstructions liable to prevent intubation.
7 Lubricate about 15–20 cm of the tube with a thin coat of lubricating jelly that has been placed on a topical swab.	To reduce the friction between the mucous membranes and the tube.

Action	Rationale
8 Insert the proximal end of the tube into the clearest nostril and slide it backwards and inwards along the floor of the nose to the nasopharynx. If an obstruction is felt, withdraw the tube and try again in a slightly different direction or use the other nostril.	To facilitate the passage of the tube by following the natural anatomy of the nose.
9 As the tube passes down into the nasopharynx, ask the patient to start swallowing and sipping water.	To focus the patient's attention on something other than the tube. The swallowing action closes the glottis, enabling the tube to pass into the oesophagus.
10 Advance the tube through the pharynx as the patient swallows until the tape-marked tube reaches the point of entry into the external nares. If the patient shows signs of distress, e.g. gasping or cyanosis, remove the tube immediately.	Distress may indicate that the tube is in the bronchus.
11 Check the position of the tube to confirm that it is in the stomach by using one of the following three methods:	
(a) Taking an X-ray of chest and upper abdomen;	To confirm placement of radio-opaque NG tube. X-ray of radio-opaque tubes is the most accurate confirmation of position and is the method of choice in patients with altered anatomy, those who are aspirating or are unconscious with no gag reflex.
(b) Aspirating 2 ml of stomach contents and testing this with pH indicator strips (Rollins 1997). When aspirating fluid for pH testing, wait at least one hour after a feed or medication has been administered (either orally or via the tube). Before aspirating, flush the tube with 20 ml of air to clear other substances (Metheny *et al.* 1993). Feeding via the tube must not begin until the position of the tube has been confirmed.	Indicator strips can distinguish between gastric acid (pH < 3) and bronchial secretions (pH > 6) (Rollins 1997). Wait at least 1 hour before aspirating to enable the feed or medication to be absorbed, otherwise an inaccurate test result will be obtained.
(c) Introducing 5 ml of air into the stomach via the tube and checking for a bubbling sound using a stethoscope placed over the epigastrium (Jones 1998).	Air can be detected by a bubbling sound when entering the stomach.
12 Secure the tube to the nostril with adherent dressing tape, e.g. elastoplast (Burns *et al.* 1995). If contraindicated, a hypoallergenic tape should be used. An adhesive patch (if available) will secure the tube to the cheek.	To hold the tube in place. To ensure patient comfort.

GUIDELINES • Care of a percutaneous endoscopically placed gastrostomy (PEG) tube

This procedure should be performed daily and should begin approximately 24 hours following insertion. This will help maintain skin integrity and detect any problems early, e.g. infection, skin breakdown.

Equipment

1 Sterile procedure pack containing gallipot, low-linting gauze.
2 9% sodium chloride or antiseptic solution.

Procedure

Action

1 Explain and discuss the procedure with the patient.

Rationale

To ensure that the patient understands the procedure and gives his/her valid consent.

Guidelines • Care of a percutaneous endoscopically placed gastrostomy (PEG) tube (cont'd)

Action	Rationale
2 Perform procedure using aseptic technique. Self-caring patients should be taught socially clean technique.	To prevent cross-infection (for further information see procedure on aseptic technique). Risk of cross-infection is greatly reduced if patients carry out self-care.
3 Remove postprocedural dressing if in place. Observe peristomal skin and stoma site for signs of infection, irritation or excoriation.	To gain access to stoma site. To detect complications early and instigate appropriate treatment.
4 Note the number of the measuring guide on the tube closest to the end of the external fixation device. Loosen the tube from the fixation device and ease fixation device away from the abdomen.	To ensure gastrostomy tube is reattached to the fixation device in the correct position. To ensure stoma site is thoroughly cleansed.
5 Clean the stoma site with a sterile solution such as 0.9% sodium chloride. Using low-linting gauze dry the area thoroughly.	To remove any exudate, to prevent infection and skin excoriation.
6 Rotate the gastrostomy tube 360°.	To prevent the tube adhering to the sides of the stoma tract.
7 Gently push the external fixation device against the abdomen.	To enable the gastrostomy tube to be reattached to the fixation device.
8 Gently but firmly pull the gastrostomy tube and attach to the fixation device.	To ensure that the tube is correctly secured.
9 Ensure the correct point on the measuring guide on the tube is placed closest to the end of the fixation device.	To ensure that the tube is correctly secured. If the patient gains weight the external fixation device should be released slightly to prevent pressure necrosis of the stoma site.
10 Do not cover the gastrostomy site with a new dressing unless there is a heavy discharge or leakage from the stoma site.	To encourage wound healing.
11 Do not use bulky dressings, particularly under the external fixation device.	This can increase the pressure on the internal retention disc or retention balloon and increase the risk of tissue necrosis and ulceration occurring in the stomach (Nutricia Clinical Care 1996).
12 Advise the patient not to use moisturizing creams or talcum powder around the stoma site.	To prevent infection and/or irritation to skin. The grease in creams can cause the external retention device to slip, allowing movement of the tube and increasing the risk of leakage and infection. Creams and talcs can affect the tube material, causing it to stretch or leak (Nutricia Clinical Care 1996).
Patients should be taught how to carry out this procedure themselves. Once the stoma site has healed (approximately 10 days postinsertion) it is no longer necessary to perform an	aseptic technique. A socially clean procedure using soap and water to cleanse the stoma site should be adopted.

Nursing care plan

Supervision of patients with swallowing difficulties is important and in some cases patients may require support at meal times, or when drinking, to carry out the recommended strategies. It is important for nurses to participate in educational programmes for patients and carers in order to encourage awareness of the implications of dysphagia. Anxieties associated with dysphagia should be allayed and confidence to undertake safe eating and drinking techniques built up. Patients may experience one or a number of the following problems.

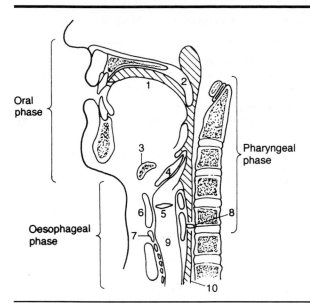

Figure 27.1 The normal swallow.
(1 tongue; 2 soft palate; 3 hyoid bone; 4 epiglottis; 5 vocal
cords; 6 thyroid cartilage; 7 cricoid cartilage; 8
pharyngoesophageal sphincter; 9 trachea; 10 oesophagus.)
The oral, pharyngeal and oesophageal phases are separate
but highly coordinated.

Problem	Cause	Prevention	Suggested action
Patient experiencing difficulties with drinking and/or eating (which may lead to dehydration, insufficient nutritional intake, and compromised airway).	(a) Mechanical. Patients who have undergone surgery and/or radiotherapy to the oral cavity, pharynx, larynx, or trachea (including temporary or permanent tracheostomy) are likely to experience swallowing difficulties of a temporary or more persistent nature (Fig. 27.1). (b) Neurological. Patients who have tumours which affect the brain stem area and thus the cranial nerves will present with symptoms of dysphagia. These symptoms will continue as long as the disease and/or treatment effects are evident. (c) Oesophageal obstruction or dysfunction. Patients who have tumours of the upper gastrointestinal tract may well experience		Refer to specialist speech and language therapist for full assessment and management plan. Refer to dietitian for nutritional assessment and management plan.

Problem	Cause	Prevention	Suggested action
	discomfort and difficulty with the oesophageal phase of the swallow. The only way to alleviate oesophageal difficulties is through medical or surgical management. Swallowing therapy is not indicated in these circumstances, although the specialist speech and language therapist may be able to offer advice to mininize difficulties experienced by the patient.		
Dehydration and/or difficulty in maintaining adequate hydration.	Thin liquids (e.g. water) are difficult for the patient with dysphagia to manage. Watery liquids do not retain their cohesion in the mouth and therefore pass swiftly into the pharynx. Patients may avoid liquids of this consistency and become dehydrated.	Identify patients who are at risk.	Seek medical advice on the appropriateness of intravenous hydration.
Difficulty in maintaining a clear airway (may be severe enough to block airway in tracheostomy patients).	Inability to manage secretions, indicated by drooling and/or gurgly voice. Tracheostomy patients may feel breathing is laboured.	Monitor patient's progress carefully and regularly and liaise with the speech and language therapist about any changes noted.	Following assessment by specialist speech and language therapist, adjusting the patient's position may help (e.g. sitting posture and head position before and after swallowing). Oral suction may be required. See Chap. 40, Tracheostomy Care and Laryngectomy Voice Rehabilitation.
Patient requires nutritional support and/or alternative feeding method.	Dysphagia and/or disease process leading to inadequate nutrition.	All patients with dysphagia should be fully assessed by a dietitian to ensure current nutritional requirements are met by nutritional support, alternative feeding method, normal diet, or a combination of these.	Nutritional support and/or alternative feeding method may be indicated following discussion with members of the multidisciplinary team. Following assessment by a specialist speech and language therapist recommendations may be made about sitting posture, head position, and consistency of food and drink. These will be

			individually tailored to the patient's needs. Nursing staff should monitor progress carefully, noting changes and reporting them to the appropriate professional.
Dysphagia in oral and/or pharyngeal stages of swallowing, related to head position and or structural or neurological deficits.	Patients with tumours of the upper gastrointestinal tract may experience difficulty with the oesophageal phase of the swallow; patients with tumours affecting the brain stem/cranial nerves will experience dysphagia.		Proceed as advised by the specialist speech and language therapist: modified head positions, e.g. turned to the affected or unaffected side, tilted to the unaffected side, or chin flexed may be appropriate. Do *not* attempt these manoeuvres without prior assessment and advice from a specialist speech and language therapist.
Selecting suitable food and/or drink.	Not all members of the multidisciplinary team and/or catering and other staff may be aware of the extent of the patient's swallowing difficulties.	Liaise with specialist speech and language therapist and dietitian.	Provide food and drink of a consistency which will not exacerbate the patient's problems. This might include soft foods, thickened liquids, or purees. Food and drink must be individually tailored to suit the patient.

(Groher 1997; Logemann 1998)

Observations

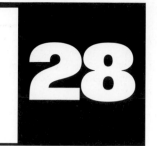

Pulse

Definition

The pulse is an impulse transmitted to arteries by contraction of the left ventricle, and customarily palpated where an artery crosses a bone, for example, the radial artery at the wrist (Roper 1995).

Indications

The pulse is taken for the following reasons:

1 To gather information on the heart rate, pattern of beats (rhythm) and amplitude (strength) of pulse.
2 To determine the individual's pulse on admission as a base for comparing future measurements.
3 To monitor changes in pulse.

Reference material

The arterial pulse rate reflects the heart rate and is influenced by activity, postural changes and emotion (Marieb 1998). Each time the heart beats, it propels blood through the arteries. This pumping action of the heart causes the walls of the arteries to expand and distend. The effect can be felt with the fingers as a wave-like sensation felt as the pulse (Timby 1989). The pulse can be felt in any arteries lying close to the body surface (Fig. 28.1) by lightly compressing the artery against firm tissue and by recording the number of beats (Timby 1989).

The pulse is palpated to note the following:

1 Rate
2 Rhythm
3 Amplitude.

Rate

The normal pulse rate varies in different client groups as age-related changes affect the pulse rate. The approximate range is illustrated in Table 28.1 (Timby 1989).

The pulse may vary depending on the posture of an individual. For example, the pulse of a healthy man may be around 66 beats per minute when he is lying down; this increases to 70 when sitting up, and 80 when he stands suddenly (Marieb 1998).

The rate of the pulse of an individual with a healthy heart tends to be relatively constant. However, when blood

volume drops suddenly or when the heart has been weakened by disease, the stroke volume declines and cardiac output is maintained only by increasing the rate of heart beat.

Cardiac output is the amount of blood pumped out by each heart ventricle in 1 minute, while the stroke volume is the amount of blood pumped out by a ventricle with each contraction. The relationship between these and the heart rate is expressed in the following equation:

$$\text{Cardiac output} = \text{heart rate} \times \text{stroke volume}$$

The heart rate and hence pulse rate are influenced by various factors acting through neural, chemical and physically induced homeostatic mechanisms (Fig. 28.2):

1 Neural changes in heart rate are caused by the activation of the sympathetic nervous system which increases heart rate, while parasympathetic activation decreases heart rate (Ganong 1995).
2 Chemical regulation of the heart is affected by hormones (adrenaline and thyroxine) and electrolytes (sodium, potassium and calcium) (Ganong 1995). High or low levels of electrolytes particularly potassium, magnesium and calcium can cause an alteration in the heart's rhythm and rate.
3 Physical factors that influence heart rate are age, sex, exercise and body temperature (Marieb 1998).

Tachycardia is defined as an abnormally fast heart rate, over 100 beats per minute in adults, which may result from a raised body temperature, increased sympathetic response due to physical/emotional stress, certain drugs or heart disease (Marieb 1998).

Bradycardia is a heart rate slower than 60 beats per minute. It may be the result of a low body temperature, certain drugs or parasympathetic nervous system activation. It is also found in fit athletes when physical and cardiovascular conditioning occurs. This results in hypertrophy of the heart with an increase in its stroke volume. These heart changes result in a lower resting heart rate but with the same cardiac output (Marieb 1998). If persistent bradycardia occurs in an individual as a result of ill health, this may result in inadequate blood circulation to body tissues. A slowing of the heart rate accompanied by a rise in blood pressure is one of the indications of raised intracranial pressure.

Rhythm

The pulse rhythm is the sequence of beats. In health, these are regular. The coordinated action of the muscles of the heart in producing a regular heart rhythm is due to the ability of cardiac muscle to contract inherently without nervous control (Marieb 1998). The coordinated action of the muscles in the heart results from two physiological factors:

1 Gap junctions in the cardiac muscles which form inter-connections between adjacent cardiac muscles and allow transmission of nervous impulses from cell to cell (Marieb 1998).

2 Specialized nerve-like cardiac cells that form the nodal system. These initiate and distribute impulses through-out the heart, so that the heart beats as one unit (Marieb 1998). These are the sinoatrial node, atrioventricular node, atrioventricular bundle and the Purkinje fibres.

The sinoatrial node is the pacemaker, initiating each wave of contraction. This sets the rhythm for the heart as a whole (Fig. 28.3). Its characteristic rhythm is called *sinus rhythm*.

Defects in the conduction system of the heart can cause irregular heart rhythms, or arrhythmias, resulting in unco-ordinated contraction of the heart.

Fibrillation is a condition of rapid and irregular contrac-tions. A fibrillating heart is ineffective as a pump (Marieb 1998). *Atrial fibrillation* is a disruption of rhythm in the atrial areas of the heart occurring at extremely rapid and uncoordinated intervals. The rapid impulses result in the ventricles not being able to respond to every atrial beat and, therefore, the ventricles contract irregularly. There are many causes of this condition, but the following are the most common: (1) ischaemic heart disease; (2) acute illness; (3) electrolyte abnormality; (4) thyrotoxicosis.

Ventricular fibrillation is an irregular heart rhythm char-acterized by chaotic contraction of the ventricles at very

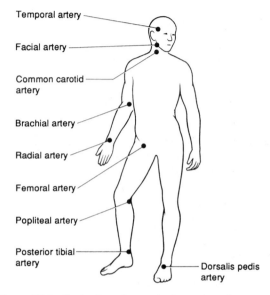

Figure 28.1 Body sites where pulse is most easily palpated. The pulse can be felt in arteries lying close to the body surface.

Table 28.1 Normal pulse rates per minute at various ages

Age	Approximate range	Average
Newborn	120–160	140
1–12 months	80–140	120
12 months–2 years	80–130	110
2–6 years	75–120	100
6–12 years	75–110	95
Adolescent	60–100	80
Adult	60–100	80

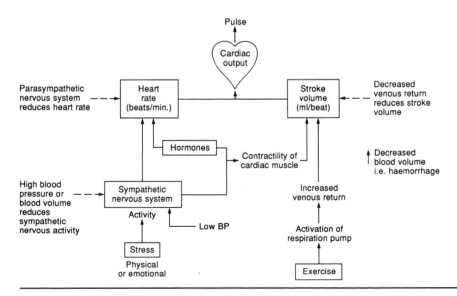

Figure 28.2 Influence of neural, chemical and physical factors on cardiac output and hence pulse.

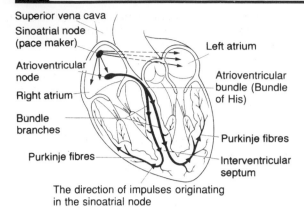

Superior vena cava
Sinoatrial node (pace maker)
Atrioventricular node
Right atrium
Bundle branches
Purkinje fibres
Left atrium
Atrioventricular bundle (Bundle of His)
Purkinje fibres
Interventricular septum
The direction of impulses originating in the sinoatrial node

Figure 28.3 Intrinsic conduction system of the heart.

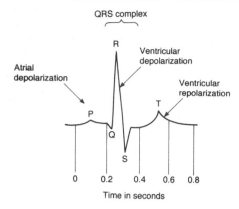

QRS complex
Atrial depolarization
Ventricular depolarization
Ventricular repolarization
R
P
Q
S
T
0 0.2 0.4 0.6 0.8
Time in seconds

Figure 28.4 An ECG tracing illustrating normal deflection waves.

rapid rates. Ventricular fibrillation results in cardiac arrest and death if not reversed with defibrillation and the injection of epinephrine. The cause of this condition is often myocardial infarction, electrical shock, acidosis, electrolyte disturbances and hypovolaemia.

Because body fluids are good conductors of electricity it is possible through electrocardiography to observe how the currents generated are transmitted through the heart. The electrocardiograph provides a graphic representation and record (electrocardiogram) of electrical activity as the heart beats. The electrocardiogram (ECG) makes it possible to identify abnormalities in electrical conduction within the heart. The normal ECG consists of a series of three distinct areas called deflection waves. The first of these is the P wave, which results from an electrical impulse in the sinoatrial node. The large QRS complex results from ventricular depolarization, and takes place prior to contraction of the heart muscles. The T wave is caused by ventricular repolarization. In a healthy heart, the size and rhythm of the deflection waves tend to remain constant (Fig. 28.4). Changes in the pattern or timing of the deflection in the ECG may indicate problems with the heart's conduction system, such as those caused by myocardial infarction (Marieb 1998). Examples of conduction abnormalities are shown in Fig. 28.5.

Amplitude

Amplitude is a reflection of pulse strength and the elasticity of the arterial wall. The flexibility of the artery of the young adult feels very different from the hard artery of the patient suffering from arteriosclerosis. It takes some clinical experience to appreciate the differences in amplitude. However, it is important to be able to recognize major changes such as the faint flickering pulse of the severely hypovolaemic patient.

Assessing gross pulse irregularity

Paradoxical pulse is a pulse that markedly decreases in amplitude during inspiration. On inspiration, more blood is

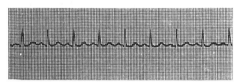

Normal sinus rhythm

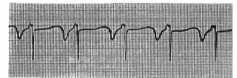

Junctional rhythm. Sinoatrial node is non-functional, P waves are absent and heart rate is paced by the AV node

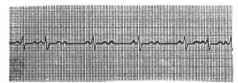

Second degree heart block. P waves are not conducted through the AV node

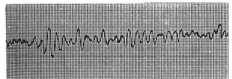

Ventricular fibrillation. Chaotic electrical conduction, grossly irregular. This is seen in an acute heart attack and electrical shock

Figure 28.5 Normal and abnormal ECG tracings.

pooled in the lungs and so decreases the return to the left side of the heart; this affects the consequent stroke volume. A paradoxical pulse is usually regarded as normal, although in conjunction with such features as hypotension and dyspnoea, it may indicate cardiac tamponade.

When there is a gross pulse irregularity, it may be useful to use a stethoscope to assess the apical heart beat. This is done by placing the diaphragm of the stethoscope over the apex of the heart and counting the beats for 60 seconds. A second nurse should record the radial pulse at the same time. The deficit between the two should be noted using, for example, different colours on the patient's chart to indicate the apex and radial rates.

Conditions where a patient's pulse may need careful monitoring are described below:

1 Postoperative and critically ill patients require monitoring of the pulse to assess for cardiovascular stability. The patient's pulse should be recorded pre-operatively in order to be able to make comparisons. Hypovolaemic shock post surgery from the loss of plasma or whole blood results in a decrease in circulatory blood volume. The resulting acceleration in heart rate causes a tachycardia that can be felt in the pulse. The greater the loss in volume the more thready the pulse is likely to feel.

2 Blood transfusions require the careful monitoring of the pulse as an incompatible blood transfusion may lead to a rise in pulse rate (Cluroe 1989) (see Chap. 41, Transfusion of Blood and Blood Products).

3 Patients with local or systemic infections or neutropenia require monitoring of their pulse to detect septicaemic shock. This is characterized by a decrease in the circulatory blood volume with a resulting rise in pulse rate.

4 Patients with cardiovascular conditions require regular assessment of the pulse to monitor their condition and the efficacy of medications.

Note: it should be noted that even where the patient has continuous ECG monitoring, such as in coronary care, A&E, ITU, it is still important to manually feel a pulse to determine amplitude and volume.

References and further reading

Birdsall, C. (1985) How do you interpret pulses? *Am J Nurs*, **85**(7), 785–6.

Cluroe, S. (1989) Blood transfusions. *Nursing*, **3**(40), 8–11.

Ganong, W.F. (1995) *Review of Medical Physiology*, 17th edn. Appelton & Lange, Norwalk, Connecticut.

Jarvis, C.M. (1980) Vital signs: a preview of problems. In: *Assessing Vital Functions Accurately*. Intermed Communications.

Hickey, J.V. (1986) *The Clinical Practice of Neurological and Neurosurgical Nursing*, 2nd edn. J.B. Lippincott, Philadelphia.

Marieb, E.M. (1998) *Human Anatomy and Physiology*, 4th edn. Benjamin Cummings, California.

Roper, N. (ed.) (1995) *Pocket Medical Dictionary*, p. 223. Churchill Livingstone, Edinburgh.

Timby, B. (1989) *Clinical Nursing Procedure*. J.B. Lippincott, Philadelphia.

Wieck, L. *et al.* (1986) *Illustrated Manual of Nursing Techniques*, 3rd edn. J.B. Lippincott, Philadelphia.

GUIDELINES · Pulse

Procedure

Action

1 Explain and discuss the procedure with the patient.

2 Measure where possible the pulse under the same conditions each time. Ensure that the patient is comfortable.

3 Place the second or third fingers along the appropriate artery and press gently.

4 Press gently against the peripheral artery being used to record the pulse.

5 The pulse should be counted for 60 sec.

6 Record the pulse rate.

Note: in children under 2 years of age, the pulse should not be taken in this way; the rapid pulse rate and small area for palpation can lead to inaccurate data. The heart rate should be

Rationale

To ensure that the patient understands the procedure and gives his/her valid consent.

To ensure continuity and consistency in recording.
To ensure that the patient is comfortable.

The fingertips are sensitive to touch. The thumb and forefinger have pulses of their own that may be mistaken for the patient's pulse.

The radial artery is usually used as it is often the most readily accessible.

Sufficient time is required to detect irregularities or other defects.

To monitor differences and detect trends; any irregularities should be brought to the attention of the appropriate personnel.

assessed by utilizing a stethoscope and listening to the apical heart beat.

12 Lead electrocardiogram (ECG)

Definition

A 12 lead ECG is a non-invasive procedure that is used to ascertain information about the electrophysiology of the heart. It is performed electively prior to various interventions such as surgery and anti-cancer chemotherapy. ECGs are also an important investigation during an acute situation, particularly in the presence of chest pain, haemodynamic disturbance or cardiac rhythm changes.

GUIDELINES • 12 Lead ECG

Equipment

1 ECG machine with chest and limb leads labelled respectively, e.g. LA to left arm, V1 to first chest lead.
2 Disposable electrodes.
3 Swabs saturated with 70% isopropyl alcohol.
4 Abrasive strips.

Procedure

Action	Rationale
1 Explain to the patient that the ECG is to be taken.	To ensure that the patient understands the procedure and gives his/her valid consent.
2 Ensure that the patient is comfortably positioned either lying or sitting.	To ensure optimal recording and comfort of the patient.
3 Clean limb and chest electrode sites (Fig. 28.6). If necessary, prepare skin by clipping hairs or use abrasive strip.	To ensure good grip and therefore good contact between skin and electrode which results in less electrical artefact.
4 Apply the ten electrodes as described in Fig. 28.6.	To obtain the ECG recording from vertical and horizontal planes.
5 Attach the ten leads from the ECG machine to the electrodes.	To obtain the ECG recording.
6 Check that the leads are connected correctly and to the relevant electrode.	To ensure the correct polarity in the ECG recording.
7 Ensure that the leads are not pulling on the electrodes or lying over each other.	To reduce electrical artefact and to obtain a good ECG recording.
8 Ask patient to relax and refrain from movement.	To obtain the optimal recording by the reduction of artefact from muscular movement.
9 Check that calibration is 10 mm/millivolt.	To ensure standard recording to aid interpretation.
10 Commence 12 lead recording.	To obtain ECG.
11 In the case of artefact or poor recording, check electrodes and connections.	To ensure optimal recording.
12 During the procedure give reassurance to the patient.	To ensure the patient feels informed and reassured.
13 If necessary, record a rhythm strip utilizing leads II and V1.	To assist with interpretation if there have been any acute rhythm disturbances.
14 Detach ECG printout and label with patient's name, hospital number, date and time.	To ensure that the ECG is labelled with the correct patient and date and time.
15 Inform patient that the procedure is now finished and help to remove the electrodes.	To ensure that the patient can relax and that the electrodes are removed.
16 Mount the ECG recording in the appropriate documentation.	To ensure that the recording does not get lost.
17 Inform medical staff that ECG has been completed and its location.	To enable relevant medical staff to use the ECG data in their care planning.

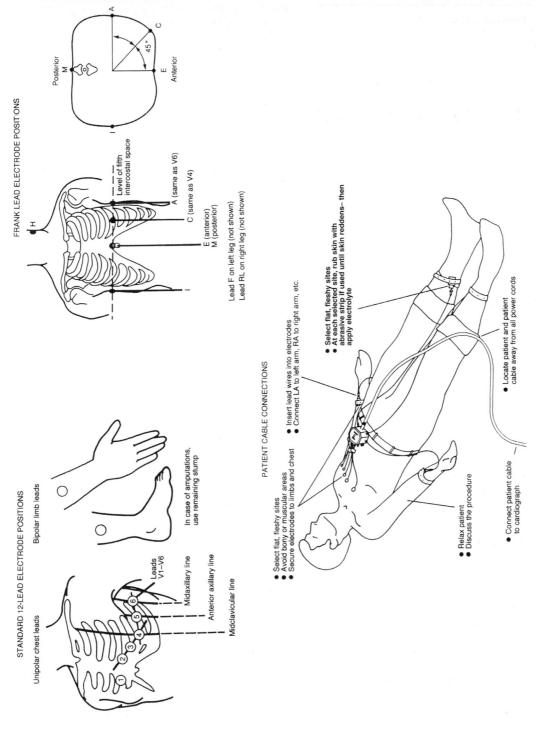

FRANK LEAD ELECTRODE POSITIONS

Posterior M

A

C

45°

E

Anterior

H

Level of fifth intercostal space

A (same as V6)

C (same as V4)

E (anterior)
M (posterior)

Lead F on left leg (not shown)
Lead RL on right leg (not shown)

STANDARD 12-LEAD ELECTRODE POSITIONS

Unipolar chest leads

Bipolar limb leads

In case of amputations, use remaining stump

Leads V1–V6

Midaxillary line

Anterior axillary line

Midclavicular line

PATIENT CABLE CONNECTIONS

- Insert lead wires into electrodes
- Connect LA to left arm, RA to right arm, etc.

- Select flat, fleshy sites
- At each selected site, rub skin with abrasive strip if used until skin reddens– then apply electrolyte

- Select flat, fleshy sites
- Avoid bony or muscular areas
- Secure electrodes to limbs and chest

- Relax patient
- Discuss the procedure

- Connect patient cable to cardiograph

- Locate patient and patient cable away from all power cords

Figure 28.6 12 lead ECG. (Courtesy of Agilent Technologies Ltd.)

Blood pressure

Definition

Blood pressure may be defined as the force exerted by blood against the walls of the vessels in which it is contained. Differences in blood pressure between different areas of the circulation provide the driving force that keeps the blood moving through the body (Marieb 1998). Blood pressure is usually expressed in terms of millimetres of mercury (mm Hg).

Indications

Blood pressure is measured for one of two reasons:

1 To determine the patient's blood pressure on admission as a baseline for comparision with future measurements.
2 To monitor fluctuations in blood pressure.

Reference material

Blood flow is defined as the volume of blood flowing through a vessel at a given time from the heart. Blood flow is equivalent to cardiac output. Resistance to the cardiac output is opposite to flow and is a measure of the friction the blood encounters as it passes through the differently sized vessels (Marieb 1998)'. There are three important sources of resistance: blood viscosity, vessel length and vessel diameter (Fig. 28.7).

Viscosity is the internal resistance to flow and may be thought of as the 'stickiness' of a fluid. Blood is more viscous than water due to the elements of plasma proteins and cells that form its constituent parts, and consequently blood moves more slowly. The longer the vessel length, the greater the resistance encountered. The relationship between vessel length and viscosity is often constant; however, blood vessel diameter changes frequently and is an important factor in altering peripheral resistance. Increased peripheral resistance occurs by altering the fluid flow. In a small blood vessel more of the fluid is in contact with the vessel walls which results in increased friction. Arterioles are the major determinants of peripheral resistance because they are small-diameter blood vessels which can expand in response to neural and chemical controls (Ganong 1995).

Normal blood pressure is maintained by neural, chemical and renal controls. The neural controls operate via reflex arcs (Marieb 1998) derived from stretch receptors found in the wall of the proximal arterial tree, especially in the region of the aortic arch and carotid sinuses. When arterial pressure rises, there is increased stimulation of these nerve endings. The increased number of impulses along the vagus and glossopharyngeal nerves leads to reflex vagal slowing of the heart and reflex release of vasoconstrictor tone in the peripheral blood vessels. The resulting fall in cardiac output and the reduction of peripheral resistance tend to restore the blood pressure to the normal

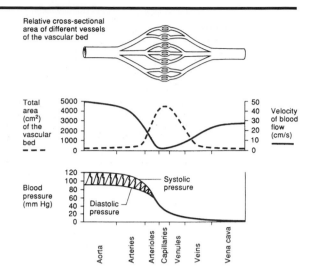

Relative cross-sectional area of different vessels of the vascular bed

Figure 28.7 Effect of vessel length and diameter on blood pressure and blood flow.

value. A fall in the arterial pressure decreases the stimulation of the arterial stretch receptors. The reflex tachycardia and vasoconstriction that ensue tend to raise the blood pressure to its normal value, forming a continuous homeostatic process (Ganong 1995). When the oxygen content of the blood drops sharply, chemoreceptors in the aortic arch transmit impulses to the vasomotor centre and reflex constriction occurs. The rise in blood pressure that follows helps to increase blood return to the heart and lungs (Marieb 1998). Renal regulation provides a major long-term mechanism of influencing blood pressure. When there is a fall in arterial pressure this results in chemical changes which lead to the release of the enzyme renin. Renin triggers a series of enzymatic reactions that result in the formation of angiotensin, a powerful vasoconstrictor chemical. Angiotensin also stimulates the adrenal cortex to release aldosterone, a hormone that increases renal reabsorption of sodium. The sodium, in turn, increases the volume of water reabsorbed by the kidneys; such retention of fluid and vasoconstriction of blood vessels raises arterial pressure (Marieb 1998).

Blood pressure varies not only from moment to moment but also in the distribution between various organs and areas of the body. It is lowest in neonates and increases with age, weight gain, with stress and anxiety (Marieb 1998). Shock, myocardial infarction and haemorrhage are factors that cause a fall in blood pressure as they reduce cardiac output and peripheral vessel resistance or they diminish venous return after fluid loss (Fig. 28.8).

Normal blood pressure

Normal blood pressure generally ranges from 100/60 to 140/90 mm Hg. Blood pressure can fluctuate within a wide range and still be considered normal.

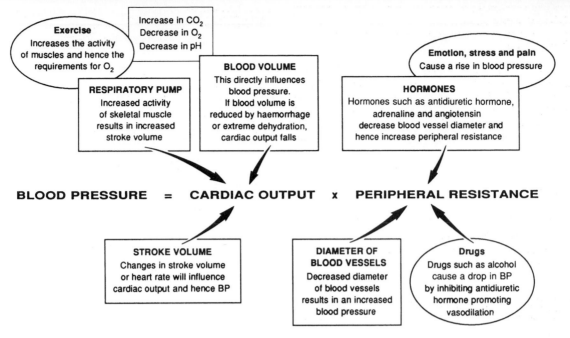

Figure 28.8 Factors that lead to a change in blood pressure.

Systolic pressure

The systolic pressure is the maximum pressure of the blood against the wall of the vessel following ventricular contraction and is taken as an indication of the integrity of the heart, arteries and arterioles (Marieb 1998).

Diastolic pressure

The diastolic pressure is the minimum pressure of the blood against the wall of the vessel following closure of the aortic valve and is taken as a direct indication of blood vessel resistance (Marieb 1998).

Hypotension or low blood pressure is generally defined in adults as a systolic blood pressure below 100 mm Hg (Marieb 1998). In many cases, hypotension simply reflects individual variations; however, it may indicate orthostatic hypotension, i.e. postural changes that result in a lack of normal reflex response leading to a low blood pressure, or it may be the first indicator of a shock condition, e.g. septic shock, cardiogenic, hypovolaemic or toxic shock syndrome.

Hypertension is defined as an elevation of systolic blood pressure. This may be a temporary response to fever, physical exertion or stress. Persistent hypertension is a common disease and approximately 30% of people over the age of 50 years are hypertensive (Marieb 1998). Persistent hypertension is diagnosed in an individual when the average of three or more blood pressure readings taken at rest, several days apart, exceeds the upper limits of what is considered normal for the patient.

Mean arterial pressure

The mean arterial pressure is the average pressure required to push blood through the circulatory system. This can be determined electronically or mathematically as well as by using an intra-arterial catheter and mercury manometer.

Mathematically, for example:

$$\text{mean arterial pressure} = \frac{1}{3} \text{ systolic pressure} + \frac{2}{3} \text{ diastolic pressure}$$

A blood pressure of 130/85 mm Hg gives a mean arterial pressure of 100 mm Hg.

Factors affecting blood pressure

The main factors that regulate blood pressure by altering peripheral resistance and blood volume are shown in Fig. 28.8.

Methods of recording and equipment

There are two main methods for recording the blood pressure: direct and indirect. *Direct* methods are more accurate than indirect methods. The most accurate method of measuring blood pressure involves the insertion of a minute pressure transducer unit into an artery for transmission of a waveform or digital display on a monitor. The most commonly used techniques involve placing a cannula in an artery and attaching a pressure-sensitive device to the external end.

Patients who need to be constantly monitored, e.g. in theatres, high-dependency and intensive care units, may require such devices to be used. In such patients it is essential to have an early knowledge of any change in the blood pressure, as this may indicate a deterioration in condition and require prompt treatment.

The *indirect* method is the auscultatory method. This procedure is used to measure blood pressure in the brachial artery of the arm.

A blood pressure reading can either be taken by the traditional method of a sphygmomanometer or electronically, using a device such as a dynamap. With any piece of equipment, adequate training should be provided, to ensure accuracy.

The sphygmomanometer

The sphygmomanometer (Fig. 28.9) consists of a compression bag enclosed in an unyielding cuff, and inflating bulb, pump or other device by which the pressure is increased, a manometer from which the applied pressure is read, and a control valve to deflate the system.

Manometer

Mercury sphygmomanometers are reliable, on the whole, and are easy to maintain. Any damaged equipment should either be repaired or disposed of. Correct disposal is important due to the risk of mercury contamination (HSE 1989). While in use, the manometer must be kept in a vertical position, otherwise substantial errors can occur (Campbell *et al.* 1990).

Cuff

The cuff is made of washable material that encircles the arm and encloses the inflatable rubber bladder. It is secured around the arm or leg by wrapping its tapering end to the encircling material, usually by Velcro.

Inflatable bladder

A bladder that is too short and/or too narrow will give falsely high pressures. The British Hypertension Society recommended in 1986 that the centre of the bladder should cover the brachial artery and that the bladder length should be 80% of the arm circumference and the width at least 40% (Gillespie & Curzio 1998).

Control valve, pump and rubber tubing

The control valve is a common source of error. It should allow the passage of air without excessive pressure needing to be applied on the pump. When the valve is closed it should hold the mercury at a constant level and, when released, it should allow a controlled fall in the level of mercury. The rubber tubing should be long (approximately 80 cm) and with airtight connections that can easily be separated.

Campbell *et al.* (1990), in reviewing the methods for sphygmomanometer inaccuracies, found that errors in

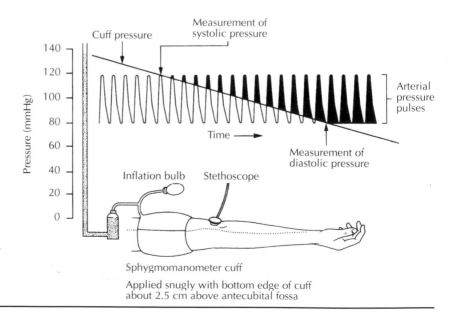

Figure 28.9 Using a sphygmomanometer, and the appearance and disappearance of Korotkoff's sounds.

technique and equipment malfunction accounted for differences in readings of more than 15 mm Hg. Problems with equipment malfunction were further supported in a study by Carney *et al.* (1995), who evaluated 463 sphygmomanometers and found that only 58% were in working order.

The stethoscope

Using the stethoscope it is possible to identify a series of five phases as blood pressure falls from the systolic to the diastolic. These phases are known as Korotkoff's sounds (Fig. 28.10).

When the cuff pressure has fallen to just below the systolic pressure, a clear but often faint tapping sound suddenly appears in phase with each cardiac contraction. The sound is produced by the transient and turbulent blood flowing through the brachial artery during the peak of each systole.

As the pressure in the cuff is reduced further, the sound becomes louder, but when the artery is no longer constricted and the blood flows freely, the sounds become muffled and then can no longer be heard. The diastolic pressure is usually defined as the cuff pressure at which the sounds disappear (Marieb 1998).

The stethoscope's diaphragm should be placed lightly over the point of maximal pulsation of the brachial artery (Petrie *et al.* 1997). The diaphragm is designed to amplify low frequency sounds such as Korotkoff's sounds (Hill & Grim 1991). Excessive pressure on the stethoscope's diaphragm may partially occlude the brachial artery and delay the occurrence of Korotkoff's sounds. For this reason the diaphragm should not be tucked under the edge of the cuff.

Korotkoff's sounds form five phases:

1 The appearance of faint, clear tapping sounds which gradually increase in intensity.
2 The softening of sounds, which may become swishing.
3 The return of sharper sounds which become crisper but never fully regain the intensity of the phase 1 sounds.
4 The distinct muffling sound which becomes soft and blowing.
5 The point at which all sound ceases.

Additional information

Much recent research has focused on the faulty techniques employed when blood pressures are taken (Campbell *et al.* 1990; Bogan *et al.* 1993; Kemp *et al.* 1994; Torrance & Serginson 1996; Gillespie & Curzio 1998). Blood pressure readings are altered by various factors that influence the patient, the techniques used and the accuracy of the sphygmomanometer. The variability of any readings can be reduced by an improved technique and by taking several readings (Campbell *et al.* 1990). In 1981 Thompson discussed the methodology of blood pressure recording and identified poor technique and observer bias as possible sources of error. He concluded that many nurses were inadequately trained in blood pressure measurement and that more attention needed to be paid to this area. In 1996 Beevers & Beevers found that observer error could be reduced if techniques for measuring blood pressure were taught repeatedly during medical and nursing training. Furthermore, the techniques should be reinforced regularly.

Similar conclusions were found in studies by Mancia *et al.* (1987), Feher & Harris St John (1992), and Torrance and Serginson (1996). Poor technique due to inadequate education can cause marked variation in the accuracy of measurements and can lead to inappropriate treatment decisions (Kemp *et al.* 1994).

Ambulatory blood pressure is increasingly regarded as superior to individual blood pressure readings (National High Blood Pressure Education Programme Coordinating Committee 1990; Perloff *et al.* 1993). Ambulatory blood pressure monitoring is expensive, time-consuming and has some risks as it can cause phlebitis (Creery *et al.* 1985). Although ambulatory blood pressure monitoring is considered more accurate, manual measurement remains the most common method (Veerman & van Monfrans 1993).

Variations in the procedure and frequency of taking blood pressure may be required in different patient groups with differing conditions. With a child it is important that the correctly sized cuff is used and that the average of repeated measurements is recorded. Low diastolic pressures are common in children and thus the pressure at muffling (Korotkoff phase 4) may be difficult to determine. Low diastolic pressures are common in elderly patients who may have atherosclerosis, and in patients with an increased cardiac output, i.e. as a result of pregnancy, exercise or hypothyroidism.

In pregnancy, changes in blood pressure may indicate

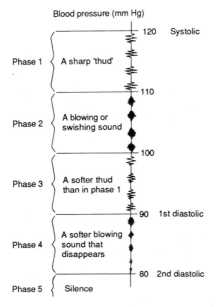

Figure 28.10 Korotkoff's sounds.

pregnancy-induced hypertension. An increase of 30 mm Hg or more systolic pressure and 15 mm Hg diastolic pressure over the previous readings may be indicative of this condition (Ferris 1990).

Patients with lines or shunts for dialysis in their arms or superior vena cava obstruction may be unsuitable for upper arm measurements of blood pressure; however, the blood pressure may be measured in the leg or forearm. For this procedure the patient lies prone and a thigh or large cuff is applied to the lower third of the thigh. The cuff is wrapped securely with its lower edge above the knee and its bladder centred over the posterior popliteal artery. The stethoscope diaphragm should be applied on the artery below the cuff. Systolic blood pressure is normally 20–30 mm Hg higher in the leg than in the arm. The right sized cuff should be used for obtaining the blood pressure using the forearm, and the bladder should be centred over the radial artery below the elbow, and the cuff wrapped in a similar manner to the normal procedure. The stethoscope diaphragm should be positioned over the radial artery about 2.5 cm above the wrist. Forearm blood pressure measurements may vary significantly from an upper arm measurement, and therefore it is important to document cuff size and location (Hill & Grim 1991).

Patients who have had breast surgery with lymph node dissections and/or radiotherapy, or have lymphoedema should not have their blood pressure recorded on the affected side. This is due to the increased sensitivity of the area and the risk of developing lymphoedema. Patients should be told to only have their blood pressure taken using the unaffected arm or legs.

Conditions where a patient's blood pressure may need careful monitoring are described below:

1 Hypertension is never diagnosed on a single blood pressure reading. Blood pressures are monitored to evaluate the condition of the patient and the effectiveness of medication (Marieb 1998).

2 Postoperative and critically ill patients require monitoring of blood pressure to assess for cardiovascular stability. The patient's blood pressure should be recorded pre-operatively in order to make significant comparisons. The reduction in cardiac diastole after surgery may result in a decreased coronary perfusion and therefore reduced cardiac output and vasoconstriction. Report immediately a falling systolic pressure as this may be an indication of hypovolaemic shock (Marini & Wheeler 1997). Haemorrhage may be primary at the time of operation or intermediary in the first few hours after surgery. The blood pressure returns to the patient's normal levels and causes loosening of poorly tied vessels and the flushing out of clots. The resulting blood loss causes a decrease in cardiac output and hypotension. Secondary haemorrhage can occur some time after surgery and can be due to infection. This also results in a fall in blood pressure (see Chap. 30, Peri-Operative Care).

3 Blood transfusions require careful monitoring of the blood pressure for several reasons. An incompatible blood transfusion may lead to agglutination and a resulting fall in the blood pressure. Circulatory overload may

lead to a rise in blood pressure, while the infusion of large quantities of blood may alter clotting factors and result in bleeding, causing a fall in blood pressure (Cluroe 1989).

4 Patients receiving intravenous infusions require blood pressure monitoring to observe for circulatory overload. Certain chemotherapy protocols use protracted amounts of intravenous fluids. In this group of patients diuretics are frequently used to reduce the increase in blood volume which results in a rise in blood pressure. Careful monitoring of blood pressure, weight, kidney function and electrolytes is imperative to prevent fluid overload and electrolyte imbalance (Marini & Wheeler 1997).

5 Patients with local or systemic infections or neutropenia require monitoring of their blood pressure in order to detect septicaemic shock. This is characterized by a change in the capillary epithelium and vasodilation due to circulating cell mediation (Bone 1996), which permits loss of blood and plasma through capillary walls into surrounding tissues. The decrease in the circulating volume of blood results in impaired tissue perfusion, culminating in cellular hypoxia (Ganong 1995).

References and further reading

Beevers, M. & Beevers, G.B. (1996) Blood pressure measurement in the next century, a plea for stability. *Blood Press Monit*, **1**(2), 117–20.

Bogan, B., Kritzer, S. & Deane, D. (1993) Nursing student compliance to standards for blood pressure measurement. *J Nurse Educ*, **32**(2), 90–92.

Bone, R.C. (1996) The pathogenesis of sepsis and rationale for new treatments. *Proceedings of the International Intensive Care Conference*, Barcelona.

Campbell, N.R. *et al.* (1990) Accurate, reproducible measurement of blood pressure. *Can Med Assoc J*, **143**(1), 19–24.

Carney, S.L., Gillies, A.H., Smith, A.J. & Smitham, S. (1995) Hospital sphygmomanometer use: an audit. *J Qual Clin Pract*, **15**(1), 17–22.

Cluroe, S. (1989) Blood transfusion. *Nursing*, **3**(40), 8–11.

Conceicao, S. *et al.* (1976) Defects in sphygmomanometers. *Br Med J*, **2**, 886–8.

Creery, T.C. *et al.* (1985) Phlebitis associated with non-invasive 24 hour ambulatory blood pressure monitor. *JAMA*, **254**, 2411.

Feher, M. & Harris St John, K. (1992) Blood pressure measurement by junior hospital doctors: a gap in medical education? *Health Trends*, **24**(2), 59–61.

Ferris, T.F. (1990) Hypertension in pregnancy. *The Kidney*, **23**(1), 1–5.

Ganong, W.F. (1995) *Review of Medical Physiology*, 17th edn. Appelton and Lange, Norwalk, Connecticut.

Gillespie, A. & Curzio, J. (1998) Blood pressure measurement: assessing staff knowledge. *Nurs Stand*, **12**(23), 35–7.

Hill, M.N. & Grim, C.M. (1991) How to take a precise blood pressure. *Am J Nurs*, **91**(2), 38–42.

HSE (1989) Control of Substances Hazardous to Health Regulations. Health and Safety Executive London.

Kemp, F., Foster, C. & McKinlay, S. (1994) How effective is training for blood pressure measurement? *Prof Nurse*, **9**(8), 521–4.

Londe, S. & Klitzner, T. (1984) Auscultatory blood pressure measurement: effect of blood pressure on the head-on stethoscope. *West J Med*, **141**(2), 193–5.

Mancia, G. *et al.* (1987) Alerting reaction and rise in blood pressure during measurement by physician and nurse. *Hypertension*, **9**, 209–215.

Marieb, E.M. (1998) *Human Anatomy and Physiology*, 4th edn., pp. 690–718. Benjamin Cummins, California.

Marini, J. & Wheeler, A. (1997) *Critical Care Medicine: The Essentials*, 2nd edn., pp. 19–43. Williams and Wilkins, Baltimore.

Maxwell, M.H. (1982) Error in blood pressure measurement due to incorrect cuff size in obese patients. *Lancet*, **2**, 33–6.

National High Blood Pressure Education Programme Coordinating Committee (1990) Report on ambulatory blood pressure monitoring. *Arch Intern Med*, **150**, 2270–80.

North, L.W. (1979) Accuracy of sphygmomanometers. *Assoc Operating Room Nurses J*, **30**, 996–1000.

Perloff, D. *et al.* (1993) The prognostic value of ambulatory blood pressures. *JAMA*, **249**, 2792–8.

Petrie, J.C., O'Brian, E.T., Litler, W.A. & deSwiet, M. (1997) *British Hypertension Society: Recommendations on Blood Pressure Measurement*, 2nd edn. British Hypertension Society, London.

Thompson, D.R. (1981) Recording patients' blood pressure: a review. *J Adv Nurs*, **6**(4), 283–90.

Torrance, C. & Serginson, E. (1996) Student nurses' knowledge in relation to blood pressure measurement by sphygmomanometry and auscultation. *Nurse Educ Today*, **16**(6), 397–402.

Veerman, D.P. & van Monfrans, G.A. (1993) Nurse measured or ambulatory blood pressure in routine hypertension care? *J Hypertens*, **11**, 287–92.

Webster, J. *et al.* (1984) Influence of arm position on measurement of blood pressure. *Br Med J*, **288**, 1574–5.

GUIDELINES • Blood pressure

Equipment

1 Sphygmomanometer
2 Stethoscope

Procedure

Action	*Rationale*
1 Explain to the patient that blood pressure is to be taken and discuss the procedure.	To ensure that the patient understands the procedure and gives his/her consent.
2 Allow the patient to rest for 3 min if the patient is supine or seated and for 1 min if the patient is standing (Petrie *et al.* 1997).	To ensure an accurate reading is obtained.
3 Ensure that the upper arm is supported and positioned at heart level, with the palm of the hand facing upwards (Hill & Grim 1991).	To obtain an accurate reading. Measurements made with the arm dangling by the hip can be 11–12 mmHg higher than those made with the arm supported and the cuff at heart level. Measurements made with the arm raised can be falsely high (Webster *et al.* 1984).
4 Ensure that tight or restrictive clothing is removed from the arm (Petrie *et al.* 1997).	To obtain a correct reading.
5 Use a cuff that covers 80% of the circumference of the upper arm (Petrie *et al.* 1997).	To obtain a correct reading.
6 Apply the cuff of the sphygmomanometer snugly around the arm, ensuring that the centre of the bladder covers the brachial artery.	To obtain a correct reading.
7 Position the manometer within 1 m of the patient, and where it can be seen at eye level (Petrie *et al.* 1997).	To prevent the cuff tubing hanging down and causing a risk of being caught by objects or by the operator. The manometer should be at eye level to obtain an accurate recording.
8 Inflate the cuff until the radial pulse can no longer be felt. This provides an estimation of the systolic pressure. Deflate the cuff completely and wait 15–30 sec before continuing to measure (Hill & Grim 1991).	A low systolic pressure may be reported in patients who have an auscultatory gap. This is when Korotkoff's sounds disappear shortly after the systolic pressure is heard, and and resume well above what corresponds to the diastolic pressure. About 5% of the population have an auscultatory gap and it is most common in those with hypertension (Hill & Grim 1991). This error can be avoided if the systolic pressure is first estimated by palpation.

Guidelines • Blood pressure (cont'd)

Action	*Rationale*
9 The cuff is then inflated to a pressure 30 mm Hg higher than the estimated systolic pressure.	Pressure exerted by the inflated cuff prevents the blood from flowing through the artery.
10 The diaphragm of the stethoscope should be placed over the point of the brachial artery.	Apply just enough pressure on the stethoscope to keep it in its place over the brachial artery. Excessive pressure can distort sounds or make them persist for longer than normal (Londe & Klitzner 1984).
11 Do not tuck the diaphragm under the edge of the cuff (Petrie *et al.* 1997).	To prevent an inaccurate result due to the pressure exerted by the cuff on the brachial artery.
12 Deflate the cuff at 2–3 mmHg per sec or per heartbeat.	At a slower rate of deflation venous congestion and arm pain can develop, resulting in a falsely low reading. At faster rates of deflation the mercury may fall too quickly, resulting in an imprecise reading (Hill & Grim 1991).
13 The measurement of systolic blood pressure is when a minimum of two clear repetitive tapping sounds can be heard. Diastolic pressure is measured at the point when the sound can no longer be heard.	To ensure that an accurate reading is obtained.
14 A record should be made of the systolic and diastolic pressures and comparisons made with previous readings. It should be recorded which arm was used to take the blood pressure. Any irregularities should be brought to the attention of the appropriate personnel.	The average of two or more blood pressure readings is often taken to represent a patient's normal blood pressure. Taking more than one measurement reduces the influence of anxiety and may provide a more accurate record (Hill & Grim 1991).
15 Remove the equipment and clean with soap and water after use.	To reduce the risk of cross-infection.

Respirations

Definition

The function of the respiratory system is to supply the body with oxygen and remove carbon dioxide. This is achieved by the diffusion of gases between the air in the alveoli of the lungs and the blood in the alveolar capillaries (Marieb 1998).

Indications

The respiration rate is evaluated:

1 To determine a baseline respiratory rate for comparisons.
2 To monitor fluctuations in respiration.
3 To evaluate the patient's response to medications or treatments that affect the respiratory system.

Reference material

The body cells require a continuous supply of oxygen to carry out their vital functions and this is provided by respiration (Marieb 1998). To accomplish respiration, four distinct events must occur:

1 Ventilation is where air is moved into and out of the lungs so that gas in the air sacs is replenished.
2 Gaseous exchange between the blood and the alveoli.
3 Oxygen and carbon dioxide are transported to and from the lungs by the cardiovascular system. This is called respiratory transportation.
4 Internal respiration is the cellular respiration that occurs in the cell where oxygen is utilized and carbon dioxide produced.

Control of respiration

Respiratory centre

The respiratory centre generates the basic pattern of breathing. It is located in the brain and is made up of groups of nerve cells in the reticular endothelial system of the medulla oblongata. Regular impulses are sent by these cells to the motor neurones in the anterior horn of the spinal cord which supply the intercostal muscles and the diaphragm (Ganong 1995). When the motor neurones are stimulated, the muscles contract and inspiration occurs. When the neurones are inhibited, the muscles relax and expiration follows.

Although the respiratory centre generates the basic rhythm, the depth and rate of breathing can be altered in response to the body's changing needs. The most important factors are those of nervous and chemical control (Fig. 28.11).

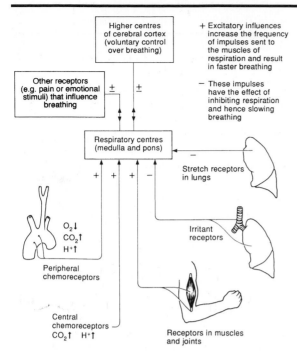

Figure 28.11 Factors influencing rate and depth of breathing.

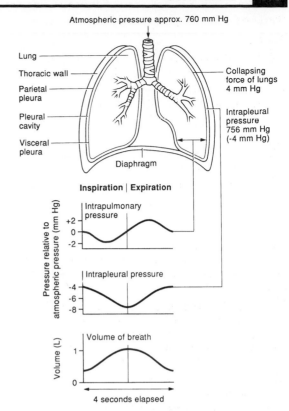

Figure 28.12 Intrapulmonary and intrapleural pressure relationships. Ventilation occurs due to pressure changes transmitted from the thoracic cavity to the lungs.

Nervous control

Lung tissue is stretched on inspiration and this stimulates afferent fibres in the vagus nerve. These impulses cause inspiration to cease and expiration occurs. Emotion, pain and anxiety also cause an increased respiratory rate (Marieb 1998).

Chemical control

An increase in the amount of carbon dioxide in the blood supplying the respiratory centre stimulates the respiratory centre and breathing becomes faster and deeper.

During exercise, carbon dioxide is produced in the muscles by the oxidation of carbohydrate. The amount of carbon dioxide in the blood increases and this stimulates the respiratory centre, producing an increase in depth and rate of respiration. More oxygen is made available in the alveoli for the blood to transport to the muscles, at the same time eliminating more carbon dioxide.

Any substance that, like carbon dioxide, lowers the pH of the blood will stimulate the respiratory centre. Figure 28.11 illustrates the factors influencing the rate and depth of breathing.

Patients with respiratory disease, e.g. emphysema and chronic bronchitis, who maintain high levels of carbon dioxide, will have arterial oxygen levels below 9 kPa (see Chap. 35, Respiratory Therapy). This is termed the 'hypoxic drive'. This chronic elevation of the partial pressure of carbon dioxide results in the chemoreceptors becoming unresponsive to this chemical stimulus. The change in respiratory drive results in respiration being stimulated by decreases in oxygen levels rather than levels of carbon dioxide (Marieb 1998). This may be detrimental to the patient's respiration if oxygen is administered therapeutically at high levels.

Ventilation

Ventilation results from pressure changes transmitted from the thoracic cavity to the lungs (Fig. 28.12). Inspiration is initiated by contraction of the diaphragm and external intercostal muscles. This results in the rib cage rising up, and the thrusting forward of the sternum. The ribs also swing outwards, expanding their diameter and hence the volume of the thorax (Marieb 1998). Because the lungs adhere tightly to the thoracic wall, attached by the layers of parietal and visceral pleura, this increases the intrapulmonary volume (Marieb 1998). Gases travel from an area of high pressure to areas of low pressure. The increased intrapulmonary volume results in a negative pressure of 1–3 mm Hg less than the atmospheric pressure (Marieb 1998). The resulting pressure gradient causes air to rush into the lungs (Fig. 28.13).

Expiration is largely passive, occurring as the inspiratory muscles relax and the lungs recoil as a result of their elastic properties (Marieb 1998). When intrapulmonary pressure exceeds atmospheric pressure this compresses the microscopic air sacs (alveoli) and an expiration of gases occurs.

Disease that affects the pleura of the individual may influence ventilation. A chest wound or rupture of the visceral pleura may allow air to enter the pleural space from the respiratory tract. The presence of air in the intrapleural space is referred to as a pneumothorax. Pleurisy, inflammation of the pleura where secretion of pleural fluid declines, causes a stabbing pain with each inspiration. Alternatively, an excessive increase in pleural secretions may hinder breathing (Marieb 1998). Air in the pleural space results in lung collapse (atelectasis). This affects the intrapulmonary pressure and hence ventilation.

The degree to which the lungs stretch and fill during inspiration and return to normal during expiration is due to the compliance and elasticity of lung tissue. Lung compliance depends on the elasticity of lung tissue and the flexibility of the thorax (Marieb 1998). When this is impaired, expiration becomes an active process, requiring the use of energy. The diseases that lower lung compliance are characterized by changes in the lung parenchyma. Examples include emphysema and fibrosing alveolitis, as a result of intrinsic or extrinsic means (Marieb 1998).

Intrinsic: severe infection
             rheumatoid arthritis
             SLE (systemic lupus erythematosus)
Extrinsic: pneumoconiosis
             psitticosis
             asbestosis
             oxygen fibrosis

In emphysema the lungs become progressively less elastic and more fibrous, which hinders both inspiration and expiration. The increased muscular activity results in greater energy required to breathe.

Compliance is diminished by any factor that:

1 Reduces the natural resilience of the lungs.
2 Blocks the bronchi or respiratory passageways.
3 Impairs the flexibility of the thoracic cage.

Friction in the air passageways causes resistance and affects ventilation (Ganong 1995). Normally, airway resistance is reduced so that minimal opposition to airflow occurs. However, any factor that amplifies airway resistance such as the presence of mucus, tumour or infected material in the airways demands that breathing movements become more strenuous (Marieb 1998).

Respiratory volumes

The amount of air that is breathed varies depending on the condition of inspiration and expiration. Information about a patient's respiratory status can be gained by measuring various lung capacities, which consist of the sum of different respiratory volumes.

The respiratory volumes shown in Fig. 28.14 represent normal values for a healthy 20-year-old male weighing about 70 kg (Marieb 1998).

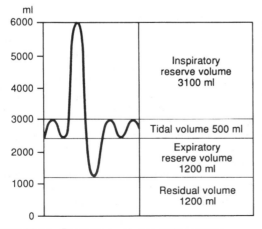

Figure 28.13   Changes in thoracic volume during breathing.

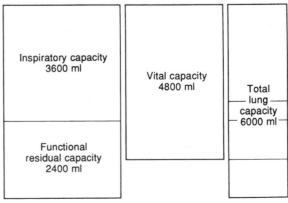

Figure 28.14   Respiratory volumes and capacities.

Tidal volume (TV)

The tidal volume is the amount of air inhaled or exhaled with each breath under resting conditions (about 500 ml).

Inspiratory reserve volume (IRV)

The inspiratory reserve volume is the amount of air that can be inhaled forcibly after a normal tidal volume inhalation (about 3100 ml).

Expiratory reserve volume (ERV)

The expiratory reserve volume is the maximum amount that can be exhaled forcibly after a normal tidal volume exhalation (about 1200 ml).

Residual volume (RV)

The residual volume is the amount of air remaining in the lungs after a forced expiration (about 1200 ml).

Respiratory capacities

Respiratory capacities are measured for diagnostic purposes. They consist of two or more respiratory lung volumes.

Total lung capacity (TLC)

The total lung capacity is the amount of air in the lungs at the end of a maximum inspiration.

$$TLC = TV + IRV + ERV + RV \ (6000 \, ml)$$

Vital capacity (VC)

The vital capacity is the maximum amount of air that can be expired after a maximum inspiration.

$$VC = TV + IRV + ERV \ (4800 \, ml)$$

Inspiratory capacity (IC)

The inspiratory capacity is the maximum amount of air that can be inspired after a normal expiration.

$$IC = TV + IRV \ (3600 \, ml)$$

Functional residual capacity (FRC)

The functional residual capacity is the amount of air remaining in the lungs after a normal tidal volume expiration.

$$FRC = ERV + RV \ (2400 \, ml)$$

Dead space

A percentage of the inspired air (about 120 ml) fills the respiratory passageways and does not contribute to gaseous exchange. This is termed the anatomical dead space.

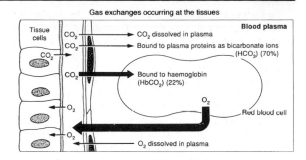

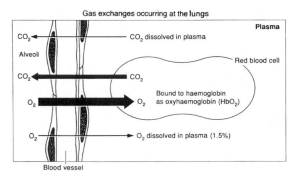

Figure 28.15 Transport and exchange of carbon dioxide and oxygen.

Table 28.2 Composition of gas in the atmosphere and alveoli

	Atmosphere inspired (%)	Alveoli (%)
Oxygen	20.9	13.7
Carbon dioxide	0.04	5.2
Nitrogen	78.6	74.9
Water	0.46	6.2

Gaseous exchange

Oxygen in the inspired air enters while carbon dioxide leaves the blood in the lungs in the process of ventilation. These gases move in opposite directions in the alveoli by the mechanism of diffusion (Marieb 1998). Adjacent to the alveoli is a dense vascular network. Oxygen moves into the alveolar capillaries and carbon dioxide moves out (Fig. 28.15). This process is called gaseous exchange. Factors influencing this process include the partial pressure gradients, the width of the respiratory membrane and the surface area available.

The gaseous composition of the atmosphere and alveoli is demonstrated in Table 28.2. The atmosphere consists almost entirely of oxygen and nitrogen; the alveoli contain more carbon dioxide and water vapour and considerably less oxygen. These different figures reflect the following processes:

1 Gaseous exchange in the lungs.
2 Humidification of air by the respiratory passageways.
3 The mixing of alveolar gas that occurs with each breath.

Respiratory transportation

Oxygen is carried in the blood in two ways, bound to the haemoglobin within the red blood cells and dissolved in plasma. Haemoglobin carries 98.5% of the oxygen from the lungs and the tissues. The amount of oxygen bound to haemoglobin depends on several factors:

1 The partial pressure of oxygen (PaO_2) and the partial pressure of carbon dioxide ($PaCO_2$) in the blood. The gradient of partial pressure influences the rates of diffusion, the oxygen gradient being steeper than that of carbon dioxide. Carbon dioxide is transported from the tissue primarily as bicarbonate ions in the plasma (70%), whereas only small amounts are transported by haemoglobin in the red blood cells (22%).
2 The blood pH influences the affinity of haemoglobin for oxygen: as the pH decreases, as in acidosis, the amount of oxygen unloaded in the tissues increases.
3 As body temperature rises above normal levels, the affinity of haemoglobin for oxygen declines, and therefore oxygen unloading is enhanced. This effect is seen in localized temperature changes such as inflammation.

Diseases that reduce the oxygen-carrying ability of the blood whatever the cause are termed anaemia. This is characterized by oxygen blood levels that are inadequate to support normal metabolism (Marieb 1998). Common causes of anaemia include:

1 Insufficient number of red cells, including destruction of red cells, haemorrhage and bone marrow failure.
2 Decreases in haemoglobin content, including iron deficiency anaemia and pernicious anaemia.
3 Abnormal haemoglobin, including thalassaemia and sickle cell anaemia (Marieb 1998).

Internal respiration

Internal respiration is the exchange of gases that occurs within the tissues between the capillaries and the cells. Carbon dioxide enters the blood and oxygen moves into the cells (Fig. 28.15).

Hypoxia is the result of an inadequate amount of oxygen delivered to body tissues. The blue coloration of tissues and mucosal membranes is termed cyanosis.

Lung defence mechanisms

The upper airway is designed to warm, humidify and filter inspired air. The nasal passages absorb noxious gases and trap inhaled particles. Smaller particles are removed by the cough reflex.

Observation of respiration

Respirations in an individual should be observed for rate, depth and pattern of breathing.

Rate

Rate and depth determine the type of respiration. The normal rate at rest is approximately 14–18 breaths per minute in adults and is faster in infants and children (Table 28.3). The ratio of pulse rate to respiration rate is approximately 5:1.

Changes in the rate of ventilation may be defined as follows. *Tachypnoea* is an increased respiratory rate, seen in fever, for example, as the body tries to rid itself of excess heat. Respirations increase by about 7 breaths per minute for every 1°C rise in temperature above normal. They also increase with pneumonia, other obstructive airway diseases, respiratory insufficiency and lesions in the pons of the brainstem (Brunner & Suddarth 1989).

Bradypnoea is a decreased but regular respiratory rate, such as that caused by the depression of the respiratory centre in the medulla by opiate narcotics, or by a brain tumour.

Depth

The depth of respiration is the volume of air moving in and out with each respiration. This tidal volume is normally about 500 ml in an adult and should be constant with each breath. A spirometer is used to measure the precise amount (see Respiratory capacities). Normal, relaxed breathing is effortless, automatic, regular and almost silent.

Dyspnoea is undue breathlessness and an awareness of discomfort with breathing. There are several types of dyspnoea:

1 Exertional dyspnoea is shortness of breath on exercise and is seen with heart failure.
2 Orthopnoea is a shortness of breath on lying down which is relieved by the patient sitting upright. This is often caused by left ventricular failure of the heart.
3 Paroxysmal, nocturnal dyspnoea is a sudden breathlessness that occurs at night when the patient is lying down and is often caused by pulmonary oedema and left ventricular failure (Brunner & Suddarth 1989).

Pattern

Changes in the pattern of respiration are often found in disorders of the respiratory control centre (Brunner & Suddarth 1989). Examples of changes in respiratory pattern follow:

Hyperventilation is an increase in both the rate and depth of respiration. This follows extreme exertion, fear and

Table 28.3 Respiratory rates (Timby 1989)

Age	Average range/minute
Newborn	30–80
Early childhood	20–40
Late childhood	15–25
Adulthood – male	14–18
Adulthood – female	16–20

anxiety, fever, hepatic coma, midbrain lesions of the brain-stem, and acid–base imbalance such as diabetic ketoacido-sis (Kussmaul's respiration) or salicylate overdose (in both of these situations the body compensates for the metabolic acidosis by increased respiration), as well as an alteration in blood gas concentration (either increased carbon dioxide or decreased oxygen). The breathing pattern is normally regular and consists of inspiration, pause, longer expiration and another pause. However, this may be altered by some defects and diseases. In adults, more than 20 breaths per minute is considered moderate, more than 30 is severe.

Apnoeustic respiration is a pattern of prolonged, gasping inspiration, followed by extremely short, inefficient expira-tion, seen in lesions of the pons in the midbrain.

Cheyne–Stokes respiration is periodic breathing, charac-terized by a gradual increase in depth of respiration fol-lowed by a decrease in respiration, resulting in apnoea (Brunner & Suddarth 1989).

Biot's respiration is an interrupted breathing pattern, like Cheyne–Stokes respiration, except that each breath is of the same depth. It may be seen with spinal meningitis or other central nervous system conditions.

Conditions where a patient's respirations may need careful monitoring are described below:

1 Patients with conditions that affect respiration, such as those described in the text, require monitoring of respi-ration to evaluate their condition and the effectiveness of medication.
2 Postoperative and critically ill patients require monitor-ing of respiration. The patient's respiration should be recorded pre-operatively in order to make significant comparisons. The breathing is observed to assess for the return to normal respiratory function.
3 Patients receiving oxygen inhalation therapy or receiv-ing artificial respiration require monitoring of breathing to assess respiratory function.

References and further reading

Bell, G.H. *et al.* (1980) *Textbook of Physiology and Biochemistry*, 10th edn. Churchill Livingstone, Edinburgh.

Boylan, A. & Brown, P. (1985) Respirations. *Nurs Times*, **81**, 35–8.

Brunner, L.S. & Suddarth, D.S. (1989) *The Lippincott Manual of Medical-Surgical Nursing*, Vol. 2. Harper & Row, London.

Ganong, W.F. (1995) *Review of Medical Physiology*, 17th edn. Appelton & Lange, New York.

Glennister, T.W.A. & Ross, R.W. (1980) *Anatomy and Physiology for Nurses*, 3rd edn. William Heinemann Medical Books, London.

Jarvis, C.M. (1980) Vital signs: a preview of problems. In: *Assessing Vital Functions Accurately*. Intermed Communications.

Kertson, L.D. (1989) *Comprehensive Respiratory Nursing: A Decision-making Approach*. W.B. Saunders, Philadelphia.

Marieb, E.M. (1998) *Human Anatomy and Physiology*, 4th edn. Benjamin Cummings, California.

Roberts, A. (1980) Systems and signs. Respiration 1, 2. *Nurs Times*, **76**, *Systems of Life*, Nos 71, 72, p. 8.

Rokosky, J.S. (1981) Assessment of the individual with altered res-piratory function. *Nurs Clin North Am*, **16**(2), 195–9.

Timby, B. (1989) *Clinical Nursing Procedure*. J.B. Lippincott, Philadelphia.

Temperature

Definition

Body temperature represents the balance between heat gain and heat loss.

Indications

Measurement of body temperature is carried out for two reasons:

1 To determine the patient's temperature on admission as a baseline for comparison with future measurements.
2 To monitor fluctuations in temperature.

Reference material

All tissues produce heat as a result of cell metabolism, and this is increased by exercise and activity (Marieb 1998). Body temperature is usually maintained between 36 and 37.5°C regardless of the environmental temperature (Marini & Wheeler 1997). Man is described as homoio-thermic, that is, having a core temperature that remains constant in spite of environmental changes. The body core generally has the highest temperature while the skin is the coolest (Fig. 28.16). Core temperature reflects the heat of arterial blood and represents the balance between the heat generated by body tissues in metabolic activity and that lost through various mechanisms.

A relatively constant temperature is maintained by homeostasis, which is a constant process of heat gain and heat loss. The body requires stability of its temperature to produce an optimum environment for biochemical and enzyme reactions to maintain cellular function. A body temperature above or below this normal range affects total body function (Marieb 1998). A temperature above 41°C can cause convulsions and a temperature of 43°C renders life unsustainable.

The hypothalamus within the brain acts as the body's thermostat, controlling the body's temperature by various physiological mechanisms (Fig. 28.17). Heat is gained through metabolic activity of the body, especially of the muscles and liver. Heat loss is achieved through the skin by the processes of radiation, convection, conduction and evaporation.

Various factors cause fluctuations of temperature:

1 The body's circadian rhythms cause daily fluctuations. The body temperature is higher in the evening than in the morning (Brown 1990). Minor & Waterhouse (1981) in a research study recorded a difference of 0.5–1.5°C between morning and evening measurements.

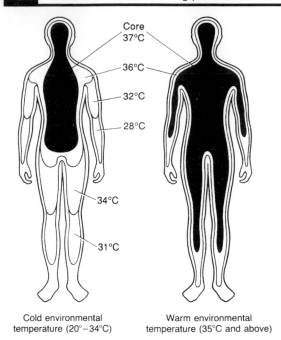

Core
37°C

36°C

32°C

28°C

34°C

31°C

Cold environmental
temperature (20°–34°C)

Warm environmental
temperature (35°C and above)

Figure 28.16 Body core and skin temperatures.

Table 28.4 Non-infectious causes of hyperthermia

Alcohol withdrawal	Malignant hyperthermia
Anticholinergic drugs	Neuroleptic malignant
Allergic drug or transfusion	syndrome
reaction	Pheochromocytoma
Autonomic insufficiency	Salicylate intoxication
Crystalline arthritis (gout)	Status epilepticus
Drug allergy	Stroke or CNS damage
Heat stroke	Vasculitis
Hyperthyroidism	Agonist drugs
Malignancy	

2 Ovulation results in a fluctuation of temperature.

3 Exercise and eating cause an elevation in temperature (Marieb 1998).

4 Extremes of age affect a person's response to environmental change. The young or elderly are unable to maintain an efficient equilibrium. Thermoregulation is inadequate in the newborn and especially in low-birth-weight babies. In old people there is an increased sensitivity to cold, and a lower body temperature generally (Howell 1972; Nakamura *et al.* 1997).

Hypothermia is where body temperature drops and mechanisms to increase heat production are ineffective. This causes a decline in the metabolic rate and a resulting decrease in all bodily functions. Clinical hypothermia is when the core temperature falls below 35°C (95°F). However, it frequently escapes detection due to the symptoms being non-specific and an oral thermometer's failure to record in the appropriate range (Marini & Wheeler 1997). Hypothermia is often multifactorial in origin and can be as a result of:

1 Environmental exposure.

2 Medications that can either alter the perception of cold, increase heat loss through vasodilation or inhibit heat generation, e.g. alcohol, paracetamol.

3 Metabolic conditions, e.g. hypoglycaemia and adrenal insufficiency.

4 During an operation and postoperatively. This is due to exposure of the body during surgery and the use of drugs which dampen the vasoconstrictor response (Marini & Wheeler 1997).

Pyrexia is defined as a significant rise in body temperature. Sudden temperature elevations usually indicate infection. However, other life-threatening non-infectious causes of fever are often overlooked (see Table 28.4).

Fever caused by pyrexia is the result of the internal thermostat resetting to higher levels. This resetting of the thermostat results from the action of pyrogens which are chemical substances now known to be cytokines. Cytokines are chemical mediators which are involved in cellular immunity. They enhance the immune response and are released from white blood cells, injured tissues and macrophages. This causes the hypothalamus to release prostaglandins which in turn reset the hypothalamic thermostat. The body then promotes heat-producing mechanisms such as vasoconstriction. Heat loss is reduced, the skin becomes cool and the person 'shivers'. This is often called a rigor (Marieb 1998). A rigor is marked by shivering and the patient complains of feeling cold. The temperature quickly rises as a result of the normal physiological response to cold. This results in the following physiological changes:

1 Thermoreceptors in the skin are stimulated, resulting in vasoconstriction. This decreases heat loss through conduction and convection.

2 Sweat gland activity is reduced to minimize evaporation.

3 Shivering occurs, muscles contract and relax out of sequence with each other, thus generating heat.

4 The body increases catecholamine and thyroxine levels, elevating the metabolic rate in an attempt to increase temperature (Damanhouri & Tayeb 1992).

All of these changes contribute to a rise in metabolism with an increase in carbon dioxide excretion and the need for oxygen. This leads to an increased respiratory rate. When the body temperature reaches its new 'set-point' the patient no longer complains of feeling cold, shivering ceases and sweating commences.

There are several grades of pyrexia, and these are described in Table 28.5.

There are different methods for lowering body temperature. Antipyretic drugs can cause a marked fall in temperature (Vane 1978; Connell 1997). It is thought that these drugs inhibit the inflammatory action of prostaglandins, affecting the hypothalamus by temporarily resetting the thermostat to normal levels. However, these drugs must be

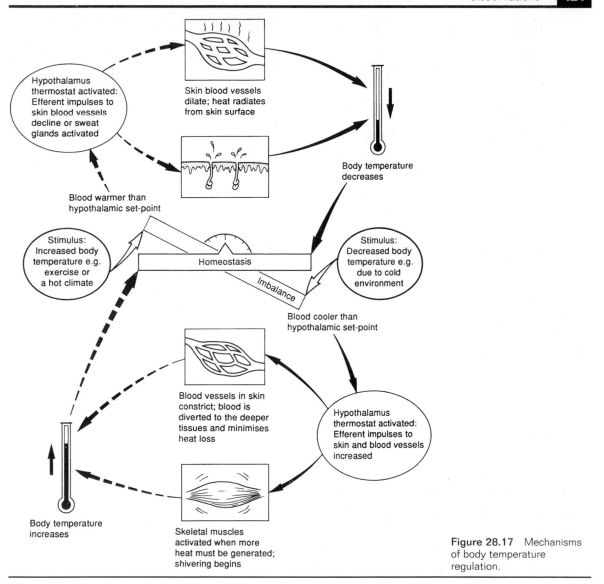

Figure 28.17 Mechanisms of body temperature regulation.

Table 28.5 Grades of pyrexia

Low-grade pyrexia	Normal to 38°C	Indicative of an inflammatory response due to a mild infection, allergy, disturbance of body tissue by trauma, surgery, malignancy or thrombosis
Moderate to high-grade pyrexia	38–40°C	May be caused by wound, respiratory or urinary tract infections
Hyperpyrexia	40°C and above	May arise because of bacteraemia, damage to the hypothalamus or high environmental temperatures

used with caution in patients with established liver disease or a history of gastric bleeding, as they can cause gastric irritation, and put increasing strain on a diseased liver to break down the drug.

Fanning is of benefit for moderate to high pyrexias.

Fanning and tepid sponging is not recommended while the patient's temperature is still rising as this will only make the patient feel colder, cause distress (Sharber 1997) and increase shivering (Krikler 1990).

Recordings of body temperature are an index of biological function and are a valuable indicator of a patient's health.

Temperature recording sites

Traditionally, the oral, axillae or rectum have been the preferred sites for obtaining temperature readings. This is due to their accessibility. With the development of new technology the use of the tympanic membrane is increasingly becoming popular, as it is less invasive and provides rapid results (Burke 1996).

Oral

To measure the temperature orally, the thermometer is placed in the sublingual pocket of tissue at the base of the tongue. This area is in close proximity to the thermoreceptors which respond rapidly to changes in the core temperature, hence changes in core temperatures are reflected quickly here (Marini & Wheeler 1997).

Oral temperatures are affected by the temperatures of ingested foods and fluids and by the muscular activity of chewing. A respiratory rate that exceeds 18 breaths per minute, together with a patient who smokes, will also reduce the core temperature values (Marieb 1998).

It is important that the thermometer is placed in the sublingual pocket and not in the area under the front of the tongue as there may be a temperature difference of up to 1.7°C between these areas. This temperature difference is due to the sublingual pockets being more protected from the air currents which cool the frontal areas (Neff et al. 1989). Oxygen therapy has been shown not to affect the oral temperature reading (Hasler & Cohen 1982; Lim-Levy 1982).

Rectal

The rectal temperature is often higher than the oral temperature because this site is more sheltered from the external environment. Rectal thermometry has been demonstrated in clinical trials to be more accurate than oral thermometry. The researchers (Jensen et al. 1994) conclude that rectal thermometry is the more accurate route for daily measurements, but is more invasive, often unacceptable for the patient and time consuming. Although this method is more precise, fever can still be detected by oral screening. If greater accuracy is required the rectal method offers greater precision. The presence of soft stool may separate the thermometer from the bowel wall and give a false reading, especially if the central temperature is changing rapidly. In infants this method is not recommended as it provides a risk of rectal ulceration or perforation.

A rectal thermometer should be inserted at least 4 cm in an adult to obtain the most accurate reading.

Axilla

The axilla is considered less desirable than the other sites because of the difficulty to achieve accurate and reliable readings as it is not close to major vessels, and skin surface temperatures vary more with changes in temperature of the environment (Woollens 1996). It is usually only used for patients who are unsuitable for, or who cannot tolerate, oral thermometers, e.g. after general anaesthetic or those patients with mouth injuries.

To take an axillary temperature reading the thermometer should be placed in the centre of the armpit, with the patient's arm firmly against the side of the chest. It is important that the same arm is used for each measurement as there is often a variation in temperature between left and right (Howell 1972).

Whichever route is used for temperature measurement, it is important that this is then used consistently, as switching between sites can produce a record that is misleading or difficult to interpret.

Time for recording temperatures

The average person experiences circadian rhythms which make their highest body temperature occur in the late afternoon or early evening, i.e. between 4 PM and 8 PM. The most sensitive time for detecting pyrexias appears to be between 7 PM and 8 PM (Angerami 1980). This should be considered when interpreting variations in 4- or 6-hourly observations, and when taking once-daily temperatures.

Types of thermometer

A variety of thermometers are now available, from clinical glass thermometers with oral or rectal bulbs to the electronic sensor thermometer to the tympanic thermometer. Mercury thermometers have been used extensively in the past, but it has been shown they are unable to detect temperatures lower than 34.5°C (94°F) or higher than 40.5°C (105°F). They are also slow to respond to temperature changes (Marini & Wheeler 1997). The use of electronic devices is therefore preferable where there are extremes of temperature or where there are temperature fluctuations. Infrared-sensing ear canal probes (tympanic membrane thermometers) have the advantages of providing rapid results, are easy to use and are convenient for both the nurse and the patient (Burke 1996). However, inconsistent study results have highlighted problems with their use (Yeo & Scarbough 1996; Thomas et al. 1997). The practitioner must understand the principles of use and the correct technique in order to obtain an accurate recording (White et al. 1994; Burke 1996).

Ideally, all variables such as site, technique and instrument should remain unchanged, but this is not always practical. Nurses are often pressurized, as they are busy and this could be one of the reasons for inconsistencies in data. With the emergence of electronic devices to measure temperature, this has gone some way to addressing these problems (Woollens 1996).

Conditions where a patient's temperature requires careful monitoring

1 Patients with conditions that affect basal metabolic rate, such as disorders of the thyroid gland, require monitor-

ing of body temperature. Hypothyroidism is a condition where an inadequate secretion of hormones from the thyroid gland results in a slowing of physical and metabolic activity; thus the individual has a decrease in body temperature. Hyperthyroidism is excessive activity of the thyroid gland; a hypermetabolic condition results, with an increase in all metabolic processes. The patient complains of a low heat tolerance. Thyrotoxic crisis is a sudden increase in thyroid hormones and can cause a hyperpyrexia (Mize et al. 1993).

2 Postoperative and critically ill patients require monitoring of temperature. The patient's temperature should be observed pre-operatively in order to make any significant comparisons. In the postoperative period the nurse should observe the patient for hyperthermia or hypothermia as a reaction to the surgical procedures (Mize et al. 1993).

3 Patients with a susceptibility to infection, for example those with a low white blood cell count (less than 1000 cells/mm^3), or those undergoing radiotherapy, chemotherapy or steroid treatment, will require a more frequent observation of temperature. The fluctuation in temperature is influenced by the body's response to pyrogens. Immunocompromised patients are less able to respond to infection. Bacteraemia means a bacterial invasion of the blood stream. Septic shock is a circulatory collapse as a result of severe infection. Pyrexia may be absent in those who are immunosuppressed or in the elderly.

4 Patients with a systemic or local infection require monitoring of temperature to assess development or regression of infection.

5 Patients receiving a blood transfusion require careful monitoring of temperature for incompatible blood reactions. Reaction to a blood transfusion is most likely to occur in the early stages and a rise in the patient's temperature is indicative of a reaction. Cluroe (1989) suggests frequent recordings of temperature in the first 15 minutes of a blood transfusion as well as general observation of the patient. Pyrexia can occur throughout a blood transfusion, and results from a reaction by recipient antibodies. It may occur as soon as 60–90 minutes after the start of blood transfusion (Cluroe 1989).

References and further reading

Angerami, E.L.S. (1980) Epidemiological study of body temperature in patients in a teaching hospital. *Int J Nurs Stud*, **17**, 91–9.

Brown, S. (1990) Temperature taking – getting it right. *Nurs Stand*, **5**(12), 4–5.

Burke, K. (1996) The tympanic membrane thermometer in paediatrics: a review of the literature. *Accid Emergency Nurs*, **4**(4), 190–193.

Cluroe, S. (1989) Blood transfusions. *Nursing*, **3**(40), 8–11.

Connell, F. (1997) The causes and treatment of fever: a literature review. *Nurs Stand*, **12**(11), 40–43.

Damanhouri, Z. & Tayeb, O.S. (1992) Animal models for heat stroke studies. *J Pharmacol Toxicol Meth*, **28**, 119–27.

Hasler, M. & Cohen, J. (1982) The effect of oxygen administration on oral temperature assessment. *Nurs Res*, **31**, 265–8.

Howell, T. (1972) Axillary temperature in aged women. *Age Ageing*, **1**, 250–254.

Jensen, B.N. et al. (1994) The superiority of rectal thermometry to oral thermometry with regard to accuracy. *J Adv Nurs*, **20**, 660–65.

Krikler, S. (1990) Pyrexia: what to do about temperatures. *Nurs Stand*, **4**(25), 37–8.

Lim-Levy, F. (1982) The effect of oxygen inhalation on oral temperature. *Nurs Res*, **31**, 150–152.

Marieb, E.M. (1998) *Human Anatomy and Physiology*, 4th edn., pp. 908–964. Benjamin Cummings, California.

Marini, J. & Wheeler, A. (1997) *Medical Care Medicine*, 2nd edn., pp. 456–64. Williams and Wilkins, London.

Minor, D.G. & Waterhouse, J.M. (1981) *Circadian Rhythms and the Human*. Wright, Bristol.

Mize, J., Koziol-McLain, J. & Lowenstein, S.R. (1993) The forgotten vital sign: temperature patterns and associations in 642 trauma patients at an urban level 1 trauma centre. *J Emergency Nurs*, **19**(4), 303–305.

Nakamura, K., Tanaka, M., Motohashi, Y. & Maeda, A. (1997) Oral temperatures in the elderly in nursing homes in summer and winter in relation to activities of daily living. *Int J Biometeorol*, **40**(2), 103–106.

Neff, J. et al. (1989) Effect of respiratory rate, respiratory depth, and open versus closed mouth breathing on sublingual temperature. *Res Nurs Health*, **12**, 195–202.

Sharber, J. (1997) The efficacy of tepid sponge bathing to reduce fever in young children. *Am J Emergency Med*, **15**(2), 188–92.

Thomas, K.A., Savage, M.V. & Brengelmann, G.L. (1997) Effect of facial cooling on tympanic temperature. *Am J Crit Care*, **6**(1), 46–51.

Vane, J.R. (1978) In: Cox et al. *Pharmacology of the Hypothalamus*. Macmillan, London.

White, N., Baird, S. & Anderson, D.L. (1994) A comparison of tympanic thermometer readings to pulmonary artery catheter core temperature recordings. *Appl Nurs Res*, **7**(4), 165–9.

Woollens, S. (1996) Temperature measurement devices. *Prof Nurse*, **11**(8), 541–7.

Yeo, S. & Scarbough, M. (1996) Exercise induced hyperthermia may prevent core temperature measurement by tympanic membrane thermometer. *J Nurs Meas*, **4**(2), 143–51.

GUIDELINES • Temperature

Equipment

1 Electronic thermometer and oral probe.
2 Disposable probe covers.

Guidelines • Temperature (cont'd)

Procedure

Action	*Rationale*
1 Explain and discuss the procedure with the patient.	To ensure that the patient understands the procedure and gives his/her valid consent.
2 Remove the probe from the stored position in the thermometer and check that the reading is 34°C.	If the readout does not register, the machine is faulty and should not be used.
3 Push the probe firmly into the probe cover.	The probe cover protects the tip of the probe and is necessary for the functioning of the instrument.
4 Ask the patient to open the mouth and insert the probe under the tongue into the 'heat pocket' at the posterior base of the tongue.	The highest oral temperature reading is at the posterior base of the tongue, which is least affected by environmental conditions.
5 Ask the patient to close the mouth.	To increase the patient's comfort and to keep the probe in place.
6 Hold the thermometer in place until an audible tone is heard and the machine signals the correct temperature.	Tissue contact must be maintained for an accurate reading to be obtained.
7 If figures on the display stop rising without an audible tone, tissue contact has been lost. Regain tissue contact and continue.	The probe must be supported outside the mouth as its top-heavy shape tends to move the sensitive tip out of the heat pocket.
8 Remove the probe from the patient's mouth when signalled by the machine and note the temperature displayed, and document on patient's records. Discuss with medical colleagues if the results are abnormal.	An audible tone indicates that the reading is complete. To ensure the documentation is accurate and to act promptly on abnormal fluctuations in temperature which may indicate a deterioration in the patient's condition.
9 Discard the probe cover into a waste bag by pressing the probe from the thumb.	Probe covers are for single use only. The discard mechanism prevents transfer of the patient's saliva to the nurse's hands.
10 Return the probe to its storage position in the thermometer, cancelling the temperature reading.	The probe is best protected from damage in this storage position.

Urinalysis

Definition

Urinalysis is the testing of the physical characteristics and composition of freshly voided urine.

Indications

The composition of urine can change dramatically as a result of disease processes. It may contain red blood cells, glucose, proteins, white blood cells, or bile (Marieb 1998). The presence of such abnormalities in urine is an important warning sign of illness and may be helpful in clinical assessment in the following ways:

1 To determine the individual's urine status on admission as a baseline for comparisons with future assessments.
2 To monitor changes in urinary constituents as a response to medication.
3 To be used as a screening test to gather information about physical status.

Reference material

Urine is formed in the kidneys which process approximately 180 litres of blood-derived fluid a day. Approximately 1.5% of this total actually leaves the body. Urine formation and the simultaneous adjustment of blood composition involves three processes (Marieb 1998) (Fig. 28.18):

1 Glomerular filtration
2 Tubular reabsorption
3 Tubular secretion.

Glomerular filtration occurs in the glomeruli of the kidney which act as non-selective filters. Filtration occurs as a result of increased glomerular blood pressure caused by the difference in diameter between afferent and efferent arterioles. The effect is a simple mechanical filter that permits substances smaller than plasma proteins to pass from the glomeruli to the glomerular capsule (Marieb 1998).

Tubular reabsorption then occurs, removing necessary substances from the filtrate and returning them to the peritubular capillaries. Tubular reabsorption is an active

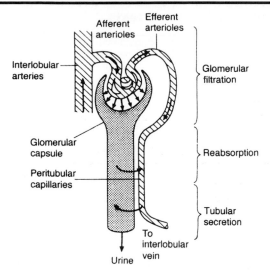

Figure 28.18 A nephron depicted diagrammatically to show the three major mechanisms by which urine is produced.

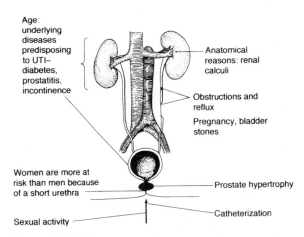

Figure 28.19 Urinary tract infections: predisposing factors.

process that requires protein carriers and energy. Substances reabsorbed include nutrients and most ions. It is also a passive process, however, driven by eletrochemical gradients. Substances reabsorbed in this way include sodium ions and water. Creatinine and the metabolites of drugs are not reabsorbed either because of their size, insolubility, or a lack of carriers. Most of the nutrients, 80% of the water and sodium ions, and the majority of actively transported ions are reabsorbed in the proximal convoluted tubules (Marieb 1998).

Reabsorption is controlled by hormones. Aldosterone increases reabsorption of sodium (and hence also water), and antidiuretic hormone (ADH) enhances reabsorption of water in the collecting tubules (Marieb 1998).

Tubular secretion is both an active and a passive process in which the tubules excrete drugs, urea, excess ions and other substances into the filtrate. It plays an important part in maintaining the acid–base balance of blood (Marieb 1998).

Regulation of urine concentration and volume occurs in the loop of Henle where the osmolarity of the filtrate is controlled. As the filtrate flows through the tubules the permeability of the walls controls how dilute or concentrated the resulting urine will be. In the absence of ADH dilute urine is formed because the filtrate is not reabsorbed as it passes through the kidneys. As levels of ADH increase, the collecting tubules become more permeable and water moves out of the filtrate back into the blood. Consequently, smaller amounts of more concentrated urine are produced (Marieb 1998).

Characteristics of urine

Urine is typically clear, pale to deep yellow in colour and slightly acidic (pH 6), though pH can change as a result of metabolic processes or diet. Vomiting and bacterial infection of the urinary tract can cause urine to become alka-line. Urinary specific gravity ranges from 1.001 to 1.035, according to how concentrated the urine is (Fillingham & Douglas 1997; Marieb 1998).

The colour of urine is due to a pigment called urochrome which is derived from the body's destruction of haemoglobin. The more concentrated urine is, the deeper yellow it becomes. Changes in colour may reflect diet (e.g. beetroot or rhubarb), or may be due to blood or bile in the urine. If fresh urine is turbid (cloudy), the cause may be an infection of the urinary tract. The urinary tract is the most common site of bacterial infection. It is thought to affect 10–20% of the female population (Mims *et al.* 1993). There are many predisposing factors (Fig. 28.19), the most common of which is instrumentation, that is, cystoscopy and urinary catheterization (Johnson 1986).

Bacteriuria is defined as the presence of bacteria in the urine. Because urine specimens can become contaminated with periurethral flora during collection, infection is distinguished by counting the number of bacteria. Significant bacteriuria is defined as a presence of more than 10^5 organisms per ml of urine in the presence of clinical symptoms (Fig. 28.20). Covert bacteriuria is the presence of more than 10^5 organisms per ml of urine without clinical symptoms. Distinguishing between counts of 10^3 and 10^5 can be difficult, making it important that urine is collected carefully and transported rapidly to the laboratory (Mims *et al.* 1993).

Fresh urine smells slightly aromatic. This can change as a result of disease processes such as diabetes mellitus, when acetone is present in the urine, giving it a fruity smell. The composition of urine can change dramatically as a result of disease, and abnormal substances may be present (see Table 28.6). Urinalysis can identify many of these substances, and should be part of every physical assessment (Cook 1996; Torrance & Elley 1998).

Renal clearance is the rate at which the kidneys clear a

particular chemical from the plasma. Studies of renal clearance provide information about renal function or the course of renal disease. There is no single test of renal function.

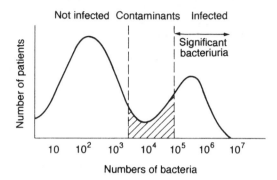

Figure 28.20 Significant bacteriuria. Specimens of urine are rarely sterile. A cut-off point is identified to distinguish true infection (significant bacteriuria) from effects of contamination from surrounding tissues.

Dipstick (reagent) tests

Strips that have been impregnated with chemicals are dipped quickly in urine and read as a means of testing urine. When dipped in urine, the chemicals react with abnormal substances and change colour. Although dipstick reagents have been primarily used as screening tools for protein or glucose in the urine, more sophisticated reagents are now available. These reagents test for nitrites and leucocyte esterase as indicators of bacterial infection. Leucocyte esterase is an enzyme from neutrophils not normally found in urine and is a marker of infection. Nitrites are produced in urine by the bacterial breakdown of dietary nitrates (Woodward & Griffiths 1993). Screening for bacteriuria can have significant cost savings for departments that routinely screen for urinary tract infection by sending samples of midstream urine (MSU) from all patients. Lowe (1986) found that by using dipstick reagents to screen for infection, it was possible to reduce by 40% microbiology workload, with subsequent cost savings. This has been substantiated in further studies by Flanagan et al. (1989) and Hiscoke et al. (1990).

The routine use of urine dipsticks for testing for infection is not widespread in the UK (Woodward & Griffiths 1993). This is mainly due to concern about the sensitivity of these sticks. Several studies have recently looked at the

Table 28.6 Changes to composition of urine and their possible causes

Substance	Name of condition	Possible causes
Glucose	Glycosuria	Diabetes mellitus
Proteins	Proteinuria	May be seen in pregnancy and high-protein diets; heart failure; severe hypertension; infection; asymptomatic renal disease
Ketone bodies	Ketonuria	Starvation; untreated diabetes mellitus
Haemoglobin	Haemoglobinuria	Transfusion reaction; haemolytic anaemia; severe burns
Bile pigments	Bilirubinuria	Liver disease, or obstruction of bile ducts
Erythrocytes	Haematuria	Bleeding in urinary tract: kidney stones, infection, or trauma
Leucocytes	Pyuria	Urinary tract infection

Table 28.7 How drugs may influence the results of reagent sticks

Drug	Reagent test	Effect on the results
Ascorbic acid	Glucose, blood, nitrite	High concentrations may diminish colour
L-dopa	Glucose Ketones	High concentrations may give a false negative reaction Atypical colour
Nalidixic acid Probenacid	Urobilinogen	Atypical colour
Phenazopyridine (pyridium)	Protein Ketones Urobilinogen, bilirubin Nitrite	May give atypical colour Coloured metabolites may mask a small reaction May mimic a positive reaction
Rifampicin	Bilirubin	Coloured metabolites may mask a small reaction
Salicylates (aspirin)	Glucose	High doses may give a false negative reaction

accuracy of using these dipstick reagents for screening for urinary tract infections (Hurlbut & Littenberg 1991). Flanagan *et al.* (1989) in a study found that the sticks had a 96.1% sensitivity to infection, while Mills *et al.* (1992) in a study of surgical patients found 91% sensitivity pre-operatively, but that sensitivity fell to 71% post-surgery. They concluded that dipstick reagents are a useful screening tool. However, specimens still need to be microbiologically examined to determine the nature and sensitivity of the infection for treatment. Overall, there is a good correlation between these biochemical tests and microscopic analysis, with reagent sticks costing approximately 18 pence in comparison with £13 for microbiological analysis (Ravichandra *et al.* 1994). When interpreting the results of reagent sticks it is important to remember the limitations of the test as false negatives are possible.

Many drugs may influence urine tests (see Table 28.7). It is therefore important to assess the patient's medication when considering the results of dipstick urinalysis. The wide range of urine tests available and the ease with which they can be used have established the use of reagent sticks throughout clinical practice. It is important to be aware, however, that they do have limitations and that manufacturer's instructions should be followed carefully, as results, especially tests for glucose and protein, can influence treatment and care decisions.

References and further reading

Bonnardeux, A. *et al.* (1994) Study of the reliability of dipstick urinalysis. *Clin Nephrol*, **41**(3), 167–72.

Cook, R. (1996) Urinalysis: ensuring accurate urine testing. *Nurs Stand*, **10**(46), 49–55.

Cooper, C. (1993) What colour is that urine specimen? *Am J Nurs*, **93**(8), 37.

Fillingham, S. & Douglas, J. (eds) (1997) *Urological Nursing*. Baillière Tindall, London.

Flanagan, P.G. *et al.* (1989) Evaluation of four screening tests for bacteriuria in elderly people. *Lancet*, **1**(8647), 1117–19.

Hiscoke, C., Yoxall, H., Greig, D. & Lightfoot, N.F. (1990) Validation of a method for the rapid diagnosis of urinary tract infection suitable for use in general practice. *Br J Gen Pract*, **40**, 403–405.

Hurlbut, T.A. & Littenberg, B. (1991) The diagnostic accuracy of rapid dipstick tests to predict urinary tract infection. *Am J Clin Pathol*, **96**, 582–8.

Johnson, A. (1986) Urinary tract infection. *Nursing*, **3**, 102–105.

Keeler, L.L. (1994) Tests to detect asymptomatic urinary tract infections. *J Am Med Assoc*, **271**(18), 1399–400.

Kunin, C.M. (1979) *Detection, Prevention, and Management of Urinary Tract Infections*. Henry Kimpton, London.

Lowe, P. (1986) Chemical screening and prediction of bacteriuria – a new approach. *Med Lab Sci*, **43**, 28–33.

Marieb, E.M. (1998) *Human Anatomy and Physiology*, 4th edn. Benjamin Cummings, California.

Mills, S.J. *et al.* (1992) Screening for bacteriuria in urological patients using reagent strips. *Br J Urol*, **70**, 314–17.

Mims, C.A. *et al.* (1993) *Medical Microbiology*, C.V. Mosby, London.

Misdraji, J. & Nguyen, P.L. (1996) Urinalysis: when and when not to order. *Postgrad Med*, **100**(1), 173–6, 181–2, 185–6.

Ravichandra, D. *et al.* (1994) Urine testing for acute lower abdominal pain in adults. *Br J Surg*, **81**, 1459–60.

Stevens, M. (1989) Screening urines for bacteriuria. *Med Lab Sci*, **46**, 194–206.

Torrance, C. & Elley, K. (1998) Urine testing 2 – urinalysis. *Nurs Times*, **94**(5), Suppl. 2.

Woodward, M.N. & Griffiths, D.M. (1993) Use of dipsticks for routine analysis of urine from children with acute abdominal pain. *Br Med J*, **306**, 1512.

GUIDELINES • Reagent sticks

Procedure

Action	*Rationale*
1 Store reagent sticks in accordance with manufacturer's instructions. This often includes any dark place or in a refrigerator.	Tests may depend on enzymatic reaction. To ensure reliable results.
2 Explain and discuss the procedure with the patient.	To ensure that the patient understands the procedure and gives his/her valid consent.
3 Obtain clean specimen of fresh urine from patient.	Urine that has been stored deteriorates rapidly and can give false results.
4 Dip the reagent strip into the urine. The strip should be completely immersed in the urine and then removed immediately and tapped against the side of the container.	To remove any excess urine.
5 Hold the stick at an angle.	Urine reagent strips should not be held upright when reading them because urine may run from square to square, mixing various reagents.
6 Wait the required time interval before reading the strip against the colour chart.	The strips must be read at exactly the time interval specified, or the reagents will not have time to react, or may be inaccurate.

GUIDELINES • Mid-stream specimen of urine

A clean-catch mid-stream specimen of urine is the most effective method of obtaining a voided specimen of urine for laboratory analysis.

Equipment

1 Sterile specimen container.

Procedure

Action

1 Explain and discuss the procedure with the patient.

2 Ask the patient to carefully clean the labia or glans with soap and water (not antiseptic).

3 Allow the first part of the urine stream to be voided and then catch the rest.

4 Specimens should be clearly labelled and sent immediately to the laboratory.

Rationale

To ensure that the patient understands the procedure and gives his/her valid consent.

This cleansing is to reduce the amount of contamination from surrounding tissues. Antiseptics can influence the result of the urinalysis (Mims *et al.* 1993).

This helps to wash out any contaminants that may be present in the urethra.

Delay allows the specimen to deteriorate, leading to inaccurate results. If it is not possible to send the specimen immediately, it should be refrigerated.

Blood glucose

Definition

The body regulates the blood glucose levels by producing insulin. Insulin's main effect is to lower the blood glucose level, but it also influences protein and fat metabolism. If the pancreas fails to produce sufficient insulin, the level of glucose in the blood will remain high. Conversely, if too much insulin is made, or given, then the level of glucose in the blood remains low. In a healthy individual the body regulates the blood glucose to be maintained between 4 and 7 mmol/l (Cowan 1997).

Indications

Blood glucose is monitored when the body is unable to maintain the blood glucose within the normal range. Conditions where a patient's blood glucose may need careful monitoring are:

1 In order to make a diagnosis of diabetes mellitus.
2 In the acute management of unstable diabetic states: diabetic ketoacidosis, hyperosmolar non-ketotic coma, and hypoglycaemia.
3 In order to make a diagnosis of hypoglycaemia.
4 Where the blood glucose level is not in keeping with the patient's clinical status.

Reference material

To maintain normal blood glucose levels, insulin and the counter-regulatory hormones, or stress hormones, must be in balance. These hormones, which include adrenaline, noradrenaline, cortisol, growth hormone and glucagon, are released in the event of stress (Sharp 1993).

During infection, major surgery or critical illness, people's regulatory hormone levels of cortisol, noradrenaline and glucagon will rise in response to the stressful event. This stimulates glycogen and fat breakdown, which causes the blood glucose levels to rise. In a healthy individual, insulin production would increase. In a person who is unable to raise his/her insulin levels, e.g. a diabetic, the result is hyperglycaemia (Curry & Weedon 1993). The majority of people who have diabetes will be known to be diabetic prior to this event. However, there may be a proportion who have had no history of such a disorder, only becoming diabetic in response to their primary illness and treatment. This diagnosis does not mean that they will remain a diabetic, but that they may need careful monitoring after their recovery.

Hypoglycaemia

Hypoglycaemia is described as a blood glucose level that is unable to meet the metabolic demands of the body (Marini & Wheeler 1997). Often young and healthy individuals can be asymptomatic during this inadequate level of glucose in the blood. Early symptoms are sweating, tachycardia and hypertension. Seizures may also be a presenting symptom, but are more common in children than in adults. The most common cause is induced by insulin when combined with alcohol consumption (Marini & Wheeler 1997). In hospital, hypoglycaemia may occur when there is renal impairment, with insufficient clearing of insulin and with irregular or insufficient food intake (Marini & Wheeler 1997).

Other causes of hypoglycaemia are:

1 Infection which can result in hepatic failure, renal insufficiency, depletion of muscle glycogen and starvation.
2 Alcohol which suppresses glyconeogenesis and nutritional intake. This induces a low insulin state, ketone production and fatty acid release.
3 Hepatic failure, which can be due to tumour infiltration, cirrhosis or hepatic necrosis.
4 Renal failure.
5 Salicylate poisoning.
6 Insulin-secreting tumours.
7 Surgery (Marini & Wheeler 1997).

Treatment should be by the administration of glucose. The route will depend on the conscious level of the individual and the treatment the patient has undergone, e.g. postoperatively it may be necessary to refrain from eating and drinking, as well as the recommendations of the medical staff.

Hyperglycaemia

When insulin is deficient or absent, blood glucose levels remain high after a meal. This is because insulin acts like a key, unlocking a door to allow glucose to enter the cell. If absent, the glucose is unable to enter most cells. When the glucose levels becomes excessive (hyperglycaemia) the person will feel nauseated, and the body will precipitate the flight or fight response. The cells are starved of glucose and the body reacts inappropriately by producing reactions usually seen in states of fasting (hypoglycaemia). Processes such as glycogenolysis (the breakdown of glycogen to release glucose), lipolysis (the breakdown of stored fats into glycerol and fatty acids), and gluconeogenesis (the conversion of glycerol and amino acids into glucose) are instigated (Marieb 1998).

The blood glucose continues to rise and some of the glucose is excreted in the urine. As the level of glucose in the kidney increases, water reabsorption by the tubules becomes inhibited. This causes the body to excrete large amounts of urine (polyuria). The person will feel thirsty and will pass urine often and in large quantities. This will lead to dehydration, a fall in blood pressure and electrolyte imbalance. The acid–base imbalance due to the loss of sodium and potassium (hypokalaemia) leads to the person complaining of abdominal pains, nausea and vomiting. As the patient's condition deteriorates, cardiac irregularities

may occur with central nervous depression (Marini & Wheeler 1997) (Fig. 28.21).

Even though there is excessive glucose in the body, the body cannot utilize it, so an alternative source of energy has to be found. To compensate, the body starts to break down fats and protein. Fats are mobilized which leads to high levels of fatty acids in the blood (lipidaemia). This can also cause sudden and dramatic weight loss. The fatty acid metabolites, known as ketones, accumulate in the blood faster than they can be excreted or used. The blood pH will fall, resulting in ketoacidosis and ketones being excreted into the urine. If ketoacidosis is allowed to continue it can become life-threatening as it disrupts all physiological processes, including oxygen transportation and heart activity. Depression of the nervous system leads to coma and death (Marieb 1998).

Diabetic ketoacidosis is a serious condition, which has a mortality rate of between 5 and 15% despite treatment (Marini & Wheeler 1997). It is a result of a deficiency of insulin and a high level of stress hormones. In the diabetic patient it is usually precipitated by a poor diet, inadequate medication and can be brought on by infection. The most prominent metabolic changes caused by ketoacidosis are metabolic acidosis and volume depletion.

Treatment involves fluid replacement, restoration of the acid–base imbalance and careful monitoring. If patients in a ketoacidotic state do not respond to fluid replacement and correction of the pH, then other conditions such as septic shock, bleeding, adrenal insufficiency, myocardial infarction and pancreatitis should be considered, and treated accordingly (Marini & Wheeler 1997).

The administration of intravenous insulin should be titrated by an infusion device, and measurements of blood glucose should be taken 1–2 hourly in order to guide the rate of delivery. If the blood glucose does not fall within the first few hours it may indicate insulin resistance and the amount of insulin may need to be increased.

Note: care needs to be taken in the rapid reversal of fluid loss and electrolyte imbalance. Excessive fluids can cause sudden acid–base shifts and exacerbate hypokalaemia. Central nervous system acidosis and arrhythmias are preventable with constant monitoring. Once urine flow is re-established, potassium should be given. Magnesium and phosphate levels in the blood should also be monitored. A common complication after aggressive treatment is hypoglycaemia.

Blood glucose monitoring

Monitoring a patient's blood glucose provides an accurate indication of how the body is controlling glucose metabolism. In the short term, monitoring can prevent hypoglycaemia and ketoacidosis, and in the long term it can reduce or prevent disorders that affect the vascular and neural pathways. Blood testing is now known to be more accurate than urine testing as the results relate to the time of testing (Cowan 1997). Blood samples can be taken from capillary, venous or arterial routes. The vessel used will depend on

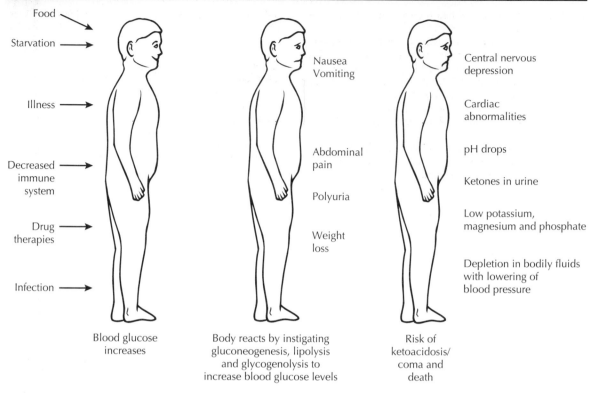

Food

Starvation

Illness

Decreased immune system

Drug therapies

Infection

Nausea Vomiting

Abdominal pain

Polyuria

Weight loss

Central nervous depression

Cardiac abnormalities

pH drops

Ketones in urine

Low potassium, magnesium and phosphate

Depletion in bodily fluids with lowering of blood pressure

Blood glucose increases

Body reacts by instigating gluconeogenesis, lipolysis and glycogenolysis to increase blood glucose levels

Risk of ketoacidosis/ coma and death

Figure 28.21   Effects of increasing glucose due to insufficient insulin production.

the accessibility of obtaining the blood sample, the frequency of testing and the condition of the patient.

It is essential that both the correct equipment is used and the operator is trained and proficient in its operation. Many different monitoring devices are currently available. Nursing and medical research has now been undertaken to identify the most accurate and practicable equipment (Harding 1993; Trajanoski *et al.* 1996; Chan *et al.* 1997; Cowan 1997; Rumley 1997; Kirk & Rheney 1998).

In 1987 the Department of Health issued a hazard warning notice following death of a patient due to an incorrect blood glucose test. This highlighted the need for formal training and strict quality control (Weedon & Willis 1991). This was further supported by a study by Almond (1986), who highlighted several potential errors from the differences shown between the laboratory true level and the meter reading. In spite of the hazard warning in 1987, Heenan (1990) continued to find inaccurate results, which were often due to incorrect timing of the test, insufficient amounts of blood taken and smearing of the sample. This led to a further safety notice being circulated by the Department of Health in 1996. Entitled 'Extra-Laboratory Use of Blood Glucose Meters and Test Strips: Contraindications, Training and Advice to Users', the report stipulates that staff undertaking 'near-patient testing' should be aware that certain patient conditions may lead to false and misleading results. The testing of blood glucose in the blood may be affected by the following:

1 Hyperlipaemia (containing abnormal fat concentrations, for example cholesterol above 56.5 mmol/l).
2 Haematocrit values. If extremely high, i.e. above 55%, and blood glucose values are above 11 mmol/l, the value may be up to 15% too low. If the haematocrit level is low, i.e. less than 35%, the value may be up to 10% too high.
3 Dialysis treatment.
4 Bilirubin values above 0.43 mmol/l, e.g. in jaundice.
5 Intravenous infusion of ascorbic acid (vitamin C).
6 When there has been peripheral circulatory failure, e.g. following severe dehydration caused by hyperglycaemic-hyperosmolar state with or without ketoacidosis, hypotension, shock or peripheral vascular disease. In these cases the results of the blood sample taken from the peripheral blood, e.g. from a finger prick, may be much lower than laboratory measurements taken from venous or arterial sources. In these cases treatment should be based on laboratory measurements only (Wickham *et al.* 1986).

The Department of Health report (1996) highlights that there must be standardization in training, reliability and quality control. In order to achieve this, the following aspects need to be considered when selecting near-patient blood glucose monitoring equipment:

1 That the equipment is designed for use by non-laboratory staff and is suitable for use in the clinical environment.

2 That all the equipment used is compatible and will give reliable results.

3 That the pathological laboratory is involved in the purchase and in the maintenance of the equipment. This may involve the purchase of one type of device from one company for the whole hospital, to reduce costs and provide standardization (Lowes 1995).

4 The product should be easy to use, and the staff should be involved in the choice of the device (Kirk & Rheney 1998).

5 The ongoing cost and maintenance of the device need to be considered, such as buying strips, control solution and replacement devices (Kirk & Rheney 1998).

6 That there are written standard operating procedures that are available and preferably kept with the device.

7 That there is training given to the operators and that records are kept. However, the training must include:
   (a) The basic principle of measurement and knowledge of what is considered normal.
   (b) That staff can demonstrate the proper use of the equipment as laid down by the operating instructions and specifications (Bayne 1997).
   (c) That staff can demonstrate the consequences of improper use.
   (d) That health and safety is maintained in the collection of blood samples, i.e. to prevent spillage and needle stick injuries.
   (e) To ensure the importance of complete documentation.
   (f) That staff use appropriate calibration and quality control techniques.
   (g) That staff undertake a series of practical procedures in order to satisfy the instructor of competency.
   (h) That blood sugar strip analysis should only be used as a guide and a tool, with diagnosis and treatment decisions being made on confirmed laboratory results.

(DoH 1996).

There is a requirement to monitor the quality of the results of the device and the person operating it. This is both a hospital and a government directive. Independent quality control should be carried out with the collaboration of the pathology laboratory. External auditing of the quality control should be undertaken and this may be provided in the package offered by the company. Problems that can occur include compliance by both patient and staff, blood sampling problems, the quality of the solution, the external

audit and the training needs of the individual (Lowes 1995).

References and further reading

Almond, J. (1986) Measuring blood glucose levels. *Nurs Times*, **82**(41), 51–4.

Bayne, C. (1997) How sweet it is: glucose monitoring equipment and interpretation. *Nurs Manag*, **28**(9), 52–4.

Chan, J., Wong, R., Cheung, C. *et al.* (1997) Accuracy, precision and user-acceptability of self blood glucose monitoring machines. *Diabetes Res Clin Pract*, **36**(2), 91–104.

Cowan, T. (1997) Blood glucose monitoring devices. *Prof Nurse*, **12**(8), 593–7.

Curry, M. & Weedon, L. (1993) Balancing act. *Nurs Times*, **89**(23), 50–52.

DHSS (1987) *Blood Glucose Measurements: Reliability of Results Produced in Extra-Laboratory Areas*. HN (Hazard) (87) 13. NHS Procurement Directorate, 14 Russell Square, London.

DoH (1990) *Lancing Devices for Multi-Patient Capillary Sampling: Avoidance of Cross Infection by Correct Selection and Use*. DEF 42/00/10003. Medical Services Directorate, 14 Russell Square, London.

DoH (1996) *Extra-Laboratory Use of Blood Glucose Meters and Test Strips: Contraindications, Training and Advice to Users*. Medical Devices Agency Adverse Incident Centre Safety Notice 9616, June.

Harding, K. (1993) A comparison of four glucose monitors in a hospital medical surgical setting. *Clin Nurse Specialist*, **7**(1), 13–16.

Heenan, A. (1990) Blood glucose measurement. *Nurs Times*, **86**(4), 65–8.

Kirk, J. & Rheney, C. (1998) Important features of blood glucose meters. *J Am Pharm Ass (Washington)*, **8**(2), 210–19.

Lowes, L. (1995) Accuracy in ward-based blood glucose monitoring. *Nurs Times*, **91**(13), 44–5.

Marieb, E.M. (1998) *Human Anatomy and Physiology*, 4th edn., pp. 586–620. Benjamin Cummings, California.

Marini, J. & Wheeler, A. (1997) *Critical Care Medicine: The Essentials*, 2nd edn., pp. 498–510. Williams and Wilkins, Baltimore.

Rumley, A. (1997) Improving the quality of near patient blood glucose measurement. *Annu Clin Biochem*, **34**(Part 2), 281–6.

Sharp, S. (1993) Blood glucose monitoring in the intensive care unit. *Br J Nurs*, **2**(4), 209–14.

Trajanoski, Z., Brunner, G., Gfrerer, R., Wach, P. & Pieber, T. (1996) Accuracy of home blood glucose meters during hypoglycaemia. *Diabetes Care*, **19**(12), 1412–15.

Weedon, L. & Willis, P. (1991) Introducing reflectance meters to hospital wards. *Pract Diabetes*, **8**(6), 228–33.

Wickham, N. *et al.* (1986) Unreliability of capillary blood glucose in peripheral vascular disease. *Pract Diabetes*, **3**, 100.

GUIDELINES · Blood glucose monitoring

Only nursing staff who have obtained a certificate of training for the equipment should undertake this task.

Equipment

1 Blood glucose monitor.
2 Test strips.

3 Control solution.
4 A device to obtain a blood sample, e.g. a lancet.

Guidelines • Blood glucose monitoring (cont'd)

Procedure

Action	*Rationale*

1 Before taking the device to the patient the monitor needs to be checked for the following:

(a) That one pack of test strips is open and that they are in date, i.e. not expired.

(b) That the monitor and the test strips have been calibrated together.

(c) That if a new pack of strips is required, the monitor is recalibrated.

(d) That the quality control test has been carried out that day, and on changing batteries, new strips and on any unusual unpredicted result.

(e) That the quality control check has been recorded in the record book and signed.

To ensure accuracy of the result. The quality control and checks have been carried out in order to ensure the safety of the patient.

2 Explain the procedure to the patient. Some patients may want to look away at the sight of a needle.

The patient should be aware of the procedure in order to allay some of his/her anxieties, and to be able to cooperate in the procedure.

3 Patients should be advised to wash their hands prior to blood sampling. The use of alcohol rub should be avoided. Encourage patients to keep their hands warm until sampling has been performed.

To ensure a non-contaminated result. To encourage good blood flow (Cowan 1997).

4 Ask the patient to sit or lie down.

To ensure the patient's safety as some patients may feel faint when blood is taken.

5 Wash your hands, and put on protective gloves.

To minimize the risk of cross-infection. To minimize the risk of contamination.

6 Use a disposable lancet. These are advised following an outbreak of hepatitis B in French and US hospitals (DoH 1990)

To minimize the risk of cross-infection.

7 Take a blood sample from the side of the finger using the lancet, ensuring that the site of piercing is rotated. Avoid frequent use of the index finger and thumb. The finger may bleed without assistance, or may need assistance by 'milking' to form a droplet of blood which is large enough to cover the test pad.

The side of the finger is used as it is less painful and easier to obtain a hanging droplet of blood. The site is rotated to reduce the risk of infection from multiple stabbing, the areas becoming toughened and to reduce pain.

8 Apply the blood to the pad in only one application. If not, then throw the pad away and start again.

If the test pad is not covered then the result will be inaccurate.

9 Dispose of lancet in a container designed for sharps.

To reduce the risk of needle stick injury.

10 Depending on the type of monitor, the procedure will differ. See individual manuals and hospital policies.

To ensure the accuracy of the result.

11 Once the result is obtained, record immediately.

To ensure the accuracy of the result.

12 Dispose of waste appropriately. Remove gloves and dispose.

To reduce the risk of cross-infection.

13 Make the patient comfortable and observe site of test for bleeding.

To ensure the patient's comfort.

14 Wash hands.

To prevent cross-infection.

Pain Assessment and Management

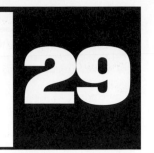

Definition

Pain is not a simple sensation but a complex phenomenon having both a cognitive (physical) and an affective (emotional) component. Because pain is subjective the favoured definition for use in clinical practice, proposed originally by McCaffery (1968), is: 'Pain is whatever the experiencing person says it is, existing whenever the experiencing person says it does.' The aim of pain assessment is to identify *all* the factors – physical and non-physical – that affect the patient's perception of pain. A comprehensive clinical assessment is essential to gain a thorough understanding of the patient's pain and as a means to evaluate the effectiveness of interventions.

Reference material

There are several ways to categorize the types of pain that occur in patients with cancer, but it is important to recognize that cancer patients may experience both acute and chronic pain. Foley (1998) describes the following types of pain, which are also recognized by McCaffery & Beebe (1989).

Acute pain

Acute pain usually has a brief duration and has a protective function. It is normally associated with injury or disease and is expected to subside when the injury or disease process has resolved.

Chronic pain

Chronic pain is usually prolonged and defined as pain that exists for more than 3 months (International Association for the Study of Pain 1996). It is often associated with major changes in personality, lifestyle and functional ability (Foley 1998).

In addition, it is essential to mention episodic, incident and breakthrough pains, which are all terms referring to 'a transitory exacerbation of pain experienced by the patient who has relatively stable and adequately controlled baseline pain' (Hanks 1983). The breakthrough pain experienced by the patient is when the regular opioid regimen used for baseline pain fails to provide adequate analgesic cover. During pain assessment it is essential that nurses include exploration of this type of pain.

Acute pain assessment for surgical patients

For surgical pain to be controlled effectively, pain must be assessed regularly and systematically. The process of pain assessment begins before surgery and continues through to discharge.

Assessment of anxiety, meaning of pain and past pain experience

A number of psychosocial factors influence an individual's pain. Patients may be anxious about the outcome of the surgery or how pain will be controlled, particularly if they have bad memories of previous pain experiences (Audit Commission 1997). Anxiety in turn exacerbates pain by increasing muscle tension. Providing patients with appropriate support and information to address these concerns can reduce both anxiety and postoperative pain (Audit Commission 1997).

Assessment of pre-existing pain

Patients who have been taking regular strong analgesics for a pre-existing chronic pain problem may require higher doses of analgesia to manage an acute pain episode. It is therefore important to take a history of pre-existing pain and analgesic use so that appropriate analgesic measures can be planned in advance of surgery.

Assessment of location and intensity of pain

Location

Many complex surgical procedures involve more than one incision site and the nature and extent of pain at each site may vary. A careful assessment of the location and type of pain is required, because each pain problem may respond to different pain management techniques.

Intensity

The effects of intervention can only be assessed and improved if some form of pain measurement is made. To achieve this, a baseline pain assessment should be carried out and repeated at regular intervals following any intervention so that its effectiveness can be evaluated against the baseline. The simplest techniques for pain measurement involve the use of either a visual analogue scale, verbal rating scale or numerical rating scale. Using one of these scales, patients are asked to match pain intensity to the scale.

Three principles apply to the use of these scales:

1 The patient should be involved in scoring his/her own pain intensity. This is because several studies have shown that professionals frequently underestimate pain intensity when compared with patients (Seers 1988; Kuhn et al. 1990; Scott 1994; Field 1996).
2 Pain intensity should be assessed on movement because patients need to be able to move comfortably to prevent immobility and its associated complications, e.g. deep vein thrombosis (Gould et al. 1992).
3 It is important to remember that a complete picture of a patient's pain cannot be derived solely from the use of a pain scale (Lawler 1997). Ongoing communication with the patient is required to uncover and manage any psychosocial factors that may be affecting the patient's pain experience.

Chronic pain assessment

The nature of chronic pain means that at times it can be difficult to assess, as patients rarely present with this one symptom. For example, approximately two-thirds of advanced cancer patients will also complain of anorexia, one-half will have a symptomatic dry mouth and constipation, and one-third will suffer nausea, vomiting, insomnia, dyspnoea, cough or oedema (Hanks 1983; Donnelly & Walsh 1995). It will be clear from these figures that chronic pain assessment cannot be seen in isolation; identification of all related symptoms is of equal importance as they will contribute to a lowered pain threshold (the least stimulus intensity at which a person perceives pain) and impaired pain tolerance (the greatest stimulus intensity causing pain that a person is prepared to tolerate). Seventy five percent of cancer patients present with pain, 33% of whom will have pain in three or more sites (Grond et al. 1996). Furthermore, chronic cancer pain is often multifocal.

A diagnosis of cancer does not necessarily mean that the malignant process is the cause of the pain. Pain in chronic cancer may be:

1 Caused by the cancer itself.
2 Caused by treatment.
3 Associated with debilitating disease, such as a pressure ulcer.
4 Unrelated to either the disease or the treatment, such as headache.

The cause of *each* pain should therefore be identified carefully; many pains unrelated to the cancer will respond to specific treatment. If the pain is due to the cancer, then it is important to determine the precise mechanism of pain because treatment will vary accordingly.

The perception of painful stimuli will always be modulated by the emotional response to that perception. Changes in mood may alter considerably the experience of pain (McCaffery & Beebe 1989). Pain assessment needs to

acknowledge this fact, and particular attention must be paid to factors that will modulate pain sensitivity (Table 29.1).

Need for pain assessment tools

Accurate pain assessment is a prerequisite of effective control and is an essential component of nursing care. In the assessment process, the nurse gathers information from the patient that allows an understanding of the patient's experience and its effect on the patient's life. The information obtained guides the nurse in planning and evaluating strategies for care. Pain is rarely static; therefore its assessment is not a one-time process but is ongoing.

Pain assessment is difficult to achieve. For example, the tendency suggested by both research and clinical practice is for the patient not to report any pain or to do so inadequately or inaccurately, minimizing the pain experience (McCaffery 1983; McCaffery & Beebe 1989). Hunt et al. (1977) found that nurses tended to overestimate the pain relief obtained from analgesia and underestimate the level of the patient's pain.

Pain charts have been considered as useful tools for assisting nurses to assess pain and plan nursing care. Raiman (1986) found that the use of a chart improved communication between staff and patients. Walker et al. (1987) found that the specific advantages of using a chart lie in promoting both the initial assessment of pain and its monitoring. It was also found that the involvement of many patients in their pain management helped to increase their confidence in it.

Use of pain assessment tools

There are numerous methods of assessing pain, and the published literature indicates that pain assessment charts can be used successfully to assess and monitor pain (McCaffery & Beebe 1989; Twycross et al. 1996). Some degree of caution, however, must be exercised in their use. The nurse must be careful to select the tool that is most appropriate for a particular type of pain experience. For example, it would not be appropriate to use a pain assessment chart that had been designed for use with patients with chronic pain, to assess postoperative pain. Furthermore, pain charts should not be used totally indiscriminately. Walker et al. (1987) found that charts appeared to have little value in cases of unresolved or intractable pain.

Table 29.1 Factors affecting pain sensitivity

Sensitivity increased:	Sensitivity lowered:
Discomfort	Relief of symptoms
Insomnia	Sleep
Fatigue	Rest
Anxiety	Sympathy
Fear	Understanding
Anger	Companionship
Sadness	Diversional activity
Depression	Reduction in anxiety
Boredom	Elevation of mood

The use of pain assessment tools for acute pain has been shown to increase both the effectiveness of nursing interventions and improve the management of pain (Scott 1994; Harmer & Davies 1998). Several pain assessment tools are available (Kitson 1994). Since many of these focus on assessing the intensity of pain, it is important that nurses do not neglect to combine their use of these tools with an assessment of the patient's psychosocial needs.

The most commonly used pain assessment tools meet the following criteria (Hancock 1996):

1 Simplicity – ease of understanding for all the patient group.
2 Reliability – reliability of the tool when used in similar patient groups.
3 Sensitivity – sensitivity of the tool to the patient's pain.
4 Accuracy – accurate recording of data through patient involvement.
5 Practicality – a practical tool is more likely to be used by patients and nursing staff.

For practical purposes, a combined pain assessment and observation chart is frequently used in the postoperative period. The Royal Marsden Hospital Postoperative Observation and Pain Assessment Chart is an example of one of these (Fig. 29.1). Patients are given an information leaflet before surgery and encouraged to record their own pain intensity (usually 4-hourly, but more frequently if pain is not controlled) on the pain scale at the bottom of the chart.

The Royal Marsden Hospital Chronic Pain Assessment Chart

A study was carried out at The Royal Marsden Hospital in order to design a chart for use with patients with chronic cancer pain and to evaluate its effectiveness (Walker *et al.* 1987). The study indicated that the chart (Fig. 29.2) was a valuable tool for pain assessment in 98% of cases. The following guidelines are written with reference to The Royal Marsden Hospital Chronic Pain Assessment Chart, but it is recognized that nurses may modify the chart to meet the needs of their own particular branch of nursing.

The need for effective pain control

There are several reasons why pain needs to be well controlled following surgery, not least that patients have a right to expect good pain control (Audit Commission 1997). Uncontrolled pain can lead to increased anxiety and muscle tension which further exacerbate pain. It can delay the recovery process by hindering mobilization and deep breathing, which increases the risk of a patient developing a deep vein thrombosis, chest infection or pressure ulcer (Macintyre & Ready 1997). With severe pain, activity of the sympathetic nervous system and the neuroendocrine 'stress response' causes platelet activation, changes in regional blood flow and stress on the heart. These can lead to impaired wound healing, and myocardial ischaemia

(Macintyre & Ready 1997). There is evidence to suggest that in the long term, poorly controlled acute pain may lead to the development of chronic pain. Tasmuth *et al.* (1996) found that patients who went on to develop chronic pain following surgically treated breast cancer remembered having more severe postoperative pain than those women who had no chronic pain.

Management of pain

The control of pain is directed by the 'Analgesic Ladder' which was presented by the World Health Organization in 1996 (Fig. 29.3). The simple principles are such that pharmacological intervention begins on the first step of the ladder and proceeds upwards as and when the pain reaches a higher level and the current analgesia is no longer effective. It is important to remember that the patient will experience different types of pain due to different aetiological and physiological changes, manifested through the cancer trajectory (e.g. bone pain, neuropathic pain). It is important to make an assessment of each pain separately, since the pain may need to be managed in a different manner and one analgesic intervention will rarely be sufficient. Often the best practice is to combine the baseline analgesia with an appropriate adjuvant treatment in order to achieve maximum pain control.

Oral administration of therapeutic interventions may not always be appropriate and consideration should be given to other routes of administration, e.g. rectal, parenteral and sublingual. The rectal route is now less commonly used in favour of subcutaneous administration via a syringe driver (see Chap. 20, Infusion Devices).

Accurate ongoing assessment is imperative for efficient and effective pain control.

Acute pain management following surgery

Since nurses, surgeons, anaesthetists, pain specialists, pharmacists and physiotherapists are all involved in the management of surgical pain, teamwork is essential. Professionals must reach clear agreement as to their individual roles so that patients receive the best possible care from pre-admission through to discharge (Audit Commission 1997).

A wide variety of pharmacological and non-pharmacological techniques are available for the management of surgical pain. The following basic principles apply to their use:

1 Tailor the treatments to:
   (a) Meet individual needs
   (b) Prevent pain, rather than allowing it to become established.
2 Whenever possible, choose the simplest and safest techniques to achieve the desired level of pain relief (McQuay *et al.* 1997).
3 Use the WHO Analgesic Ladder (Fig. 29.3) to select the most appropriate analgesics for mild, moderate and severe acute pain.

The Royal Marsden Hospital

Patient Name: _____ Hosp. No.: _____ C.U./Consultant: _____

POST OPERATIVE OBSERVATION AND PAIN ASSESSMENT CHART

Date				
Time				
Temp				
40°C				
39°C				
38°C				
37°C				
36°C				
35°C				

220- 210- 200- 190- 180- 170- 160- 150- 140- 130- 120- 110- 100- 95- 90- 85- 80- 75- 70- 65- 60- 85- 80- 75- 70-

B L O O D   P R E S S U R E

P U L S E

+20 +15 C +10 +5 V 0 -5 P

R 40 E 35 S 30 P. 25

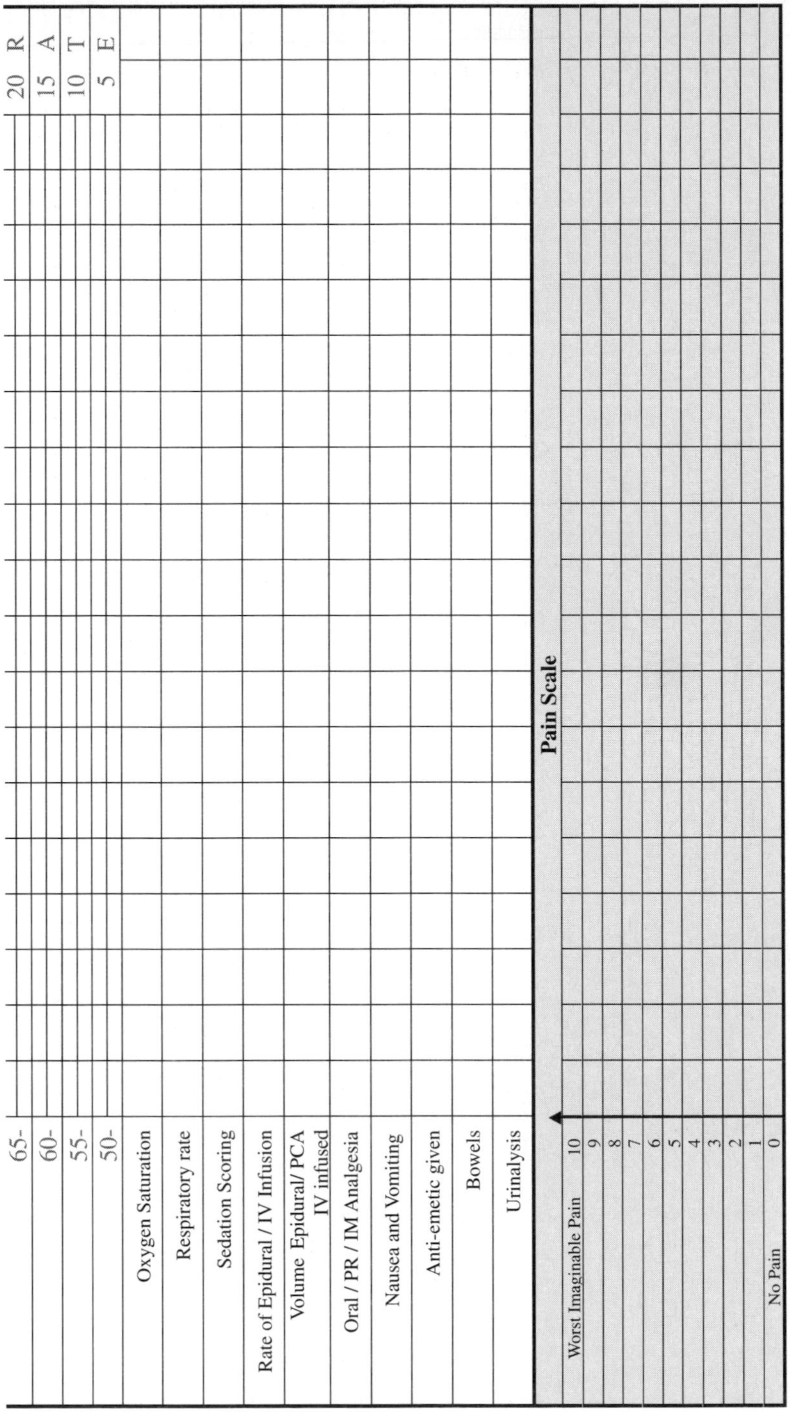

		65-																											
20 R		60-																											
15 A		55-																											
10 T		50-																											
5 E																													
		Oxygen Saturation																											
		Respiratory rate																											
		Sedation Scoring																											
		Rate of Epidural / IV Infusion																											
		Volume Epidural/ PCA IV infused																											
		Oral / PR / IM Analgesia																											
		Nausea and Vomiting																											
		Anti-emetic given																											
		Bowels																											
		Urinalysis																											
Pain Scale	Worst Imaginable Pain 10																												
	9																												
	8																												
	7																												
	6																												
	5																												
	4																												
	3																												
	2																												
	1																												
	No Pain 0																												

Figure 29.1 The Royal Marsden Hospital Postoperative Observation and Pain Assessment Chart.

The Royal Marsden Hospital

Chronic Pain Assessment Chart

Surname:

First name:

Hospital no.

Date:

Initial Assessment

Patient's own description of the pain(s):

What helps relieve the pain?

What makes the pain worse?

Do you have pain

1 At night?   Yes/No (comment if required)

2 At rest?   Yes/No (comment if required)

3 On movement?   Yes/No (Comment if required)

Pain sites

Please draw on the body outlines below to show where you feel pain. Label each site of pain with a letter A,B,C, etc.

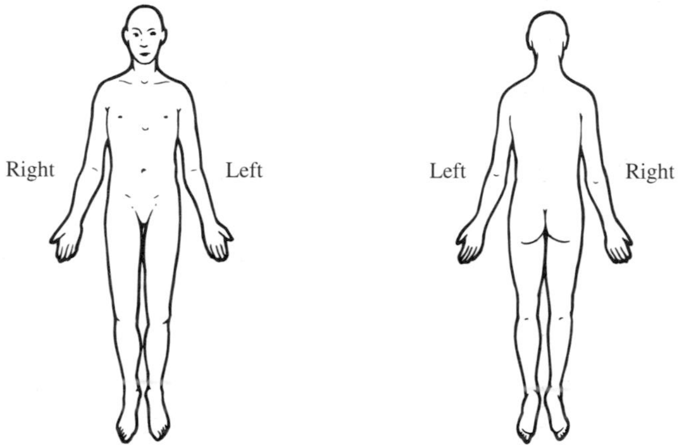

Right   Left   Left   Right

Key to pain intensity: Continuation no:

0 = no pain   4 = very severe pain

1 = mild pain   5 = intolerable/overwhelming pain

2 = moderate pain

3 = severe pain   s = sleeping

It may be easier to determine the intensity of pain by looking at the pain scale below.

no pain	0	1	2	3	4	5	intolerable/ overwhelming pain
		mild pain	moderate pain	severe pain	very severe pain		

Date	Times	Pain sites								Analgesia name, route and dose	Patient activity and comments
		A	B	C	D	E	F	G	H		

Figure 29.2   The Royal Marsden Hospital Chronic Pain Assessment Chart.

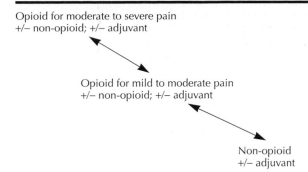

Opioid for moderate to severe pain
+/– non-opioid; +/– adjuvant

Opioid for mild to moderate pain
+/– non-opioid; +/– adjuvant

Non-opioid
+/– adjuvant

Figure 29.3   The Analgesic Ladder. (Modified from World Health Organization 1996.)

4 Give analgesics orally, unless swallowing, gastric absorption or a patient's condition dictates otherwise.
5 Combine techniques to provide balanced analgesia and enhance overall pain control (Kehlet & Jorgen 1993).
6 Ensure patients receive regular anti-emetics to control postoperative nausea and vomiting. Vomiting increases muscle tension and exacerbates pain.

Pharmacological techniques

Opioid analgesics

Opioids are the first-line treatment for pain that follows major surgery. The key principle for the safe and effective use of opioids is for the dose to be titrated to achieve pain relief while minimizing any unwanted side effects (McQuay *et al.* 1997; see 'Chronic pain' below for further details on side effects).

A number of opioids are used for controlling pain following surgery. These include morphine, diamorphine and fentanyl. The most common routes of opioid administration are either intravenous, epidural, subcutaneous, intramuscular or oral.

Intravenous analgesia

Continuous intravenous infusions of opioids such as morphine, diamorphine and fentanyl are effective for controlling pain in the immediate postoperative period. Their use is often restricted to high-dependency units where patients can be closely monitored because of the potential risk of respiratory depression (Macintyre & Ready 1997).

Patient controlled analgesia (PCA) is an alternative and safer technique for giving intravenous opioids (usually morphine) in the ward environment (Sidebotham *et al.* 1997). With PCA, patients self-administer intermittent doses of opioids, by using an infusion pump and timing device. When in pain, the patient presses a button connected to the pump and a set dose of opioid is delivered (usually intravenously but it may also be given subcutaneously) to the patient. By using a PCA pump, patients can administer analgesia as soon as pain occurs and titrate the dose of analgesia according to increases and decreases in the pain stimulus. This is particularly helpful for controlling more intense pain during movement. Because the PCA pump is designed to deliver small frequent doses of analgesia at timed intervals, the risk of respiratory depression is less than with a continuous infusion. For further details about the use of PCA pumps please refer to Chap. 20, Infusion Devices.

Epidural analgesia

Low concentrations of local anaesthetics and opioids can be infused directly into the epidural space using a catheter. Giving analgesia epidurally is a particularly valuable technique for the prevention of postoperative pain in patients undergoing major thoracic, abdominal and lower limb surgery (Yarde 1989). Commonly used opioids for epidural analgesia include fentanyl and diamorphine. Further details of this technique are given in Chap. 15.

Subcutaneous analgesia

Opioids are often given subcutaneously to manage chronic cancer pain. More recently, there has been an increase in the use of subcutaneous opioids for postoperative pain control. Both PCA- and nurse-administered opioid injections of morphine and diamorphine via an indwelling subcutaneous cannula have been used successfully to manage postoperative pain (Vijayan 1997). An advantage of giving analgesia subcutaneously is that it avoids the problems associated with maintaining intravenous access.

Intramuscular analgesia

Until the early 1990s regular 3–4 hourly intramuscular injections of opioids such as pethidine, morphine or preparations containing morphine (Omnopon) were routinely used for the management of postoperative pain. Because alternative techniques such as PCA and epidural analgesia are available, intramuscular analgesia is now used less frequently. Some useful algorithms have been developed to give guidance on titrating intramuscular analgesia (Gould *et al.* 1992; Macintyre & Ready 1997; Harmer & Davies 1998).

Oral analgesia

Oral opioids are used less frequently in the immediate postoperative period because most patients are nil by mouth for a period of time. Often this route is used if patients require strong analgesics following discontinuation of epidural or intravenous analgesia. Morphine is an ideal oral preparation because it is available as a tablet (Sevredol) or elixir (Oramorph).

Non-opioid analgesics

Paracetamol and paracetamol combinations

The use of non-opioid analgesics such as paracetamol or

paracetamol combined with a weak opioid such as codeine is recommended for managing pain following minor surgical procedures or when the pain following major surgery begins to subside (McQuay *et al.* 1997). Paracetamol can also be given rectally if the oral route is contraindicated.

Paracetamol taken in the correct dose of not more than 4 g per day is relatively free of side effects. When used in combination with codeine preparations, the most frequent side effect is constipation.

Non-steroidal anti-inflammatory drugs

Non-steroidal anti-inflammatory drugs have been shown to provide better pain relief than paracetamol combinations for acute pain (McQuay *et al.* 1997). These drugs can be used alone or in combination with both opioid and non-opioid analgesics. The non-steroidal anti-inflammatory drug diclofenac can also be administered rectally, whilst piroxicam can be taken as a melt which is placed on the tongue and absorbed via the oral mucosa. These alternative routes can be used when fluid intake is restricted. Unfortunately there are side effects associated with non-steroidal anti-inflammatory drugs and these limit their use in cancer patients. These include coagulation problems, renal impairment and gastrointestinal disturbances.

Nitrous oxide (Entonox)

Inhaled nitrous oxide provides analgesia that is short-acting and works quickly. It has a special role in managing pain associated with wound dressings and drain removal (see Chap. 14 on the use of Entonox).

Local anaesthetics

In addition to epidural analgesia, local anaesthetics may be used to block individual or groups of peripheral nerves during surgical procedures and to infiltrate surgical wounds at the end of an operation (Carroll & Bowsher 1993).

Non-pharmacological techniques

Non-pharmacological methods for managing postoperative pain include psychological and physical techniques. These measures can be particularly helpful when used to supplement pharmacological techniques.

Psychological techniques

Psychological techniques include the following.

Procedural and sensory information

For the majority of patients, information before surgery about details of the procedure, expected discomforts and ways to decrease pain can help to minimize anxiety and enhance patient control (Hayward 1975; Boore 1976). However, because some patients may find the same information increases their anxiety, it has been suggested that it is important to give patients the choice of how much information they would like (Mitchell 1997).

Cognitive behavioural techniques such as relaxation and distraction

There is increasing evidence that teaching patients relaxation techniques prior to surgery can reduce postoperative pain, improve coping skills and enhance recovery (Johnston & Vogele 1993). Simple relaxation techniques for surgical patients include deep-breathing exercises and progressive muscle relaxation. The use of music in the immediate postoperative period has also been shown to relax patients and function as a distractor from pain (Heiser *et al.* 1997).

Support and reassurance

Patients should be provided with ongoing support and reassurance from all members of the multidisciplinary team.

Physical techniques

A number of physical techniques have been used in conjunction with analgesic measures to control pain. These include simple measures such as careful body positioning, the use of soft and therapeutic mattresses, heat and cold, massage, exercise, transcutaneous electrical nerve stimulation (TENS) and acupuncture (Lewith & Kenyon 1984; McCaffery 1990; Ballard 1997).

Many of these interventions can improve pain control by simply increasing patient comfort and wellbeing. Unfortunately there is limited research evidence for their efficacy in pain management, with the exception of TENS which has not been shown to reduce postoperative pain (McQuay *et al.* 1997). In chronic pain management, Horrigan (1993) wrote about the positive effects of TENS, acupuncture, massage and relaxation and how these interventions may even lead to a reduction in their general analgesic requirements.

Despite the lack of research evidence to support the use of these therapeutic interventions, they continue to have a psychological benefit to patients and their families, especially relating to maintaining control of their lives. Acceptance by health professionals of these additional therapies may lead to an increase in compliance and trust between the staff and the patient.

Chronic pain

Using the WHO Analgesic Ladder (1996)

Step 1: non-opioid drugs

Examples of non-opioid drugs include paracetamol and aspirin. These drugs are effective in mild to moderate pain, especially musculoskeletal and visceral pain (Twycross *et al.* 1990).

Step 2: weak opioids

Examples of weak opioids include co-codamol (codeine 30 and paracetamol 500) and dihydrocodeine (also available in long-acting form). These drugs are used when adequate pain management is not achieved with the use of non-opioids and are usually used in combination formulations. They are equivalent to small doses of opioid drugs.

Tramadol has proved to be useful in the treatment of chronic pain and also has a role in neuropathic pain. It tends to be well tolerated and it is a useful step for those patients who are reluctant to commence morphine (see below), but who have several pain problems. It is available in immediate and slow-release preparations (Budd 1995).

Step 3: strong opioids

Morphine

A large amount of information and research are available concerning morphine and therefore it tends to be the drug of choice within this category (Hanks & Cherny 1998). All strong opioids require careful titration from an expert practitioner. It is better to begin with a small dose, usually one that is equivalent to the previous medication, and increase gradually in conjunction with careful assessment of its effectiveness (Hanks et al. 1996). Titration begins with the immediate-release form which is available in tablet (Sevredol) or elixir (Oramorph) preparations, and once pain control is achieved the patient can be converted to the long-acting sustained release form that acts over a 12- or 24-hour period (MST or MXL respectively).

Breakthrough analgesia is administered using the equivalent 4-hourly dose of the immediate-release form and subsequent adjustments can be made to the long-acting form if the patient is requiring more than three breakthrough doses in a 24-hour period.

Patients should be warned of potential side effects such as constipation, nausea and increased sleepiness, in order to allay any fear. The patient should also be told that nausea and drowsiness are transitory and normally improve within 48 hours, but that constipation can be an ongoing problem and it is recommended that a laxative should be prescribed at the same time as the opioid is started (Hanks et al. 1996).

Patients often have many concerns about commencing strong drugs such as morphine. Frequent fears centre around addiction and believing that its use signifies the terminal phase of the illness (Twycross 1994). Time should be taken to reassure patients and their families and provide verbal and written information.

Many new drugs are now available for use in chronic pain which allow the practitioner to carefully assess the patient on an individual basis and make an informed decision about the most appropriate drug/route to use.

Transdermal durogesic (fentanyl)

Fentanyl is a strong opioid, available in a patch, which is recommended in patients who have stable pain requirements. It is reported to have an improved side effect profile in comparison to morphine (Ahmedzai & Brooks 1997), although some patients experience nausea and mild drowsiness (BMA/Royal Pharmaceutical Society of Great Britain 1999) and occasionally patients may develop a reaction to the adhesive in the patch (Ling 1997). Use of the patch has increased because it allows the patient freedom from taking tablets.

Changing of the patch is recommended every 3 days, and steady plasma levels are reported to be reached after 8–16 hours (Zech et al. 1994), although in some patients it may be necessary to change it more frequently. The patch should be applied to skin that is free from excess hair and any form of irritation and should not be applied to irradiated areas. It is advisable to change the location on the body to avoid an adverse skin reaction. Occasionally difficulties arise relating to the titration of the patch as each patch is equivalent to a range of morphine (see Table 29.2). There is currently no fentanyl breakthrough medication, although trials are beginning in the UK using an immediate-release fentanyl lozenge which has been proven to be effective in the USA (Fine et al. 1991). The present drug of choice for breakthrough medication is immediate-release morphine (tablet or elixir).

Palladone (hydromorphone)

Palladone (hydromorphone) has only recently become available in the UK. It is mostly used when patients experience unacceptable drowsiness with morphine. It is similar to morphine in its pharmokinetic profile and it is approximately 5–7.5 times more potent than morphine. It is available in immediate-release and sustained-release preparations and titration occurs in the same manner as morphine (Hays et al. 1994).

The side effects are similar to those of morphine (Ellershaw 1998).

Phenazocine

Phenazocine is also an effective alternative to morphine preparations. It is generally used when patients have unacceptable levels of drowsiness or nausea on morphine, although many centres do not use it due to the availability of newer preparations.

It is only available in 5-mg tablets (which is equivalent to 25 mg morphine) and this makes its use somewhat limited. It is administered every 4–6 hours and there is no sustained-release preparation. Breakthrough pain is treated with the equivalent 4-hourly dose in the same manner as morphine.

Table 29.2   Oral morphine conversion to durogesic (fentanyl patch)

Four-hourly oral morphine dose (mg)	Durogesic patch strength (g/h)	24-hour oral morphine dose (mg)
20	25	135
25–35	50	135–224
40–50	75	225–314
55–65	100	315–404
70–80	125	405–494
85–95	150	495–584
100–110	175	585–674
115–125	200	675–764

Methadone

Methadone is a drug that has not been used frequently in the management of pain; however, its use is now increasing. The reluctance to use methadone arose from the difficulties experienced in titrating the drug due to its long half life (15 hours) which caused accumulation to occur, especially in the elderly (Gannon 1997). There are different methods of achieving effective titration (Gannon 1997), for example, one regimen is to administer methadone on an 'as required' basis initially (usually not more often than 3-hourly) and then to calculate the dosage required over a 24-hour period after 5–6 days. This dose can then be divided and given as a 2 or 3 times daily regimen and this avoids the buildup of methadone within the body. Titration is recommended within a hospital setting to ensure accurate administration. This can be difficult for patients because they have to experience pain before they are administered a dose of methadone in the titration period.

Methadone is particularly useful in patients with renal failure. Morphine is excreted via the kidneys and if renal failure occurs this may lead to the patient experiencing severe drowsiness as a result of culmination of morphine metabolites (Gannon 1997).

Oxycodone

The oral form of oxycodone is not available in the UK at the present time, although trials are currently being set up to examine its use in the chronic pain setting. There is, however, a limited availability of the suppository form for named patients from the drug company (NAPP).

It has similar properties to morphine, but when adjusted orally it is more potent (1.5–2 times) and it is usually given 6-hourly because of having a plasma half life of 3.5 hours (Narcessian 1997). It has similar side effects to morphine, although oxycodone has been found to cause less nausea (Heiskanen et al. 1996) and significantly less itchiness (Mucci-LoRusso et al. 1998).

Breakthrough analgesia

'Stat', 'rescue' or 'breakthrough' doses of analgesia are given if the background dose of the drug is not sufficient to adequately control pain levels and an additional dose is required. There should not be a time limit on this type of prescription because it would need to be given when and if the patient demonstrated any signs of discomfort or pain (with the exception of renal failure where dosages would need to be limited).

Breakthrough doses are calculated on a 4-hour equivalence; for example, if a patient was prescribed 60 mg MXL (a long-acting form of morphine given once a day), the equivalent breakthrough dose would be 10 mg of the immediate-release formulation. If several breakthrough doses are required within a 24-hour period, then the background analgesia (long-acting form) would have to be increased.

Adjuvant drugs (co-analgesics)

Adjuvant drugs are drugs whose primary indication is for conditions other than pain, but which have a role in the management of chronic pain. The action of traditional analgesics has been shown to be enhanced when used in conjunction with adjuvant agents (Bonica 1994). Examples of this category of drugs include non-steroidal anti-inflammatory drugs, steroids, antibiotics and anticonvulsants (Portenoy 1998).

The World Health Organization Analgesic Ladder recommends the use of these drugs in combination with non-, weak and strong opioids.

Cancer treatment interventions

In addition to pharmacological and non-pharmocological strategies, treatment of cancer pain may be managed most effectively with radiotherapy, surgery, chemotherapy, hormonal manipulation and bisphosphonates. Most palliative care units/hospices may not have access to these interventions and, indeed, careful consideration must be given to ensure that the advantages achieved from any proposed treatment are not outweighed by the potential side effects and consequent poor quality of life. The aim of these treatments would be to reduce the overall size of the tumour(s), and therefore to improve symptom control, and this must be clearly indicated to the patient.

Anaesthetic interventions

Sometimes it is difficult to attain and maintain adequate pain control and it is in situations such as this that anaesthetic interventions may be of benefit.

Effective control can be achieved by epidural and/or local blocks, especially for pelvic pain and postradiation brachial plexopathy. These interventions can be useful, but careful consideration and assessment must be given to the patient's current condition and the prognosis, as many of these treatments can leave the patient severely limited in his or her activities (McQuay 1990; see Chap. 15, Epidural Analgesia).

Conclusion

The management of acute and chronic pain is a constant challenge to the health care professional. Accurate assessment of the type and site of each pain, accompanied by careful monitoring of any intervention are essential in order to provide care that benefits the patient and does not impinge on his or her quality of life.

Nurses are in an ideal situation to promote a trusting relationship with the patient by encouraging the patient to express any concerns, thus allowing the patient adequate opportunities to work in partnership and be an active participant in his or her pain management programme.

References and further reading

Ahmedzai, F. & Brooks, D. (1997) *Transdermal fentanyl versus oral morphine in cancer pain: preference: efficacy and quality of life*. On behalf of TTS – Fentanyl Comparative Group, Publ. 13, pp 254–61.

Audit Commission (1997) *Anaesthesia Under Examination*. Audit Commission, Oxon.

Ballard, K. (1997) Pressure-relief mattresses and patient comfort. *Prof Nurse*, **13**(1), 27–32.

BMA/Royal Pharmaceutical Society of Great Britain (1999) *British National Formulary*. Pharmaceutical Press, Oxford.

Bonica, J. (1994) *Effective Pain Management for Cancer Patients*. Simms Medical Systems, Deltec.

Bonica, J., Ventafridda, V. & Twycross, R. (1990) Management of cancer pain. In: *The Management of Pain* (ed. J. Bonica), 2nd edn., pp. 400–460. Lea & Febiger; Philadelphia.

Budd, K. (1995) Tramadol – a step towards the ideal analgesia? *Eur J Palliat Care*, **2**(2), 56–60.

Carr, E. (1990) Post-operative pain: patient expectations and experiences. *J Adv Nurs*, **15**(1), 89–100.

Carroll, D. & Bowsher, D. (1993) *Pain; Management and Nursing Care*. Butterworth-Heinemann, Oxford.

Carroll, D. & Bowsher, D. (1995) *Pain Management and Nursing Care*. Butterworth Heinemann, Oxford.

Caunt, H. (1992) Reducing the psychological impact of post-operative pain. *J Nurs*, **1**(1), 13–19.

Cherny, N.I. & Portency, R.K. (1993) Cancer pain management current strategy. *Cancer*, Suppl. **72**(11).

Choiniere, M. & Amsel, R. (1996) A visual analogue thermometer for measuring pain intensity. *J Pain Symptom Manag*, **11**(5), 299–311.

Coda, B., O'Sullivan, B., Donaldson, G. *et al.* (1997) Comparative efficacy of patient-controlled administration of morphine, hydromorphone, or sufentil for the treatment of oral mucositis following bone marrow transplantation. *Pain*, **72**(3), 333–46.

Diamond, A. & Coniam, S. (1993) *The Management of Chronic Pain*. Oxford University Press, Oxford.

Dicks, B. (1990) Programmed instruction, cancer pain. *Cancer Nurs*, **13**(4), 256–61.

Donnelly, S. & Walsh, D. (1995) The symptoms of advanced cancer. *Semin Oncol*, **22**(2), Suppl. 3, 67–72.

Doyle, D., Hanks, G. & MacDonald, N. (eds) (1998) *Oxford Textbook of Palliative Medicine*, 2nd edn. Oxford Medical Publications, Oxford.

Ellershaw, J. (1998) Hydromorphone: a new alternative to morphine. *Prescriber*, **9**(4), 21–7.

Field, L. (1996) Are nurses still underestimating patient's pain post-operatively? *Br J Nurs*, **15**(13), 778–84.

Fine, P.G., Marcus, M., De Boer, A.J. & Van der Oord, B. (1991) An open label study of oral transdermal fentanyl citrate (OTFC) for the treatment of breakthrough cancer pain. *Pain*, **45**, 149–53.

Foley, K. (1998) Pain assessment and cancer pain syndromes. In: *Oxford Textbook of Palliative Medicine* (eds D. Doyle, G. Hanks & N. MacDonald), 2nd edn., pp. 310–31. Oxford Medical Publications, Oxford.

Foley, K.M. (1989) Controversies in cancer pain. Medical perspectives. *Cancer*, Suppl. **63**, 2259–65.

Gannon, C. (1997) The use of methadone in the care of the dying. *Eur J Palliat Care*, **4**(5), 152–8.

Gould, T., Crosby, D., Harmer, M. *et al.* (1992) Policy for controlling pain after surgery: effect of sequential changes in management. *Br Med J*, **305**(6863), 1187–93.

Grond, S., Zech, D., Diefenbach, C., Radbruch, I. & Lehmann, K.

(1996) Assessment of cancer pain: a prospective evaluation. *Pain*, **64**(1), 107–14.

Hancock, H. (1996) The complexity of pain assessment and management in the first 24 hours after cardiac surgery. *Intens Crit Care Nurs*, **12**(6), 346–53.

Hanks, G. & Cherny, N. (1998) Opioid analgesic therapy. In: *Oxford Textbook of Palliative Medicine* (eds D. Doyle, G. Hanks & N. MacDonald), 2nd edn., pp. 331–54. Oxford Medical Publications, Oxford.

Hanks, G. & Expert Working Group of the European Association for Palliative Care (1996) Morphine in cancer pain: modes of administration. *Br Med J*, **3**(12), 823–6.

Hanks, G.W. (1983) Management of symptoms in advanced cancer. *Update*, **26**, 1691–702.

Harmer, M. & Davies, K. (1998) The effect of education, assessment and a standardised prescription on postoperative pain management. *Anaesthesia*, **53**(5), 424–30.

Hays, H. *et al.* (1994) Comparative clinical efficacy and safety of immediate release and controlled release hydromorphone for chronic severe pain. *Cancer*, **74**(6), 1808–16.

Hayward, J. (1975) *Information, a Prescription Against Pain, the Study of Nursing Care*. Research Project, Series 2, (5). RCN, London.

Heiser, R., Chiles, K., Fudge, M. & Gray, S. (1997) The use of music during the immediate postoperative recovery period. *AORN J*, **65**(4), 777–85.

Heiskanen, T., Ruismaki, P. & Kelso, E. (1996) Double blind, randomised repeated dose crossover comparison CR oxycodone and CR morphine tablets in cancer pain; 1 & 2, pharmacodynamic profile. *8th World Congress of Pain*, Vancouver, abstract 49 & 50.

Horrigan, C. (1993) Alternative nursing interventions. In: *Pain: Management and Nursing Care* (D. Carroll & D. Bowsher), pp. 136–45. Butterworth Heinemann, Oxford.

Hoskin, P.J. & Dicks, B. (1988) Symptom control. In: *Oncology for Nurses and Health Care Professionals* (eds R. Tiffany & P. Webb), vol. 2, 2nd edn. Harper & Row, London.

Hunt, J.M. *et al.* (1977) Patients with protracted pain; a survey conducted at the London Hospital. *J Med Ethics*, **3**(2), 61–73.

International Association for the Study of Pain (1996) Classification of chronic pain. *Pain*, Suppl. **3**, 51–226.

Johnston, M. & Vogele, C. (1993) Benefits of psychological preparation for surgery: a meta-analysis. *Ann Behav Med* **15**(4), 245–56.

Kehlet, H. & Jorgen, B. (1993) The value of 'multimodal' or 'balanced analgesia' in postoperative pain treatment. *Anes Analg* **77**(5), 1048–56.

Kitson, A. (1994) Post-operative pain management: a literature review. *J Clin Nurs*, **3**(1), 7–18.

Kuhn, S., Cooke, K., Collins, M. *et al.* (1990) Perceptions of pain relief after surgery. *Br Med J*, **300**(6741), 1687–90.

Lawler, K. (1997) Pain assessment. *Prof Nurs Study*, Suppl., **13**(1), S5–8.

Lewith, G. & Kenyon, J. (1984) Physiological and psychological explanations for the mechanism of acupuncture as a treatment for chronic pain. *Soc Sci Med*, **19**(2), 1367–78.

Liebeskind, J. & Melzack, R. (1954) The International Pain Foundation. Meeting a need for education in pain management. *Pain*, **30**, 1–2.

Ling, J. (1997) The use of transdermal fentanyl in palliative care. *Int J Palliat Nurs*, **3**(2), 65–8.

Macintyre, P. & Ready, L. (1997) *Acute Pain Management. A Practical Guide*. W.B. Saunders, London.

McCaffery, M. (1968) *Nursing practice theories related to cognition, bodily pain, and man–environment interactions*. University of California, Los Angeles.

McCaffery, M. (1990) Nursing approaches to non-pharmacological pain control. *Int J Nurs Stud*, **27**(1), 1–5.

McCaffery, M. & Beebe, A. (1989) *Pain: Clinical Manual for Nursing Practice*. Mosby, St Louis.

McQuay, H. (1990) The logic of alternative routes. *J Pain Sympt Manag*, **5**(2), 75–7.

McQuay, H., Moore, A. & Justins, D. (1997) Treating acute pain in hospital. *Br Med J*, **314**(7093), 1531–5.

Melzac, R. & Dennis, S.G. (1980) Phylogenetic evolution of pain expression in animals. In: *Pain and Society* (eds H.W. Kosterlitz & L.Y. Teranius). Chomie, New York.

Mitchell, M. (1997) Patients' perceptions of pre-operative preparation for day surgery. *J Adv Nurs*, **26**(2), 356–63.

Mucci-LoRusso, P., Berman, B., Silberstein, P., Citron, M. & Bressler, L. (1998) Controlled release oxycodone compared with controlled release morphine in the treatment of cancer pain: a randomised, double-blind, parallel group study. *Eur J Pain*, **2**, 239–49.

Narcessian, E. (1997) CR oxycodone in clinical practice. *Satellite Symposium: 5th Congress of the European Association for Palliative Care*, Barbican Centre, London.

Portenoy, R. (1998) Adjuvant analgesics in pain management In: *Oxford Textbook of Palliative Medicine* (eds D. Doyle, G. Hanks & N. MacDonald), 2nd edn., pp. 361–90. Oxford Medical Publications, Oxford.

Raiman, J. (1986) Pain relief – a two way process. *Nurs Times*, **82**(15), 24–8.

Royal College of Surgeons and Anaesthetists (1990) *Commission on the Provison of Surgical Services*. Report of Working Party on Pain After Surgery, London.

Russell, K. (1998) Nursing management of pain in advanced cancer. *J Nurs Care*, Spring, 8–10.

Saunders, C. & Sykes, N. (1993) *The Management of Terminal Malignant Disease*, 3rd edn. Hodder & Stoughton, Boston.

Schofield, P. (1995) Using assessment tools to help patients in pain. *Prof Nurse*, **10**(11), 703–706.

Scott, I. (1994) Effectiveness of documented assessment of post operative pain. *Br J Nurs*, **3**(10), 494–501.

Seers, K. (1988) Factors affecting pain assessment. *Prof Nurse*, **3**(6), 201–205.

Sidebotham, D., Monique, R., Dijkhuizen, R. & Schug, S. (1997) The safety and utilization of patient controlled analgesia. *J Pain Symp Manag*, **14**(4), 202–209.

Tasmuth, T., Estlandberg, A. & Kalso, E. (1996) Effect of present pain and memory of past post-operative pain in women treated with surgery for breast cancer. *Pain*, **68**(2–3), 343–7.

Twycross, R. (1994) *Pain Relief In Advanced Cancer*. Churchill Livingstone, New York.

Twycross, R. (1997) *Symptom Management in Advanced Cancer*, 2nd edn. Radcliffe Medical Press, Oxford.

Twycross, R.G. & Fairfield, S. (1982) Pain in far advanced cancer. *Pain*, **14**, 303–310.

Twycross, R., Harcourt, J. & Bergl, S. (1996) A survey of pain in patients with advanced cancer. *J Pain Symp Manag*, **12**(5), 273–82.

Twycross, R. & Lack, S. (1990) *Therapeutics in Terminal Cancer*, 2nd edn. Churchill Livingstone, Edinburgh.

Vijayan, R. (1997) Subcutaneous morphine – a simple technique for postoperative analgesia. *Int J Acute Pain*, **1**(1), 21–6.

Walker, V.S. *et al.* (1987) Pain assessment charts in the management of chronic cancer pain. *Palliat Med*, **1**, 111–16.

Williams, A. (1995) Pain measurement in chronic pain management. *Pain Rev*, **2**(1), 39–63.

World Health Organization (1996) *Cancer Pain Relief*. WHO, Geneva.

Yarde, A. (1989) Epidural analgesia. *Prof Nurse*, **4**(12), 608–13.

Zech, D., Lehmann, A. & Grond, S. (1994) A new treatment option for chronic cancer pain. *Eur J Palliat Care*, **1**(1), 26–30.

GUIDELINES · Patient assessment and preparation before surgery: optimizing pain control

Procedure

Action	*Rationale*
1 If patient has had previous surgery, ask for details of: (a) Previous and current pain control methods (drug and non-drug) (b) Effectiveness of these methods (c) Experience of side effects, such as nausea and vomiting.	To ensure previous experiences are taken into consideration when planning pain control. To allay any fears based on previous experience. To ensure care is planned to minimize side effects and nausea and vomiting.
2 Assess patient for pre-existing long-term pain problems. Obtain information on: (a) Pain type, location and intensity (b) Use of analgesics.	To plan in advance of surgery the pain control methods that will be used to manage both the patient's long-term and anticipated postoperative pain.
3 Check patient suitability for various pain control methods: e.g. renal function, clotting abnormalities, dexterity, visual impairment.	To avoid the use of inappropriate pain control methods, e.g. (a) Diclofenac in renal impairment (b) Epidural analgesia with clotting abnormalities (c) PCAs, if lack of dexterity or visual impairment makes the patient incapable of pressing the demand button which is connected to the pump.
4 Liaise with multidisciplinary team and patient to select most appropriate pain control method(s).	To ensure effective collaboration between the patient and team in order to optimize postoperative pain control.

5 Explain and discuss with patient:
   (a) How pain will be assessed and the use of a pain scale.
   (b) How pain will be controlled
   (c) Goals for pain control at rest and on movement.

To allay anxiety and promote patient wellbeing and control. To encourage active involvement in pain control. To give patients a chance to ask questions. To ensure the patient understands the rationale for pain control during deep breathing and movement. This will help prevent postoperative complications, e.g. chest infections.

6 Provide patient with written information about pain control.

To support verbal information.

7 Where appropriate, demonstrate the use of pain control methods before surgery.

To ensure the patient has the skill and knowledge to effectively use the pain control methods chosen, e.g. PCAs.

GUIDELINES • Using a Chronic Pain Chart

Procedure

Action

1 Explain the purpose of using the chart to the patient.

2 Encourage the patient, where appropriate, to identify pain himself/herself.

3 When it is necessary for the nurse to complete the chart, ensure that the patient's own description of his/her pain is recorded.

4 (a) Record any factors that influence the intensity of the pain, e.g. activities or interventions that reduce or increase the pain such as distractions or a heat pad.
   (b) Record whether or not the patient is pain-free at night, at rest or on movement.

5 Index each site (A to H, Fig. 29.2) in whatever way seems most appropriate, e.g. shading or colouring of areas or arrows to indicate shooting pains.

6 Give each pain site a numerical value according to the key to pain intensity or the pain scale and note time recorded.

7 Record any analgesia given and note route and dose.

8 Record any significant activities that are likely to influence the patient's pain.

Note: fixed times for reviewing the pain have been omitted intentionally to allow for flexibility. It is suggested that, initially, the patient's pain be reviewed every 4 h. When a

Rationale

To ensure that the patient understands the procedure and gives his/her valid consent and cooperation.

The body outline (Fig. 29.2) is a vehicle for the patient to describe his/her own pain experience.

To reduce the risk of misinterpretation.

Ascertaining how and when the patient experiences pain enables the nurse to plan realistic goals. For example, relieving the patient's pain during the night and while he/she is at rest is usually easier to achieve before relief from pain on movement.

This enables individual pain sites to be located.

To indicate the intensity of the pain at each site.

To monitor efficacy of prescribed analgesia.

Extra pharmacological or non-pharmacological interventions might be indicated.

patient's level of pain has stabilized, recordings may be made less frequently, e.g. 12-hourly or daily. The chart should be discontinued if a patient's pain becomes totally controlled.

Peri-Operative Care

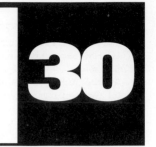

Peri-operative care refers to the nursing care delivered to a patient before (pre), during (intra) and after (post) surgery.

Pre-operative care

Definition

Pre-operative care is the preparation and assessment, physical and psychological, of a patient before surgery.

Objectives

Physical

1 To minimize postoperative complications, e.g. by teaching the patient deep breathing exercises and the relevance after surgery to wellbeing.
2 To assess the physical condition of the patient so that potential problems can be anticipated and prevented.
3 To ensure that the patient is in an optimum physical condition before surgery.

Psychological

1 To ensure that the patient understands the nature of the surgery to be undergone.
2 To teach the patient what to expect postoperatively, e.g. about any drains, catheters and so on that may be necessary afterwards.
3 To assess areas of anxiety that the patient may have and discuss them, using nursing interventions if appropriate e.g. loss of part of body.

Reference material

Patient education and postoperative pain

Much research and discussion have been devoted to the subject of postoperative pain and the ways in which pre-operative patient education can influence the pain experience. Since pain and anaesthesia are often the patient's greatest fears (Carnevali 1966), it is necessary to address this cause of anxiety in the pre-operative period.

Reducing patient anxiety by giving pre-operative information has been shown to reduce postoperative pain (Hayward 1975; Bray 1986). It also results in the patient requiring less analgesia. The reduction of anxiety and pro-moting postoperative recovery can be achieved in several ways. The fragmentation of nursing care could account for some patient anxiety (Copp 1988), and pre-operative visiting by nurses from theatres is being undertaken in many hospitals. It has been found that this can 'help the patient to manage his anxiety, not least by providing a continuity of care in collaboration with other members of the surgical teams' (Leonard & Kalideen 1985; Carter & Evans 1996). Copp (1988) also found that teaching patients recovery exercises decreased their feelings of helplessness and, therefore, reduced anxiety, and that the use of cognitive coping methods is an effective way of reducing anxiety.

Further research (Balfour 1989) has shown that 'patients continue to suffer unrelieved pain following abdomen surgery' and that 'nurses continue to underadminister prescribed analgesics'. Jackson (1995) suggested that 50% of patients have pain for most of the 72 hours after surgery. Postoperative analgesia is often administered on a *pro re nata* (as required) basis so that patients request it when they are in pain. One strategy is to use methods to maintain a constant drug concentration in the blood via a continuous infusion. This often reduces side-effects, such as nausea, while providing good analgesic cover. Use of patient-controlled analgesia (PCA) gives the patient a sense of autonomy which may decrease anxiety, and which will in turn influence the patient's pain perception (Carr 1989) (See Chap. 29, Pain Assessment and Management).

Skin preparation

Before surgery the patient is required to have a bath or shower. The aim of a pre-operative bath or shower is to reduce the risk of postoperative wound infection.

Recent research into the use of antiseptic preparations to be used in the pre-operative bath or shower certainly supports this practice. Byrne *et al.* (1990) recommend that three pre-operative showers with 4% chlorhexidine detergent would reduce the risk of infection. This is further supported by McCorkey *et al.* (1990) who suggested a comprehensive infection control programme which includes chlorhexidine showers, and discontinuation of shaving contributes significantly to reducing infection in coronary artery bypass graft surgery. Wells *et al.* (1983) found that a single bath using chlorhexidine did not reduce postoperative infections in patients undergoing open heart surgery. This is supported by Leigh *et al.* (1983), who found that a single chlorhexidine bath eliminated the skin carriage of *Staphylococcus aureus* but did not reduce postoperative wound infection rates.

Hayek *et al.* (1987) studied the effects of two pre-operative baths comparing the use of chlorhexidine against ordinary soap and a placebo. The findings indicated that the two pre-operative chlorhexidine showers reduced the postoperative infection rate in 'clean' surgery. In the clean group, chlorhexidine use reduced the incidence of *Staphylococcus* by 50%; in the clean/contaminated surgery group there was some reduction of staphylococcal infections. Although chlorhexidine caused a reduction of overall infection in the contaminated wounds, it was not statistically significant.

Shaving is also a common pre-operative procedure. Studies suggest that there is a direct relationship between wound infection and hair removal, with the lowest wound infection rates obtained in cases where no hair was removed and the highest infection rate occurring when a razor was used (Alexander *et al.* 1983; Willford 1983). However, there is no suggestion that anything less than three shaves would significantly affect rate of infection. Therefore a comprehensive disinfection programme could significantly reduce the rate of infection.

One alternative method is to use a depilatory cream, which has demonstrated lower postoperative infection rates when the absence of hair from the operation site is required (Goeau-Brissonniere *et al.* 1987). Winfield (1986) found that although depilatory cream is more expensive than shaving, it can save nursing time as most patients can apply the cream themselves. Similarly, although skin irritation can occur (in 9% of cases), it compares favourably with skin irritation from razors (13%), including grazes and small cuts.

Pre-operative fasting

Any patient presenting for anaesthesia may have undigested food in the stomach. For elective surgery the patient is usually 'nil by mouth' for long enough to allow the stomach to empty. Research by Hung (1992) has revealed that patients often did not know why they were fasting, and that they were often deprived of food and drink for longer than the recommended time of 6 hours and maximum time of 12 hours. Patients on an afternoon theatre list were less likely to be starved for as long as those on the morning list, who were frequently starved from midnight.

Stomach emptying on average takes 6 hours for solid food and 4 hours for fluids (Carrie & Simpson 1988). However, gastric emptying may be delayed by anxiety or the action of some drugs, e.g. opiates. Atropine and hyoscine are sometimes prescribed as part of the patient's premedication, primarily to reduce saliva production. However, they also have a blocking action on the parasympathetic nervous system, which reduces motility of the digestive tract and therefore reduces the likelihood of vomiting (Green 1986).

Antiembolic stockings

Deep vein thrombosis, if it occurs, is usually diagnosed 3–14 days postoperatively. The incidence is highest in middle-aged and elderly patients, those on prolonged bedrest, and after major surgery of the lower abdomen, pelvis or hip joints. Patients with a history of coronary artery disease are also at risk (Carrie & Simpson 1988). Once high-risk patients have been identified, prophylactic treatment can begin.

One such treatment is the use of anti-embolic stockings (Jefferey & Nicolaides 1990). Carmen *et al.* (1990) give specific recommendations on a number of issues in venous thromboembolism and one of these is the use of compression stockings. These contribute in reducing incidences of deep vein thrombosis if appropriately used. Thomas (1992) further supports this idea and goes one step further to emphasize the reuse of some embolic stockings, i.e. washing of stockings does not reduce the pressure and consistency remains the same. Thomas studied ten different stockings and found that Brevet came in the top two. These stockings work by promoting venous flow and reducing stasis. They increase the velocity of flow, not only in the legs but also in the pelvic veins and inferior vena cava (Drinkwater 1989).

During surgery the use of heel supports which reduce the pressure on the calves on the operating table will also encourage venous return. The use of intermittent calf compression air boots which promote venous flow during surgery has also been reported to be effective (Pierce 1994). Good pain control will encourage patients to mobilize early and carry out postoperative exercises, which are also important in preventing serious postoperative complications.

References and further reading

Alexander, J.W. *et al.* (1983) The influence of hair removal methods on wound infections. *Arch Surg*, **118**, 347–52.

Balfour, S.E. (1989) Will I be in pain? Patient and nurse attitudes to pain after abdominal surgery. *Prof Nurse*, **1**(5), 28–33.

Biley, F.C. (1989) Nurse perception of stress in pre-operative surgical patients. *J Adv Nurs*, **14**, 575–81.

Bray, C.A. (1986) Post-operative pain. Altering the patient's experience through education. *AORN J*, **43**(3), 679–83.

Brown, S.A. (1983) Venous thrombosis: another complication of cancer (care plan). *Oncol Nurs Forum*, **10**(2), 41–7.

Byrne, D.J., Napier, A. & Cushin, A. (1990) Rationalization of whole body disinfection. *J Hosp Infect*, **15**(2), 183–97.

Carmen, T.L. & Fernandez, B.B.J. (1999) Issues and controversies in venous thromboembolism. *Clin J Med*, **66**(2), 113–23.

Carnevali, D.L. (1966) Pre-operative anxiety. *Am J Nurs*, **66**(7), 1536–8.

Carr, F. (1989) Waking up to post-operative pain. *Nurs Times*, **85**(3), 38–9.

Carrie, L.E.S. & Simpson, P.J. (1988) *Understanding Anaesthesia*. William Heinemann, London.

Carter, L. & Evans, T. (1996) Surgical nurse pre-operative visiting: a role for theatre nurses. *Br J Nurs*, **5**(4), 919–20, 922, 924–5.

Clarke, J. (1983) The effectiveness of surgical skin preparations. *Nurs Times, Theatre Nurs Suppl*, 28 Sep, **79**(39), 8–17.

Copp, G. (1988) Intra-operative information and pre-operative visiting. *Surg Nurse*, **1**(2), 27–8.

Davis, P.S. (1988) Changing nursing practice for more effective control of post-operative pain through a staff-initiated educational programme. *Nurse Educ Today*, **8**, 325–31.

Drinkwater, K. (1989) Management of deep vein thrombosis. *Surg Nurse*, **2**(1), 24–6.

Goeau-Brissonniere, O. *et al.* (1987) Pre-operative skin preparation: a prospective study comparing a depilatory agent in shaving. *Presse Med*, **16**(31), 1517–19.

Gooch, J. (1989) Who should manage pain – patient or nurse? *Prof Nurse*, **4**(6), 295–6.

Green, J.H. (1986) *Basic Clinical Physiology*, 3rd edn. Oxford University Press, Oxford.

Hayek, L.J. *et al.* (1987) A placebo-controlled trial of the effect of pre-operative baths or showers with chlorhexidine detergent on postoperative wound infection rates. *J Hosp Infect*, **10**(2), 165–72.

Hayward, J. (1975) *Information: A Prescription Against Pain*. Royal College of Nursing (Research Series), London.

Hung, P. (1992) Pre-operative fasting. *Nurs Times*, 25 Nov–1 Dec, 57–60.

Jackson, J. (1995) Acute pain: its physiology and the pharmacology of analgesia. *Nurs Times*, **91**(16), 27–8.

Jefferey, P.C. & Nicolaides, A.N. (1990) Graduated compression stocking in the prevention of post-operative deep vein thrombosis. *Br J Surg*, **77**(4), 380–383.

Johnson, A. (1989) Preparing for elective surgery. *Nurs Stand*, **3**(23), 22–4.

Leigh, D.A. *et al.* (1983) Total body bathing with 'Hibiscrub' (chlorhexidine) in surgical patients. A controlled trial. *J Hosp Infect*, **4**(3), 229–35.

Leonard, M.D. & Kalideen, P. (1985) 'So you're going to have an operation.' *Nat Assoc Theatre Nurses News*, **22**(2), 12–21.

Lore, C. (1990) Deep vein thrombosis: threat to recovery. Part 1. *Nurs Times*, **86**(5), 40–43.

McConnell, E.A. (1990) Clinical do's and don'ts: applying antiembolism stockings (pictoral, protocol). *Nursing*, **20**(10), 92.

McCorkey, S.J., L'Ecuyer, P.B., Murphy, P.M. *et al.* (1999) Results of a comprehensive infection control program for reducing surgical site infections in coronary artery bypass graft surgery. *Infect Control Hosp Epidemiol*, **20**(8), 538–8.

Pierce, L.A. (1994) Patient positioning during surgical procedures. *Plast Surg Nurs*, **14**(4), 242–3.

Thomas, A.E. (1987) Pre-operative fasting – a question of routine? *Nurs Times*, **83**(49), 46–7.

Thomas, S. (1992) *Graduated External Compression and the Prevention of DVT*. Surgical Materials Test Laboratory, Bridgend.

Wells, F.C. *et al.* (1983) Wound infection in cardiothoracic surgery. *Lancet*, **1**, 1209–10.

Willford, P.S. (1983) Hair removal – shave, preps, depilation, and other pre-operative considerations. Are they really necessary? *J Operat Room Res Inst*, **3**(3), 26–8.

Winfield, V. (1986) Too close a shave? *Nurs Times, J Infect Control Nurs*, **82**(10), 64–8.

GUIDELINES • Pre-operative care

Equipment

1 Theatre gown.
2 Labelled denture container if necessary.
3 Hypo-allergenic tape to cover wedding rings.
4 Any equipment and documents required by law and hospital policy if a pre-medication has been prescribed.

Procedure

Action

1 Ensure the patient is wearing an identification bracelet with the correct information.

2 Assess the pre-operative education received by the patient and ensure that it is complete and understood.

3 Record the patient's pulse, blood pressure, respirations, temperature and weight.

4 Check that the patient has undergone relevant procedures, e.g. X-ray, ECG, blood tests and that these results are included with the patient's notes.

5 Instruct the patient on showering or bathing.

6 Assist the patient to change into a theatre gown after having a shower.

7 Long hair should be held back with, for example, a non-metallic tie.

Rationale

To ensure correct identification and prevent possible problems.

To ensure that the patient understands the nature and outcome of the surgery and reduce anxiety and possible post-operative complications.

To provide data for comparison postoperatively. The weight is recorded so that the anaesthetist can calculate the dose of drugs to be used.

To ensure all relevant information is available to the nurses, anaesthetists and surgeons. Absence of results may delay or cause cancellation of an operation.

To minimize risk of postoperative wound infection.

8 Ensure that patients undergoing major surgery or abdominal/pelvic surgery, the elderly, frail or bedbound patients or those with a previous history of emboli or other high-risk factors have antiembolic stockings applied correctly. The use of intermittent calf compression boots should be considered.

To reduce the risk of post-operative deep vein thrombosis or pulmonary emboli.

9 Complete the pre-operative check list by asking the patient and checking records and notes before giving any premedication.

(a) Check when patient last had food or drink and ensure that it was at least 6 h before.

(b) Check whether patient micturated before premedication.

(c) Note whether the patient has dental crowns, bridge work or loose teeth.

(d) Ensure prostheses, dentures and contact lenses are removed.

(e) Spectacles may be retained until the patient is in the anaesthetic room. Hearing aids may be retained until the patient has been anaesthetized. (These may be left in position if a local anaesthetic is being used.) Any prosthesis should then be labelled clearly and retained in the recovery room.

(f) All jewellery (apart from wedding ring), cosmetics, nail varnish and clothing, other than the theatre gown, are to be removed.

Note: questioning premedicated patients is not a reliable source of checking information as the patient may be drowsy and/or disorientated.

To reduce the risk of regurgitation and inhalation of stomach contents on induction of anaesthetic.

To prevent urinary incontinence and embarrassment. To allow better access to abdominal cavity for abdomen or pelvic surgery if a catheter is not to be used.

The anaesthetist needs to be informed to prevent accidental damage. Loose teeth or a dental prosthesis could be inhaled by the patient when an endotracheal tube is inserted.

To promote patient safety during surgery, e.g. dentures may obstruct airway, contact lenses can cause corneal abrasions.

To allow patient to see and hear, thus reducing anxiety and enabling the patient to understand any procedures carried out.

Metal jewellery may be accidentally lost or may be cause of harm to patient, e.g. diathermy burns. Facial cosmetics can make the patient's colour difficult to assess. Nail varnish makes the use of the pulse oximeter, used to monitor the patient's pulse and oxygen saturation levels, impossible and masks peripheral cyanosis.

10 Valuables should be placed in the hospital's custody and recorded according to the hospital policy.

To prevent loss of valuables.

11 Check the consent form is correctly completed, signed and dated.

To comply with legal requirements and hospital policy.

12 Check the operation site is marked correctly.

To ensure the patient undergoes the correct surgery for which he/she has consented.

13 Check that the patient has undergone pre-anaesthetic assessment by the anaesthetist.

To ensure that the patient can be given the most suitable anaesthetic.

14 Give the premedication, if prescribed, in accordance with the anaesthetist's instructions and conforming to legal requirements and hospital policy.

Different drugs may be prescribed to complement the anaesthetic to be given, e.g. temazepam to reduce patient anxiety by inducing sleep and relaxation.

15 Advise the patient to remain in bed once the premedication has been given and to use the nurse call system if assistance is needed.

To reduce the risk of accidental patient injury as the premedication may make the patient drowsy and disorientated.

16 Ensure the patient is supported fully on the canvas, especially the head, when transferred from the ward bed to the trolley.

To reduce the risk of injury to the neck, etc. during transfer from the ward to the operating theatre.

17 Ensure that all relevant information, e.g. X-rays, notes, blood results, accompany the patient to the operating theatre.

To prevent delays which can increase the patient's anxiety, and to ensure that the anaesthetist and surgeon have all the information they require for the safe treatment of the patient.

Guidelines • Pre-operative care (cont'd)

Action	*Rationale*
18 The patient should be accompanied to the theatre by a ward nurse who remains until the patient is anaesthetized.	To reduce the patient's anxiety.
19 The ward nurse should give a full handover to the anaesthetic nurse or operating department assistant on arrival of the patient at the anaesthetic room.	To ensure the patient has the correct operation. To ensure continuity of care by exchanging all relevant information.

Intra-operative care

Definition

Intra-operative care is the physical and psychological care given to the patient in the anaesthetic room and theatre until transferral to the recovery room.

Objectives

1 To ensure that the patient understands what is happening at all times in order to minimize anxiety.
2 To ensure that the patient has the surgery for which the consent form was signed.
3 To ensure patient safety at all times and minimize postoperative complications by:
  (a) Giving the required care for the unconscious patient.
  (b) Ensuring no injury is sustained from hazards associated with the use of swabs, needles, instruments, diathermy and power tools.
  (c) Minimizing postoperative problems associated with patient positioning, such as nerve or tissue damage.
  (d) Maintaining asepsis during surgical procedures to reduce the risk of postoperative wound infection in accordance with hospital policies on infection control.

Reference material

Diathermy

Diathermy is used routinely during many operations to control haemorrhage by cauterizing blood vessels or cutting or fulgerizing body tissues. Diathermy is potentially hazardous to the patient if used incorrectly. It is important that all theatre nurses know how to test and use all diathermy equipment in their department to prevent patient injury (Theatre Safeguards 1988; AORN 1994).

The main risk when using diathermy is of thermoelectrical burns. The most common cause is incorrect application of the patient plate or a break in the connecting lead (Moakes 1991). If this occurs when using an isolated diathermy machine then the current output will stop. However, if a grounded diathermy machine is used then the electrical current will find an alternative route back to the diathermy machine (Wainwright 1988). If the patient

is in contact with any metal, e.g. on the operating table (3M 1986, p. 4; Wicker 1997) then loss of plate contact using a grounded unit could result in a serious burn.

Other causes of burns include skin preparation solutions or other liquids pooling around the plate site (DoH 1990). With alcohol-based skin preparations especially, the skin should be allowed to dry before diathermy is used, as the alcohol can ignite (Wainwright 1988). If the patient's position is changed during the operation the patient plate should be rechecked to ensure that it is still in contact and that the connecting clamp or lead is not causing pressure in the new position.

Use of diathermy and the plate position should be noted on the nursing care plan, and the patient's skin condition should be checked postoperatively.

Patient positioning

The position of the patient on the operating table must be such as to facilitate access to the operation site(s) by the surgeon, taking into account the patient's airway, monitoring equipment or intravenous choices. Nor should it compromise the patient's circulation, respiratory system or nerves (AORN 1990). Pre-operative assessment will identify patients with particular needs which may be influenced by factors such as weight, nutritional state, age, skin condition and pre-existing disease. All these factors may indicate the need for extra precautions during positioning. Consideration by and the cooperation of all theatre personnel can help prevent many of the pre-operative complications related to intra-operative positioning.

All equipment that may be needed to support the patient during surgery, e.g. the table, arm supports, lithotomy poles and securing straps, should be checked to ensure that they are in working order, clean and free from sharp edges. Metal parts that may come into contact with the patient should be covered as there is an increased risk of burns if diathermy is used (Wainwright 1988). Padding should be placed at the patient's elbows and heels, and pillows positioned between the legs if the patient is lying in a lateral position. Special consideration should also be given to areas such as the back of the head and ears. The use of a warm air mattress on the operating table can also help to reduce pressure on vulnerable areas such as the hips or sacrum, as well as reducing the risk of hypothermia (Atkinson & Kohn 1986).

When a patient is transferred between the trolley or bed

and operating table, adequate personnel should be present to ensure patient and staff safety (AORN 1990). It is recommended that an approved rolling or sliding device is used to transfer patients from trolley to operating table, in compliance with legislation on manual handling. Safe manual handling and the safety of the patient depend on the participation of the correct number of staff in the specified handling manoeuvre.

All movements of the limbs of the unconscious patient should take into account the anatomy and natural planes of movement of that limb to avoid stretching and pressure on the related nerve planes (Theatre Safeguards 1988). Hyperabduction of the arm when placed on a board, for example, could stretch the brachial plexus, causing some postoperative loss of sensation and reduced movement of the forearm, wrist and fingers. The ulnar and radial nerves may be affected by direct pressure as a result of insufficient padding on arm supports or lack of care when inserting poles into the canvas and hitting the elbows.

Pre-existing conditions such as backache or sciatica can be exacerbated, particularly if the patient is in the lithotomy position as the sciatic nerve can be compressed against the poles (Underwood & Jameson 1990). Most postoperative palsies are due to improper positioning of the patient on the operating table (Nightingale 1985; Ulrich et al. 1997).

Control of infection and asepsis in operating theatres

The term asepsis means the absence of any infectious agents. The aseptic technique is the foundation on which contemporary surgery is built (Gruendemann & Meeker 1983). The aim of operating theatres is to provide an area free from infectious agents. Large quantities of bacteria are present in the nose, mouth, on the skin, hair and on the attire of personnel; therefore people entering the operating theatres wear clean scrub suits and lint-free surgical hats to eliminate the possibility of these bacteria, hair or dandruff being shed (Hambraeus & Laurell 1980). Sterile gowns and gloves are worn to prevent cross-infection. It is recommended that waterproof footwear is worn by staff (Ayliffe et al. 1992). Face masks are worn to prevent droplets falling from the mouth into the operating field. The extent to which face masks are capable of preventing droplet spread is disputed. A new mask should be worn for each operation, and masks that become damp must be replaced. The use of masks in the operating room has been greatly debated and it has been suggested that perhaps these should only be used within the immediate vicinity of the operating site (NATN 1998). Orr (1981) found no increase in the infection rate when masks were not worn during general surgery. It is, however, accepted that masks offer protection to the wearer from blood splashes and for safety reasons should be worn by the scrub team.

The scrubbing procedure is essential to the maintenance of asepsis in the operating theatre. An antiseptic soap or detergent preparation, such as 4% chlorhexidine solution, e.g. Hibiscrub or povidone-iodine (e.g. Betadine, Disadine), should be used. A 5-minute scrub is recommended, and any visible dirt or blood must be removed from the skin and from under fingernails (Ayliffe et al. 1992). The closed method of donning sterile surgical gloves is preferred.

Universal precautions should be taken in theatres to minimize the risk of infection from blood and body fluids. These include the wearing of gloves, masks, barrier gowns and aprons. Protective eyewear or face shields should be worn during procedures likely to cause splashes or droplets of blood or generate bone chips (Ayliffe et al. 1992). Instruments must be handled carefully, and needle holders and forceps used to manipulate sutures to minimize the risk of needlestick or sharps injury.

Laparoscopic surgery

Laparoscopy has evolved from a diagnostic modality into a widespread surgical technique. Advantages for the patient include: a shorter stay in hospital, reduced post-operative pain and a shorter recovery period (Hulka 1985; Netherson & Wood 1991). Laparoscopic surgery is now common in operating departments, and it is important that potential complications are identified and steps taken to minimize risk to the patient, both during surgery and in the recovery period. Patients should be prepared psychologically and physically for an open procedure, which may be undertaken under certain circumstances. Instruments and supplies for an open procedure must be readily available in the operating theatre.

Laparoscopy involves insufflation of the abdomen with carbon dioxide (CO_2). Prolonged insufflation can cause hypothermia, as thermal loss due to CO_2 is known to occur at the rate of 0.3°C per 40–50 litres of gas (Williams & Murr 1993). Holzman et al. (1992) refer to the increased risk of hypercarbia and surgical emphysema during insufflation with CO_2. Careful monitoring and recording of the patient's vital signs, including oxygen saturation and expiratory gas levels, are therefore essential during laparoscopy.

Haemorrhage can occur during the procedure and may be difficult to detect because surgeons have a limited view of the area being operated upon. Electrosurgical injuries to organs may occur as a result of capacitive coupling (Tucker et al. 1992) (capacitive coupling is the transfer of electrical currents from the active electrode through coupling of stray currents into other conductive surgical equipment). Theatre staff must be aware of potential complications and ensure that equipment is used safely and according to the manufacturer's instructions.

The equipment used for laparoscopic surgery is very specialized and can be daunting for theatre staff. The Association of Operating Room Nurses (1994) recommends that all equipment is regularly and competently maintained and a maintenance record kept in a log. Policies and procedures should be developed for the checking procedure, and all staff thoroughly instructed in the operation of laparoscopic equipment.

References and further reading

Association of Operating Room Nurses (1990) Proposed recommended practices; positioning the surgical patient. *AORN J*, **51**(1), 216–22.

Association of Operating Room Nurses (1994) Proposed recommended practices: endoscopic minimal access surgery. *AORN J*, **59**(2), 507–514.

Atkinson, L.J. & Kohn, M.L. (1986) *Berry and Kohn's Introduction to Operating Room Technique*. McGraw Hill, New York.

Ayliffe, G. *et al.* (1992) *Control of Hospital Infection: A Practical Handbook*, 3rd edn. Chapman & Hall, London.

DoH (1990) Ignition of spirit based skin cleaning fluid by surgical diathermy, setting fire to disposable surgical drapes resulting in patient burns. *HC (Hazard)*, (90), 25.

Gillette, M.K. & Cansico, C.C. (1989) Intra-operative tissue injury, major causes and preventative measures (study). *AORN J*, **50**(1), 66–8.

Gruendemann, B. & Meeker, H.M. (1983) *Alexander's Care of the Patient in Surgery*, 7th edn. Mosby, St Louis.

Hambraeus, A. & Laurell, G. (1980) Protection of the patient in the operating suite. *J Hosp Infect*, **1**, 5.

Holzman, M. *et al.* (1992) Hypercarbia during carbon dioxide gas insufflation for therapeutic laparoscopy: a note of caution. *Surg Laparosc Endosc*, **2**(1), 11–14.

Hulka, J.F. (1985) *Textbook of Laparoscopy*. Gruene & Stratton, Orlando.

Joint Memorandum by Medical Defence Union and Royal College of Nursing (1978) *Safeguards Against Failure to Remove Swabs and Instruments From Patients*.

Lamp (cover story) (1990) There's more in the wash than dirty linen! *Lamp*, **47**(3), 12.

3M (1986) *Safety in Diathermy*. 3M Health Care Ltd., Loughborough.

Moakes, E. (1991) Electrosurgical unit safety. *AORN J*, **53**(3), 744–52.

Netherson, L. & Wood, R. (1991) Laparoscopy in the 1990s. In: *Surgery*, pp 2096–2100. The Medical Group.

NATN (1998) *Principles of Safe Practice in the Peri-Operative Environment*. National Association of Theatre Nurses, Harrogate.

Nightingale, K. (1985) Hazards to patients during surgery. *Nat Assoc Theatre Nurses News*, January, 13–16.

Orr, N. (1981) Is a mask necessary in the operating theatre? *Ann R Coll Surg Engl*, **63**, 390.

Theatre Safeguards (1988) Joint report by MDU, RCN, NATN.

Tucker, R.D. *et al.* (1992) Capacitive coupled stray currents during laparoscopic and endoscopic electrosurgical procedures. *Biomed Instrum Technol*, **26**(4), 303–311.

Ulrich, W. *et al.* (1997) Damage due to patient positioning in anaesthesia and surgical medicine. *Anaesthesiol Intens Med Notfallmed Schmerzther*, **32**(1), 4.

Underwood, M.J. & Jameson, J. (1990) Preventing nerve injuries. *Technic*, **83**, 11–13.

Wainwright, D. (1988) Diathermy – how safe is it? *Nat Assoc Theatre Nurses News*, **25**(1), 7–8.

Wicker, C.P. (1997) Electrosurgery. In: *Principles of Safe Practice in the Operating Theatre*. National Association of Theatre Nurses, Harrogate.

Williams, M.D. & Murr, P.C. (1993) Laparoscopic insufflation of the abdomen depresses cardiopulmonary function. *Surg Endosc*, **7**, 12–16.

GUIDELINES · Intra-operative care

Procedure

Action	Rationale
1 Greet the patient by name. Confirm with the ward nurse that it is the correct patient for the scheduled operation.	To make the patient feel welcome. To ensure that the patient is safeguarded against problems related to misidentity.
2 Identify the patient by checking the name bracelet and number against the patient's notes and the operating list.	To question the premedicated patient can be unreliable (Theatre Safeguards 1988; NATN 1998).
3 Examine the pre-operative checklist (Fig. 30.1).	To ensure that all of the listed measures have been completed and that any additional information has been recorded.
4 Check that the blood results, X-rays, etc. are present in the patient's notes.	To ensure that all of the required results are available for the medical team's use.
5 Maintain a calm, quiet environment and explain all the procedures to the patient.	To reduce anxiety and enhance the smooth induction of anaesthesia.
6 When the patient is anaesthetized ensure that the eyes are closed and hypoallergenic tape is applied.	To prevent corneal damage due to drying or accidental abrasion.
7 Ensure that there are adequate staff to transfer the patient to the operating table. Ensure the brakes on the trolley and operating table have been applied. Ensure the patient's head and limbs are supported when transferring to the operating table.	To ensure that the patient receives no injury during the transfer.
8 Check with anaesthetist before moving patient.	To ensure airway is protected.

9   Ensure all limbs are supported and secure on the table. Ensure adequate padding and cushioning of bony prominences. The patient's position will be dictated by the nature of the surgery but must take into account the requirements of the anaesthetist and the physical, psychological and social needs of the patient.

If the patient is unconscious and unable to maintain a safe environment, support is necessary to prevent injury. The patient is especially at risk from damage due to pressure and stretching, so measures to maintain the skin's integrity are vital. Nerve damage due to compression or stretching must be prevented.

10   Ensure the patient is covered by the gown or blanket. These items should only be removed immediately before surgery.

To maintain the patient's dignity. To help prevent a reduction in body temperature or accidental hypothermia.

11   Use a warm air mattress on the operating table. Ensure all fluids used are warmed if possible.

To help maintain the patient's body temperature and prevent postoperative complications due to hypothermia.

12   Ensure all the equipment to be used is checked and in working order before the operating list commences, including suction, the anaesthetic machine, medical gases, monitoring equipment, diathermy and operating table.

To prevent accidental injury due to faulty equipment and to ensure all equipment necessary to the patient's treatment is present.

13   Ensure diathermy patient plate is attached securely in accordance with the manufacturer's instructions and hospital policy.

To ensure that no injury is sustained from the use of diathermy during surgery.

14   Follow hospital policy for the checking of swabs, needles and instruments.

To ensure that swabs, needles and instruments are accounted for at the end of the operation (Joint Memorandum by MDU and RCN 1978; NATN 1998).

15   Follow hospital policy for the disposal of sharps and clinical waste.

To reduce the risk of injury to the patient and staff.

16   Ensure the surgeon is informed that the number of swabs, needles and instruments is correct.

It is the responsibility of the nurse and surgeon to check that nothing is accidentally left inside the patient on completion of surgery.

17   The scrub nurse accompanies the patient with the anaesthetist to the recovery area. A handover is given that includes:

To ensure continuity of care of the patient.

(a) What procedure was performed.
(b) The presence, position and nature of any drains, infusions or intravenous or arterial devices.

To ensure that the recovery nurse has all the information required to assess the patient's recovery needs.

(c) Information including allergies or pre-existing medical conditions, such as diabetes mellitus.
(d) The patient's cardiovascular state and pattern of anaesthesia used.
(e) Specific instructions from the anaesthetist for postoperative care.

To assist the recovery nurse in the assessment of postoperative problems with which the patient may present.

(f) Information about any anxieties of the patient expressed before surgery such as a fear of not waking after anaesthesia or fear about coping with pain.
(g) All information is to be recorded on the theatre nursing care plan.

To ensure appropriate action can be taken as the patient regains consciousness and to enable an assessment of the efficacy of nursing interventions used.
To provide a written record of nursing intervention for use by recovery staff and ward nursing staff.

THE ROYAL MARSDEN HOSPITAL

Date ....Patient Name ....Hospital No. ....

Consultant .... Ward ....

PRE-OPERATIVE ASSESSMENT
(Relevant information to include potential medical/physical and communication problems e.g. Diabetes, Blindness/Deafness, Language differences etc.)

PATIENT WEIGHT:

T.P.R. B/P

ALLERGIES:

PRE-OPERATIVE CHECKLIST

	YES/NO	INITIAL
SECTION A – To be checked by observing/asking patient		
Identiband present and correct	....	....
Time food or drink last taken	....	....
Urine passed prior to pre-medication	....	....
Dental crowns /bridge work / loose teeth	....	....
Dentures removed (with patient)	....	....
Hearing Aid (with patient)	....	....
Contact lenses removed	....	....
Patient correctly prepared for theatre –		
e.g. shaved if necessary	....	....
Jewellery removed (rings taped)	....	....
Cosmetic and clothing removed	....	....
Valuables placed in hospital custody	....	....
SECTION B – To be checked from nursing/medical notes		
Consent to anaesthetic/operation form signed	....	....
Operation site marked if appropriate	....	....
Patient has undergone pre-anaesthetic examination	....	....
Pre-medication given at	(time)....................	....
Case notes accompany patient –	....	....
X-rays accompany patient –	....	....

TIME IN ANAESTHETIC ROOM ....SIGNATURE WARD NURSE ....

SIGNATURE OF CHECKING ODA / NURSE ....

Figure 30.1 The Royal Marsden Hospital theatre care document.

DOCUMENTATION OF CARE

TIME IN THEATRE. . . . .

TEMP (18 - 21C)	YES/NO
HUMIDITY (30% - 50%)	YES/NO
EQUIPMENT CHECKED	YES/NO

PATIENT CARE

identification / consent   YES/NO

POSITION OF PATIENT: Supine   Prone   Lateral   Lithotomy   Trendelenburg

Other (please specify) ....

Apparatus used for safe positioning of patient:

Arm supports   Heel support   Gamgee   Arm Boards   Head Ring

Other (please specify) ....

Hot air mattress   Yes/No   TED Stockings/Venous stimulators

Position of Diathermy Plate ....

Catheter (size/type/balloon size) ....

Skin preparation   Iodine – Aqueous / Alcoholic

                        Chlorhexidine – Aqueous / Alcoholic

                        Other (please specify) ....

Throat pack ....

Tourniquet times   on.....................off ....

SURGEON(S) ....

SCRUB PERSON(S) ....CIRCULATING PERSON(S)..

                 ....

ANAESTHETIST.. ODA/NURSE ....

LA   /   GA

PROCEDURE PERFORMED ....

Swab / Needle / Instrument Count ....

Condition of patient's skin at end of surgery ....

Diathermy site checked (Initial) ....

Skin Closure : Sutures (Interrupted / Continuous) – Type ....

                Staples   Other (please specify) ....

Drains :   Vacuum   Silicone   Yeates / Corrugated   Other (specify) ....

Dressings: ....   Packs   vaginal / nasal ....

Specimens – Histology (Formalin / Fresh / Frozen Section) Microbiology Cytology

Signature of Scrub Person ....

Figure 30.1 *Continued.*

THEATRE RECOVERY

TIME IN ....

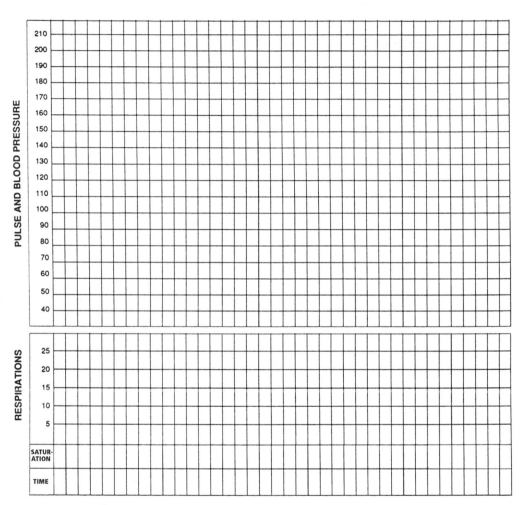

RESPIRATORY FUNCTION –

AIRWAY – observe, assess and ensure patency

BREATHING – record respiratory rate, observe
chest movement

Give O_2 as prescribed

Record O_2 saturation

ACTION & EVALUATION

Figure 30.1 The Royal Marsden Hospital theatre care document (*cont'd*).

CARDIOVASCULAR FUNCTION

Record Pulse & Blood Pressure

Observe skin/ mucosa for temperature and perfusion

Observe wound sites, dressings and drains

LEVEL OF CONSCIOUSNESS
Observe responsiveness, orientation & mobility

FLUID BALANCE
Observe and record all input/drainage from IVIs, catheters, NG tubes etc.

MEDICATION
Record all drugs given, time of administration and effect

COMMENTS AND INSTRUCTIONS SPECIFIC TO PATIENT

ACTION & EVALUATION

....

SIGNATURE OF RECOVERY NURSE

Figure 30.1   *Continued.*

Postanaesthetic recovery

Definition

Postanaesthetic recovery involves the short-term critical care required by patients during their immediate postoperative period until they are stable, conscious and orientated.

Indication

All patients undergoing surgery and anaesthesia.

Reference material

The postanaesthetic recovery room is an area within the operating department specifically designed, equipped and staffed for the support, monitoring and assessment of patients through the reversing stages of anaesthesia.

The recovery period is potentially hazardous. Therefore, when the patient arrives in the postanaesthetic recovery room, individual nursing care is required until patients are able to maintain their own airway (Miller 1994). While the majority of patients can be expected to achieve uneventful recovery, 24% of all patients have complications (Hines *et al.* 1992). Although nausea and vomiting are high on the list of complications (9.8%; Hines *et al.* 1992), the

most notable are respiratory and circulatory complications. Obstruction of the upper airway is the most common respiratory complication in the immediate postoperative period. Close observation and appropriate action can prevent the sequence of respiratory obstruction resulting in hypoxia leading to cardiac arrest (Campbell & Spence 1990).

Guedel's classification of general anaesthesia

Guedel first published his systemization of the signs of inhalation anaesthesia, based on the description of patients under open-drop ether anaesthesia in 1920. Current practice does not depend on the use of a single agent administered in this way and the effects of opiates and muscle relaxants will affect the signs of the stages of anaesthesia as formulated in his classification. However, the system can still be used as a framework within which to assess the progress of postanaesthetic recovery as long as other factors influencing the return of consciousness are taken into consideration (Table 30.1). With modern anaesthetic agents particulary propofol (Diprivan), rapid and symptom-free recovery from anaesthesia is seen and the frequency of nausea and vomiting, headaches and confusion/restlessness has been shown to be reduced (Grant & Mackenzie, 1985). This type of anaesthetic is commonly used in day surgery.

Table 30.1 Guedel's classification of general anaesthesia (Guedel 1937; Lunn 1982)

Stage I	Analgesia or the stage of disorientation from induction of anaesthesia to loss of consciousness
Stage II	Excitement: reflexes remain and coughing, vomiting and struggling may occur; respiration can be irregular with breath-holding
Stage III	Surgical anaesthesia, divided into four planes: Plane I – eyelid reflex lost, swallowing reflex disappears, marked eyeball movement but loss of conjunctival reflex Plane II – eyeball movement ceases, laryngeal reflex lost although inflammation of the upper respiratory tract increases reflex irritability, corneal reflex disappears, secretion of tears increases, respiration automatic and regular, movement and deep breathing as a response to skin stimulation disappears Plane III – diaphragmatic respiration, progressive intercostal paralysis, pupils dilated and light reflex abolished. The laryngeal reflex lost in plane II can still be initiated by stimuli arising in the anus or cervix Plane IV – complete intercostal paralysis to diaphragmatic paralysis
Stage IV	Medullary paralysis with respiratory arrest and vasomotor collapse as a result of anaesthetic overdose

Assessment for discharge

The length of any patient's stay in the recovery room is dependent on the patient's condition and the rate at which that patient returns to a physical, mental and emotional state where he or she can be left unattended between routine observations.

Minimum criteria for discharge are:

1 The patient is conscious and orientated and all protective reflexes have returned to normal.
2 Respiratory function is adequate and good oxygenation is being maintained.
3 Pulse and blood pressure are within normal pre-operative limits on consecutive observation.
4 There is no persistent or excessive bleeding from wound or drainage sites.
5 Patients with urinary catheters have passed adequate amounts of urine (more than 0.5 ml/kg/hour) (Eltringham et al. 1989).
6 Satisfactory analgesia has been provided for the patient, prescribed by the anaesthetist.

Wherever possible, a prior knowledge of patients gained from pre-operative contact is of great value in assessing their return to a normal state. It also has the advantage of helping their orientation to time and place, as familiarity generates a degree of security and confidence.

Local and regional anaesthesia

Patients having surgical procedures performed under local or spinal anaesthesia, whether intra- or extra- (cpi-) dural, will require a period of postoperative observation, although the priorities of their care will be geared towards different considerations, such as hypotension, headaches and dizziness.

Layout of equipment

While a greater part of the nursing procedures carried out in the recovery room will of necessity be of a routine and repetitive nature, the reason for their performance is for the detection of potential as well as actual complications and the initiation of appropriate interventions. The need for speed, efficiency and economy of movement is essential when time becomes a critical factor in the ultimate safety of the patient. Thus, the basic equipment for monitoring airway maintenance and assisted ventilation must be available at the patient's head in each recovery bay. Equipment must be arranged for ease of access and always be clean and in full working order. Further support equipment should be available centrally, whenever possible being stored on trolleys for ease of transportation.

Summary

Postanaesthetic care can best be described and understood as a series of many nursing procedures performed in sequence and simultaneously on patients who are in an artificially induced and traumatized condition. These patients will display varying degrees of responsiveness and physical and emotional states. It is important to establish a rapport with each individual to prevent the feeling of 'conveyor-belt processing' and gain the patient's confidence and cooperation. It is also necessary to understand that when emerging from the final stage of anaesthesia, some patients can behave in an emotional and disinhibited fashion, at variance with their normal behaviour (Eckenhoff et al. 1961). These displays are always transient and fortunately patients seldom have any recollection of them. While most patients can be expected to achieve an uneventful recovery, the duration and extent of surgery and anaesthesia are indicators of the pattern of recovery from the procedure and it can be judged to be uneventful only from hindsight. Physical and psychological recovery can be unpredictable at times.

References and further reading

Andrews, S.J. (1979) The recovery room as a nursing service. *J R Soc Med*, **72**, 275–7.
Atkinson, R.S. *et al.* (1982) *A Synopsis of Anaesthesia*, 9th edn. John Wright, Bristol.

Asbury, A.J. (1981) Problems of the immediate post-anaesthesia period. *Br J Hosp Med*, **25**, 159–63.

Association of Anaesthetists of Great Britain and Ireland (1985) *Postanaesthetic Recovery Facilities – Working Party Recommendations*. AAGBI, London.

Bales, R. (1988) Hypothermia, a postoperative problem that's easy to miss. *Reg Nurse*, **51**(4), 42–3.

Bowers Feldman, M.E. (1988) Inadvertent hypothermia, a threat to homeostasis in the postanaesthetic patient. *J Postanaes Nurs*, **3**(2), 82–7.

Campbell, D. & Spence, A.A. (1990) *Norris and Campbell's Anaesthetics, Resuscitation and Intensive Care*, 7th edn. Churchill Livingstone, Edinburgh.

Crayne, H.E. *et al.* (1988) Thermoresuscitation for postoperative hypothermia using reflective blankets. *AORN J*, **47**(1), 222–3, 226–7.

Drummond, G.B. (1991) Keep a clear airway. *Br J Anaes*, **66**, 153–66.

Eckenhoff, J.E., Kneale, D.H. & Dripps, R.D. (1961) The incidence and aetiology of postanaesthetic excitement. *Anaesthesiology*, **22**, 667.

Eltringham, R. (1979) Complications in the recovery room. *J R Soc Med*, **72**, 278–80.

Eltringham, R. *et al.* (1989) *Post-Anaesthetic Recovery: A Practical Approach*, 2nd edn. Springer, Berlin.

Fallacaro, M. *et al.* (1986) Inadvertent hypothermia – etiology, effects and preparation. *AORN J*, **44**(1), 54–61.

Farman, J.V. (1978) The work of the recovery room. *Br J Hosp Med*, **19**, 606–616.

Farman, J.V. (1979) Do we need recovery rooms? *J R Soc Med*, **72**, 270–72.

Grant, J.S. & Mackenzie, N. (1985) Recovery following propofol ('Diprivan') anaesthesia. A review of three different anaesthetic techniques. *Postgrad Med J*, **61**(3), 133–7.

Guedel, A.E. (1937) *Inhalation Anaesthesia: A Fundamental Guide*. Macmillan, New York.

Hines, R., Beresh, P.G., Watrous, G. *et al.* (1992) Complications occurring in the postanaesthesia care unit: a survey. *Anaesthes Analg*, **74**, 503.

Hudson, R.B.S. (1979) Pattern of work in the recovery room. *J R Soc Med*, **72**, 273–5.

Levinson, B.W. (1965) States of awareness during general anaesthesia. Preliminary communication. *Br J Anaes*, **37**(7), 544–6.

Lunn, J.N. (1982) *Lecture Notes on Anaesthetics*, 2nd edn. Blackwell Scientific Publications, Oxford.

Mallett, J. (1990) Communication between nurses and postanaesthetic patients. *Intens Care Nurs*, **6**, 45–53.

Miller, R.D. (1994) *Anasthesia*, Vol. 2, 4th edn. Churchill Livingstone, Edinburgh.

Nimmo, W.S. *et al.* (eds) (1994) *Anaesthesia*, 2nd edn. Blackwell Science, Oxford.

White, H.E. *et al.* (1987) Body temperature in elderly surgical patients. *Res Nurs Health*, **10**(5), 317–21.

GUIDELINES • Postanaesthetic recovery

Equipment

1 Theatre trolley bed, which must incorporate the following features:
   (a) Oxygen supply.
   (b) Trendelenburg tilt mechanism.
   (c) Adjustable cot sides.
   (d) Adjustable back rest.
   (e) Brakes.
   (f) Radio translucency.
2 Basic equipment required for each patient:
   (a) Oxygen supply, preferably wall-mounted with tubing, face masks (with both fixed and variable settings), a T-piece system and full range of oropharyngeal and nasopharyngeal airways.
   (b) Suction – regulatable with tubing, and a range of nozzles and catheters.

Note: spare oxygen cylinders with flowmeters and an electrically powered portable suction machine should always be available in case of pipeline failure.

   (c) Sphygmomanometer and stethoscope. Automatic blood pressure recorders are a valuable means of saving time and of minimizing disturbance to patients, especially those in pain or disorientated, and leaving the nurse's hands free to attend to other needs. However, such equipment can be nonfunctioning in certain cases, e.g. shivering or profoundly bradycardic patients, and is subject to electrical and mechanical failure.
   (d) Pulse oximeter, whenever possible.
   (e) Miscellaneous items: receivers, tissues, disposable gloves, sharps container and waste receptacle.
3 Essential equipment centrally available for respiratory and cardiovascular support:
   (a) Self-inflating resuscitator bag, e.g. Ambu bag and/or Mapleson C circuit with face mask.
   (b) Full intubation equipment: laryngoscopes with spare bulbs and batteries, range of endotracheal tubes, bougies and Magill's forceps, syringe and catheter mount.
   (c) Anaesthetic machine and ventilator.
   (d) Wright respirometer.
   (e) Cricothyroid puncture set.
   (f) Range of tracheotomy tubes and tracheal dilator.

Guidelines • Postanaesthetic recovery (cont'd)

(g) Intravenous infusion sets and cannulae, range of intravenous fluids.
(h) Central venous cannulae and manometer.
(i) Emergency drug box – contents in accordance with current hospital policy.
(j) Defibrillator.
4 Standard equipment for routine nursing procedures.

Procedure

The following recommended actions are not necessarily listed in order of priority. Many will be carried out simultaneously and much will depend on the patient's condition, surgery and level of consciousness. All actions must be accompanied by commentary and explanation regardless of the apparent responsiveness as the sense of hearing returns before the patient's ability to respond (Lambrechts & Parkhouse 1961; Levinson 1965).

Action	*Rationale*
1 Assess the patency of the airway by feeling for movement of expired air.	To determine the presence of any respiratory depression or neuromuscular blockade. Observe chest and abdominal movement, respiratory rate, depth and pattern (Drummond 1991).
(a) Listen for inspiration and expiration. Apply suction if indicated. Observe any use of accessory muscles of respiration and check for tracheal tug.	To ensure absence of material in the airway, i.e. blood, mucus, vomitus. To ascertain absence of laryngeal spasm.
(b) If indicated, support the chin with the neck extended.	In the unconscious patient the tongue is liable to fall back and obstruct the airway and protective reflexes are absent.
(c) Apply a face mask and administer oxygen at the rate prescribed by the anaesthetist. If an endotracheal tube or laryngeal mask is in position, check whether the cuff or mask is inflated and administer oxygen by means of a T-piece system.	To maintain adequate oxygenation. Oxygen should be administered to all patients in the recovery room (Nimmo *et al*. 1994).
(d) Observe skin colour and temperature. Check the colour of lips and conjunctiva, then peripheral colour and perfusion.	Central cyanosis indicates impaired gaseous exchange between the alveoli and pulmonary capillaries. Peripheral cyanosis indicates low cardiac output (Nimmo *et al*. 1994).
2 Feel the pulse. The patient's position will probably mean that the head, carotid, facial or temporal arteries will offer the easiest access. Note the rate, rhythm and volume and record.	To assess cardiovascular function and establish a postoperative baseline for future observations.
3 Obtain full information about anaesthetic technique, potential problems and the patient's general medical condition.	To plan subsequent treatment.
4 Obtain full information about the surgical procedure and any drains, packs, blood loss and specific postoperative instructions.	To ensure intervention is based on informed observation.

Note: the information gained from points 3 and 4 will be recorded on the anaesthetic chart and the nursing care document (Fig. 30.1), but an initial verbal handover will ensure that there is no delay in providing care that may be needed before all relevant information can be gathered from documentation.

5 Take and record blood pressure on reception and at a minimum of 5-minute intervals. Record the pulse and respiratory rate at the same interval unless patient's condition dictates otherwise.	To enable any fluctuations or gross abnormalities in observations to be established quickly. Accurate records are of medico-legal importance in the event of an enquiry.
6 Hypothermia. Check the temperature of the patient, especially those who are at high risk of hypothermia, e.g. the elderly, children, those who have undergone long surgery or where large amounts of blood or fluid replacement therapy have been used. Check patients who are shivering, restless, confused or with respiratory	More than 90% of patients undergoing surgery experience some degree of postoperative hypothermia (Fallacaro *et al*. 1986; White *et al*.1987). The symptoms of hypothermia can mimic those of other postoperative complications, which may result in inappropriate treatment. Some of the symptoms such as

depression (hypothermia interferes with the effective reversal of muscle relaxants: Bowers Feldman 1988). Use 'space' (reflective) blankets and warm blankets to warm the patient.

7 Check wound site(s) and observe dressings and any drains. Note and record drainage.

8 Ensure any intravenous infusions are running at the prescribed rate. Check the prescription chart for any medications prescribed for administration during the immediate postoperative period.

9 Remain with the patient at all times. Assess level of consciousness during reversing stages of anaesthesia, observing for returning reflexes, i.e. swallowing, tear secretion and eyelash and lid reflexes and response to stimuli – both physical (*not* painful) and verbal (do not shout).

10 Orientate the patient to time and place as frequently as is necessary.

11 Suction of the upper airway is indicated if gurgling sounds are present on respiration and if blood secretions or vomitus are evident or suspected, and the patient is unable to swallow or cough either at all or adequately. Suction must be applied with care to avoid damage to mucosal surfaces and further irritation or initiation of a gag reflex or laryngeal spasm.

12 Endotracheal suction is performed following the same procedure as that for suction of tracheostomy tubes. (For further information see the procedure on tracheostomy, Chap. 40).

13 Give mouth care. (For further information, see Guidelines·Mouth care, Chap. 24.)

14 After regional and/or spinal anaesthesia, assess the return of sensation and mobility of limbs. Check that the limbs are anatomically aligned.

shivering put an increased demand on cardiopulmonary systems as oxygen consumption is increased (Bowers Feldman 1988). Other complications such as arrhythmias or myocardial infarct can result (Bales 1988), and the longer the duration of the postoperative hypothermia, the greater the patient mortality (Crayne et al. 1988).

To be aware of any changes or bleeding and take appropriate action, e.g. inform the surgeon.

To ensure correct treatment is given.

To ascertain progress towards normal function.

To alleviate anxiety, provide reassurance, gain the patient's confidence and cooperation. Premedication and anaesthesia can induce a degree of amnesia and disorientation.

Foreign matter can obstruct the airway or cause laryngeal spasm in light planes of anaesthesia. It can also be inhaled when protective laryngeal reflexes are absent. Vagal stimulation can induce bradycardia in susceptible patients (Atkinson et al. 1982, p. 819).

To maintain the patency of the tube and remove secretions.

Pre-operative fasting, drying gases and manipulation of lips, etc. leave mucosa vulnerable, sore and foul tasting.

To prevent inadvertent injury following sensory loss.

Nursing care plan

Note: no observation of cardiovascular function is informative when taken in isolation. Full assessment must be made of respiratory function in conjunction with observations of pulse, blood pressure, emotional state and significant medical history.

Problem	Cause	Suggested action
Airway obstruction.	Tongue occluding the airway.	Support chin forward from the angle of the jaw. If necessary insert a Guedel airway. Use a nasopharyngeal airway if the teeth are clenched or crowned.
	Foreign material, blood, secretions, vomitus.	Apply suction. Always check for the presence of throat pack.
	Laryngeal spasm.	Increase the rate of oxygen. Assist ventilation with an Ambu bag and face

Problem	Cause	Suggested action
		mask. If there is no improvement, inform anaesthetist and have intubation equipment ready. Offer the patient reassurance.
Hypoventilation.	Respiratory depression from opiates, inhalations, agents, barbiturates.	Inform the anaesthetist and have available naloxone (opiate antagonist) and doxapram (respiratory stimulant). *Note*: if naloxone is given it can reverse the analgesic effects of opiates and has a duration of action of only 20–30 minutes. The patient must be observed for signs of returning hyperventilation. (Nimmo *et al.* 1994)
	Decreased respiratory drive from a low partial pressure of carbon dioxide ($PaCO_2$), loss of hypoxic drive in patients with chronic pulmonary disease.	With chronic pulmonary disease, give oxygen using, e.g., a Venturi mask with graded low concentrations (Atkinson *et al.* 1982).
	Neuromuscular blockade from continued action of nondepolarizing muscle relaxants, potentiation of relaxants caused by electrolyte imbalance, impaired excretion with renal or liver disease.	Inform the anaesthetist, have available neostigmine and glycopyrolate, or atropine potassium chloride and 10% calcium chloride. Often the degree of blockade is mild and will wear off in minutes without treatment, but it is extremely frightening and patients will need continuous reassurance that their condition is not unnoticed and is resolving and that they will not be left alone.
Hypotension.	Hypovolaemia.	Take central venous pressure (CVP) readings if catheter is in place. Give oxygen. Lower the head of the trolley unless contraindicated, e.g. hiatus hernia, gross obesity. Check the record of anaesthetic agents used which might cause hypotension, e.g. enflurane, halothane, beta-blockers, nitroprusside, opiates, droperidol, sympathetic blockade following spinal anaesthesia. Check the peripheral perfusion. If the CVP is low, increase intravenous infusion unless contraindicated, e.g. congestive cardiac failure. Check drains and dressings for visible bleeding and haematomata. Inform the anaesthetist or surgeon.
Hypertension.	Pain, carbon dioxide retention.	Treat pain with prescribed analgesia. Pain from certain operation sites can also be alleviated by changing the patient's position.
	Distended bladder.	Offer a bedpan or urinal.
	Some anaesthetic drugs.	Check the prescription chart for those patients on regular antihypertensive therapy. If the

		situation is not resolved inform the anaesthetist.
Bradycardia.	Very fit patient, opiates, reversal agents, beta-blockers, pain, vagal stimulation, hypoxaemia from respiratory depression.	Check the prescription chart and anaesthetic sheet. Connect the patient to the ECG monitor to exclude heart block. Inform the anaesthetist.
Tachycardia.	Pain, hypovolaemia, some anaesthetic drugs, septicaemia, fear, fluid overload.	Provide analgesia. Check the anaesthetic chart. Connect the patient to the ECG monitor to exclude ventricular tachycardia.
Pain.	Surgical trauma, worsened by fear, anxiety and restlessness.	Provide prescribed analgesia and assess its efficacy. Reassure and orientate the patients, who can be unaware that surgery has been performed, in which case their pain is more frightening. Try positional changes where feasible, e.g. experience has shown that after breast surgery some relief can be obtained from raising the back support by 20–40°; patients with abdominal or gynaecological surgery can be more comfortable lying on their side; elevate limbs to reduce swelling where appropriate. Unless significant relief is obtained, inform the anaesthetist.
Nausea and vomiting.	Opiates, hypotension, abdominal surgery, pain; some patients are prone to vomiting.	Offer antiemetics if the patient is conscious. Encourage slow, regular breathing. If the patient is unconscious, turn onto the side, tip the head down and suck out pharynx, give oxygen. *Note*: have wire-cutters available if the jaws are wired.
Hypothermia.	Depression of the heat-regulating centre, vasodilatation, following abdominal surgery, large infusions of blood and fluids.	Use extra blankets or a 'space blanket'. Monitor the patient's temperature.
Shivering.	Some inhalational anaesthetics, especially halothane, hypothermia.	Give oxygen, reassure the patient and take patient's temperature.
Hyperthermia.	Infection, blood transfusion reaction.	Give oxygen, use a fan or tepid sponging if this is warranted.
	Malignant hyperpyrexia.	Medical assessment of antibiotic therapy. Malignant hyperpyrexia is a medical emergency and a malignant hyperpyrexia pack with the necessary drugs should be readily available.
Oliguria.	Mechanical obstruction of catheter, e.g. clots, kinking.	Check the patency of the catheter.
	Inadequate renal perfusion, e.g. hypotension, systolic pressures under 60 mm Hg, hypovolaemia, dehydration.	Take blood pressure and CVP if available. Increase intravenous fluids. Inform the anaesthetist.
	Renal damage, e.g. from blood transfusion, infection, drugs, surgical damage to the ureters.	Refer to the anaesthetist or surgeon.

GUIDELINES • Postoperative recovery

Procedure

After discharge from the recovery room to the ward, the nursing care given during the postoperative period is directed towards the prevention of those potential complications resulting from surgery and anaesthesia which might be anticipated to develop over a longer period of time.

Consideration of the psychological and emotional aspects of recovery will of necessity be altered by the changed state of consciousness, awareness and knowledge of patients and their differing responses to surgery, diagnosis and treatment.

Potential respiratory complications

Action	*Rationale*
1 Observe respirations, noting rate and depth and any presence of dyspnoea or orthopnoea. (a) Observe chest movement for equal, bilateral expansion. (b) Observe colour and perfusion. (c) Position the patient to facilitate optimum lung expansion and reinforce pre-operative teaching of deep breathing exercises and coughing.	Respiratory function postoperatively can be influenced by a number of factors: increased bronchial secretions from inhalation anaesthesia; decreased respiratory effort from opiate medication; pain or anticipation of pain from surgical wounds; surgical trauma to the phrenic nerve; pneumothorax as a result of surgical or anaesthetic procedures. All factors limiting the adequate expansion of the lung and the ejection of bronchial secretions will encourage the development of atelectasis and consolidation of the affected lung tissue.
2 Change position of patients on bedrest every 2–3 h.	To prevent and monitor formation of pressure sores and tissue viability.
3 Provide adequate prescribed analgesia.	Patients in pain are more likely to be disorientated and show signs of high blood pressure and tachycardia (Nimmo *et al.* 1994).
4 Record temperature and pulse. If sputum produced, observe nature and quantity for culture.	If infection follows there may be a rise in temperature, pulse and respiratory rate.

Potential circulatory problems

Deep venous thrombosis and pulmonary embolus

Action	*Rationale*
1 Encourage early mobilization where patient's condition allows. For patients on bedrest, encourage deep breathing and exercises of the leg – flexion/extension and rotation of the ankles.	Patients are at increased risk of developing deep venous thrombosis as a result of muscular inactivity, postoperative respiratory and circulatory depression, abdominal and pelvic surgery, prolonged pressure on calves from lithotomy poles, etc., increased production of thromboplastin as a result of surgical trauma, pre-existing coronary artery disease.
2 Where worn, ensure that antiembolic stockings are of the correct size and fit smoothly.	Incorrect sizing causes swelling and bruising to ankles and can constrict blood supply.
3 Advise against crossing of legs or ankles.	To prevent constriction of blood supply and swelling.
4 Record temperature.	
5 Report any complaints of calf or thigh pain to medical staff.	To monitor for signs of deep vein thrombosis.
6 Observe for any dyspnoea, chest pain or signs of shock.	To monitor for signs of pulmonary embolism.

Haemorrhage

Action	Rationale
1 Observe dressings, drains and wound sites, and quantity and nature of drainage. Observe pulse, blood pressure, respirations and colour.	Early haemorrhage may occur as the patient's blood pressure rises. Record postoperatively re-establishing blood flow or blood as a result of the slipping of a ligature or the dislodging of a clot.
2 Observe wound for redness, tenderness and increased temperature.	Secondary haemorrhage may occur after a period of days as a result of infection and sloughing.

Potential fluid and electrolyte imbalance and malnutrition

Action	Rationale
1 Maintain accurate records of intravenous infusions, oral fluids, wound and stoma drainage, nasogastric drainage, vomitus, urine and urological irrigation.	Pre-operative fasting and dehydration, increased secretion of antidiuretic hormone, blood loss and paralytic ileus all contribute to potential fluid and electrolyte imbalance. Vomiting and stasis of intestinal fluid may lead to potassium depletion.
2 Observe nature and quantity of all drainage, aspirate, faeces, etc.	To monitor and replace fluid loss.
3 Give prescribed antiemetics if nausea or vomiting occur.	
4 Observe state of mouth for coating, furring and dryness.	To maintain oral hygiene and to assess for thrush and hydration.
5 Encourage oral fluids as soon as the patient is able to take them unless the nature of the surgery contraindicates this.	To encourage hydration, and promote diuresis and digestion.
6 Encourage early resumption of diet.	Return to an adequate nutritional state is necessary for wound healing (see Chap. 47, Wound Management); it is particularly important that diabetic patients should return to their pre-operative insulin/diet regime to avoid increased risk of metabolic disturbance.

Potential problem of pain

Action	Rationale
1 Observe the patient, noting physiological signs indicative of pain, e.g. sweating, tachycardia, hypotension, pallor or flushed appearance.	These are the first indications of pain related to intra-operative trauma and postoperative complications.
2 Note restlessness, immobility and facial expressions.	Continuous severe pain can cause restlessness, anxiety, insomnia and anorexia, and may thus interfere with recovery by impeding deep breathing, mobilization and nutrition.
3 Listen to the patient and ascertain the location and nature of the pain. If necessary, use a pain scale chart (see Chap. 29).	Communication skills are necessary for the effective assessment and alleviation of pain as there may be multiple contributory factors, both physical and emotional in origin.
4 Administer prescribed analgesia and observe effect.	To relieve and control pain and if necessary to review pain relief available.
5 Try changing position of patient. Give attention, information and reassurance; assist with relaxation exercises.	To promote comfort and reduce anxiety due to pain.

Peritoneal Dialysis and Continuous Venovenous Haemodiafiltration

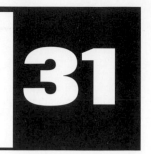

Definition

Dialytic therapies are procedures used for patients with inadequate renal function who are unable to rid the body of waste products. These products are the waste by-products of metabolism, such as urea, creatinine and salts, e.g. potassium and sodium as well as excess body water. To effect dialysis, an alternative membrane or filter is used. In the case of peritoneal dialysis it is the peritoneal membrane itself that is used. In all other forms of dialysis an artificial filter is used. Dialytic therapies may be instituted when there is an acute problem with renal function and can also be used in the chronic situation if renal transplantation is not possible or is delayed.

Reference material

Dialysis is possible because of the properties of substances that permit diffusion, osmosis and convection. Diffusion is the force acting on gaseous, solid or liquid molecules to spread them from a region of high concentration to a region of lower concentration.

Osmosis is the passage of a solvent through a semi-permeable membrane that separates solutions of different concentrations. The force that causes this movement of solvents is osmotic pressure and this varies directly with the concentration of the solution. As the solvent moves across the membrane, it tends to pull certain amounts of solute with it. This is known as the solvent drag effect. Equilibration is the achievement of equalization of solute and solvent concentrations on both sides of the membrane. As equilibration is achieved, dialysis ceases and solvents and solutes can be absorbed back into the bloodstream (Fig. 31.1). Convection is the use of hydrostatic pressure to force water and solutes through a semipermeable membrane.

Types of dialytic therapies

Several dialytic therapies are available:

1 Haemodialysis
2 Peritoneal dialysis
3 Continuous venovenous haemodiafiltration
4 Ultrafiltration.

The choice of procedure is determined by a patient's clinical needs, resources and manpower implications.

If the patient has chronic renal failure and transplantation is not possible, the optimum procedure is haemodialy-sis. This is usually performed 2–3 times a week either in the patient's home or in the chronic dialysis unit. Many patients and their families learn this technique. Haemodialysis is rarely used in the acute setting even if patients are hypercatabolic as most acutely ill patients cannot tolerate the changes in haemodynamic status and the volume of fluid shifts.

Peritoneal dialysis and the continuous slow filtration therapies are both performed outside specialist renal centres and will therefore be discussed in greater detail.

Peritoneal dialysis (PD)

Indications

Peritoneal dialysis may be selected for the following reasons (Oh 1995):

1 Widespread availability
2 Technical simplicity
3 Because the patient's biochemistry can be kept stable and patients often feel better as a result.
4 Patients may remain ambulant; and require less visits to hospital, thus achieving greater independence of medical care.
5 Low maintenance costs.

Reference material

In 1926 Rosenak, basing his work on that of Ganter, conceived the possibility of using the peritoneum of humans as a dialysing membrane (Blumenkrantz & Roberts 1979). The use of peritoneal dialysis reached a peak in 1959 with the introduction of commercial dialysis solutions and tubing. In the 1960s advances in peritoneal dialysis were being made by Tenckhoff (Warren 1989), and long-term access now became a reality. More recently, vast improvements have been made in the design, efficacy and portability of continuous ambulatory peritoneal dialysis devices. At this time the technique of haemodialysis was introduced and the two treatments are now used widely (Warren 1989).

Anatomy and physiology

The peritoneum is the largest serous membrane of the body. In adults it has a surface area of approximately 2.2 m^2. It is a closed unit consisting of two parts:

1 The parietal peritoneum that lines the inside of the abdominal wall.
2 The visceral peritoneum that is reflected over the viscera.

The space between the two parts is the peritoneal cavity. This cavity is normally a potential space containing only a small amount of serous fluid. The serous fluid lubricates the viscera and allows them to move freely upon one another and the parietal peritoneum (Marieb 1996).

The visceral peritoneum consists of five layers of fibrous and elastic connective tissue and a sixth layer called the mesothelium. Blood and lymphatic capillaries are found only in the deepest layer of tissue in adults. A substance that passes from the bloodstream into the peritoneal cavity must pass through the capillary endothelium, the mesothelium and the five layers of the visceral peritoneum. The mesothelium represents the major barrier to mass transfer for most substances (Marieb 1996).

For peritoneal dialysis to achieve maximum efficacy, fresh solutions must be instilled at the point of equilibration to prevent reabsorption of water and uraemic toxins. It should be noted that solvent drag enhances the efficiency of peritoneal dialysis.

Solution concentrations

The osmotic pressure of dextrose is utilized in peritoneal dialysis to remove water and solutes from the patient. The composition of most commercially available peritoneal dialysis solutions falls into the following three groups:

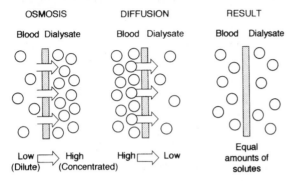

Figure 31.1 The process of osmosis and diffusion. (From *Nursing Times*, 22 April 1987, p. 41, with permission.)

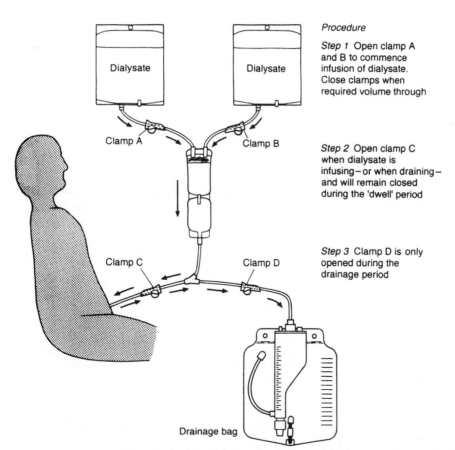

Procedure

Step 1 Open clamp A and B to commence infusion of dialysate. Close clamps when required volume through

Step 2 Open clamp C when dialysate is infusing – or when draining – and will remain closed during the 'dwell' period

Step 3 Clamp D is only opened during the drainage period

Figure 31.2 Using the Y-type administration set.

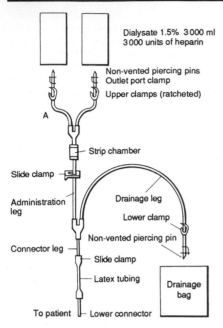

Dialysate 1.5% 3000 ml
3000 units of heparin

Non-vented piercing pins
Outlet port clamp
Upper clamps (ratcheted)

A

Strip chamber

Slide clamp

Administration leg

Drainage leg

Lower clamp

Non-vented piercing pin

Connector leg

Slide clamp

Latex tubing

Drainage bag

To patient — Lower connector

Figure 31.3 Peritoneal dialysis system setup. (Courtesy of Abbott Renal Care.)

1 The solution's electrolyte composition approximates to normal extracellular fluid, i.e. its potassium concentration is 4 mmol/l and its glucose concentration is 1.3–1.5%.
2 As solution 1, but contains no potassium.
3 Hypertonic solution with a glucose concentration of 6.3% and the same potassium concentration as solution 1.

The choice of dialysate solution will depend on the primary aim of dialysis and the patient's baseline plasma electrolyte levels (Bloe 1990).

Dialysis cycle

Normally, a cycle consists of three stages (Fig. 31.2).

Stage 1 (inflow)

The dialysis solution at body temperature is infused into the peritoneal cavity to initiate the dialysis. The fluid infuses by gravity and its rate can be controlled by raising or lowering the container in relation to the patient's abdomen or by releasing or compressing the occluding clamp on the tubing.

Stage 2 (dwell time)

The dwell time is the time that the fluid remains in the peritoneal cavity to allow for equilibration. Different dwell times may be established to remove substances of differing

molecular weights. The dwell time is relevant to the molecular weight of the solute and how much needs to be removed.

Stage 3 (drainage)

The drainage stage is that of emptying the equilibrated solution from the peritoneal cavity to complete dialysis or to prepare for the infusion of fresh solution. Drainage is also dependent on gravity.

Types of peritoneal dialysis

Intermittent

For peritoneal dialysis used in the acute situation, a manual system is usually used to effect a quick and gentle dialysis (Fig. 31.3). Optimal dialysis is achieved with short dialysis cycles of about 1 hour each, with a dwell time of 30 minutes and drainage time of 20 minutes. Specific numbers of exchanges are prescribed and dialysis is then discontinued temporarily, with initiation recurring as uraemia increases (Bloe 1990).

Continuous ambulatory peritoneal dialysis (CAPD)

The CAPD technique was first introduced in 1975. It is a closed, continuous system of peritoneal dialysis and allows the patient the independence of a life free from dialysis machines. The regime practised is usually four exchanges per day, with the last staying in the peritoneal cavity overnight. Many devices have been developed to assist patients in their own homes to cope with the treatment while remaining free from the danger of infection and peritonitis (Warren 1989).

Clear outlines of CAPD can be found in Shoemaker (1995) and Zappacosta & Perras (1984).

Continuous filtration methods

Definition

Continuous filtration methods mimic the filtration that would occur in the glomerulus of the kidney. Water and solutes are forcibly moved from the plasma through a semipermeable membrane. Membranes are synthetic and vary in terms of the size of molecular solutes they filter out. Selection of the filter depends on the clinical situation. Continuous filtration therapies involve the production of large volumes of filtrate (300–800 ml/hour). This output must be balanced by the administration of electrolyte solutions (Oh 1995).

Reference material

The use of continuous filtration methods has increased significantly since the late 1980s with advances in technology

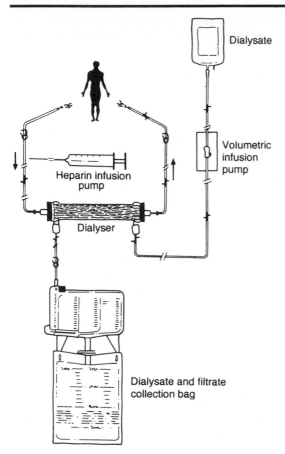

Dialysate

Volumetric
infusion
pump

Heparin infusion
pump

Dialyser

Dialysate and filtrate
collection bag

Figure 31.4 Schematic representation of CVVHD.
(Reproduced by permission of Fresenius Medical Care Ltd.)

and the training of critical care nurses. These methods are
used in particular in high-dependency or intensive therapy
settings because of their ability to provide excellent clearance of solutes and fluid whilst avoiding haemodynamic
instability that can result from conventional haemodialysis
(Tinker & Zapol 1992). Several methods are available,
including:

1 Ultrafiltration (UF)
2 Slow continuous ultrafiltration (SCUF)
3 Continuous arteriovenous haemofiltration (CAVH)
4 Continuous venovenous haemodiafiltration (CVVHD).

CVVHD is the therapy with the widest application to a
variety of clinical situations and is therefore examined in
greater detail here.

CVVHD

Continuous venovenous haemodiafiltration combines convection and diffusion. The convection of ultrafiltration utilizes a large hydrostatic pressure gradient which means that
up to 2 litres of water an hour can be removed from the
plasma via the filter. Diffusion of the solutes (i.e. urea,
creatinine and potassium) is achieved by blood flow
through the filter, while dialysate is administered in a
counter current using an infusion device.

In CVVHD the 'artificial kidney' used ensures effective
clearance of solutes with small and middle-sized molecular
weights. Because blood flows through an extracorporeal
circuit and over a filter there is a danger of blood clots
forming in the patient circuit. An anticoagulant is therefore administered continuously. For a diagrammatic representation of the circuit, see Fig. 31.4.

Note: because CVVHD runs continuously it is essential
to calculate concomitant drug therapy utilizing the literature available. Some drugs are effectively cleared by the
filters while others are only partially cleared (Pittrow &
Penk 1998; Bunn & Ashley 1999).

References and further reading

Ahmad, S. *et al.* (1988) Center and home chronic hemodialysis.
In: *Diseases of the Kidney* (eds R.W. Scrier & C.W. Gottschalk).
Little, Brown & Co, Boston.

Arenz, R. (1982) Continuous ambulatory peritoneal dialysis.
AORN J, **35**(5), 946, 948, 950, 952, 954.

Barton, I., Barton J. & Chesser, A.M. (1997) Haemofiltration: how
to do it. *Br J Hosp Med*, **57**(5), 188–93.

Bloe, C.G. (1990) Peritoneal dialysis. *Prof Nurse*, **5**(7), 345–9.

Blumenkrantz, M.J. & Roberts, M. (1979) Progress in peritoneal
dialysis: an historical prospective. *Contrib Nephrol*, **17**, 101–110.

Bunn, R. & Ashley, C. (1999) *The Renal Drug Handbook*. Radcliffe
Medical Press, Oxford.

Hilton, P.J., Taylor, J., Forni, L.G. & Treacher, D.F. (1998)
Bicarbonate-based haemofiltration in the management of acute
renal failure with lactic acidosis. *Q J Med*, **91**(4), 279–83.

Marieb, E.N. (1996) *Human Anatomy and Physiology*. Benjamin
Cummings, California.

Oh, T.E. (1995) *Intensive Care Manual*. Butterworth,
Sydney.

Pittrow, L. & Penk, A. (1998) Pharmacokinetics and dosage of
fluconazole in continuous haemofiltration and haemodialysis.
Mycoses, **41**, Suppl 2, 86–8.

Shoemaker, W.C., Ayres, S.M., Grenisk, A. & Holbrook, P.R.
(1995) *Textbook of Critical Care*, pp. 1029–40 W.B. Saunders,
Philadelphia.

Stansfield, G. (1985) Coping with CAPD. *Nurs Mirror*, **161**(14),
28–9.

Tinker, J. & Zapol, W. (1992) *Care of the Critically Ill Patient*.
Springer, London.

Warren, H. (1989) Changes in peritoneal dialysis nursing. *ANNA
J*, **16**(3), 237–41.

Zappacosta, A. & Perras, S. (1984) *CAPD*. J.B. Lippincott,
Philadelphia.

GUIDELINES · Peritoneal dialysis

Equipment

1 Dialysis Y-type administration set and drainage bag.
2 Sterile peritoneal set containing forceps, blade and holder, topical swabs, towels, suturing equipment.
3 Sterile gown, gloves.
4 Peritoneal catheter stylet or trocar and drainage bag.
5 Local anaesthetic (1–2% lignocaine hydrochloride).
6 Syringe, needle.
7 Chlorhexidine in 70% alcohol.
8 Supplementary drugs as prescribed.
9 Peritoneal dialysis fluid, as prescribed, warmed to 37°C.

Procedure

Action	Rationale
1 Explain and discuss the procedure with the patient. An acutely ill patient may be confused and restless, but every effort should be made to inform patient of what is about to happen.	To ensure that the patient understands the procedure and gives his/her valid consent. Some hospitals require a patient to sign a consent form before the procedure can be carried out.
2 Ask the patient to micturate and defaecate before the procedure begins.	To avoid perforation of the bladder and/or rectum when the trocar is introduced into the peritoneum.
3 Record the patient's vital signs before the procedure begins.	To assess physical/psychological state and to monitor changes.
4 Weigh the patient before the procedure begins and then daily.	To assess hydration and to monitor any fluid losses.
5 Assist the patient to lie in the semirecumbent position.	To ensure that the patient is in the best position for the procedure's requirements.
6 Continue to observe and reassure the patient throughout the procedure.	To assess and monitor any physical/psychological changes.
7 Assist the doctor as required.	To facilitate a smooth and effective procedure for the patient.

Insertion of catheter

Action	Rationale
1 Using aseptic technique, the doctor prepares the abdomen surgically and injects the skin and subcutaneous tissues with a local anaesthetic.	To reduce the risk of contamination and infection. To minimize the pain of the incision.
2 A small incision is made in the abdominal wall 3–5 cm below the umbilicus. The trocar is inserted through the incision. The patient is asked to raise the head from the pillow after the trocar is introduced.	This tightens the abdominal muscles and permits easier penetration of the trocar without danger of injury to the internal organs.
3 When the peritoneum is punctured, the trocar is directed to the left side of the pelvis. The stylet is removed and the catheter is inserted through the trocar and gently manoeuvred into position.	To prevent the omentum from adhering to the catheter or occluding its opening.
4 Once the trocar is removed, the skin may be sutured and a sterile dressing placed around the catheter.	To prevent the loss of the catheter in the abdomen. To prevent leakage of peritoneal fluid onto the surrounding skin.
5 The tubing is flushed with the dialysis fluid.	To prevent air from entering the peritoneal cavity.

Preparation of dialysis fluid

Action	Rationale

Action

1 Wash hands with bactericidal soap and water or bactericidal alcohol hand rub. Proceed using aseptic technique.

2 The dialysis fluid should have been warmed to body temperature (37°C).

3 Add any drugs, e.g. heparin, to the dialysis fluid if prescribed.

4 Attach the dialysis fluid to the administration set via luer lock connections.

5 Attach the catheter connector to the administration set.

6 Allow the dialysis fluid to flow freely into the peritoneal cavity. (This normally takes from 5 to 10 minutes.)

7 Allow fluid to remain in the peritoneal cavity for the prescribed time. Prepare the next exchange while the first container of fluid is in the peritoneal cavity.

8 Unclamp the drainage tube. Drainage time will vary with each patient but, on average, should be completed in 10 minutes.

9 Clamp off the drainage tube when outflow ceases and begin infusing the next exchange, again using aseptic technique.

10 Record the following:
(a) Time of commencement and completion of each exchange and the start and finish of the drainage stage
(b) Amount of fluid infused and recovered
(c) Fluid balance after each complete exchange
(d) Any medication added to the dialysis fluid.

11 Take and record the vital signs:
(a) Blood pressure and pulse every 15 minutes during the first exchange and hourly thereafter, depending on the patient's condition.
(b) Temperature every 4 h, or more frequently if condition demands.

12 Record fluid balance accurately.

13 Dialysis is usually continued until blood chemistry levels are satisfactory.

Rationale

To reduce risk of infection.

For the patient's comfort. To prevent abdominal pain. Heating causes dilation of the peritoneal vessels and increases clearance of urea. Cold fluid would decrease rate of removal of large molecular solutes and can cause abdominal cramp pain.

Heparin prevents fibrin clots from occluding the catheter.

To ascertain whether the catheter is in the required position. The flow should be steady and brisk. If not, the tip of the catheter may be buried in the omentum or it may have been occluded by a blood clot.

The fluid must remain in the peritoneal cavity for the prescribed dwell time so that potassium, urea and other waste products may be removed. The solution is most effective over the first 5–10 minutes when the concentration gradient is at its greatest (Tinker & Zapol 1992).

To rid the body of the required products. The abdomen is drained by a siphon effect through the closed system. Drainage is normally straw-coloured.

To enable the next cycle to begin. To reduce the risk of local and/or systemic infection.

To detect and monitor trends and fluctuations and to identify any outflow obstruction.

Hypotension may be indicative of excessive fluid loss due to the glucose concentration of the dialysis fluid. Changes in pulse may indicate impending shock or overhydration. To monitor for any signs of infection. Infection is more likely to become evident after dialysis has been discontinued.

To prevent complications such as circulatory overload and hypertension that may occur if most of the fluid is not recovered during the drainage stage. The fluid balance should be about even or show slight fluid loss, unless the reason for treatment was to remove excess fluid.

The duration of dialysis is related to the severity of the condition and the size and weight of the patient. The usual time is about 12–36 h, giving between 24 and 28 exchanges.

Guidelines • Peritoneal dialysis (cont'd)

Action	Rationale
14 Ensure that the patient is comfortable during dialysis by attending to pressure area care and altering the patient's position as required. Assist the patient to sit in a chair for short periods as the condition allows.	The period of dialysis is lengthy and often exhausts the patient.
15 Send a daily specimen of peritoneal fluid for microscopy and culture.	To monitor for any infections, etc.

Nursing care plan

Problem	Cause	Suggested action
Peritonitis, indicated by fever, persistent abdominal pain and cramping, abdominal fullness, abdominal rigidity, slow dialysis drainage, cloudy and offensive-smelling drainage, swelling and tenderness around the catheter and increased white blood cell count.	Poor aseptic technique during catheter insertion or dialysis.	If peritonitis is suspected, notify the doctor immediately. Send a peritoneal fluid sample to the laboratory for fluid analysis, culture and sensitivity testing, Gram staining and cell count. Antibiotics may be prescribed by the doctor either locally or systemically in severe cases. Monitor vital signs; careful pain control is required.
Infection at the site of entry, indicated by redness, swelling, rigidity, tenderness and purulent drainage around the catheter.	Poor aseptic technique during catheter insertion or dialysis, or incomplete healing around the site of entry.	Notify a doctor. Obtain a specimen of the drainage fluid and send it to the laboratory. Antibiotics and pain control may be prescribed as above. Monitor vital signs.
Subcutaneous tunnel infection with cuffed catheter indicated by redness, rigidity and tenderness over subcutaneous tunnel.	Poor aseptic technique during catheter insertion or dialysis, or incomplete healing in subcutaneous tunnel.	Notify a doctor. Antibiotics may be prescribed as above. Monitor vital signs.
Perforation of the bladder or the bowel, indicated by signs and symptoms of peritonitis, bright yellow dialysis fluid drainage (if bladder is perforated) or faeces in drainage (if bowel is perforated).	Catheter inserted when the patient had a full bladder or bowel.	If perforation is suspected, stop dialysis and notify a doctor immediately. Monitor vital signs. Only minimal oral fluids should be given in case surgery is required.
Bleeding through the catheter.	Minor trauma to the abdomen or minor trauma to the subcutaneous tunnel (with a cuffed catheter) or perforation of a major abdominal blood vessel during surgery.	Bleeding usually stops spontaneously. If it does not, notify the doctor, who may order blood transfusions. One-litre hourly dialysis exchanges may be ordered until the drainage fluid is clear.
Dialysis fluid leaking around the catheter.	Excessive instillation of dialysis fluid. Incomplete healing around the cuff of the catheter. Catheter obstruction. Catheter dislodged or positioned improperly.	Instil less dialysis fluid at exchanges. Drain the patient's abdomen completely during outflow. Use small volumes of dialysis fluid in exchanges through a new catheter. Irrigate the catheter with sterile 0.9% sodium chloride solution. Inform a doctor, who will replace the catheter or revise its position surgically.
Kinking of the cuffed catheter.	Subcutaneous tunnel too short or scarring in the subcutaneous tunnel.	Inform a doctor, who will remove the catheter and implant a new one.

Lower back pain.	Pressure and weight of dialysis fluid in the abdomen (particularly so in CAPD patients).	Doctor may order analgesics. Exercises to strengthen the patient's muscles and improve posture may also be ordered.
Abdominal or rectal pain (with possible referred pain in shoulder).	Improperly positioned catheter tip causing irritation. Dialysis fluid accumulating under the diaphragm. Dialysis fluid not at 37°C. With 2 litres of 6.36% solution, severe shoulder pain can occur. If air enters the peritoneal cavity, pain may occur.	Catheter position to be revised surgically. Drain the abdomen completely during outflow. Ensure that the fluid is infused at the correct temperature. If hypertonic dialysis fluid is used, only one container should be used per cycle. Maintain a closed system.
Paralytic ileus indicated by sharp pain in abdomen, constipation, abdominal distension, nausea and vomiting, and diarrhoea.	Catheter manipulated excessively during insertion.	Notify the doctor immediately as signs and symptoms may indicate peritonitis. A nasogastric tube to suction the stomach may be ordered. Cholinergic medication, such as neostigmine, may be prescribed. Administer fluids and electrolytes as prescribed. If general condition allows, encourage patient to walk, unless advised otherwise by the doctor. Prepare the patient for surgery, as advised by the doctor. The condition may disappear spontaneously after 12 h.
Cramping.	Dialysis fluid warmer or cooler than 37°C. Too rapid infusion or drainage. Pressure from excess dialysis fluid in the abdomen. Chemical irritation. Air in the abdomen.	Adjust the temperature of the dialysis fluid to 37°C before infusion. Decrease the infusion or drainage rate to a regime the patient can tolerate. Infuse less dialysis fluid at exchanges to a total volume that the patient can tolerate. Use a dialysis fluid with a dextrose concentration lower than 7%. Clamp off the dialysis tubing before the dialysis fluid empties completely into the abdomen.
Excessive fluid loss.	Use of dialysis fluid with too great a dextrose concentration for the patient or inadequate sodium intake or inadequate fluid intake.	Monitor the patient's weight and blood pressure. Ensure that the patient is receiving dialysis fluid with the correct dextrose concentration. The doctor may prescribe a reduced dextrose concentration.
Fluid overload.	Use of dialysis fluid with an osmotic pressure that is too low for the patient or excessive sodium intake or excessive fluid intake.	Monitor the patient's weight and blood pressure. The doctor will order a reduced fluid and sodium intake. The doctor may also order increased use of dialysis fluid with a 4.25% dextrose concentration.
Metabolic disturbance usually affects plasma levels of glucose, potassium or sodium.	Continued use of inappropriate dialysate fluid.	Monitor relevant plasma levels pre- and postdialysis. If patient has pre-existing diabetes mellitus or insulin deficiency, insulin dosage should be titrated carefully.

Problem	Cause	Suggested action
Respiratory difficulties.	Pressure from the fluid in the peritoneal cavity and upward displacement of the diaphragm or 'splinting' of the diaphragm, resulting in shallow breathing.	Elevate the head of the bed. Encourage breathing exercises and coughing. Involve the physiotherapist to establish respiratory care.

GUIDELINES • Preparation of equipment for continuous venovenous haemodiafiltration (CVVHD) utilizing a CVVHD machine

Note: when using the CVVHD method of filtration, the patient access is gained by a single or double-lumen catheter. This will be inserted into a central vein, usually the internal jugular, sub-clavian or femoral vein. The catheter will then be flushed with a heparinized solution and capped off ready to commence CVVHD.

Equipment

1 Fluid-warming infusion device.
2 Volumetric pumps ×2.
3 CVVHD machine.
4 Artificial kidney/filter.
5 Set of dialysate tubing: 1 red, 1 blue.
6 Intravenous infusion sets ×2.
7 Y-connector.
8 Fluid-warming insert.
9 20-ml luer lock syringe.
10 10-ml luer lock syringe.
11 Plastic clamps ×5.
12 Gloves.
13 Chlorhexidine in 70% alcohol.
14 Low-linting gauze swabs.

Procedure

Action	Rationale
1 Discuss patient's condition with the multidisciplinary team and establish treatment plan.	To ensure all medical and nursing teams are aware of patient's biochemistry and haematological profiles and the plan for treatment.
2 Collect all equipment together as above.	To ensure that all the equipment is available before commencing the procedure.
3 Instil 2000 units of heparin into each litre of 0.9% sodium chloride.	To anticoagulate the tubing and the filter to provide prophylactic cover against clotting in the extracorporeal circuit.
4 Lace up the machine with the two sets of tubing: one red and one blue.	To form the CVVHD circuit.
5 Connect the spiked end of the red tubing to one of the heparinized litres of saline and apply a plastic clamp to the tubing.	To be ready to commence priming the filter tubing. To stop fluid infusion until the circuit is ready.
6 Attach the bell-shaped end of the blue-marked tubing to the nozzle on the machine situated just below the housing for bubble trap – this is the venous pressure manometer.	To ensure the venous pressure is accurately monitored.
7 Attach a 20-ml luer lock syringe to the open end of the blue tubing next to the bubble trap.	This will be used to draw air out or push air in to the bubble trap, thus maintaining the fluid at the correct level in the bubble trap.
8 Undo the clamp on the red tubing that is attached to the litre of heparinized saline.	To have everything ready to commence priming the tubing.
9 Turn on the blood pump to a speed of 75–100 ml/h.	To commence circulation of heparinized saline.

Action	Rationale
10 As the fluid circulates and enters the bubble trap, draw air gently out of the trap until fluid is at a level with the mark an inch below the top of the trap.	To ensure that there is enough fluid to allow trapping of bubbles in the circulating fluid.
11 Continue circulating fluid until there is only about 200 ml left in the litre bag. Clamp the tubing and stop the pump.	The circulation of the first litre will have primed the tubing and started to fill the filter and expand the fibres. The pump needs to be stopped before the end of the litre to ensure that no further air enters the circuit.
12 Attach the second heparinized litre to the red spike. Undo the clamp and start the pump at a speed of 75–100 ml/h.	To further prime the tubing and completely saturate the fibres in the filter.
13 As the second litre is running, gently rotate the filter.	To ensure good filling and flow throughout the filter.
14 When there is about 200 ml left in the litre bag, clamp the tubing and stop the pump. Turn off the machine.	The priming is now complete and stopping the pump before the bag is completed prevents air entering the circuit.
15 Disconnect the red spiked end from the litre bag and attach to the small blue patient end of the dialysate tubing.	To prepare the patient circuit.
16 Attach the dialysate fluid via the fluid warmer to the now free port on the filter.	To provide access for the warmed dialysate fluid into the filter to achieve movement of solutes.
17 Decide on anticoagulant regimen and if appropriate attach syringe containing anticoagulant to the free tubing on the red side and feed through the dedicated heparin pump.	To ensure delivery of anticoagulant as prophylaxis against the circuit or filter clotting and blocking.
18 The system is now ready to use.	

GUIDELINES • Commencement of CVVHD

Procedure

Action	Rationale
1 Explain and discuss the procedure with the patient and his/her family.	To ensure that the patient understands the procedure and gives his/her valid consent.
2 Ensure that all information concerning the patient's blood biochemistry, full blood count and clotting profile are available.	To have a baseline from which to work and to monitor any change in the patient.
3 Ensure that the patient's mean arterial pressure is above 60 mm Hg or that physician's guidelines have been provided.	During the first 2 h of CVVHD there is usually a large fluid drainage, which can result in a sudden drop in blood pressure.
4 Ensure that baseline recordings of weight, temperature, heart rate, blood pressure, respiratory rate, tissue oxygen saturation (SaO_2) and central venous pressure (CVP) have been recorded.	To have a baseline from which to work and to monitor any change in the patient.
5 Ensure that the patient is attached to a haemodynamic monitor.	CVVHD can cause cardiac instability, although this is rare (Oh 1995).
6 Ensure that a treatment programme has been agreed with the multidisciplinary team and review regularly	To ensure that the plan for cycling and the total fluid removal has been discussed and that it is altered according to patient status.
7 Prepare the appropriate fluid replacement.	There is a rapid fluid loss with CVVHD and patients often require replacement of this loss.

Guidelines • Commencement of CVVHD (cont'd)

Action	Rationale
8 Prepare a sterile field and apply gloves.	To reduce the risk of infection and provide protection for the nurse.
9 While keeping the patient catheter clamped, remove the bungs from both lumens and clean with chlorhexidine in 70% alcohol.	To reduce the risk of infection and to prevent haemorrhage.
10 Flush each lumen with heparinized saline.	To ensure that the patient's catheter is patent.
11 Apply plastic clamps to the patient ends of the red and blue tubing and separate from each other. Clean with chlorhexidine in 70% alcohol.	To prevent air entering the tubing and to reduce the risk of infection.
12 Connect red tubing to the red lumen and blue tubing to the blue lumen of the catheter.	To complete patient circuit.
13 Undo catheter clamps and plastic clamp on tubing.	To ensure free flow.
14 Ensure that there are no clamps left on and that all connections are secure.	To ensure that there is no obstruction to flow and no risk of fluid leakage.
15 Turn on machine and start blood pump at 75–100 ml/h.	To commence CVVHD at a gentle speed.
16 Observe patient, monitors and dialysis circuit carefully.	To ensure that any alteration in patient condition is noted immediately.
17 As blood circulates, ensure bubble trap fluid level stays constant.	To ensure trapping of bubbles.
18 If everything is stable, increase speed to appropriate level, probably between 100 and 150 ml/h.	To ensure good filtration.
19 Observe fluid drainage. Once the colour changes from clear to straw, empty the drainage bag.	To ensure correct fluid balancing.
20 Commence dialysate fluid infusion at appropriate rate, usually between 1 and 2 litres/h.	To provide the counter-current and achieve movement of solutes.
21 Continue monitoring patient – hourly heart rate, rhythm, BP, CVP, SaO_2 and respiratory rate or more frequently if required.	To ensure any change in patient condition is noted immediately and dealt with as appropriate.
22 Maintain accurate fluid balancing.	To ensure patient is protected from large positive or negative fluid shifts.
23 Send regular blood samples for biochemical analysis.	To adjust dialysate fluid and electrolyte replacement therapy as appropriate.
24 Send regular blood samples for clotting profile.	To provide appropriate anticoagulant therapy.
25 Ensure patient tubing and circuit are easily visible and free from obstruction.	To protect patient from sudden disconnection or obstruction to tubing.
26 Review patient's condition regularly with multidisciplinary team.	To ensure optimum patient monitoring and evaluation of care to enable appropriate treatment.
27 Ensure optimum recording in documentation of venous pressure, pump speeds and drainage.	To ensure information exchange between members of nursing team.

Personal Hygiene

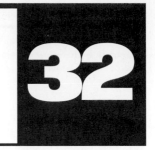

Definition

The science of hygiene can be described as 'a condition or practice, such as cleanliness, that is conducive to the preservation of health' (Weller & Wells 1995). The aspect of personal hygiene refers to 'individual measures taken to preserve one's own health' (Weller & Wells 1995), which pertains to the person taking responsibility to meet this fundamental need. The prevention of infection is also pertinent and will be referred to within the text (see Chap. 4, Barrier Nursing).

Reference material

'Cleanliness is not a luxury in a highly developed country, it is . . . a basic human right' (Young 1991). When an individual becomes ill, he or she may depend on others to perform this elementary intervention. If this occurs, it is important that the nurse is able to appropriately observe and assess the patient.

Hygiene is a personal entity and everyone will have their own individual requirements and standards of cleanliness. In this way, 'nurses must take care not to impose their own norms on patients and clients and should respect their autonomy in decisions concerning care' (Spiller 1992). When assessing personal considerations, the patient's religious and cultural beliefs should be taken into account. Various examples of this will be given throughout the text.

In Western culture, privacy is of the utmost importance and considered to be a basic human right. In some cultures, modesty is crucial, e.g. for Moslems, and can cause problems in the hospital setting (Neuberger 1987). Patients will feel a great deal of embarrassment having to depend on another person to help/assist them with this extremely private act and consideration should be given to their personal needs (Wagnild & Manning 1985; Spiller 1992). It is therefore surprising to find that such little reference is made to these elements in the literature. The nurse's role is 'the maintenance of an acceptable level of cleanliness' (Young 1991) which promotes 'comfort, safety and well-being' (Heath 1995) for the patient. Frequently, the time taken to attend to personal hygiene will provide ample opportunity for communication. Wilson (1986) states:

> . . . a bedbath facilitates listening and enables the nurse to pick up cues to a patient's anxieties and fears. It provides the time and opportunity for the nurse to offer support and encouragement when difficult situations have to be confronted, solutions sought and decisions made.

However, the emergence of the role of the Health Care Assistant (HCA) has meant that some practical tasks have been taken away from qualified nurses. The National Vocational Qualification (NVQ) means that HCAs are being trained to attend to patients' basic care needs (Carr-Hill *et al.* 1992) and to 'gain practical skills that complement those of the qualified nurse' (Workman 1996).

Controversy has arisen in light of these tasks being taken on because nurses sometimes view HCAs as depriving them of 'their real nursing roles' and see them as a threat to their profession (Workman 1996).

Nursing models, which provide a conceptual framework for practice, all make some reference to meeting the patient's hygiene needs. Roper *et al.* (1981) adapted Henderson's original concept of nursing (Henderson 1966) to develop a model reflecting the activities of daily living. This model is still generally used in Project 2000 nurse training.

Another example was given by Orem (1980) who focused on the ability of the patient to self-care and refers to the universal self-care requisites of the 'condition of the skin, nails and hair' and the 'usual patterns of hygiene'. The assessment process will show if there is a 'deficit' and then an appropriate nursing intervention can result.

The assessment should allow the nurse to carry out the appropriate intervention(s) and evaluate the effectiveness of care given.

Areas of care

Skin care

Maintaining the skin's integrity is essential to the prevention of infection and the promotion of health. The skin has several functions:

1 Maintenance of temperature
2 Protection
3 Excretion
4 Sensation.

It is made up of three layers: the epidermis, dermis and the deep subcutaneous layer.

The *epidermis* is the outer coating of the skin and contains no blood vessels or nerve endings. The cells on the surface are continually being rubbed off and replaced by new cells which have arisen from deeper layers. The epidermis has hairs, sweat glands and the ducts of sebaceous glands passing through it.

The *dermis* is the thicker layer which contains blood

vessels, nerve fibres, sweat and sebaceous glands and lymph vessels. It is made up of white fibrous tissue and yellow elastic fibres which give the skin its toughness and elasticity.

The *subcutaneous layer* contains the deep fat cells (areolar and adipose tissue) and provides the heat regulation factor for the body. It is also the support structure for the outer layers of the skin (Ross & Wilson 1998).

The skin will go through many changes in the course of development, e.g. temperature, texture, elasticity, and has a great ability to adapt to changes in the environment and stimuli. Its integrity, continuity and cleanliness are essential to maintain its physiological functions.

In elderly people the skin structure becomes thinner and the growth of epidermal and dermal cells slows down. This results in the skin becoming dryer and increasingly brittle, thus leading to an increased risk of tissue breakdown (see Chap. 47, Wound Management). The skin will also become more permeable to infection (Armstrong-Esther 1981), so extra care and vigilance should be taken when washing and drying elderly patients.

An initial assessment using observational skills is essential to ascertain the skin's general condition. Several factors may influence the appearance of the tissue.

1 Hydration state – dehydration will cause loss of elasticity and drying of the skin. Oedema will cause stretching and thinning of the skin.
2 The individual's age, health and mobility status (Gooch 1989), e.g. presence of pressure ulcers (see Chap. 47, Wound Management).
3 Treatment therapies, e.g. radiotherapy (skin may become moist and cracked), chemotherapy (some cytotoxic agents such as methotrexate can cause erythematous rashes, and continuous infusions of 5-fluorouracil (5-FU) can cause a condition called palmer-plantar erythrodysesthesia syndrome which presents with cracking and epidermal sloughing of the palms and soles (Lokich & Moore 1984). A low platelet count can lead to an increased risk of bruising and a decrease in the white blood cells can influence the rate of healing. Steroids may cause the skin to become papery and fragile. (See Chap. 33, Radioactive Source Therapy: Sealed Sources, and Chap. 47, Wound Management).
4 Any concurrent skin conditions, e.g. eczema, psoriasis.

Frailty and the presence of pressure ulcers, redness, abrasions, cuts, papery skin and open wounds should prompt the nurse to take extra care in the bathing procedure. Involving patients in their care plans ensures that correct and/or preferred lotions are used. For example, some people prefer not to apply soap to the facial area and others will need to use a particular soap which does not contain perfumes. Persistent use of some soaps can alter the pH of the skin, leading to drying and cracking (Gooch 1989). In addition, patients may like to use moisturizers and this should be respected and applied accordingly. Care should be taken with skin folds and crevices, paying particular attention to thorough drying of the areas and observing for any breaks in the skin.

Frequently, patients may have intravenous devices and wound drains inserted as part of their therapy and these should be handled with caution to prevent the hazards of introducing infection or of 'pulling' the tubes.

Each patient will require assessment of their individual needs (Heath 1995) and encouragement to promote rehabilitation as appropriate. If a full blanket bath is needed then the nurse must respect the patient's privacy and comfort. A refreshing change to the original version of the bed bath was researched by Lisa Wright, a ward sister at Sheffield Hospital. After obtaining a bursary to enable her to visit the USA she was able to observe the nurses performing a towel bath which consisted of using a large bath towel and a no-rinse skin-cleansing product. This alternative practice ensured the patient's privacy and comfort and was well evaluated by staff and patients (Wright 1990).

Patients who require minimal assistance may be able to have a bath or shower depending on the level of dependence, e.g. equipment they may be attached to and particular preferences. Attention should be given to religious and cultural needs, for example European and Asian people prefer to sit under running water as opposed to sitting in a bath (Sampson 1982). Other patients may need a full blanket bath.

Perineal/perianal care

Perineal care is probably the area most likely to produce embarrassment and humiliation (Heath 1995). It is, however, important to be meticulous with this area, especially for those people who may be more prone to infection, e.g. patients with indwelling urinary catheters (see Chap. 43, Urinary Catheterization), and people who suffer from incontinence.

Problems arising from treatment therapy, for example radiotherapy, fistulae, diarrhoea, constipation, urinary tract infections, require additional vigilance with cleanliness and patients should be encouraged at every opportunity to perform this themselves (see Chap. 33, Radioactive Source Therapy: Sealed Sources; Haisfield Wolfe 1998).

Ideally, perineal hygiene should be attended to after the general bath or, at the very least, the water and wipes should be changed and clean ones utilized (Gooch 1989; Gould 1994) due to the large colonies of bacteria that tend to live in or around this area (Gould 1994). It is generally acknowledged that soap and lotions administered improperly to the perineum/perianal area can cause irritation and infection (Heidrick et al. 1984; Ravnskov 1984; Charmorro 1990). Many nurses will use soap or a similar chemical derivative in order to promote and ensure thorough cleaning, but frequently lack of knowledge can lead to further problems and discomfort for the patients (Lindell & Olsson 1989). It was suggested that warm water alone be used to avoid irritating the mucous membranes which become sensitive during the ageing process. Care should be taken to maintain privacy and reduce embarrassment at all times, especially with regard to cultural influences.

Hair care

The way a person feels is often related to their appearance. Hair care can be complex – consideration should be given to the patient's personal preferences.

Washing of the hair can be difficult if a patient is bed-bound, but there are several ways to manage this. One example is by manoeuvring the patient to the top of the bed and hanging the head over the end (Wells & Trostle 1984). If hair washing is not possible, due to pain for example, then the use of an aerosol dry shampoo can be beneficial. Shampooing frequency depends on the patient's wellbeing and his/her hair condition.

Care of the beard and moustache is also important. Excess food can often become lodged here so regular grooming is essential for hygiene and comfort purposes. Beard trimmers can be used as appropriate.

Grooming the hair provides an ideal opportunity to observe for dandruff, psoriasis, flaky skin and head lice. Hair lice are extremely infectious so it is imperative to treat the hair with a medicated shampoo from the pharmacy as soon as possible. Careful washing of towels is necessary, and a separate towel should be used for each patient to avoid an outbreak of lice (Stichele et al. 1995).

A patient's cultural and religious beliefs should always be taken into consideration when attending to hair. Some religions do not allow hair washing or brushing, while others may require the hair to be covered by a turban. Similarly, in some countries facial hair is significant and should never be removed without the patient's/relatives' consent. Always establish any preferences before beginning care.

In the oncology setting chemotherapy is an established treatment and some cytotoxic drugs can cause alopecia (loss of hair). This is a particularly sensitive and traumatic event and skilled advice is required regarding adjustment to hair loss and the correct fitting of a wig (Tierney 1987). A shampoo with a neutral pH is recommended for patients who are at risk of alopecia. Prevention of alopecia is discussed further in Chap. 36, Scalp Cooling.

Regular brushing and combing can avoid tangling and matting of the hair.

Care of the nails and feet

The feet and nails require special care in order to avoid pain and infection occurring. Nails should be trimmed correctly. Specialist advice from a chiropodist can be useful. Chronic diseases such as diabetes and the long-term use of steroids can result in problems such as pressure ulcers, breakdown of the skin integrity and delays in the healing process. Special attention should be paid to cleaning the feet and in between the toes to avoid any fungal infection. Powders and creams are available that help with the treatment of infections and odour management.

Care of the ears and nose

Lack of attention to cleaning the ears and nose can lead to impairment of the senses. Usually these small organs require minimal care, but observation for a buildup of wax in the ears and deposits in the nose is essential to maintain patency and efficacy.

Cotton buds and tap water are useful for gently cleaning the areas. Special care should be taken to avoid pushing too hard in the aural cavity, with a risk of piercing the ear drum.

Patients undergoing enteral feeding and oxygen therapy should have regular nasal care to avoid excessive drying and excoriating of the delicate air passages. Gentle cleaning of the nasal mucosa with cotton buds and water is recommended and application of a thin coating of vaseline to prevent discomfort can be beneficial. Patients who have had piercing of the ears or nose will require cleansing of the holes to avoid the risk of infection. Body piercing is common practice in many countries now.

Eye care

Specific aspects of eye care, e.g. irrigation, are referred to in Chap. 17, Eye Care.

In general, the eye structure and delicate surface are protected by the tears that maintain the eye's moistness, but in a patient who is unconscious, drying of the eye may occur (Ross & Wilson 1998). Gentle cleansing with low-linting gauze and 0.9% sodium chloride will be sufficient to prevent infection and will keep the eyes moist. The eye is an important organ of communication and consideration should always be given to a patient's sight aids, e.g. glasses, contact lenses. Assistance may be required to help clean these aids and advice regarding the most appropriate method should be sought, preferably from the patient.

Some patients may have an artificial eye and care should be taken to ensure this remains clean. Advice regarding the ideal method of removal and insertion should be sought.

Mouth care

Most aspects of mouth care, e.g. cleaning and infection control, are referred to in Chap. 24, Mouth Care.

Cleaning of equipment

Within an establishment, the environment and the shared use of equipment will lead to a potential risk of infection, e.g. beds, lifting aids, commodes.

One study involving three wards in a general hospital showed the movement of three marked bowls, one in each ward. Regular observations were made regarding the drying and storage of these bowls and the results demonstrated clearly that drying and storage were haphazard and many bowls were contaminated (Greaves 1985). The same study also looked at the misuse of face cloths. They were shown to be a source of infection as they were used for several patients and not washed sufficiently in between use. Recommendations from the survey were that either patients should be supplied with their own bowls or the bowls in general use should be thoroughly cleaned and dried and stacked pyramid fashion (Greaves 1985; Gould 1994).

It is also important that patients are taught to realize the significance of personal hygiene and handwashing. A recent study illustrated that the lack of good personal hygiene and environmental cleanliness can lead to the outbreak of infection, especially within high-dependency units (Chadwick *et al.* 1996). This is particularly relevant when patients are independent and are using shared toilet and bathroom facilities. Vigorous cleaning with hot soapy water is recommended for shared facilities (see Chap. 4, Barrier Nursing).

If possible, each patient should have his or her own toiletries and towels which should be laundered regularly (Gould 1994).

Summary

The patient is an individual who will depend on others to assist them in times of ill health. 'Whenever possible, patients should be enabled to perform their own hygiene, so that they can continue their usual practice' (Gooch 1989). In this way, patients will be able to maintain their own comfort and privacy for something that is a 'basic human right' (Young 1991).

Care should be taken to observe the patient's cultural and religious beliefs and advice can be sought from the patient and relatives (Muftic 1997).

Attention should be paid to the cleaning of the equipment to avoid cross-infection. Personal hygiene is a simple procedure that can be performed for patients, but considerable thought should be given to individual preferences and patient comfort.

It is clearly evident from the lack of research that more work is required in this area to improve and raise standards of patient care.

References and further reading

Armstrong-Esther, C.A. (1981) Skin introduction. *Nursing*, Series 1, 1115.

Carr-Hill, R., Dixon, P. & Gibbs, I. (1992) *Skill Mix and the Effectiveness of Nursing Care*. York Publications, Centre for Health Economics, University of York.

Chadwick, P., Oppenheim, B., Fox, A., *et al.* (1996) Epidemiology of an outbreak due to glycopeptide resistant *Enterococcus faecum* on a leukaemia unit. *J Hosp Infect*, **34**, 171–82.

Charmorro, T. (1990) Cancer of the vulva and vagina. *Semin Oncol Nurs*, **6**(3), 198–205.

Edwards, M. (1997) The nurse's aide: past and future necessity. *J Adv Nurs*, **26**, 237–45.

Frederiksen, A.M. (1997) Education – mouth care and bedbath. *Sgeplejeskolen*, **97**(15), 26–7.

Gooch, J. (1989) Skin hygiene. *Prof Nurse*, October, 13–17.

Gould, D. (1994) Helping the patient with personal hygiene. *Nurs Stand*, **8**(34), 30–32.

Greaves, A. (1985) We'll just freshen you up, dear. *J Infect Control Nurs*, *Nurs Times* Suppl., 6 March, 3–8.

Haisfield Wolfe, M.E. (1998) Providing effective perineal–rectal skin care to patients with cancer. *Oncol Nurs Forum*, **25**(3), 472.

Haugen, V. (1997) Perineal skin care for patients with frequent diarrhoea or faecal incontinence. *Gastroenterol Nurs*, **20**(3), 87–90.

Heath, B.M.H. (ed.) (1995) *Potter and Perry's Foundation in Nursing Theory and Practice*, pp. 505–518. Mosby Wolfe, London.

Heidrick, F.E., Beurg, A.O. & Bergman, J. (1984) Clothing factors and vaginitis. *J Family Pract*, **19**(4), 491–4.

Henderson, V. (1966) *The Nature of Nursing*. Collier Macmillan, London.

Kershaw, B. & Salvage, J. (1992) *Models for Nursing* p. 27. John Wiley, London.

Lindell, M. & Olsson, H. (1989) Lack of care givers' knowledge causes unnecessary suffering in elderly patients. *J Adv Nurs*, **14**, 976–9.

Lokich, J.J. & Moore, C. (1984) Chemotherapy associated palmar plantar erythrodysesthesia syndrome. *Ann Intern Med*, **101**, 798–800.

Muftic, D. (1997) Maintaining cleanliness and protecting health as proclaimed by Koran texts and hadiths of Mohammed SAVS. *Med Arh*, **51**(1–2), 41–3.

Neuberger, J. (1987) *Caring for Dying People of Different Faiths*, 2nd edn., p. 26. Mosby, London.

Orem, D. (1980) *Nursing – Concepts of Practice*, 2nd edn. McGraw Hill, New York.

Pearson, A. & Vaughan, B. (1988) *Nursing Models for Practice*. Heinemann, Oxford.

Rasero, L., Errico, A., Puccetti, M. & Tellarino, G. (1996) The role of measures of personal hygiene in the prevention of infections in autologous bone marrow transplantation. Results of a randomised prospective study. *Riv Inferm*, **15**(3), 127–30.

Ravnskov, U. (1984) Soap is the major cause of dysuria. *Lancet*, **5**, 1027.

Roper, N. *et al.* (1981) *Learning to Use the Process of Nursing*. Churchill Livingstone, Edinburgh.

Ross, J. & Wilson, K. (1998) *Foundations of Anatomy and Physiology*. Churchill Livingstone, Edinburgh.

Sampson, C. (1982) *The Neglected Ethic; Religious and Cultural Factors in the Care of Patients* p. 36. McGraw-Hill, London.

Spiller, J. (1992) For whose sake – patient or nurse? *Prof Nurse*, April, 431–4.

Stichele, V. *et al.* (1995) Systemic review of clinical efficacy of topical treatments for headlice. *Br Med J*, **311**(7005), 604–608.

Tierney, A.J. (1987) Preventing chemotherapy induced alopecia in cancer patients: is scalp cooling worthwhile? *J Adv Nurs*, **12**, 303–310.

Wagnild, G. & Manning, R.W. (1985) Convey respect during bathing procedures. *J Gerontol Nurse*, **11**(12), 6.

Weller, B. & Wells, R. (1995) *Baillière's Nurses Dictionary*, 22nd edn. Baillière Tindall, London.

Wells, R. & Trostle, K. (1984) Creative hairwashing techniques for immobilized patients. *Nursing*, **14**(1), 47.

Wilson, M. (1986) Personal cleanliness. *Nursing*, **3**(2), 80–82.

Workman, B. (1996) An investigation into how the Health Care Assistants perceive their role as 'support workers' to the qualified staff. *J Adv Nurs*, **23**, 612–19.

Wright, L. (1990) Bathing by towel. *Nurs Times*, **86**(4), 36–9.

Young, L. (1991) The clean fight. *Nurs Stand*, **5**(35), 54–5.

GUIDELINES • Bed bathing a patient

Procedure

Action	*Rationale*
1 Assess the patient's needs.	To plan care.
2 Plan care with the patient, noting his or her personal preferences.	To encourage participation and independence. To ensure patient comfort during procedure.
3 Collect all equipment by bedside:	To avoid leaving the patient during procedure.
(a) Clean bedlinen	
(b) Fleecy drawsheet or bath towel	To cover patient during procedure.
(c) Laundry skip	
(d) Towel(s) and flannel(s)	It may be necessary to provide disposable flannel if the patient does not use a separate flannel for face and body. The patient may, however, not wish this.
(e) Soap and toiletries as preferred by patient	To meet patient's preference.
(f) Clean clothes	
(g) Washbasin – reserved for patient – and warm water	To reduce risk of cross-infection (Greaves 1985).
4 Clear area around bed; ensure that it is private and draught-free.	To ensure space to carry out procedure and patient comfort.
5 Offer patient a urinal, bedpan or commode.	To reduce possibility of disruption to procedure and prevent any discomfort.
6 Cover patient with drawsheet or bath towel. Loosen top covers at foot of bed and fold back bed clothes.	To ensure bed clothes remain dry and patient remains warm.
7 Ask patient if he or she uses soap on the face. Wash, rinse and dry face, neck and ears. Some patients may wish to do this themselves. Note: if additional care is required for the eyes and nose, carry out on completion of bedbath. (Refer to section on care of eyes and nose.)	Many patients prefer plain water on the face. To promote cleanliness. To maintain independence. To ensure patient comfort and cleanliness.
8 Remove top half of night clothes, and if an intravenous device is in situ or an extremity is injured remove night clothes on unaffected side first.	Leaving lower half of body clothed aids patient privacy and warmth. Removal of night clothes on unaffected side first is easier and more comfortable for the patient.
9 Wash, rinse and dry top half of body. Start with side furthest away from you. Care needs to be taken not to wet drains/dressings and IV devices. Apply toiletries as required by patient. Replace night clothes. Change the water during procedure if cold and/or scummy.	To promote patient wellbeing and cleanliness. To minimize risk of infection. To ensure patient comfort and provide sufficient clean water to rinse off soap which might otherwise have a drying effect on the skin (Gooch 1989).
10 Wash, rinse and dry legs and back. Start with side furthest away from you – cover area that is not being washed. Observe pressure areas. Replace clothes Change bottom sheet while patient is being turned, if patient is to remain in bed. Change water to wash genitalia. Patients may prefer to do this themselves. Use another flannel. Take care with any indwelling catheters (see Chap. 43, Urinary Catheterization).	To promote cleanliness. To preserve dignity. To prevent and treat pressure ulcers. To preserve dignity. To reduce unnecessary activity for the patient and nurse. To minimize the risk of infection. To preserve dignity.
11 Provide appropriate equipment and assist patient, if required, to brush teeth and/or rinse mouth.	To freshen mouth and minimize plaque buildup (see Chap. 24, Mouth Care).
12 Help patient to sit or lie in desired position.	To promote patient comfort. To reduce risk of pressure ulcers (see Chap. 47, Wound Management).

Guidelines • Bed bathing a patient (cont'd)

Action	*Rationale*
13 Comb patient's hair as desired.	To promote positive body image.
14 Remake bed.	To enhance patient comfort.
15 Remove equipment from bedside. Replace patient's possessions in their appropriate place. Place locker, bedside table and call bell within reach.	To clear working environment for patient and nurse. To promote patient independence.
16 Wash hands.	To reduce risk of cross-infection.

Prior to each part of the procedure, explain and obtain agreement from the patient. The procedure can allow time and opportunity for communication and interaction between the nurse and patient.

Radioactive Source Therapy: Sealed Sources

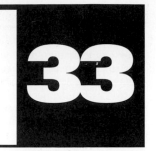

Sealed radioactive source therapy

Definition

Sealed radioactive sources are usually powders or solids enclosed in a casing which is inserted into the patient. Generally, there is little risk of spreading radioactive contamination from these sources, unless the casing is cracked during sterilization. Radioactive iridium-198 is a solid metal which may be made into alloy wires and used for direct insertion into tissues or cavities. Although not sealed in a metal casing, the methods applied to the use of sealed sources are also applied to this substance. The principles of radiation protection – distance, time and shielding, which minimize personal exposure to radiation – must be applied when working with sealed sources to ensure that all unnecessary exposure is avoided (Wootton 1993).

Indications

Permanent or temporary insertions of small, sealed sources are used to deliver very high doses of radiation into tumours or tumour-bearing tissue while giving rapidly diminishing doses to adjacent structures. This will limit the damage caused to normal tissue. A specific dose of radiation will be received by the cancer. This is delivered continuously over a period of minutes, hours or days.

Reference material

Measures of radiation

Radiation kills by causing ionization within living cells. The activity of radioisotopes was at one time measured in millicuries (mc), but the standard unit is now the becquerel (Bq) (Wootton 1993). A becquerel is the Système International (SI) unit of activity and is 1 disintegration per second.

$$k \text{ (kilo)} = 1 \times 10^3$$
$$M \text{ (mega)} = 1 \times 10^6, \text{ e.g. megabecquerel (MBq)}$$
$$G \text{ (giga)} = 1 \times 10^9$$

The half-life of a radioactive substance is the time taken for half of the original number of radioactive atoms to decay and lose their radioactivity. The sensitive target appears to be deoxyribonucleic acid (DNA) in the nucleus of the cell. The ionizing radiation thus passes through the cells and tissues, and the dose of radiation received is measured in terms of energy absorbed. The unit of absorbed dose is the gray:

$$100 \text{ centigray (cGy)} = 1 \text{ gray (Gy)}$$

For the purposes of radiation protection the dose to the whole body must be known. Whereas the absorbed dose is measured in gray, the dose to the whole body is measured in *sieverts*. For instance, for staff over 18 who are not pregnant, wearing a monitoring badge to monitor exposure to radiation, the annual dose limit is 20 millisieverts, but doses allowed to staff should be kept below 6 millisieverts (Health and Safety Executive 1999).

Ionizing radiation regulations

The use of ionizing radiation is governed by strict regulations. The principles of distance, shielding and time limitation must be observed to minimize radiation exposure in accordance with *The Ionising Radiation Regulations 1999* (Health and Safety Executive 1999). An important principle for staff to observe is to keep all radiation exposure 'as low as reasonably achievable' (the ALARA principle).

The safety of patients exposed to ionizing radiation is regulated by the *Ionising Radiation Regulations (Protection of Persons Undergoing Medical Examination or Treatment) (POPUMET)* (DHSS 1988). These regulations require that all staff who clinically (practitioners) or physically (operators) direct a medical exposure to ionizing radiation are adequately trained in the use of radiation protection. The knowledge they have acquired should be appropriate to their activities in accordance with the requirement of the above regulations.

Radioactive isotopes used as sealed sources

Most radioactive isotopes used as sealed sources for brachytherapy emit both beta (β) and gamma (γ) radiation. Brachytherapy is where there is a very short distance between the radiation source and the tumour. It is either intracavitary, where radioisotope sources are placed in pre-existing body cavities, such as the uterine cavity or vagina, or interstitial, where radioisotope sources are inserted directly into the tissues in tubes or needles (Blake *et al.* 1998).

The radiation useful in treating malignant disease includes X-rays, produced artificially by electron bombardment of a metal target, and gamma rays, a natural emission in the nuclear decay of radioisotopes. They are sometimes referred to as 'photon' radiation. Beta particles are also capable of ionization; these are distinguishable from electromagnetic radiation by their characteristic of carrying a negative electrical charge. Beta particles result when a neutron within the nucleus disintegrates to form a proton and an electron. The electron is ejected from the nucleus, producing beta radiation (Holmes 1988).

Caesium-137

Caesium-137 is a radioisotope that can be used in the form of interstitial implants or in intracavitary applicators. It has a half-life of 30 years and has largely replaced radium as a source of brachytherapy.

Oral implants

Caesium-137 can be used in a needle-like implant that is inserted directly into the tissue surrounding the tumour. This is a fairly common treatment for early lesions of the cheek, lip and anterior two-thirds of the tongue. If bone involvement is suspected, e.g. in the mandible, alternative external treatment will be given.

The sources (Fig. 33.1) are inserted in theatre under a general anaesthetic. They are inserted individually in a predetermined pattern so that the implant covers the whole growth, with a safety margin of at least 1 cm. Each needle is positioned by pushers so that its eye, through which silk is threaded, is just visible beneath the mucosal surface. Each silk is then stitched to the tongue with a single suture. When all the needles have been inserted, the silks are counted and gathered together. They are threaded through a piece of rubber to prevent friction and trauma to the mouth. The silks are strapped to the cheek to prevent any needle being swallowed should it work loose. Small beads are attached to the ends of the threads to facilitate counting the needles. X-rays are always taken to check the positions of the needles and to enable estimation of the dose distribution.

Gynaecological applicators

Caesium-137 can be used in applicators. The most common malignancies treated by the use of radioactive applicators are tumours of the female genital tract. Intracavitary applicators are used which deliver a high dose to the region of the cervix, the paracervical tissue, the upper part of the vagina and the uterine body.

Iridium-192

Iridium-192 is a radioisotope which can be used in the form of pins or wires in interstitial therapy. Its half-life is 74.2 days. Iridium-192 is an ideal choice because of the low energy of its gamma emission, which simplifies radiation protection, and because in the form of a platinum-iridium alloy it can be drawn into thin flexible wires. The wires consist of an active platinum-iridium alloy core encased in a sheath of platinum 10 μm thick, which screens out the beta radiation from the iridium-192.

Iridium-192 can now be made with a very high specific activity, that is, in a very radioactive form. High activity sources of iridium are used in high dose-rate remote afterloading systems, which reduce the amount of radiation to which clinical oncologists and other staff are exposed.

Iridium-192 implants are used under the following circumstances:

1 As a treatment for small primary lesions, especially tongue or breast lesions.
2 As a 'boost' dose after external radiotherapy for larger primary tumours or where nodes are also involved.
3 To treat recurrence.

Iridium-192 hair pin and single pin types of implants are usually used intraorally (Fig. 33.2). They are slotted into tissue using steel guides to obtain accurate alignment. Radiological examination is used to check the position of the guides before the iridium is inserted. The pins are held in place by sutures.

The staff of the physics department are normally responsible for calculating how long a radioactive implant is to stay in place. This is usually about 6 days, depending on the size of the tumour. Removal is carried out in theatre by the clinical oncologist.

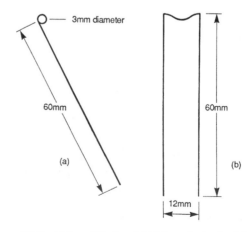

Figure 33.2 Iridium-192 pins. (a) Iridium single pin. (b) Iridium hair pin.

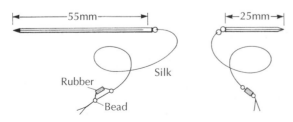

Figure 33.1 Caesium-137 needles.

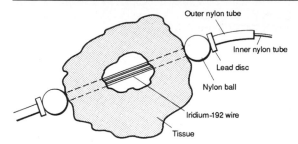

Figure 33.3 Iridium-192 wire in polythene cannula. Typical assembly in tissue.

Iridium-192 wires are usually used for breast lesions or lesions of the vulva or perineum (Fig. 33.3). Polythene or metal cannulae are inserted under a general anaesthetic. In the case of breast lesions, both ends of each tube protrude through the skin. Correct alignment is established often with the aid of a Perspex template which fits over the breast and holds the metal cannulae in the correct alignment. In the case of vulval or perineal insertions, only one end of the tube protrudes. For these, alignment of the sources may be achieved by using a Perspex template and vaginal obturator.

The iridium wire source is afterloaded, usually on the ward, and the wires are held in the cannulae with crimped lead washers. The tiny size of the high activity iridium-198 source in high dose rate machines may allow some interstitial brachytherapy to be given as a few treatments of several minutes each, in contrast to the single treatment of many hours' duration which is necessary with low-activity iridium wire.

The clinical oncologist is responsible for calculating how long a radioactive implant should stay in place. This is usually for 3–6 days, depending on the size of the tumour. Removal of the implant is usually carried out on the ward.

Iodine-125

Seeds of iodine-125 have replaced those of gold-198 which was used for many years after the withdrawl of radon seeds on the grounds of safety. The half-life of iodine-125 is 60 days. Some therapists believe that there is a radiobiological advantage to this long half-life in treating slowly growing tumours such as carcinoma of the prostate.

Seeds are inserted into the tissue that is to be irradiated under ultrasound or image intensifier control. The patient requires a general anaesthetic for the insertion.

The disadvantage of this method is that large numbers of seeds are required, which means that more precautions must be taken in order to achieve a regular geometrical arrangement to ensure satisfactory distribution of the dose.

Application of sources

Small sealed sources inserted into the body may take the form of:

1 *Intracavitary applicators*, i.e. sources that are placed in natural cavities and usually held in place by packing.
2 *Interstitial implants*, i.e. sources that are inserted directly into the tumour-bearing tissue.

(*Note*: sources held in plastic surface applicators or moulds are applied directly to superficial cancers.)

Intracavitary applicators and interstitial implants can be used in three forms:

1 The source is preloaded in the applicator before it is placed in the patient for a fixed length of time, e.g. caesium-137 needles and iridium-192 hair pins.
2 Permanent insertion in the case of iodine-125 seeds, which, once inserted, would be difficult to remove.
3 Afterloading systems – where the applicator is placed in position and the radioactive source is inserted when the position of the applicator and the condition of the patient are satisfactory. Insertion of the sealed source can be undertaken manually in the case of iridium-192 wires or by remote control as in the case of the low dose rate Selectron machine and the microSelectron high dose rate machine.

Afterloading techniques have the advantage of allowing the source carrier to be accurately positioned (Cooper 1993), and for the sources to be withdrawn to a radiation-proof safe during patient care, sparing staff from radiation exposure.

Historically, cervical cancer was one of the first tumours to be treated with radiotherapy, when radium was inserted into the endocervical canal and vagina to irradiate local disease. Techniques were developed in several centres, notably Paris, Stockholm and Manchester, which allowed consistency of treatment and, therefore, enabled the effectiveness and morbidity of treatment to be measured. A technique in common use today is the *Manchester* technique, in which an intrauterine tube and two vaginal ovoids are placed in the uterus and lateral vaginal fornices (Fig. 33.4a). The proportions of radioisotope (initially radium and latterly caesium) within the intrauterine tube and the vaginal ovoids were calculated to give a constant dose rate to a geometrical point A when using different lengths of intrauterine tube and different sizes of vaginal ovoids. This constancy of dose rate when using applicators of different sizes is an important aspect of the Manchester system.

Active sources

The radioisotope initially used for intracavitary brachytherapy was radium, which, because of its gaseous daughter-product radon, is hazardous. Radium has, therefore, been replaced by caesium, but the hazards of handling active sources have largely led to the development of afterloading techniques minimizing source handling and staff exposure.

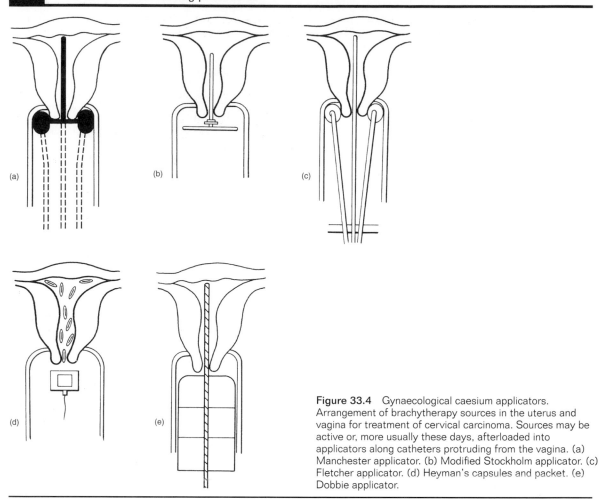

Figure 33.4 Gynaecological caesium applicators. Arrangement of brachytherapy sources in the uterus and vagina for treatment of cervical carcinoma. Sources may be active or, more usually these days, afterloaded into applicators along catheters protruding from the vagina. (a) Manchester applicator. (b) Modified Stockholm applicator. (c) Fletcher applicator. (d) Heyman's capsules and packet. (e) Dobbie applicator.

Afterloading brachytherapy

The basis of afterloading brachytherapy is that applicators are placed within the cervix and vaginal fornices, and that the radioisotope is only introduced into these when the applicators are correctly positioned, check radiographs have been taken and the patient is comfortable and in a protected environment. The sources may then be inserted either manually or by remote control. Manual methods are common and have the advantage of being cheap, but do not entirely protect staff as the sources have to be inserted by staff and cannot be removed for short periods while a patient's needs are attended to. Remote systems have the advantage of complete protection of staff, but have the disadvantage of high cost and the need for interlocking mechanisms. These ensure that the correct source has been inserted into the correct applicator for the programmed length of time.

Remote afterloading systems allow the dose rate of brachytherapy to be increased. Classically, the dose rate with the Manchester system was approximately 50 cGy/hour to point A. With modern engineering methods, caesium pellets can be produced which will allow a dose rate of between 150 and 200 cGy/hour to point A. Many systems now use sources that allow a higher than standard dose rate to be delivered. This has the advantage of reducing treatment time, but does have radiobiological consequences, necessitating a small reduction in dose (Brenner & Hall 1991).

If the concept of increasing dose rate is taken further, high dose rate brachytherapy, delivering doses at rates in excess of 1 Gy/minute to point A, offers the possibility of very short treatment times. This allows complete geometrical stability of the applicator during the treatment and makes a higher patient throughput possible. However, there is considerably less time for repair of radiation damage to normal tissues in a high dose rate treatment and, therefore, such treatments have to be fractionated over several days, in contrast to the continuous treatment given by a low dose rate brachytherapy implant. Early clinical results show no difference between treatment at low dose rate and at high dose rate (Fu & Phillips 1990), although mathematical modelling indicates that there is an increased risk of late tissue damage from fractionated high dose rate brachytherapy compared with a continuous low dose rate insertion.

Intracavitary applicators

Intracavitary applicators are inserted under a general anaesthetic, and the position of the applicator is checked by X-ray before the patient returns to the ward. A urinary catheter is also inserted in theatre to reduce the risk of the sources becoming dislodged by the patient when micturating.

Several different types of applicator are available and choice is usually determined by the site of the tumour, the anatomy of the patient and the preference of the treatment centre. The most commonly used types of applicator are described below (also see Fig. 33.4).

Manchester applicator

Manchester applicators are briefly described above. In their original form they were live sources enclosed in intra-uterine tubes of varying lengths and vaginal applicators (ovoids) of varying sizes. The applicators were inserted under general anaesthetic and held in place by a gauze pack. More recently, the applicators have been modified for either manual or remote afterloading at either low or high dose rate, but the principle of the three applicator system remains. Removal of the applicators or, if still used, the live sources is carried out on the ward and may require administration of Entonox for analgesia.

Stockholm applicator

This is used for carcinoma of the body of the uterus or cervix. Usually a uterine tube and two vaginal packets are inserted. Occasionally, if the vaginal vault is small, one packet is omitted or replaced by a vaginal tube. The radioactive material is held in place with a proflavine-soaked gauze pack. It is usually left in place for 22 hours. Tubes and packets have strings attached for removal and colour-coded beads indicate which should be removed first.

Modified Stockholm applicator

This is used for carcinoma of the body of the uterus and cervix. It consists of a uterine tube and a square box which connect together by a point and a hole. The vagina is then packed with gauze saturated with proflavine. They are usually left in place for 20 hours. The box should be removed first.

Fletcher applicator

This is used for carcinoma of the corpus or cervix, but the patient needs to have a fairly capacious vaginal vault. Hollow applicators, a uterine tube and two vaginal ovoids are inserted in theatre and loaded with the radioactive sources later, on the ward, by the radiotherapist. The apparatus is held in place with a proflavine pack. Long ends project through the vulva so that afterloading can be done.

These insertions are usually left in place for 60–72 hours. No strings are needed as the apparatus itself projects from the vulva.

Heyman's capsules

These are used for carcinoma of the corpus where there is enlargement of the uterus and an expanded uterine cavity. They consist of small metal capsules, each of which contains a small, radioactive source. As many capsules as possible are placed into the uterus. Usually two vaginal packets are used as well. They are held in place by a proflavine gauze pack and are left in for about 12–18 hours. Each capsule has a flexible wire attached, strapped to the thigh, for removal, and a numbered tag to indicate the order of removal.

Heyman's capsules are rarely used now as improvements in anaesthetics allow the great majority of patients with endometrial cancer to undergo hysterectomy.

Dobbie applicator

This is used to irradiate the whole vagina. A Perspex cylindrical applicator, with radioactive sources in the centre, is inserted into the vagina and sutured in place to the vulva. It may be used with low or high dose rate sources. Strings are attached to the applicator for removal.

Manual afterloading systems

Manual afterloading systems are largely being replaced by remote systems, but they are still used in a few centres and are widely used in developing countries.

The plastic applicator tubes follow the pattern of the Manchester system with an intrauterine tube and two vaginal ovoids. The plastic tubes are designed to be disposed of after a single use. Insertion of the tubes takes place under general anaesthetic, after which confirmatory X-rays are taken with dummy sources in place. As with the classical Manchester system there are varying lengths of intra-uterine tube and sizes of ovoids.

If the X-rays are satisfactory and the dosimetry has been calculated, the radioactive caesium sources are introduced on their carrying rods using long-handled forceps. Once in place inside the plastic tube a silver metal cap is screwed over the end of the plastic tube to hold the sources securely.

Manual afterloading does not permit, for reasons of staff safety, the use of high activity sources and treatment may last many hours or even several days. When treatment is complete the caps are removed from the tubes and the sources are withdrawn and placed immediately in a lead storage vessel. The plastic applicator tubes are then removed.

It is particularly important to observe for displacement or extrusion of the applicator tubes over the long treatment times. It is customary to mark the thigh level with the end of the applicator tubes and to compare this alignment at regular intervals as the treatment progresses. In addition, the silver metal caps should be monitored regularly for any loosening or displacement.

Remote afterloading

Definition

Remote-controlled afterloading machines transfer active sources from a radiation-proof safe to the patient only when it is safe to do so. The transfer may be pneumatic or cable-driven. The low dose rate Selectron machine operates pneumatically, whereas the high dose rate microSelectron is cable driven (Wilkinson *et al.* 1983).

Indications

Remote-controlled afterloading machines are gradually replacing conventional intracavitary caesium applicators as well as other manual and mechanical afterloading techniques.

The low dose rate Selectron is used predominantly for the treatment of gynaecological cancers. While the high dose rate microSelectron is also regularly used in the treatment of gynaecological cancers, in some cases it may also be useful in the treatment of bronchial or oesophageal or other intraluminal carcinomas (Bomford *et al.* 1993).

Reference material

The low dose rate Selectron

The Selectron unit comprises a lead-shielded safe containing caesium-137 sources in the form of small spherical pellets, a microprocessor, keyboard, display unit and printer (Fig. 33.5). Leading from the Selectron unit are either three or six flexible plastic transfer tubes corresponding to numbered treatment channels. Each tube ends in a fragile plastic catheter which is inserted into the appropriately numbered applicator and secured by a coupling device. The unit has a supply of compressed air and it is air pressure that the system uses to transfer the sources from the safe within the unit to the applicators along the connecting tubes. Operation of the unit is initiated from a remote-control unit situated outside the protected treatment area. Together, these components form the basis of the remote-controlled afterloading system (Blake *et al.* 1998).

The Selectron provides an accurate and safe method of radiotherapy treatment for cancers of the cervix, uterus and upper part of the vagina.

The advantages of the Selectron system are threefold:

1 Remote afterloading eliminates contact with radioactive material and protects personnel.
2 It allows highly accurate dosimetry.
3 The activity of the caesium-137 sources is such [up to 40 millicurie (mc)] that treatment times for patients are considerably shorter than with conventional techniques.

Patients have hollow, lightweight stainless steel applicators positioned in the operating theatre under a general anaesthetic. These are usually modified Manchester or Fletcher type applicators consisting of a uterine tube and

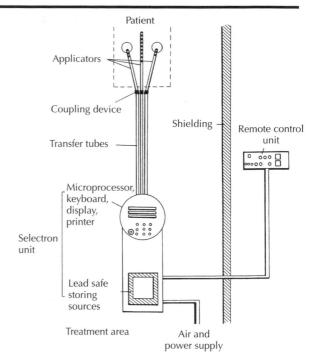

Figure 33.5 Selectron unit.

two vaginal ovoids held in place with a proflavine-soaked vaginal packing. However, several other applicators are available. Accurate positioning of the applicators is confirmed by taking X-rays with dummy sources in situ and the optimum source configuration is selected, taking account of individual anatomical variations.

The Selectron is programmed by the physicist. For each treatment channel being used, active source pellets are interspersed with inactive stainless steel spacer pellets to achieve the desired dose distribution. The treatment time required to reach the prescribed dose is also entered. With a six-channel Selectron unit it is possible to treat two patients with three applicators each simultaneously. The radiotherapist is responsible for connecting the transfer tubes to the applicators. The transfer tubes are led over a bed bracket which supports the weight of the tubes and prevents traction being applied to the applicators in the patient. If the wrong catheter is connected to the applicator, the system will fail to operate.

Operating the Selectron

Treatment is commenced by activation of the remote control unit when all staff have left the treatment area. While treatment is in progress it can be interrupted and restarted from the remote control unit by pressing the stop and start buttons. The display panel indicates which channels are being used for treatment and which are unused with red and green lights respectively. The time of the longest treatment is displayed in decimal hours and a telephone intercom system allows for communication with the patient without the need to interrupt treatment.

Interrupting the treatment by pressing the green stop button results in the sources being withdrawn into the Selectron unit and stops the timer. This allows nursing staff to enter the treatment area in safety and give routine or specific care to the patient. Pressing the red start button transfers the sources back into the applicators and restarts the timer. The red lights demonstrate that the channels are operating again satisfactorily.

The system has built-in safety features. In the event of a failure in the system, treatment stops automatically. An audible and visual alarm at the remote control unit alerts staff to a problem and indicates whether this is a fault related to the air or power supply, the pellets or the timer. There is an optional nurse station display unit with a similar alarm indicator which also emits an audible signal when treatment has been interrupted. This helps to prevent treatment being inadvertently left interrupted for long periods.

A record of any break in treatment is shown on the print-out from the unit itself, together with any programming or system fault. These appear as an error code and can be identified by reference to the Selectron users' manual.

At the end of the treatment time, all sources will be withdrawn automatically from the applicators back into the Selectron unit. When two patients are being treated simultaneously termination of the treatment of one patient may be some time before that of the other. This means the timer will register the longer treatment time, but the indicator lights for the channels used for the first patient will have changed from red to green.

Additional safety features include a door switch facility to retract sources immediately if the door to the treatment area is opened when treatment is in progress, and/or Geiger dose meters visible when entering the treatment area and approaching the patient, which indicate when there are radioactive sources either in the patient or in the connecting tubes.

The high dose rate (HDR) microSelectron

The operating principles of the HDR microSelectron are similar to those of the low dose rate Selectron. Low dose rate Selectron applicators are afterloaded with active sources interspersed with inactive spacers to produce the correct isodose pattern. HDR microSelectron machines, on the other hand, achieve the desired isodose pattern with a single iridium-192 source which moves within the applicators and stops at preset positions for predetermined dwell times.

The HDR microSelectron delivers radiation at approximately 100 times the rate of the LDR Selectron and treatment times are therefore much shorter. It has the added advantage of applicators with a smaller diameter which can be put in place under local anaesthetic in the outpatients' department (Blake 1989).

Once in position, HDR microSelectron intracavitary applicators are fixed to the treatment couch by means of an adjustable clamp (Patel et al. 1994). Movement of the applicators is therefore minimal and dosimetry calculations accurately represent actual treatment (Crook & Esche 1993). In addition, more constant and reproducible geometry of source positioning is possible (Perez et al. 1992).

Treatment protocols generally consist of two treatments but can involve as many as five. Following explanation and support for the patient, the procedure, which lasts between 20 and 30 minutes, is carried out under local anaesthetic (Blake 1989). For the first treatment a urinary catheter is passed and the balloon inflated with dilute contrast medium. Check radiographs are taken once the applicator tubes are in place to collect information which is fed into the Selectron planning computer and used to calculate the treatment time.

The HDR microSelectron follows the same principles for programming and treatment as the LDR Selectron. When treatment is complete the applicators and catheter are removed and the patient is free to go home. A study by Blake (1989) found that patients undergoing treatment with the HDR microSelectron for gynaecological cancer have found the experience acceptable, and responded positively to being treated as outpatients.

Adequate preparation of the patient is essential. Brown (1990) suggests that time spent preparing the patient increases tolerance of the implant procedure, and that badly prepared patients may be more anxious and less able to follow instructions. An assessment of patients' physical and emotional needs must be made prior to each treatment to identify if any aspect of the treatment is problematic.

The advantages of the HDR microSelectron are threefold:

1 The shorter treatment time reduces variations in the patient's position and allows more accurate dosimetry (Perez et al. 1992).
2 Treatment lasts only minutes, minimizing the need for immobilization and reducing discomfort and the risk of complications associated with bed-rest.
3 Treatment can be offered on an outpatient basis with a consequent reduction in cost (Blake 1989).

Complications of intracavitary radiotherapy for gynaecological cancers

Radiation-induced early complications of intracavitary treatment are generally mild. They include proctitis and cystitis. Severe reactions are rare, but may include severe or prolonged proctitis in patients with pre-existing bowel disease, and urgency and freqency of micturition, nocturia and dysuria. Late complications may include bowel and bladder strictures, ulceration and, occasionally, fistula formation (Sutton 1986). Perez et al. (1992), following a review of the research literature, found that major rectal complications were reported in 1.4% to 10% of cases, whereas minor or moderate complications were found in

0.7–24% of cases. Bladder complications were reported in 0.3–4% of cases.

Preparation of patient

Information about radiation therapy should be given to patients and carers when therapy is first discussed to allay fears and misconceptions about radiotherapy. Verbal information should be reinforced with written material to prepare the patient, reduce anxiety and promote coping. A contact name and telephone number are useful for patients who wish to obtain further information at a later date.

Information for gynaecological patients receiving radiotherapy can be divided into three categories: disease and treatment, short- and long-term side-effects and sexuality.

It should be explained that patients will require an indwelling urinary catheter and that they will be connected to the Selectron unit with flexible plastic tubes. Movement in bed will be restricted. Patients should be prepared for the noises made by the Selectron system, especially when sources are being transferred in and out of the applicators. Some patients find the prospect of treatment alarming and may prefer to receive regular sedation for the duration of the treatment. It is reassuring for patients to know that they will be monitored closely by nursing staff using a closed-circuit television system. A personal telephone line and a nurse call system must also be provided to enable patients to communicate with staff.

Vaginal care following intracavitary treatment

Because the vaginal canal is included in the radiation field, vaginal stenosis, fibrosis, loss of elasticity and lubrication, and a decrease in sensation may develop after treatment if prophylactic measures are not taken (Jenkins 1986).

To help prevent changes due to radiation, women who are sexually active should continue to have regular intercourse after any discomfort caused by an acute radiation reaction has resolved. Alternatively, a dilator can be used to keep the vagina open and stretched. Water-soluble lubricants may alleviate the dry mucosa, and hormone therapy, if appropriate, may be given orally or vaginally to increase natural lubrication (Blake et al. 1998).

Women should begin using a dilator 2 weeks after treatment has finished. Initially, the dilator should be inserted into the vagina daily for 5–10 minutes (removing and reinserting three or four times). A water-soluble lubricant should be used to ensure ease of insertion (Dolan 1987; Martin & Braly 1991). Following advice from a doctor or nurse specialist, frequency of dilatation can be reduced to between three times and once per week. However, dilatation should continue for life if the patient wishes to maintain vaginal patency (Dolan 1987). Dilatation should maintain vaginal patency and allow follow-up vaginal examination and smears to be performed without undue discomfort. It should also help comfortable resumption of intercourse.

Some clinical oncologists additionally recommend douching during radiotherapy and following brachytherapy, continuing for up to 8 weeks, to avoid infections and the formation of adhesions. Douching should not be carried out, however, if there is a risk of haemorrhage from a persistent tumour (Blake et al. 1998).

Patients are encouraged to douche once a day using a disposable douche and tap water. Douching should continue until symptoms have resolved and advice has been given by a doctor or nurse specialist.

Follow-up care

Remote-controlled afterloading brachytherapy is a safe and effective treatment for cervical cancer, and has the added advantage of eliminating radiation exposure to staff, visitors and other patients. However, side-effects can occur (Rogers et al. 1999), including complications to the bladder (Wang et al. 1997; Fujikawa et al. 1999), rectum (Clark et al. 1997; Wang et al. 1997; Uno et al. 1998), vagina (Bergmark et al. 1999) and signs and symptoms associated with menopause in premenopausal women (Feldman 1989).

In a study by Cull et al. (1993), women with cervical cancer reported the concerns they had, including the fear of recurrent disease. These women felt that they required more information about cancer, its treatment and how they could help themselves to cope with their illness. The authors suggest that the emotional status of women with cervical cancer could be improved by giving more attention to their psychological concerns. This is supported by a study to evaluate patient disclosure of psychosocial problems, where a 51% disclosure rate was found. These authors suggest that disclosure can be increased by adding one or two questions about mood and interpersonal problems into more general conversation (Robinson & Roter 1999), and emphasize the need for nurses to assess their patients carefully.

It has been suggested that the majority of patients will return to the same precancer psychological and behaviour status, except in the area related to sexual function which continues to be associated with significant morbidity (Anderson 1996). Cancer treatment can cause persistent changes to the vagina which results in considerable distress by compromising sexual activity (Bergmark et al. 1999); patients need to be reassured that many women regain their capacity for sexual activity and enjoyment. Bruner et al.'s (1993) study found that 43% of women reported sexual activity post-treatment, compared with 31% pretreatment, whilst 22% of the women reported a decrease in sexual frequency and 37% reported a decrease in sexual satisfaction. Sexual counselling may improve outcome. Counselling should focus on self-esteem, body image and sexuality (Feldman 1989). Although vaginal dilation is widely recommended to maintain vaginal health and good sexual functioning, it appears that compliance is poor. However, this can be improved when the patient is given assistance in overcoming her fears and taught how to use the dilator (Robinson et al. 1999).

Male partners of women with cancer reported difficulty in knowing how to behave and how to communicate with their partners (Lalos *et al.* 1995). Almost all male partners were given the news of the diagnosis exclusively by their ill partner, which provoked feelings of anger and bitterness (Lalos 1997). Coping improved if the men were integrated in the patient's care from the time the diagnosis of cancer was made (Lalos *et al.* 1995).

Discharge of the patient

Patients are usually discharged on the day of completion of brachytherapy. They must void urine normally following removal of the urinary catheter. Patients are sometimes unsteady on their feet after prolonged bed rest and may require assistance. They should be informed that normal bowel actions may not return for a day or so; advice on managing diarrhoea or constipation should be given. Light spotting or discharge from the vagina is normal. If patients experience pain or any more marked bleeding, hospital staff should be contacted immediately. Symptoms of urinary tract infection such as dysuria and/or elevated temperature should also be reported.

References and further reading

Anderson, B.L. (1994) Yes, there are sexual problems: now, what can we do about them? *Gynecol Oncol*, **52**(1), 10–13.

Anderson, B.L. (1996) Stress and quality of life following cervical cancer. *J Natl Cancer Inst Monger*, **21**, 65–70.

Baker, J. (1979) Implants and applications. In: Scan-technology in nursing – radiotherapy (ed. R. Tiffany). *Nurs Times*, **148**, Suppl., part 10, 37–40.

Bergmark, K. *et al.* (1999) Vaginal changes and sexuality in women with a history of cervical cancer. *N Engl J Med*, **340**(18), 1383–9.

Blake, P.R. (1989) Intracavitary therapy and the use of the micro-Selectron-HDR at the Royal Marsden Hospital, London. *Activity. The Selectron Users' Newsl*, **2**, 4–7.

Blake, P.R. (1991) Radiotherapy and chemotherapy in the treatment of gynaecologic cancer. In: *Textbook of Gynaecology* (ed. R. Varma). Edward Arnold, London.

Blake, P.R. *et al.* (1998) *Gynaecological Oncology*. Oxford University Press, Oxford.

Bomford, C.K. *et al.* (1993) *Textbook of Radiotherapy*. Churchill Livingstone, Edinburgh.

Brenner, D.J. & Hall, E.J. (1991) Fractionated high dose rate versus low dose rate regimens for intracavitary brachytherapy of the cervix. *Br J Radiol*, **64**, 133–41.

Brown, D. (1990) The role of the nurse in brachytherapy. *Activity*, **4**(3), 53–5.

Bruner, D.W. *et al.* (1993) Vaginal stenosis and sexual function following intracavitary radiation for the treatment of cervical and endometrial carcinoma. *Int J Radiat Oncol Biol Phys*, **27**(4), 825–83.

Clark, B.G. *et al.* (1997) The prediction of late rectal complications in patients treated with high dose rate brachytherapy for carcinoma of the cervix. *Int J Radiat Oncol Biol Phys*, **38**(5), 989–93.

Cooper, J.S. (1993) Carcinomas of the oral cavity and oropharynx. In: *Moss' Radiation Oncology. Rationale, Techniques, Results* (eds D. Cox & J.D. Cox), 7th edn. Mosby, St Louis.

Crook, J. & Esche, B.A. (1993) The uterine cervix. In: *Moss' Radi-*

ation Oncology. Rationale, Techniques, Results (eds D. Cox & J.D. Cox), 7th edn., pp. 617–82. Mosby, St Louis.

Cull, A. *et al.* (1993) Early stage cervical cancer: psychosocial and sexual outcomes of treatment. *Br J Cancer*, **68**(6), 1216–20.

Dean, E.M. *et al.* (1988) Gynaecological treatments using the Selectron remote afterloading system. *Br J Radiol*, **61**(731), 1053–7.

DHSS (1988) *Ionising Radiations Regulations (Protection of Persons Undergoing Medical Examination or Treatment)*. Stationery Office, London.

Dolan, M.E. (1987) Sexuality in gynaecological patients undergoing radiation therapy treatments. In: *Radiation Therapy of Gynaecological Cancers* (eds D. Nori & B.S. Helias), pp. 399–407. Alan Liss, New York.

Dudjak, L. (1988) Radiation therapy nursing care record: a tool for documentation. *Oncol Nurs Forum*, **15**(6), 763–77.

Dunne-Daly, C.F. (1994) Education and nursing care of brachytherapy patients. *Cancer Nurs*, **17**(5), 434–45.

Eardley, A. (1992) Standards of care for the patient having radiotherapy: can they be achieved? *J Cancer Care*, **1**, 151–5.

Feldman, J.E. (1989) Ovarian failure and cancer treatment: incidence and intervention for premenopausal women. *Oncol Nurs Forum*, **16**(5), 651–7.

Flay, L.D. & Matthews, J.H. (1995) The effects of radiotherapy and surgery on the sexual function of women treated for cervical cancer. *Int J Radiat Oncol Biol Phys*, **31**(2), 399–404.

Frith, B. (1991) Giving information to radiotherapy patients. *Nurs Stand*, **5**(34), 33–5.

Fu, K. & Phillips, T. (1990) High dose rate versus low dose rate intracavitary brachytherapy for carcinoma of the cervix. *Int J Radiat Oncol Biol Phys*, **19**, 791–6.

Fujikawa, K. *et al.* (1999) Spontaneous rupture of the urinary bladder is a rare complication of radiotherapy for cervical cancer: report of six cases. *Gynecol Oncol*, **73**(3), 439–42.

Gibbs, J. (1991) Radiation hazards. *Nurs Times*, **87**(27), 46–7.

Hassey, K.M. (1987) Principles of radiation safety and protection. *Semin Oncol Nurs*, **3**(1), 23–9.

Health and Safety Executive (1999) *The Ionising Radiation Regulations 1999*. Stationery Office, London.

Hodt, H.J. *et al.* (1952) A gun for interstitial implantation of radioactive gold grains. *Br J Radiol*, **25**, 419–21.

Holmes, S. (1988) *Radiotherapy. The Lisa Sainsbury Foundation Series*. Austen Cornish, London.

Horwich, A. (1995) *Oncology: A Multidisciplinary Textbook*. Chapman & Hall Medical, London.

Hussey, K. (1985) Demystifying the care of patients with radioactive implants. *Am J Nurs*, **85**, 789–92.

Jenkins, B. (1986) Sexual healing after pelvic irradiation. *Am J Nurs*, **86**(8), 920–22.

Jenkins, B. (1988) Patients' reports of sexual changes after treatment for gynaecological cancer. *Oncol Nurs Forum*, **15**(3), 349–54.

Klevenhagen, S.C. (1986) The role of the physicist in radiotherapy. In: *Radiotherapy in Clinical Practice* (ed. H.E. Hope-Stone), pp. 411–32. Butterworths, London.

Lalos, A. (1997) The impact of diagnosis on cervical and endometrial cancer patients and their spouses. *Eur J Gynaecol Oncol*, **18**(6), 513–19.

Lalos, A. *et al.* (1995) Experience of the male partner in cervical and endometrial cancer – a prospective interview study. *J Psychosom Obstet Gynaecol*, **16**(3), 153–65.

Lamb, M.A. (1990) Psychosexual issues: the women with gynaecological cancer. *Semin Oncol Nurs*, **6**(3), 237–43.

Martin, L.F. & Braly, P.S. (1991) Gynaecological cancers. In: *Cancer Nursing* (eds S.B. Baird *et al.*), pp. 502–535. W.B. Saunders, Philadelphia.

Martin, A. & Harbinson, S. (1979) *An Introduction to Radiation Protection*, 2nd edn. Chapman & Hall, London.

Nucletron Engineering (1981) *Selectron Users' Manual*. Nucletron Engineering, Chester.

Paine, C.H. (1972) Modern afterloading methods for interstitial radiotherapy. *Clin Radiol*, **23**, 263–72.

Patel, F.D. *et al.* (1994) Low dose vs high dose rate brachytherapy in the treatment of carcinoma of the uterine cervix: a clinical trial. *Int J Radiat Oncol Biol Phys*, **28**, 335–41.

Perez, C.A. *et al.* (1992) Clinical applications of brachytherapy. In: *Principles and Practice of Radiation Oncology* (eds C.A. Perez & L.W. Brady). J.B. Lippincott, Philadelphia.

Pierquin, B. *et al.* (1978) The Paris system in interstitial radiation therapy. *Acta Radiolog Oncol, Radiat, Phys Biol*, **17**(1), 33–48.

Robinson, J.W. & Roter, D.L. (1999) Psychosocial problem disclosure by primary care patients. *Soc Sci Med*, **48**(10), 1353–62.

Robinson, J.W., Faris, P.D. & Scott, C.B. (1999) Psychoeducational groups increase vaginal dilation for younger women and reduce fears for women of all ages with gynecological carcinoma treated with radiotherapy. *Int J Radiat Oncol Biol Phys*, **44**(3), 497–506.

Rogers, C.L., Freel, J.H. & Speiser, B.L. (1999) Pulse low dose rate brachytherapy for uterine cervix carcinoma. *Int J Radiat Oncol Bio Phys*, **43**(1), 95–100.

Royal College of Nursing (1991) *Standards of Care for Cancer Nursing*. RCN Cancer Nursing Society, London.

Royal Marsden Hospital (1994) *Local Rules for the Protection of Ward and Theatre Staff Against Ionising Radiation Arising from Patients Administered with Radioactive Material*. Royal Marsden Hospital, London.

Rushton, M. (1991) Nursing patients with gynaecological malignancies. In: *Oncology for Nurses and Health Care Professionals* (eds R. Tiffany & D. Borley), 2nd edn., pp. 340–65, Harper & Row, Beaconsfield.

Shell, J. & Carter, J. (1987) The gynaecological implant patient. *Semin Oncol Nurs*, **3**(1), 54–66.

Shepherd, J.H. & Monaghan, J.M. (1990) *Clinical Gynaecological Oncology*, 2nd edn. Blackwell Scientific Publications, Oxford.

Souhami, R. & Tobias, J. (1995) *Cancer and its Management*. Blackwell Science, Oxford.

Sutton, M.L. (1986) Gynaecological radiotherapy. In: *Radiotherapy in Clinical Practice* (ed. H.F. Hope-Stone), pp. 203–237. Butterworths, London.

Thranov, I. & Klee, M. (1994) Sexuality among gynecologic cancer patients: a cross-sectional study. *Gynecol Oncol*, **52**(1), 14–19.

Tiffany, R. (1979) *Cancer Nursing – Radiotherapy*. Faber & Faber, London.

Uno, T. *et al.* (1998) High dose rate brachytherapy for carcinoma of the cervix: risk factors for late rectal complications. *Int J Radiat Oncol Biol Phys*, **40**(3), 615–21.

Wang, C.J. *et al.* (1997) High-dose-rate intracavitary brachytherapy (HDR-IC) in treatment of cervical carcinoma: five year results and implication of increased low-grade rectal complication on initiation of an HDR-IC fractionation scheme. *Int J Radiat Oncol Biol Phys*, **38**(2), 391–8.

Welby-Allen, M. (1982) Selectron treatment in gynaecology. *Nurs Times*, **78**(46), 1948–50.

West, M. (1993) The principles of dose limitation and the various means of dose reduction to the patient, including protection of the gonads. In: *Radiation Protection of Patients* (ed. R. Wootton), pp. 58–65. Cambridge University Press, London.

Whale, Z. (1991) A threat to femininity? Minimising side-effects in pelvic irradiation. *Prof Nurse*, **6**(6), 309–311.

Wilkinson, J.M. *et al.* (1983) The use of Selectron afterloading equipment to simulate and extend the Manchester system for intracavitary therapy of the cervix uteri. *Br J Radiother*, **56**, 409–414.

Wootton, R. (1993) *Radiation Protection of Patients*. Cambridge University Press, London.

GUIDELINES • Care of patients with insertions of sealed radioactive sources

Action	Rationale
1 When transferring patients from theatre to ward, the nurse and porter should remain at the head and foot of the bed and at least 120 cm from the centre of the bed in in the event of any delay in the transfer. If the source is intra-oral, the nurse should stand at the foot of the bed.	To minimize the risk of exposure to radiation.
2 A yellow radiation hazard board should accompany the the patient back from theatre. This must remain at the bottom of the bed or outside the cubicle until the source is removed.	To warn everybody that the patient has a radioactive source.
3 Nursing staff must calculate the time allowed with the patient in any 24-h period. This time should be written on the yellow hazard notice on the bed or cubicle door.	To minimize exposure to radiation.
4 A Geiger counter should be available on the ward.	To monitor radioactivity if a dislodged source is suspected, e.g. in the bed linen.
5 One nurse should be delegated responsibility for the nursing care of the patient. The time spent with the patient should be shared between all of the staff on duty. and time spent in nursing procedures must be kept to a minimum.	To minimize the risk of overexposure to radiation.

6 Every nurse must wear a radiation badge above the level of the lead shield.

To record the extent of exposure to radiation.

7 All bed linen and waste materials removed from the patient area should be monitored before being removed from the ward.

To prevent loss of an accidentally dislodged source.

8 If a source becomes dislodged, use the long-handled forceps to put the source into a lead pot. Care should be taken not to damage the source. It must never be handled directly with the fingers.

To minimize the dose of radiation received.

9 Visitors must remain at least 120 cm away from the patient. The visit should not last longer than the time shown on the warning notice. No children or pregnant women are allowed to visit.

To minimize the risk of overexposure to radiation.

10 When the patient needs to visit another department, for example to X-ray, the following must be ensured:
  (a) That the receiving department is aware of the hazard of exposure to radioactivity.

In order that medical care can continue to be provided while the patient is receiving radioactive sealed source therapy. To allow the appointment to be made when the department is quiet, thus ensuring waiting time is kept to a minimum and to minimize exposure to others.

  (b) One porter and a nurse should accompany the patient in a wheelchair; two porters and a nurse should accompany the patient on a trolley. In the event of any delays, the nurse and porters should remain at the head and foot of the bed and at least 120 cm from the centre of the bed; if the source is intra-oral, the nurse should stand at the foot of the bed.

To minimize the risk of exposure of staff to radiation.

  (c) A radiation warning hazard sign should accompany the patient.

To warn all staff that the patient has a radioactive source in situ.

  (d) Unless the patient is likely to be in the department a long time the nurse and porter should stay with the patient.

To ensure time distance, shielding and segregation restrictions are maintained.

  (e) If the source becomes dislodged during transfer, the porter must ring the switchboard who will send out an emergency call to the physics department. The nurse must ensure the area around the patient is kept clear of other patients, staff and visitors. A member of staff from the ward should take a lead pot, forceps and a monitor to the nurse who will place the source in the lead pot and monitor the area to ensure it is free of radioactivity.

To minimize the risk of exposure to radiation.

To contain the radioactive source and minimize risk of exposure.

  (f) The Radiation Protection Adviser and supervisor should be informed of incident.

To evaluate the incident, and to prevent it recurring.

11 *In the event of a cardiac arrest*, an Ambu bag or similar device must be used, and the physics department must be informed immediately.

To minimize exposure.

12 *In the event of a fire*, the Fire policy must be followed. Following evacuation, the appropriate distance between the radioactive patient and other staff should be maintained; help should be sought from the physics department.

To minimize exposure.

13 *In the event of a patient's death*
  Remove sources:
  (a) The radiation sources should be removed by the radiotherapist. Inform the physics department.

Remove radioactivity to allow last offices to be undertaken as normal.

  Non-removable sources:
  (a) When a source cannot be removed, e.g. iodine-125 seeds, inform the physics department immediately.

In order for the physics department staff to begin making the necessary arrangements for removal of the body to the mortuary. To contain seeds if they become dislodged.

Guidelines • Care of patients with insertions of sealed radioactive sources (cont'd)

Action	Rationale
(b) The body should be placed in a cadaver bag.	
(c) Transfer of the body should be arranged by the physics department.	The physics staff will supervise the transfer of the body.
14 *In the event of bleeding*, in order to stem bleeding in the vicinity of the implant, apply pressure using at least four thick dressing pads. The padding should only be compressed for 15 min by any single person.	To minimize exposure.
15 Only staff who have received training and have been authorized may enter a controlled area. A list of suitably trained staff should be kept by the domestic and catering managers and by the ward's local Radiation Protection Supervisor. A domestic or catering supervisor should undertake tasks if the ward-based employee is not trained.	To keep all radiation exposure as low as can be reasonably achievable.
Domestic and catering staff should not remove items such as cleaning equipment and crockery until it has been monitored by a nurse.	To prevent sources being removed from the room.

GUIDELINES • Care of patients with intra-oral sources

Preparation of patient

Dental assessment of the patient is usually carried out before oral brachytherapy so that caries, mouth infections and dental extractions may be dealt with in case of the oral blood supply being impaired by the treatment. The patient is usually admitted 24 hours before the implant, during which time the nature of the procedure and the implications of having a radioactive source should be explained to the patient. The patient should be nursed in a single room away from other patients to reduce the amount of radiation exposure to other people.

Action	Rationale
1 Encourage frequent mouth care. The patient should void the solution into a bowl and not into a handbasin.	To reduce the risk of infection. To prevent the loss of a dislodged source.
2 Provide a soft, puréed or liquid diet.	To reduce the risk of the patient biting into the source or tongue. Eating is often difficult when implants are present.
3 Avoid spicy and/or hot foods. Discourage the patient from smoking and/or drinking alcohol.	To prevent exacerbation of local reaction or soreness.
4 Encourage ingestion of carbonated drinks.	To alleviate dryness.
5 Provide crushed ice for the patient to suck and/or soluble aspirin as a mouthwash.	To minimize oral pain and discomfort.
6 Give steroids as prescribed.	To prevent and/or minimize swelling.
7 Provide writing equipment for the patient.	To reduce the need for oral communication. This is liable to increase soreness and alter the distribution of the sources.
8 Provide paper tissues and a bowl for saliva.	The patient may have difficulty in swallowing due to soreness and oedema.
9 The sources should be checked at regular intervals, e.g. at the beginning of a span of duty.	To make sure that the sources have not become dislodged.
10 The patient must be confined to the room.	To minimize the risk of radiation exposure to other people on the ward.

Discharge of the patient

The patient is usually discharged the day after the removal of the implant. The patient should be warned about the painful local reaction that may be experienced due to rapid cell breakdown induced by the radiation. In order to minimize the risk of infection or soreness, the patient should be taught how to care for the treated area, e.g. oral toilet 4-hourly when awake and after meals.

GUIDELINES · Care of patients with gynaecological sources

Preparation of patient

The patient is usually admitted 12–48 hours before the procedure so that any pre-anaesthetic investigations may be performed. An enema or suppositories are usually given to reduce the chance of the patient having a bowel action while the sources are in place, which could dislodge the sources. Some patients, however, have diarrhoea on admission due to previous radiotherapy and will need regular medication, such as codeine phosphate, both before and during the application of the sources. A full explanation should be given to the patient along with information about the implications of having a radioactive source inside her and informed consent obtained. The patient should be bathed before any premedication is administered.

Action	*Rationale*
1 The patient must remain in bed in a recumbent or semirecumbent position while the applicators or implants are in place.	To prevent the applicators becoming dislodged or changing their position in relation to the internal organs.
2 Rolling from side to side is permitted and should be encouraged if the patient is at risk of developing a pressure sore.	To promote comfort and to relieve prolonged pressure on any one area.
3 On return from theatre, the sanitary towel should be checked for discharge. Disposable pants may be worn. Check that the catheter is correctly positioned to allow drainage.	To secure the position of the sanitary towel. To ensure that urine is draining freely.
4 Observe for any blood or other discharge from the vagina. Check the temperature and pulse 2-hourly.	To monitor haemorrhage, shock and other postoperative complications.
5 Administer prescribed analgesics, antiemetics and antidiarrhoeal agents.	For the patient's comfort.
6 Encourage fluid intake as soon as the patient is allowed to drink. If the source is to be in for longer than 24 h: (a) Encourage a fluid intake of 50–100% a day over and above the patient's normal intake. (b) A low-residue diet may be taken.	To ensure adequate hydration. To reduce the risk of urinary tract infection. To prevent the stimulation of a bowel action.

GUIDELINES • Removal of gynaecological caesium

The removal of applicators is usually performed by suitably qualified and competent nursing staff.

Equipment

1 Sterile gynaecological pack containing large receiver, green towel, paper towel, long dissecting forceps, sanitary towel, cotton wool balls.
2 Equipment for the administration of Entonox.
3 Solutions of choice for swabbing, e.g. 0.9% sodium chloride.

4 Gloves.
5 Sterile scissors or stitch cutter.
6 Clean draw sheet.
7 Geiger counter.

Procedure

Action	Rationale
1 Explain and discuss the procedure with the patient.	To ensure that the patient understands the procedure and gives her valid consent.
2 Check the date and time for removal on the form that was received from the physics department when sources were inserted.	The accurate timing of the removal is essential for the administration of the correct therapeutic dose of radiation.
3 Check that any pre-removal drugs (e.g. sedatives, analgesics) have been administered.	
4 Check, with another nurse, the exact time of removal and the number of applicators.	To reduce the risk of error.
5 Ensure that: (a) The lead shield is suitably positioned beside the patient. (b) The lead pot is also suitably positioned with the lid removed.	To shield the nurse from exposure to radiation. So that sources can be placed in the pot immediately after removal.
6 Begin the administration of Entonox at least 2 min before commencing the procedure.	To allow time for the effects of the gas to be felt. (For further information on Entonox administration, see Chap. 14.)
7 Prepare a trolley, put on gloves and open the pack before going to the bedside.	This is a clinically clean, not an aseptic procedure. To reduce the time spent in close proximity to the source.
8 Working from behind the lead shield, assist the patient into the dorsal position with knees apart. Remove the sanitary towel.	To obtain access to the sources.
9 Remove any sutures, if present. Remove the vaginal packing.	
10 Remove the caesium sources in reverse order of insertion. Contact the clinical oncologist immediately if difficulty is encountered in removing a source. Place the removed sources in a lead pot immediately and cover with the lid.	To prevent damage to the vagina. To contain radioactivity.
11 Remove the lead pot to a designated area, e.g. an isotope sluice or safe. Ensure that the lid of the pot or the sluice door is locked.	To remove the radioactive source from the ward area. To prevent unauthorized access to the source.
12 Monitor the patient's level of radioactivity.	To ensure that no sources remain inside the patient.
13 Remove the urinary catheter.	

14 Swab the vulva and perineal area with a solution such as 0.9% sodium chloride. Ensure that the patient has a a clean sanitary towel in position and is made comfortable.

To promote patient hygiene and comfort.

15 Monitor the bed linen, paper bags, vaginal packing and other waste material. (Two nurses should monitor the the patient independently.)

To ensure that no source has been lost or remains inside the patient.

16 The patient should remain in bed until the physics department staff are satisfied that all sources are accounted for.

To ensure that all sources have been accounted for before the patient moves around.

17 Remove the radiation warning notice.

Nursing care plan

Problem	Cause	Suggested action
Patient has a bowel action.		Inform the radiotherapist.
Patient removes caesium source herself.	Confusion, e.g. postanaesthetic.	Using long-handled forceps place the source in the lead container or safe. Inform the radiotherapist and the physics department.
Pyrexia.	Pelvic cellulitis or abscess. Reaction to the proflavine pack. Urinary infection. Physiological reaction to the breakdown of the tumour. Chest infection. Peritonitis due to perforation of the uterus.	If the patient's temperature remains over 37.5°C for two consecutive readings, inform the radiotherapist. The caesium may have to be removed if the pyrexia persists.

GUIDELINES • Care of patients undergoing Selectron treatment

Action	Rationale
1 Nurse the patient on a pressure-relieving mattress or with a foam wedge under her buttocks.	To promote comfort and to relieve backache since rolling is not permitted.
2 Ensure the plastic transfer tubes are supported securely in the bed bracket, leaving slight slack.	To enable the patient to change position slightly without putting traction on the applicators.
3 Limit the frequency and duration of interruption to treatment. Visitors are discouraged unless the patient is markedly distressed.	To prevent unnecessary prolongation of treatment time.
4 Unless otherwise indicated by the patient's physical or psychological mental condition, check 2-hourly: (a) Temperature, pulse and vaginal loss. (b) Contents of catheter drainage bag. (c) Assist patient to adjust her position.	 To monitor for haemorrhage, shock or other postoperative complications. To ensure urine is draining freely. To promote comfort and relieve prolonged pressure on any one area.

Guidelines • Care of patients undergoing Selectron treatment (cont'd)

Action	Rationale
5 Administer prescribed analgesics, antiemetics, antidiarrhoeal and sedative agents as appropriate and evaluate effect.	To promote the patient's comfort and wellbeing.
6 Encourage fluid intake as soon as the patient is able to drink.	To ensure adequate hydration and reduce the risk of urinary tract infection.
7 If the patient wishes to eat, a light, low-residue diet may be taken.	To prevent stimulation of a bowel action.

GUIDELINES • Removal of Selectron applicators

If two patients are being treated simultaneously, removal of the applicators may be delayed until both patients have finished treatment, depending on the individual treatment times.

Equipment

As for removal of other gynaecological applicators, see Guidelines • Removal of gynaecological caesium, above, (items 1–7) plus:

8 Rubber caps for the applicators.

Procedure

Action	Rationale
1 Check treatment has been terminated by: (a) Ensuring the appropriate channel lights are green. If the other patient's treatment is continuing, interrupt treatment. (b) Ensure time display on the Selectron unit reads zero for the appropriate channels. (c) Ensure the print-out indicates treatment has stopped for those channels.	The applicators should be removed only on completion of treatment.
2 Record the finish time on the patient's dosimetry sheet.	This is kept as a record in the patient's notes.
3 Check that the closed-circuit television camera is not focused on the patient.	To ensure privacy.
4 Explain and discuss the procedure with the patient.	To ensure that the patient understands the procedure and gives her valid consent.
5 Ensure any pre-removal drugs have been administered.	To allow analgesic or sedative to be effective.
6 Assist the patient into a comfortable position with her knees apart.	To allow access to the applicators.
7 Uncouple the plastic transfer tubes by rotating the black coupling anticlockwise in the direction of the arrow and very carefully store the tubes on the plastic supporting mantle attached to the Selectron unit.	To prevent the plastic catheter becoming damaged or kinked.
8 Place rubber caps on the ends of the applicators.	To ensure no fluid or debris is allowed to enter the applicator tubes.
9 Commence administration of Entonox (see Chap. 14) at least 2 min before removal of the applicators.	To allow the effect of the gas to be felt.

10 Prepare the equipment and put on gloves.	The procedure is clinically clean and not aseptic.
11 Remove the vulval dressing pads, any sutures and vaginal packing.	These must be removed before the applicators can be eased out.
12 Dismantle the applicators by loosening the screws holding them together.	To promote ease of removal.
Remove the uterine tube first, ensuring it is taken out complete with its small white flange, followed by the ovoids.	To prevent the flange being left in the patient's vagina.
13 Remove the catheter, swab the vulval area and ensure the patient has a clean sanitary pad and a fresh sheet.	To promote cleanliness and patient comfort.
14 The patient can then be assisted into a comfortable position and is permitted up to have a bath.	The patient is reassured that the procedure has been completed, that she is no longer radioactive and can resume normal activities.

Applicators are retained carefully for cleaning in accordance with local policies. Remaining treatment can then be given to the second patient.

Nursing care plan

See also 'Nursing care plan' for conventional gynaecological sources, above.

Problem	Cause	Suggested action
Patient removes the applicators herself.	Confusion, e.g. postanaesthetic.	Interrupt treatment. Deposit applicators and attached tubing in the lead pot. Inform radiotherapist and physicist. Restart treatment if two patients are being treated.
Applicator is partially dislodged.	Patient may have moved too much or too vigorously.	Interrupt treatment. Inform physicist and radiotherapist. The applicator may have to be removed as above.
Alarm sounding at nurse station.	Treatment has been interrupted and inadvertently left off.	Check patient is unattended and recommence treatment.
Sources are not transferred to the applicators.	Incorrect coupling or loose connection.	Check print-out to identify which channel is at fault. Tighten appropriate coupling device.
Alarm activated at remote control unit.	Failure in the system.	Check the error code on the print-out with the Selectron users' manual. Rectify as indicated in the manual or seek technical assistance from the physics department.
Pellets stuck in the applicator or transfer tubing.	A damaged or kinked catheter.	Inform the physics department. Withdraw the plastic catheter using long-handled forceps and deposit in the protected container until technical assistance can be provided. Reassure the patient.

GUIDELINES • Caring for the patient with radioactive seeds (e.g. iodine-125)

Preparation of the patient

The patient is usually admitted at least 1 day before treatment: patients should be nursed ideally in a single room but, more importantly, in a bed away from the main thoroughfare.

Seeds are implanted permanently into the tissue and therefore the patient must agree to stay in hospital until the physics staff state that the radioactivity is at a legally permissible level for discharge.

Breast and lymph node implantation

Action

1 Leave the dressing securely in position unless special instructions are given by the radiotherapist.

2 If dressing becomes dislodged, leave it at the bedside, preferably in a lead pot, and inform the physics staff.

3 If there is any possibility that the sources have become detached, inform physics department staff immediately and do not remove anything from the room.

Rationale

Sources may became detached, dressings will prevent them from becoming lost.

If sources have became detached and are in the dressings physics staff will take the necessary action.

It is important that the source is not lost as this could result in contamination of the environment. The patient's total dose will be altered and the medical staff will need to be informed.

Lung implantation

Action

1 Check all sputum and drainage from the chest with the Geiger counter. If no radioactivity is found the sputum and drainage may be disposed of in the usual way unless special instructions are given by the physics department or radiotherapy staff.

2 If radioactivity is detected, inform physics department staff immediately. Save the sputum or drainage for them to deal with.

Rationale

To check for radioactivity in case any sources are coughed up or expelled in the drainage.

To prevent contamination of the hospital environment.

Bladder and prostate implantation

Action

1 Check all urine with the Geiger counter. If no radioactivity is found the urine may be disposed of in the usual way.

2 If radioactivity is detected, inform physics staff immediately and save urine for them to deal with.

3 Leave suspect urine in a safe place at the bedside, e.g. under the bed.

Rationale

To check for radioactivity in case any sources are expelled in the urine.

To prevent contamination of the hospital environment.

To prevent accidental disposal.

GUIDELINES • Care of patients with breast sources

Preparation of patient

The patient will usually be admitted for local excision of the breast tumour and an axillary clearance. Drains are inserted and these are usually removed before the iridium wire sources are loaded 24–48 hours after surgery. When the sources are loaded, the patient should be nursed in a single room.

Action	*Rationale*
1 Leave any dressing undisturbed for the duration of treatment.	To minimize the time spent in proximity to the patient.
2 Confine the patient to the room.	To minimize the risk of radiation to other people on the ward.
3 Administer prescribed analgesia as required throughout the treatment period and before removal.	For the patient's comfort.

Discharge of the patient

The patient should normally be discharged the day after the removal of the implant. The patient should be warned about the painful local reaction which she may experience due to the rapid cell breakdown induced by the radiation. In order to minimize the risk of infection or soreness, the patient should be taught how to care for the treated area.

Radioactive Source Therapy and Diagnostic Procedures: Unsealed Sources

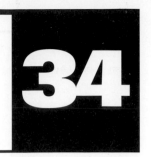

Definition

Unsealed radioactive sources are radionuclides supplied in liquid or colloidal form, systemically administered orally or by injection. They are used in the diagnosis and treatment of disease (Horwich 1995; Souhami & Tobias 1995).

Definition of terms

1 *Radiopharmaceutical:* this is a specially formulated sterile compound consisting of two main components: the pharmaceutical, which primarily determines the distribution profile of the compound around the body's organs, and a radionuclide, which enables the distribution of the radiopharmaceutical to be determined (Saha 1992).
2 *Radionuclide:* a nuclide of an element which possesses an unstable configuration of protons and neutrons within the nucleus, and which achieves stability by undergoing a radioactive decay process (Wootton 1993).
3 *Imaging:* images that show the distribution of radiopharmaceutical within the patient and are obtained using a gamma camera.
4 *Scanning:* the measurement of the distribution of radioactivity over an area of the body by counting the rate at which the radiation is received (count rate) by a detector moved over the body surface (Perkins 1995).

Reference material

Unsealed sources are used to concentrate a radioisotope in a particular part of the body. Unsealed sources carry an additional risk of environmental contamination and therefore protective measures are required to prevent contamination of staff, visitors and other patients and the environment (Wootton 1993). For example, unsealed sources may concentrate in body fluids, which will then contain radioactivity, and when eliminated reduce the amount of radioactivity in the patient (Martin & Harbinson 1997), but increase the risk of contact by staff.

Radionuclides used for diagnosis of disease in the nuclear medicine department and four unsealed sources will be discussed here.

Radionuclides used in nuclear medicine department

Unsealed radionuclides are used in nuclear medicine for the diagnosis of disease, using both imaging and non-imaging investigations. The important properties that make them useful for diagnostic purposes include:

1 The physical half-life
2 Decay characteristics
3 Ease of incorporation into radiopharmaceuticals
4 Availability of radionuclide.

A desirable radionuclide should have a half-life just long enough to allow for the preparation, administration and concentration in the region of interest (Langmead 1983), but short enough for radiation to effectively disappear after the test (Wootton 1993). Imaging studies commonly performed in a nuclear medicine department include:

1 Assessment of structures and/or function of organs
2 Sites of infection
3 Presence of tumours.

Common non-imaging studies include investigations into red cell mass and plasma volume, gastrointestinal tract and renal function.

Radiopharmaceuticals are legally categorized as prescription only medicines (POMS), and, in addition to the standard legislation surrounding the administration of such drugs, are subject to regulations related to their radioactive content. In the UK, a statutory committee called the Administration of Radioactive Substances Advisory Committee (ARSAC) has been established to give ionizing radiation advice to health ministers and to manage the certification process for administration of radiopharmaceuticals. This committee issues certificates which authorize individuals to administer radiopharmaceuticals to patients. It also lists the maximum permissible doses of radioactivity that may be administered to adult patients, and appropriately reduced adult doses for children, according to a child's body weight or body surface area.

A radionuclide investigation involves administration of the appropriate radiopharmaceutical, and dynamic imaging or waiting a predetermined time to allow the dose to be taken up in the organ to be investigated. The patient is then positioned and is required to keep still during the scan, because movement causes artefacts which reduce diagnostic accuracy. The scan may last 15–60 minutes (Perkins 1995). Most procedures require little physical patient preparation (Table 34.1).

Table 34.1   Radionuclide investigations

Investigation/ target organ	Radiopharmaceutical	Procedures and clinical interventions
Imaging studies		
Bone scan Used to assess bone function in which malignancy, fractures and diseases such as osteomalacia and Paget's disease can be diagnosed (Smith 1989)	Technetium ($^{99}Tc^m$) phosphate and phosphonate compounds, including methylene diphosphonate (MDP) and hydroxymethylene diphosphonate (HDP)	Patient to drink 5–6 cups of fluid and to empty bladder regularly while waiting for scan. This is to enhance soft tissue clearance and minimize absorbed radiation dose to the bladder
Renogram (dynamic renal study) Used to assess renal function by monitoring clearance of radiopharmaceutical via kidneys (Testa & Prescott 1996)	$^{99}Tc^m$ MAG$_3$ Benzoylmercaptoacetyltriglycine $^{99}Tc^m$ DTPA Diethylenetriamine pentaacetic acid	Patients to drink approximately 600 ml of fluid and to empty bladder prior to scan, which takes approximately 1 h. Intravenous diuretic is to be administered to patient during the scan to diagnose obstructive uropathy (Smith & Gemmell 1989)
Static renal study Used to assess size, shape and position and function of kidneys (Testa & Prescott 1996). Used to diagnose renal scarring in children (Smith 1989)	$^{99}Tc^m$ DMSA Dimercaptosuccinic acid	No preparation
Perfusion lung scan Used to assess blood supply to alveolar tree. Provides complementary information to a ventilation lung scan. Used to diagnose pulmonary embolism (Buxton-Thomas 1989)	$^{99}Tc^m$ MAA Macroaggregated albumin	Radiopharmaceutical is administered as a slow bolus intravenous injection. Patient to lie supine and breathe deeply while injection is being given. This is to enhance even distribution of MAA through lung capillary bed. If patient is pregnant, administered activity needs to be reduced
Ventilation lung scan Provides complementary information to a perfusion lung scan in diagnosis of pulmonary embolism. Used to assess patency of airways	$^{99}Tc^m$ Technegas, $^{99}Tc^m$ aerosol, $^{81}Kr^m$ gas, ^{133}Xe gas (Owunwanne *et al.* 1995)	A chest X-ray performed within the preceding 24 h is required prior to scan, to assist with interpretation of lung scan. Patient breathes the radiopharmaceutical through a special mouthpiece while scan is being performed
Cardiac studies – perfusion imaging Used to assess areas of viable perfused myocardium. This is a two-part test with myocardial perfusion monitored under stress and subsequently at rest. Stress may be exercise- or pharmocologically induced (Nowotnik 1995). Often performed on patients with suspected coronary artery disease, recent myocardial infarction or those who have undergone coronary artery bypass surgery	$^{99}Tc^m$ MIBI, $^{99}Tc^m$ tetrafosmin, ^{201}Tl thallous chloride	Patient needs to be closely monitored during postexercise period because there is the potential risk of triggering a myocardial infarction after stress This test is usually performed within a cardiology unit with appropriately trained personnel and equipment. Patient is usually kept in the department until he/she has been assessed by a clinician
Cardiac – left ventricular ejection fraction (LVEF)/multiple gated acquisition scan (MUGA) Used to evaluate cardiac function in patients prior to and during courses of chemotherapy containing cardiotoxic agents (Owunwanne *et al.* 1995)	$^{99}Tc^m$ labelled red blood cells	Current weight of patient is required for calculation of dose of a red bood cell labelling agent, which ensures red blood cells are labelled with required radioactivity (Feiglin 1989). This volume calculated is then administered intravenously 20–30 min prior to scan. Patient lies supine for 30–40 min

Table 34.1 (continued)

Investigation/ target organ	Radiopharmaceutical	Procedures and clinical interventions
Thyroid scan May be used to confirm presence of one or more nodules within the thyroid, or to identify functional characteristics of nodule(s) (Sandler et al.1989)	^{99}Tc^m pertechnetate, ^{123}I/^{124}I/^{131}I sodium iodide	Patient to avoid foods containing iodine (including seasalt, seafood, cod liver oil, mineral tablets and kelp) for 3 days prior to test. These foods decrease uptake of radiopharmaceutical within thyroid bed. Patient to discontinue thyroid medication for between 3 days and 3 weeks prior to test, depending on specific instructions given by clinician
Parathyroid scan Used to diagnose parathyroid adenomas in patients with primary hyperparathyroidism (Sandler et al. 1989)	^{99}Tc^m pertechnetate, ^{201}Tl thallous chloride	This is a two-part test, comprising a thyroid scan which is completed prior to the parathyroid scan. Patient should follow instructions for thyroid test
Tumour imaging Used to differentiate between metabolically active tumours and space-occupying lesions, or for the diagnosis of unknown primary tumours	^{18}F FDG 2-Fluorodeoxyglucose	Patient to fast for up to 6 h prior to injection, with only water to be taken. Patients may experience a metallic taste in the mouth immediately after administration. Waiting interval between injection and scan is 30 min, scan being performed with a positron emission tomography (PET) camera
Used to diagnose infection and diagnose and stage cancers such as lung, Hodgkin's disease and lymphomas (McDonagh 1991)	^{67}Ga gallium citrate	Due to excretion of gallium citrate via the GI tract, patients should be given laxatives or encouraged to increase fibre and fluid intake to avoid constipation. There are specific radiation protection precautions to be adhered to
Used to diagnose and assess patients with neuroectodermal tumours including phaeochromocytomas, neuroblastomas, carcinoid, medullary thyroid cancers and paragangliomas (Perkins 1989)	^{123}I *m*IBG meta-iodobenzylguanidine	Patient must take Lugol's iodine or potassium iodide for 2 days prior to and for 3 days after day of administration. *m*IBG may cause hypertension and is administered slowly over a 10-min period. On occasions, patients may experience some discomfort at the injection site. This may be relieved by applying heat to area of discomfort and reducing rate of infusion. For paediatric patients, it is preferable to administer *m*IBG via a central venous catheter. Some drugs that act on the adrenergic system may interfere with uptake of *m*IBG
Often used in conjunction with *m*IBG scans to assist with localization of the primary tumour and sites of metastatic spread in the aforementioned diseases (Bomanji et al. 1995)	^{111}In Octreotide DTPA-D-Phe-1-Octreotide	Patients with insulinoma should have their blood sugar levels monitored pre- and post-injection. An i.v. solution containing glucose should be available in case of hypoglycaemia. Patients should be encouraged to increase fluid and fibre intake to avoid constipation
Sites of infection To identify areas of lymphocyte localization in patients with either acute or chronic inflammatory infections	Labelled white blood cells	50 ml of blood is taken from patient using a 19G needle. Labelled blood is reinjected after approximately 2 h, following which patient is scanned later the same day and/or the following day
Gastrointestinal tract To determine cause of gastrointestinal bleeding, including Meckel's diverticulum (McDonagh 1991)	^{99}Tc^m pertechnetate	Patients (usually children) need to fast for 4–6 h before scan; adults to fast from midnight

Table 34.1   (continued)

Investigation/ target organ	Radiopharmaceutical	Procedures and clinical interventions
Non-imaging studies *Kidney function* Measurement of glomerular filtration rate (GFR) provides an assessment of renal function. Often used in renal transplant patients, in compromised renal function due to long-term use of certain drugs (e.g. cyclosporin) or in patients with systemic lupus erythematosus (Smith 1989). Oncology patients often have renal function assessed prior to chemotherapy, particularly if regimen includes platinum-based cytotoxic agents	^{51}Cr EDTA Ethylenediaminetetra-acetic acid	Renal clearance of administered radiopharmaceutical is assessed from residual radioactivity in blood samples taken from patient at either 3 h, or at 2, 3 and 4 h post-injection. Patient's height and weight are required to enable GFR to be calculated accurately. It is important that no hydration or blood products are commenced during the test as this may alter results of test
Red cell mass/plasma volume Often used to diagnose *polycythaemia vera* in patients with cardiovascular disease (Merrick 1984)	^{125}I human serum albumin, ^{51}Cr or ^{99}Tc^{m} labelled red blood cells	10 ml of blood is taken from patient using a 19G needle. Labelled blood is reinjected after approximately 1.5 h, following which patient's blood is taken at 10-min intervals for 40 min. Patient's height and weight are recorded
Schilling test To investigate patients with suspected pernicious anaemia	^{57}Co /^{58}Co vitamin B$_{12}$ Cyanocobalamin	Patient to fast 8–10 h before administration of radioactive B$_{12}$ capsule (McDonagh 1991). ^{57}Co/^{58}Co labelled vitamin B$_{12}$ is administered orally, prior to intramuscular injection of unlabelled vitamin B$_{12}$. Patient should empty bladder prior to test, and a 24-h urine sample should be collected following administration of oral vitamin B$_{12}$

Four unsealed sources will be discussed:

1 Rhenium-186 hydroxyethylidene diphosphonate (Re186 HEDP), used in the treatment of bone metastases.
2 Iodine-131 (I-131), used in the treatment of thyroid disorders.
3 Meta-iodobenzylguanidine (mIBG), used in the treatment and diagnosis of neuroblastoma and other neuroectodermal tumours.
4 Monoclonal antibodies labelled with iodine-131, used in the treatment of recurrent cystic glioblastoma.

Rhenium-186 hydroxyethylidene diphosphonate (Re186 HEDP)

Definition

Rhenium-186 forms a stable diphosphonate chelate with hydroxyethylidene diphosphonate (HEDP) forming rhenium-186 hydroxyethylidene diphosphonate (Re186 HEDP) (Lewington 1993). The linking of the radionuclide rhenium-186 to a suitable chemical compound produces a radiopharmaceutical which is localized in metastatic foci in

bone (Donald *et al.* 1989). Rhenium-186 HEDP is a beta-gamma-emitting radionuclide with a maximum beta energy of 1.07 MeV (megaelectron volts), and has a gamma ray emission of 137 keV (Maxon *et al.* 1988).

The beta particles travel only short distances and, therefore, their energy deposition is localized in metastatic foci in bone, delivering a therapeutic radiation dose directly to the metastases while delivering a much lower dose to normal bone marrow. Because Re186 HEDP also emits gamma rays, which can be located by diagnostic imaging techniques, it is possible to verify its location in areas of metastatic disease, and to measure the dose of radiation delivered to the tumour and bone marrow (Maxon *et al.* 1992).

Use

Bone metastases are the most common cause of cancer pain, and can lead to immobility, pathological fractures, bone marrow failure, neurological symptoms and hypercalcaemia (Lewington 1993). Approximately 80% of patients with prostate cancer develop bone metastases (Maxon *et al.* 1991) in spite of surgery, hormone therapy, external beam radiotherapy and chemotherapy (Maxon *et al.* 1988).

In 1991 prostate cancer was the second most common cause of death from malignant disease in men (Dearnaley 1994). Studies using Re186 HEDP as targeted radiotherapy have shown that it can provide prompt and significant relief of pain in approximately 80% of patients (Maxon *et al.* 1990). It has also been shown to increase patients' mobility, improve quality of life, and reduce the rate at which new painful sites develop, which in turn reduces requirements for additional radiation therapy and lifetime management costs (McEwan 1997).

Re186 HEDP has advantages over conventional external beam radiotherapy because it is tumour specific with relative sparing of surrounding healthy tissue (Lewington 1993). While thrombocytopenia is a dose-limiting toxicity, leucopenia is less severe (de Klerk *et al.* 1994), although in a study by Holle (1997) an 87% response rate was achieved with no myelosuppressive effects. It is also possible to adjust the dosage to each patient to avoid unacceptable toxicity (de Klerk *et al.* 1996). A mild transient increase in pain may occur within a few days of administering Re186 HEDP (Maxon *et al.* 1992).

Re186 HEDP is administered by intravenous injection. Because Re186 HEDP is excreted in the urine, urinary catheterization is carried out prior to treatment to ensure that the bladder remains empty and the radiation dose to the bladder is minimized. Therefore caution must be exercised when emptying the catheter bag (see 'Preparation of therapy room', below). Because the half-life of Re186 HEDP is only 90 hours (Maxon *et al.* 1988), patients may only need to be segregated after it has been administered for between 24 and 48 hours (Maxon *et al.* 1988).

Iodine-131

Definition

Radioactive iodine-131 is a beta-gamma emitter with a half-life of 8 days, and is used mainly in the form of iodide solution. The beta radiation gives a high, local dose in iodine concentrating tissue. The gamma component is useful for external measurement and scanning (Pointon 1991).

Use

Thyroid tissue selectively concentrates iodide, which enables iodine-131 to be used in the diagnosis and treatment of thyroid disorders. These patients usually have a good prognosis (Harmer 1996):

1 Thyrotoxicosis. Usually treatments of between 75 and 400 megabecquerels (MBq) activity of iodine-131 can be given, often on an outpatient basis.
2 Well-differentiated thyroid cancers (papillary and follicular) and metastases that function similarly to the thyroid tissue. Treatment is usually on an inpatient basis because of the higher activities involved.

Iodine-131 is normally administered as a capsule taken orally by the patient, followed by a hot drink. It can also be administered in liquid form either intravenously or orally.

Treatment programme for carcinoma of the thyroid

Surgical removal of the thyroid

Normal thyroid tissue concentrates iodine more efficiently than malignant tissue, and some malignant tissues concentrate iodine-131 only after removal of normal tissue (Pointon 1991). It is recommended, therefore, that a surgical near-total thyroidectomy is performed before administration of iodine-131.

Iodine-131 treatment

This is one of the most specific therapies available that has few adverse effects (O'Doherty & Coakley 1998). Following thyroidectomy an ablation dose of, typically, 3 GBq of iodine-131 is administered to ablate the remnants of thyroid tissue. Further treatments of 5.5 GBq may be necessary to destroy deposits in local lymph nodes and distant metastases.

Preparation of patient before admission

1 *Twenty-one days before admission*: patients taking tetraiodothyronine (T_4) (thyroxine) must stop taking this medication.
2 *Ten days before admission*: patients taking triiodothyronine (T_3) must stop taking this medication.
3 *Three days before admission*: occasionally, to enhance the uptake of iodine-131, three daily injections of thyroid-stimulating hormone are administered.

Principles of protection policies

Iodine-131 is excreted rapidly in patients who have had a thyroidectomy via all body fluids, especially the urine. In those patients who have not undergone thyroidectomy, excretion is rapid initially, slowing as the iodine-131 is bound by the thyroid tissue. Consequently, great care must be taken with all body fluids, especially during the first few days.

Meta-iodobenzylguanidine (mIBG)

Definition

Meta-iodobenzylguanidine is a synthetic physiological guanethidine analogue which is structurally similar to both the neurotransmitter hormone norepinephrine and the ganglionic blocking drug guanethidine. mIBG will localize in a wide variety of neuroendocrine tumours including neuroblastomas and phaeochromocytomas (Barry *et al.* 1990) yet in relatively few normal cells (Kemshead *et al.* 1990).

mIBG can be linked to iodine-131 and iodine-123 (a radionuclide) to produce the radiopharmaceutical I-131 mIBG or I-123 mIBG. A radiopharmaceutical is a radionuclide linked to a suitable chemical compound whose biochemical properties allow the radionuclide to be localized in the desired tissue (Donald *et al.* 1989).

Use

I-131 mIBG can be used as a safe, effective, non-invasive method of localizing both primary and metastatic neuroendocrine tumours (Barry *et al.* 1990). Therapeutic doses of I-131 mIBG can be given to patients in whom standard surgical and chemotherapeutic treatments have failed to control primary tumours, or can be used as an adjuvant to these treatments to prevent recurrence of the tumour (Fielding *et al.* 1991). In the treatment of neuroblastoma, response rates of 75% can be initially achieved using induction chemotherapy and stem cell rescue, although only 25% of patients will survive long term (Meller 1997). I-131 mIBG has been found to be equally effective but with considerably less toxicity (Hoefnagel *et al.* 1995).

Prior to therapy patients undergo scanning investigations using a tracer dose of I-123 or I-131 mIBG which allows calculation of the treatment dose. Therapeutic doses of I-131 mIBG are custom-synthesized for each patient and kept chilled or frozen from the time of synthesis until the dose is administered to reduce the risk of autoradiolysis. The solution is thawed and infused intravenously over 30–60 minutes using a shielded delivery system. During infusion pulse and blood pressure are monitored (Barry *et al.* 1990).

Side-effects include anorexia and mild nausea and vomiting, which can be controlled with antiemetics and an adequate intake of fluids. The major toxicities are to bone marrow, with a higher incidence of significant thrombocytopenia than neutropenia (Hoefnagel *et al.* 1987), and to the bladder (Fielding *et al.* 1991).

Preparation of patient

To prevent the uptake of any free iodine-131, the uptake of radioactive iodine by the thyroid gland is blocked by giving patients excess oral iodine continually from 3 days before until 3 weeks after administration of mIBG for therapy doses while for diagnostic investigations the Lugols iodine is taken over 5 days, commencing 2 days before the injection of I-123 mIBG.

As mIBG stimulates noradrenaline, drugs that act as antagonists (e.g. phenothiazines) are contraindicated during treatment (Shulkin & Shapiro 1990).

Monoclonal antibodies labelled with iodine-131 for recurrent cystic glioblastoma

Definition

Monoclonal antibodies specific to glioma antigens can be radiolabelled with iodine-131 and administered as therapy for patients with cystic gliomas. The tumour is targeted by the monoclonal antibodies which deliver the radiation dose to the tumour. Because the antibodies are specific to glioma tissue, the exposure of normal tissues is limited (Lashford *et al.* 1988).

An antibody is a protein which is produced as a result of the introduction of an antigen. It has the ability to combine with the antigen that stimulated its production. Monoclonal antibodies are identical copies of a single antibody (Stites & Terr 1991). It is possible to produce monoclonal antibodies that are specific to tumour cells, which can be labelled with a radioisotope. When administered to the patient, the labelled monoclonal antibody seeks, attaches itself to, and then as the radioisotope decays, emitting radiation, it destroys malignant cells which carry the appropriate specific antigen (Epenetos 1993).

Use

High-grade malignant gliomas are at present not curable with conventional treatment (surgery, radiotherapy and chemotherapy) (Brada 1989). Small studies of monoclonal antibodies labelled with iodine-131 administered intrathecally have shown that some patients have a significant and lasting therapeutic response without significant immediate or lasting toxicity (Lashford *et al.* 1988).

The procedure consists of surgically inserting a catheter into the tumour, and then administering a diagnostic dose of monoclonal antibody labelled with iodine-124. Following positron emission tomography (PET), a technique for imaging the distribution of radiolabelled pharmaceuticals (Horwich 1995), it is possible to calculate the therapeutic dose of antibody labelled with iodine-131. The therapeutic dose is administered slowly into the catheter by the patient's physician.

Following administration, it is important to carry out careful neurological observations to identify complications related to placement of the catheter, allergic reactions to the monoclonal antibody labelled with iodine-131 or possible toxicities associated with instillation of intracystic therapies.

The principles of protection policies must be followed. Education and support for patients and carers are particularly important because of the nature of this rarely used therapy.

Principles of radiation protection

The following radiation protection policies and nursing guidelines are written to conform with the *Ionizing Radiation (Medical Exposure) Regulations 2000* and associated guidance notes. They are applicable where dedicated single-bed treatment rooms with en suite toilet and bathing facilities are available.

Further precautions may be necessary when these conditions are not met. The advice of the radiation protection adviser must always be sought.

When patients are treated with radioactive sources it may be necessary to limit the time staff and others spend in close proximity to the patient. A controlled area notice with a radiation trefoil and a *no unauthorized entry* sign is displayed to restrict access to the patient. Entry to this controlled area is governed by a written work protocol supported by local rules which are compiled and employed to ensure that all persons entering a controlled area adopt safe working procedures. Radiation protection supervisors are appointed to each controlled area to ensure local rules are followed (DHSS 1985).

Nurses must follow the procedures set out for the period when controlled area restrictions apply. This, and careful planning of work, will ensure that exposure to radiation is minimized in a way that is compatible with good nursing care. Patients are cared for in a shielded room using the radiation protection principles of distance, shielding and time minimization, as for iodine-131 therapy (see below).

Controlled area

The entrance to the controlled area must be marked with a warning sign. Information is displayed to indicate the following:

1 The radioactive material and activity administered.
2 The nursing time allowed per day:
  (a) Essential nursing procedures only should be carried out and unnecessary time must not be spent in close proximity to the patient while the sign is displayed.
  (b) The time given is such that a nurse remaining at a distance of approximately 60 cm from the patient for the time indicated each day would, after 5 consecutive days, receive the maximum permissible dose for the working week.

Appropriate barriers, i.e. lead shields, should be placed at the entrance to:

1 Prevent inadvertent entry by unauthorized personnel.
2 Reduce radiation exposure to visitors and staff.

Patients treated with unsealed radioactive sources should be confined to their rooms, except for special medical or nursing procedures, when they must be accompanied by suitably trained staff.

Therapeutic unsealed sources generate a significant amount of liquid radioactive waste. This can be from the patient's shower and toilet. However, the amount of radioactive waste that enters the sewage system is governed by local regulations. Multiple holding tank systems can be employed where waste can be held to allow decay to occur before being released into the main waste drainage system (Leung & Nikolic 1998).

Film badges

Film badges should be worn at all times when on duty.

Contamination control

With unsealed sources, it is important to guard against contamination both of personnel and the hospital environment by the correct use of protective gloves, gowns and overshoes. The patient's body fluids are highly radioac-

tive, especially in the days immediately after iodine-131 has been administered. The application of cosmetics, eating, drinking or smoking while there is any possibility that the hands are contaminated are prohibited.

In the event of any incident involving radioactive material, the physics department must be advised immediately, even if the incident occurs outside normal working hours.

Preparation of therapy room

Equipment

Equipment should be kept to a minimum. It must be checked to ensure that it is in working order, as maintenance staff will only be allowed into the room in exceptional circumstances.

Bed linen and disposable items (gloves, aprons, overshoes, cutlery and crockery) should be kept in a utility room or anteroom along with the patient's treatment chart and a radiation monitor.

Personal items

Nurses should be sensitive to the psychological implications for patients of being labelled 'radioactive' and confined in isolation. Although patients may want to bring some personal belongings with them, they should be advised to keep these to a minimum, as items may become contaminated and need to be stored until radioactivity has decayed.

Protective floor covering

Plastic-backed absorbent paper, kept in place by adhesive tape, is used to retain accidental urine spills or splashes on the floor immediately surrounding the toilet. Each patient is assessed to decide if further floor covering is necessary, e.g. catheterized patients will require floor covering below a catheter bag.

Cleaning the treatment room

During occupancy of the treatment room by the patient, cleaning of the room is kept to a minimum and should be supervised by the physics staff. After the patient is discharged, monitoring and any necessary decontamination of the room will be arranged by the physics department, which will inform the relevant personnel when this has been completed. Only then may the room be entered and thoroughly cleaned.

Preparation of patient

Consent

Patients are required to sign a consent form agreeing to treatment, following a full explanation from the treating clinician. This is to comply with medical, ethical and legal requirements and local hospital policy. Consent is usually obtained in the outpatient clinic before ordering the radioactive material.

On admission

Before the administration of unsealed sources, any symptoms of diarrhoea or constipation must be remedied. Diarrhoea could result in contamination of the treatment area. Constipation not only inhibits the elimination of radioactivity but also could obscure radiological investigations, e.g. scanning.

Patients and relatives should be educated about the principles of radiation protection and the procedures with which the patient has to comply while in isolation. It is important to identify potential anxieties before administration while the nurse is able to reassure the patient and is unconstrained by time limits.

The patient must also agree to stay in hospital until the physics department advises that the level of radioactivity permits discharge.

Discharge of patient

A patient should not be discharged from hospital until the activity retained has fallen below recommended levels. This level will depend on several factors, including:

1 Mode of transport on leaving hospital
2 Journey time involved
3 Personal circumstances, i.e. young children or pregnant women at home.

Patients will be assessed individually for radiation clearance by the physics department before discharge. The treating physician will then be advised of the results of the assessment. Advice will be given to patients on issues such as return to work and visits to public places. Patients who are discharged with more than 150 MBq of radioactivity retained will be given appropriate information in the form of an instruction card carrying details of precautions to be taken. This card must be signed by the treating clinician.

It must be emphasized that this card is to be carried and the instructions followed until the latest date shown so that, for instance, staff would be alerted should the patient be readmitted to hospital. Additional verbal instructions may be necessary.

Regulations

Ionizing Radiations Regulations (1985). Stationery Office, London. *Ionizing Radiations (Protection of Persons Undergoing Medical Examination or Treatment) Regulations* (1988). Stationery Office, London. *Ionizing Radiations (Medical Exposure) Regulations* 2000. Stationery Office, London.

References and further reading

Barry, L. *et al.* (1990) Radioiodinated metaiodobenzylguanidine (MIBG) in the management of neuroblastomas. In: *Neuroblas-*

toma Tumor Biology and Therapy (ed. C. Pochedly). CRC Press, Boston.

Bomanji, J.B., Britton, K.E. & Clarke, S.E.M. (1995) *Oncology, Clinicians' Guide in Nuclear Medicine* (ed. P.J. Ell). British Nuclear Medicine Society, London.

Brada, M. (1989) Back to the future: radiotherapy in high grade gliomas. *Br J Cancer*, **60**, 14.

Buxton-Thomas, M. (1989) The lungs. In: *Practical Nuclear Medicine* (eds. P.F. Sharp, H.G. Gemmell & F.W. Smith). IRL Press, Oxford.

Datz F.L. (1993) *Handbook of Nuclear Medicine*. Mosby, Missouri.

Dearnaley, D.P. (1994) Cancer of the prostate. *Br Med J*, **308**, 780–84.

De Klerk, J.M. *et al.* (1994) Evaluation of thrombocytopenia in patients treated with rhenium-186-HEDP: guidelines for individual dosage recommendations. *J Nucl Med*, **35**(9), 1423–8.

De Klerk, J.M. *et al.* (1996) Bone marrow absorbed dose of rhenium-186 HEDP and the relationship with decreased platelet counts. *J Nucl Med*, **37**(1) 38–41.

DHSS (1985) *Ionizing Radiation Regulations*. Stationery Office, London.

Donald, R.B. *et al.* (1989) *Nuclear Medicine Technology and Techniques*. C.V. Mosby, Baltimore.

Epenetos, A.A. (1993) *Monoclonal Antibodies: Two Applications in Clinical Oncology*. Chapman & Hall Medical, London.

Feiglin, D. (1989) The cardiovascular system. In: *Practical Nuclear Medicine* (eds. P.F. Sharp, H.G. Gemmell & F.W. Smith). IRL Press, Oxford.

Fielding, S.L. *et al.* (1991) Dosimetry of 131 I MIBG for treatment of resistant neuroblastoma: results of a UK study. *Eur J Nucl Med*, **18**, 308–16.

Goldstone, K.E., Jackson, P.C., Myers, M.C. & Simpson, A.E. (1997) *Radiation Protection in Nuclear Medicine and Pathology*. Institute of Physics and Engineering in Medicine, York.

Harmer, C.L. (1996) Radiotherapy in the management of thyroid cancer. *Ann Acad Med Singapore*, **25**(3), 413–19.

Hoefnagel, C.A. *et al.* (1987) Radionuclide diagnosis and therapy of neural crest tumors using 131 I MIBG. *J Nucl Med*, **28**, 308–14.

Hoefnagel, C.A., De Kraker, J., Valdes Olmos, R.A. & Voute, P.A. (1995) 131-I MIBG as a first line treatment in advanced neuroblastoma. *J Nucl Med*, **39**(4), Suppl. 1, 61–4.

Holle, L.H. (1997) Palliative treatment for pain in osseous metastasized prostatic carcinoma with osteotropic rhenium-186 hydroxyethylidene diphosphonate. *Urologe A*, **36**(6), 540–47.

Horwich, A. (ed.) (1995) *Oncology: A Multidisciplinary Textbook*. Chapman & Hall Medical, London.

International Commission on Radiological Protection (1990) *Publication 57: Radiological Protection of the Worker in Medicine and Dentistry*. Pergamon Press, Oxford.

Kemshead, J.T. *et al.* (1990) Neuroblastoma: perspectives for future research. In: *Neuroblastoma Tumor Biology and Therapy* (ed. C. Pochedly). CRC Press, Boston.

Langmead, W.A. (1983) *Radiation Protection of the Patient in Nuclear Medicine. A Manual of Good Practice*. Oxford University Press, Oxford.

Lashford, L.S. *et al.* (1988) A pilot study of iodine-131 monoclonal antibodies in the therapy of leptomeningeal tumours. *Cancer*, **61**, 857–68.

Leung, P.M. & Nikolic, M. (1998) Disposal of therapeutic 131 I waste using a multiple holding tank system. *Health Phys*, **75**(3), 315–21.

Lewington, V.J. (1993) Targeted radionuclide therapy for bone metastases. *Eur J Nucl Med*, **20**, 66–74.

McDonagh, A. (1991) Getting your patient ready for a nuclear medicine scan. *Nursing*, **21**(2), 53–7.

McEwan, A.J. (1997) Unsealed source therapy of painful bone metatases an update. *Semin Nucl Med*, **2**, 165–82.

Martin, A. & Harbinson, S. (1977) *An Introduction to Radiation Protection.* Chapman & Hall Medical, London.

Maxon, H.R. *et al.* (1988) Re-186 HEDP for treatment of multiple metastatic foci in bone: human biodistribution and dosimetric studies. *Radiology*, **166**, 505–507.

Maxon, H.R. *et al.* (1990) Re-186 treatment of painful osseous metastases: initial clinical experience in 20 patients with hormone resistant prostate cancer. *Radiology*, **176**, 155–9.

Maxon, H.R. *et al.* (1991) Rhenium-186 HEDP for treatment of painful osseous metastases: results of a double-blind crossover comparison with placebo. *J Nucl Med*, **32**, 1877–81.

Maxon, H.R. *et al.* (1992) Rhenium–186 hydroxyethylidene diphosphonate for the treatment of painful osseous metastases. *Semin Nucl Med*, **22**(1), 33–40.

Mayes, J. *et al.* (1989) *Neuroblastoma: MIBG in its Diagnosis and Management.* Springer, London.

Meller, S. (1997) Targeted radiotherapy for neuroblastoma. *Arch Dis Child*, **77**(5), 389–91.

Merrick, M.V. (1984) The blood and reticuloendothelial system. In: *Essential Nuclear Medicine*, pp. 180–91. Churchill Livingston, Edinburgh.

Mould, R.F. (1985) *Radiation Protection in Hospitals.* Adam Hilger, Bristol and Boston.

National Council for Radiation Protection (1989) *Report 105. Radiation Protection for Medical and Allied Health Personnel.* NCRP, Bethseda, Maryland.

National Radiological Protection Board (1988) *Guidance Notes for the Protection of Persons Against Ionizing Radiations Arising from Medical Use.* Stationery Office, London.

Nowotnik, D.P. (1995) *Textbook of Radiopharmacy*, 2nd edn. (ed. C.B. Sampson), pp. 40–41. Gordon and Breach Science Publishers, Switzerland.

O'Connor, M.K. (1996) *The Mayo Clinic Manual of Nuclear Medicine.* Churchill Livingstone, Edinburgh.

O'Doherty, M.J. & Coakley, A.J. (1998) Drug therapy alternatives in the treatment of thyroid cancer. *Drugs*, **55**(6), 801–812.

Owunwanne, A., Patel M. & Sadek, S. (1995) *The Handbook of Radiopharmaceuticals*, pp. 73–6. Chapman & Hall Medical, London.

Perkins, A.C. (1989) Tumour imaging. In: *Practical Nuclear Medicine* (eds. P.F. Sharp, H.G. Gemmell & F.W. Smith). IRL Press, Oxford.

Perkins, A.C. (1995) *Nuclear Medicine Science and Safety.* John Libby, London.

Pinkerton, P.T. (1991) *Treatment Strategies in Paediatric Cancers.* Gardiner-Caldwell Communication, UK.

Pointon, R.C.S. (1991) *The Radiotherapy of Malignant Disease.* Springer, London.

Saha, G.B. (1992) *Fundamentals of Nuclear Pharmacy.* Springer, New York.

Sandler, M.P., Shapiro, B., Gross, M. & Partain (1989) Thyroid, parathyroid and adrenal gland imaging. In: *Practical Nuclear Medicine* (eds. P.F. Sharp, H.G. Gemmell & F.W. Smith). IRL Press, Oxford.

Sharp, C., Shrimpton, J.A. & Bury, R.F. (1998) *Diagnostic Medical Exposures: Advice on Exposure to Ionising Radiation During Pregnancy.* National Radiological Protection Board, Didcot.

Shulkin, B.L. & Shapiro, B. (1990) Radioiodinated MIBG in the management of neuroblastoma. In: *Neuroblastoma Tumor Biology and Therapy* (ed. C. Pochedly). CRC Press, Boston.

Sisson, J.C. *et al.* (1984) Radiopharmaceutical treatment of malignant phaeochromocytoma. *J Nucl Med*, **24**, 197–206.

Smith, F.W. (1989) The skeletal system. In: *Practical Nuclear Medicine* (eds. P.F. Sharp, H.G. Gemmell & F.W. Smith). IRL Press, Oxford.

Smith, F.W. & Gemmell, H.G. (1989) The urinary tract. In: *Practical Nuclear Medicine* (eds P.F. Sharp, H.G. Gemmell & F.W. Smith). IRL Press, Oxford.

Souhami, R. & Tobias, J. (1995) *Cancer and its Management.* Blackwell Science, Oxford.

Stites, D.P. & Terr, A.I. (1991) *The Basis of Human Immunology.* Prentice-Hall International, London.

Testa, H.J & Prescott, M.C. (1996) *Nephrourology, Clinician's Guide in Nuclear Medicine* (ed. P.J. Ell). British Nuclear Medicine Society, London.

Tiffany, R. (ed.) (1987) *Cancer Nursing: Radiotherapy.* Faber and Faber, London.

Tiffany, R. (ed.) (1988) *Oncology for Nurses and Health Care Professionals*, Vols 1 and 2. George Allen & Unwin, London.

Troncone, L., Rufini, V., Luzi, S., Mastrangelo, R. & Riccardi, R. (1995) The treatment of neuroblastoma with 131-I MIBG at diagnosis. *J Nucl Med*, **39**(4), Suppl. 1, 65–8.

Walter, J. (1977) *Cancer and Radiotherapy.* Churchill Livingstone, Edinburgh.

Wootton, R. (1993) *Radiation Protection of Patients.* Cambridge University Press, Cambridge.

GUIDELINES · Care of patient before administration of iodine-131

Action	Rationale
1 Explain and discuss the procedure with the patient.	To ensure that the patient understands the procedure and gives his/her valid consent.
2 The patient is to be fasted for 2 h before and after administration of an iodine-131 dose. Offer a light diet for the remainder of the day.	To reduce the risk of nausea and/or vomiting.
3 Administer a prophylactic antiemetic 30 min before scheduled administration of the dose.	To prevent nausea and vomiting.
4 Check that the preparation of the room and the patient is complete. Ensure that any surplus items have been removed.	To prevent contamination of extraneous equipment.
5 Remove jewellery except wedding rings.	Jewellery may become contaminated.

GUIDELINES • Care of the patient receiving iodine-131 thyroid treatment

Action	Rationale
1 Explain and discuss the procedure with the patient.	To ensure that the patient understands the procedure and gives his/her valid consent.
2 Assist the patient to remove dentures/bridges, if dose is administered in liquid form.	To prevent radioactive material being trapped behind dental plates.
3 The patient swallows the capsule or drinks the iodine-131 through a straw, physically directed by an authorized physicist in the presence of the clinician directing treatment.	Drinking through a straw reduces the amount of radioactive material left around the mouth. To meet current regulations.
4 Offer the patient a drink of water to rinse out the mouth. (This must be swallowed.) Assist the patient to replace dentures.	To remove any iodine-131 from inside the mouth.
5 Physics staff place the radiation warning sign at the entrance to the therapy room.	To identify the room as a controlled area.

GUIDELINES • Care of the patient receiving iodine-131 mIBG treatment

Action	Rationale
1 Explain and discuss the procedure with the patient.	To ensure that the patient understands the procedure and gives his/her valid consent.
2 Apply a vital signs monitor with a variable time setting mode to the patient that will be visible to staff from outside the room.	Following the administration of mIBG, a transient rise in blood pressure and pulse may occur.
3 Check that the patient has been cannulated, and commence prescribed intravenous fluids 3 h before iodine-131 mIBG administration.	Iodine-131 mIBG is administered intravenously through a three-way tap attached to the intravenous administration set.
4 The clinician will set up iodine-131 mIBG infusion and give it over 30–60 min.	To minimize transient rise in blood pressure and pulse.
5 Monitor blood pressure and pulse at least: (a) Every 5 min during infusion (b) Every 10 min for the first 45 min post-infusion (c) Hourly for 4 h (d) Four-hourly; or more frequently if required. (e) Monitor whole body retention measurements as directed by physics.	To detect and monitor any change.
6 Continue intravenous hydration for 24 h post-infusion and simultaneously encourage oral fluids.	To increase the urinary output and elimination of radioactivity from the bladder.

GUIDELINES • Care of the patient after administration of unsealed source therapy

Entering the room

Action	Rationale
1 Put on disposable gloves.	To prevent contamination of the hands.
2 Put on disposable overshoes.	To prevent spread of contamination outside the treatment area.

Guidelines • Care of the patient after administration of unsealed source therapy (cont'd)

Action	Rationale
3 Put on a suitable protective gown:	
(a) Long-sleeve cotton gown, e.g. for lifting patient.	To protect against low levels of contamination, e.g. from the patient's skin.
(b) Disposable plastic apron, e.g. for dealing with vomit or incontinence.	To protect against high levels of contamination.
4 Plan work before entering the controlled area and then work quickly and efficiently, keeping within the time allowance stated.	To minimize radiation exposure, as consistent with good nursing care.
5 Only use disposable crockery and cutlery to present meals to patients.	China crockery and cutlery may become contaminated.

Maintaining patient comfort and hygiene

Action	Rationale
1 Encourage the patient to bathe/shower frequently at least once a day.	To reduce any radioactive perspiration on the skin.
2 Encourage the patient to wash the hands thoroughly after each possible contact with bodily fluids, e.g. cleaning teeth, going to the toilet, etc.	To remove radioactivity from the hands.
3 The patient should regularly remove any dentures and clean under running water.	To remove radioactive saliva from around dentures.
4 The patient should regularly remove any contact lenses and rinse in their usual cleaning fluid.	To remove any radioactive tears from lenses.
5 Encourage a good fluid intake of between 2 and 3 litres per day.	To increase the urinary output and elimination of radioactivity from the bladder.
6 Ensure that the patient has own personal toilet facilities and flushes the toilet twice after use.	To reduce contamination of others and of the environment. Urine of patients treated with iodine-131 is initially highly radioactive.
7 Bedbound patients should be catheterized before the dose is given. Empty the catheter bag every 4–6 h, or more frequently if necessary.	Catheterization reduces the nursing time spent with the patient and the likelihood of contamination. Frequent emptying of the bag reduces the radiation level in the room.
8 If the patient requires a bedpan or urinal, this item must be kept solely for this patient's use. The bedpan or urinal must be handled carefully and the contents disposed of in the toilet, which is flushed twice. The bedpan or urinal may be washed in the bedpan washer. It should be sealed in a plastic bag for the journey to and from the sluice.	To reduce contamination of the environment and of other patients and staff.
9 If leakage occurs from injection sites, wound sites, etc., the nurse should contact the medical staff and the physics department immediately. Any contact with the dressing should be done with long-handled forceps.	It must be remembered that all body fluids are potentially radioactive.
10 Gloves and a protective gown must be worn whenever handling soiled bed linen.	To prevent contamination.
11 All used linen must be deposited in a special bag provided for this purpose.	Used linen must be monitored for contamination before going to the laundry.
12 Collection of laboratory specimens should, if possible, be deferred. If collections are unavoidable, a radiation warning sticker must be attached to the specimen and request card and the specimen delivered to the laboratory following consultations with the physics department.	To reduce the risk of contamination of the laboratory and its staff.

Visitors

Action	Rationale
1 Visiting time is limited as advised by the physicist during the first day following administration of an unsealed source.	The patient is highly radioactive during this period.
2 On subsequent days, visiting is unlimited, providing visitors remain outside the room behind the lead screen.	To minimize the exposure of visitors to radiation.
3 Physical contact with the patient or bed linen is not allowed as protective clothing is not available to visitors.	To prevent contamination of visitors.
4 Children under 16 years of age and pregnant women should be discouraged from visiting.	Radiation exposure of children and the unborn must be kept as low as practicable.

On leaving the room

Action	Rationale
1 Remove overshoes, taking care not to touch the shoes worn underneath.	These are removed first while gloves are still being worn to prevent the spread of contamination to hands or the floor outside the room.
2 Remove the plastic apron, by holding the front of apron and breaking the neck and waist ties.	
3 Remove gloves by peeling them off the hands, taking care not to touch the outside surfaces with bare hands, and discard them in the clinical waste bag provided.	To prevent transfer of contamination from the gloves' outer surfaces to the hands.
4 Wash hands thoroughly using soap and water.	To remove any contamination.
5 Use the radiation monitor each time when leaving the room and monitor for contamination of the hands, feet and clothing. If contamination has occurred, inform the physics department immediately and follow the decontamination procedure.	To ensure that the nurse is not contaminated.
6 The physics department will advise if further whole body monitoring is required.	To check for internal or external contamination.

GUIDELINES · Care of the patient receiving unsealed sources for diagnostic investigations

Action	Rationale
1 Explain and discuss the procedure with the patient, and, if relevant, with the relative accompanying the patient.	To ensure the patient is physically and psychologically prepared for the procedure and understands the procedure and gives his/her informed consent.
2 Preparation of patients (special considerations):	
(a) Provide effective pain control for those patients with pain.	Patients should be pain-free so that immobility during scan time can be maintained.
(b) Pregnant women will generally not be scanned. When essential tests must be undertaken, the patient must sign a consent form and receive a reduced dose of radionuclide.	To avoid unnecessary irradiation to the abdominal/pelvic region which will include the embryo or fetus.
(c) The person accompanying the patient should not be pregnant, or bring young children or babies with them.	To avoid unnecessary exposure in the time period immediately after the radionuclide administration.

Guidelines • Care of the patient receiving unsealed sources for diagnostic investigations (cont'd)

Action	Rationale
(d) In women of reproductive age, the possibility of pregnancy must be excluded and the patient asked if her menstrual period is late. Patients receiving I-131 or other radioactive agent with a long half-life should not become pregnant for a minimum of 3 months (Sharp *et al.* 1998).	To avoid unnecessary irradiation to the abdomen of a women who may be pregnant.
(e) With breastfeeding mothers, seek advice from the radiation protection adviser.	Radioactivity can be excreted in breast milk. Therefore breast feeding may need to be suspended and the mother encouraged to avoid unnecessary cuddling of the child during this time.
(f) If the patient is incontinent, incontinence pads should be worn and universal precautions are to be adopted.	To limit the spread of contamination. Disposable gloves and apron should be worn and handwashing performed following patient contact, as these will prevent contamination of staff in close contact with the patient.
(g) Empty urine bags regularly.	To remove the radioactivity away from the patient area.
(h) Debilitated patients may require prolonged close contact. Nursing staff should share the care of these patients, by regular rotation of staff.	To keep doses to staff as low as possible, by avoiding prolonged exposure to any one member of staff.

Action	Rationale
3 Administering radionuclides:	
(a) Follow guidelines for drug administration in Chap. 12.	To comply with national and professional guidelines for the administration of drugs.
(b) Follow aseptic techniques guidelines in Chap. 3.	To reduce the risk of contamination.
(c) Follow radiation protection precautions, which include:	To reduce the possible contamination of self and the environment.
• Wear thermoluminescent (TLD) finger-dose meter and film badge.	To measure radiation doses received by member of staff.
• Wear disposable gloves and plastic apron, which are discarded after use.	To reduce the risk of contamination.
• Draw up the dose behind a lead shield, and place the syringe in a lead syringe shield.	To reduce exposure to radiation.
• Dispose of all used syringes and needles in a designated radioactive sharps disposal bin which is stored within a lead shield.	To contain radioactivity and allow safe disposal.
• Wash hands at end of procedure.	To remove any possible radioactive contamination.
• Monitor hands at end of procedure and before leaving the room.	To check for possible radioactive contamination.
• Monitor the room for radioactive contamination at the end of each day or if contamination may have occurred.	To establish whether contamination has occurred.

Action	Rationale
4 Avoid urine, faecal and blood sample collection for laboratories other than nuclear medicine, for 24 h. If collection is unavoidable, a radiation warning sticker must be attached to the specimen and request card, and the specimen taken to the laboratory under the supervision of the physics departmental staff (see Chap. 37, Specimen Collection).	To prevent contamination of the laboratory and its staff, as specimens taken within 24 h of some scans may contain radioactivity.
5 Avoid bone marrow and stem cell harvests for 24 h. Seek advice from the physics department.	Cells may contain radioactivity.
6 Seek advice from physics staff if the patient is to undergo a procedure in the operating theatre within 24 h of a scan.	To prevent theatre equipment from becoming contaminated with radioactivity.
7 Place soiled bed linen used within the first 24 h of certain scans, i.e. bone scan, within a plastic bag and inform the physics departmental staff.	To prevent contamination of the environment.

GUIDELINES • Emergency procedures

In an emergency, the safety and medical care of the patient must take precedence over any potential radiation hazards to staff. Written radiation safety instructions must be available in all radiation areas where an emergency may arise. These instructions must contain a detailed description of how to manage a patient in the event of a medical emergency and the action required in other emergency situations, such as fire. The course of action in an emergency procedure depends on local circumstances and the nature of the emergency.

An incident occurring within the first 24 hours of iodine-131 being administered is obviously a greater hazard than a similar incident on the day of discharge. Movement of the patient to other wards or areas i.e. X-ray or HDU, must only be undertaken following the physics department's advice.

Major spillage of radioactive blood or body fluids, i.e. incontinence and/or vomiting

Action	Rationale
1 Inform the physics department immediately.	So that the physics department can advise on radiation protection as soon as possible.
2 If physics department staff are not immediately available, use a radiation monitor to assess the extent of the spillage.	To define extent of contamination and determine what further measures need to be taken.
3 Put some absorbent material on top of all the radioactive wet area.	To absorb contamination.
4 Follow the advice of the physics department staff in clearing spillage.	To prevent spread of contamination.

Contamination of bare hands

Action	Rationale
1 Wash hands in warm soapy water, paying special attention to the areas around the fingernails, between the fingers and on the outer edges of the hands. Continue washing until contamination is below the permissible limits indicated by local monitoring protocols.	To remove radioactive material from any areas where it might be trapped.
2 If a wound is produced in a contamination accident, wash thoroughly under running water, opening the edges of the cut. This should be continued until physics department staff can demonstrate that no residual radioactivity remains in the wound.	To stimulate bleeding and permit thorough flushing of the cut.

Death

Action	Rationale
1 Inform the physics department immediately.	So that the physics department staff can begin making the necessary arrangements for removal of the body to the mortuary.
2 Two nurses wearing gloves, plastic aprons, gowns and overshoes should perform last offices. All orifices must be packed carefully. Any vomit, blood, faeces or urine must be cleaned from the body.	To avoid contamination with body fluids. Minimal handling of the body reduces the risk of contamination.
3 The body should be totally enclosed in a plastic cadaver bag.	To avoid contamination of the porters and the mortuary staff.
4 Transfer of the body should be arranged with the physics department.	The physics department will supervise the transfer of the body.

Guidelines • Emergency procedures (cont'd)

Cardiac arrest

Action	Rationale
1 The switchboard must be told to inform the physics department as soon as possible after alerting the emergency resuscitation team.	So that the physics department can advise on radiation protection as soon as possible.
2 Do not use mouth-to-mouth resuscitation. All areas must be supplied with an Ambu bag for this purpose.	Mouth-to-mouth contact could result in contamination of the resuscitator.
3 Overshoes, gloves and gowns must be put on as soon as it is practicably possible.	To minimize personal contamination.
4 All emergency equipment must be monitored and decontaminated as necessary before being returned to general use.	To prevent contaminated equipment leaving the controlled area.

Fire

Action	Rationale
1 Every effort should be made to contact the physics department without compromising the patient's safety.	To help in the evacuation of the patients treated with iodine-131.
2 Following evacuation, patients treated with iodine-131 should be kept at a distance from other patients and staff.	To minimize exposure of others to radiation.

Respiratory Therapy

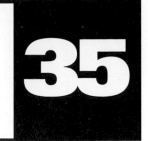

Definition

Respiratory therapy is the administration of or methods to supplement or augment oxygen when tissue oxygenation is impaired. Oxygen is essential to allow aerobic metabolism to produce energy from the intake of food.

If tissue oxygenation becomes inadequate, anaerobic metabolism will lead to lactic acidosis and cell death (Oh 1997).

Indications

There are many indications for respiratory therapy. The major ones are listed below:

1 Acute respiratory failure – this can be subdivided into two groups, i.e. with or without carbon dioxide retention:
   (a) With carbon dioxide retention – the most common causes are chronic bronchitis, chest injuries, e.g. flail segment and rupture of the diaphragm, drug overdose leading to coma, postoperative hypoxaemia and the neuromuscular diseases.
   (b) Without carbon dioxide retention – the most common causes are asthma, infective conditions, e.g. pneumonia and legionella, pulmonary oedema and pulmonary embolism (Oh 1997).
2 Acute myocardial infarction.
3 Cardiac failure.
4 Shock, particularly haemorrhagic, bacteraemic and cardiogenic.
5 A hypermetabolic state induced, for example, by major sepsis, trauma or burns.
6 States where there is a reduced ability to transport oxygen, e.g. anaemia.
7 Inability to utilize the oxygen carried, as in cyanide poisoning (Foss 1990).
8 During cardiorespiratory resuscitation.
9 During anaesthesia for surgery.

Reference material

Physiology (see also Chap. 28, Observations)

Tissue oxygenation is reliant on the following factors:

1 The oxygen cascade
2 Association and dissociation of haemoglobin and oxygen
3 Cardiac output (Oh 1997).

An understanding of these factors and their interaction is essential in understanding the physiology of oxygen transport and transfer in the body.

The movement of oxygen from the alveoli in the lungs to the pulmonary blood is effected rapidly due to the pressure gradient that exists. The partial pressure of oxygen (PaO_2) in the alveoli is 13.7 kilopascals (kPa) as compared to 5.3 kPa in the pulmonary capillaries. This allows a swift exchange of oxygen through diffusion. Similarly, oxygen is easily given up by the arterial blood to the tissues, again because of the steep pressure gradient. The partial pressure of arterial blood is 13.3 kPa and that of the tissues 2.7 kPa (Marieb 1996). Table 35.1 and Fig. 35.1 show the various pressure gradients in the oxygen cascade.

Oxygen is carried in the blood in the following two ways: dissolved in plasma; and bound to the haemoglobin within the red blood cells. Only about 1.5% of oxygen is carried in the plasma as oxygen is poorly soluble in water. Therefore, 98.5% of oxygen is transported around the body in a loose chemical alliance with haemoglobin (Marieb 1996). Haemoglobin is made up of four polypeptide chains, each of which is bound to a haem group that contains iron. The iron groups bind to oxygen, and therefore each molecule of haemoglobin can combine with four molecules of oxygen. A haemoglobin molecule is said to be fully saturated with oxygen when all four haem groups are attached to oxygen. When less than four are so attached, haemoglobin is said to be partially saturated (Marieb 1996).

The action of the four polypeptide molecules and their relationship to oxygen is interlinked so that when one molecule has taken up a molecule of oxygen, the others are facilitated to do the same. The same is also true for the opposite action when haem molecules unload their oxygen molecules to the tissues (Marieb 1996).

The timing of haemoglobin uptake and release of oxygen is affected by the following factors:

1 The partial pressure of oxygen (PaO_2)
2 Temperature
3 Blood pH
4 Partial pressure of carbon dioxide ($PaCO_2$) (Marieb 1996).

Table 35.1 Oxygen cascade. Pressure gradients for oxygen transfer (kPa) from inspired gas to tissue cells

Inspired air	20.0	Capillary	6.8
Alveolar	13.7	Tissue	2.7
Arterial	13.3	Mitochondrial	0.13–1.3

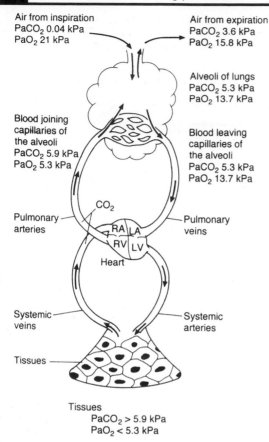

Figure 35.1 Gas movement in the body is facilitated by partial pressure differences. Top of figure illustrates pressure gradients that facilitate oxygen and carbon dioxide exchange in the lungs. Bottom of figure shows pressure gradients that facilitate gas movements from systemic capillaries to tissues.

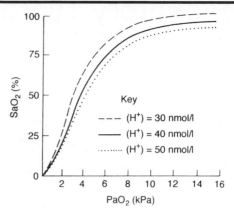

Figure 35.2 The oxygen dissociation curve, illustrating the normal curve at 40 nmol/l.

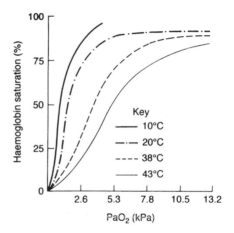

Figure 35.3 The oxygen dissociation curve and effect of temperature changes. As the temperature rises the curve shifts to the right, illustrating that oxygen unloading is accelerated as temperature rises.

The oxygen dissociation curve

The oxygen dissociation curve illustrates the factors affecting tissue oxygenation (Figs. 35.2, 35.3 and 35.4).

Haemoglobin and oxygenation

The extent of oxygen binding to haemoglobin depends on the PaO_2 of the blood, but the relationship is not precisely linear (see Fig. 35.2). The slope is steeply progressive between 1.5 and 7 kPa and then plateaus out between 9 and 13.5 kPa. This is important for oxygen therapy because it illustrates that haemoglobin is almost completely saturated at 9 kPa and therefore further increases in the partial pressure of oxygen will cause only a slight rise in oxygen binding.

The most rapid uptake and delivery of oxygen to and from haemoglobin occurs during the steep portion of the curve (Marieb 1996).

Haemoglobin, temperature and oxygen

As body temperature rises the affinity of haemoglobin for oxygen is reduced and less oxygen is bound while more oxygen is unloaded (Marieb 1996) (Fig. 35.3).

Haemoglobin, pH and oxygen

As the pH of the blood declines (acidosis) the affinity of haemoglobin for oxygen decreases and more oxygen will be unloaded to the tissues. This is known as the Bohr effect. The same effect occurs when the partial pressure of carbon

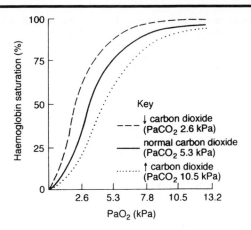

Figure 35.4 The oxygen dissociation curve and effect of carbon dioxide changes. As the $PaCO_2$ rises the curve shifts to the right, illustrating that oxygen unloading is accelerated as $PaCO_2$ rises.

dioxide rises as this will also lead to a fall in blood pH and acidosis (Marieb 1996) (Fig. 35.4).

Generally, a shift in the oxygen dissociation curve to the right will favour unloading of oxygen to the tissues, and a shift to the left will favour reduced tissue oxygenation. Factors that would influence a shift to the right are changes in temperature and pH. Factors that would influence a shift to the left are temperature and $PaCO_2$ changes (Oh 1997).

Cardiac output

The final factor influencing tissue oxygenation is the cardiac output. When this is severely reduced, for example in shock states, there will be a severely reduced amount of oxygen available to the tissues (Tinker & Zapol 1992).

Oxygen consumption

At rest the normal oxygen consumption is approximately 200–250 ml/min. As the available oxygen per minute in a normal man is about 700 ml, this means there is an oxygen reserve of 450–500 ml/min. Factors that increase the above consumption of oxygen include fever, sepsis, shivering, restlessness and increased metabolism (Oh 1997). It is difficult to say at which absolute level oxygen therapy is necessary as each situation should be judged by the requirements for oxygen and the availability of oxygen. Therefore, all of the above information needs to be taken into account together with the measurement of the arterial blood gases.

Generally, additional oxygen will be required when the PaO_2 has fallen to 8 kPa or less (Oh 1997). Oxygen saturation level in the tissues is also useful and can be measured using a pulse oximeter, which works by emitting narrow shafts of red and infrared light through the tissue of a finger, toe or earlobe. Different amounts of light rays are absorbed

by the arterial blood depending on its saturation with oxygen. The final oxygen saturation (SaO_2) is then calculated by computer (Ehrhardt & Graham 1990).

Hazards of respiratory therapy

Carbon dioxide narcosis

Carbon dioxide is the chemical that most directly influences respiration by its direct effect on the efficiency of alveolar ventilation. The normal partial pressure of carbon dioxide in the blood is 4.0–5.5 kPa. When this level rises, the pH of the cerebrospinal fluid drops which in turn causes excitation of the central chemoreceptors, and hyperventilation occurs (Marieb 1996).

In people who always retain carbon dioxide, and are therefore usually hypercapnic because of chronic pulmonary disease such as chronic bronchitis, the chemoreceptors are no longer sensitive to a raised level of carbon dioxide. In these cases the falling PaO_2 becomes the principal respiratory stimulus (the hypoxic drive) (Marieb 1996). Therefore, if a high level of supplementary oxygen was delivered to such patients, severe respiratory depression would ensue and ultimately unconsciousness and death.

Oxygen toxicity

Pulmonary toxicity following prolonged higher percentages of oxygen therapy is recognized clinically, but there is still much to be learnt about the condition. The pattern is one of decreasing lung compliance as a result of a sequela of haemorrhagic interstitial and intra-alveolar oedema, leading ultimately to fibrosis (Oh 1997).

It is thought that, where possible, long periods (that is 24 hours or more) of oxygen therapy above 50% should be avoided, although clinically it seems that there is much variance in the response of individual patients (Higgins 1990).

Retrolental fibroplasia

Retrolental fibroplasia is a disease affecting premature babies that weigh under 1200 g (about 28 weeks' gestation) if they are exposed to high concentrations of oxygen within the first 3–4 weeks of life. It appears that the oxygen stimulates immature blood vessels in the eye to vasoconstrict and obliterate, which results in neovascularization, accompanied by haemorrhage, fibrosis and then retinal detachment and blindness (Oh 1997).

General considerations

1 Oxygen is an odourless, tasteless, colourless, transparent gas that is slightly heavier than air.
2 Oxygen supports combustion; therefore there is always a danger of fire when oxygen is being used. The following safety measures should be remembered:

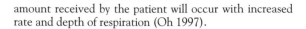

(a) Oil or grease around oxygen connections should be avoided.

(b) Alcohol, ether and other inflammatory liquids should be used with caution in the vicinity of oxygen.

(c) No electrical device must be used in or near an oxygen tent.

(d) Oxygen cylinders should be kept secure in an upright position and away from heat.

(e) There must be no smoking in the vicinity of oxygen.

(f) A fire extinguisher should be readily available.

(g) Care should be taken with high concentrations of oxygen when using the defibrillator.

Equipment necessary to administer respiratory therapy

Any oxygen delivery system will include these basic components:

1 Oxygen supply, either from a piped supply or a portable cylinder. All medical gas cylinders have to conform to a standardized colour coding: oxygen cylinders are black with a white shoulder and are labelled 'Oxygen' or 'O$_2$'.

2 A reduction gauge – to reduce the pressure to that of atmospheric pressure.

3 Flowmeter – a device that controls the flow of oxygen in litres per minute.

4 Tubing – disposable tubing of varying diameter and length.

5 Mechanism for delivery – a mask or nasal cannulae.

6 Humidifier – to warm and moisten the oxygen before administration (Allan 1988).

Methods of administration

Simple semirigid plastic masks (Fig. 35.5)

Simple semirigid plastic masks are low-flow masks which entrain the air from the atmosphere and therefore are able to deliver a variable oxygen percentage (anything from 21 to 60%) (Allan 1988). Large discrepancies between the delivered fractional inspired oxygen (FiO$_2$) and the actual

amount received by the patient will occur with increased rate and depth of respiration (Oh 1997).

Nasal cannulae catheter (Fig. 35.6)

Nasal cannulae catheters provide an alternative to a mask, but again there are great discrepancies between the delivered FiO$_2$ and the actual oxygen percentage received by the patient. When used at low flow rates, for example 2 l/min, they are well tolerated and afford the patient more freedom than a mask. At high flow rates, above 8 l/min, they may cause discomfort and dryness of the nasal mucosa. Nasal cannulae cannot be attached satisfactorily to an external humidification device (Allan 1988), but the nasal passages will aid humidification.

Fixed performance masks or high-flow masks (Venturi-type masks) (Fig. 35.7)

With fixed performance masks it is possible to achieve an unvarying mixture of gases and a known concentration of oxygen using the high air flow oxygen enrichment principle. These masks derive their name from the Venturi barrel in which a relatively low flow rate of oxygen is forced through a narrow jet. There are side holes in the barrel and this jet causes the air to be drawn in at a high rate. As the

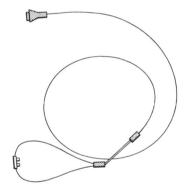

Figure 35.6 Nasal cannulae.

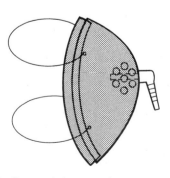

Figure 35.5 Semirigid plastic mask.

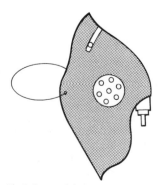

Figure 35.7 High-flow mask.

mixture of gas created is at a flow rate above that of inspiration, the mixture will be constant (Foss 1990). There are many Venturi-type masks available, but the larger-capacity masks are the most accurate and therefore the safest when a known concentration of oxygen is required or when efficient elimination of carbon dioxide is essential, for example, to provide respiratory therapy for the patient with chronic respiratory disease (Allan 1988).

T-piece circuit

The T-piece circuit is a simple, large-bore, non-rebreathing circuit which is attached directly to an endotracheal or tracheostomy tube. Humidified oxygen is delivered through one part of the T, and expired gases leave through the other part. This device may be used as part of the weaning process when a patient has been ventilated previously by a mechanical ventilator (Oh 1997).

Continuous positive airway pressure (CPAP)

Definition

CPAP therapy is the maintenance of a positive airway pressure greater than ambient pressure throughout inspiration and expiration. It can be delivered through a face mask, nasal mask, mouthpiece or through an endotracheal or tracheostomy tube (Oh 1997).

Indications

1 In acute respiratory failure in a spontaneously breathing patient who is able to maintain his or her own airway.
2 As a method of weaning a patient from mechanical ventilation.
3 After major surgery as a means of improving gaseous exchange.
4 As a supportive measure in patients where intubation and mechanical ventilation are not considered appropriate (Greenbaum et al. 1976).
5 Acute hypoxia with a normal $PaCO_2$.
6 Acute respiratory distress syndrome (ARDS).
7 Postoperatively (following major abdominal or thoracic surgery) prophylactically to prevent atelectasis.
8 Pulmonary oedema.
9 In patients with sleep apnoea.
10 In neonates with respiratory distress syndrome/hyaline membrane disease.

Reference material

Use of the CPAP circuit dates back at least to 1912, when Bunnell used a primitive circuit during thoracic surgery. The first recorded use in intensive care was by Poulton and Oxon in 1936. In the 1940s increased interest in CPAP was prompted by research into respiratory support in high altitude flying. Further developments occurred in the 1950s and 1960s, and in 1976 Greenbaum et al. reported the use of CPAP with a face mask in adult respiratory distress syndrome (ARDS). In 1972 Williamson & Modell successfully used CPAP for selected spontaneously breathing patients with acute respiratory failure.

The aim of CPAP therapy is to improve gas exchange (oxygen and carbon dioxide) within the lungs and improve the work of breathing. CPAP is able to do this by:

1 Increasing the functional residual capacity (FRC), which is the amount of gas left in the lungs at the end of normal expiration which is available for pulmonary gas exchange. In acute lung injury where gaseous exchange is severely inhibited CPAP increases the FRC by improving ventilation in poorly or non-ventilated alveoli (Miller & Semple 1991).
2 Decreasing intrapulmonary shunting and thereby improving the ventilation to perfusion mismatch in patients with pulmonary oedema (Lenique et al. 1997).

Disadvantages of CPAP therapy

1 With any circuit that includes the use of positive end expiratory pressure (PEEP) there is the possibility of reduction in cardiac output; however, spontaneous ventilation decreases both the incidence and severity of this complication (Oh 1997).
2 There is a danger of vomiting and aspiration of gastric contents due to gastric insufflation, although this is minimized when used in awake patients, or by the insertion of an oro/nasogastric tube (Schumaker et al. 1996).
3 Damage to skin integrity due to pressure from the tightly fitting face mask; the sites particularly vulnerable are the bridge of the nose and over the ears.

Paediatric circuits

A child's compliance with oxygen masks or cannulae may be limited, requiring other devices to be used. Some examples of these are listed below:

1 *Headbox or hood.* Oxygen can be delivered to infants and small children using a headbox or hood. The clear plastic box is fitted carefully over the child's head, encasing the head and neck. It is essential to monitor the oxygen concentration near the face to enable an accurate assessment of FiO_2 (Oh 1997).
2 *Oxygen tent/cot.* An oxygen tent can be used to supply oxygen therapy to larger children. The child is placed in a clear plastic tent which fits over the bed. The humidified oxygen supply is then directed into the tent. The advantages with the oxygen tent are that the child has freedom from any device over the face, and high degrees of humidity can be reached which may be especially useful in obstructive conditions, e.g. croup (Allan 1988). The main disadvantages are the difficulty in maintaining a constant oxygen concentration (Oh 1997) and decreased access to the child for the family and carers.

Tracheostomy mask

Tracheostomy masks perform in a similar way to the simple semirigid plastic face mask, outlined above. The mask is placed over the tracheostomy tube or stoma, and the patient will receive less oxygen than is delivered as it will be diluted by room air (Oh 1997).

Mechanical ventilation

Mechanical ventilation is indicated when there is reversible acute respiratory failure. The decision to use mechanical ventilation will be made after an assessment of respiratory mechanics, oxygenation and ventilation (Oh 1997). A wide range of ventilators are available and they all have slight differences of application but fall into two major groups:

1 Positive pressure ventilators – these are the most widely used for the acute treatment of adults and children.
2 Negative pressure ventilators – these are used much more rarely (usually for patients with chronic neurological problems such as poliomyelitis and some forms of muscular dystrophy) (Hinds 1988). (For a detailed outline of respiratory therapy using mechanical ventilation, see Hinds 1988; Oh 1997.)

Hyperbaric respiratory therapy

Hyperbaric respiratory therapy is used mainly in the treatment of skin lesions and soft tissue injury and has also been used more recently for the patient with multiple sclerosis. The therapy is designed to administer 100% oxygen at a range of pressures greater than atmospheric pressure.

Hyperbaric therapy can be used topically or systemically depending on the patient's need, and the treatment is usually intermittent over a period of weeks or months (Oh 1997).

Humidification

Humidity is the amount of water vapour present in a gaseous environment (Oh 1997). For the purpose of clinical application, humidity is usually divided into absolute and relative humidity. Absolute humidity is a measurement of the total mass of water in a specified volume of gas at a known temperature. Relative humidity is the ratio (expressed as a percentage) of the mass of water in a given volume of gas (as above) to the mass of water required to saturate the same volume of gas at a given temperature (Oh 1997).

Normally, the air travelling through the airways is warmed, moistened and filtered by the columnar mucus-secreting epithelial cells of the nasopharynx (Foss 1990). The air entering the trachea will have a relative humidity of about 90% and a temperature of between 32 and 36°C. The humidification and warming process then continues down the airways so that at the alveoli it is fully saturated at 37°C (Oh 1997).

The humidification pathway is necessary to compensate for the normal loss of water from the respiratory tract (about 250 ml under resting conditions) (Oh 1997). If the humidification apparatus is impaired due to disease such as upper respiratory tract infection or dehydration, alternative methods of humidification may need to be considered (Schumaker *et al.* 1996).

Respiratory therapy will compound these problems because the added gas will cause further dehydration of the mucous membranes and pulmonary secretions, making it more difficult for the patient to expectorate (Foss 1990). External humidification is essential when respiratory therapy is being delivered to a patient whose physiological humidification has been bypassed by an endotracheal or tracheostomy tube (Oh 1997).

Methods of humidification

Many devices can be used to supply humidification; the best of these will fulfil the following requirements:

1 The inspired gas must be delivered to the trachea at a room temperature of 32–36°C and should have a water content of 33–43 g/m^3 (Oh 1997).
2 The set temperature should remain constant; humidification and temperature should not be affected by large ranges of flow.
3 The device should have a safety and alarm system to guard against overheating, overhydration and electric shocks.
4 It is important that the appliance should not increase resistance or affect the compliance to respiration.
5 It is essential that whichever device is selected, wide-bore tubing (elephant tubing) must be used to allow efficient formation of water vapour.

Devices for humidification

1 *Condensers*. These are also known as heat and moisture exchangers or 'Swedish nose'. They perform the function of the nasopharynx, retaining the heat and water from expired gas through condensation and returning them to the inspired gas. A new range of disposable condensers are now widely used to humidify oxygen delivered through an endotracheal or tracheostomy tube, but heated humidifiers may still be preferred for long-term use (Oh 1997).
2 *Cold water bubble humidifier*. This device delivers partially humidified oxygen that is about 50% relative humidity. Its use is not advised as it is so inefficient (Oh 1997).
3 *Water bath humidifiers*. With these devices, inspired gas is forced over or through a heated reservoir of water. To achieve an adequate humidity for the patient, the water bath must reach temperatures of 45–60°C. The gas will then cool as it moves down the breathing circuit to the patient, and a relative humidity of 100% will be reached. Hot water bath humidifiers are therefore very efficient and useful in the care of the immobile patient, particularly to humidify when the patient is receiving mechani-

cal ventilatory support. However, they have four main disadvantages:

(a) Danger of overheating and causing damage to the trachea.
(b) Their efficiency can alter with changes in gas flow rate, surface area and the water temperature.
(c) Condensation and collection of water in the oxygen delivery tubes.
(d) The possibility of microcontamination of stagnant water (Tinker & Zapol 1992).

4 *Aerosol generators.* These devices are not governed by temperature, but provide microdroplets of water suspended in the gas (Oh 1997). The gas provided through aerosol devices can be very highly saturated with water, especially when ultrasonic nebulizers are used. There are three main types of aerosol humidifier:

(a) Gas-drive nebulizer
(b) Mechanical (spinning disc) nebulizer
(c) Ultrasonic nebulizer.

These devices are useful for the spontaneously breathing patient with chronic chest disease.

References and further reading

Allan, D. (1988) Making sense of oxygen delivery. *Nurs Times*, **83**(18), 40–42.

Allison, R.C. (1991) Initial treatment of pulmonary oedema: a physiological approach. *Am J Med Sci*, **302**(6), 385–91.

Beaumont, M., Lejeune, D., Marlotte, H. & Lofaso, F. (1997) Effects of chest wall counter pressures on lung mechanics under high level of CPAP in humans. *J Physiology*, **83**(2), 591–8.

Edwards, D. (1988) Principles of oxygen transport. *Care Crit Ill*, **4**(5), 13–16.

Ehrhardt, B.S. & Graham, M. (1990) Making sense of oxygen delivery. *Nursing* (US), March, 50–54.

Foss, M.A. (1990) Oxygen therapy. *Prof Nurse*, January, 180–90.

Greeg, R.W. *et al.* (1990) Continuous positive airway pressure by face mask in *Pneumocystis carinii* pneumonia. *Crit Care Med*, **18**(1), 21–4.

Greenbaum, D.M., Synder, J.V., Grenvik, A.K.E. & Safar, P. (1976) Continuous positive airways pressure without tracheal intubation in spontaneously breathing patients. *Chest*, **69**, 615–20.

Gregg, R.W., Bruce, C., Fieldman, M.D. *et al.* (1990) Continuous positive airway pressure by face mask in *Pneumocystis carinii* pneumonia. *Crit Care Med*, **18**(1), 21–4.

Higgins, J. (1990) Pulmonary oxygen toxicity. *Physiotherapy*, **76**(10), 588–92.

Hinds, C.J. (1988) *Intensive Care. A Concise Textbook*. Baillière Tindall, London.

Keilty, S.E. & Bott, J. (1992) Continuously positive airway pressure. *Physiotherapy*, **78**(2), 90–92.

Lenique, F., Habis, M., Lofasof, F. *et al.* (1997) Ventilatory and haemodynamic effects of continuous positive airway pressure in heart failure. *Am J Resp Crit Care Med*, **155**, 500–505.

Lin, E. & Hanning, C.D. (1994) Artificial ventilation of the lungs. *Anaesthesia*, **1**, 526–52.

Marieb, E.N. (1996) *Human Anatomy and Physiology*. Benjamin Cummings, California.

Miller, R. & Semple, S. (1991) Continous positive airway pressure ventilation for respiratory failure associated with *Pneumocystis carinii* pneumonia. *Resp Med*, **85**, 133–8.

Oh, T.E. (1997) *Intensive Care Manual*. Butterworths, Sydney.

Placer, B. (1997) Using airway pressure. *Nurs Times*, **93**(31), 42–4.

Romand, J.A. & Donald, F. (1995) Physiological effects of continuous positive airway pressure ventilation in the critically ill. *Care Crit Ill*, **11**(6), 239–42.

Schumaker, W.C., Ayres, S.M., Grevik, A. & Holbrook, P.R. (1996) *Textbook of Critical Care*, pp. 628–952. W.B. Saunders, Philadelphia.

Smith, C.E., Mayer, L.S., Metsiker, C. *et al.* (1998) Continuous positive airway pressure patient caregivers learning needs and barriers to use. *Heart Lung*, **27**(2).

Stock, M.C., Downs, J.B. & Corkran, R.R.T. (1984) Pulmonary function before and after prolonged continuous positive airway pressure by mask. *Crit Care Med*, **12**(11), 973–4.

Tinker, J. & Zapol, W. (1992) *Care of the Critically Ill Patient*. Springer, New York.

Williamson, D.C. & Modell, J.H. (1972) Intermittent continuous airways pressure by mask – its use in the treatment of atelectasis. *Arch Surg*, **177**, 970–72.

GUIDELINES · Pre-continuous positive airway pressure (CPAP)

Procedure

Action	Rationale
1 Explain the principle of CPAP to the patient and where possible show the patient the CPAP system.	To minimize anxiety and aid in patient compliance.
2 Observe and record the following: (a) Patient's respiratory function and his or her ability to maintain own airway	To obtain a baseline of respiratory function.
(b) Colour, skin, etc.	To observe for any change in respiratory function.
(c) Respiratory rate (d) Oxygen saturation.	
3 Check if arterial catheter is in situ.	In order to take sample to measure gas analysis.
4 Observe and record the patient's cardiovascular function, including:	To obtain a baseline in order to assess any change in conditions (see Chap. 28, Observations).

Guidelines • Pre-continuous positive airway pressure (CPAP) (cont'd)

Action	Rationale
(a) Heart rate	
(b) Blood pressure.	
5 Assess patient's conscious level.	To obtain a baseline and to be able to assess for change in condition (see Chap. 26, Neurological Observations).
6 Assess patient's level of anxiety.	To enable an assessment to be made and, where necessary, a referral to medical staff.

GUIDELINES • Setting up continuous positive airway pressure (CPAP)

Equipment

1 Oxygen supply.
2 Compressed air supply.
3 Flow generator.
4 Oxycheck.
5 Prepared CPAP circuit.
6 Y-connector.
7 T-piece.

8 Humidifier.
9 Temperature probe.
10 Water trap.
11 CPAP mask.
12 Headstrap.
13 PEEP valves (2.5/5.0/7.5/10.0 cm).

See diagram of circuits (Fig. 35.8).

Action	Rationale
1 Set up CPAP circuit.	
2 Ensure patient is in a comfortable position, sitting up in bed, well supported by a pillow.	To promote comfort and aid lung expansion and breathing.
3 Ensure patient is comfortable in surrounding environment.	To promote comfort and aid in compliance with using CPAP.
4 Explain to patient how the mask is to be applied. Apply mask gently, applying pressure as the patient adapts to the tight fitting mask. Hold mask until patient is comfortable and settled.	To relieve anxiety and to reassure patient. To aid patient's compliance with CPAP.
5 Once the patient is settled with mask, apply the headstrap. Ensure mask and headstrap are comfortable for the patient; alter position as required.	To retain mask in place and aid patient comfort.
6 Ensure a good seal and that no leaks are present.	To ensure a tight seal in order that the system functions optimally.
7 Apply protective field dressing around vulnerable pressure points: nose, ear, back of head and neck.	To alleviate pressure and prevent tissue breakdown.

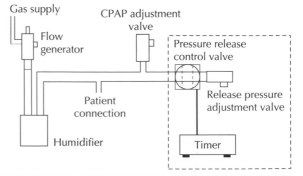

Figure 35.8 Diagram of circuits.

8 Give further explanation to family/next of kin of how CPAP works and the importance of their presence and participation in communication.

To relieve anxiety.

9 Reassure the patient constantly.

10 Discuss with doctor use of medication that might aid the patient in compliance with CPAP therapy.

To relieve patient anxiety and promote cooperation.

Nursing care plan

Problem	Cause	Suggested action
Maintenance of airway.	Deteriorating respiratory function. Physical tiring.	Continuously monitor respiratory function: skin colour; breathing pattern; respiratory rate; oxygen saturation; blood gases if arterial catheter in situ. Report changes to medical or anaesthetic staff.
Cardiovascular instability.	Hypotension. Arrhythmias. Decreasing central venous pressure. Decreasing cardiac output due to CPAP.	Continuously monitor cardiovascular function: heart rate; blood pressure. Continuously monitor central venous pressure. Report changes to medical staff.
Dehydration	Decreased oral intake. Decreased circulating volume. Nausea and vomiting.	Maintain an accurate fluid balance chart measuring input of both oral and intravenous fluids. Check overall balance on an hourly basis. Report to medical staff who may order intravenous fluid therapy. Prescribe antiemetic.
Fluid overload: May present with pulmonary oedema. Retention of urine.	Sepsis. Cardiac failure.	Observe and assess patient. Maintain accurate fluid balance chart. Report to medical staff, who may order a diuretic. Undertake further assessment of fluid balance. Catheterize patient if unable to pass urine. Carry out accurate assessment of output.
Inadequate dietary intake.	Gastric distension due to CPAP. Loss of appetite. Difficulty in eating; distress caused by respiratory status and CPAP. Nausea and vomiting	Encourage diet of oral supplementary fluids. If unable to take orally, refer to dietitian and doctor; an alternative method of feeding may be considered, e.g. nasogastric feeding. Administer antiemetic. Encourage and reassure patient.
Aspiration, if unable to maintain own airway.	Inability to maintain own airway. Continuous pressure from CPAP system. Insufflation of air.	Observe and assess patient closely. After discussion with medical staff the following actions should be considered: insert nasogastric tube; use clear CPAP mask.
Gastric distension and discomfort may cause nausea and vomiting.	Continuous pressure from CPAP system. Insufflation of air.	Encourage patient to belch to relieve air if it aids comfort. Insert nasogastric tube.
Dry mouth.	CPAP system utilizes a very high oxygen flow which has a drying effect.	Carry out regular mouth care (see Chap. 24, Mouth Care). Give patient regular sips of water, ice to suck or drinks as

Problem	Cause	Suggested action
		patient is able to take. Humidify, as in CPAP circuit.

Eyes
  Dry
  Sore
  Conjunctival oedema.
	Mask – air leak.
	High flow oxygen.
	Facial pressure from mask – causing oedema.
		Ensure mask is well sealed with no leaks. Apply pressure-relieving padding around mask. Apply regular eye care (see Chap. 17, Eye Care).
		Adjust mask to facial contour.
		Alter and position mask as comfortable. Loosen mask every couple of hours to relieve pressure.
		Apply square of granuflex to bridge of nose to protect skin.

Tissue integrity problems with sacrum, elbows, heels.	Continued bed rest. Difficulty in moving. Fear of moving.	Change patient's position in bed regularly. Nurse patient on alternate sides. Patient may sit out of bed if able. Consider alternate pressure-relieving mattress if patient immobile or has high Waterlow score (see Chap. 47).
Mask incorrectly sealed.		Alter mask position to correct and ensure comfort. Ensure mask is correct size. Alter position as required to ensure correct seal.
Anxiety.	Tight-fitting mask. Feeling of claustrophobia and isolation. Fear of dying.	Reassure patient. Inform patient that nurse is present at all times and able to see patient. Inform patient of any changes taking place. Communicate with the patient's family, keep them informed and involve them in care and communication with patient. Inform doctor of patient's anxiety level. Administer anxiolytic agent if required.
Maintenance of safety of patient and environment.		Ensure nurse present with patient at all times.
Communication. Inability to communicate effectively.		Observe patient and CPAP system closely to ensure equipment is working adequately and there is no failure of the system. Reassure patient and ensure he or she is comfortable.

Scalp Cooling

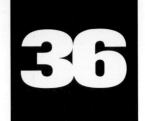

Definition

Scalp cooling is a method of reducing scalp temperature and causing constriction of blood vessels, thus decreasing the amount of drug that can pass into the hair follicles and reducing cellular uptake of the drug.

Indications

The effectiveness of scalp cooling has been demonstrated satisfactorily with doxorubicin, epirubicin and docetaxel (Dean et al. 1979; Middleton et al. 1982; Robinson 1987; Lemanager et al. 1995). Patients receiving other cytotoxic drugs which may cause alopecia, such as vindesine and vincristine, have undergone the procedure, although there are insufficient data to evaluate its effectiveness with these drugs. However, scalp cooling requires the consultant's permission as the procedure may protect scalp micrometastases, especially where there is the possibility of circulating cancer cells, e.g. in cases of leukaemia and lymphoma (Witman et al. 1981). In spite of this, scalp cooling has been used successfully in patients with relapsed lymphoma (Keller & Blausey 1988; Pirohit et al. 1992). Dean et al. (1983), drawing on evidence from 7800 women with breast cancer, found that only two experienced recurrence of disease on the scalp, suggesting that the risk of scalp metastases was minimal. They concluded that scalp cooling should not be contraindicated and could be used routinely with a wide variety of solid tumours. Nevertheless, patients with advanced metastatic disease have been found to develop scalp metastases during scalp cooling and Middleton et al. (1985) argued strongly against the use of scalp cooling in this group. The most recent study found no scalp metastases at follow-up (Ron et al. 1997).

The issues relating to scalp metastases are controversial. This dilemma, along with the recent media coverage (Wilson 1994; Carr 1998), have led some practitioners to question whether scalp cooling should be offered. Patients have highlighted how they feel about hair loss (Carr 1998) and also the need to provide more comfortable and effective scalp cooling in all cancer units and centres (Wilson 1994). In addition, an extensive review of the literature concluded that scalp cooling was effective and should be offered to all patients for whom it was appropriate (Crowe et al. 1998). This was supported by the views of many nurses who felt that the use of scalp cooling with chemotherapy protocols which are associated with hair loss can effectively prevent alopecia and result in improved quality of life for patients (Lemanager et al. 1998).

Reference material

Alopecia has been singled out as the most distressing side-effect of cancer chemotherapy (Tierney 1987; Carr 1998). It has been identified as such a devastating prospect that some patients may refuse to accept treatment (Tierney 1987). Hair loss can also result in changes to the patient's body image which may not be improved by the regrowth of hair (Munstedt et al. 1997). Several techniques have been tested to prevent chemotherapy-induced hair loss, the first being scalp tourniquets. These were used to minimize the contact the drug had with the hair follicles by occluding, using pressure, the superficial blood vessels supplying the scalp (Maxwell 1980). However, while some investigators found scalp tourniquets effective, others reported this method to be time-consuming, uncomfortable or ineffective (Parker 1987). Research findings indicate that scalp hypothermia may be simpler, less traumatic and more effective as a means of preventing alopecia when compared with the scalp tourniquet (David & Speechley 1987). Scalp cooling has an advantage over the scalp tourniquet in that it inhibits the cellular uptake of a drug that is temperature dependent (Dean et al. 1979).

The scientific rationale for scalp cooling

The rationale is based on characteristics of hair growth, the effect of cytotoxic drugs on hair follicles, physiological changes in scalp circulation and pharmacokinetics (Keller & Blausey 1988). Ninety percent of all scalp hair is in an active phase of growth. The growth phase is characterized by significant mitotic activity, thus rendering the hair bulb especially sensitive to chemotherapeutic agents (Parker 1987). Scalp hypothermia produces changes in the scalp circulation by causing vasoconstriction of superficial vessels. Decreased blood flow to the scalp reduces the amount of the drug reaching the hair follicles and thus minimizes damage to the scalp hair (Kennedy et al. 1983; Parker 1987). Its success is also related to the metabolic effects of cooling, i.e. slowing the metabolic rate (Bulow et al. 1985), and it also appears that the degree of hair loss is temperature dependent. In order to prevent alopecia the temperature of the scalp must be reduced to at least 24°C but preferably 22°C (Gregory et al. 1982). The cap should be kept in a freezer overnight (Robinson 1987) in order to reach temperatures of −18 to −20°C (Anderson et al. 1981; Kennedy et al. 1983; Robinson 1987; Giacone 1988). Then when the cap is placed on the head the scalp temperature will drop from 37°C to 23–24°C within the first 15 minutes (Hallet 1981; Guy *et al.* 1982; Tollenaar *et al.* 1994). This is why a preinjection scalp cooling time of 20–30 minutes is said to be required (Anderson *et al.* 1981; Kennedy *et al.* 1983; Satterwhite & Zimm 1984; Middleton *et al.* 1985; Robinson 1987; Giacone 1988).

Types of drugs

Doxorubin is commonly used in cancer chemotherapy and has a uniquely short half-life of approximately 30 minutes (compared to other drugs, such as cyclophosphamide which has a plasma half-life of over 6 hours). This factor makes prophylactic scalp cooling feasible because it need only be utilized during peak plasma levels (Cline 1984). This is particularly important since doxorubicin results in a consistently high incidence of alopecia (80–90% of all patients), often leading to total hair loss (Welch & Lewis 1980). The involvement of doxorubicin, whether used alone or in combination, is a feature of most of the reported scalp cooling studies. In some studies, there was less success in maintaining hair with increasing doses of doxorubicin and/or liver metastases (Dean *et al.* 1983; David & Speechley 1987), but this may be resolved by extending the time the cap remains in place following chemotherapy administration.

Scalp cooling has also been used during the administration of epirubicin, as a single agent, with good results (Robinson 1987), although doses may influence outcomes (Adams *et al.* 1992). Subsequent studies have investigated combination regimens containing epirubicin and other drugs such as cyclophosphamide and 5-fluorouracil, with results of mild to moderate hair loss. However, when intravenous cyclophosphamide is added to any single agent anthracycline, the success rate is reduced from 80% of patients keeping most of their hair to about 50–60% of patients (Middleton *et al.* 1985; David & Speechley 1987). Some authors have therefore concluded that when combinations of cyclophosphamide and anthracyclines are given, scalp cooling had no place at all (Tollenaar *et al.* 1994). A relatively new group of drugs known as the taxanes also have the unfortunate side-effect of total alopecia; however, evidence has been produced to show that using scalp cooling in patients receiving docetaxel can prevent complete hair loss (Lemanager *et al.* 1995, 1997).

Techniques

Initially scalp cooling was achieved using crushed ice in plastic bags (Dean *et al.* 1979). A study of the efficacy of using a moulded prefrozen ice cap handmade from cryogel bags was conducted at The Royal Marsden Hospital (Anderson *et al.* 1981). The project involved 31 patients, 29 of whom had advanced breast cancer; 22 of the 28 patients who continued scalp cooling after the first cycle achieved what was described as 'socially acceptable hair protection', i.e. they did not require a wig. Failures were attributed in part to liver function abnormality and success

to the emphasis on consistency and rigour with the scalp cooling techniques. In addition, an analysis of data from 180 patients at The Royal Marsden Hospital (David & Speechley 1987) confirmed that severe alopecia was consistently prevented in patients on doxorubicin alone (70%), with encouraging results for patients on other combinations of cytotoxic drugs. Most of the studies that used an ice cap method of scalp cooling used a 'homemade' or commercial cap (Anderson *et al.* 1981; Dean *et al.* 1983; David & Speechley 1987; Lemanager *et al.* 1997).

Commercial caps

The first commercial cap (Kold Kap) was successful in reducing hair loss, particularly with higher doses of doxorubicin (Dean *et al.* 1981, 1983). A three-layer cap (inner cotton, middle cryogel, outer lamb's wool) was also reported to prevent total hair loss (Howard & Stenner 1983). However, Wheelock *et al.* (1984) found that most patients suffered from severe hair loss even with the use of the Kold Kap.

Recent attempts have been made to produce an alternative type of cap that would improve effectiveness of scalp cooling, in particular to achieve a temperature that ensures a sufficiently low and constant reduction in scalp temperature that would endure during the entire procedure. Two types of scalp cooling machines have been designed: (1) a thermocirculator system with a more reliable temperature control (coolant pumped between two layers of a lightweight cap) initially produced encouraging results in combination therapy (Guy *et al.* 1982). However, in spite of using this machine, it has been found that in patients receiving fluorouracil, epirubicin and cyclophosphamide (FEC) as a combination there was still a 50% chance of total alopecia occurring (Tollenaar *et al.* 1994). (2) The use of refrigerated air passed over the patient's scalp via a hair-drying helmet was reported to be beneficial in over 50% of patients, with most experiencing no hair loss or slight hair loss and six requiring a wig (Symonds & McCormick 1986). However, other authors found that the system was only successful at lower doses of epirubicin (Adams *et al.* 1992).

Most recent work has involved the use of the Chemocap (a commercially made cryogel cap), which has been used by patients receiving single agent and combinations of anthracyclines, as well as those receiving docetaxel and has been very successful (Lemanager *et al.* 1995, 1997). There have also been good results using an electrically cooled cap in patients receiving CMF (cyclophosphamide methotrexate fluorouracil) chemotherapy (Ron *et al.* 1997).

The success of all these methods in preventing hair loss varies and the amount of hair loss experienced by the patient is dependent on a number of factors:

1 Involvement of the liver with metastatic disease leads to elevated plasma levels of doxorubicin for a longer period. Extension of the cooling period does not seem to improve the results (Satterwhite & Zimm 1984).
2 Inadequate cooling because of exceptionally thick hair may lead to partial loss. It has been demonstrated that

maximum cooling occurs 20 minutes after the cap has been placed in position. The weight of the cap (as well as the temperature) is a factor, as this ensures that the contact is maintained over the complete scalp (Hunt *et al.* 1982). Success does not appear to be dose dependent, as was first thought (David & Speechley 1987).

3 It seems likely that when anthracyclines are used in combination with other drugs that cause alopecia (e.g. etoposide and cyclophosphamide) the success rate is not as high as with anthracyclines alone (Middleton *et al.* 1985; Tierney 1991).

Patient selection

All patients with solid tumours receiving doxorubicin, epirubicin or docetaxel as a single agent or in combination should be offered scalp cooling. However, scalp cooling should not be offered to:

1 Patients with haematological disease unless the consultant feels it is appropriate to offer scalp cooling on the basis of quality of life;
2 Patients receiving drugs that cause hair loss, e.g. etoposide, vincristine, paclitaxel, where there is no research or evidence of the effectiveness of scalp cooling;
3 Patients who have already received a first course of chemotherapy which may induce hair loss but who were not offered or declined scalp cooling.

Patients must consent when they have been fully informed about the nature and length of the procedure, and the chances of success. Scalp cooling can be a long and uncomfortable procedure and should not be offered unless it is beneficial or the patient insists on undergoing the procedure even after a full explanation regarding the lack of any benefit. Patients must also be informed that they may discontinue the procedure at any time if they find it too physically or psychologically traumatic (Tierney 1987) or if they fail to retain hair.

Research shows that scalp cooling can be very distressing (Tierney *et al.* 1989), and work has now been carried out into how patients feel about the procedure and whether they find it worthwhile. In a small study (n = 30), 50% of patients found scalp cooling worthwhile and 70% would undergo the procedure again in order to prevent hair loss (Dougherty 1996). Patients have reported adverse effects during and following treatment, such as headaches, claustrophobia and 'ice phobias' (Tierney *et al.* 1989).

Patients who have relapsed and are undergoing further chemotherapy which causes alopecia may find the loss of hair a second time to be more devastating (Gallagher 1996). It is important therefore to ensure that if a patient fails to retain hair or decides not to undergo scalp cooling, adequate time is spent helping the patient to adapt to the hair loss physically, psychologically and socially. This can be partly achieved by ensuring that the patient sees the surgical appliance officer as soon as possible, in order to obtain a wig that can be matched to the patient's desired hair style and colour. Advice can be given on hair care and various ideas of hats, turbans and scarves, and reinforced with a hair care information booklet.

References and further reading

Adams, L. *et al.* (1992) The prevention of hair loss from chemotherapy by the use of cold air scalp cooling. *Eur J Cancer Care*, **15**, 16–18.

Anderson, J. *et al.* (1981) Prevention of doxorubicin-induced alopecia by scalp cooling in patients with advanced breast cancer. *Br Med J*, **282**, 423–4.

Baxley, K.O. *et al.* (1984) Alopecia: effect on cancer patients' body image. *Cancer Nurs*, December, 499–503.

Bulow, J. *et al.* (1985) Frontal subcutaneous blood flow and epi- and subcutaneous temperatures during scalp cooling in normal man. *Scand J Clin Lab Invest*, **45**, 505–508.

Carr, K. (1998) How I survived the fall out. *You Magazine, Mail on Sunday*, 10 May, 61–7.

Cline, B.W. (1984) Prevention of chemotherapy-induced alopecia; a review of the literature. *Cancer Nurs*, June, 221–8.

Crowe, M., Kendrick, M. & Woods, S. (1998) *Is scalp cooling a procedure that should be offered to patients receiving alopecia induced chemotherapy for solid tumours?* Proceedings of 10th International Conference on Cancer Nursing, Jerusalem, Abstract, p. 64.

David, J.A. & Speechley, V. (1987) Scalp cooling to prevent alopecia. *Nurs Times*, **83**(32), 36–7.

Dean, J.C. *et al.* (1979) Prevention of doxorubicin-induced hair loss with scalp hypothermia. *New Engl J Med*, **301**, 1427–9.

Dean, J.C. *et al.* (1981) Scalp hypothermia: a comparison of ice packs and the Kold Kap in the prevention of adriamycin induced alopecia. *Proc 17th Annu Meeting Am Soc Clin Oncol*, **22**, 253–4.

Dean, J.C. *et al.* (1983) Scalp hypothermia: a comparison of ice packs and the Kold Kap in the prevention of doxorubicin induced alopecia. *J Clin Oncol*, **1**(1), 33–7.

Dougherty, L. (1996) Scalp cooling to prevent hair loss in chemotherapy. *Prof Nurse*, **11**(8), 1–3.

Freedman, T.G. (1994) Social and cultural dimensions of hair loss in women treated for breast cancer. *Cancer Nurs*, **17**(4), 334–41.

Gallagher, J. (1996) *Women's experiences of hair loss associated with chemotherapy – longitudinal perspective.* Proceedings of 9th International Conference on Cancer Nursing, Brighton, Abstract, p. 52.

Giacone, G. *et al.* (1988) Scalp hypothermia in the prevention of doxorubicin induced hair loss. *Cancer Nurs*, **11**(3), 170–73.

Gregory, R.P. *et al.* (1982) Prevention of doxorubicin induced alopecia by scalp hypothermia: relation to degree of cooling. *Br Med J*, **284**, 1674.

Guy, R. *et al.* (1982) Scalp cooling by thermocirculator. *Lancet*, 24 April, 937–8.

Hallett, N. (1981) Preventing fall out. *Nurs Mirror*, 5 March, 32–3.

Howard, N. & Stenner, R.W. (1983) Technical notes – an improved 'ice cap' to prevent alopecia caused by adriamycin (doxorubicin). *Br J Radiol*, **56**, 963–4.

Hunt, J. *et al.* (1982) Scalp hypothermia to prevent adriamycin-induced hair loss. *Cancer Nurs*, **5**(1), 25–31.

Keller, J.F. & Blausey, L.A. (1988) Nursing issues and management in chemotherapy-induced alopecia. *Oncol Nurs Forum*, **15**(5), 603–607.

Kennedy, M. *et al.* (1983) The effects of using Chemocap on occurrence of chemotherapy induced alopecia. *Oncol Nurs Forum*, **10**(1), 19–24.

Lemanager, M. *et al.* (1995) Docetaxel induced alopecia can be prevented. *Lancet*, **346**, 371–2.

Lemanager, M. *et al.* (1997) Effectiveness of cold cap in the prevention of docetaxel induced alopecia. *Eur J Cancer*, **33**(2), 297–300.

Lemanager, M. *et al.* (1998) Alopecia induced chemotherapy – a controllable side effect. *Oncol Nurs Today*, **3**(2), 18–20.

Maxwell, M.B. (1980) Scalp tourniquets for chemotherapy-induced alopecia. *Am J Nurs*, **5**, 900–902.

Middleton, J. *et al.* (1982) Prevention of doxorubicin-induced alopecia by scalp hypothermia: relation to degree of cooling. *Br Med J*, **284**, 1674.

Middleton, J. *et al.* (1985) Failure of scalp hypothermia to prevent hair loss when cyclophosphamide is added to doxorubicin and vincristine. *Cancer Treat Rep*, **69**(4), 373–5.

Munstedt, K. *et al.* (1997) Changes in self concept and body image during alopecia induced cancer chemotherapy. *Supp Care Cancer*, **5**, 139–43.

Parker, R. (1987) The effectiveness of scalp hypothermia in preventing cyclophosphamide induced alopecia. *Oncol Nurs Forum*, **14**(6), 49–53.

Pirohit, O.P. *et al.* (1992) A six week chemotherapy regimen for relapsed lymphoma efficacy results and the influence of scalp cooling. *Ann Oncol*, **3** (Suppl. 5), 126.

Robinson, M.H. (1987) Effectiveness of scalp cooling in reducing alopecia caused by epirubicin treatment of advanced breast cancer. *Cancer Treat Rep*, **71**, 913–14.

Ron, I.G. *et al.* (1997) Scalp cooling in the prevention of alopecia in patients receiving depilating chemotherapy. *Supp Care Cancer*, **5**, 136–8.

Satterwhite, B. & Zimm, S. (1984) The use of scalp hypothermia in the prevention of doxorubicin-induced hair loss. *Cancer*, **54**, 34–7.

Symonds, R.P. & McCormick, C.V. (1986) Adriamycin alopecia prevented by cold air scalp cooling. *Am J Clin Oncol*, **9**(5), 454–7.

Tierney, A.J. (1987) Preventing chemotherapy-induced alopecia in cancer patients: is scalp cooling worthwhile? *J Adv Nurs*, **12**, 303–310.

Tierney, A.J. (1991) Chemotherapy-induced hair loss. *Nurs Stand*, **5**(38), 29–31.

Tierney, A.J. *et al.* (1989) *A Study to Inform Nursing Support of Patients Coping with Chemotherapy for Breast Cancer.* Report prepared for the Scottish Home and Health Department.

Tollenaar, R.A.E.M. *et al.* (1994) Scalp cooling has no place in the prevention of alopecia in adjuvant chemotherapy in breast cancer. *Eur J Cancer*, **30A**(10), 1448–53.

Wagner, L. & Bye, M.G. (1979) Body image and patients experiencing alopecia as a result of cancer chemotherapy. *Cancer Nurs*, **2**, 365–9.

Welch, D. & Lewis, K. (1980) Alopecia and chemotherapy. *Am J Nurs*, **80**, 903–905.

Wheelock, J.B. *et al.* (1984) Ineffectiveness of scalp hypothermia in the prevention of alopecia in patients treated with doxorubicin and cisplatin combinations. *Cancer Treat Rep*, **68**, 1387–8.

Wilson, C. (1994) The ice cap that could help save your hair. *Daily Mail*, September 20, 36–7.

Witman, G. *et al.* (1981) Misuse of scalp hypothermia. *Cancer Treat Rep*, **65**(5–6), 507–508.

GUIDELINES • Scalp cooling

Equipment

1 A scalp cooling cap:
   (a) Commercial make.
   (b) Homemade from eight hot/cold packs. These must be taped together and moulded around a wig stand (Fig. 36.1). When bandaged in position, the cap is placed in a deep freeze (temperature approximately −18°C) for 24 h.

2 Ear protection – gauze, cotton wool pads.
3 Two crepe bandages (10 and 15 cm wide).
4 Two towels.
5 Comfortable chair (recliner) or bed.
6 Extra pillows and blankets as required.

Procedure

Action	Rationale
1 Before beginning, it is important to explain and discuss the procedure fully with the patient. The patient should understand that the scalp cooling can be discontinued at any time and that it will not jeopardize the chemotherapy.	To ensure that the patient understands the procedure and what the success rate is likely to be depending on the type of chemotherapy regimen he/she is receiving. To ensure that the patient gives his/her valid consent and knows

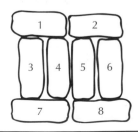

Figure 36.1 Format of hot/cold packs prior to moulding.

		that if the scalp cooling does not work, he/she can obtain a wig.
2	Check the cap has been in the deep freeze for 24 h.	To ensure the cap is cold enough to be effective.
3	Wet patient's hair thoroughly.	To aid conduction of coldness and to aid with fitting of cap.
4	Place the ear protection in position.	To prevent cold injury.
5	Soak one crepe bandage in cold water and use it to bandage the patient's head tightly. The bandage should be applied evenly and should provide a thin layer over the scalp.	To compress the hair and prevent any air being trapped between the cap and scalp. To aid conduction of coldness.
6	Place the cap on the patient's head, making sure it fits closely and covers the whole hairline.	To ensure cooling over the head, including all the hair roots.
7	Add supplementary packs if necessary.	To ensure adequate cooling of the scalp.
8	Bandage the cap in place.	To maintain even and close contact of the cap to the scalp.
9	Add pillows, etc. as required.	To provide support for the patient's head and neck and to reduce the effect of the heaviness of the cap (approximately 2–3 kg).
10	Place a dry towel around the patient's shoulders.	To catch any water as the cap defrosts.
11	Offer the patient the use of a blanket.	To provide the patient with some protection against the feeling of cold.
12	Leave the patient for at least 15 min before injection of the drug.	To obtain initial cooling of the scalp.
13	Administer the drug by intravenous injection as per prescription.	To administer treatment as appropriate.
14	On completion of the drug (i.e. the one likely to cause alopecia, e.g. doxorubicin), leave the patient for a further 45 min.	To maintain cooling until the plasma levels of drug have fallen (Hunt *et al.* 1982).
15	When sufficient time has elapsed, remove the cap and bandages carefully.	To prevent damage to the scalp and hair.
16	Encourage the patient to rest, if desired.	To prevent faintness due to the weight being lifted off.
17	Towel the patient's hair dry.	To prevent damage to the hair. To ensure that the patient is comfortable and has a chance to rearrange hair before leaving hospital.
18	Ensure the patient is given a hair care information booklet in order to care for hair correctly between treatments.	To reinforce verbal information given during procedure.

Nursing care plan

Problem	Cause	Suggested action
Inadequate cooling.	Poorly fitting cap. Cap not sufficiently cooled.	Follow the procedure carefully. Ensure the cap size is correct and that the hair roots are covered. If the patient has very thick hair, use the heaviest cap available. Check the cap has been cooled to the corrected temperature.
Excess cooling.	Thin hair.	Use extra layers of bandages between the cap and scalp. If it is still painful then discontinue the procedure.

Problem	Cause	Suggested action
Complaints of headache.	Weight and coldness of cap.	Provide physical support to the neck and shoulders and blankets as required.
Distressed patient.	Claustrophobia.	Support and reassure the patient. If necessary, remove the cap.
	Ice phobia.	Be aware of this possible problem; encourage the patient to discuss feelings.
Hair loss.	Scalp cooling was not successful.	Offer the patient the opportunity to discontinue the scalp cooling. Make arrangements for the patient to see the appliance officer and obtain a wig. Discuss care of hair and scalp and give patient information booklet.

Specimen Collection for Microbiological Analysis

Definition

Specimen collection is the collection of a required amount of tissue or fluid for laboratory examination, to allow for the isolation and identification of micro-organisms that cause disease, and to determine their antibiotic sensitivity to guide the doctor with the selection of appropriate antibiotic therapy (Woods & Washington 1995).

Indications

Specimen collection is required when microbiological, biochemical or other laboratory investigations are indicated. Nursing staff should be able to identify the need for microbiological investigations and, if appropriate, initiate the taking of specimens (Papasian & Kragel 1997). Specimen collection is often a first crucial step in investigations that define the nature of the disease and determine diagnosis and the mode of treatment.

The clinical microbiology laboratory plays a fundamental role in the diagnosis of infection. Its importance increases in immunosuppressed patients because the usual signs and symptoms may be absent (Kiehn *et al.* 1989) and because infection is the cause of significant morbidity and mortality (Sandin & Rinaldi 1996).

Reference material

General principles

Successful laboratory diagnosis depends on the collection of specimens at the appropriate time, using the correct technique and equipment and transporting them to the designated laboratory safely without delay. For this to be achieved, good liaison is essential between medical, nursing, portering and laboratory staff.

The first step in the accurate diagnosis of infectious disease is to obtain adequate specimens for microbiological examination. Therefore the sample must be representative of the disease process (Thys *et al.* 1994). Signs of infection such as fever should trigger a careful clinical assessment to ensure the most useful laboratory samples are obtained (O'Grady *et al.* 1998).

The nurse's role is:

1 To identify the need for and importance of microbiological investigation.
2 To initiate, if appropriate, the taking of a swab or specimen, e.g. during wound dressing it is usually the nurse who identifies signs of infection.
3 To know the appropriate investigation to be undertaken so as to avoid indiscriminate specimen collection which wastes time and money.
4 To collect the desired material in the correct container.
5 To arrange prompt delivery to the laboratory.

Close communication between the doctor and the laboratory is important, especially when unusual infections are suspected or the patient is immunosuppressed, as the infection may be caused by unusual organisms whose identification requires special techniques (Kiehn *et al.* 1989).

Collection of specimens

If specimens of poor quality are sent to the microbiology department, then the results may be of little or no clinical utility (Wilson 1996). The greater the quantity of material sent for laboratory examination, the greater the chance of isolating a causative organism. Other considerations include (1) the type of organisms and (2) their growth requirements. Aerobic bacteria will grow in the presence of air (Nicas & Eisenstein 1995). Anaerobic bacteria fail to grow in air, preferring an atmosphere reduced of oxygen. Facultative bacteria can grow either in the presence or absence of air. Fastidious bacteria require selective plating media to encourage growth (Finegold 1995), and may not survive prolonged storage or may be overgrown with less fastidious organisms, before cultures can be made (Woods & Washington 1995).

There are many types of specimen collection tools, for example, swabs and pots. Advice should be sought from the microbiology department with regards to the best type of container required for unusual specimens. It is essential that the specimen and its transport container are appropriate for the infection being investigated, to ensure that adequate quantity of material is obtained to allow complete microbiological examination. Material from skin and mucous membranes can be collected by a swab, which generally contains transport medium. This is designed to preserve micro-organisms, while preventing the multiplication of rapidly growing organisms, which makes identification easier. Unfortunately only a limited amount of material can be collected by this means; therefore pus should be collected in a syringe which can be transferred to a sterile container (Wilson 1995). Biopsy material, pus, fluid or tissue removed surgically provide ideal material in adequate quantities for appropriate microbiological smears and cultures (Wood & Washington 1995).

Specimens are readily contaminated by poor technique.

Cultures taken from such specimens often result in confusing or misleading results. Aseptic technique must be used when collecting specimens to avoid inadvertent contamination of the site of sample or the specimen (Macleod 1992). Specimens must be collected in sterile containers with close-fitting lids and swabs must never be removed from their sterile containers until everything is ready for taking the sample.

Ideally, samples should be collected before beginning any treatment, e.g. antibiotics or antiseptics. If the patient is receiving such treatment at the same time the specimen is collected, the laboratory staff must be informed. Both antibiotics and antiseptics may destroy organisms that are, in fact, active in the patient and will affect the outcome of the laboratory test. Specimens should also be obtained using safe technique and practices (Hart 1991). For example, gloves should always be worn when handling all body fluids.

Documentation

Requests for microbiological investigations must include the following information:

1 Patient's name, ward and/or department.
2 Hospital number.
3 Date specimen collected.
4 Time specimen collected.
5 Diagnosis.
6 Relevant signs and symptoms.
7 Relevant history, e.g. recent foreign travel.
8 Any antimicrobial drug being taken by the patient.
9 Type of specimen.
10 Consultant's name.
11 Name of the doctor who ordered the investigation, as it may be necessary to telephone the result before the typed report is dispatched.

Without full information, it is impossible to examine a specimen adequately or to report it accurately.

Incorrectly or unlabelled specimens will normally be discarded (Health Services Advisory Committee 1991).

Transportation of specimens

Guidelines are now available on the labelling, transport and reception of specimens (Health Services Advisory Committee 1991). Specimens that need to be transported outside the hospital, e.g. by van, car, taxi or by post, must be transported in an adequate leak-proof primary container, a leak-proof secondary container and an outer box to comply with United Nations Packing Instructions 602 (1996). Laboratory technicians will undertake this task, following local written instructions relating to containment, labelling and transport boxes (Health Services Advisory Committee 1991).

The sooner a specimen arrives in the laboratory, the greater is the chance of organisms present surviving and being identified. Delays will cause changes that may radically alter the result. The laboratory count of bacteria in a delayed specimen could be significantly different to that of the specimen when it was collected.

If specimens cannot be sent to a laboratory immediately, they should be stored as follows:

1 Blood culture samples in a 37°C incubator.
2 All other specimens in a specimen refrigerator at a temperature of 4°C, where the low temperature will slow the bacterial growth (Higgins 1995).

In diagnostic pathology it is likely that at any given time there will be a number of specimens that present a risk of infection. Every health authority, therefore, must ensure that medical, nursing, phlebotomy, laboratory, portering and any other staff involved in handling specimens are trained to do so. The person collecting the specimen must ensure that the specimen container used is an appropriate one for the purpose, is properly closed and has not been externally contaminated by the contents (Health Services Advisory Committee 1991). Any accidental spillage must be cleaned up immediately by staff, who should wear gloves to prevent contamination. Ideally, all specimens should be placed in a double self-sealing bag with one compartment containing the request form and the other the specimen. Specimens should be transported to the laboratory in washable baskets or trays.

It is essential to remember that there will always be patients or specimens that have not been identified as presenting a particular risk of infection. If a specimen is suspected or known to present an infectious hazard, the person taking the specimen has the responsibility to ensure that the form and containers are correctly labelled with a biohazard label, to enable those handling the specimen to take appropriate precautions (Health Services Advisory Committee 1991).

Specimens from patients who have recently been treated with toxic therapy, i.e. gene therapy, drugs, radioactivity or active metabolites, need to be handled with caution. Local rules must be compiled, which will outline how such specimens should be labelled, bagged and transported to the laboratory. For example, in the case of gene therapy the specimen must be labelled with a biohazard label, double bagged and transported to the laboratory in a secure transport box with a fastenable lid. Each box must carry a warning label, be made of smooth impervious material such as plastic or metal which will retain liquid and can be easily disinfected and cleaned in the event of leakage of the specimen. (See Chap. 34 for further information related to unsealed sources and specimen collection.)

Types of investigation

Bacterial

A wide range of methods are available for obtaining cultures and identifying organisms from a specimen or swab. To employ all these tests would be time consuming and costly. Testing, therefore, tends to be selective. It is at this stage that the laboratory request form plays a particularly important part. A faecal specimen, for example, from a patient with diarrhoea who also has a recent history of foreign travel, would be investigated for organisms not normally looked for in faecal specimens from patients without such a history.

The majority of specimens undergo microscopic investigation. This is valuable as an early indication of the causative organisms in an infection. The specimen is often cultured for 24–48 hours longer in the case of blood cultures. Prolonged incubation (up to 21 days) may be required for growth of some organisms, e.g. *Brucella* species (Mims *et al.* 1993). This is followed by antibiotic sensitivity testing on any pathogenic organisms that are isolated. This involves the application of paper discs impregnated with antibiotics onto the agar plates. After overnight incubation during which time the growth of bacteria may be inhibited by the antibiotic disc, the zones of inhibition can be observed for the degree of sensitivity of the organism (Mims *et al.* 1993).

Viral

Three types of technique are available for the diagnosis of viral infections:

1 Electron microscopy
2 Culture
3 Serology.

For culture specimens the use of viral transport media and speed of delivery to the laboratory are important as viruses do not survive well outside the body. With good liaison, the nursing personnel should obtain the specimen when the laboratory staff have the transport ready to take it to the virus laboratories. If delays occur, the specimen should be refrigerated at a temperature of 4°C.

The time at which specimens are collected for viral investigations is important. Many viral illnesses have a prodromal phase during which the multiplication and shedding of the virus are at a peak and the patient is most infectious (Mims & White 1984).

Serological

Serological testing for the presence of antigens and antibodies is used when it is not possible to isolate the organism from the patient's tissue easily. By demonstrating serum antibodies to suspected organisms it is inferred that the patient is, or has been, infected with the organism. A single test is inadequate as if the titres (the concentration of the substance being measured) are raised it is impossible to determine whether this is due to past or present infection. Two tests need to be carried out, both of which involve the collection of 10 ml of blood once at the beginning of the illness and again 10–14 days later. If a rising titre level is demonstrated it suggests the patient's infection is current (Mims *et al.* 1993).

Mycosis

Although many pathogenic fungi will grow on ordinary bacteriological culture media, they grow better and with less risk of bacterial overgrowth on special mycological media. The presence of fungi in clinical specimens is difficult to interpret, as *Candida albicans*, for example, is commonly present in the upper respiratory, alimentary and female genital tract and on the skin of healthy people (Meunier 1988).

Mycobacteriological

For further information, please refer to the procedure on tuberculosis (Chap. 4).

Protozoa

Most protozoa do not cause disease, but those that do, e.g. malaria, make a formidable contribution to human illness (Akinola 1984). Laboratory investigations depend on direct microscopy which necessitates specimens being delivered to the laboratory as quickly as possible, while the protozoa are mobile and therefore visible.

Blood

When blood specimens are obtained from existing intravenous devices it is essential that the device is flushed thoroughly before use and that the first sample is discarded to prevent erroneous results (Johnston & Messina 1991).

Blood cultures

Bacteraemia and fungaemia are indications of the failure of the host's immune system to localize infection at its primary focus (Weinstein 1994) and are associated with significant morbidity and mortality (Smith-Elekes & Weinstein 1993). Accurate and speedy microbiological detection of infection using blood cultures is of paramount importance to determine the cause and guide the treatment of infection (see Chap. 4, Barrier Nursing). Success in gaining information from blood cultures relies on the accurate timing of the specimen and obtaining the correct volume of blood. Most bacteraemias are intermittent. Therefore blood cultures should be taken when the signs of infection are present (Woods & Washington 1995); these may include fever, chills, rigors, changes in mental status and lethargy.

Failure to use an aseptic technique when obtaining blood cultures can result in the diagnosis of a pseudobacteraemia, due to bacteria originating outside the patient's bloodstream, contaminating the culture. This could result in inappropriate antibiotic therapy being administered and a significant waste of health care resources (Jumaa & Chattopadhyay 1994).

The needle used to obtain blood for blood culture investigation should be changed prior to the inoculation of the blood into the blood culture bottle. This is because studies have shown an increase in contamination rates when the needle is not changed (Spitalnic *et al.* 1995).

The reliability of blood cultures obtained from an indwelling central venous catheter (CVC) is controversial.

Henderson (1995) highlights that there is a risk of the specimen being contaminated. However, if a CVC-associated infection is suspected these cultures may provide valuable information.

Some catheters facilitate microbial adherence, which will increase in proportion to the time the catheter is in situ (Henderson 1995). However, Wormser *et al.* (1990) suggest that if an aseptic technique is used to obtain blood from a catheter that has been in place for a relatively short time then reliable results can still be achieved.

Quantitative analysis of drugs in blood

Therapeutic drug monitoring by blood analysis is now technically feasible for a wide variety of antibiotics. The therapeutic range and dosage regimen for each antibiotic has been established, based on its known pharmacokinetics and from animal and human treatment studies (Dawson & Reeves 1997). Precise dosages of some antibiotics can be regulated by monitoring drug concentration in the blood (Reeves 1980).

With drugs that possess a narrow therapeutic range in serum, as with the aminoglycoside antibiotics (Barza *et al.* 1978), if the serum levels are too low the patient is jeopardized by the probable lack of efficacy. However, if the serum concentration is excessive, the patient may suffer serious toxicity. In the case of gentamicin, exposure to high serum levels for a prolonged period may cause renal impairment or ototoxicity (Cipolle *et al.* 1981). However, when the serum levels are within the normal range, the incidence of dose-related side-effects is minimal in most patients (Koch-Weser 1972).

In order to correctly individualize drug dosage, and then to monitor the drug effectively, the doctor needs to be familiar with the metabolic processes and relationships between a drug dose and drug concentration in biological fluids (Greenblatt *et al.* 1975). This is affected by many factors, such as route of administration (Riegelman 1973) and age (Rane *et al.* 1976). Disease processes, for example liver (Blaschke 1977) and renal disease (Peters *et al.* 1978), will also affect metabolism and excretion of the drug.

Drug monitoring is time consuming and costly. However, it is important to evaluate the cost of the test in the light of the information it yields both to ensure that therapeutic concentrations of the drug are achieved and to prevent toxicity (Mims *et al.* 1993). Therapeutic drug monitoring begins with the appropriate timing of the collection and continues through the analytical process to the integration of the results, which can be used to guide the doctor's treatment options (Hammett-Stabler & Johns 1998).

Analysis involves laboratory testing of blood serum. Although this knowledge can be gained from random sampling, most benefit will be obtained by the correct timing of sample collection. This will provide a direct relationship to drug administration, and therefore give the correct interpretation of the serum concentration results.

Ideally, a trough sample just before the next scheduled dose, plus a peak level at a set time following the adminis-tration of the drug, will provide the most useful information (Mims *et al.* 1993). Abnormally elevated drug levels may be obtained if the blood samples are taken from a CVC through which the drug has been administered. This is more likely if the catheter has not been flushed correctly following administration of the drug (Johnston & Messina 1991) or the first 10 ml of blood has not been discarded. Occasionally the CVC may have to be used, for example, for paediatric patients or when only poor or limited venous access is available. If a multilumen CVC is in place, a different lumen from the one used to administer the drug must be used to obtain the blood specimen. If scrupulous attention to policy is adhered to, blood levels obtained from CVC can compare favourably with specimens taken from peripheral veins (Shulman *et al.* 1998).

If blood samples have to be taken from a CVC because peripheral vein access is not available, this information must be written onto the microbiology request card (Shulman *et al.* 1998).

A 6-year audit of gentamicin drug monitoring to establish optimal regimens found that in those patients who achieved therapeutic drug levels, the average duration of antibiotic therapy was statistically shorter than in those patients who failed to achieve therapeutic peak concentrations. During this audit, 7% of patients' blood levels was found to be in the toxic range. This audit indicated that drug monitoring leads to improved drug administration (Ismail *et al.* 1997) by preventing toxicity and improving outcome.

In the procedure guidelines below two examples of drug analysis have been discussed; the laboratory will supply specific times for blood sampling for other drugs.

For further information on the collection of blood see the procedure for venepuncture (Chap. 45).

Urine

Urine is normally sterile, while the distal urethra of both men and women is normally colonized with a large number of bacteria (Woods & Washington 1995) and even a carefully taken urine specimen may contain a few bacteria. As urine is such a good culture medium, any bacteria present at the time of collection will continue to multiply in the specimen container, resulting in a falsely raised bacteriuria (Higgins 1995), which will then result in misleading information (Stokes & Ridgway 1980; Woods & Washington 1995).

It was thought that cleansing of the area around the urinary meatus prior to the collection of a midstream specimen of urine would reduce genital secretion contamination by removing loose epithelial cells and adherent bacteria. However, studies have suggested that such cleansing makes no difference to contamination rates (Holliday *et al.* 1991), although perineal and penile cleansing may be of benefit to those patients whose personal hygiene is poor.

The principle for obtaining midstream collection of urine is that any bacteria present in the urethra are washed away in the first portion of urine voided (Higgins 1995).

References and further reading

Akinola, J. (1984) Malaria. *Nurs Times*, **80**(38), 40–43.

Ayton, M. (1982) Microbiological investigations. *Nursing*, **2**(8), 26–9, 232.

Barton, S. & Jenkins, D. (1989) An exploration for the problems of the false negative cervical smear. *Br J Obstet Gynaecol*, **96**, 492–9.

Barza, M. *et al.* (1978) Why monitor serum levels of gentamicin? *Clin Pharmacokinetics*, **3**, 202–215.

Blaschke, T.F. (1977) Protein binding and kinetics of drugs in liver disease. *Clin Pharmacokinetics*, **2**, 32–44.

Cipolle, R.J. *et al.* (1981) Therapeutic use and serum concentration monitoring. In: *Individualizing Drug Therapy: Practical Applications of Drug Monitoring* (eds W.J. Taylor & A.L. Finn). Gross, Townsend & Frank, New York.

Dawson, S.J. & Reeves, D.S. (1997) Therapeutic monitoring, the concentration–effect relationship and impact on the clinical efficacy of antibiotic agents. *J Chemother*, **9**(Suppl. 1), 84–92.

Finegold, S.M. (1995) Anaerobic bacteria: general concepts. In: *Principles and Practice of Infectious Diseases* (eds G.L. Mandell, J.E. Bennett & R. Dolin), 4th edn., pp. 2156–73. Churchill Livingstone, New York.

Greenblatt, D.J. *et al.* (1975) Clinical pharmacokinetics. *New Engl J Med*, **293**, 964–70.

Hammett-Stabler, C.A. & Johns, T. (1998) Laboratory guidelines for monitoring of antimicrobial drugs. National Academy of Clinical Biochemistry. *Clin Chem*, **44**(5), 1129–40.

Hargiss, C.O. & Larson, E. (1981) How to collect specimens and evaluate results. *Am J Nurs*, **81**, 2166–74.

Hart, S. (1991) Blood and body fluid precautions. *Nurs Stand*, **5**, 25–7.

Health Services Advisory Committee (1991) *Safety in Health Services Laboratories: The Labelling, Transport and Reception of Specimens*. Stationery Office, London.

Henderson, D.K. (1995) Bacteremia due to percutaneous intravenous devices. In: *Principles and Practice of Infectious Diseases* (eds G.L. Mandell, J.E. Bennett & R. Dolin), 4th edn., pp. 2587–99. Churchill Livingstone, New York.

Higgins, C. (1995) Microbiological examination of urine in urinary tract infection. *Nurs Times*, **91**(11), 33–5.

Holliday, G., Strike, P.N. & Masterton, R.G. (1991) Perineal cleansing and mid stream urine specimen in ambulatory women. *J Hosp Infect*, **18**(1), 71–5.

Ismail, R. *et al.* (1997) Therapeutic drug monitoring of gentamicin: a 6-year follow-up audit. *J Clin Pharm Ther*, **22**(1), 21–5.

Johnston, J.B. & Messina, M. (1991) Erroneous laboratory values obtained from central catheters. *J Intraven Nurs*, **14**(1), 13–15.

Jumaa, P.A. & Chattopadhyay, B. (1994) Pseudobacteraemia. *J Hosp Infect*, **27**(3), 167–77.

Kiehn, T.E., Ellner, P.D. & Budzko, D. (1989) Role of the microbiological laboratory in care of the immunosuppressed patient. *Rev Infect Dis*, **11**(Suppl. 7), S1706–10.

Koch-Weser, R.J. (1972) Serum drug concentration as therapeutic guides. *New Engl J Med*, **287**, 227–31.

Macleod, J.A. (1992) Collecting specimens for the laboratory tests. *Nurs Stand*, **6**(20), 36–7.

Meunier, F. (1988) Fungal infection in the compromised host. In: *Clinical Approach to Infection in the Compromised Host* (eds R.H. Rubin & L.S. Young), pp. 193–212. Plenum, New York.

Mims, C.A. & White, D.O. (1984) *Viral Pathogenesis and Immunology*. Blackwell Science, Oxford.

Mims, C.A. *et al.* (1993) *Medical Microbiology*. C.V. Mosby, St Louis.

Nicas, T.I. & Eisenstein, B.I. (1995) Bacterial disease introduction. In: *Principles and Practice of Infectious Disease* (eds G.L. Mandell, J.E. Bennett & R. Dolin), 4th edn., pp. 1752–4. Churchill Livingstone, New York.

O'Grady, N.P. *et al.* (1998) Practice guidelines for evaluating new fever in critically ill adult patients. *Clin Infect Dis*, **26**(5), 1042–59.

Papasian, C.J. & Kragel, P.J. (1997) The microbiology laboratory's role in life-threatening infections. *Crit Care Nurse*, **20**(3), 44–59.

Parker, M.J. (1982) *Microbiology for Nurses*, 6th edn. Baillière Tindall, London.

Peters, U. *et al.* (1978) Digoxin metabolism in patients. *Arch Intern Med*, **138**, 1074–6.

Rane, A. *et al.* (1976) Clinical pharmacokinetics in infants and children. *Clin Pharmacokinetics*, **1**, 2–24.

Reeves, D.S. (1980) Therapeutic drug monitoring of aminoglycoside antibiotics. *Infection*, **8**(Suppl. 3), S313–20.

Riegelman, S. (1973) Effects of route of administration on drug disposition. *J Pharmacokinetics Biopharm*, **1**, 419–34.

Sandin, R.L. & Rinaldi, M. (1996) Special consideration for the clinical microbiology laboratory in the diagnosis of infections in the cancer patient. *Infect Dis Clin North Am*, **10**(2), 413–30.

Shulman, R.J. *et al.* (1998) Central venous catheter versus peripheral veins for sampling blood levels of commonly used drugs. *J Parenteral Enteral Nutr*, **22**(4), 234–7.

Singer, A. *et al.* (1994) *Lower Genital Tract Pre-cancer*. Blackwell Science, Oxford.

Smith, A.L. (1985) *Principles of Microbiology*, 10th edn. C.V. Mosby, St Louis.

Smith-Elekes, S. & Weinstein, M.P. (1993) Blood cultures. *Infect Dis Clin North Am*, **7**(2), 221–34.

Spitalnic, S.J., Woolard, R.H. & Mermel, L.A. (1995) The significance of changing needles when inoculating blood cultures: a meta-analysis. *Clin Infect Dis*, **21**(5), 1103–106.

Stokes, E.J. & Ridgeway, G.L. (1980) *Clinical Bacteriology*, 5th edn. Edward Arnold, London.

Thys, J.P., Jacobs, F. & Bye, B. (1994) Microbiological specimen collection in the emergency room. *Eur J Emerg Med*, **1**(1), 47–53.

Weinstein, M.P. (1994) Clinical importance of blood cultures. *Clin Lab Med*, **14**(1), 9–16.

Wilson, J. (1995) *Infection Control in Clinical Practice*. Baillière Tindall, London.

Wilson, M.E. & Mizer, H.E. (1969) *Microbiology in Nursing Practice*. Macmillan, London.

Wilson, M.L. (1996) General principles of specimen collection. *Clin Infect Dis*, **22**(5), 766–77.

Woods, G.L. & Washington, J.A. (1995) The clinician and the microbiology laboratory. In: *Principles and Practice of Infectious Diseases* (eds G.L. Mandell, J.E. Bennett & R. Dolin), 4th edn., pp. 169–99. Churchill Livingstone, New York.

Wormser, G.P. *et al.* (1990) Sensitivity and specificity of blood cultures obtained through intravenous catheters. *Crit Care Nurs*, **18**(2), 152–6.

GUIDELINES • Specimen collection

Procedure

Action

1 Explain and discuss the procedure with the patient and ensure privacy while the procedure is being carried out.

2 Wash hands using bactericidal soap and water or bactericidal alcohol hand rub.

3 Place specimens and swabs in the appropriate, correctly labelled containers.

4 Dispatch specimens promptly to the laboratory with the completed request form.

Rationale

To ensure that the patient understands the procedure and gives his/her valid consent.

Hand washing greatly reduces the risk of infection transfer.

To ensure that only organisms for investigation are preserved.

To ensure the best possible conditions for any laboratory examinations.

Eye swab

Action

1 Using either a plastic loop or a cotton wool-covered wooden stick, hold the swab parallel to the cornea and gently rub the conjunctiva in the lower eyelid.

2 If possible, smear the conjunctival swab on an agar plate at the bedside.

Rationale

To ensure that a swab of the correct site is taken. To avoid contamination by touching the eyelid.

Eye swabs are often unsatisfactory because of the action of tears, which contain the enzyme lysozyme which acts as an antiseptic. Conjunctival scrapings are preferable. This procedure is usually performed by medical staff.

Nose swab

Action

1 Moisten the swab beforehand with sterile water.

2 Move the swab from the anterior nares and direct it upwards into the tip of the nose (Fig. 37.1).

3 Gently rotate the swab.

Rationale

To prevent discomfort to the patient. The healthy nose is virtually dry and a dry swab may cause discomfort.

To swab the correct site and to obtain the required sample.

Perinasal swab (for whooping cough)

Action

1 Using a special soft-wire mounted swab, pass it along the floor of the nasal cavity to the posterior wall of the nasopharynx (Fig. 37.1).

2 Rotate the swab gently.

Rationale

To minimize trauma to nasal tissue. To obtain a swab from the correct site.

Sputum

Action

1 Use a specimen container that is free from organisms of respiratory origin. This need not, therefore, be a sterile container.

2 Care should be taken to ensure that the material sent for investigations is sputum, not saliva.

Rationale

Sputum is never free from organisms since material originating in the bronchi and alveoli has to pass through the pharynx and mouth, areas that have a normal commensal population of bacteria.

To obtain the required sample.

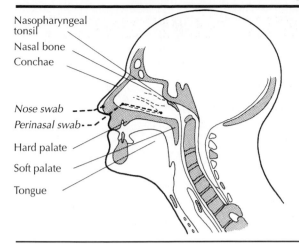

Nasopharyngeal tonsil
Nasal bone
Conchae

Nose swab
Perinasal swab
Hard palate
Soft palate
Tongue

Figure 37.1 Area to be swabbed when sampling the nose.

3 Encourage patients who have difficulty producing sputum to cough deeply first thing in the morning. Alternatively, a physiotherapist should be called to assist.	To facilitate expectoration.
4 Send any sputum specimen to the laboratory immediately.	The bacterial population alters rapidly and rapid dispatch should ensure accurate results.

Throat swab

Action	Rationale
1 Ask the patient to sit in such a position that he/she is facing a strong light source. Depress the patient's tongue with a spatula.	To ensure maximum visibility of the area to be swabbed. The procedure is one that is likely to cause the patient to gag and the tongue will move to the roof of the mouth, contaminating the specimen.
2 Quickly, but gently, rub the swab over the prescribed area, usually the tonsillar fossa or any area with a lesion or visible exudate (Fig. 37.2).	To obtain the required sample.
3 Avoid touching any other area of the mouth or tongue with the swab.	To prevent contamination by other organisms.

Ear swab

Action	Rationale
1 No antibiotics or other chemotherapeutic agents should have been used in the aural region 3h before taking the swab.	To prevent collection of traces of such therapeutic agents.
2 Place the swab into the outer ear as shown in Fig. 37.3. Rotate the swab gently.	To avoid trauma to the ear. To collect any secretions.

Wound swab

Action	Rationale
1 Take any swabs required before cleaning procedure begins.	To collect the maximum number of micro-organisms and to prevent collection of any therapeutic agents that may be employed in the dressing procedure.
2 Rotate the swab gently.	To collect samples. It is preferable to send samples of purulent discharge instead of swabs.

Note: the use of disposable gloves is recommended in the following procedures in order to prevent cross-infection.

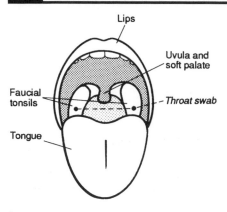

Figure 37.2 Area to be swabbed when sampling the throat.

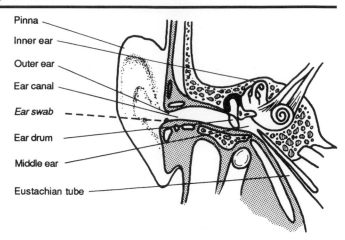

Figure 37.3 Area to be swabbed when sampling the outer ear.

Guidelines • Specimen collection (cont'd)

Vaginal swab

Action	Rationale
1 Introduce a speculum into the vagina to separate the vaginal walls. Take the swab as high as possible in the vaginal vault.	To ensure maximum visibility of the area to be swabbed. To ensure that the swab is taken from the best site. If infection by *Trichomonas* species is suspected, a charcoal-impregnated swab is recommended as this organism survives longer in this medium.

Penile swab

Action	Rationale
1 Retract prepuce.	To obtain maximum visibility of area to be swabbed.
2 Rotate swab gently in the urethral meatus.	To collect any secretions.

Rectal swab

Action	Rationale
1 Pass the swab, with care, through the anus into the rectum.	To avoid trauma. To ensure that a rectal and not an anal sample is obtained.
2 Rotate gently.	To avoid trauma.
3 In patients suspected of suffering from threadworms, take the swab from the perianal region.	Threadworms lay their ova on the perianal skin.

Faeces

Action	Rationale
1 Ask the patient to defaecate into a clinically clean bedpan.	To avoid unnecessary contamination from other organisms.
2 Scoop enough material to fill a third of the specimen container using a spatula or a spoon, often incorporated in the specimen container.	To obtain a usable amount of specimen. To prevent contamination.
3 Examine the specimen for such features as colour, consistency and odour, and record your observations.	To monitor any fluctuations and trends.
4 Segments of tapeworm are seen easily in faeces and any such segments should be sent to the laboratory for identification.	Unless the head is dislodged, the tapeworm will continue to grow. Laboratory confirmation of the presence of the head is essential.
5 Patients suspected of suffering from amoebic dysentery should have any stool specimens dispatched to the laboratory immediately.	The parasite causing amoebic dysentery exists in a free-living non-motile cyst. *Both* are characteristic in their fresh state but are difficult to identify when dead.

Urine

Action	Rationale
1 Specimens of urine should be collected as soon as possible after the patient wakens in the morning and at the same time each morning if more than one specimen is required.	The bladder will be full as urine has accumulated overnight. If specimens are taken at other times, the urine may be diluted. All specimens will be comparable if taken at the same time each morning.
2 Dispatch all specimens to the laboratory as soon after collection as possible.	Urine specimens should be examined within 2 h of collection or 24 h if kept refrigerated at a temperature of 4°C. At room temperature overgrowth will occur and lead to misinterpretation.

Midstream specimen of urine: male

Action	Rationale
1 Retract the prepuce and clean the skin surrounding the urethral meatus with soap and water, 0.9% sodium chloride solution or a solution that does not contain a disinfectant.	To prevent other organisms contaminating the specimen. Disinfectants may irritate or be painful to the urethral mucous membrane.
2 Ask the patient to direct the first and last part of his stream into a urinal or toilet but to collect the middle part of his stream into a sterile container.	To avoid contamination of the specimen with organisms normally present on the skin.

Midstream specimen of urine: female

Action	Rationale
1 If necessary, clean the urethral meatus with soap and water, 0.9% sodium chloride solution or a solution that does not contain a disinfectant.	To prevent other organisms contaminating the specimen. Disinfectants may irritate or be painful to the urethral mucous membrane.
2 (a) Use a separate cotton-wool swab for each swab. (b) Swab from the front to the back.	To prevent cross-infection. To prevent perianal contamination.
3 Ask the patient to micturate into a bedpan or toilet. Place a sterile receiver or a wide-mouthed container under the stream and remove before the stream ceases.	To avoid contamination of the specimen with organisms normally present on the skin.
4 Transfer the specimen into a sterile container.	

Guidelines • Specimen collection (cont'd)

Specimen of urine from an ileal conduit

For further information see the relevant section in the procedure on stoma care (Chap. 39).

Catheter specimen of urine

For further information see the relevant section in the procedure on urinary catheterization (Chap. 43).

24-hour urine collection

Action	Rationale
1 Request the patient to void the bladder at the time appointed to begin this procedure. Discard this specimen.	To ensure the urine collected is that produced in the 24 h stated.
2 All urine passed in the next 24 h is collected in a large specimen bottle. The final specimen is collected at exactly the same time the bladder was voided 24 h earlier.	Body chemistry alters constantly. A 24-h collection will accommodate all the variables within a representative period.
3 Care must be taken to ensure the patient understands the procedure in order to eliminate the risk of an incomplete collection.	A 24-h collection will not be obtained if one sample is lost, and the results will be invalid.

Semen

Action	Rationale
1 Sexual intercourse should not have taken place for 3–4 days before the specimen is collected.	To ensure the sperm count will be at maximum levels. It takes between 3 and 4 days for the sperm count to return to normal after ejaculation.
2 A fresh masturbated specimen must be collected in a sterile container and delivered to the laboratory within 2 h of the collection of the specimen.	Sperm will die if there is a delay in testing. Specimens must not be collected in a condom as sperm die when in contact with materials such as rubber.

Cervical scrape

Action	Rationale
1 The ideal time for smear testing is mid-cycle.	To allow for accuracy of results as the cervix is usually free of contamination from menstrual flow at this time.
2 The menses should be avoided.	This is less uncomfortable for the patient.
3 The smear must be taken before a vaginal examination is carried out.	To ensure that normal tissue samples are obtained.
4 Label the ground glass end of the slide with the patient's name.	To ensure patient identification.
5 Expose the cervix by using a dry speculum or one moistened with warm tap water.	To ensure maximum visibility. Greasy lubricants inhibit specimen collection.
6 Using the bilobed end of the cervical spatula, scrape firmly but gently around the squamocolumnar junction of the cervix. If the os is splayed open or scarred, a wider sweep with the broad end of the spatula may be necessary.	To obtain a usable amount of specimen.

7 Smear both sides of the spatula evenly on the slide with one stroke from each side of the spatula.

To ensure complete specimens.

8 Fix immediately.

To preserve the specimen and ensure accurate results.

9 Allow the fixing agents to dry.

Dry specimens are less likely to be damaged.

10 Place the slides in a transport container.

To safeguard delicate glass slides.

11 Small endocervical lesions, which could be missed by the use of a spatula, may be sampled using an endocervical plastic brush (Singer *et al.* 1994).

This brush with its narrow tip can be inserted into the cervical canal, improving the quality of smear taken from the endocervix (Barton & Jenkins 1989).

12 Identify the lesion and insert and gently rotate the brush in the cervical canal.

To obtain a usable amount of specimen.

13 Withdraw the brush and gently smear the brush evenly on the slide (treat slide as above; see 8, 9 and 10).

To ensure a complete specimen.

14 Send, with a completed cervical cytology request form, to the appropriate laboratory.

GUIDELINES • Analysis of drug levels in blood

Procedure

Action

1 Following venepuncture guidelines (Chap. 45), withdraw 10 ml of blood to obtain specimen for clotted sample to provide trough-level serum using a new needle or wing infusion device. Clearly label blood specimen container 'pre-drug administration blood'.

Rationale

To obtain a blood sample safely that is not contaminated by previous administration of drug residue, which could provide an inaccurate result.

2 Administer intravenous antibiotic as patient's prescription states (following procedure for administration of drugs by direct injection, bolus, or push; see Guidelines, Chap. 12) via patient's established vascular device.

To continue with patient's prescribed drug regime.

3 One hour after administration of drug withdraw 10 ml of blood to obtain specimen for clotted sample to provide peak-level serum following venepuncture guidelines, Chap. 45. Clearly label blood specimen container 'post-drug administration blood'.

Time gap allows for even distribution of the drug through the blood and for peak blood levels to be achieved.

4 Rarely but occasionally when only poor and limited venous access is available, the blood specimens may have to be obtained from the patient's existing device. The device must be flushed thoroughly before taking the blood sample (see Chap. 46).
The blood specimen container and request form must be labelled to indicate this deviation from the usual procedure.

The possibility of these specimens being contaminated with residue drug is high.

Contamination can be reduced by thorough flushing of the device.
The clinician interpreting the result will then be aware of the method of obtaining the blood specimen.

Spinal Cord Compression Management

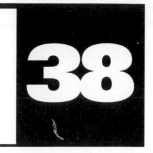

Definition

Spinal cord compression is the compression of the spinal cord and nerve roots.

Reference material

Spinal cord compression (SCC) can be caused by a number of factors including extradural or intradural tumours. The majority of extradural tumours are metastatic in nature. Intradural, extramedullary tumours are roughly evenly divided between primary and metastatic tumours, while intradural, intramedullary tumours are most often primary gliomas.

Spinal cord compression due to primary or metastatic tumour is an oncological emergency. Prompt action is required both in the diagnosis and its management so as to prevent neurological deterioration which can make the difference between the patient being paralysed or functionally independent. As such, the maintenance of neurological function is paramount in order to ensure an improvement in the patient's quality of life. Patients at risk of developing SCC should be made aware of potential signs. Professionals have an important proactive role in educating or raising awareness in this area (British Association of Surgical Oncology 1999).

In the context of cancer therapy and rehabilitation the management of SCC differs from that of the young individual whose spinal cord has been damaged as a result of trauma, and although many problems will be similar for both groups of patients, this chapter will deal with the former.

Incidence and aetiology

The spine is the most common site for bone metastases. It is estimated that 3–5% of patients with cancer and 10–15% of patients with spinal metastases may develop compression during the course of their illness (Hillier & Wee 1997), while approximately 5% of patients with systemic cancer will have SCC on autopsy (Posner 1995). Primary tumours of the spinal cord are relatively uncommon, while secondary involvement of the central nervous system is more common (Sharpe 1998). In the adult population, approximately 50% of all metastases in the spine causing epidural SCC arise from breast, lung or prostate carcinoma. In children, the primary pathology is usually Ewing's sarcoma, neuroblastoma, osteogenic sarcoma or rhabdomyosarcoma (Britton & Ng 1998).

In SCC there is oedema and decreased blood supply to the spinal cord and mechanical damage to the neural tissue, which can lead to a hemiparesis or hemiplegia (Dyck 1991).

Classification

Tumours of the spine are classified according to their relationship to the dura and the spinal cord itself (Addison & Shah 1998):

1 Extradural lesions, that is lesions of the osseous spine, epidural space and paraspinal soft tissues; these tumours compress the dural and spinal cord.
2 Intradural extramedullary lesions, which are inside the dura but outside the spinal cord.
3 Intramedullary lesions, which are within the spinal cord itself.

(Britton & Ng 1998)

Clinical presentation

The signs and symptoms of SCC may be evident several weeks before cord compression actually occurs (Held & Peahota 1993). Clinical presentation of SCC includes the following:

1 Pain. This is usually the earliest presenting symptom. The onset of pain is usually mild and becomes more severe with time. However, the absence of pain does not mean an absence of SCC (Posner 1995).
2 Motor deficits, that is, weakness of the extremities. Motor deficits may progress to ataxia, loss of coordination and paralysis (Dyck 1991).
3 Sensory loss. This may include decreased sensation, pain and temperature, pins-and-needles and numbness of the toes and fingers. These symptoms can ascend to the level of SCC (Held & Peahota 1993). It is worth noting that sensory complaints without pain are rare with SCC (Posner 1995).
4 Autonomic nervous system problems. These include the symptoms of constipation and urinary retention. Often, constipation is aggravated in those patients receiving opiates and, therefore, appropriate bowel management must be observed.

Early diagnosis is essential in order to ensure prompt treatment. The success of treatment is dependent on the patient's general condition and mobility. Studies indicate that patients who are not mobile at presentation do not generally regain the ability to walk (Held & Peahota 1993; Ingham *et al.* 1993).

Investigations

Investigations can include plain X-rays (cervical, lumbar and thoracic), bone scan, computerized tomography (CT) and magnetic resonance imaging (MRI). Such investigations are often dependent on what imaging techniques are available. However, if available, MRI is the investigation of choice (Britton & Ng 1998).

At present, one of the disadvantages of MRI is slower image acquisition; it can take up to four times as long to image a patient with suspected SCC compared with CT scans. The MRI scanner is a more enclosed space than a CT scanner. This, coupled with the time taken for the scan, needs to be considered for those patients in pain. It should be noted that recent autopsy studies suggest that about 25% of spinal lesions are not identifiable by plain X-rays (Posner 1995).

It is important that there is a clear established route of rapid diagnosis and management for the optimum treatment of SCC, including assessment by an orthopaedic surgeon or neurosurgeon skilled in managing spinal disease. To facilitate expert medical/clinical or surgical oncology assessment, there may be a need for the transfer of images (e.g. scans) to a regional cancer centre (British Association of Surgical Oncology 1999).

Treatment

Treatment should be commenced as soon as possible once a diagnosis has been established to maximize recovery chances and minimize functional deficits (Janjan 1996). Treatment can be a combination of steroids, surgery, radiotherapy and/or chemotherapy. For those patients presenting with pain, proper analgesia coupled with steroids should also be considered as an integral part of treatment.

Steroids

Steroids are used primarily for the control and reduction of brain and spinal cord oedema (this may result in a decrease in neurological deficits) and for the relief of spinal pain (Posner 1995). Steroids have both glucocorticoid (anti-inflammatory) and mineralocorticoid (water and mineral) effects. Steroids have multiple side-effects, many of which can be unpleasant and may take from weeks to months to subside after completion of therapy (Evans & Guerrero 1998).

Surgery

Surgery in the form of laminectomy to decompress the spinal cord or vertebral body resection to allow for removal of the tumour can be considered. The surgical approach for spinal tumours depends on whether the tumour is extradural, intradural or intramedullary (Addison & Shah 1998). Other factors that need to be taken into account are the patient's age, his or her performance status, as well as any other pre-existing medical condition. In the context of malignant disease, radiation and steroids are often preferred treatments over surgery because of the added risks of surgery in patients with advanced metastatic cancer (Peterson 1993).

Radiotherapy

Radiation therapy is the mainstay of treatment for malignant epidural compression (Ingham *et al.* 1993). Radiotherapy is considered as effective as decompression laminectomy and will also relieve pain in about three quarters of patients (Ingham *et al.* 1993). Radiotherapy should be commenced immediately once SCC has been diagnosed to prevent further neurological deterioration. However, patients with complete paralysis rarely respond to radiotherapy (Hillier & Wee 1997).

Chemotherapy

For patients with SCC from chemoresponsive tumours, such as small cell lung cancer and lymphomas, treatment with the cytotoxic drug appropriate for the tumour may be considered (Guerrero 1998).

Rehabilitation

Rehabilitation must commence on diagnosis and must encompass the skills of various professionals. No one professional intervention would be wholly effective in isolation (Robinson 1998). An effective team does not just provide a better programme for the patient's rehabilitation needs but also very importantly allows for colleague support and advice from other team members when dealing with complex cases (Robinson 1998).

In the context of SCC due to metastatic cancer, the rehabilitation team should take a palliative care approach as this group of patients generally have a poor prognosis. The emphasis should therefore be on the improvement of quality of life, not just for the patient but also for those managing his or her care. Home adaptation, appropriate lifting, special mattresses and wheelchairs may be indicated and therefore the involvement of the primary health care, palliative care teams and social services should be sought at an early stage of care. Their psychosocial and sexual needs also need to be addressed and both the patient and family provided with appropriate counselling if and when required. Families should be encouraged to participate in care, where appropriate or acceptable to the patient, whether the patient is in hospital or at home, and techniques such as the management of indwelling catheters, bowel care and appropriate scheduling of medication should be taught. Such measures are important in order to encourage independence and avoid the development of future crisis. This should also ensure that families feel that they have been consulted and involved in care throughout the illness experience. Such involvement may help family members when coping with future bereavement.

References and further reading

Addison, C. & Shah, S. (1998) Neurosurgery. In: *Neuro-Oncology for Nurses* (ed. D. Guerrero), pp. 124–50. Whurr, London.

Barker, S.J. (1995) Anaesthesia in the high-risk patient. In: *Textbook of Critical Care* (eds W.C. Shoemaker, M.A. Ayres, A. Grenvik & P.R. Holbrook), 3rd edn. W.B. Saunders, Philadelphia.

Borgman-Gainer, M.F. (1996) Independent function: movement and mobility. In: *Rehabilitation Nursing: Process and Application*, (ed. S. Hoeman) 2nd edn., pp. 225–69. Mosby, New Jersey.

British Association of Surgical Oncology (1999) The management of metastatic bone disease in the United Kingdom. The Breast Speciality Group of the BASO. *Eur J Surg Oncol*, **25**(1), 3–23.

Britton, J. & Ng, V. (1998) Clinical neuro-imaging. Chapter 4. In: *Neuro-Oncology for Nurses* (ed. D. Guerrero), pp. 81–123. Whurr, London.

Carson, M., Williams, T., Everett, A. & Barker, S. (1997) The nurse's role in the multidisciplinary team. *Eur J Palliat Care*, **4**(3), 96–8.

Cooper, J. (1997) Occupational therapy in specific symptom control and dysfunction. In: *Occupational Therapy in Oncology and Palliative Care* (ed. J. Cooper), pp. 59–87. Whurr, London.

Davidhizar, R. (1997) Disability does not have to be the grief that never ends: helping patients adjust. *Rehab Nurs*, **22**(1), 32–5.

Delaney, T. & Oldfield, E. (1989) Spinal cord compression. In: *Cancer Principles and Practice of Oncology* (eds D.E. Vita, V. Hellman & S. Rosenberg), 3rd edn., pp. 1978–86. Lippincott, Philadelphia.

Dyck, S. (1991) Surgical instrumentation as a palliative treatment for spinal cord compression. *Oncol Nurs Forum*, **18**(3), 515–21.

Evans, C. & Guerrero, D. (1998) Medication used in the symptom management of CNS tumours. In: *Neuro-Oncology for Nurses* (ed. D. Guerrero), pp. 201–220. Whurr, London.

Faithfull, S. (1998) Fatigue in patients receiving radiotherapy. *Prof Nurse*, **13**(7), 459–61.

Gender, A.R. (1996) Bowel regulation and elimination. In: *Rehabilitation Nursing: Process and Application* (ed. S. Hoeman), 2nd edn., pp. 452–75. Mosby, New Jersey.

Guerrero, D. (1998) Radiotherapy. In: *Neuro-Oncology for Nurses* (ed. D. Guerrero), pp. 151–78. Whurr, London.

Hardy, J. (1998) Corticosteroids in palliative care. *Eur J Palliat Care*, **5**(2), 46–50.

Hatcliffe, S. & Dawe, R. (1996) Monitoring pressure sores in a palliative care setting. *Int J Palliat Nurs*, **2**(4), 182–6.

Held, J.L. & Peahota, A. (1993) Nursing care of the patient with spinal cord compression. *Oncol Nurs Forum*, **20**(10), 1507–16.

Hickey, J.V. (1997) Vertebral and spinal cord trauma. In: *The Clinical Practice of Neurological and Neurosurgical Nursing*, 4th edn. Lippincott, London.

Hillier, R. & Wee, B. (1997) Palliative management of spinal cord compression. *Eur J Palliat Care*, **4**(6), 189–92.

Hunter, M. (1998) Rehabilitation in cancer care: a patient-focused approach. *Eur J Palliat Care*, **7**(7), 85–7.

Ingham, J., Beveridge, A. & Cooney, N.J. (1993) The management of spinal cord compression in patients with advanced malignancy. *J Pain Sympt Manage*, **8**(1), 1–7.

Janjan, N.A. (1996) Radiotherapeutic management of spinal metastases. *J Pain Sympt Manage*, **11**(1), 47–56.

Kirkbridge, P. (1995) The role of radiation therapy in palliative care. *J Palliat Care*, **11**(1), 19–26.

Kramer, J.A. (1992) Spinal cord compression in malignancy. *Palliat Med* **6**(6), 202–211.

Linstadt, D.E. (1999) Spinal cord. In: *Textbook of Radiation Oncology* (eds S.E. Leibel & T.L. Phillips), pp. 404–411. W.B. Saunders, Philadelphia.

Penson, J. & Fisher, R. (eds) (1995) *Palliative Care for People with Cancer*. Edward Arnold, London.

Peterson, R. (1993) A nursing intervention for early detection of spinal cord compressions in patients with cancer. *Cancer Nurs*, **16**(2), 113–16.

Pires, M. (1996) Bladder Elimination and Continence. In: *Rehabilitation Nursing: Process and Application* (ed. S. Hoeman) 2nd edn., pp. 417–45. Mosby, New Jersey.

Posner, J. (1995) *Neurologic Complications of Cancer*. F.A. Davis, Philadelphia.

Raney, D. (1991) Malignant spinal cord tumours: a review and case presentation. *J Neurosci Nurs*, **1**(23), 44–9.

Robinson, S. (1998) Multidisciplinary teamwork. In: *Neuro-Oncology for Nurses* (ed. D. Guerrero), pp. 221–52. Whurr, London.

Sharpe, G. (1998) Pathological and clinical aspects of CNS tumours. In: *Neuro-Oncology for Nurses* (ed. D. Guerrero), pp. 66–80. Whurr, London.

Thompson, E. & Hicks, F. (1998) Intrathecal baclofen and homeopathy for the treatment of painful muscle spasms associated with malignant spinal cord compression. *Palliat Med*, **6**(12), 119–21.

Twycross, R. & Back, I. (1998) Nausea and vomiting in advanced cancer. *Eur J Palliat Care*, **5**(2), 39–45.

Wilkowski, J. (1986) Spinal cord compression; an oncologic emergency. *J Emerg Nurs*, **12**(1), 9–12.

GUIDELINES • Care of patients with spinal cord compression

Initial care

Action	Rationale
1 Explain and discuss the procedure(s) with the patient.	To ensure that the patient understands the procedure and gives his/her valid consent.
2 Reassure patient and significant others that assessment will be performed.	To decrease pain associated with anxiety.
3 Ensure adequate psychological and physical preparation for tests and procedures by giving accurate explanations and instructions.	To ensure patient is informed of any procedures and possible action plans.
4 Reinforce that the aims of any intervention will be the relief of pain and the restoration of function if possible (Wilkowski 1986; Hillier & Wee 1997).	To provide hope.

5 Assist with and explain details of ongoing investigations, e.g. X-rays, bone scan, CT scan, MRI scan.

To ensure patient is aware of each stage of the procedure as it occurs and to decrease anxiety.

Moving and handling

Action

1 Ensure that assessment for manual handling is carried out [see Chap. 25, Moving and Handling (Manual Handling) Patients].

2 Maintain the patient on bed rest until he/she has received an initial assessment and evaluation of his or her condition by the medical team. When the patient needs to be moved (for example, to use a bed pan), the patient should be moved very carefully using the safe principles of manual handling to prevent twist or torsion to the spine (Dyck 1991). If a hard cervical collar is indicated this should be fitted by the appropriately trained professional.

3 A fuller assessment of the patient's condition and ability to mobilize should be conducted by the multiprofessional team including the physiotherapist, medical team, nurse and importantly the patient; all these individuals should be involved in decisions and discussions regarding moving and handling.

Rationale

To maintain staff and patient safety. To avoid the risk to the patient of further complications resulting from injury.

To stabilize any vertebral instability and minimize the risk of further damage to the vertebrae and spinal cord. The fragile status of vertebrae may result in a crush fracture to the body of a vertebra and/or a spinal cord transection.

Individual risk assessment and agreeing safest practice requires a multiprofessional perspective which should additionally cover patient transfers, positioning and mobilization. This approach may assist the patient with pain control and comfort.

Assessment

Action

1 Monitor and document vital signs (see Chap. 28, Observations), maintaining awareness of signs of spinal shock (see Nursing Care Plan, this chapter). Report any signs of spinal shock to the medical team immediately.

2 Assess the patient's neurological status including limb strength, sensation, bladder and bowel function.

3 Monitor blood chemistry and patient for signs of hypercalcaemia, such as confusion, drowsiness and lethargy.

If patient is hypercalcaemic then
(a) Administer intravenous hydration and pharmacological agents prescribed to lower serum calcium as instructed calcium as instructed by medical team.
(b) Monitor and care for vascular device (see Chap. 44, Vascular Access Devices: Insertion and Management).

4 Assess alterations in elimination of urine and/or faeces defined in terms of urgency, frequency, level of control over function, retention, constipation and incontinence.

Rationale

To provide information with regard to the patient's condition and to ensure treatment and care are planned and implemented. Spinal shock requires immediate review by the medical team. These complications are more commonly associated with spinal injury patients, but may also exist in spinal cord compression patients.

To establish patient's level of consciousness (see Chap. 26, Neurological Observations).

To ascertain any evidence of increasing spinal cord compression, as indicated by motor dysfunction, weakness, ataxia, paraparesis, sensory loss, numbness, tingling, loss of sensation to pain and temperature, and constipation and urinary retention.

To correct fluid and electrolyte imbalance. Elevated calcium levels may be associated with bone metastasis causing the spinal cord compression.

To promote patient safety and comfort and to maximize/ facilitate patient's understanding of investigations and treatment plan.

Early autonomic and nervous system involvement results in constipation and urinary retention. Bowel and bladder incontinence develop with advanced autonomic nervous system involvement and carries a poor prognosis (Held & Peahota 1993).

Guidelines • Care of patients with spinal cord compression (cont'd)

Action	Rationale
Monitor blood chemistry results.	Raised urea and other electrolytes may be associated with urinary retention (Penson & Fisher 1995).
5 Urinary catheterization may be necessary if urinary retention is present.	Approximately half of patients with spinal cord compression present with bladder distention that requires catheterization (Held & Peahota 1993).
If appropriate, conduct procedure using aseptic technique; provide and teach regular catheter care (see Chap. 43, Urinary Catheterization).	To allow voiding of urine. To reduce risk of infection.
6 Assess patient's pain (see Chap. 29, Pain Assessment and Management). This should include factors such as duration, location, type, intensity and quality of pain.	To assist in identifying possible level of spinal cord involvement and to assist in the appropriate prescribing of analgesia and interventions designed to minimize pain. Information concerning pain will provide an indication of underlying pathology. For example, local pain occurs over the area of the tumour and may be constant. Radicular pain (pain caused by nerve root compression) may travel down the extremity associated with the area of compression and may be worsened by sneezing, coughing or straining. Thoracic pain is often described as a tight band around the chest or upper abdomen. Medullary pain is referred pain, which is often described as 'burning' or 'shooting' in nature and may be poorly localized (Raney 1991).
Document on Pain Assessment Chart (see Chap. 29 Pain Assessment and Management).	To provide for continuity of care, accurate documentation and for future review. To ensure pain assessment and analgesic requirements are reviewed on a regular basis, as patient's needs may alter as treatment and rehabilitation progress. To allow for comparative reassessment and evaluation of interventions.
If required, administer analgesia as prescribed, noting effects and any side-effects; report to medical team as necessary. Consider use of non-pharmacological interventions such as relaxation, therapeutic massage and adjusting patient's position.	Adequate pain control is essential for comfortable mobilization. Relaxed muscles will facilitate better movement. Narcotics are not always sufficient to control nerve root pain and additional medications prescribed by experts in pain control, such as anticonvulsants, steroids and tricyclic antidepressants, may help to ease pain (Hillier & Wee 1997). The role of complementary therapies has yet to be explored fully, but they may prove useful in reducing pain in particular patients.
7 Assess skin condition (see also Chap. 47, Wound Management).	Pressure ulcers may develop if the patient has spent time in bed, due to pain and poor physical status.
Change position (see Chap. 47, Wound Management and Chap. 42, The Unconscious Patient) as required to promote tissue integrity. The appropriateness of using pressure-relieving aids, e.g. therapeutic beds (Hatcliffe & Dawe 1996), should be assessed on an *individual basis* and balanced with the risk of spinal cord transection.	Sensory deficits may mean that stimuli of pain and pressure are not received by the patient (Dyck 1991). This means that they are more likely to develop pressure ulcers. There is no research evidence to indicate whether a firm or pressure-relieving/reducing mattress is most appropriate for the care of patients with spinal cord compression – the greatest risk posed to the patient from either vertebral instability and subsequent spinal cord transection or pressure ulcer development should be assessed jointly with the nursing and medical teams and physiotherapist.
Good body alignment must be maintained while facilitating frequent change of positioning.	Good body alignment should be maintained at all times to minimize risk of further injury to the spine as much as possible.

8 Facilitate any family discussion on treatment options together with the medical team.

9 Assess patient's understanding of any information given by the multiprofessional team following any investigations, the patient's diagnosis and treatment plan. Gently reinforce details imparted and discuss according to patient's needs.

10 Document complete assessment and care in nursing records.
Reassessments should be carried out at least once every 8 h and more often if deterioration occurs (Dyck 1991).

To ensure patient and family are aware of the extent and possible effects of any intervention.

For some patients, spinal cord compression means a new cancer diagnosis. However, for the majority of patients it is a reminder of the cancer's progression and of their own mortality. It is, therefore, important to assess and monitor the patient's understanding of the information received and to facilitate understanding of the treatment programme (Hillier & Wee 1997) and provide support as necessary. It is essential for the team to be honest, but tactful, for example, patients with dense paraplegia rarely recover.

To act as a baseline for noting any changes on reassessment and following any interventions.
To monitor and report any changes in function, so that rapidity of deterioration or improvement is noted. To provide an accurate record for any future use and evaluation.

Treatment(s)

Action

1 *Neurosurgery*
If the patient undergoes neurosurgery, provide appropriate pre- and postoperative care (e.g. breathing exercises, pain management, log-rolling, recording of vital signs and neurological function, bowel and bladder care) (see Chap. 31, Peri-Operative care).

2 *Radiotherapy*
If the patient requires radiotherapy:
(a) Prepare patient to receive radiotherapy by providing information and education.

(b) Prepare patient for daily treatments.

(c) Monitor and care for side-effects (administering treatment, such as drugs as prescribed) depending on area affected as follows:
  • Skin – erythema over treated area (see Chap. 47, Wound Management).
  • Oesophagitis – administer as prescribed – usually analgesia and antacids; provide a soft diet.
  • Nausea and vomiting – administer as prescribed – usually antiemetics (Twycross & Back 1998).
  • Diarrhoea – provide a low fibre diet; administer as prescribed antidiarrhoeal agents, e.g. Imodium (see Chap. 6, Bowel Care).

Rationale

Surgery in the form of a decompression laminectomy and debulking of tumour, with or without the stabilization of metal rods or bone graft, may be a treatment option (Dyck 1991; Hickey 1997) and is influenced by:
(a) The site of the tumour
(b) The degree of spinal instability
(c) The likely prognosis
(d) The extent of spinal disease.
Many postoperative measures concerning monitoring of spinal cord compression remain the same as during presurgery. This can be the case for days or weeks postsurgery.

Radiotherapy alone is effective in over 85% of cases of spinal cord compression and is used in combination with steroids. Radiotherapy may also be used in combination with surgery, depending on location and extent of neurological compromise (Janjan 1996). Radiotherapy may be commenced as an emergency treatment to preserve as much neurologic function as possible (Kirkbridge 1995).

Radiotherapy is administered over an average of 5–7 days at an average dose of 20 Gy in five fractions. Higher total doses of radiotherapy can only be tolerated by the spinal cord when small fractions of radiation are separated by 24 h (Kirkbridge 1995).

Radiation field usually extends two vertebral bodies above and below the spinal cord compression. A number of symptoms may occur as a result of using radiotherapy and as a particular consequence of the area irradiated, that is the cervical/thoracic/lumbar area of the spine.

Nausea, vomiting, diarrhoea and dysuria occur as the result of irradiation to the thoracic/lumbar spine (Kirkbridge 1995).

Guidelines • Care of patients with spinal cord compression (cont'd)

Action	Rationale
• Dysuria – exclude urinary tract infection by culturing MSU (midstream specimen of urine) and increase fluid intake.	
• Fatigue – provide and encourage rest periods.	The development of fatigue may be related to radiobiological action, with metabolites from cell destruction and normal tissue damage accumulating to give rise to fatigue (Faithfull 1998).
3 *Chemotherapy* If the patient requires chemotherapy, where appropriate, assist the patient's understanding of information regarding the rationale for chemotherapy and possible side-effects.	Chemotherapy may be administered if extradural spinal cord compression is present, e.g. lymphoma, myeloma, teratoma, but also in cases where SCC is the first presentation of cancer (Held & Peahota 1993). Each case is assessed individually for appropriateness of treatment. Side-effects will impact on the rehabilitation process, due to fatigue, bone marrow depression, skin fragility, constipation, altered appetite.

Rehabilitation care

Action	Rationale
1 Begin rehabilitation as soon as possible, taking into consideration any limitations associated with the stability of the spine and pain. Refer to physiotherapist as soon as diagnosis of spinal cord compression is suspected or confirmed.	If the spine is not stable and medical stabilization procedures are inappropriate the patient may need to have completed radiotherapy (to reduce the tumour) before mobilization; close liaison with the medical and physiotherapy team is necessary to plan appropriate mobilization.
2 Refer to the multiprofessional team as appropriate. This should include: (a) Physiotherapist (b) Occupational therapist (c) Social worker (d) Community liaison nurse specialist (e) Dietician and (f) Specialist palliative care physicians and nurses. Regular multidisciplinary team meetings should be held to assess progress.	Nurses play a key role in facilitating effective teamwork. The successful delivery of rehabilitation demands excellent internal organization and multidisciplinary approaches (Carson *et al.* 1997). To ensure continuous care and a consistent approach to care.
3 Set short-term attainable goals to achieve the best possible quality of life.	Patients may have a first presentation of their disease with spinal cord compression. Therefore the nurse's role is to promote self-care activities since prognosis may be longer term. If spinal cord compression is the result of metastatic disease, then rehabilitation would take a functional approach, as the patient may still survive for months, depending on the primary cancer type and histology, etc.
A rehabilitation programme with regular assessment and intervention should be initiated.	Goals are based on a patient's entire situation and lifestyle (Hunter 1998). To restore confidence and self-esteem, to give structure to the patient's day and to increase understanding of realistic aims of rehabilitation.
Goals need to be flexible.	The degree of patient functioning cannot always be anticipated (Cooper 1997).
4 Assess and monitor patient's and family's psychological status and adaptation to diagnosis and implications on lifestyle. Encourage patient to express feelings. Do not give false reassurance but communicate empathy for patient's feelings. Promote the use of a	Rehabilitation starts with helping the patient to confront the existence of a disability and may continue as the grief process proceeds. Feelings of helplessness, hopelessness and depression are common. Bedbound patients become withdrawn and lose motivation (Hillier & Wee 1997).

variety of coping techniques. Cultivate a positive and realistic outlook on life (Davidhizar 1997).

The degree of the patient's motivation will influence the rehabilitation process (Davidhizar 1997). The skill in managing this condition is to provide a level of care, without sacrificing patient autonomy and control.

5 Maximize potential for mobilization by the following:

    (a) Work as an integral part of the rehabilitation team to ensure that rehabilitation is continuous.

To maintain and increase patient's independence in activities requiring motor performance. To help patient to adjust and adapt to altered mobility. To facilitate participation in social and occupational activities.

    (b) Assist the patient to perform an active or passive range of movement exercises, based on physiotherapy assessment, patient assistance and instructions.

Active and passive range of movement exercises help to prevent complications associated with decreased movement and will also increase muscle strength. However, joint damage, due to decreased or lack of sensation, is possible with these exercises.

    (c) Reinforce transfer techniques proposed and formulated by the physiotherapist and occupational therapist.

To ensure safety of patient and nursing team and to ensure consistency of approach across the multidisciplinary team.

    (d) A home assessment may be needed to ensure that correct equipment is fitted appropriately (Borgman-Gainer 1996).

For safety and independence (Hillier & Wee 1997).

6 Monitor pressure areas continuously; it may be necessary to provide a therapeutic mattress and cushions as well as appropriate manual handling equipment.

It is essential to be aware that this group of patients differ to spinal injury patients; due to immunosuppressive treatments and overall physical condition, the predisposition to shearing forces and pressure sores may be greater (Cooper 1997).

7 Assess and promote optimal urinary elimination pattern, once transfer techniques have been established.

To establish degree of bladder function and to retrain bladder function. The degree of bladder dysfunction depends on the degree of damage to the sensory and motor tracts of the spinal cord, which sends messages between the bladder and the supraspinal centre. The presence of spinal shock, autonomic neurogenic bladder, sensory paralytic bladder and motor paralytic bladder are influential on management techniques.

Insert indwelling catheter or teach intermittent catheterization to the patient or relative if appropriate.

Catherization may be necessary to assist with elimination for those patients who experience a loss of bladder motor function (Pires 1996). Long-term catheterization may be an option and will require significant patient/family teaching (see Chap. 43, Urinary Catheterization).

If the patient is incontinent, treat sensitively and promote hygiene and skin integrity.

The patient may be very embarrassed and upset by this condition. To minimize the risk of any associated complications.

8 Promote and encourage optimal bowel care (see Chap. 6, Bowel Care). If patient is incontinent, promote dignity and physical hygiene.

Bowel activity is influenced by decreased mobility, spinal innervation, narcotics and other analgesics, and anorexia (Gender 1996).

9 Acknowledge and assess effects of diagnosis and disability on sexual function. Facilitate discussion with patient and partner, if appropriate.

Sexuality is often overlooked by professional carers who are focusing on the more obvious physical effects of spinal cord compression, rather than the psychosocial issues (Hillier & Wee 1997).

10 Begin discharge planning as soon as level of functioning is ascertained. Work closely with the rehabilitation team and the patient and family in conjunction with GPs and community teams, hospitals, hospices, voluntary services and charitable organizations (see Chap. 11, Discharge Planning).

To offer realistic care packages to enable the patient to return home quickly where appropriate. The coordination required to discharge and support these patients at home is complex and challenging (Hillier & Wee 1997).

Nursing care plan

Problem	Cause	Preventative action	Suggested action
Neurogenic or 'spinal' shock, characterized by hypotension and bradycardia.	Spinal shock is caused by a disruption of sympathetic outflow and manifests as low vascular resistance with increased intravascular capacity. The patient is functionally hypovolaemic even if no blood has been lost (Barker 1995).	Care with manual handling to prevent further injury to spine as outlined previously.	Assess vital signs and contact medical team urgently. Carry out IV fluid resuscitation to correct hypovolaemia. Patient may require transfer to critical care area. Bladder catheterization – to assess fluid volume status (Barker 1995).
'Autonomic dysreflexia' indicated by an acute rise in blood pressure, bradycardia, visual blurring, flushing above injury level and pallor below, and seizures.	Complication associated with compression of spinal cord at T6–8 or higher; caused by an imbalance between sympathetic and parasympathetic innervation. It is indicated by an abnormally strong sympathetic response and is triggered by an internal stimulus, such as a distended bladder.	If left untreated, condition may be lethal and thus the first line of treatment is prevention or removal of the stimulus (i.e. drainage of distended bladder). The medical team should be informed immediately (Dyck 1991).	
Low blood pressure.	Dehydration associated with nausea and vomiting (possibly associated with hypercalcaemia).		
Raised blood pressure.	Pain and anxiety.	Provide interventions to avoid or minimize pain.	
Altered respiratory status.	Diaphragmatic paralysis can be associated with cervical and/or thoracic spine involvement (*note*: breathing pattern may be altered due to pain).	Monitor respiratory rate and pattern when recording vital signs on admission. To assess patient and to establish baseline measurement for comparison with future measurements. Encourage patient to report any altered sensation or difficulty with breathing to note any changes immediately.	Respiratory function monitoring should be observed and documented as often as clinical assessment demands. If the patient is for full resuscitation, early communication with ITU and anaesthetic staff is essential, as this event necessitates urgent transfer for assisted ventilation (Dyck 1991). However, if the emphasis of treatment is palliative, mechanical ventilation may not be deemed appropriate by the multidisciplinary team. Provide the family with information and support.

| Urgency to eliminate urine. | Presence of indwelling catheter and/or urinary infection. | Consider removal of indwelling catheter. Assess the degree and type of sensation present, e.g. distention. Establish a timed voiding schedule and teach behavioural techniques such as pelvic floor exercises and relaxation exercises. |

Stoma Care

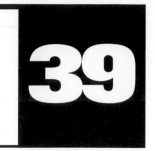

Definition

'Stoma' is a word of Greek origin meaning 'mouth' or 'opening' (Black 1994a). A bowel or urinary stoma is usually created by bringing a section of bowel out on to the abdominal wall as a diversionary procedure because the urinary or colonic tract beyond the position of the stoma is no longer viable.

Indications

Stoma care is required for the following purposes:

1 To collect urine or faeces in an appropriate appliance.
2 To achieve and maintain patient comfort and security.
3 To maintain good skin and stoma hygiene (Black 1997).

Reference material

Types of stoma

Colostomy

In a colostomy the stoma may be formed from any section of the large bowel, e.g. 'end' or 'terminal' sigmoid colostomy (usually permanent; Fig. 39.1). A temporary (usually transverse) colostomy may be raised to divert the faecal output, thus allowing healing of an anastomosis further along the colon. With a defunctioning loop colostomy, a rod or bridge may be used to maintain a hold on the abdominal surface. Such a rod or bridge is removed 5–10 days after insertion (Fig. 39.2). Once the stoma/cutaneous margin has healed a further operation will be required to close this stoma when it is no longer needed, i.e. when the anatomized bowel has healed. The term 'defunctioning' is used to indicate that the bowel distal to the stoma is being rested (Borwell 1994; Myers 1996).

Ileostomy

In an ileostomy the ileum is brought out onto the abdominal wall (Fig. 39.2), as when, for example, the large colon is affected by inflammatory disease. Many patients with ulcerative colitis are offered an ileo-anal pouch and therefore do not have to have a permanent stoma. For this operation a colectomy (removal of the whole colon) is performed and the terminal ileum is made into a reservoir (pouch) and brought down and attached to the anus. A temporary ileostomy allows the pouch to heal.

Ileal loop, ileal conduit or urostomy

The performance of such operations (when the bladder is removed or diseased) requires the ureters to be transplanted from the bladder into a length, approximately 15 cm, of ileum which has been isolated, along with its mesentery, from the remainder of the small bowel. One end of the ileum, with the resected ureters, remains inside the abdomen, while the other is brought out on to the abdominal wall and everted to form a slightly protruding stoma (Fig. 39.3) (Borwell 1997a; Nicholls & Williams 1998).

Other types of urinary diversion

Other types of urinary diversion include ureterostomy, a procedure that brings the ureters out onto the abdominal wall together (one stoma) or separately (two stomas). It may be possible for some patients with bladder disease to have a continent pouch or 'new' bladder formed internally. One example of this is the 'Mitrofanoff' technique (Gelister & Woodhouse 1991; Horn 1991; Leaver 1996). For further information on these continent urinary diversions, see Chap. 9.

Indications for bowel stoma

1 Cancer of the bowel
2 Cancer of the pelvis
3 Trauma
4 Neurological damage
5 Congenital disorders
6 Ulcerative colitis
7 Crohn's disease
8 Diverticular disease
9 Familial polyposis coli
10 Intractable incontinence
11 Radiation enteritis.

Indications for urinary stoma

1 Cancer of the bladder
2 Cancer of the pelvis
3 Trauma
4 Congential disorders
5 Neurological damage
6 Intractable incontinence

(Black 1994a.)

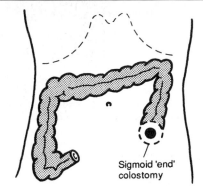

Figure 39.1   Sigmoid 'end' colostomy.

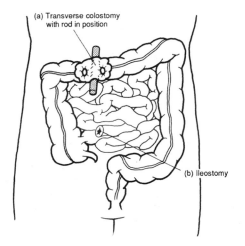

Figure 39.2   (a) Transverse colostomy and (b) ileostomy.

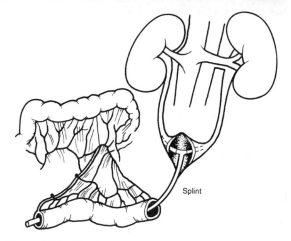

Figure 39.3   Urostomy.

Pre-operative preparation for stoma surgery

Physical preparation of the patient will vary according to the type of operation and the policies of individual surgeons and hospitals. This will involve the usual preparation for anaesthesia (Chap. 30, Peri-Operative Care), preparation of the area of the body involved and of the bowel. Other specific procedures may also be included (Winkley 1998).

Psychological preparation of the individual facing stoma surgery should begin as soon as surgery has been considered, preferably by utilizing the skills of a trained stoma care nurse. Boore (1978), Hayward (1978), Ivimy (1997) and Beddows (1997) have illustrated the importance of pre-operative information and explanation in reducing postoperative physical and psychological stress. Information-giving and discussion with patients about their stoma and lifestyle start pre-operatively and continue throughout the patient's stoma experience. The aims of these interactions are as follows:

1 To help the individual with a stoma to return to his or her previous place in society whenever possible.
2 To help in the process of adapting to a changed body image (Price 1990; Salter 1997).
3 To reduce anxiety. The patient's perception of life with a stoma may have a positive or detrimental influence on rehabilitation. There may be myths and wrong information to dispel, and the patient's awareness of the experiences of another ostomate to discuss (Salter 1992; Bryant 1993).
4 To explain that the presence of a stoma need not adversely affect any previous quality of life such as hobbies, work, social life or any other interests, although the underlying disease might (Salter 1992).
5 To prepare the patient for the appearance and likely behaviour pattern of the stoma (Pullen 1998).
6 To reassure patients that they will be able to manage an appliance whatever the environment (Salter 1995).
7 To assure patients that they will be supported fully while in hospital and will not be discharged until they are confident about the stoma's care and that continuing support will be available in the community (Salter 1995; Pullen 1998).

Such pre-operative education has been shown to increase cooperation and trust and reduce anxiety, the length of time the patient remains in hospital and the amount of postoperative analgesia required (Wade 1989). It should be borne in mind that any information given should be relevant to the patient's needs. Family and/or close friends may also be involved, when appropriate, on agreement with the patient (Price 1996).

Diet

All patients should be encouraged to eat a wide variety of foods. Explanations of how the gut functions, how it has been changed since surgery and the effects certain foodstuffs may cause should be given. For example, colostomy and ileostomy formation means the loss of the anal sphincter so passage of wind cannot be controlled. High-fibre foods such as beans and pulses produce wind as they are broken down in the gut; hence individuals who eat large quantities of these foodstuffs may be troubled by wind.

Colostomy

Certain foods, e.g. large portions of fruit and vegetables (onions, sprouts, cabbage, etc.), may cause loose stools or excess flatus. It is suggested that rather than eliminate these items from the diet, the foods identified should be tried again in smaller portions. No food item affects everyone in the same way and it is best for the individual to experiment (Black 1998; Blackley 1998; Wood 1998). It might be preferable to reduce the portion and prepare for the consequences. Beer and fizzy drinks may cause excess flatus. Beer and other forms of alcohol will affect the ostomate as they do everyone else (Little 1989).

Ileostomy

Certain foods will cause excess flatus. Pulses, dried fruit, peanuts and coconut are digested slowly and so they will need to be masticated well before swallowing.

If these foods are taken in excess and not masticated well they could swell in the gut and cause a 'bolus' obstruction. Some foods, e.g. tomato skins or pips, may pass into the appliance unaltered due to a more rapid transit time (Hulten & Palselius 1996; Black 1997; Blackley 1998). Care should also be taken by patients using oral contraception as absorption may be impaired (Black 1994b).

Urostomy

There are no dietary restrictions with urostomy. It must be stressed, however, that an adequate fluid intake must be maintained to minimize the risk of urinary infection. Approximately 2 litres is the recommended minimum (Black 1997). The slow return of both a normal appetite and bowel function is a common feature following this operation (due to bowel handling in surgery) and it gives cause for much anxiety. The patient should be warned of this and advised to take small, light meals supplemented by nutritious drinks. Normal appetite may not return for 2 or 3 months after the operation.

Fear of malodour

This is a common fear for patients with bowel stomas, often based on hearsay or experience with other ostomists in hospital or the community. Appliances are odour free when fitted correctly. Flatus may be released via charcoal filters and deodorizers are available. The individual must be reassured, however, that any problems that occur postoperatively will be investigated, with a good possibility of them being solved by such means as the use of alternative appliances (Bryant 1993; Black 1997).

Sex and the ostomate

The possibility of sexual impairment for both men and women after stoma surgery depends on the nature of the operation, the ensuing damage to the nerves and tissues involved. The psychological impact of the surgery and its effect on the individual's body image must also be taken into consideration. Surgery that results in physical sexual disability will have psychological repercussions, while some sexual difficulties may be of psychological origin (Bryant 1993; Salter 1996). Impairment may be permanent or temporary. In the latter case, resolution of the difficulty may take anything up to 2 years. Pre- and postoperative counselling should be offered for both patient and partner. In cases of male erectile dysfunction a number of treatment options are available. These include the insertion of penile implants, vacuum constriction devices, intracavernosal injections or intraurethral applications of alprostadil, a prostaglandin E_1 (Caverject or Medicated Urethral Systems for Erection, MUSE) and oral sildenafil (Viagra) (Ashford 1998; Newey 1998; Wagner & Saenz de Jejada 1998; *ABPI Compendium* 1999–2000).

Female patients may experience dyspareunia; this may be due to narrowing or shortening of the vagina or a reduction in the volume of vaginal secretions (Schover 1986). The use of a lubricant, adopting different positions during lovemaking or encouraging greater relaxation by extending foreplay may help resolve painful intercourse (Topping 1990; Bryant 1993).

Useful references on the psychological and sexual aspects of care may be found in Van De Wiel *et al.* (1991), Anders (1993), Borwell (1997b) and Huish *et al.* (1998).

Personnel who may be expected to provide information

1 Medical staff
2 Stoma care nurse
3 Nursing staff on ward
4 Primary health care team
5 Another suitable ostomate. 'Visitors' are trained by the voluntary associations and, ideally, should be of similar age, sex and background to the patient to enable the patient to discuss problems of adapting to life with a stoma (Rheaume & Gooding 1991; Mowdy 1998).

Useful aids

1 Information booklets
2 Samples of the various appliances
3 Diagrams
4 Audio tapes
5 Video tapes.

These aids are valuable to reinforce and clarify the verbal information.

Pre-operative assessment

It is important to determine whether a patient will be able to manage a stoma by assessing the following:

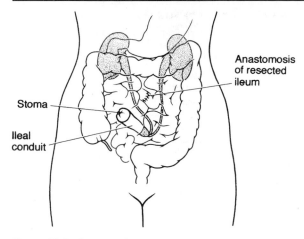

Figure 39.4   Position of stoma.

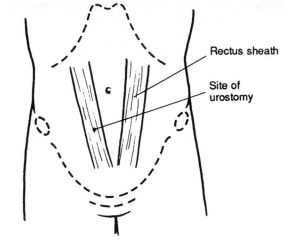

Figure 39.5   Site of urostomy.

1 Eyesight
2 Manual dexterity
3 The presence of other debilitating diseases, e.g. Parkinson's disease or arthritis
4 Mental state
5 Loss of an upper limb
6 Skin conditions
7 Abnormal contours, e.g. the changes that occur with spina bifida (Stevens 1996).

Siting of the stoma is one of the most important preoperative tasks to be carried out by the doctor, stoma care nurse or experienced ward nurse (Figs 39.4 and 39.5). This minimizes future difficulties such as interference by the stoma with clothes, or skin problems caused by leakage of the appliance due to a badly sited stoma (e.g. on the waistline or in a body crease) (Crooks 1994; Myers 1996). When siting the stoma, consideration should be given to the following:

1 A flat area of the skin to facilitate safe adhesion of the appliance.
2 Avoidance of bony prominences such as hips and ribs which may interfere with the adhesion of the appliance, or pendulous breasts which may obscure the stoma from the patient's view, making self-care impossible.
3 Avoidance of skin creases, especially in the region of the groin or the umbilicus, to avoid urine or faecal matter tracking along the skin creases.
4 Avoidance of scars, which may cause skin creases which may lead to leakages.
5 Avoidance of waistline or belt areas, as patient's clothing may put pressure on the stoma which may lead to leaks or trauma.
6 Maintenance of the stoma within the rectus sheath, as this reduces the risk of herniation later (Ortiz *et al.* 1993; Kelly 1995; Myers 1996). The muscle may be identified by asking the patient to lie flat, then to raise the head. The muscle may also be palpated and easily felt when the patient coughs.

7 Ideally, the patient should be able to see the stoma site (Blackley 1998).

The patient must be observed while lying, sitting in a comfortable chair, with the abdominal muscles relaxed, and standing. Consideration must be given to any bending or lifting involved with the patient's work and any other activities in which the patient partakes. Account must also be taken of any weight gain or loss in the postoperative period, as this may change the contours of the abdomen and hence the position of the stoma.

Postoperative period

Control of stoma action

Ileal loop

Urine will dribble from the stoma every 20–30 seconds. The output may be slightly less after periods of reduced fluid intake, e.g. at night. An appliance has to be worn at all times.

Ileostomy

Once the stoma starts to act a few days after surgery, the fluid output, normally 500–850 ml every 24 hours, takes on a porridge consistency when a normal intake of food is established. The effluent contains enzymes that will excoriate the skin if contact is allowed. While the effluent cannot be controlled, the ostomist may find that the stoma is more active after main meals (Myers 1996; Black 1997).

Colostomy

Due to its position, only a small amount of water will be reabsorbed from the faecal matter which is passed via a transverse colostomy; therefore the effluent will be unformed. Patients with a sigmoid colostomy may find that wholemeal foods assist in producing a formed stool once or twice daily (Myers 1996; Black 1998).

Medications that reduce peristaltic action, e.g. codeine phosphate, may also be used to control diarrhoea. The only means of controlling a sigmoid colostomy, however, is by regular irrigation or by use of a Conseal plug system. Stoma care nurses will need to assess patients before teaching them how to perform irrigation procedure or use of Conseal plugs.

Irrigation

Irrigation is a method of controlling the output of a colostomy by means of washing out the stoma with warm tap water (with the use of a coned irrigation set), every 24–48 hours.

The advantage of successful colostomy irrigation is that there is no stool leakage between irrigations (De-Hong 1991; Davis 1996).

Postoperative stages

Stage I

In theatre, an appropriately sized skin-protective wafer should be applied around the stoma, followed by a drainable, transparent appliance, which should be left on for approximately 2 days. For the first 48 hours postoperatively, observe stoma colour (a pink and healthy appearance indicates a good blood supply), size and stoma output (bearing in mind that it may take a few days for a bowel to act). The drainable appliance should always be emptied frequently, gas should be allowed to escape and the appliance should not be allowed to get more than half full with effluent. If the appliance becomes too full, leaks may occur and the weight from the effluent or the pressure from gas may cause the appliance to fall off (Black 1997).

Immediately postoperatively patients would not be expected to perform their own stoma care but would be encouraged to observe the nurse caring for them and may discuss it with the nurse. Viewing the stoma may be difficult for the patient, who may be very aware of other people's reaction to it (Price 1993).

Stage II

As the patient's condition improves, a demonstration change of the appliance will be given with full explanation of the principles of stoma care. This will be followed by further opportunities to discuss any problems or raise new queries. Provided the patient agrees, it is useful to involve the patient's partner or close friends or relatives at this stage. Their acceptance of the stoma may encourage the patient and help to restore the patient's self-esteem (Salter 1995). In the following days, patients will be encouraged to participate in and gradually assume responsibility for their own stoma care. They may now be ready to discuss appliances and choose the one that they wish to use at home. Preparation for discharge will be discussed (Black 1994c; Heywood Jones 1994).

Stage III

Ideally, the patient should now be independent, eating a normal diet, be ready for discharge and should be confident in stoma care.

If the family or close friends are closely involved during all stages and are supportive, patients are better able to adapt to the threat of mutilating surgery and altered pattern of elimination (Price 1993). The family or close friends are also likely to require support and information so that they are in a position to help the ostomate. Acceptance of the stoma is a gradual process and, on discharge from hospital, patients may only be beginning to adapt to life with a stoma (Salter 1997).

Specific discharge plans

Follow-up support

The patient is discharged with adequate supplies until a prescription is obtained from the general practitioner. Written reminders are provided of how to care for the stoma, how to obtain supplies of appliances, and any other information that may be required. The patient should have details of non-medical stoma clinics, details about the relevant agencies and information about voluntary associations. Arrangements should also have been made for a home visit from the stoma care nurse and/or the community nurse (Blackley 1998).

Obtaining supplies

All NHS patients with a permanent stoma are entitled to free prescriptions for their stoma care products, and should complete the relevant forms for exemption from payment. Appliances can then be obtained from the local chemist, a free home delivery service or directly from the appropriate manufacturers.

Stoma appliances and accessories

Many of the appliances now available are very similar in style, colour and efficiency and often there is very little to choose between them when the time comes for the ostomate to decide what to wear.

The aim of good stoma care is to return patients to their place in society (Black 1994c). One of the ways in which this can be facilitated is to provide them with a safe, reliable appliance. This means that there must be no fear of leakage or odour and the appliance should be comfortable, unobtrusive and easy to handle. The ostomate should be allowed a choice of bag from a selection of appropriate appliances. It is also necessary to ensure that there are no problems with the stoma or peristomal skin.

Choosing the right size of appliance

Bags are labelled according to the size of the opening that fits around the stoma. To keep the skin unblemished, it must be protected from the stoma output. The size chosen, therefore, should be one that fits snugly around the stoma to within 0.5 cm of the stoma edge. This narrow edge of skin is left exposed to prevent any of the adhesives, some of which are more rigid than others, rubbing against the stoma. The appliances usually come with measuring guides to allow for correct choice of size. During the first weeks the oedematous stoma will reduce in size and the bags or flange of the two-piece type appliances will have to be changed accordingly.

Types of appliance

Although some people whose stomas were created several years ago are wearing non-disposable rubber bags, most appliances used today are made of a specially designed laminate composed of three types of plastic. This should ensure that the appliances are:

1 Leak proof
2 Odour proof
3 Unobtrusive
4 Noiseless
5 Disposable.

The appliances differ slightly according to the stoma for which they are meant. All types, however, fall within one of two broad categories:

1 One-piece. This comprises a bag with an adhesive wafer that fits around the stoma. When the bag is renewed, the adhesive is removed from the skin. Its advantage is that it is easy to handle, e.g. by an ostomate suffering from arthritis.
2 Two-piece. This comprises a flange for the skin that fits around the stoma and a bag that clips on to the flange. It can be used with sore and sensitive skin as when bags are removed from the flange, the skin is left undisturbed. However, the patient must have the dexterity to clip the bag securely onto the flange (Willis 1995; Heenan 1996).

Drainable bags

1 Bowel stoma bags (Fig. 39.6a).
   Suitable for: ileostomy, transverse colostomy.
   Stoma output: fluid to semiformed (volume is too great for closed bags).
   Use: emptied frequently, taking care to rinse outlet afterwards; may be left on for up to 3 days.
   Additional features: specially designed flatus filters are being fitted to some bags. These are less likely to become obstructed by faecal fluid or leak via the small opening. The outlet may have a separate clip or fixed 'roll-up' closure.
   Colour: clear, opaque.
2 Urinary stoma bags (Fig. 39.6b).
   Suitable for: urostomy.
   Stoma output: urine.
   Use: emptied frequently via a fixed tap; may be left on for up to 3 days.
   Additional features: may be used with large collecting bag and tubing for night drainage.
   Colour: clear, semi-opaque or opaque.

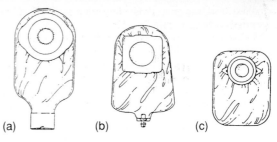

Figure 39.6   Stoma equipment. (a) Bowel stoma bag; (b) urinary stoma bag; (c) closed bag.

3 Closed bags (Fig. 39.6c).
   Suitable for: sigmoid colostomy.
   Stoma output: a formed stool.
   Use: changed once or twice a day.
   Additional features: some have incorporated flatus filters that allow the release of flatus through charcoal patches that absorb the odour.
   Colour: clear or opaque.

Some drainage bags may be fitted with protective adhesive especially for sensitive skin and many now have a cotton-weave backing to reduce and absorb perspiration and to prevent the plastic from sticking to the skin.

Accessories

The specific products in this section have been mentioned as examples of what aids are available and reference to them is not necessarily intended as a recommendation.

Solutions for skin and stoma cleaning

Mild soap and water, or water only, are sufficient for skin and stoma cleaning. Detergents, disinfectants and antiseptics cause dryness and irritation and should not be used. The stoma is not a wound or a lesion and should be regarded as a resited urethra or anus.

Skin barriers

1 Creams.
   Unless made specifically for use on peristomal skin, creams should not be used, as the residual surface film of grease prevents adherence of the appliance. Creams usually have a soothing and moisturizing effect.
   Use: for sensitive skin, as a protective measure.
   Method: use sparingly; massage gently into the skin until completely absorbed; excess grease may be wiped off with a soft tissue.
   Example: Chiron barrier cream (aluminium chlorohydrate 2% in an emulsified base) (*ABPI Compendium* 1999–2000).
   Precaution: not to be used on broken or sore skin.
2 Skin gels/sealants.
   Use: act as a film on the skin, first to prevent irritation and, second, to give protection as it is removed with the

adhesive of the bag, thus preventing removal of the stratum corneum of the skin.
Method: pat onto the skin gently; dries quickly.
Examples: Skin Gel, Skin Prep.
Precaution: should not be used on broken skin as they contain alcohol and cause stinging (*ABPI Compendium* 1999–2000).

3 Protective wafers.
Use: these are hypoallergenic and are designed to cover and protect skin, and allow healing if the skin is sore or broken. May be useful in cases of skin reaction or allergy to the adhesive or an appliance.
Method: the wafers may be cut with the aid of a template (pattern) to the required shape and fitted on to the skin. The appliances are then attached to the wafer. The rim of the wafer should not press against the stoma but should fit to 0.5 cm around it.
Examples: Stomahesive or Comfeel type of wafers. Stomahesive is composed of gelatin, pectin, sodium carboxymethycellulose, and polyisobutylene (Martindale 1993); it adheres painlessly to normal, erythematous, moist or broken skin; it is available in three sizes.
Precautions: allergy may occur, but rarely.

4 Protective rings.
Use: protective rings are used to provide skin protection around the stoma; they will protect a smaller area than the wafers mentioned above. They are also useful to fill in 'dips' or 'gulleys' in the skin.
Method: like the wafers, they have an adhesive side and may be applied directly to the skin. They form an integral part of some of the appliances.
Example: Salts Cohesive seals.
Precautions: as for protective wafers above.

5 Pastes.
Use: useful to fill in crevices and 'gulleys' in the skin to provide a smooth surface for an appliance.
Method: *Stomahesive* – either leave for 60 seconds after applying to the skin, when the surface will be dry, making the paste easier to mould into the skin contour, or apply with a spatula, or wet the finger first to prevent the paste sticking and mould the paste immediately. Will sting on raw areas as it contains alcohol. Apply a little Orahesive powder to these areas first. *Orabase* – similar to Stomahesive in composition but with the addition of liquid paraffin. Used to protect raw areas. Does not contain alcohol so will not cause local irritation.
Examples: Stomahesive paste, soft paste and Orabase paste.

6 Powders.
Use: for protection of sore or raw areas without impeding adhesion of the appliance.
Method: sprinkle on affected areas.
Example: Orahesive powder.

Adhesive preparations

1 Lotions.
Use: only required when appliance does not adhere well to the skin, e.g. because of leakage, uneven site, or if abdominal fistulae present.

Method: the individual products differ considerably in their method of application and it is recommended that the user consults the manufacturer's instructions.
Example: Saltair solution.

Convex devices

Use: these devices are designed to be used with retracted stomas. The convex shape allows a greater seal round the stoma by filling in any crevices caused by retraction, scars or skin creases.
Method: convexity may be achieved by fitting specially designed plastic inserts into the baseplate of a two piece appliance or by using appliances with built in convexity.
Examples: convex inserts, Impression range of appliances.

Deodorants

1 Aerosols.
Use: to absorb odour.
Method: one or two puffs into the air before emptying or removal of appliance.
Examples: Atmacol, Limone, Naturcare.

2 Drops and powders.
Use: for deodorizing bag contents.
Method: before fitting pouch or after emptying and cleaning drainable pouch, squeeze tube two or three times.
Examples: Ostobon deodorant powder, Chironair odour control liquid.

3 Flatus filters (charcoal filled) usually incorporated into the bag.
Use: to allow gradual release of flatus from the bag while allowing absorption of odour by the charcoal. The charcoal may only be effective for between 6 and 12 hours, depending on brand of filter.

Useful addresses

1 Association for Spina Bifida and Hydrocephalus (ASBAH), 42 Park Road, Peterborough PE1 2UQ (Tel: 01733 555988).
2 British Colostomy Association, 13–15 Station Road, Reading, Berkshire RG1 1LG (Tel: 0118 9391537 or 0800 3284257).
3 IA (Ileostomy and Internal Pouch Support Group), PO Box 132, Scunthorpe, DN15 9YW (Tel: 01724 720150 or 0800 0184724).
4 Urostomy Association, 'Buckland', Beaumont Park, Danbury, Essex CM3 4DE (Tel: 0124 5224294).

References and further reading

ABPI Compendium of Data Sheets and Summaries of Product Characteristics 1999–2000. Datapharm Publications, London.
Allison, M. (1995) Comparing methods of stoma formation. *Nurs Stand*, 9(24), 26–8.
Anders, K. (1993) Open communication can restore self-esteem: sexuality issues related to cystectomy for stoma formation. *Prof Nurse*, 8(10), 638–43.

Ashford, L. (1998) Erectile dysfunction. *Prof Nurse*, **13**(9), 603–608.

Beddows, J. (1997) Alleviating pre-operative anxiety in patients: a study. *Nurs Stand*, **11**(37), 35–8.

Black, P.K. (1994a) Stoma care: a practical approach. *Nurs Stand*, **8**(34), RCN *Nurs Update*, Learning Unit 045.

Black, P.K. (1994b) Hidden problems of stoma care. *Br J Nurs*, **3**(14), 707–711.

Black, P.K. (1994c) Choosing the correct stoma appliance. *Br J Nurs*, **3**(11), 545–6, 548, 550.

Black, P.K. (1997) Practical stoma care. *Nurs Stand*, **11**(47), 49–55.

Black, P.K. (1998) Update. Colostomy. *Prof Nurse*, **13**(12), 851–7.

Blackley, P. (1998) *Practical Stoma, Wound and Continence Management.* Research Publications, Australia.

Boore, J.R.P. (1978) *A Prescription for Recovery: The Effect of Preoperative Preparation of Surgical Patients on Postoperative Stress, Recovery and Infection.* RCN, London.

Borwell, B. (1994) Colostomies and their management. *Nurs Stand*, **8**(45), CE article 332.

Borwell, B. (1997a) Ileo-anal pouch surgery and its after-care. *Commun Nurse*, August.

Borwell, B. (1997b) The psychosexual needs of a stoma patient. *Prof Nurse*, **12**(4), 250–55.

Broadwell, D.C. (1987) Peristomal skin integrity. *Nurs Clin North America*, **22**(2), 321–32.

Bryant, R.A. (1993) Ostomy patient management: care that engenders adaptation. *Cancer Invest*, **11**(5), 565–77.

Caldwell, K. (1995) Homesexuality: a neglected issue in stoma care. *Br J Nurs*, **4**(17), 1009–1012.

Crooks, S. (1994) Foresight that leads to improved outcome: stoma care nurses' role in siting stomas. *Prof Nurse*, **10**(2), 89–92.

Davies, K. (1990) Impotence after surgery. *Nursing*, **4**(18), 13–26.

Davis, K. (1996) Irrigation technique. In: *Stoma Care Nursing – A Patient-Centred Approach* (ed. C. Myers). Arnold, London.

De-Hong, Y. (1991) An assessment of colostomy irrigation. *Ostomy Int*, **11**(2), *Nursing* (1st series), **17**, 727–9.

Dickenson, C. (1995) The bladder: cystectomy and ileo-conduit to treat cancer. *Nurs Times*, **91**(42), 34–5.

Etnyre, W. (1990) Meeting the needs of gay and lesbian ostomates. *Proc 8th Bien Cong World Council Enterost Ther*, Toronto, 15–20 July. Hollister, Illinois.

Faller, N. & Lawrence, K. (1992) A pictorial workshop: 'Tips on clips: hints on tail closures', 'Ideas sobre pinzas'. *World Council Enterost Ther J*, **12**(4), 26–7.

Fillingham, S. & Douglas, J. (1997) *Urological Nursing.* Baillière Tindall, London.

Gelister, J.F. & Woodhouse, C.R. (1991) Role of continent suprapubic diversion in pelvic cancer. *Br J Urol*, **68**, 376–9.

Hayward, J. (1978) *Information – A Prescription Against Pain.* RCN, London.

Heenan, A.L.J. (1996) Two piece stoma systems. *Prof Nurse*, **11**(5), 313–14.

Heywood Jones, I. (1994) Skills update. Stoma care. *Commun Outlook*, December.

Horn, S. (1991) Nursing patients with a continent urinary diversion. *Nurs Stand*, **4**(21), 24–6.

Huish, M., Kumar, D. & Stones, C. (1998) Stoma surgery and sex problems in ostomates. *Sex Marital Ther*, **13**(3), 311–28.

Hulten, L. & Palselius, I. (1996) Are dietary restrictions necessary for ileostomy surgery? *Eurostoma*, **13**, 20.

Ivimy, A. (1997) Postoperative recovery is influenced by preoperative care. *Eurostoma*, **17**, 8–9.

Kelly, L. (1995) Patients becoming people. *J Community Nurs*, August, 12–16.

Klopp, A. (1990) Body image and self-concept among individuals with stomas. *J Enterost Ther*, **17**(3), 98–105.

Krasner, D. (1993) Six steps to successful stoma care. *Reg Nurse*, July.

Leaver, R. (1996) Continent urinary diversions: the Mitrafanoff principle. In: *Stoma Care Nursing – A Patient-Centred Approach* (ed. C. Myers). Arnold, London.

Little, G.R. (1989) The dietary implications of having a stoma. *Surg Nurse*, **2**(6), Suppl., vi–ix.

MacDonald, K. & Joels, J. (1990) Stoma care: which appliance to choose? *Surg Nurse*, **3**(1), i–vi.

Martindale (1993) *The Extra Pharmacopoeia* (ed. J.E.F. Reynolds), 13th edn. Pharmaceutical Press, London.

Mowdy, S. (1998) The role of the WOC nurse in an ostomy support group. *J Wound Ostomy Continence Nurses*, **25**, 51–4.

Myers, C. (1996) *Stoma Care Nursing – A Patient-Centred Approach.* Arnold, London.

Newey, J. (1998) Causes and treatment of erectile dysfunction. *Nurs Stand*, **12**(47), 39–40.

Nicholls, R.J. & Williams, J. (1998) *Ulcerative Colitis.* Convatec, Uxbridge.

Ortiz, H. *et al.* (1993) Does the frequency of colostomy hernia depend on the colostomy location in the abdominal wall? *World Council Enterost Ther J*, **13**(2), 13–14.

Price, B. (1990) *Body Image Nursing: Concepts and Care.* Prentice Hall, New York.

Price, B. (1993) Profiling the high risk altered body image patient. *Sen Nurse*, **13**(4), 17–21.

Price, B. (1994) Understanding the experience of an altered body image. *Eurostoma*, **5**, 10–11.

Price, B. (1996) Practical support roles for relatives of stoma patients. *Eurostoma*, **16**, 10–11.

Pullen, M. (1998) Support role. *Nurs Times*, **94**(47).

Rheaume, A. & Gooding, B.A. (1991) Social support, coping strategies, and long term adaptation to ostomy among self-help group members. *J Enterost Ther*, **18**, 11–15.

Salter, M. (1992) Body image: the person with a stoma, Part 1. *Wound Manag*, **2**(2), 8–9.

Salter, M. (1995) Guest editorial: some observations on body image. *World Council Enterost Ther*, **15**(3), 4–7.

Salter, M. (1996) Sexuality and the stoma patient. In: *Stoma Care Nursing – A Patient-Centred Approach* (ed. C. Myers). Arnold, London.

Salter, M. (1997) *Altered Body Image: the Nurse's Role.* Baillière Tindall, London.

Schover, L.R. (1986) Sexual rehabilitation of the ostomy patient. In: *Ostomy Care and the Cancer Patient* (eds D.B. Smith & D.E. Johnson). Grune & Stratton, Orlando.

Stevens, P.J. (1996) Never divorce the hole from the whole. *Proc 11th Bien Cong World Council Enterost Ther*, Jerusalem, 23–28 June. Hollister, Illinois.

Tomaselli, N. & Morin, K. (1991) Body image in patients with stomas: a critical review of the literature. *J Enterost Ther*, **18**(3), 95–9.

Topping, A. (1990) Sexual activity and the stoma patient. *Nurs Stand*, **4**(41), 24–6.

Van De Wiel, H.B.M. *et al.* (1991) Sexual functioning after ostomy surgery. *Sex Marital Ther*, **6**(2), 196–209.

Wade, B. (1989) Nursing care of the stoma patient. *Surg Nurse*, **2**(5), Suppl., ix–xii.

Wade, B. (1990) Patients' fears after stoma surgery. *Nurs Stand*, **55**(3).

Wagner, G. & Saenz de Jejada, I. (1998) Update on male erectile dysfunction. *Br Med J*, **316**, 678–81.

Wells, R. (1990) Sexuality: an unknown word for patients with a stoma? *Proc 2nd Int Symp Supportive Care in Cancer Patients*, St Gallen, 28 Feb–3 Mar (unpublished paper).

White, C. (1998) Psychological management of stoma-related concerns. *Nurs Stand*, 12(36), 35–8.

White, C.A. & Hunt, J.C. (1997) Psychological factors in post-operative care adjustment to stoma surgery. *Ann R Coll Surg Engl*, 79, 3–7.

Willis, J. (1995) Stoma care principles and product type. *Nurs Times*, 91(2), 43–5.

Winkley, M. (1998) Pre-operative fasting. *Nurs Times*, 94(40).

Wood, S. (1998) Nutrition and stoma patients. *Nurs Times*, 94(48).

GUIDELINES • Stoma care

These procedural guidelines contain the basic information needed for changing a stoma appliance. Modifications may be made according to the following factors:

1 The place of change, i.e. bathroom, bedside, availability of sink, etc.
2 The person changing the appliance, i.e. nurse, patient or carer.
3 Type of appliance used, e.g. one- or two-piece, closed or drainable.
4 Any accessories used, e.g. flatus filters, hypoallergenic tape, barrier creams, etc.

Equipment

1 Clean tray holding:
   (a) Tissues.
   (b) New appliances.
   (c) Disposal bags for used appliances and tissues.
   (d) Relevant accessories, e.g. flatus filters, tape, etc.
2 Bowl of warm water.
3 Soap.
4 Jug for contents of appliance.
5 Gloves. (It is now common practice and, in many cases, hospital policy, to wear gloves when dealing with blood and body fluids due to risk of infections. Thus they should be worn for cleaning stomas. It is recognized that it could be difficult to attach an appliance with gloves in situ (due to adhesive), but once stoma has been cleaned of excreta and blood, gloves may be removed to apply bag.) This practice should be explained to patients so that they do not feel it is just because they have a stoma that gloves are worn.

Procedure

Action	*Rationale*
1 Explain and discuss the procedure with the patient.	To ensure that the patient understands the procedure and gives his/her valid consent.
2 Explain the procedure.	To familiarize the patient with the procedure.
3 Ensure that the patient is in a suitable and comfortable position where the patient will be able to watch the procedure; if well enough, a mirror may be used to aid visualization.	To allow good access to the stoma for cleaning and for secure application of the stoma bag. The patient will become familiar with the stoma and will also learn much about the care of the stoma by observation of the nurse (Bryant 1993).
4 Use a small protective pad to protect the patient's clothing from drips if the effluent is fluid and apply gloves for nurse's protection.	Avoids the necessity for renewing clothing or bedclothes and demoralization of the patient as a result of soiling.
5 If the bag is of the drainable type, empty the contents into a jug before removing the bag.	For ease of handling the appliance and prevention of spillage.
6 Remove the appliance. Peel the adhesive off the skin with one hand while exerting gentle pressure on the skin with the other.	To reduce trauma to the skin. Erythema as a result of removing the appliance is normal and quickly settles (Broadwell 1987).
7 Remove excess faeces or mucus from the stoma with a damp tissue.	So that the stoma and surrounding skin are clearly visible.
8 Examine the skin and stoma for soreness, ulceration or other unusual phenomena. If the skin is unblemished and the stoma is a healthy red colour, proceed.	For the prevention of complications or the treatment of existing problems (see Nursing care plan).

9 Wash the skin and stoma gently until they are clean.

To promote cleanliness and prevent skin excoriation.

10 Dry the skin and stoma gently but thoroughly.

The appliance will attach more securely to dry skin.

11 Apply a clean appliance.

12 Dispose of soiled tissues and the used bag. Rinse the bag through in the sluice with water, wrap it in a disposable bag and place it in an appropriate plastic bin. At home the bag should be emptied into the toilet; a closed bag may be cut at the lower end using scissors especially reserved for this purpose, then rinsed using a jug or by holding it under the flushing water. Wrap the bag in newspaper, tie it in a plastic bag and dispose of it in a rubbish bag.

Faecal material in waste bags is a potential source of infection. Excreta should be disposed of down the sluice or toilet.

13 Wash hands thoroughly using bactericidal soap and water or bactericidal alcohol hand rub.

To prevent spread of infection by contaminated hands.

GUIDELINES • Collection of a specimen of urine from an ileal conduit or urostomy

Equipment

1 Sterile dressing pack.
2 Soft catheter – Nelaton type, not larger than 12 or 14 Fr.
3 Disposable plastic apron.
4 Universal specimen container.

5 Skin-cleansing solution.
6 Bactericidal alcohol hand rub.
7 Clean stoma appliance.

Procedure

Action

1 Explain and discuss the procedure with the patient.

Rationale

To ensure that the patient understands the procedure and gives his/her valid consent.

2 Ensure that the patient is in a comfortable position, e.g. sitting up, supported by pillows, and that the stoma is easily accessible.

For patient comfort and to allow access to stoma.

3 Screen the bed, then wash hands using bactericidal soap and water or bactericidal alcohol hand rub and dry them.

For the patient's privacy and to reduce the risk of cross-infection (see Chap. 3, Aseptic Technique). Curtains are drawn at this stage so that dust and airborne organisms disturbed by the curtains do not settle on the sterile trolley.

4 Prepare the trolley and take it to the patient's bedside.

To ensure equipment is easily available.

5 Put on a disposable plastic apron.

To reduce risk of cross-infection.

6 Remove the sterile dressing pack, catheter and receiver from their outer wrappings. Place them on the top shelf of the trolley.

To prepare equipment.

7 Remove the appliance from the stoma and cover the stoma with a clean topical swab.

To absorb any spillage from the stoma.

8 Clean hands with a bactericidal alcohol hand rub, and put on clean disposable gloves before opening the sterile field on the trolley.

To reduce the risk of introducing infection into the stoma during the procedure.

Guidelines • Collection of a specimen of urine from an ileal conduit or urostomy (cont'd)

Action	Rationale
9 Remove the non-linting gauze with forceps, check and discard it. Arrange a towel to absorb spillage from the stoma.	To keep the areas as clean as possible and to protect the patient and the bedclothes from spilled urine.
10 Clean around the stoma with water or saline, from the centre outwards.	Good cleansing of the area reduces the risk of introduction of surface pathogens into the ileal loop.
11 Apply gentle skin traction to allow stomal opening to be more visible. Insert the catheter tip gently to a depth of 2.5–5 cm only and wait for urine to drain through. Collect the sample in the specimen container. The recommended volume is 3–5 ml.	To avoid catheter coming into contact with external surfaces of stoma. Gentle handling reduces the risk of ileal perforation and is more comfortable for the patient. To ensure adequate sample of urine for bacteriological assessment.
12 Remove the catheter and seal in the specimen container. Remove gloves and attend to stoma care and apply a pouch as usual. Make the patient comfortable.	To prevent spillage of sample. To ensure patient comfort.
13 Dispose of equipment.	
14 Wash hands with bactericidal soap and water and dry.	To reduce risk of cross-infection.
15 Check that the specimen is labelled correctly and dispatch it to the laboratory with the appropriate forms.	

Nursing care plan

Problem	Cause	Suggested action
Leakage of urine or faeces.	Ill-fitting appliance.	Remeasure stoma and ensure a snug-fitting appliance. Prepare template for future use.
	Skin creases or 'gulleys' preventing correct application of adhesive.	Build up indented areas and fill in gulleys to create a smooth surface, e.g. using paste.
	Infrequent emptying of drainable bag leading to stress on adhesion.	Drainable bags should be emptied frequently, e.g. 2- to 3-hourly if necessary.
Sore skin.	Leakage.	As above.
	Skin reaction to adhesive.	Change to an appliance from another manufacturer or apply a protective square between skin and adhesive. Anti-inflammatory agents may be required for very severe reactions.
	Poor hygiene.	Improve the technique of nurses, patient or carers.
Odour.	Ill-fitting appliance; lack of seal between skin and adhesive.	Fit the appliance with care. Consider a change of the type of appliance.
	Poor hygiene.	Improve the technique of nurses, patient or carers.
	Poor technique, e.g. when emptying drainable bag.	Empty the bag, then rinse the end with water to ensure that it is clean before closing.

Urostomy specimen

Problem	Cause	Suggested action
Stoma specimen of urine contaminated.	Contaminants introduced during specimen collection.	Take a repeat specimen, observing aseptic procedure and cleaning the stoma well.
Ileum perforated during specimen collection.	Catheter too hard or inserted too roughly.	Report to a doctor immediately.
Difficulty passing catheter into conduit.	Small degree of retraction of ileum.	Apply gentle pressure to the area around the stoma to make it protrude.
	Unpredictable direction of ileum.	Gently insert your little (gloved) finger into the stoma to determine the direction of the conduit. Insert the catheter tip along this line.

Tracheostomy Care and Laryngectomy Voice Rehabilitation

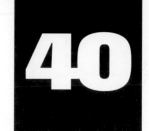

Tracheostomy care

The care of patients with a tracheostomy varies from one hospital to another. The changing of a tracheostomy tube will usually be undertaken by a doctor or a trained nurse who has been instructed in this procedure. It is important, however, that nurses are aware of the procedures and basic principles and know how to respond in an emergency situation.

Definition

A tracheostomy is a surgical opening in the anterior wall of the trachea (Fig. 40.1a; Allan 1987).

Indications

Tracheostomy may be carried out:

1 To provide and maintain a patent airway.
2 To enable the removal of tracheobronchial secretions.

A tracheostomy may be performed as a temporary or permanent procedure (Hooper 1996), or in an emergency situation (Corbridge 1998).

General care of tracheostomy patients

1 When caring for a tracheostomy patient the following should always be at the bedside or accessible if the patient is self-caring or ambulant:
   (a) Humidified oxygen with tracheostomy mask.
   (b) Suction machine with a selection of suction catheters.
   (c) Covered bowl of sodium bicarbonate (1 teaspoon to 500 ml sterile water) to clear suction tubing of secretions when suctioning has been performed.
   (d) Clean disposable gloves (Hooper 1996) and individually packaged, sterile, disposable gloves (Ward *et al.* 1997).
   (e) Disposable plastic apron and eye protection (Ward *et al.* 1997).
   (f) Two cuffed tracheostomy tubes, one the same size as the patient is wearing, the other a size smaller, in the event of an emergency tracheostomy tube change.
   (g) One 10 ml syringe to inflate cuff on tracheostomy tube.
   (h) Tracheal dilators, in the event of tracheostomy tube falling out or being removed and inability to insert another tube. Tracheal dilators can be used to keep stomal opening patent until medical assistance arrives.
2 Tracheostomy tube changes are mostly dependent on the type of secretions the patient has, for example, a patient with copious, tenacious secretions will need a daily tube change, sometimes twice a day, as this will be the only way of ensuring that the stoma and tube are free from any accumulation of secretions. If the patient has minimal secretions then the necessity to change the tube decreases until some patients need to have their tube changed only weekly.

Sometimes if the patient has a wound area up to the stoma edge, the tracheostomy tube has to be removed to gain access for cleaning the wound and observing its general status.

The tracheostomy dressing can be renewed without removing the tube and this should be done twice a day and as necessary. This ensures that any secretions are cleared, and do not lay wet against the skin, causing excoriation and resulting in wound breakdown (Minsley & Wrenn 1996).

Reference material

Types of tracheostomy

Temporary

A temporary tracheostomy (Fig. 40.1b) is performed for patients as an elective procedure, e.g. at the time of major surgery such as a partial glossectomy.

Permanent

A permanent tracheostomy is the creation of a tracheostomy following a total laryngectomy (Fig. 40.1c). The top three tracheal cartilages are brought to the surface of the skin and sutured to the neck wall to form a stoma. The 'end' tracheostomy is permanent and the rigidity of the tracheal cartilage keeps the stoma open. The patient will breathe through this stoma for the remainder of his/her life. As a result, there is no connection between the nasal passages and the trachea.

Emergency

A tracheostomy may be performed as an emergency procedure when a patient has an obstructed airway. Among the

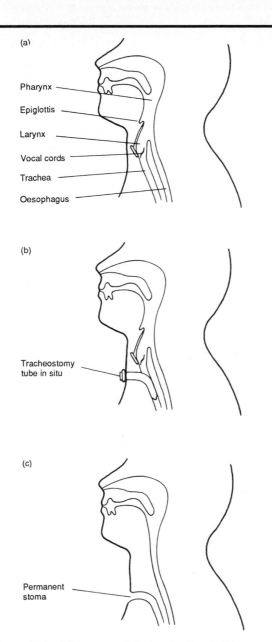

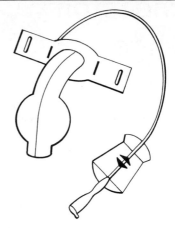

Figure 40.2 Portex cuffed tube.

Figure 40.1 (a) Anatomy of the head and neck. (b) Temporary tracheostomy. (c) Permanent tracheostomy (total laryngectomy).

more common conditions causing obstruction are trauma to the airway or neck, poisoning, infections or neoplasms.

Types of tubes

Experience has shown that the choice of tracheostomy tube depends on the type of operation performed; the patient's ability to tolerate the tube depends on various external factors. A selection of tubes is listed below.

Portex cuffed tracheostomy tube

This is a disposable plastic tracheostomy tube with an introducer and inflatable cuff to give an airtight seal (Fig. 40.2). The cuff prevents blood from reaching the lungs and the seal facilitates ventilation at the time of surgery.

It is an anaesthetic tube which is usually in situ for 24–48 hours. Depending on the patient's condition and the operation performed, the Portex tube will be removed and the stoma left exposed, e.g. total laryngectomy, or a more suitable sturdier tube will be inserted, such as a Shiley tracheostomy tube.

Shiley plain tracheostomy tube (Fig. 40.3a)

This is a plastic tube with an introducer and two inner tubes. One inner tube has an extension at its upper aspect. This facilitates connection to other equipment, e.g. nebulizers and speaking valves.

This tube is usually used for the following reasons:

1 To keep the tracheostomy tract patent if the patient is going to have further surgery.
2 In place of a metal tracheostomy tube if the patient is going to have radiotherapy to the neck area when a metal tube would cause tissue reaction (Holmes 1996).
3 For a laryngectomy patient who has a benign or malignant stenosis of the trachea and requires a longer tube than the regular length laryngectomy tube to keep the stenosis patent.

Shiley cuffed tracheostomy tube (Fig. 40.3b)

This is a plastic tube with an introducer and one inner tube. The inner tube has an extension at its upper aspect to facilitate connection to other equipment. The outer tube has an inflatable cuff to give an airtight seal. The cuff prevents secretions from reaching the lungs. The seal facilitates ventilation.

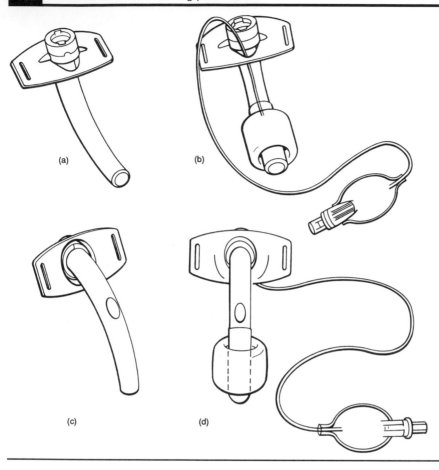

Figure 40.3 Shiley's tracheostomy tubes.
(a) Shiley plain tube.
(b) Shiley cuffed tube.
(c) Shiley plain fenestrated tube.
(d) Shiley cuffed fenestrated tube.

This is often used for the immediate postoperative phase, i.e. 24–72 hours. Large volume, low pressure cuffs have now been devised by manufacturers which do not damage the tracheal mucosal wall (Allan 1987). For those patients who require a cuffed tracheostomy tube for lengthy periods, a cuff manometer should be used to check cuff pressure. In order to prevent tracheal injury or aspiration, cuff pressures should be maintained between 18 and 20 mmHg (Crimlisk *et al.* 1996).

Shiley fenestrated tube (Fig. 40.3c)

This is a plastic tube with an introducer and two inner tubes. One inner tube has an extension at its upper end to facilitate connection to other apparatus. The other inner tube has a fenestration in the middle which, when inserted, lines up with the fenestration in the outer tube. This is to encourage the passage of air and secretions into the oral and nasal passages. It is useful when attempting to encourage a return to normal function following long-term use of a temporary tracheostomy.

The fenestrations enable this type of tube to be most suitable for the weaning method. A cap is inserted onto the tube, occluding the artificial airway. This enables the patient to become used to breathing via the oral and nasal passages again. The cap can be left in situ for certain periods of time until the patient can tolerate the tube occluded for a full uninterrupted 24 hours. Only then can removal of the entire tube, known as decannulation, be considered (Bull 1996).

Shiley cuffed fenestrated tube (Fig. 40.3d)

This is a plastic tube with an introducer and two inner tubes. One inner tube has an extension at its upper aspect to facilitate connection to other apparatus, while the other has a fenestration midway down the tube. This tube can also be occluded with a cap, to assess the patient's oral and nasal airway, first ensuring that the cuff has been completely deflated and that the fenestrated inner tube is in situ. The outer tube has a fenestration in the middle of the cannula, again to encourage a return to normal function. The outer tube also has an inflatable cuff to give an airtight seal. The cuff prevents secretions from reaching the lungs. This tube is useful for patients with swallowing problems but who are starting to return to normal function.

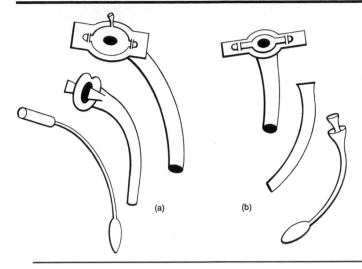

Figure 40.4 (a) Jackson's silver tube.
(b) Negus's silver tube.

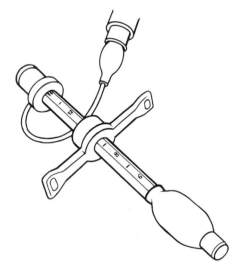

Figure 40.5 Kapitex Bivona Hyperflex cuffed tracheostomy tube.

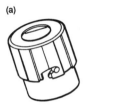

Figure 40.6 (a) Rusch speaking valve. (b) Decannulation plug.

Jackson's silver tracheostomy tube

This is a silver tube with an introducer and inner tube (Fig. 40.4a). The inner tube is locked in position by a small catch on the outer tube and may be removed and cleaned as necessary without disturbing the outer tube.

Negus's silver tracheostomy tube

This is a silver tracheostomy tube with an introducer and a choice of inner tubes, with and without speaking valves (Fig. 40.4b). The outer tube does not have a safety catch; consequently the inner tube may be coughed out inadvertently.

Kapitex Bivona Hyperflex tube

This is a silicone, wire-reinforced cuffed tracheostomy tube (Fig. 40.5). It has an adjustable flange and is a longer length tube, thereby accommodating unusual airway anatomy. The cuff is totally flat when deflated, which makes the insertion and removal less traumatic. An introducer is provided to aid insertion. It is essential that tracheostomy care is maintained scrupulously in order to prevent obstruction as no inner tube is provided with this product.

Speaking valve

This is a plastic device with a two-way valve which fits onto the extended aspects of the Shiley inner tube (Fig. 40.6a). When breathing, the valve stays open but when the patient attempts to speak the valve closes, thus redirecting air up through the normal air passages and allowing the production of voice.

Kapitex Tracoetwist fenestrated tube

This is a plastic tube with an introducer and two inner tubes (Fig. 40.7). One of these inner tubes has an extension at its upper end to facilitate connection to other apparatus. The other inner tube has a fenestration midway down the tube.

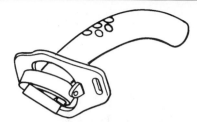

Figure 40.7 Kapitex Tracoetwist fenestrated tube.

The outer tube also has a fenestration consisting of a series of small holes. This helps to reduce the risk of granulation tissue growing through the fenestration and enables suction catheters to slide down the tube more easily when performing suction. The neck plate or flange moves in a vertical and horizontal direction enabling the plate to move as the patient moves. An inner tube with integrated speaking valve can be ordered separately. From the author's experience, this inner tube can be difficult to clean because the speaking valve is permanently attached.

A variety of other tubes are available in this series, including both cuffed and plain tracheostomy tubes.

Decannulation plug

This is a small plastic plug which fits into the outer fenestrated tube. (Fig. 40.6b). It is used to encourage patients to breathe via the oral and nasal air passages before removal of the tracheostomy tube. Alternatively, a small plastic plug (Kapitex) or a blind hub (Shiley) can be fitted into or over the inner fenestrated tube. This is particularly useful for patients who are still producing tenacious secretions as the plug or hub can be removed to enable the inner tube to be cleaned.

Colledge silver laryngectomy tube

This is a silver laryngectomy tube with an introducer (Fig. 40.8a). It is often used to dilate a laryngectomy stoma which has stenosed. These tubes can be cleaned, autoclaved and reused.

Shiley laryngectomy tube

This is a plastic tube with an introducer and inner tube (Fig. 40.8b). It is shorter in length than a tracheostomy tube, thereby conforming to the slightly shorter trachea in the patient who has undergone a total laryngectomy. The inner tube may be removed and cleaned frequently without disturbing the outer tube. It is sometimes worn postoperatively while the stoma is healing to help facilitate a good shaped stoma.

Shaw's silver laryngectomy tube

This is a silver laryngectomy tube with an introducer and an inner tube beyond both lower and upper aspects of the outer tube (Fig. 40.8c). Thus pressure dressings may be secured without occluding the stoma. The silver catch on the outer tube keeps the inner tube in position.

Stoma button

This is a soft Silastic 'button' (Fig. 40.8d). It may be used in place of a laryngectomy tube. It is very light and comfort-

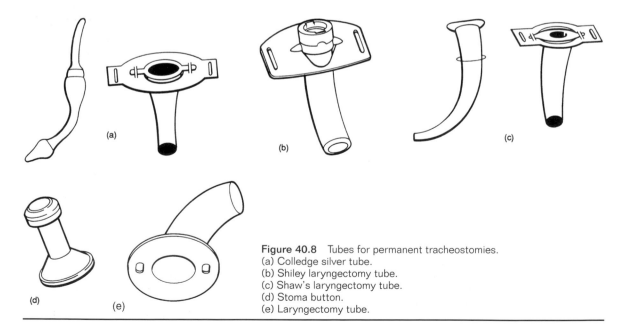

Figure 40.8 Tubes for permanent tracheostomies.
(a) Colledge silver tube.
(b) Shiley laryngectomy tube.
(c) Shaw's laryngectomy tube.
(d) Stoma button.
(e) Laryngectomy tube.

able to wear and is the appliance of choice when the patient has a Blom–Singer speaking valve in situ. In order to facilitate the use of the Blom–Singer speaking valve a diamond-shape is cut out of the Silastic.

Laryngectomy tube

This is a slightly opaque Silastic tube which is longer in length in comparison to the stoma button. These tubes are 36 and 55 mm in length and are available in a variety of different sizes (Fig. 40.8e). This tube is most suitable for patients who experience a degree of stenosis further down the trachea (see 'Stoma buttons and vents' later in this chapter for further information).

References and further reading

Allan, D. (1987) Making sense of tracheostomy. *Nurs Times,* **83**(45), 36–8.

Beall Harris, R. & Bernstein Hyman, R. (1984) Clean vs. sterile tracheotomy care and level of pulmonary infection. *Nurs Res,* **33**(2), 80–85.

Becker Weilitz, P. & Dettenmeier, P.A. (1994) Back to basics. Test your knowledge of tracheostomy tubes. *Am J Nurs,* **94**(2), 46–50.

Bull, P.D. (1996) (ed.) *Lecture Notes on Diseases of the Ear, Nose and Throat,* 8th edn., pp 172–80. Blackwell Science, Oxford.

Clarke, L. (1995) A critical event in tracheostomy care. *Br J Nurs,* **4**(12), 676, 678–81.

Coltart, L. (1998) Voice restoration after laryngectomy. *Nur Stand,* **13**(12), 36–40.

Corbridge, R.J. (ed.) (1998) *Essential ENT Practice. A Clinical Text,* pp 40–60. Arnold, London.

Creamer, E. & Smyth, E.G. (1996) Suction apparatus and the suctioning procedure: reducing the infection risks. *J Hosp Infect,* **34**, 1–9.

Crimlisk, J.T., Horn, M.H., Wilson, D.J. & Marino, B. (1996) Artificial airways: a survey of cuff management practices. *Heart Lung J Acute Crit Care,* **25**(3), 225–35.

De Carle, B. (1985) Tracheostomy care. *Nur Times,* **81**(6), 50–54.

Edels, Y. (1983) *Laryngectomy – Diagnosis to Rehabilitation.* Croom Helm, London.

Fiorentini, A. (1992) Potential hazards of tracheobronchial suctioning. *Intens Crit Care Nurs,* **8**(4), 217–26.

Forfar, J.O. & Arneil, G.C. (1984) *Textbook of Paediatrics,* Vol. 1, 3rd edn., pp 26–70. Churchill Livingstone, Edinburgh.

Fowler, S., Knapp-Spooner, C. & Donohue, D. (1995) The ABCs of tracheostomy care. *J Pract Nurs,* **45**(1), 44–8.

Griggs, A. (1998) Tracheostomy: suctioning and humidification. *Nurs Stand,* **13**(2), 49–56.

Holmes, S. (1996) *Radiotherapy.* Radiation induced side effects, pp. 67–78. Austin Cornish, London.

Hooper, M. (1996) Nursing care of the patient with a tracheostomy. *Nurs Stand,* **10**(34), 40–43.

Hudak, M. & Bond-Domb, A. (1996) Post operative head and neck cancer patients with artificial airways: the effect of saline lavage on tracheal mucous evacuation and oxygen saturation. *ORL Head Neck Nurs,* **14**(1), 17–21.

Inwood, H. & Cull, C. (1998) Advanced airway management. *Prof Nurse,* **13**(8), 509–513.

Longman Family Dictionary (1986) Chancellor Press, London.

Martin, L.K. (1989) Management of the altered airway in the head and neck cancer patient. *Semin Oncol Nurs,* **5**(3), 182–90.

McEleney, M. (1998) Endotracheal suction. *Prof Nurse,* **13**(6), 373–6.

Minsley, M.A.H. & Wrenn, S. (1996) Long-term care of the tracheostomy patient from an outpatient nursing perspective. *ORL Head Neck Nurs,* **14**(4), 18–22.

Schoeffel, R.E., Anderson, S.D. & Altounyan, R.E. (1981) Bronchial hyperreactivity in response to inhalation of ultrasonically nebulised solutions of distilled water and saline. *Br Med J,* **283**, 1285–7.

Seay, S.J. & Gay, S.L. (1997) Problem in tracheostomy patient care: recognising the patient with a displaced tracheostomy tube. *ORL Head Neck Nurs,* **15**(2), 10, 11.

Shekleton, M.E. & Nield, M. (1987) Ineffective airway clearance related to artificial airway. *Nurs Clin N Am,* **22**(1), 167–78.

Sigler, B.A. (1989) Nursing care of patients with laryngeal carcinoma. *Semin Oncol Nurs,* **5**(3), 160–165.

Somerson, S.J., Husted, C.W., Somerson, S.W. & Sicilia, M.R. (1996) Mastering emergency airway management. *Am J Nurs,* **96**(5), 24–30.

Thurston-Hookway, F. & Seddon, S. (1989) Care after laryngectomy. *Nursing,* **3**(35), 5–10.

Ward, V., Wilson, J., Taylor, L., Cookson, B. & Glynn, A. (1997) Supplement to *Hospital-Acquired Infection: Surveillance, Policies and Practice. Preventing Hospital-Acquired Infection. Clinical Guidelines.* Public Health Laboratory Service, London.

Whitaker, K. (1997) *Comprehensive Perinatal and Paediatric Respiratory Care,* 2nd edn., pp 193–238. Delmar Publishers, New York.

Young, C. (1984) Recommended guidelines for suction. *Physiotherapy,* **70**(3), 106–108.

Laryngectomy voice rehabilitation

Definition

A voice prosthesis is a one-way silicone valve that slots into a surgically created fistula reconnecting the trachea to the pharynx following surgical removal of the larynx. The valve, once fitted, allows air to be directed from the lungs and trachea into the pharynx when the patient wishes to speak. This airflow causes the pharyngeal muscles to vibrate, producing the sound or voice for speech (Fig. 40.9). Since the valve is one-way it also prevents food and drink passing from the pharynx into the trachea and down

the airway. A valve which begins to leak food and/or drink may be defective, worn-out, or ill-fitting.

The fistula for the voice valve may be created at the time of the total laryngectomy operation. Hence the terms *primary surgical voice restoration* (at the time of laryngectomy) and *secondary surgical voice restoration* (i.e. procedure carried out later) are used.

Reference material

Voice prostheses for patients undergoing laryngectomy have been available in Britain since the early 1980s (Blom

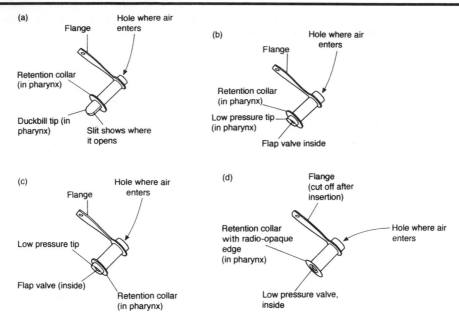

Figure 40.9 Laryngectomy voice rehabilitation. (a) Duckbill valve. (b) Low pressure valve, 16 Fr gauge. (c) Low pressure valve, 20 Fr gauge. (d) Indwelling valve, 20 Fr gauge.

& Singer 1980). There are a number of different types of prosthesis on the market, including Blom–Singer, Bivona, Provox and Gröningen. All work according to the same principle. The Blom–Singer prosthesis, developed in the USA by Eric Blom, a speech pathologist, and Mark Singer, an otolaryngologist, will be described in detail here.

Types of valves (Fig. 40.9)

Although there are many different makes of voice valve, most have a diameter of either 16 or 20 Fr. All makes of valve are available in a series of different lengths (1.4–3.6 cm) to fit the depth of the tracheopharyngeal wall, which varies from patient to patient. Initially, the patient should be measured and fitted with a prosthesis by an experienced and specialized practitioner who will select the most suitable type of valve, taking into account the patient's fitness and individual needs.

Duckbill valve/Blom–Singer type voice prosthesis

This prosthesis is named after its design: the valved end of the prosthesis opens like a duck's bill to allow air to pass into the pharynx. Talking with the prosthesis requires a little more effort than talking prior to laryngectomy. The device has a rounded end, making it easy to insert, and is less susceptible to infection by *Candida albicans* than the low pressure model. The duckbill valve requires more effort

to use than the low pressure type as it creates greater resistance to the airflow.

Low pressure valve/Blom–Singer type voice prosthesis

The Blom–Singer low pressure device has a flatter posterior aspect than the duckbill with a small hinged flap acting as the one-way valve. It can sometimes be more difficult to insert though new insertion techniques help to minimize problems. Its design makes it more susceptible to infection with *Candida albicans*. Talking with the prosthesis requires approximately the same amount of effort as talking prior to laryngectomy.

Low pressure valve/Blom–Singer type voice prosthesis (20 Fr gauge)

This is a special wide-diameter prosthesis recommended for patients with specialized needs. The decision to fit this lies with the specialist ENT doctor and/or specialist speech and language therapist.

Indwelling valve/Blom–Singer type voice prosthesis (20 Fr gauge)

This type of prosthesis has been available in Britain since late 1994. The main advantage is that it can last for about

6 months, providing the patient uses prophylactic antifungal treatment to counteract fungal infection of the valve. It has to be inserted and removed by a specialist speech and language therapist, ENT doctor experienced in fitting and managing voice prostheses or a nurse trained in the procedure.

Economy duckbill valve/Bivona type voice prosthesis (economy)

This is another duckbill valve, similar to the Blom–Singer device. It is made of flesh-tone silicone and is available in a full range of sizes, including the extra long 4 cm size.

Bivona type voice prosthesis (ultra-low resistance)

The Bivona ultra-low voice prosthesis functions with little resistance like the Blom–Singer type, low pressure model. The valved part of the prosthesis is a small, blue, hinged flap within the main body of the device. The posterior aspect is hooded to divert food and drink away. This device is susceptible to infection by *Candida albicans*.

Provox type indwelling voice prosthesis

This device is more difficult to insert as it has to be passed through the mouth and pharynx. This can be done under local anaesthetic, although for some patients a general anaesthetic is preferable. Once inserted it remains in place for an average of 4–6 months. This device is susceptible to infection by *Candida albicans*. The Provox 2 voice prosthesis has more recently become available and can be inserted and removed via the tracheostoma. It has a wider diameter than the Blom–Singer type prosthesis.

Gröningen type voice prosthesis

In most cases this prosthesis is inserted under general anaesthetic. It is currently used at only one centre in the UK. Once inserted it remains in place for approximately 6 months. This device is susceptible to infection by *Candida albicans*.

Stoma buttons and vents

To prevent stenosis of the stoma created for the voice prosthesis, patients may need to wear a stoma button, especially in the first few weeks after surgery. Although the stoma would not close completely, it may become so narrow that breathing is restricted and care of the voice prosthesis difficult.

Stoma buttons, made of soft Silastic, are available in a range of diameters: 10, 12 and 14 mm. For patients with voice prostheses, 12 or 14 mm is most suitable, so that the stoma is wide enough for the patient to clean the prosthesis. If a voice prosthesis is used with a stoma button, a hole is cut in the button to allow air to pass through the valve during speech. An experienced, specialized practitioner is required to adapt the button in this way. (For further information see 'Stoma button' above.)

Bivona type vent and Forth Medical type laryngectomy tube for use with a voice prosthesis

These devices are made of a softer plastic than the traditional Shiley type laryngectomy tube, making them more comfortable and more appropriate for long-term use (beyond the postoperative period and on a continuing basis providing they are kept clean). Some patients find the stoma consistent enough in diameter to dispense completely with a vent or button some 6 months to 1 year after the laryngectomy. Other patients need to continue wearing either a vent or a button all the time. They are available in a range of three diameters, and two different lengths: 36 or 55 mm. If a voice prosthesis is used at the same time as either of these two devices, an aperture is made in the upper side to allow air to pass through the valve. The Forth tube is made with an indentation to mark the site of the aperture.

Indications for replacing a voice prosthesis

1 *Voice prosthesis showing signs of wear and tear.* In most cases, experience indicates that a voice prosthesis will last for 6–8 weeks. After that time patients may find it harder to use it to make voice, when previously they had no difficulty. This deterioration is gradual.
2 *Voice prosthesis is leaking.* Valves are made of silicone and are therefore susceptible to fungal infection by *Candida albicans*. Micro-organisms burrow into the silicone and interfere with the functioning of the posterior (internal) end of the prosthesis. The effect of this is to cause saliva and drinks to leak in small drops through it, causing the patient to cough. Leakage such as this is a very common problem and can shorten the life of the prosthesis considerably.
3 *Drink and/or food are leaking around the valve.* This problem is less common. It indicates that the diameter of the fistula has become greater than the diameter of the valve, probably as a result of infection. A specialist speech and language therapist or a nurse or doctor with the ENT training required to fit and manage voice prostheses should be contacted for advice.
4 *Patient cannot make any sound with the voice prosthesis.* It is possible that patients may suddenly find that they can no longer make any sound with the prosthesis, or sound may be intermittent. The prosthesis must be removed and inspected, and almost certainly needs to be changed. A specialist speech and language therapist, or a nurse or doctor with the ENT training required to fit and manage voice prostheses should be contacted for advice.

Indications for replacing a 'lost' or dislodged voice prosthesis

The voice prosthesis is held in position by a silicone retention collar which is an integral part of the whole device. It is therefore possible for it to become accidentally dislodged. Patients are told that this might happen, and shown how to insert a Jacques 14 Fr red rubber catheter or a white Silastic 14 Fr Foley catheter through the fistula to keep it open. If patients are able to perform this procedure when a voice prosthesis is accidentally dislodged, the fistula remains open and a new prosthesis is inserted after removal of the catheter. If the voice prosthesis is ejected and the patient is unable to insert a catheter satisfactorily a speech and language therapist or doctor with experience in fitting and managing voice prostheses should be contacted for advice.

References and further reading

Blom, E.D. (1988) Tracheo-oesophageal valves: problems, solutions and directions for the future. *Head Neck Surg*, 10, 5142–5.

Blom, E.D. & Singer, M. (1980) An endoscopic technique for the restoration of voice after laryngectomy. *Ann Otol Rhinol Laryngol*, 89(6), 529–33.

Blom, E. & Singer, M. (1998) *Tracheo-Oesophageal Voice Restoration Following Total Laryngectomy*. Singular Publishing, San Diego.

Edels, Y. (1983) *Laryngectomy: Diagnosis to Rehabilitation*. Croom Helm, London.

Evans, E. (1990) *Working with Laryngectomees*. Winslow, Oxford.

Garth, R.J.N. *et al.* (1991) Tracheo-oesophageal puncture: a review of problems and complications. *J Laryngol Otol*, 105, 750–54.

Lund, V. *et al.* (1987) Blom–Singer puncture: practicalities in everyday management. *J Laryngol Otol*, 101, 164–8.

GUIDELINES · Changing a tracheostomy dressing

Equipment

1 Sterile dressing pack.
2 Tracheostomy dressing or a keyhole dressing.
3 Cleaning solution, such as 0.9% sodium chloride.

4 Tracheostomy tape.
5 Bactericidal alcohol hand rub.

Procedure

Action	*Rationale*
1 Explain and discuss the procedure with the patient.	To ensure that the patient understands the procedure and gives his/her valid consent.
2 Screen the bed or cubicle.	To ensure the patient's privacy.
3 Wash hands using bactericidal soap and water or bactericidal alcohol hand rub, and prepare the dressing tray or trolley.	To reduce the risk of infection.
4 Perform the procedure using aseptic technique.	To prevent infection.
5 Remove the soiled dressing around the tube and clean around stoma with 0.9% sodium chloride.	To avoid discomfort to the patient. To remove secretions and crusts.
6 Replace with a tracheostomy dressing or a comfortable keyhole dressing.	To ensure the patient's comfort. To avoid pressure from the tube.
7 Renew tracheostomy tapes, checking that one finger can be placed between the tapes and neck.	To secure the tube. To ensure that the tapes are not too tight or too loose (Allan 1987).

GUIDELINES • Suction and tracheostomy patients

The aim of suction is to maintain an airway and to prevent the formation of crusts. The frequency of suction varies with individual patients, according to their needs.

Equipment

1 Suction machine (wall source or portable).
2 Aero-flow sterile suction catheters (assorted sizes; see action 5).
3 Individually packaged, sterile, disposable gloves (Ward et al. 1997) and clean, disposable gloves (Hooper 1996).
4 Jug of sodium bicarbonate solution (1 teaspoon in 500 ml sterile water). The receptacle must be sterile initially and changed every 24 h (Ward et al. 1997) to prevent the growth of bacteria.
5 ENT spray containing sterile 0.9% sodium chloride.
6 Disposable plastic apron.
7 Eye protection, e.g. goggles.
8 Bactericidal alcohol hand rub.

Procedure

Action	Rationale
1 Instruct the patient to use the spray every 2 h or more frequently if secretions are tenacious, i.e. two or three sprays directly into the tracheostomy.	Suction will not be achieved if the secretions become too tenacious or dry. Regular administration of 0.9% sodium chloride will assist in loosening secretions (Becker Weilitz & Dettenmeier 1994; Hudak & Bond-Domb 1996).
2 Suctioning should be taught if the patient is able to perform his/her own suction. Otherwise inform the patient what is to be done.	To obtain the patient's cooperation and to help him or her relax. The procedure is unpleasant and can be frightening for the patient. Reassurance is vital. Self-control of the patient's suction is preferable if the patient is able to manage it.
3 Wash hands with bactericidal soap and water or bactericidal alcohol hand rub, and put on a disposable plastic apron, and eye protection.	To reduce the risk of cross-infection. Some patients may accidently cough directly ahead at the nurse; standing to one side with tissues at the patient's tracheostomy minimizes this risk.
4 Check that the suction machine is set to the appropriate level.	In general, suction pressure should not exceed 120 mm Hg in adults (Shekleton & Nield 1987), with an acceptable suction pressure of between 80 and 120 mm Hg (Somerson et al. 1996). In neonates this should be between 50 and 80 mm Hg and in paediatrics 80 and 100 mm Hg, (Whitaker 1997). The paediatric age range is defined as 1–15 years, with adolescence overlapping at 13–19 years of age (Forfar & Arneil 1984). Sputum which is more tenacious requires more powerful suction, the maximum level being 200 mmHg. If pressures up to and above 200 mmHg are used, then vacuum-interrupted suctioning techniques are recommended to prevent pressure buildup should the catheter become occluded (Young 1984).
5 As a guide, to calculate the appropriate suction catheter size, divide the tracheostomy tube's internal diameter by two, then multiply this result by three to obtain the French gauge (Fg) (Griggs 1998). Open the end of the suction catheter pack and use the pack to attach the catheter to the suction tubing. Keep the rest of the catheter in the sterile packet.	The size of suction catheter is dependent on tenacity and volume of secretions, that is, the thicker the secretions and the larger the volume, the greater the bore of the tube. Ideally, catheter size should be less than half the tracheal diameter (Young 1984). This ensures that hypoxia does not occur while suctioning. To reduce the risk of transferring infection from hands to the catheter and to keep the catheter as clean as possible.

Guidelines • Suction and tracheostomy patients (cont'd)

Action	Rationale
6 For new surgically formed tracheostomy and laryngectomy stomas, use an individually packaged, sterile, disposable glove on the hand manipulating the catheter (Ward *et al.* 1997). (A clean disposable glove can be used on the other hand.) Clean, disposable gloves can be used for subsequent admissions or for established stomas.	Gloves minimize the risk of infection transfer to the catheter or from the sputum to the nurse's hands.
7 Withdraw the catheter from the sleeve and introduce the catheter to about one-third of its length and apply suction by placing the thumb over the suction port control.	Gentleness is essential; damage to the tracheal mucosa can lead to trauma and respiratory infection. The catheter should go no further than the carina to prevent trauma.
8 Withdraw the catheter gently with a rotating motion. Do not suction the patient for more than 10 sec at a time (Martin 1989; Fiorentini 1992).	To remove secretions from around the mucous membranes. Prolonged suction will result in infection if the mucous membranes are traumatized, and the patient may experience a choking sensation.
9 Wrap catheter around gloved hand, then pull back glove over soiled catheter, thus containing catheter in glove, then discard.	Catheters are used only once to reduce the risk of introducing infection.
10 Rinse the connection by dipping its end in the jug of sodium bicarbonate solution with the suction turned on to clear secretions into the receptacle.	To loosen secretions that have adhered to the inside of the tube.
11 If the patient requires further suction, repeat the above actions using new gloves and a new catheter.	
12 Repeat the suction until the airway is clear.	

Humidification

Definition

Humidification may be defined as increasing the moisture or dampness in the atmosphere (*Longman Family Dictionary* 1986). In health, inspired air is filtered, warmed and moistened by the ciliated lining, and mucus is produced in the upper respiratory pathways. Because the upper respiratory pathways are bypassed in patients with a tracheostomy, they need artificial humidification to ensure that these pathways remain moist (Corbridge 1998).

GUIDELINES • Humidification

Procedure

Immediate postoperative care, i.e. the first 24–48 h

Action	Rationale
1 Fill a suitable nebulizer with sterile water and attach it to the air or oxygen supply. Set the air or oxygen rate as recommended by the manufacturer. Give a constant supply of humidified air or oxygen for 24–48 h.	Constant humidification is required while the new stoma adapts to the outside environment (especially for laryngectomy patients). Humidification also prevents the formation of crusts which are liable to obstruct the airway. The use of sterile water reduces the risk of infection (Somerson *et al.* 1996). This should be discarded and renewed every 24 h.
2 Spray 0.9% sodium chloride into the trachea as necessary, using a spray.	To loosen secretions prior to suction and to stimulate the cough reflex. To keep secretions moist.
3 For patients in cubicles, a room humidifier may be placed at the bedside.	

Subsequent care

Action	Rationale
1 Give humidified oxygen as required. Usually, patients need about 10–15 min of humidification every 4 h. This may be adapted according to the patient's needs, e.g. throughout the night, according to time.	Patients begin to adapt to breathing through their tracheostomy after the first 24–48 h. Some humidification is required according to individual needs and to prevent crust formation in the airway.
2 If the patient does not require oxygen, blow humidifiers may be used.	These provide humidified air without the need for an oxygen supply.
3 Teach the patient to keep the tracheostomy moist by using a spray containing 0.9% sodium chloride, before suctioning.	To loosen secretions and to prevent crust formation. To prevent contamination. 0.9% sodium chloride is supplied in small bottles or sachets which, if not used within 24 h, should be changed to prevent infection. The spray should be washed and dried each day and resterilized once the patient is discharged.
4 Provide laryngeal stoma protectors, e.g. Lyofoam, Buchanan bib or Romet covers.	To protect the airway.

GUIDELINES · Changing a tracheostomy tube

With a newly formed tracheostomy, tube changing should be avoided where possible for the first 2 or 3 days to enable the tract to become well established (Bull 1996).

Equipment

1 Sterile dressing pack.
2 Tracheostomy dressing or a keyhole dressing.
3 Tracheostomy tape.
4 Cleaning solution, such as 0.9% sodium chloride.
5 Barrier cream.
6 Lubricating jelly.
7 Disposable plastic apron.
8 Bactericidal alcohol hand rub.
9 Eye protection.

Procedure

Action	Rationale
1 Explain and discuss the procedure with the patient.	To ensure that the patient understands the procedure and gives his/her valid consent.
2 Wash hands using bactericidal soap and water or bactericidal alcohol hand rub, and prepare a dressing trolley.	To prevent contamination.
3 Screen the patient's bed.	To ensure the patient's privacy.
4 Perform the procedure using clean technique.	To prevent contamination.
5 Assist the patient to sit in an upright position, supported by pillows with the neck extended.	To ensure the patient's comfort and to maintain a patent airway. If the neck is not extended, skin folds may occlude the tracheostomy when the tube is removed.
6 Remove the dressing pack from its outer wrappings and open the tracheostomy dressing.	Technique should be clean to reduce the risk of cross-infection.
7 Put on a disposable plastic apron.	
8 Clean hands with bactericidal alcohol hand rub.	

Guidelines • Changing a tracheostomy tube (cont'd)

Action	Rationale
9 Put on clean disposable plastic gloves.	To prevent infection.
10 Prepare the tracheostomy tube as outlined in steps 11–14.	So that the tube is ready for immediate insertion when required.
11 Thread on piece of tape through the slits in the flanges so that the tape passes behind the flange next to the stoma.	The tape is kept behind the flange to prevent it occluding the passage of air into the tracheostomy tube.
Alternatively, secure tracheostomy ties to both flanges.	These are made of Velcro and are more comfortable to wear and easy to adjust.
12 Put the tracheostomy dressing around the tube.	To prevent abrasion of the patient's skin by the tube.
13 Lubricate the tube sparingly with a lubricating jelly.	To facilitate insertion.
14 Remove the soiled tube from the patient's neck while asking the patient to breathe out.	Conscious expiration relaxes the patient and reduces the risk of coughing. Coughing can result in unwanted closure of the tracheostomy.
15 Clean around the stoma with 0.9% sodium chloride and dry gently. Apply barrier cream with topical swabs. (An aqueous cream may be used if the patient is having the site irradiated.)	To remove superficial organisms and crusts. Skin around the stoma is at risk of breakdown due to the constant presence of moisture in this area (Allan 1987). Meticulous skin care is therefore essential in order to prevent infection.
16 Insert a clean tube with introducer in place, using an 'up and over' action.	Introduction of the tube is less traumatic if directed along the contour of the trachea.
17 Remove the introducer immediately.	The patient cannot breathe while the introducer is in place.
18 Place the inner tube in position.	The inner tube can be changed as necessary when the outer tube is in position, thus minimizing the risk of trauma to trachea and stoma. The quantity of secretions present will determine the frequency with which the inner tube is changed.
19 Tie the tape securely at the side of the neck.	To secure the tube. Place the tie in an accessible place, at the same time ensuring that it will not cause discomfort to the patient.
20 Remove gloves and ask the patient to breathe out onto the palm of your hand.	Flow of air will be felt if the tube is in the correct position.
21 Ensure that the patient is comfortable.	
22 Clear away the trolley and equipment.	
23 Scrub the soiled tube with a brush under cold running water. If the tube is very soiled then use sodium bicarbonate to remove debris. The tube must be rinsed thoroughly and stored dry at the patient's bedside.	To remove debris that may occlude the tube and/or become a source of infection.

Note: plastic tubes should not be soaked in solutions as there is a danger that the material may absorb the solution which could then cause irritation of the trachea.

Nursing care plan

Problem	Cause	Suggested action
Profuse tracheal secretions.	Local reaction to tracheostomy tube.	Suction frequently, e.g. every 1–2 h.
Lumen of tracheostomy tube occluded.	Tenacious mucus in tube.	Spray frequently with 0.9% sodium chloride, e.g. every 1–3 h, and

		suction. Change the inner tube regularly, e.g. 1- to 3-hourly.
	Dried blood and mucus in the tube, especially in the postoperative period.	Provide humidified air. (For further information, see 'Guidelines: Humidification', above.)
Tracheostomy tube dislodged accidentally.	Tapes not secured adequately.	Put in spare tube. This should be clean and ready at the bedside. *Note*: tracheal dilators must be kept at the bedside of patients with tracheostomies.
Unable to insert clean tracheostomy tube.	Unpredicted shape or angle of stoma.	Remain calm since an outward appearance of distress may cause the patient to panic and lose confidence. Lubricate the tube well and attempt to reinsert at various angles. If unsuccessful, attempt to insert a smaller-size tracheostomy tube. If this is impossible, keep the tracheostomy tract open using tracheal dilators and inform the doctor.
	Tracheal stenosis due to patient coughing, very anxious or because the tube has been left out too long.	Insert a smaller-size tracheostomy tube. If insertion still proves difficult, do not leave the patient but ask for a tube to be brought to the bed. Keep the tracheostomy patent with tracheal dilators if stenosis is pronounced until the tube is reinserted.
Tracheal bleeding following or during change of the tube.	Trauma due to suction or to the tube being changed. Presence of tumour. Granulation tissue forming in fenestration of tube.	Change the tube as planned if bleeding is minimal. For profuse bleeding, insert a cuffed tube and inflate. Inform the doctor. Perform tracheal suction to remove the blood from the trachea.
Infected sputum.	Nature of surgery and condition of patient often predispose to infection.	Encourage the patient to cough up secretions and/or suction regularly. Change the tube and clean the stoma area frequently, e.g. 4-hourly. Protect permanent stomas with a bib or gauze
		Following result of sputum specimen, commence appropriate antibiotics as needed.

GUIDELINES · Changing a Blom–Singer type non-indwelling voice prosthesis

Nurses must wear gloves and eye protection (to prevent phlegm/blood entering the eyes) when carrying out this procedure. The area must be well lit to illuminate the stoma.

Equipment

1 Clinically clean tray or receiver.
2 Correct replacement voice prosthesis and introducer.
3 Red rubber Foley catheter (16 Fr gauge).
4 White plastic stent or dilator with correct diameter.

5 Lubricant jelly, e.g. KY jelly or similar.
6 Tissues.
7 Blenderm transparent hypoallergenic tape or Micropore tape.

Guidelines • Changing a Blom-Singer type non-indwelling voice prosthesis (cont'd)

Procedure

Action

1 Explain and discuss the procedure with the patient.

2 Settle the patient in a chair and arrange lighting to illuminate stoma.

3 Place a little KY jelly on the tip of the red rubber catheter and/or stent, and on the voice valve and introducer.

4 Ask the patient to keep his/her lips apart as the old valve is removed; hold flange where it joins the body of the valve.

5 Swiftly insert red rubber catheter (or dilator) 20 cm into the fistula.

6 Place valve on introducer, securing with flange.

7 Remove catheter or stent and replace with valve. A slight click will be felt as the retention collar on the valve passes into the pharynx.

8 Check valve is correctly inserted by pulling it gently: it will move slightly, then resist.

9 Place 5 cm length of Blenderm tape over flange to secure it to the patient's neck.

Rationale

To ensure that the patient understands the procedure and gives his/her valid consent.

To ensure the patient is comfortable and well supported.

To ease insertion.

To minimize amount of saliva entering fistula and reduce the risk of coughing.

To keep fistula open. To ascertain the shape and direction of the fistula.

To prevent valve dislodging from introducer during insertion.

To insert valve.

To ensure valve is correctly positioned.

To keep flange neatly out of way.

Transfusion of Blood, Blood Products and Blood Substitutes

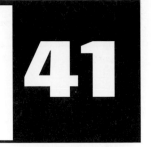

Definition

A transfusion consists of the administration of whole blood or any of its components to correct or treat a clinical abnormality.

Reference material

Blood donation and testing

Safety of both the donor and the potential recipient is an important criterion in the selection of blood donors. As well as microbiological testing of the donated blood, reliance is placed on the donor to answer questions on his or her general health, medical history and any drugs taken (Hewitt *et al.* 1990). Prevention of transmission of infection is determined by donor selection criteria and laboratory testing. In the UK, mandatory screening is done for antibodies to HIV 1 and 2, *Treponema pallidum* (syphilis) and hepatitis C and hepatitis B surface antigen (Hoffbrand & Pettit 1994; Hewitt & Wagstaff 1998).

Following donation, blood products have varying shelf lives. Red blood cell products have a shelf life of 35 days if kept at 4°C (Hoffbrand & Pettit 1994; Davies & Williamson 1998), whereas platelets can only be stored for up to 96 hours at room temperature after donation and concentration (Hoffbrand & Pettit 1994; Brozović *et al.* 1998). Table 41.1 describes the different blood products.

Cross matching – ABO and Rh

Landsteiner in 1901 discovered that human blood groups (the ABO system) existed and this marked the beginning of safe blood transfusion (Waters 1991). There are four main blood groups: A, B, AB and O. These are based on antigens on the red cells and antibodies in the serum. There is racial variation in the frequency of these within a population (Waters 1991). Apart from the ABO system, most of the other red cell antigens are detected by antibodies stimulated by transfusion or pregnancy (Waters 1991). Previous transfusions or pregnancies may immunize the patient against blood group antigens (Hoffbrand & Pettit 1994). The introduction of cells carrying A or B antigens results in immediate intravascular lysis in anyone with IgM antibodies to these antigens (Hoffbrand & Pettit 1994).

In 1940 the rhesus system was discovered. This is the second most important system in transfusion therapy (Weinstein 1993) and is also an antigen found on the red cell. Approximately 15% of the UK population do not express the rhesus antigen on their red blood cells (Hoffbrand & Pettit 1994). Transfusion of positive cells will result in immunization and the appearance of anti-D antibodies (Hoffbrand & Pettit 1994).

Full laboratory compatibility testing for cross matching of red blood cell transfusion can usually be done within 1 hour (Hoffbrand & Pettit 1994; Table 41.1).

Blood groups in haemopoietic stem cell transplantation

The human leucocyte antigen (HLA) is used to determine compatibility for organ transplantation including bone marrow and peripheral blood stem cells. Unfortunately, because ABO blood groups and HLA tissue types are determined genetically, it is not uncommon to find a well matched HLA donor who is ABO incompatible with the recipient. Major transfusion reactions can be avoided by red cell and/or plasma depletion of the donor cells in the laboratory before reinfusion. Very occasionally, if the recipient has a very high titre of anti-A or anti-B lytic antibody and the donor marrow or peripheral blood stem cells are blood group A, B or AB, then plasmapheresis of the recipient is performed to lower the titre of this antibody to safe limits. This is necessary because it is not possible to remove all the red cells from the donor product and those remaining may cause a major transfusion reaction in this situation.

Indications

The range of products currently available, those most widely used, indications for use and recommendations for administration are listed in Table 41.1.

It may be unnecessary to correct a cytopenia or clotting deficiency to normal levels. Instead, physiological levels should be restored (Kickler & Ness 1993). A rise of approximately 10 g/l of haemoglobin may be expected from each transfused unit of red blood cells (Davies & Brozovic 1990).

Delivery of blood and blood products

The transfusion of stored blood exposes the patient to the possible infusion of particulate matter (Lowe 1981), i.e. the presence of fibrin particles, clumps of white blood cells, disintegrating platelets and small clots (Fantus & Schirmir 1938). After transfusion this may result in clinical

Table 41.1 Blood and products used for transfusion

Type	Description	Indications	Cross-matching	Shelf life	Average infusion time	Technique	Special considerations
Whole blood	Complete unadulterated blood, approx. 510 ml including anticoagulant	To restore blood volume lost due to massive, acute haemorrhage whatever the cause	ABO and Rh	28–35 days at 4–6°C (dependent on anticoagulant)	2–4 hours/unit	Give via a blood administration set	If loss and replacement exceed twice the blood volume, abnormalities of haemostasis may occur
Plasma reduced blood (packed red blood cells)[a]	Whole blood minus approx. 200 ml plasma, and anticoagulant; haematocrit 60–65%	To correct red blood cell deficiency and improve oxygen-carrying capacity of the blood	ABO and Rh	21 days at 4–6°C	2–4 hours/unit	As above	—
Red cells in optimal additive solutions	Red cells minus all plasma: 100 ml fluid used as replacement to give optimal red cell preservation; haematocrit 60–65%	As above	ABO and Rh	35 days at 4–6°C	1–2 hours/unit	As above	An example of a replacement solution is 0.9% sodium chloride/ adenine/ glucose/ mannitol
Concentrated red cells[a]	Plasma removed to produce a haematocrit of 70% plus	To correct anaemias when expansion of blood volume will not be tolerated	ABO and Rh	21 days at 4–6°C	1–2 hours/unit	As above	Availability varies
Washed red blood cells[a]	Red cells centrifuged free of plasma and resuspended in 0.9% sodium chloride	To increase red cell mass and prevent tissue antigen formation in: 1 Immunosuppressed patients 2 Patients with previous transfusion reactions	ABO and Rh	Use within 12 hours or preferably, immediately	1–2 hours/unit	As above	—
Frozen red blood cells	1 Cells from normal healthy donor with very rare blood group 2 Patient's own cells taken in anticipation of later illness (autologous blood transfusion)	To treat transplant patients or patients with atypical antibodies which react with almost the entire population To increase safety of tranfusion therapy	ABO and Rh	Stored frozen cells: 3 years. Use within 12 hours of thawing	2–3 hours/unit	As above	Available from a few centres. Freezing process and recovery are time consuming and expensive
Leucocyte-poor blood[b]	Red cells from which accompanying leucocytes have been removed	To prevent further reactions in patients who have had febrile attacks when receiving whole or plasma reduced blood	ABO and Rh	4–6°C. Time stated on pack. Usually within 12 hours of preparation, preferably immediately	2–3 hours/unit	As above	Frozen red cells may be used as an alternative
White blood cells (leucocyte concentrate)[b]	Mainly granulocytes obtained by leucophoresis or by 'creaming off' the buffy layers from packs of fresh blood	To treat patients with life-threatening granulocytopenia, e.g. due to chemotherapy	ABO and HLA (human leucocyte group A antigen)	24 hours after collection. Stored at 5°C	60–90 minutes/unit	Administer via a blood administration set. Usually 1 unit only	White blood cell infusion *induces* fever, may cause hypotension, rigors and confusion. Treat symptoms and reassure patient. Preparation may

Table 41.1   *Continued*

Type	Description	Indications	Cross-matching	Shelf life	Average infusion time	Technique	Special considerations
							be irradiated to prevent initiation of graft versus host (GVH) disease in bone marrow transplant patients. *Do not* give to patients receiving amphotericin B. Indications for granulocyte transfusions should be when possible benefits are thought to outweigh considerable hazards of the treatment option (Brozović *et al.* 1998)
Platelets[a]	Platelet sediment from platelet-rich plasma, resuspended in 40–60 ml plasma	To treat thrombocytopenia due to 1 Decreased production 2 Increased destruction 3 Functionally abnormal platelets 4 Dilutional problems following massive transfusions 5 DIC (critically ill patients receiving supportive therapies such as ventilation/haemofiztrations)	ABO and rhesus compatibility preferred	Up to 5 days after collection at 22°C, with continuous gentle agitation; best within 6 hours	20–30 minutes/unit	Administration using a component set is preferred. Do not use micro-aggregate filters	General guide to use: 1 Count less than 10×10^9/litre 2 Count 10–20×10^9/litre with haemorrhage and/or persistent pyrexia 3 Count 20–50×10^9/litre or on chemotherapy may need platelets Prophylactic use in the absence of haemorrhage is controversial
Plasma: fresh or fresh frozen (FFP)	Citrated plasma separated from whole blood. All coagulation factors preserved for several months	To treat a clotting factor deficiency, when specific concentrates are unavailable or precise deficiency is unknown, e.g. DIC	ABO compatibility; Rh preferred	Fresh: within 6 hours after collection. FFP: 12 months at –25°C. Use immediately after thawing	15–45 minutes/unit (approx. 200 ml)	Administer rapidly via a blood administration set	FFP should be considered if patient has received more than 6 units of blood to prevent dilutional hypocoagulability
Albumin 4.5% (plasma protein fraction)	Solution of selected proteins from pooled plasma in a buffered, stabilized 0.9% sodium chloride diluent. Usually 400-ml bottle	To treat hypovolaemic shock or hypoproteinaemia due to burns, trauma, surgery or infection. *Note:* current medical opinion is altering regarding the *use* of plasma rich products and potential relationship and risks with TSEs and other infective agents	Unnecessary	5 years at 2°C, 3 years at 25°C; store in the dark	30–60 minutes/unit	Administer via a standard solution administration set	Heated at 60°C for 10 hours to inactivate hepatitis virus. The solution should be crystal clear with no deposits

Table 41.1 Blood and products used for transfusion (*cont'd*)

Type	Description	Indications	Cross-matching	Shelf life	Average infusion time	Technique	Special considerations
Salt-poor human albumin 20%	Heat-treated, aqueous, chemically processed fraction of pooled plasma	To treat hypovolaemic shock or hypoproteinaemia due to burns, trauma, surgery or infection. To maintain appropriate electrolyte balance. *Note*: current medical opinion is altering regarding the *use* of plasma rich products and potential relationship and risks with TSEs and other infective agents	Unnecessary	5 years at 2°C, 3 years at 25°C; store in the dark	30–60 minutes/unit	Administer via a blood administration set undiluted or diluted with 0.9% sodium chloride or 5% glucose solution. Slower administration is advised if a cardiac disorder is present to avoid gross fluid shift	Heated at 60°C for 10 hours to inactivate hepatitis virus. The solution should be crystal clear with no deposits
Factor VIII (cryoprecipitates, dried antihaemophilic globulin concentrates)	Cold-insoluble portion of plasma recovered from FFP – amount of factor VIII varies. Potency in freeze-dried concentrates can be assayed more reliably	To control bleeding disorders due to lack of factor VIII or fibrinogen, e.g. haemophilia, Von Willebrand's disease	ABO compatibility between donor plasma and recipient's red blood cells	Cryoprecipitates at –30°C for 1 year. Use immediately after thawing. Freeze-dried concentrates at +4°C. Reconstitute at room temperature and use immediately	15–30 minutes via infusion, 10–15 minutes via intravenous push	Administer rapidly via syringe or blood component set.	Heat treated at 80°C for 72 hours to eliminate risk of hepatitis or HIV contamination, as multiple donors and imported for preparation; limited availability
Dried factor IX concentrate	Preparation contains factor IX, prothrombin and factor X. Some may contain factor VII	To correct bleeding disorders due to lack of these factors, e.g. Christmas disease	Unnecessary	Refer to specific expiry dates	15–30 minutes	Administer via a blood administration set. Dose varies	As above. Limited availability

[a]Most commonly used blood products.
[b]See Leucocyte depletion, below.
DIC Disseminated intravascular coagulation.

problems including non-haemolytic febrile reactions and respiratory impairment caused by pulmonary micro-emboli. These problems are more commonly associated with large transfusions of 6 units and above.

The variable size (between 10 and 200 microns) and number of micro-aggregates are dependent on two main factors:

1 The storage time: in general the older the blood the more micro-aggregates it contains.
2 The anticoagulant used to prevent the blood clotting.

Inline blood filters

Filters are used to remove micro-aggregates and leucocytes present in the blood to be transfused.

Micro-aggregate filters

Micro-aggregate or microparticle filters are used mainly to filter out red cell debris, platelets, white blood cells and fibrin strands that have clumped together. The filter compartment of commonly used blood administration sets will only remove particles of 170–200 microns and above.

Three types of filter are available:

1 Screen or surface filters, which effectively sieve the blood. The size of the particle removed will depend on the pore size on the surface. These filters tend to become more efficient the more blood flows through them. They remove particles of 40 microns or above.
2 Depth filters: these work by absorbing the particles into the layers of fibre. They tend to be effective for the removal of smaller particles, but their efficiency diminishes as the number of units used increases. They also tend to slow the rate at which blood can be administered. These filters remove particles of 10–20 microns or above.
3 Combination filters, which consist of a surface filter above and a depth filter below.

The use of additional inline blood filters is not indicated for the majority of transfusions, and is contraindicated with certain products such as platelets, as they remove the desired components.

Leucocyte depletion filters

Sensitization from white cells or HLA antigens present in transfusion products is a major problem for recipients, as they can cause minor or major adverse reactions. Specific filters are designated for the transfusion of red cells, platelets or fresh frozen plasma (FFP). National blood transfusion services in the UK and around the world are now working towards universal leucodepletion at source to try to reduce transfusion reactions. Leucodepletion of all blood products at source is now standard practice in the UK (Williamson *et al.* 1999). Bedside filters have been withdrawn from the clinical area. Note: if products are not leucodepleted at source, bedside filters are still not advocated as safe practice as it is considered an unreliable method in preventing infusion of leucocytes (Wallington 1998).

Blood warming devices

The warming of blood and blood products is not recommended as it is of limited benefit and potentially dangerous. Use of blood warmers is only indicated when:

1 Massive, rapid transfusion could result in cooling of cardiac tissue, causing dysfunction. In an adult if the rate of transfusion is greater than 50 ml/kg per hour, or in children if the rate is greater than 15 ml/kg per hour, blood warming devices should be used (McClelland 1996).
2 Frozen plasma or other components are prescribed and must be thawed before administration.
3 Transfusion is required by patients with cold agglutination disease.
4 Exchange transfusion is indicated in the newborn (Weinstein 1997).
5 Transfusion of cryopreserved stem cells (blood or marrow).

Both water baths and dry heat blood warmers are available. However, whichever device is chosen the temperature should be maintained below 38°C. Warming in excess of this can cause haemolysis of red cells and can denature proteins while increasing risks of bacterial infection (see manufacturer's guidelines).

The optimum effectiveness of dry heat blood warmers is reached when the rate of delivery to the patient is 150–160 ml per minute. This means that their use is restricted, and because of the greater flexibility of water baths these are more frequently used. Whenever there is water, there is a risk of bacterial contamination of blood products, particularly with *Pseudomonas*. For the patient this could result in a fatal systemic infection. Therefore certain safety measures must be adhered to:

1 Water baths must be cleaned before and after use with disinfectant or sent to the Central Sterile Services Department for decontamination.

2 The blood warmer should be drained after each use and must be stored dry and empty.
3 When needed they should be refilled with sterile water.
4 A protective sterile over-bag to thaw blood and blood products reduces the entry of contaminants through microscopic punctures or breaks in the seal.
5 The blood product should be used immediately after it has been thawed.

All devices should be serviced at per hospital health and safety policies, Medical Device Authorities' (MDA) and manufacturers' guidelines.

Transfusion reactions

Knowledge in the field of immunohaematology continues to grow with improvements in collection and storage methods, which aim to increase the safety of transfusion therapy. Yet risks still exist with the infusion of any blood product; therefore the importance of complying with National Transfusion Policies is critical for the safe administration of all blood products (Cook 1997a,b). Transfusion reactions are either immunologic or non-immunologic and can be either immediate or delayed.

1 *Immunologic*: this is the body's response to foreign proteins, or an antigen/antibody reaction from red blood cells, platelets or plasma proteins.
2 *Non-immunologic*: these are reactions caused by external factors where an antigen/antibody reaction is not present.

Immediate reactions

These reactions can happen in minutes or hours after transfusion therapy.

Acute haemolytic reactions

These are directly related to incompatibilities in the ABO blood group system. Antigen/antibody reactions occur when the recipient's antibodies react with donor erythrocytes. This reaction causes a cascade of events within the recipient. The complement system is activated, causing intravascular haemolysis and the kinin system produces bradykinin, which increases capillary permeability, dilates arterioles and subsequently causes a drop in systemic blood pressure. The coagulation system is also activated and stimulates the intrinsic clotting cascade, causing small clots and triggering disseminated intravascular coagulation (DIC). DIC can lead to formation of thrombi within the microvasculature and can be fatal (Hoffbrand & Pettit 1994; Kickler & Ness 1993; Terry *et al.* 1995; Cook 1997a; Weinstein 1997).

Signs and symptoms

Chills, facial flushing, pain/oozing at cannula site, burning along the vein, chest pain, lumbar or flank pain, or shock (Weinstein 1997). Patients often express a feeling of doom, which may be associated with cytokine activity (Weir 1995; Terry *et al.* 1995). Haemolytic shock can occur after only a few millilitres of blood has been infused.

Action

Stop infusion immediately, maintain patency of venous access device and contact medical personnel immediately. Check patient identity against donor unit. Treatment is often vigorous to reverse hypotension, and aid adequate renal perfusion and renal flow to reduce potential damage to renal tubules, and appropriate therapy for DIC reactions (Provan *et al.* 1998). Heparin therapy is controversial in the event of DIC, because of the underlying causative factors and existing bleeding problems. It is important to remember that most acute haemolytic reactions are preventable, caused by clerical error or checking errors at the bedside (Hoffbrand & Pettit 1994; Cook 1997a).

Anaphylactic reactions

These are rare and usually occur after only a few millilitres of blood or plasma has been infused.

Signs and symptoms

Bronchial spasm, respiratory distress, abdominal cramps, shock and potential loss of consciousness.

Action

Stop infusion and begin immediate resuscitation of the patient.

Acute respiratory distress syndrome (ARDS)

Where recipients receive large amounts of red blood cells, the micro-aggregate debris, which forms during storage, can lead to pulmonary insufficiency, and this in turn can be fatal.

Air embolism

Air embolism remains a risk with any intravenous therapy (see Chap. 44, Vascular Access Devices).

Circulatory overload

Circulatory overload can occur when blood or any of its components are infused rapidly or administered to a patient with an increased plasma volume, causing hypervolaemia. Patients at risk are those with renal or cardiac deficiencies, the young and elderly (Cook 1997a; Weinstein 1997).

Signs and symptoms

An alteration in vital signs, dyspnoea, constriction of the chest, coughing and a change in pallor (Hoffbrand & Pettit 1994; Weinstein 1997).

Action

Stop infusion immediately and contact medical colleagues. This complication is preventable by ensuring accurate monitoring during infusion of blood or any of its components, especially in at-risk recipient groups, such as the critically ill, neonates and young children (see Chap. 44, Vascular Access Devices).

Febrile non-haemolytic reactions

These reactions are due to the recipient's antileucocyte antibody response to the transfusion of cellular components such as donor leucocytes. Specific patient groups are at risk of greater sensitization to leucocytes, for example, critically ill patients, those receiving anticancer therapies or patients requiring multiple transfusion therapy (Weinstein 1997; Williamson *et al.* 1999).

Signs and symptoms

Facial flushing, palpitations, chest tightness, and increase in body temperature with associated chills and/or rigors, and a rapid pulse.

Action

Administer antipyretic agents such as paracetamol (Contreras & Mollison 1998). Notify medical colleagues and document reaction. Leucodepleted products are recommended for those patients who are considered immunocompromised and require regular supportive transfusion therapy (Weinstein 1997; Wallington 1998). Note: all blood and blood products in the UK and internationally are working towards universal leucodepletion. All blood and blood products in the UK are leucodepleted at source (Wallington 1998; Williamson *et al.* 1999).

Hypothermia

Infusing large quantities of cold blood rapidly can cause hypothermia. Patients likely to suffer from this reaction are those who have suffered massive blood loss due to trauma, haemorrhage, clotting disorders, or thrombocytopenia (Cook 1997b).

Signs and symptoms

Alteration in vital signs, changes in pallor and observed chills.

Action

Use a blood warmer (see above). Blood should *never* be warmed using hot water, radiators or microwaves.

Sepsis

This is caused when bacteria enter the blood or blood product that is to be infused. Bacteria can enter at any point from the time of collection, during storage through to administration to the patient. Organisms implicated in transfusion-related sepsis include gram-negative *Pseudomonas*, *Yersinia* and *Flavobacterium* (Provan *et al.* 1998).

Signs and symptoms

Fever, hypotension, tachycardia and septic shock.

Action

Notify medical colleagues immediately, correct hypotension, take blood cultures and commence intravenous antibiotics.

Transfusion-related acute lung injury (TRALI)

This is caused from antileucocyte antibodies reacting against donor leucocytes. This reaction can result in 'leucoagglutination'. Leucoagglutinins can in turn become trapped in the pulmonary microvasculature, causing severe respiratory distress without evidence of circulatory overload or cardiac failure (Contreras & Mollison 1998).

Signs and symptoms

Respiratory distress, chills and fever, cyanosis and hypotension.

Action

Discontinue transfusion and notify medical colleagues immediately; begin respiratory supportive treatment.

Urticaria

This is an uncommon reaction caused by the recipient reacting to protein in donor plasma (Davies & Williamson 1998).

Signs and symptoms

Localised erythema, hives and itching.

Action

Stop infusion and administer prescribed antihistamine therapy. The infusion can then be recommenced. However, if symptoms continue with either a body rash and/or fever, the infusion should be discontinued.

Delayed effects

Some of these reactions can occur days, months or even years after a transfusion.

Citrate toxicity

This is a problem associated with the infusion of large quantities of whole blood and/or fresh frozen plasma in the newborn or patients who have liver disease (Cook 1997a; Davies & Williamson 1998).

Signs and symptoms

Tingling in extremities, muscle-cramps, hypotension, possible convulsions and cardiac arrest.

Action

Interrupt rate of infusion, check for abnormal blood chemistry and administer calcium chloride or calcium gluconate solutions as prescribed. Monitor the recipient closely for any alteration in vital signs.

Delayed haemolytic reactions

These reactions are caused when immune antibodies react to a foreign antigen. Reactions are classified as primary or secondary. A *primary* reaction is often mild, occurring days or weeks after initial transfusion, and may be indicated by no clinical alteration in haemoglobin following transfusion therapy (Cook 1997a). *Secondary* reactions occur with re-exposure to the same antigen, and on rare occasions may be associated with ABO incompatibilities (Cook 1997a).

Signs and symptoms

Fever, mild jaundice and unexplained decrease in haemoglobin value (McClelland 1996).

Action

Antiglobulin testing.

Hyperkalaemia

Hyperkalaemia is a rare complication associated with trauma and the subsequent infusion of large quantities of blood. Potassium is known to leak out of red cells during storage, thereby increasing circulatory levels in recipients receiving blood products (Cook 1997b). The process is exacerbated if products are kept too long at room temperature or gamma irradiated (Davies & Williamson 1998). Transfusion of a unit of blood should not exceed 5 hours (McClelland 1996; Davies & Williamson 1998).

Signs and symptoms

Irritability, anxiety, abdominal cramps, diarrhoea and weakness in the extremities (Cook 1997b).

Action

Notify medical colleagues and administer corrective drugs as prescribed.

Iron overload

A unit of blood contains 250 mg iron, which the body is unable to excrete, and as a result patients receiving large volumes of blood are at risk of iron overload (Davies & Williamson 1998).

Signs and symptoms

Poor growth, pigment changes, hepatic cirrhosis, hypoparathyroidism, diabetes, arrhythmia, cardiac failure and death.

Action

Administer desferrioxamine, which induces iron excretion (Davies & Williamson 1998; *British National Formulary* 1999).

Transfusion-associated graft versus host disease (TAGVHD)

Although this is a rare complication, it presents serious complications for recipients, and is often fatal. It is usually caused by the infusion of immunocompetent T lymphocytes in blood and blood products to severely immuno-compromised recipients. The donor T lymphocytes engraft and multiply, react against the foreign tissue of the host/recipient and cause TAGVHD (Davies & Williamson 1998).

It is not commonly associated with FFP or cryoprecipitate. Onset can be from 4 to 30 days after transfusion.

Signs and symptoms

High fever followed by nausea and vomiting, generalized erythroderma, and profuse diarrhoea. Morbidity and mortality is 75–90% of affected patients, with infection and bone marrow suppression the main causes of death (Terry *et al.* 1995).

Preventative measures

Irradiation (25 gray) of blood and blood products, to inactivate T lymphocytes. This is especially important in the following recipients:

1 Fetuses receiving intrauterine transfusions.
2 Patients undergoing or who have undergone blood or bone marrow progenitor cell transplantation.
3 Immunocompromised recipients.

Infectious complications of blood, blood products and blood substitutes

(See also Chap. 4, Barrier Nursing.)

Bacterial infections

Contamination of blood, blood products and blood substitutes can occur during donation, collection, processing, storage and administration. Despite strict guidelines and procedures, the risk of contamination remains. Most common contaminating organisms are skin contaminants such as staphylococci, diphtheroids and micrococci, which enter the blood at the time of venesection (Barbara & Contreras 1998; Provan *et al.* 1998).

Signs and symptoms

Signs and symptoms are usually quick to develop and include chills and rigors, fever, nausea, vomiting, pain and hypotension, and can be fatal (Weinstein 1997; Davies & Williamson 1998; Provan *et al.* 1998).

Note: bacterial contamination can present an identical clinical picture to acute haemolytic transfusion reactions.

Action

Stop the transfusion, treat symptoms, take blood cultures and administer prescribed antibiotics.

Viral infections

Viruses transmissible via blood transfusions can be either plasma borne or cell associated (Barbara & Contreras 1998; Williamson *et al.* 1998). Plasma-borne viruses include hepatitis B, hepatitis C, hepatitis A (rarely), serum parvovirus B19, HIV-1 and HIV-2. Cell-associated viruses include cytomegalovirus (CMV), Epstein–Barr virus, human T-cell leukaemia/lymphoma viruses (HTLV-1/HTLV-2), and human immunodeficiency viruses (HIV-1/HIV-2). (See Chap. 4, Barrier Nursing.)

Human T-leukaemia/lymphoma virus type 1 (HTLV-1)

HTLV-1 is an oncogenic retrovirus, associated with the white cells that cause adult T-cell leukaemia, and is connected with several neuromuscular wasting syndromes. The retrovirus is endemic in Japan, the Caribbean Basin and parts of Africa (Polesky 1989; Barbara & Contreras 1998). The enzyme-linked immunosorbent assay (ELISA) test has been recommended because of concerns relating to the transmission of the virus via blood transfusion, and the associated long incubation period of adult T-cell leukaemia. In the UK, routine testing for HTLV is currently not mandatory (Barbara & Contreras 1998).

Cytomegalovirus (CMV)

CMV is classified as part of the herpes family and hence has the ability to establish latent infection with reactivation during periods of immunosuppression (Barnes 1992; Barbara & Contreras 1998). Approximately 50% of the population in the UK has antibodies to CMV. Therefore it is recognized that the virus may be transmitted by transfusion, although it poses little threat to immunologically intact recipients. However, CMV infection in vulnerable patient groups can cause significant morbidity and mortality, e.g. CMV pneumonitis carries an 85% mortality rate in blood and bone marrow transplant recipients (Barnes 1992). Screening of donors and the use of CMV-*seronegative* or leukocyte-depleted blood and blood products are seen as essential for neonates and immuno-compromised recipients who have tested negative to CMV (Prentice *et al.* 1998).

Hepatitis B (HBV)

Screening for hepatitis B surface antigen in donor blood (HBsAg) is mandatory as approximately 1 in 23 000 donations in the UK is detected as having HBsAg (Hewitt & Wagstaff 1998).

Hepatitis C (HCV)

Screening for hepatitis C using the ELISA test is mandatory in the UK. Hepatitis C is transmitted primarily via contact with blood or blood products (Crowe 1994; Hewitt & Wagstaff 1998).

Human immunodeficiency virus (HIV-1 and HIV-2)

HIV is a retrovirus that infects and kills helper T cells also known as CD4-positive lymphocytes. Transmission of the virus can be via most blood products including red cells, platelets, fresh frozen plasma, and factor VIII and IX concentrates. These viruses are not known to be transmitted in albumin, immunoglobulins or antithrombin III products (Barbara & Contreras 1998). The retrovirus invades cells and slowly destroys the immune system, rendering the individual susceptible to opportunistic infections. Since 1983, when it was recognized that the virus could be transmitted via transfusion, actions were developed to safeguard blood supplies from transmitting the virus that caused AIDS. These include careful screening of donors and testing of donated blood. It is mandatory in the UK, USA and Canada for transfusion services to test for HIV-1 and HIV-2 (Franceschi et al. 1995; Legge 1997; Weinstein 1997; Barbara & Contreras 1998).

Parvovirus B19

Although this is non-pathogenic, there still remains the potential risk of aplastic crisis in recipients with chronic haemolytic anaemias, e.g. individuals with sickle cell anaemia. Infected plasma can contaminate batches of factor VIII. Heat treatment of freeze-dried factor VIII is at 80°C for 72 hours which inactivates most if not all of the virus (Barbara & Contreras 1998).

Other infective agents

Parasites

Plasmodium falciparum is the most dangerous of the human malarial parasites (Barbara & Contreras 1998). Prevention is by questioning of donors about foreign travel, especially those who have visited areas in which the disease is endemic (Hewitt et al. 1990).

Prion diseases

Known as transmissible spongiform encephalopathies (TSEs), these are a rare group of conditions which cause progressive neurodegeneration in humans and some animal species. Prion diseases are believed to be caused by the presence of an abnormal form of a cellular protein (Aguzzi & Collinge 1997; Barbara & Contreras 1998;

Vamvakas 1999). These abnormal proteins have an altered cellular shape, and become infectious and multiply by converting normal cellular protein to the irregular form. This irregular form is resistant to digestion and breakdown, and, once accumulation occurs, can result in the formation of plaque in brain tissue. Transmission is thought to be by direct contact with infected brain or lymphoreticular tissue (Aguzzi & Collinge 1997; Barbara & Contreras 1998; Vamvakas 1999).

1 *Prion diseases in animal species:*
   (a) Scrapie, a disease of sheep
   (b) Bovine spongiform encephalopathy (BSE)
   (c) Feline spongiform encephalopathy (FSE)
   (d) Chronic wasting disease of deer, mule and elk
2 *Prion diseases in humans:*
   (a) Sporadic – classical Creutzfeldt–Jakob disease (CJD)
   (b) Inherited – CJD, Gerstmann–Sträussler–Scheinker disease, fatal familial insomnia (FFI)
   (c) Acquired – kuru, new variant (nvCJD)

There is evidence to suggest that in TSEs, of which nvCJD is one, leucocytes, particularly lymphocytes, are the key cells in the transportation of the putative infectious agent to the brain (Aguzzi & Collinge 1997; Bradley 1999). Leucodepletion of all blood and blood components is viewed as a sensible yet precautionary action to reduce any risk of blood-borne infection. All products in the UK are now leucodepleted at source (Wallington 1998). Currently, all plasma products are brought in from the USA, except FFP and cryoprecipitate which are leucodepleted at source in the UK.

Modified techniques in blood transfusion therapy

Conservation of blood and blood products is now an important issue in medical practice, as awareness increases of the associated risks involved with allogeneic blood transfusions (Chernow et al. 1996; Nelson 1998).

Autologous transfusions

Autologous transfusion is the collection, filtration and reinfusion of one's own blood, making the donor and recipient the same person. It is intended to avoid transmission of infection from the current method of allogeneic red blood cell transfusions (Brown 1998; Gillian & Thomas 1998; van Duijn et al. 1998; Nelson 1999). There are four methods of collecting:

1 A pre-deposits programme, which collects blood prior to an operation (Provan et al. 1998).
2 Haemodilution, where blood is collected and stored until the end of a surgical procedure, then reinfused into the patient.
3 Intra-operative salvage, which involves collecting blood from an operation site, washing and anticoagulating the blood, then returning it to the patient during or at the end of the surgical procedure. This method is commonly

used in cardiovascular, hepatic, neurologic, orthopaedic, and thoracic surgery, including transplants (Weinstein 1997; Provan *et al.* 1998). Postoperative complications can occur from infusion of shed blood; therefore strict medical indications for reinfusion are necessary (Dinse & Deusch 1996; Oeltjen & Santrach 1997; Provan *et al.* 1998; Porter 1999).

4 Postoperative salvage, whereby shed blood is collected from patients following cardiac, orthopaedic, plastic surgery or trauma, making this a safe, simple and cost-effective technique.

Programmes such as these have been developed to conserve blood and prevent such reactions as isoimmunization and the transmission of infective agents. Administration procedures and monitoring of recipients remains the same as with allogeneic transfusions (Lee & Napier 1990; Dinse & Deusch 1996; Oeltjen & Santrach 1997; Weinstein 1997; Gillian & Thomas 1998; Provan *et al.* 1998; Porter 1999).

Irradiation of blood and blood products

Irradiation of blood and blood products is used to prevent the transfusion of cells/viruses capable of replication. In immunocompromised recipients, especially transplant patients, lymphocytes may proliferate and have the potential to cause graft versus host disease or rejection of transplanted organs. Irradiated products may also be used routinely in patients who are undergoing bone marrow suppressive or ablative therapies (Patterson 1992).

Infusion of cryopreserved bone marrow and peripheral blood stem cells

Stem cells from either the bone marrow or peripheral blood are cryopreserved between collection (harvesting) and reinfusion. Stem cells can be either an autologous or an allogeneic transfusion. Thawing of the cells is carried out using a large-volume water bath. Care should be taken as heating may cause cellular damage, and there is an increased risk of bacterial contamination. Aseptic techniques should be adopted during administration to reduce any possibility of contamination in a recipient group who is already immunocompromised (McClelland 1996).

Red cell substitutes

Minimizing the use of allogeneic blood would both benefit recipients and aid transfusion services where demand often outweighs supplies (Garwood & Knowles 1998). Currently, clinical trials are in progress using haemoglobin and perfluorochemical-based materials. However, their circulatory survival times are short and therefore they remain a poor substitute for the treatment of chronic anaemia. It is anticipated that red blood cell substitutes for use in transfusion medicine and other related biomedicine will emerge once they are immunologically inert, isotonic and safe (Lowe 1998; Urbaniak & Robinson 1998; Porter 1999).

References and further reading

Aguzzi, A. & Collinge, J. (1997) Post exposure prophylaxis after accidental prion inoculation. *Lancet*, **350**, 1519.

AuBochen, J.P. (1996) Cost effectiveness of preoperative autologous blood donation for orthopedic and cardiac surgeries. *Am J Med*, **101**(2a), 38–42.

Barbara, J.A.J. & Contreras, M. (1998) Infectious complications of blood transfusion: bacteria and parasites. In: *ABC of Transfusion*, (ed. M. Contreras), 3rd edn. British Medical Journal Publishing, London.

Barbara, J.A.J. & Contreras, M. (1998) Infectious complications of blood transfusion: viruses. In: *ABC of Transfusion* (ed. M. Contreras), 3rd edn. British Medical Journal Publishing, London.

Barnes, R. (1992) Infections following bone marrow transplantation. In: *Bone Marrow Transplantation in Practice* (eds J. Treleavan & J. Barrett), pp. 281–8. Churchill Livingstone, Edinburgh.

Bradley, R. (1999) BSE transmission studies with particular reference to blood. *Dev Biol Standard*, **99**, 35–40.

British National Formulary (1999) No. 38, Sept. British Medical Association and The Royal Pharmaceutical Society of Great Britain, London.

Brown, P. (1998) Transmission of spongiform encephalopathy through biological products. *Dev Biol Standard*, **93**, 73–8.

Brozović, B., Hows, J. & Contreras, M. (1998) Platelet and granuloctye transfusion. In: *ABC of Transfusion* (ed. M. Contreras), 3rd edn. British Medical Journal Publishing, London.

Chernow, B., Jackson, E., Miller, J.A. & Wiese, J. (1996) Blood conservation in acute care and critical care. *Am Assoc Crit Care Nurses*, **7**(2), 191–7.

Contreras, M. & Mollison, P.L. (1998) Immunological complications of transfusion. In: *ABC of Transfusion* (ed. M. Contreras), 3rd edn. British Medical Journal Publishing, London.

Contreras, M. & Mollison, P.L. (1998) Testing before transfusion and red cell ordering policies. In: *ABC of Transfusion* (ed. M. Contreras), 3rd edn. British Medical Journal Publishing, London.

Cook, L.S. (1997a) Blood transfusion reactions involving an immune response. *J Intraven Nurs*, **20**(1), 5–14.

Cook, L.S. (1997b) Non-immune transfusion reactions: when type and crossmatch aren't enough. *J Intraven Nurs*, **20**(1), 15–22.

Crowe, H.M. (1994) Forum: a perspective on hepatitis. *Asepsis*, **16**(2), 13–17.

Davies, S. & Brozovic, M. (1990) Transfusion of red cells. In: *ABC of Transfusions* (ed. M. Contreras), pp. 9–24. British Medical Journal Publications, London.

Davies, S.C. (1995) Reforming England's blood transfusion service. *Br Med J*, **311**, 1383–4.

Davies, S.C. & Williamson, L.M. (1998) Transfusion of red cells. In: *ABC of Transfusion* (ed. M. Contreras), 3rd edn. British Medical Journal Publishing, London.

De Silva, M., Contreras, M. & Warwick, R. (1998) Blood transfusion support. In: *The Clinical Practice of Stem Cell Transplantation* (eds J. Barrett & J. Treleaven). ISIS Medical Media, Oxford.

Dinse, H. & Deusch, H. (1996) Sepsis following autologous blood transfusion. *Anaesthetist*, **45**(5), 460–63.

DoH (1995) *Hepatitis C and Blood Transfusion Look Back 1995*. PL CMO (95)1. Stationery Office, London.

Dougherty, L. & Lamb, J. (eds) (1999) *Intravenous Therapy in Nursing Practice*. Churchill Livingstone, Edinburgh.

Editorial (1985) Warming of blood and blood products. *Can Intraven Nurses Assoc J*, **1**(2), 5.

Evatt, B.L. (1998) Prions and haemophilia: assessment of risk. *Haemophilia*, **4**(4), 628–33.

Fantus, B. & Schirmir, E.H. (1938) The therapy of the Cook County Hospital – blood preservation technique. *J Am Med Assoc*, **111**, 317.

Foster, P.R. (1999) Assessment of the potential of plasma fractionation processes to remove causative agents of transmissible spongiform encephalopathy. *Transfusion Med*, **9**(1), 3–14.

Franceschi, S., Dal Maso, L. & La Vecchia, C. (1995) Trends in incidence of AIDS associated with transfusion of blood and blood products in Europe and the United States, 1985–93. *Br Med J*, **311**, 1534–6.

Fratantoni, J.C. (1998) Creutzfeldt-Jakob disease and blood products: FDA policy. *Biologicals*, **26**(2), 133–4.

Garwood, P.A. & Knowles, S.E. (1998) Supply and demand of blood and blood components. In: *ABC of Transfusion* (ed. M. Contreras), 3rd edn. British Medical Journal Publishing Group, London.

Gillian, J. & Thomas, D.W. (1998) Autologous transfusion. In: *ABC of Transfusion* (ed. M. Contreras), 3rd edn. British Medical Journal Publishing, London.

Hewitt, P.E. & Machin, S.J. (1998) Massive blood transfusion. In: *ABC of Transfusion* (ed. M. Contreras), 3rd edn. British Medical Journal Publishing, London.

Hewitt, P.E. & Wagstaff, W. (1998) The blood donor and tests on donor blood. In: *ABC of Transfusion* (ed. M. Contreras), 3rd edn. British Medical Journal Publishing, London.

Hewitt, P.E. et al. (1990) The blood donor and tests on donor blood. In: *ABC of Transfusions* (ed. M. Contreras), pp. 1–4. British Medical Journal Publications, London.

Hoffbrand, A.V. & Pettit, J.E. (1994) *Essential Haematology*, 3rd edn. Blackwell Science, Oxford.

Kickler, T.S. & Ness, P.M. (1993) Blood component therapy. In: *Hematological and Oncological Emergencies* (ed. W.R. Bell), pp. 125–40. Churchill Livingstone, Edinburgh.

Lee, D. & Napier, J.A.F. (1990) Autologous transfusion. In: *ABC of Transfusions* (ed. M. Contreras), pp. 18–21. British Medical Journal Publications, London.

Legge, A. (1997) Direct HIV testing of donated blood is inevitable. *Br Med J*, **314**, 1437.

Lloyd, G.M. & Marshall, L. (1986) Blood micro-aggregates: their role in transfusion reactions. *Intens Care World*, **3**(4), 119–22.

Lowe, G.D. (1981) Filtration in IV therapy. Part III: Clinical aspects of blood filtration. *Br J Intraven Ther*, September, 28–38.

Lowe, K.C. (1998) Red cell substitutes. In: *ABC of Transfusion* (ed. M. Contreras), 3rd edn. British Medical Journal Publishing, London.

McClelland, B. (1996) *Handbook of Transfusion Medicine*, 2nd edn. Stationery Office, London.

Nelson, C.L. (1998) Use of allogeneic transfusions (editorial). *Clin Orthopaed*, Dec (357), 2–3.

Oeltjen, A.M. & Santrach, P.J. (1997) Autologous transfusion techniques. *J Intraven Nurs*, **20**(6), 305–10.

Patterson, K. (1992) Bone marrow harvesting and preparation of harvested marrow. In: *Bone Marrow Transplantation in Practice* (eds J. Treleavan & J. Barrett), pp. 219–26. Churchill Livingstone, Edinburgh.

Polesky, H.F. (1989) Transfusion transmitted viruses. In: *Modern Blood Banking and Transfusion Practices* (ed. D. Harmening), 2nd edn. F.A. Davis, Philadelphia.

Porter, H. (1999) Blood transfusion therapy. In: *Intravenous Therapy in Nursing Practice* (eds L. Dougherty & J. Lamb). Churchill Livingstone, Edinburgh.

Prentice, G., Grundy, J.E. & Kho, P. (1998) Cytomegalovirus. In: *The Clinical Practice of Stem Cell Transplantation* (eds J. Barrett & J. Treleaven). ISIS Medical Media, Oxford.

Provan, D., Chisholm, M., Duncombe, A., Singer, C. & Smith, A. (1998) *Oxford Handbook of Clinical Haematology*. Oxford University Press, Oxford.

Smith, D.S. (1987) The appropriate use of diagnostic services: a guide to blood transfusion practice. *Health Trends*, **19**, 12–16.

Terry, J., Baranowski, L., Lonsway, R.A. et al. (1995) *Intravenous Therapy: Clinical Principles and Practice*. W.B. Saunders, Philadelphia.

Urbaniak, S.J. & Robinson, E.A. (1998) Therapeutic apheresis. In: *ABC of Transfusion* (ed. M. Contreras), 3rd edn. British Medical Journal Publishing Group, London.

Vamvakas, E.C. (1999) Risk of transmission of Creutzfeldt-Jakob disease by transfusion of blood, plasma, and plasma derivatives. *J Clin Apheresis*, **14**(3), 135–43.

van Duijn, C.M., Delasnerie-Laupretre, N., Masullo, C. et al. (1998) Case-control study of the risk factors of Creutzfeldt-Jakob disease in Europe during 1993–95. EU Collaborative Study Group of Creutzfeldt-Jakob disease. *Lancet*, **351**(9109), 1081–5.

Waters, A.H. (1991) Platelet and granulocyte antigens and antibodies. In: *Practical Haematology* (eds J. Dacie & S.M. Lewis), 7th edn., pp. 441–54. Churchill Livingstone, Edinburgh.

Weinstein, S.H. (1997) *Plumer's Principles and Practice of Intravenous Therapy*, 6th edn. J.B. Lippincott, New York.

Weir, J. (1995) Blood component therapy. In: *Intravenous Therapy – Clinical Principles and Practice* (eds J. Terry, L. Baranowski, R.A. Lonsaway & C. Hendrick), pp. 165–87. W.B. Saunders, Philadelphia.

Williamson, L.M., Lowe, S., Love, E. et al. (1998) *Serious Hazards of Transfusion (SHOT). Summary of Annual Report 1996–97*. The SHOT Office, Manchester.

Williamson, L.M., Rider, J.R., Swann, I.D. et al. (1999) Evaluation of plasma and red cells obtained after leucocyte depletion of whole blood. *Transfusion Med*, **9**(1), 51–61.

Nursing care plan

Nurses involved in the transfusion of blood and/or blood products need to develop knowledge and skills to ensure safe administration and effective nursing care of those receiving transfusion therapy. The transfusion of any blood product carries with it the potential of reaction and risk (Cook 1997a; Porter 1999).

Safety checks prior to commencing any blood therapy

1 Check that the product has been stored correctly as per national transfusion guidelines (McClelland 1996).

2 Check patient's name, date of birth, hospital reference number, expiry of product, irradiation and CMV status (specific to immunocompromised recipient groups) with cross match form and the prescription chart.

3 Check patient consent or, in the case of patients less than 16 years, parental consent. Potential risks should be highlighted to the patient that disease transmission cannot be ruled out despite transfusion policies and practices.

4 Ensure product is administered via the correct administration set (see Table 41.1).

5 Record baseline observations prior to administration, then at 30-min intervals during the transfusion.

6 Blood transfusions should be completed within 5 h. Administration sets should be changed after the second unit of blood.

Problems frequently encountered with blood and blood products therapy when infusion slows or stops

1 The infusion slows or stops shortly after commencing the unit of blood via a peripheral cannula. This is often due to venous spasm as a result of a cold solution being infused. This can be relieved by applying a warm compress (as per hospital policy) to dilate the vein and increase the blood flow.

2 The infusion slows or stops due to occlusion of the device. Maintenance of continuous flow is important. Early recog-

nition of this problem is essential. Flush device gently with 0.9% sodium chloride and then resume infusion. If some minutes have elapsed it may be necessary to prime a new administration set with 0.9% sodium chloride to re-establish flow. If there is an occlusion of the peripheral cannula, consider resiting (see Chap. 44, Vascular Access Devices). Keeping the patient warm and relaxed will increase peripheral circulation and prevent problems.

Potential problem	Cause	Preventive measure	Suggested action
Elevated temperature after the commencement of a unit of blood, with temperature falling if the blood is slowed.	Pyrogenic reaction.	Observation of the patient's temperature, pulse and blood pressure during the transfusion dependent on patient's condition and especially at the start of each unit. If patient has had multiple transfusions or experienced this type of reaction previously, ensure that 'cover' of hydrocortisone and chlorpheniramine is written up and administered before commencement of therapy.	Slow blood transfusion rate. Inform medical staff.
A high temperature associated with fever and rigor during a transfusion.	White cell antibody reaction.	Observation as above.	Stop transfusion. Maintain patency of device by flushing with 0.9% sodium chloride. Inform medical staff.
Slightly elevated temperature with associated rash, may be severe with oedema round the eyes and larynx and shortness of breath.	Allergic reaction to protein in the plasma.	Observation as above. Ensure patient is aware of symptoms to report, e.g. appearance of a rash or breathlessness. Close observation of patient for swollen eyes and signs of breathlessness.	If mild, slow the rate of transfusion. Inform medical staff. If severe, stop transfusion. Change administration set and commence flushing device with 0.9% sodium chloride to keep vein open, or flush device and discontinue any infusion. Lie patient flat, treat as for shock. Inform medical staff.

Patient complains of feeling hot, with chest and abdominal pain. Fall in blood pressure; patient's temperature subnormal at first and later rising to a pyrexia.

Infection introduced either from bacteria in the blood or during the cannulation or connection set changes.

Adhere to strict aseptic technique when handling the blood bags and intravenous device.
Use blood within 30 min of removal from refrigerator.
Regular observations, as above.
Adhere to recommended delivery time for each unit of blood; discard if hanging for 5 h (McClelland 1996).

Stop transfusion.
Change administration set and commence flushing device with 0.9% sodium chloride slowly to keep vein open. Inform medical staff and institute prescribed treatment, e.g. steroids, antibiotics.
Return remaining blood for examination by the bacteriology department.

Patient complaining of feeling a hot flush along the vein, facial flushing and lumbar pain. The patient may become shocked with a fall in the blood pressure and the urine output may fall.

Blood not cross-matched.
Urgent cross-match completed and blood not fully compatible.
Blood administered to wrong patient.
Cross-matched blood sample wrongly labelled or taken from wrong patient.

Ensure blood cross-matching forms are completed correctly. If taking blood sample, check carefully that the name and number on the form match the patient. Ensure that a unit is checked against the cross-match form for blood group, patient's name, patient's number, ward, Rh factor, unit number of blood, when blood taken, and expiry date. Begin transfusion slowly and observe the patient carefully at the start of each unit.

Stop transfusion. Change administration set and commence flushing device with 0.9% sodium chloride to keep vein open. Lay patient flat and treat as for shock. Inform medical staff.

Transfusion risks associated with administration of large volumes of blood include:

1 Abnormal bleeding tendencies, including DIC.
2 Hypocalcaemia.
3 Risk of development of acute respiratory distress syndrome.

4 Potassium intoxication.
5 Elevated blood ammonia level.
6 Haemosiderosis.
7 Hypothermia.

Massive transfusion refers to quantities in excess of 6 units and specific texts should be consulted in these circumstances.

The Unconscious Patient

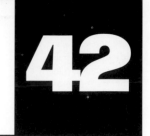

42

Definition

Consciousness is defined as a general awareness of oneself and the surrounding environment. It is a dynamic state and is therefore subject to change (Rengachary & Duke 1994; Aucken & Crawford 1998).

Introduction

There are three properties of consciousness which can be individually affected by the disease process (Jennett 1992):

1 Arousal or wakefulness (i.e. eyes open to command).
2 Alertness and awareness (i.e. orientation and communication).
3 Appropriate voluntary motor activity (i.e. obeying commands).

In coma an individual's awareness, as well as those responses essential to comfort and self-preservation, no longer operate (Wong *et al.* 1984).

This chapter deals mainly with the patient who is unconscious for a period of time and not with the patient whose coma is controlled (i.e. ventilated/sedated/anaesthetized patients).

Complete care of the unconscious patient presents a special challenge to the nurse because the patient is totally dependent on the nurse's expert skills – for his/her comfort needs and indeed for his/her life. This inability to respond must spur efforts to include the patient and the family or close friends in reorientation programmes, by using stimuli associated with the patient's previous physiological and social experiences.

The normal reflexes protecting the conscious person are lost and their protective function is assumed by the nurse until the patient can function to maximum potential. In order to do so it would be necessary to:

1 Establish and maintain a clear airway.
2 Assess the level of consciousness (see Chap. 26, Neurological Observations).
3 Record and evaluate vital signs.
4 Maintain fluid and electrolyte balance.
5 Carry out nursing care as appropriate to the patient's condition.
6 Involve relatives and/or friends in care from the beginning.

If the patient is unconscious in the terminal phase of an illness, emphasis of care should be focused on keeping the patient comfortable.

Reference material

Causes of unconsciousness

Causes of unconsciousness are numerous, and may dictate the length of the coma period. It is important to ascertain the cause of the coma so that appropriate treatment can be provided. The nurse should be observant for indications as to the reason for unconsciousness, for example, signs of head injury, needle marks on the lower limbs and evidence of tongue biting (Lindsay *et al.* 1997). Tongue biting may be the result of an epileptic fit, while needle marks on the lower limbs and abdomen could indicate that the patient is a diabetic (Fuller 1993). Some patients may recover spontaneously, e.g. after a seizure (also referred to as fit/convulsion), while others remain unconscious until their death.

The following list of causes of unconsciousness is not exhaustive, nor can it indicate the outcome of the comatosed state.

Poisons and drugs

1 Alcohol.
2 General anaesthetics.
3 Overdose of drugs, including solvents.
4 Gases, e.g. carbon monoxide.
5 Heavy metals, e.g. lead poisoning.

Vascular causes

1 Postcardiac arrest.
2 Ischaemia.
3 Hypertensive encephalopathy.
4 Haemorrhage – intracerebral or subarachnoid.
5 Sudden reduction in circulating blood volume.

Infections

1 Septicaemia.
2 Viruses, e.g. herpes, encephalitis, HIV.
3 Meningitis.
4 Protozoan infections, e.g. malaria.
5 Fungal, e.g. aspergillosis.
6 Abscess.
7 Encephalitis.

Seizures

1 Idiopathic or post-traumatic epilepsy.
2 Eclampsia.

Metabolic disorders

1 Hypoglycaemia.
2 Hypoxia.
3 Renal failure.
4 Hepatic failure.

Other causes

1 Neoplasm, primary, e.g. glioma, or secondary tumour from other body primary, e.g. lung and breast.
2 Trauma, e.g. head injury or trauma resulting in haematoma.
3 Cardiac failure.
4 Tetany.
5 Degenerative diseases, e.g. multiple sclerosis.

Note: intracranial haematomas can cause rapid unconsciousness due to brain compression while cerebral tumours will firstly produce confusion and drowsiness followed by coma when there is compression of the brain stem (Jennett 1992).

Emergency management

Acute emergency management of consciousness is of vital importance (see Chap. 8, Cardiopulmonary Resuscitation). For example, the patient's airway must be inspected, and if the patient vomits the head should be turned to one side to prevent aspiration. Depending on the circumstances, an oral airway, nasal airway, endotracheal tube or tracheostomy tube may be necessary. Whether to place the patient on a ventilator depends on the blood gases, tidal volume, rate of respirations, oxygen saturation and level of consciousness (Rengachary & Duke 1994).

Recording the level of consciousness

There are many methods of assessing and recording a patient's level of consciousness. One of the most commonly used in the UK is the Glasgow Coma Scale (Jennett & Teasdale 1974; Allan 1986). See Chap. 26, Neurological Observations.

One of the major advantages of the Glasgow Coma Scale is that it is validated and internationally recognized, thus providing a standardized tool. It promotes consistent and concise documentation so that any deterioration is detected at the earliest moment (Aucken & Crawford 1998).

Attitudes of nurses

Leon and Snyder (1980) explored the psychosocial problems in caring for head-injured patients and concluded that, in general, nurses accepted unconscious patients and were challenged by them. The phase of management appears to affect the attitude of the nursing staff, e.g. critical care, postemergent care and continuing care. Bell (1986) discusses the hopelessness, guilt, ambivalence, frustration and depression felt by nurses in some situations. The involvement of families and friends of the patient may lead the nurse to experience professional, moral and ethical problems, depending on the likely outcome of the coma and the length of the comatosed state.

All nurses must recognize that 'it is difficult to provide constant and continuous excellent care to the comatosed (head-injured) patient when the professional rewards are minimal' (Flaherty 1982). Peer support in units or wards caring for the unconscious patient is vital, particularly perhaps where the patient is a child, or the patient is brain dead (Rudy 1982; Pallis 1983). The needs of the patient's family and friends must also be addressed by the nursing staff. Grieving is a natural and necessary process for family and friends of the terminally ill or long-term unconscious patient, and they must be supported through and prepared for the eventual outcome (Allan 1988; Penson 1988).

Conclusion

For the nurse, caring for the unconscious patient poses a major challenge. She/he is dealing not only with the preservation of life and the avoidance of further disabilities (if appropriate), but also with the psychological effects of the coma on the other members of the family. Often the involvement of other multidisciplinary team members provides an opportunity in providing patient and family care and addressing the needs of the professionals. Support is crucial, whether in the acute or terminal setting, and especially where nurses are working in an environment that is physically and psychologically challenging. Sometimes it is impossible not to become very close to patients and their families and, therefore, the nurse also suffers pain, which often goes ignored (Kibler 1998).

References and further reading

Ackerman, L.L. (1993) Alterations in level of responsiveness. Nurs Clin North Am, **28**(4), 729–45.
Allan, D. (1986) Nursing the unconscious patient. Prof Nurse, **2**(1), 15–17.
Allan, D. (1988) The ethics of brain death. Prof Nurse, **3**(8), 295–8.
Aucken, S. & Crawford, B. (1998) Neurological observations. In: Neuro-Oncology for Nurses, (ed. D. Guerrero). Whurr, London.
Bell, T.N. (1986) Nurses' attitudes in caring for comatose head-injured patients. J Neurolog Nurs, **18**(5), 279–89.
Flaherty, M. (1982) Care of the comatose: complex problems faced alone. Nurs Manage, **13**(10), 44–6.
Fuller, G. (1993) Neurological Examination Made Easy. Churchill Livingstone, Edinburgh.
Gooch, J. (1985) Mouth care. Prof Nurse, **1**(3), 77–9.
Hickey, J.V. (1986) The Clinical Practice of Neurological and Neurosurgical Nursing, 2nd edn. Lippincott, Philadelphia.
Jennett, B. (1992) Coma. In: Medicine International Neurology, part 2 of 3, pp. 4120–23. The Medicine Group (Journals) Ltd.

Jennett, B. & Teasdale, G. (1974) Assessment of coma and impaired consciousness. A practical scale. *Lancet*, **2**, 81–3.

Kibler, S. (1998) Psychological care. In: *Neuro-Oncology for Nurses* (ed. D. Guerrero). Whurr, London.

Leon, M. & Snyder (1980) The psychosocial aspects of the care of long-term comatose patients. *J Neurosurg Nurs*, **11**(4), 235–7.

Lindsay, K.W., Bone, I. & Callander, R. (1997) *Neurology and Neurosurgery Illustrated*, 3rd edn. Churchill Livingstone, Edinburgh.

Mangiardi, J.R. (1990) Initial management of head injury. *Top Emerg Med*, **11**(4), 11–23.

Nikas, D. (1982) Altered states of consciousness. *Focus Crit Care*, Part I – **10**(5), 10–14; Part II – **10**(6), 10–13; Part III – (1984), **11**(1), 54–8.

Pallis, C. (1983) *ABC of Brain Stem Death*. British Medical Association, London.

Payne-James, J. *et al.* (eds) (1995) *Artificial Nutritional Support in Clinical Practice*. Arnold, London.

Penson, J. (1988) The needs of the terminally ill patient's family. *Prof Nurse*, **3**(5), 153–5.

Podurgiel, M. (1990) The unconscious experience: a pilot study. *J Neurosci Nurs*, **22**(1), 52–3.

Rengachary, S.S. & Duke, D.A. (1994) Impaired consciousness. In: *Principles of Neurology* (eds S.S. Rengachary & R.H. Wilkins). Wolfe, London.

Rudy, E. (1982) Brain death. *Dimensions Crit Care Nurs*, **1**(3), 178.

Scherer, P. (1986) Assessment: the logic of coma. *Am J Nurs*, **86**(5), 542–9.

Taylor, S.J. (1988) A guide to nasogastric feeding. *Prof Nurse*, **3**(11), 439–43.

Taylor, S.J. (1989a) Preventing complications in internal feeding. *Prof Nurse*, **4**(5), 247–9.

Taylor, S.J. (1989b) A guide to internal feeding. *Prof Nurse*, **4**(4), 195–8.

Wong, J. *et al.* (1984) Care of the unconscious patient: a problem-orientated approach. *J Neurosurg Nurs*, **16**(3), 148–50.

de Young, S. (1987) Coma recovery program. *Rehab Nurs*, **12**(3), 121–4.

GUIDELINES • Care of the unconscious patient

Equipment

At the bedside:
(Equipment 1, 2 and 3 depending on cause and expected outcome.)

1 Airway (of correct size).
2 Suction.
3 Oxygen mask.
4 Intravenous infusion equipment.
5 Personal hygiene equipment:
 (a) Eye toilet pack.
 (b) Oral toilet pack.
 (c) Catheter care pack.
6 Cot sides (to be assessed on an individual basis).

7 Observation charts depending on cause and expected outcome:
 (a) Neurological.
 (b) Intake and output.
8 Feeding equipment (as necessary).

Easy access to:

1 Ambu-bag with valve and mask; or intubation (and tracheostomy) equipment.
2 Neurological observation tray, thermometer and electronic blood pressure monitor.

Procedure

Action	Rationale
1 Call the patient by preferred name. Introduce yourself; explain each procedure before starting; talk to patient; tell patient date, time, etc.	Hearing often remains intact in the unconscious patient. To prevent sensory deprivation and promote orientation.
2 The room or ward area should be warm, and adequately ventilated, with easy access to the patient.	To facilitate rapid assessment of the patient at a glance, e.g.: (a) Colour of skin – cherry red after carbon monoxide poisoning, frost in uraemia, yellow in hepatic failure, blue in cyanosis. (b) Smell – alcohol; 'toasted almonds' after cyanide poisoning, the sickly sweet smell of diabetic ketoacidosis (Mangiardi 1990).
3 Nurse the patient in a bed with a firm base and a detachable bed head (and cot sides if deemed necessary).	To facilitate cardiac massage and intubation if required. (To prevent self-injury if the patient shows signs of agitation).
4 Insert a bed cradle, if required.	To allow unhampered limb movements and prevent pressure on limbs/feet. To enhance view of limbs if leg is in plaster or on traction (as in multiple injuries).

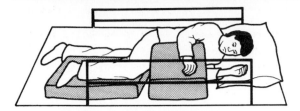

Figure 42.1   Positioning the unconscious patient.

---

5 Place patient in lateral or semi-prone position (unless patient is intubated).

To prevent occlusion of airway by tongue falling back against the pharyngeal wall.
To encourage drainage of respiratory secretions, and prevent pooling of same in throat.

Note: if a patient's injuries or other conditions prevent him/her from being nursed from side to side or prone, then a nurse should be in attendance at all times while there is an airway hazard.

6 Pass nasogastric tube.

To empty gastric contents regularly. Paralytic ileus occurs frequently in the unconscious patient and this may lead to aspiration of stomach contents.

7 Place the limbs as follows (Fig. 42.1) (dictated by patient's changing condition):
  (a) Head: put the patient's head on a pillow.
  (b) Trunk: keep the spine straight and place pillows at the patient's back for support.
  (c) Upper limb: bring the uppermost arm forward in front of the patient.
      Bend the elbow slightly, but keep the wrist extended. Support the arm on a pillow and bring the bottom arm alongside the face with the palm facing upwards.
  (d) Lower limbs: flex the uppermost leg and bring it forward. Support it on pillows.
      Keep the lower leg extended straight and in line with the spine. Make sure the patient's uppermost leg does not rest on the lower leg.
  (e) Consult with physiotherapist and anaesthetist about positioning exercises to enhance pulmonary function.
  (f) Institute passive physiotherapy exercises and observe colour, temperature and pulses of limbs.
  (g) Apply antiembolism stockings as ordered.

To promote comfort and maintain proper alignment of the body.

To prevent oedema by inappropriate pressure on venous flow.

To prevent internal rotation of the hip.

To avoid pressure ulcers on bony prominences.

To effect optimal respiratory function and gaseous exchange.

To prevent deep vein thrombosis formation; to recognize early signs of limb deformity.
To aid venous return to the heart and prevent formation of clots.

8 (a) Remove all dental prostheses and note caps, loose teeth, bleeding gums, etc.
  (b) Clean patient's nostrils.
  (c) Insert an airway (either oral or nasal) as appropriate.

To obtain and maintain clear airway and assess condition of oral cavity.

9 Perform neurological assessment as frequently as patient's condition dictates.

To note changes in condition and act on changes as appropriate.

10 (a) Administer intravenous fluids as prescribed and record.
  (b) Strict asepsis must be maintained when carrying out proceedings involving puncture sites of vascular access devices or sterile ends of intravenous infusion sets.

To maintain electrolyte and fluid balance.

To minimize the risk of infections – local or systemic.

Guidelines • Care of the unconscious patient (cont'd)

Action	Rationale
11 Maintain feeding regime either by nasogastric tube (see Chap. 27, Nutritional Support) or by fine bore continuous tube feeding or by central venous catheter (see Chap. 20, Infusion Devices)	To maintain metabolic stasis. To prevent weight loss (Taylor 1988; 1989a, b; Payne-James *et al.* 1995).
12 Touch the patient gently and describe boundaries and environment, e.g. place patient's hand on the bedside, blankets, locker and explain what each item is, describe the room.	Through touch, individuals establish (and maintain) their body boundaries and relationships with others, and their environment. Being denied opportunities to touch can impair physiological, psychological and social development (de Young 1987; Podurgiel 1990).
13 Maintain patient's general hygiene (see Chap. 32, Personal Hygiene).	To ensure patient's skin is kept clean, dry and supple (Gooch 1985).
14 Carry out eye care (see Chap. 17, Eye Care).	The blink reflex is absent during unconsciousness (or the patient's eyes may be open all the time). This may lead to corneal drying, irritation and ulceration.
15 Carry out mouth care (see procedure on mouth care, Chap. 24).	To maintain a clean, moist mouth, to prevent the accumulation of oral and postnasal secretions and to prevent the development of mouth infections (Gooch 1985).
16 Observe the patient for signs of bladder distension (or urinary bypass of catheter; see Chap. 43, Urinary Catheterization).	To minimize risk of urinary complication. In males, an external sheath may be used and catheterization may become necessary. In females, catheterization may be immediately necessary.
(a) Read catheter information carefully.	To minimize risk of overdistending the balloon and damaging the urethra.
(b) Perform regular catheter care.	To minimize risk of infection.
17 Carry out bowel care.	To prevent constipation and/or diarrhoea.
18 Change the patient's position every 2 h or as dictated by condition.	To relieve pressure areas and minimize risk of pressure ulcers occurring. To prevent respiratory complications by allowing for postural drainage, and for each side of the chest to receive a period free of compression by body weight when it can expand fully.
19 Keep relatives and friends informed of changes in the patient's condition and involve them in caring for the patient as appropriate.	To help family and friends adjust to the situation and (depending on prognosis) facilitate 'anticipatory grief' (Penson 1988).

Nursing care plan

Problem	Cause	Suggested action
Restlessness and/or confusion.	A degree of restlessness may indicate that the patient is regaining consciousness. During this time there may be a clouding of consciousness with confusion, aggression, uncooperative behaviour and disorientation. Restlessness may also indicate brain damage, cerebral anoxia (when there is a partially obstructed airway), a full bladder, bowel pain, discomfort or generalized pain.	Ascertain, where possible, the cause of the discomfort and rectify as appropriate. Summon help if the patient becomes aggressive or violent. Ensure the patient does not inflict self-injury, e.g. place cot sides in position on the bed.
Seizures	An unconscious patient is at risk of seizures.	Maintain a clear airway. Protect the patient from self-injury. Observe the

		patient during the seizure and record observations on a seizure chart. Observe for signs of injury. Administer prescribed drugs.
Cerebrospinal fluid leakage through nose or ears.	May be indicative of base of skull fracture, or some dural damage (Nikas 1982).	Place sterile swab against nose and ears and collect fluid. Test drainage for sugar (it will be positive if CSF is present). Inform medical staff.
Vomiting.	The unconscious patient is prone to paralytic ileus, or medulla oblongata may be involved.	Maintain a clear airway. Keep stomach empty until ileus resolves.
Distended bladder.	See Chap. 43, Urinary Catheterization, for problems associated with catheterization.	
Inability to maintain own nutritional intake.	See Chap. 27, Nutritional Support, for problems associated with this type of nutrition.	

Urinary Catheterization

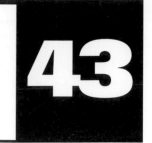

43

Definition

Urinary catheterization is the insertion of a special tube into the bladder, using aseptic technique, for the purpose of evacuating or instilling fluids.

Indications

Male

In the male, urinary catheterization may be carried out for the following reasons:

1 To empty the contents of the bladder, e.g. before or after abdominal, pelvic or rectal surgery and before certain investigations.
2 To determine residual urine.
3 To allow irrigation of the bladder.
4 To bypass an obstruction.
5 To relieve retention of urine.
6 To introduce cytotoxic drugs in the treatment of papillary bladder carcinomas.
7 To enable bladder function tests to be performed.
8 To measure urinary output accurately, e.g. when a patient is in shock, undergoing bone marrow transplantation or receiving high-dose chemotherapy.
9 To relieve incontinence when no other means is practicable.

Female

In the female, urinary catheterization may be carried out for the nine reasons listed above and for two further reasons:

10 To empty the bladder before childbirth, if thought necessary.
11 To avoid complications during intracavitary insertion of radioactive caesium.

Reference material

Catheter selection

New materials and improvements in design have allowed manufacturers to offer a wide range of urinary catheters. Careful assessment of the most appropriate material, size and balloon capacity will ensure that the catheter selected is as effective as possible, and that complications are minimized (Pomfret 1996). Types of catheters are listed in Table 43.1, together with their applications. Catheters should be used in line with the manufacturer's recommendations, in order to avoid product liability (RCN 1994).

Balloon size

A catheter with a 30 ml balloon was designed by Dr Frederick Foley in the 1920s. The sole purpose of this catheter was to prevent haemorrhage following prostatectomy. The 30 ml balloon has become associated with leakage of urine (Kennedy *et al.* 1983), and a study by Kristiansen *et al.* (1983) found that the large balloon caused damage to the neck of the bladder.

Consequently, a 5–10 ml balloon is recommended for adults, and a 3–5 ml balloon for children. Care should be taken to use the correct amount of water to fill the balloon because too much or too little may cause distortion of the catheter tip, leading to irritation and trauma to the bladder wall. One or more of the drainage eyes may also become occluded (Bard Ltd, 1987; Pomfret 1996).

Catheter size

Urethral catheters are measured in charrières (ch). The charrière is the outer circumference of the catheter in millimetres and is equivalent to three times the diameter. Thus a 12 ch catheter has a diameter of 4 mm.

Potential side-effects of large-gauge catheters include:

1 Pain and discomfort.
2 Pressure ulcers, which may lead to stricture formation.
3 Blockage of paraurethral ducts.
4 Abscess formation (Edwards *et al.* 1983; Crow *et al.* 1986; Roe & Brocklehurst 1987; Blandy & Moors 1989; Winn 1998).

The most important guiding principle is to choose the smallest size of catheter necessary to maintain adequate drainage (McGill 1982). If the urine to be drained is likely to be clear, a 12 ch catheter should be considered. Larger gauge catheters may be necessary if debris or clots are present in the urine (Pomfret 1996; Winn 1998).

Length of catheter

Until 1979 only one length of urethral catheter (41–45 cm) was available for both men and women (Crummey 1989). A shorter catheter (20–25 cm) is now available for women.

Table 43.1   Types of catheters

Catheter type	Material	Uses
Balloon (Foley) two-way catheter: two channels, one for urine drainage; second, smaller channel for balloon inflation	Latex, PTFE coated latex, silicone elastomer coated, 100% silicone, hydrogel coated	Most commonly used for patients who require bladder drainage (short-, medium- or long-term)
Balloon (Foley) three-way irrigation catheter: three channels, one for urine; one for irrigation fluid; one for balloon inflation	Latex, PTFE coated latex, silicone, plastic	To provide continuous irrigation (e.g. after prostatectomy). Potential for infection is reduced by minimizing need to break the closed drainage system (Gilbert & Gobbi 1989; Mulhall *et al.* 1993)
Non-balloon (Nelaton) or Scotts, or intermittent catheter (one channel only)	PVC and other plastics	To empty bladder or continent urinary reservoir intermittently; to instil solutions into bladder

It is more discreet than the longer catheter, and less likely to cause trauma or infections because movement in and out of the urethra is reduced. Infection may also be caused by the longer catheter looping or kinking. In obese women, however, the inflation valve of the shorter catheter may cause soreness by rubbing against the inside of the thigh, and the catheter is more likely to pull on the bladder neck (Britton & Wright 1990; Pomfret 1996).

Tip design

Several different types of catheter tip are available in addition to the standard round tip. Each tip is designed to overcome a particular problem:

1 The *Tieman-tipped catheter* has a curved tip with one to three drainage eyes to allow greater drainage. This catheter has been designed to negotiate the membranous and prostatic urethra in patients with prostatic hypertrophy.

2 The *Whistle-tipped catheter* has a lateral eye in the tip and eyes above the balloon to provide a large drainage area. This design is intended to facilitate drainage of debris, e.g. blood clots.

3 The *Roberts catheter* has an eye above and below the balloon to facilitate the drainage of residual urine.

Catheter material

A wide variety of materials are used to make catheters. The key criterion in selecting the appropriate material is the length of time the catheter is expected to remain in place. Three broad time scales have been identified:

1 Short-term (1–14 days).
2 Short- to medium-term (2–6 weeks).
3 Medium- to long-term (6 weeks–3 months).

The principal catheter materials are as follows:

1 *Polyvinylchloride (PVC)*. Catheters made from PVC or plastic are quite rigid. They have a wide lumen, which allows a rapid flow rate; however, their rigidity may cause some patients discomfort. They are mainly used for intermittent catheterization or postoperatively. They are recommended for short-term use only (Pomfret 1996).

2 *Latex*. Latex is a purified form of rubber and is the softest of the catheter materials. It has a smooth surface, with a tendency to allow crust formation. Latex has been shown to cause urethral irritation (Wilksch *et al.* 1983) and therefore should only be considered when catheterization is likely to be short-term. Hypersensitivity to latex has been increasing in recent years (Woodward 1997) and latex catheters have been the cause of some cases of anaphylaxis (Young *et al.* 1994). Woodward (1997) suggests that patients should be asked if they have ever had an adverse reaction to rubber products in the past before catheters containing latex are utilized.

3 *Teflon or silicone elastomer coatings*. A Teflon or silicone elastomer coating is applied to a latex catheter to render the latex inert and reduce urethral irritation (Slade & Gillespie 1985). Teflon or silicone elastomer coated catheters are recommended for short- or medium-term catheterization.

4 *All silicone*. Silicone is an inert material which is less likely to cause urethral irritation. Silicone catheters are not coated, and therefore have a wider lumen. The lumen of these catheters, in cross-section, is crescent or D-shaped, which may induce formation of encrustation (Pomfret 1996). Because silicone permits gas diffusion, balloons may deflate and allow the catheter to fall out prematurely (Studer 1983; Barnes & Malone-Lee 1986). Silicone catheters are recommended for long-term use.

5 *Hydrogel coatings*. Catheters made of an inner core of latex encapsulated in a hydrophilic polymer coating have recently been developed. The polymer coating is well tolerated by the urethral mucosa, causing little irritation. Hydrogel coated catheters become smoother when rehydrated, reducing friction with the urethra. They are inert (Nacey & Delahunt 1991), and are reported to be resistant to bacterial colonization and encrustation (Roberts *et al.* 1990; Woollons 1996). Hydrogel coated catheters are recommended for long-term use.

The *conformable catheter* is designed to conform to the shape of the female urethra, and allows partial filling of the bladder. The natural movement of the urethra on the catheter, which is collapsible, is intended to prevent obstructions (Brocklehurst *et al.* 1988). They are made of latex and have a silicone elastomer coating. Conformable catheters are approximately 3 cm longer than conventional catheters for women.

Anaesthetic lubricating gel

The use of anaesthetic lubricating gels is well recognized for male catheterization, but there is some controversy in their use for female catheterization. In males the gel is instilled directly into the urethra and then external massage is used to move the gel down its length. In female patients the anaesthetic lubricating gel or plain lubricating gel is applied to the tip of the catheter only, if it is used at all. It has been suggested that most of the lubricant is wiped off the catheter at the urethral introitus so therefore it fails to reach the urethral tissue (Muctar 1991).

These differences in practice imply that catheterization is a painful procedure for men but is not so for women. This assumption is not based on any empirical evidence or on any biological evidence. Other than the differences in length and route, the male and female urethra are very similar except for the presence of lubricating glands in the male urethra (Tortora & Grabowski 1993). The absence of these lubricating glands in the female urethra suggests that there is perhaps a greater need for the introduction of a lubricant. Women have complained of pain and discomfort during catheterization procedures (Mackenzie & Webb 1995), suggesting that the use of anaesthetic lubricating gels must be reconsidered. Since there is a lack of research to clarify the efficacy of lubricating gels, practice must be based on the research evidence that is available and the physiology and anatomy of the urethra.

Common sites of cross-infection

The common sites of cross-infection in a catheterized patient are illustrated in Fig. 43.1. To reduce the risk of cross-infection, particular care should be taken when obtaining urine specimens. All specimens should be taken from the rubber cuff which is specially designed to occlude the puncture hole when the needle is withdrawn (Wilson & Coates 1996; Lowthian 1998). Reference should be made to the manufacturer's instructions as to the number of times the cuff can be punctured safely. Some manufacturers indicate that cuffs can be punctured up to 50 times (e.g. Simpla). With other drainage systems this may not be possible.

Meatal cleansing

Cleaning the urethral meatus, where the catheter enters the body, is a nursing procedure intended to minimize infection of the urinary tract. There is no consensus about the value of this procedure, or about which cleansing solu-

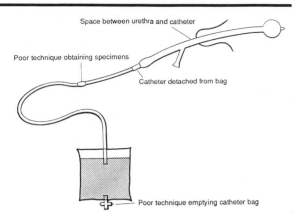

Figure 43.1 Common sites of cross-infection in a catheterized patient.

tions, if any, should be used. Antiseptics do not appear to check the development of urinary tract infections; indeed, they have been implicated in the development of multiresistant organisms (Dance *et al.* 1987). Simple meatal cleansing with soap, water and clean wash cloths is recommended (Roe 1992; Falkiner 1993; Rigby 1998).

Drainage bags

A wide variety of drainage systems are available. Selecting a system involves consideration of the reasons for catheterization, the intended duration, the wishes of the patient and infection control issues (Wilson & Coates 1996).

The highest risk of cross-infection occurs when the bag is emptied or changed (Crow *et al.* 1986). Reid *et al.* (1982) recommend weekly bag changes, on the grounds that more frequent changes do not positively influence infection rates. The Department of Health *Drug Tariff* (DoH 1999) recommends changing bags every 5–7 days.

At home, patients reuse their drainage bags (Roe 1993). This practice is currently the subject of research. Until further research evidence is available, it is recommended that patients be given a choice between disposing of used drainage bags and reusing them after thorough cleaning and drying (Roe 1993).

Leg drainage bags

A variety of supports are available for use with these bags, including sporran waist belts, leg holsters, knickers/pants and leg straps (Roe 1992).

Catheter valves

Catheter valves, which eliminate the need for drainage bags, are becoming increasingly popular. The valve allows the bladder to fill and empty intermittently, and is particularly appropriate for patients who require long-term catheterization, as they do not require a drainage bag.

Catheter valves are only suitable for patients who have good cognitive function, sufficient manual dexterity to manipulate the valve and an adequate bladder capacity. It is important that catheter valves are released at regular intervals to ensure that the bladder does not become overdistended. As catheter valves preclude free drainage they are unlikely to be appropriate for patients with uncontrolled detrusor overactivity, ureteric reflux or renal impairment (Fader *et al.* 1997).

Catheter valves are licensed by the Department of Health to remain in situ for 5–7 days and this corresponds with most manufacturers' recommendations (Pomfret 1996). Little research into the advantages and disadvantages of catheter valves has been completed.

Suprapubic catheterization

Suprapubic catheterization is the insertion of a catheter through the anterior abdominal wall into the dome of the bladder. The procedure is performed under general or local anaesthesia, using a percutaneous system (Kirkwood 1999). A number of different suprapubic catheters are available. A trocar is used with all types of catheters in order to make the tract through which the catheter is threaded. Specifically designed catheters incorporate a fixing plate, which requires sutures to secure the catheter to the skin of the abdomen. For long-term use a Foley catheter is adequate. Large charrière size (18–22 ch) hydrogel coated or 100% silicone are recommended (Winder 1994).

Suprapubic catheterization does offer some advantages over urethral catheterization. There is a reduction in the risk of patients developing urinary tract infection. Urethral integrity is retained and it allows for the resumption of normal voiding after surgery. Clamping the suprapubic catheter allows urethral voiding to occur, and the clamp can be released if voiding is incomplete. Patient satisfaction is increased as, for some, their level of independence is increased and sexual intercourse can occur with less impediment (Hammarsten & Lindquist 1992; Barnes *et al.* 1993; Fillingham & Douglas 1997; Wilson 1998).

Caring for a suprapubic catheter is the same as for a urethral catheter. Immediately following insertion of a suprapubic catheter, aseptic technique should be employed to cleanse the insertion site. Dressings may be required if secretions soil clothing, but they are not essential. Once the insertion site has healed (7–10 days), the site and catheter can be cleansed during bathing using soap, water and a clean cloth (Fillingham & Douglas 1997).

Intermittent self-catheterization (ISC)

This is not a new technique, although it has become noticeably more popular in recent years.

The procedure involves the episodic introduction of a catheter into the bladder to remove urine. After this the catheter is removed, leaving the patient catheter-free between catheterizations. The patient should perform the catheterization as often as necessary to prevent incontinence or to prevent prolonged retention of urine (usually four or five times a day) (Seth 1987).

The advantages of intermittent catheterization over indwelling urethral catheterizations include improved quality of life, greater patient satisfaction and greater freedom to express sexuality. In addition, urinary tract complications are minimized (Webb *et al.* 1990; Bakke & Malt 1993; Chai *et al.* 1995; Bakke *et al.* 1997; Getliffe 1997).

Patients suitable for intermittent self-catheterization include:

1 Those who can comprehend the technique.
2 Those with a reasonable degree of manual dexterity.
3 Those who are highly motivated.
4 Those who have a willing partner to perform the technique (i.e. if agreeable to both).
5 Those who can position themselves to attain reasonable access to the urethra (especially females) (Seth 1987).

In 1970, Lasides, in the USA, found that patients using a clean rather than a sterile technique did not encounter problematic urinary tract infection. The catheters used for intermittent self-catheterization are technically described as semidisposable, i.e. they are designed to be washed and reused for a limited period only, usually 1 week.

They should always be rinsed in running water and properly dried after use; between uses they should be kept in a container such as a plastic envelope (Simcare 1989).

References and further reading

Association for Continence Advisers (1995) *Suprapubic Catheters: A Guide for Nurses.* ACA, London.

Bakke, A. & Malt, U.F. (1993) Social functioning and general well being in patients treated with clean intermittent catheterisation. *J Psychosomatic Res*, **37**(4), 371–80.

Bakke, A., Digranes, A. & Hoisaeter, P.A. (1997) Physical predictors of infection in patients treated with clean intermittent catheterisation: a prospective 7-year study. *Br J Urol*, **79**(1), 85–90.

Bard Ltd (1987) *You, Your Patients, and Urinary Catheters.* Bard Ltd, Crawley.

Barnes, D.G., Shaw, P.J.R., Timoney, A.G. & Tsokos, N. (1993) Management of the neuropathic bladder by supra-pubic catheterisation. *Br J Urol*, **72**, 169–72.

Barnes, K.E. & Malone-Lee, J. (1986) Long-term catheter management: minimising the problem of premature replacement due to balloon deflation. *J Adv Nurs*, **11**, 303–307.

Blandy, J.P. & Moors, J. (1989) *Urology for Nurses.* Blackwell Science, Oxford.

Blannin, J.P. & Hobden, J. (1980) The catheter of choice. *Nurs Times*, **76**, 2092–3.

Britton, P.M. & Wright, E.S. (1990) Catheters: making an informed choice. *Prof Nurse*, **5**(4), 194, 196–8.

Brocklehurst, J.C. *et al.* (1988) A new urethral catheter. *Br J Med*, **296**, 1691–3.

Chai, T., Chung, A.K., Belville, W.D. & Faerber, G.J. (1995) Compliance and complications of clean intermittent catheterisation in the spinal-cord injured patient. *Paraplegia*, **33**(3), 161–3.

Crow, R. *et al.* (1988) Indwelling catheterization and related nursing practice. *J Adv Nurs*, **13**(4), 489–95.

Crow, R.A. *et al.* (1986) *A Study of Patients with an Indwelling*

Catheter and Related Nursing Practice. Nursing Practice Unit, University of Surrey.

Crummey, V. (1989) Ignorance can hurt. *Nurs Times Nurs Mirror*, **85**, 67–8, 70.

Dance, D.A.B. *et al.* (1987) A hospital outbreak caused by chlorhexidine and antibiotic resistant *Proteus mirabilis. J Hosp Infect*, **10**, 10–16.

DoH (1999) *Drug Tariff.* Stationery Office, London.

Edwards, L.E. *et al.* (1983) Post-catheterisation urethral strictures: a clinical and experimental study. *Br J Urol*, **55**, 53–6.

Fader, M., Pettersson Brooks, R., Dean, G. *et al.* (1997) A multi-centre comparative evaluation of catheter valves. *Br J Nurs*, **6**(7), 359–67.

Falkiner, F.R. (1993) The insertion and management of indwelling urethral catheters – minimising the risk of infection. *J Hosp Infect*, **25**, 79–90.

Fillingham, S. & Douglas, J. (1997) *Urological Nursing*, 2nd edn. Baillière Tindall, London.

Getliffe, K. (1997) Catheters and catheterisation. In: *Promoting Continence: A Clinical and Research Resource* (eds K. Getliffe & M. Dolman). Baillière Tindall, London.

Gilbert, A. & Gobbi, M. (1989) Making sense of bladder irrigation. *Nurs Times*, **85**(16), 40–42.

Hammarsten, J. & Lindquist, K. (1992) Supra-pubic catheter following transurethral resection of the prostate: a way to decrease the number of urethral strictures and improve the outcome of operation. *J Urol*, **147**, 648–52.

Heenan, A. (1990) Indications for long-term catheterization. *Nurs Times*, **86**, 70–71.

Jenkins, S.C. (1998) Digital guidance of female urethral catheterization. *Br J Urol*, **82**, 589–90.

Kennedy, A.P. *et al.* (1983) Factors related to the problems of long-term catheterisation. *J Adv Nurs*, **8**, 207–12.

Kirkwood, L. (1999) Taking charge. *Nurs Times*, **95**(6), 63–4.

Kohler-Ockmore, J. & Feneley, R.C.L. (1996) Long-term catheterization of the bladder: prevalence and morbidity. *Br J Urol*, **77**, 347–51.

Kristiansen, P. *et al.* (1983) Long-term urethral catheter drainage and bladder capacity. *Neurol Urodyn*, **2**, 135–43.

Lowthian, P. (1989) Preventing trauma (in patients with indwelling catheters). *Nurs Times Nurs Mirror*, **85**, 73–5.

Lowthian, P. (1998) The dangers of long-term catheter drainage. *Br J Nurs*, **7**(7), 366–79.

Mackenzie, J. (1993) Questioning the assumption that urinary catheterisation is a pain free event for women. *J Clin Nurs*, **2**, 64–5.

Mackenzie, J. & Webb, C. (1995) Gynopia in nursing practice: the case of urethral catheterization. *J Clin Nurs*, **4**, 221–6.

MacSweeney, P. (1989) Self-catheterization – a solution for some incontinent people. *Prof Nurse*, **4**(8), 399–401.

McGill, S. (1982) Catheter management: it's size that's important. *Nurs Mirror*, **154**, 48–9.

Muctar, S. (1991) The importance of a lubricant in transurethral interventions. *Urologue [B]*, **31**, 153–5 [translation].

Mulhall, A. (1990) Bacteria, biofilm and bladder catheters. *Nurs Times*, **86**, 57.

Mulhall, A.B., King, S., Lee, K. & Wiggington, E. (1993) Maintenance of closed urinary drainage systems: are practitioners aware of the dangers? *J Clin Nurs*, **2**, 135–40.

Nacey, J.N. & Delahunt, B. (1991) Toxicity study of first and second generation hydrogel-coated latex catheters. *Br J Urol*, **67**, 314–16.

Oliver, H. (1988) Continence supplement. The treatment of choice. *Nurs Times Nurs Mirror*, **84**, 70.

Pomfret, I.J. (1996) Catheters: design, selection and management. *Br J Nurs*, **5**(4), 245–51.

RCN (1994) *Guidelines on Male Catheterisation: The Role of the Nurse.* Royal College of Nursing, London.

RCN (1996) *Suprapubic catheterisation: A Guide for Nurses*, 2nd edn. Royal College of Nursing, London.

Reid, R.I. *et al.* (1982) Comparison of urine bag changing regimes in elderly catheterised patients. *Lancet*, **2**, 754–6.

Rigby, D. (1998) Long-term catheter care. *Prof Nurse Study Suppl*, **13**(5), S14–15.

Roberts, J.A. *et al.* (1990) Bacterial adherence to urethral catheters. *J Urol*, **144**, 264–9.

Roe, B.H. (1992) Use of indwelling catheters. In: *Clinical Nursing Practice: The Promotion and Management of Continence* (ed. B.H. Roe). Prentice Hall, Hemel Hempstead.

Roe, B.H. (1993) Catheter associated urinary tract infection: a review. *J Clin Nurs*, **2**(4), 197–203.

Roe, B.H. & Brocklehurst, J.C. (1987) Study of patients with indwelling catheters. *J Adv Nurs*, **12**, 713–18.

Sallam, S.B.F. & Wrightson, P.G. (1997) Accountability in urinary catheter management. *Prof Nurse*, **12**(10), 697–700.

Seth, C. (1987) Catheters ring the changes. *Nurs Times Nurs Mirror*, **84**, *Commun Outlook*, **12**, 14.

Simcare (1989) *Intermittent Self-Catheterization – A Guide for Patients' Families.* Simcare, Lancing.

Slade, N. & Gillespie, W.A. (1985) *The Urinary Tract and the Catheter: Infection and Other Problems.* John Wiley, Chichester.

Stickler, D.J. & Chawla, J.C. (1987) The role of antiseptics in the management of patients with long-term indwelling bladder catheters. *J Hosp Infect*, **10**(3), 219–28.

Stoller, M. (1995) Retrograde instrumentation of the urinary tract. In: *Smith's General Urology* (eds E.A. Tanagho & J.W. McAninch). Prentice-Hall, London.

Studer, U.E. (1983) How to fill silicone catheter balloons. *Urology*, **22**, 300–302.

Tortora, G.V. & Grabowski, S.R. (1993) *Principles of Anatomy and Physiology*, 7th edn. Harper Collins College Publishers, New York and San Francisco.

Webb, R.J., Lawson, A.L. & Neal, D.E. (1990) Clean intermittent self-catheterisation in 172 adults. *Br J Urol*, **65**(1), 20–23.

Welford, K. (1999) Lessons in self-support. *Nurs Times*, **95**(6), 64–70.

Wilksch, J. *et al.* (1983) The role of catheter surface morphology and extractable cytotoxic material in tissue reactions to urethral catheters. *Br J Urol*, **55**, 48–52.

Wilson, C., Sandhu, S.S. & Kaisary, A.V. (1997) A prospective randomized study comparing a catheter-valve with a standard drainage system. *Br J Urol*, **80**, 915–17.

Wilson, M. (1998) Infection control. *Prof Nurse Study Suppl*, **13**(5), S10–13.

Wilson, M. & Coates, D. (1996) Infection control and urine drainage bag design. *Prof Nurse*, **11**(4), 245–52.

Winder, A. (1994) Suprapubic catheterisation. *Commun Outlook*, **4**(12), 25–6.

Winn, C. (1996a) Catheterisation: extending the scope of practice. *Nurs Stand*, **10**(52), 49–56.

Winn, C. (1996b) Basing catheter care on research principles. *Nurs Stand*, **10**(18), 38–40.

Winn, C. (1998) Complications with urinary catheters. *Prof Nurse Study Suppl*, **13**(5), S7–10.

Winn, C. & Thompson, J. (1998) Urinary catheters for intermittent use. *Prof Nurse*, **13**(8), 541–5.

Winson, L. (1997) Catheterization: a need for improved patient management. *Br J Nurs*, **6**(21), 1229–52.

Woodward, S. (1997) Complications of allergies to latex urinary catheters. *Br J Nurs*, **6**(4), 786–93.

Woollons, S. (1996) Urinary catheters for long-term use. *Prof Nurse*, **11**(12), 825–32.

Wright, E. (1988a) Catheter care: the risk of infection. *Prof Nurse*, 3(12), 487–8, 490.

Wright, E. (1988b) Minimising the risks of UTI. *Prof Nurse*, 4(2), 63–4, 66–7.

Young, A.E., Macnaughton, P.D., Gaylard, D.G. & Weatherly, C. (1994) A case of latex anaphylaxis. *Br J Hosp Med*, **52**(11), 599–600.

GUIDELINES • Urinary catheterization

Equipment

1 Sterile catheterization pack containing gallipots, receiver, low-linting swabs, disposable towels.
2 Disposable pad.
3 Sterile gloves.
4 Selection of appropriate catheters.
5 Sterile anaesthetic lubricating jelly.
6 Universal specimen container.
7 0.9% sodium chloride or antiseptic solution.
8 Bactericidal alcohol hand rub.
9 Gate clip.
10 Hypoallergenic tape.
11 Scissors.
12 Sterile water.
13 Syringe and needle.
14 Disposable plastic apron.
15 Drainage bag and stand or holder.

Procedure

Male

Action	Rationale
1 Explain and discuss the procedure with the patient.	To ensure that the patient understands the procedure and gives his valid consent.
2 (a) Screen the bed.	To ensure patient's privacy. To allow dust and airborne organisms to settle before the field is exposed.
(b) Assist the patient to get into the supine position with the legs extended.	To ensure the appropriate area is easily accessible.
(c) Do not expose the patient at this stage of the procedure.	To maintain patient's dignity and comfort.
3 Wash hands using bactericidal soap and water or bactericidal alcohol hand rub.	To reduce risk of infection.
4 Put on a disposable plastic apron.	To reduce risk of cross-infection from micro-organisms on uniform.
5 Prepare the trolley, placing all equipment required on the bottom shelf.	The top shelf acts as a clean working surface.
6 Take the trolley to the patient's bedside, disturbing screens as little as possible.	To minimize airborne contamination.
7 Open the outer cover of the catheterization pack and slide the pack onto the top shelf of the trolley.	To prepare equipment.
8 Using an aseptic technique, open the supplementary packs.	To reduce the risk of introducing infection into the bladder.
9 Remove cover that is maintaining the patient's privacy and position a disposable pad under the patient's buttocks and thighs.	To ensure urine does not leak onto bedclothes.
10 Clean hands with a bactericidal alcohol hand rub.	Hands may have become contaminated by handling the outer packs.
11 Put on sterile gloves.	To reduce risk of cross-infection.
12 Place sterile towels across the patient's thighs and under buttocks.	To create a sterile field.

Guidelines • Urinary catheterization (cont'd)

Action	Rationale
13 Wrap a sterile topical swab around the penis. Retract the foreskin, if necessary, and clean the glans penis with 0.9% sodium chloride or an antiseptic solution.	To reduce the risk of introducing infection to the urinary tract during catheterization.
14 Insert the nozzle of the lubricating jelly into the urethra. Squeeze the gel into the urethra, remove the nozzle and discard the tube. Massage the gel along the urethra.	Adequate lubrication helps to prevent urethral trauma. Use of a local anaesthetic minimizes the discomfort experienced by the patient.
15 Squeeze the penis and wait approximately 5 minutes.	To prevent anaesthetic gel from escaping. To allow the anaesthetic gel to take effect.
16 Grasp the penis behind the glans, raising it until it is almost totally extended. Maintain grasp of penis until the procedure is finished.	This manoeuvre straightens the penile urethra and facilitates catheterization (Stoller 1995). Maintaining a grasp of the penis prevents contamination and retraction of the penis.
17 Place the receiver containing the catheter between the patient's legs. Insert the catheter for 15–25 cm until urine flows.	The male urethra is approximately 18 cm long.
18 If resistance is felt at the external sphincter, increase the traction on the penis slightly and apply steady, gentle pressure on the catheter. Ask the patient to strain gently as if passing urine.	Some resistance may be due to spasm of the external sphincter. Straining gently helps to relax the external sphincter.
19 Either remove the catheter gently when urinary flow ceases, or:	
(a) When urine begins to flow, advance the catheter almost to its bifurcation.	Advancing the catheter ensures that it is correctly positioned in the bladder.
(b) Gently inflate the balloon according to the manufacturer's direction, having ensured that the catheter is draining properly beforehand.	Inadvertent inflation of the balloon in the urethra causes pain and urethral trauma.
(c) Withdraw the catheter slightly and attach it to the drainage system.	
(d) Support the catheter, if the patient desires, either by using a specially designed support, e.g. Simpla G-Strap, or by taping the catheter to the patient's leg. Ensure that the catheter does not become taut when patient is mobilizing or when the penis becomes erect. Ensure that the catheter lumen is not occluded by the fixation device or tape.	To maintain patient comfort and to reduce the risk of urethral and bladder neck trauma. Care must be taken in using adhesive tapes as they may interact with the catheter material (Pomfret 1996).
20 Ensure that the glans penis is clean and then reduce or reposition the foreskin.	Retraction and constriction of the foreskin behind the glans penis (paraphimosis) may occur if this is not done.
21 Make the patient comfortable. Ensure that the area is dry.	If the area is left wet or moist, secondary infection and skin irritation may occur.
22 Measure the amount of urine.	To be aware of bladder capacity for patients who have presented with urinary retention. To monitor renal function and fluid balance. It is not necessary to measure the amount of urine if the patient is having the urinary catheter routinely changed.
23 Take a urine specimen for laboratory examination, if required (see Chap. 37, Specimen Collection).	For further information, see the procedure on collection of a catheter specimen of urine, below.
24 Dispose of equipment in a yellow plastic clinical waste bag and seal the bag before moving the trolley.	To prevent environmental contamination. Yellow is the recognized colour for clinical waste.
25 Draw back the curtains.	

26 Record information in relevant documents; this should include reasons for catheterization, date and time of catheterization, catheter type, length and size, amount of water instilled into the balloon, batch number, manufacturer, any problems negotiated during the procedure, and a review date to assess the need for continued catheterization or date of change of catheter.

To provide a point of reference or comparison in the event of later queries.

Female

Action

Rationale

1 Explain and discuss the procedure with the patient.

To ensure that the patient understands the procedure and gives her valid consent.

2 (a) Screen the bed.

To ensure patient's privacy. To allow dust and airborne organisms to settle before the sterile field is exposed. To enable genital area to be seen.

(b) Assist the patient to get into the supine position with knees bent, hips flexed and feet resting about 60 cm apart.

(c) Do not expose the patient at this stage of the procedure.

To maintain the patient's dignity and comfort.

3 Ensure that a good light source is available.

To enable genital area to be seen clearly.

4 Wash hands using bactericidal soap and water or bactericidal alcohol hand rub.

To reduce risk of cross-infection.

5 Put on a disposable apron.

To reduce risk of cross-infection from micro-organisms on uniform.

6 Prepare the trolley, placing all equipment required on the bottom shelf.

To reserve top shelf for clean working surface. (Also, see section on catheter selection.)

7 Take the trolley to the patient's bedside, disturbing screens as little as possible.

To minimize airborne contamination.

8 Open the outer cover of the catheterization pack and slide the pack on the top shelf of the trolley.

To prepare equipment.

9 Using an aseptic technique, open supplementary packs.

To reduce risk of introducing infection into the urinary tract.

10 Remove cover that is maintaining the patient's privacy and position a disposable pad under the patient's buttocks.

To ensure urine does not leak onto bedclothes.

11 Clean hands with a bactericidal alcohol hand rub.

Hands may have become contaminated by handling of outer packs, etc.

12 Put on sterile gloves.

To reduce risk of cross-infection.

13 Place sterile towels across the patient's thighs.

To create a sterile field.

14 Separate the labia minora so that the urethral meatus is seen. Using low-linting swabs, one hand should be used to maintain labial separation until catheterization is completed.

This manoeuvre provides better access to the urethral orifice and helps to prevent labial contamination of the catheter.

15 Clean around the urethral orifice with 0.9% sodium chloride or an antiseptic solution, using single downward strokes. Change gloves.

Inadequate preparation of the urethral orifice is a major cause of infection following catheterization. To reduce the risk of cross-infection.

16 Insert the nozzle of the lubricating jelly into the urethra. Squeeze the gel into the urethra, remove the nozzle and discard the tube.

Adequate lubrication helps to prevent urethral trauma. Use of a local anaesthetic minimizes the patient's discomfort.

Guidelines • Urinary catheterization (cont'd)

Action	Rationale
17 Place the catheter, in the receiver, between the patient's legs.	To provide a temporary container for urine as it drains.
18 Introduce the tip of the catheter into the urethral orifice in an upward and backward direction. If there is any difficulty in visualizing the urethral orifice due to vaginal atrophy and retraction of the urethral orifice, the index finger of the 'dirty' hand may be inserted in the vagina, and the urethral orifice can be palpated on the anterior wall of the vagina. The index finger is then positioned just behind the urethral orifice. This then acts as a guide, so the catheter can be correctly positioned (Jenkins 1998). Advance the catheter until 5–6 cm has been inserted.	The direction of insertion and the length of catheter inserted should bear relation to the anatomical structure of the area.
19 Either remove the catheter gently when urinary flow ceases, or:	
(a) Advance the catheter 6–8 cm.	This prevents the balloon from becoming trapped in the urethra.
(b) Inflate the balloon according to the manufacturer's directions, having ensured that the catheter is draining adequately.	Inadvertent inflation of the balloon within the urethra is painful and causes urethral trauma.
(c) Withdraw the catheter slightly and connect it to the drainage system.	
(d) Support the catheter, if the patient desires, either by using a specially designed support, e.g. Simpla G-Strap, or by taping the catheter to the patient's leg. Ensure that the catheter does not become taut when patient is mobilizing. Ensure that the catheter lumen is not occluded by the fixation device or tape.	To maintain patient comfort and to reduce the risk of urethral and bladder neck trauma. Care must be taken in using adhesive tapes as they may interact with the catheter material (Pomfret 1996).
20 Make the patient comfortable and ensure that the area is dry.	If the area is left wet or moist, secondary infection and skin irritation may occur.
21 Measure the amount of urine.	To be aware of bladder capacity for patients who have presented with urinary retention. To monitor renal function and fluid balance. It is not necessary to measure the amount of urine if the patient is having the urinary catheter routinely changed.
22 Take a urine specimen for laboratory examination if required.	For further information, see the procedure on collection of a catheter specimen of urine (below).
23 Dispose of equipment in a yellow plastic clinical waste bag and seal the bag before moving the trolley.	To prevent environmental contamination. Yellow is the recognized colour for clinical waste.
24 Draw back the curtains.	
25 Record information in relevant documents; this should include reasons for catheterization, date and time of catheterization, catheter type, length and size, amount of water instilled into the balloon, batch number, manufacturer, any problems negotiated during the procedure and a review date to assess the need for continued catheterization or date of change of catheter.	To provide a point of reference or comparison in the event of later queries.

Note: beware of patient having a vasovagal attack. This is caused by the vagal nerve being stimulated so that the heart slows down, leading to a syncope faint. If it happens, lie the patient down in the recovery position. Inform doctors.

GUIDELINES FOR PATIENTS • Intermittent self-catheterization

Equipment

1 Mirror (for female patients).
2 Appropriately sized catheters for male/female patients.

3 Lubricating gel.
4 Clean container (e.g. plastic envelope) for catheter.

Procedure

Female

Action	Rationale
1 Wash hands using bactericidal soap and water or bactericidal alcohol hand rub.	To reduce risk of cross-infection.
2 Take up a comfortable position, depending on mobility (e.g. sitting on toilet; standing with one foot placed on toilet seat).	To facilitate insertion of intermittent catheter.
3 Spread the labia and wash the genitalia from front to back with soap and water, then dry and insert the catheter, using lubricant if necessary. A mirror may be used to make genitalia more visible.	To reduce risk of introducing infection. For ease of insertion.
4 Drain the urine into a toilet or suitable container.	
5 Remove the catheter when flow has ceased.	
6 If catheter is to be re-used, wash through with tap water. Allow to drain and dry. Store in a dry container.	To remove urine.
7 Wash hands using bactericidal soap and water.	To reduce the risk of infection.

Male

Action	Rationale
1 Wash hands using bactericidal soap and water or bactericidal alcohol hand rub.	To prevent infection.
2 Stand in front of a toilet or a low bench with a suitable container if it is easier.	To catch urine.
3 Clean glans penis with plain water. If the foreskin covers the penis it will need to be held back during the procedure.	To reduce risk of infection.
4 Hold penis with left hand (if right-handed), three forefingers underneath and the thumb on top. The penis should be held straight out. Coat the end of the catheter with lubricating gel.	To prevent trauma to the penoscrotal junction; this also allows easier observation of procedure.
5 Pass the catheter gently with the right hand (or left, if left-handed); it can be felt as it passes the fingers holding the penis. There will be a change of feeling as the catheter passes through the prostate gland and into the bladder. It may be a little sore on the first few occasions only. If there is resistance, do not continue; withdraw the catheter and contact a nurse or doctor.	The prostate gland surrounds the urethra just below the neck of the bladder and consists of much firmer tissue. This can enlarge and cause obstruction, especially in older men.

Guidelines for patients • Intermittent self-catheterization (cont'd)

Action	Rationale
6 Urine will drain as soon as the catheter enters the bladder, so have the end positioned over the toilet or a suitable container.	To keep the area clean.
7 Withdraw catheter slowly so that all the urine is drained. The catheter will slide out easily.	To prevent stasis of residual urine.
8 Wash catheter through if it is reusable and store in a clean container.	To reduce risk of infection.
9 Wash hands and dry them.	To reduce risk of infection.
10 A mirror to stand in front of is helpful for patients with a large abdomen.	For ease of observation.

GUIDELINES • Collection of a catheter specimen of urine

Equipment

1 Swab saturated with isopropyl alcohol 70%.
2 Gate clip.

3 Sterile syringe and needle.
4 Universal specimen container.

Procedure

Action	Rationale
1 Explain and discuss the procedure with the patient.	To ensure that the patient understands the procedure and gives his/her valid consent.
2 Screen the bed.	To ensure the patient's privacy.
3 Only if there is no urine in the tubing, clamp the tubing below the rubber cuff until sufficient urine collects. (An access point is now available on catheter bags.)	To obtain an adequate urine sample.
4 Wash hands using bactericidal soap and water or bactericidal alcohol hand rub.	To reduce risk of infection.
5 Clean the access point with a swab saturated with 70% isopropyl alchohol.	To reduce risk of cross-infection.
6 Using a sterile syringe and needle (if necessary), aspirate the required amount of urine from the access point (Fig. 43.2).	If the catheter bag or tubing is punctured it causes leakage of urine and aspiration of air inwards, carrying organisms with it. Specimens collected from the catheter bag may give false results due to organisms proliferating there.
7 Reclean access point with a swab saturated with 70% isopropyl alchohol.	To reduce contamination of access point and to reduce risk of cross-infection.
8 Place the specimen in a sterile container.	To ensure that only organisms for investigation are preserved.
9 Wash and dry hands with bactericidal soap and water.	To reduce risk of cross-infection.
10 Unclamp if necessary.	To allow drainage to continue.
11 Make the patient comfortable.	

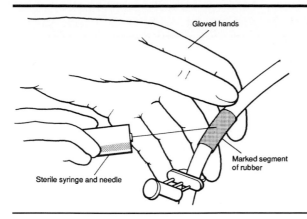

Gloved hands

Marked segment
of rubber

Sterile syringe and needle

Figure 43.2   Taking a specimen.

12 Label the container and dispatch it (with the completed request form) to the laboratory as soon as possible after sample is taken to allow more accurate results from culture.

To ensure the best possible conditions for laboratory tests.

GUIDELINES · Emptying a catheter bag

Equipment

1 Swabs saturated with 70% isopropyl alcohol.
2 Clean jug.

3 Disposable gloves.
4 Sterile jug.

Procedure

Action

1 Explain and discuss the procedure with the patient.

2 Wash hands using bactericidal soap and water or bactericidal alcohol hand rub, and put on disposable gloves.

3 Clean the outlet valve with a swab saturated with 70% isopropyl alcohol.

4 Allow the urine to drain into the appropriate jug.

5 Close the outlet valve and clean it again with a new alcohol-saturated swab.

6 Cover the jug and dispose of contents in the sluice, having noted the amount of urine if this is requested for fluid balance records.

7 Wash hands with bactericidal soap and water.

Rationale

To ensure that the patient understands the procedure and gives his/her valid consent.

To reduce risk of cross-infection.

To reduce risk of infection.

To empty drainage bag and accurately measure volume of contents.

To reduce risk of cross-infection.

To reduce risk of environmental contamination.

To reduce risk of infection.

GUIDELINES • Removing a catheter

Equipment

1 Dressing pack containing sterile towel, gallipot, foam swab or non-linting gauze.
2 Disposable gloves.
3 Needle and syringe for urine specimen, specimen container.

4 Syringe for deflating balloon.
5 Chlorhexidine solution to clean gloves.

Procedure

Action	Rationale
1 Catheters are usually removed early in the morning.	So that any retention problems can be dealt with during the day.
2 Explain procedure to patient and inform him or her of postcatheter symptoms, i.e. urgency, frequency and discomfort which are often caused by irritation of the urethra by the catheter. Symptoms should resolve over the following 24–48 hours. If not, further investigation may be needed. Encourage patient to exercise and to drink 2–3 litres of fluid per day.	So that patient knows what to expect, and can plan daily activity. For adequate flushing of bladder, especially to dilute and expel debris and infected urine, if present.
3 Wearing gloves, use saline to clean the meatus and catheter, always swabbing away from the urethral opening. In women, never scrub from the perineum/vagina towards the urethra.	To reduce risk of infection. To help reduce the risk of bateria from the vagina and perineum contaminating the urethra.
4 Clean/change gloves. Only if there is no urine in the tubing, clamp below the access point until sufficient urine collects. Take a catheter specimen of urine using the access point.	To obtain an adequate urine sample and to assess if postcatheter antibiotic therapy is needed.
5 Release leg support.	For easier removal of catheter.
6 Having checked volume of water in balloon (see patient documentation), use syringe to deflate balloon.	To confirm how much water is in the balloon. To ensure balloon is completely deflated before removing catheter.
7 Ask patient to breathe in and then out; as patient exhales, gently – but quickly – remove catheter. Male patients should be warned of discomfort as the deflated balloon passes through the prostate gland.	To relax pelvic floor muscles.
8 Clean meatus, tidy away equipment, and make the patient comfortable.	

Nursing care plan

With catheter in place

Problem	Cause	Suggested action
Urinary tract infection introduced during catheterization.	Faulty aseptic technique. Inadequate urethral cleansing. Contamination of catheter tip.	Inform a doctor. Obtain a catheter specimen of urine.

Urinary tract infection introduced via the drainage system.	Faulty handling of equipment. Breaking the closed system. Raising the drainage bag above bladder level.	Inform a doctor. Obtain a catheter specimen of urine.
No drainage of urine.	Incorrect identification of external urinary meatus (female patients). Blockage of catheter.	Check that catheter has been sited correctly. In the female if catheter has been wrongly inserted in the vagina, leave the catheter in position to act as a guide, re-identify the urethra and catheterize the patient. Remove the inappropriately sited catheter.
	Empty bladder.	When changing the catheter, clamp the catheter 30 min before the procedure. On insertion of the new catheter, urine will drain.
Urethral mucosal trauma.	Incorrect size of catheter. Procedure not carried out correctly or skillfully. Movement of the catheter in the urethra. Creation of false passage as a result of too rapid insertion of catheter.	Recatheterize the patient using the correct size of catheter. Check the catheter support and apply or reapply as necessary. Nurse may need to remove the catheter and wait for the urethral mucosa to heal.
Inability to tolerate indwelling catheter.	Urethral mucosal irritation.	Nurse may need to remove the catheter and seek an alternative means of urine drainage.
	Psychological trauma.	Explain the need for and functioning of the catheter.
	Unstable bladder. Radiation cystitis.	
Inadequate drainage of urine.	Incorrect placement of a catheter. Kinked drainage tubing.	Resite the catheter. Inspect the system and straighten any kinks.
	Blocked tubing, e.g. pus, urates, phosphates, blood clots.	If a three-way catheter, such as Foley, is in place, irrigate it. If an ordinary catheter is in use, milk the tubing in an attempt to dislodge the debris; then replace it with a three-way catheter.
Fistula formation.	Pressure on the penoscrotal angle.	Ensure that correct strapping is used.
Penile pain on erection.	Not allowing enough length of catheter to accommodate penile erection.	Ensure that an adequate length is available to accommodate penile erection.
Paraphimosis.	Failure to retract foreskin after catheterization or catheter toilet.	Always retract the foreskin.
Formation of crusts around the urethral meatus.	Increased urethral secretions, due to irritation of urothelium by the catheter, collect at the meatus and form crusts (Fillingham & Douglas 1997).	Correct catheter toilet.
Leakage of urine around catheter.	Incorrect size of catheter.	Replace with the correct size, usually 2 ch smaller.
	Incorrect balloon size. Bladder hyperirritability.	Select catheter with 10-ml balloon. Use Roberts tipped catheter. As a last resort, bladder hyperirritability can be reduced by giving diazepam or anticholinergic drugs.

Problem	Cause	Suggested action
Unable to deflate balloon.	Valve expansion. Valve displacement. Channel obstruction.	**1** Check the non-return valve on the inflation/deflation channel. If jammed, use a syringe and needle to aspirate by means of the inflation arm above the valve. **2** Obstruction by a foreign body can sometimes be relieved by the introduction of a guidewire through the inflation channel. **3** Inject 3.5 ml of dilute ether solution (diluted 50/50 with sterile water or 0.9% sodium chloride) into the inflation arm. **4** Alternatively, the balloon can be punctured suprapubically using a needle under ultrasound visualization. **5** Following catheter removal the balloon should be inspected to ensure it has not disintegrated, leaving fragments in the bladder. *Note:* steps 2 to 4 should be attempted by or under the directions of a urologist. The patient may require cystoscopy following balloon deflation to remove any balloon fragments and to wash the bladder out.

After removal of the catheter

Problem	Cause	Suggested action
Dysuria.	Inflammation of the urethral mucosa.	Ensure a fluid intake of 2–3 litres per day. Advise the patient that dysuria is common but will usually be resolved once micturition has occurred at least three times. Inform medical staff if the problem persists.
Retention of urine.	May be psychological.	Encourage the patient to increase fluid intake. Offer the patient a warm bath. Inform medical staff if the problem persists.
Urinary tract infection.		Encourage a fluid intake of 2–3 litres a day. Collect a specimen of urine. Inform medical staff if the problem persists. Administer prescribed antibiotics.

Vascular Access Devices: Insertion and Management

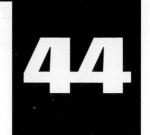

Definition

A vascular access device (VAD) is a device that is inserted into either a vein or an artery, via the peripheral or central vessels, to provide for either diagnostic [blood sampling, central venous pressure (CVP) reading] or therapeutic (administration of medications, fluids and/or blood products) purposes. There is now a comprehensive range of VADs available which allow for patients' device, therapy and quality of life needs. Table 44.1 summarizes descriptions of the main types of VADs.

Reference material

Principles of care

Regardless of the type of VAD used, the principles of care remain the same:

1 To prevent infection.
2 To maintain a 'closed' intravenous (IV) system with few connections to reduce risk of contamination.
3 To maintain a patent device.
4 To prevent damage to the device and associated intravenous equipment.

Each of these principles will be discussed generally and then in more detail under each type of access device.

Prevention of infection

Aseptic technique and compliance with recommendations for equipment and dressing changes are essential if microbial contamination is to be prevented (see Chap. 3, Aseptic Technique). Whenever the insertion site is exposed or the IV system is broken, aseptic technique should be practised. Where blood or body fluids may be present, gloves should be worn to comply with safe practice.

Cleaning solutions

Chlorhexidine in 70% alcohol has been shown to be the most effective agent for skin cleansing around the VAD insertion site prior to insertion and between dressing changes (Maki et al. 1991; Perucca 1995). 70% alcohol acts by denaturing protein and so has excellent properties for destruction of Gram-positive and -negative bacteria, as well as being active against fungi and viral organisms. Alcohol concentration between 70 and 92% provides the

most rapid and greatest reduction in microbial counts on skin but does not have any residual activity (Larson 1988). This is where chlorhexidine has an advantage over alcohol used alone, as it has excellent residual activity for 4–6 hours after application (Larson 1988; Perucca 1995; ONS 1996). Drying of any cleaning solution is vital in order for disinfection to be completed, and in the case of alcohol, which is a plasticisor, it ensures that plastic equipment will not 'glue together'.

Insertion site and cleaning of equipment

Cleaning solutions should be used not only on insertion sites, but also to clean junctions and connections, etc. It is recommended that injection caps should be cleaned vigorously with appropriate cleansing agents (Salzman et al. 1993; Brown et al. 1997). Frequency of cleaning the insertion site is debatable; peripheral sites are rarely cleaned once the device is sited because of their short duration in situ. However, central venous access sites, e.g. peripherally inserted central catheters, may be cleaned weekly (at dressing change) and short-term central venous catheters may be cleaned daily or more frequently (being associated with highest infection risk). The insertion site should be checked regularly for signs of phlebitis (erythema, pain and/or swelling) or for signs of infection (for further actions see Chap. 12, Drug Administration). Complaints of soreness, unexpected pyrexia and damaged, wet or soiled dressing are reasons for immediate inspection and renewal of the dressing.

Dressings

When the dressing is changed the insertion site should be inspected for inflammation and/or discharge, and the condition of the skin noted. An intravenous dressing is applied to minimize the contamination of the insertion site and provide stability of the device. Therefore the ideal intravenous dressing should: provide an effective barrier to bacteria; allow the catheter to be securely fixed; be sterile and easy to apply and remove; and be comfortable for the patient (RCN and Infection Control Nurses' Association 1992; Treston-Aurend et al. 1997). A dry, sterile, low-linting dressing secured with the minimum of hypoallergenic tape is most suitable for patients with skin that is prone to allergy or is thin and tears easily, as transparent dressings can damage the skin if not removed correctly. Transparent dressings have the added advantage of allow-

Table 44.1   Vascular access devices

Type of device	Material	Features	Common insertion site (veins)	Recommended indwelling life and common uses
Peripheral cannulae	Teflon Vialon	Winged Non-winged Ported	Cephalic Basilic Dorsal venous network	48–96 hours for short-term access
Midline catheters	Silicone Polyurethane	Single lumen Dual lumen	Basilic Median cubital Cephalic	Used for 1–6 weeks or longer for short- to intermediate-term access
Peripherally inserted central catheter (PICC)	Polyurethane Silicone	Dual lumen Valved	Antecubital fossa	Used primarily for patients requiring several weeks or months of intravenous access
Short-term percutaneous central venous catheter (non-tunnelled)	Polyurethane Silicone	Multiple lumen Antimicrobial collagen cuff Heparin, antibiotic and antiseptic coatings	Jugular Subclavian	Intended for days to weeks of intravenous access
Skin-tunnelled catheters	Polyurethane Silicone	Valved Antimicrobial collagen cuff Multiple lumen	Cephalic Axillary Subclavian	Indefinite. Used for long-term intermittent, continuous or daily intravenous access. May be appropriate for short-term use if reliable access needed
Implantable ports	*Catheter* Silicone *Port* Titanium Stainless steel Plastic	Dual ports Peripheral ports Valved	Antecubital fossa Subclavian	Indefinite. Used for long-term intermittent, continuous or daily intravenous access

ing inspection of the insertion site while the dressing is in situ and therefore do not require removal, and most are waterproof (Baranowski 1993; Keenleyside 1993).

Recent research has investigated the infection risks and frequency of dressing changes of both sterile gauze and transparent dressings. While some studies indicate that there is no significant difference between the two types of dressings in these respects (Petrosino *et al.* 1988), others describe slightly higher levels of bacterial colonization with non-permeable transparent dressings (Hoffman *et al.* 1992). An important factor related to infection is moisture – the collection of moisture enhances the proliferation of micro-organisms so it is essential to maintain a dry, sterile, intact IV site dressing (Perucca 1995). Moisture-permeable dressings allow moisture vapour transmission and appear to require only weekly dressing change. When these dressings are compared with sterile gauze, it has been shown that there is no significant difference in infection rates, but that they may result in a reduction in infection (Maki & Ringer 1987; Keenleyside 1993; Treston Aurend *et al.* 1997). Consequently, choice of dressing depends on which is most suitable for a particular VAD site or type of skin, and on information emerging from ongoing research.

Maintaining a closed IV system

If equipment becomes accidentally disconnected, air embolism or profuse blood loss may occur, depending on the condition and position of the patient (Ostrow 1981). Accidental disconnection poses a greater risk in patients with central venous access devices (CVADs) than in those with peripheral devices. This is because of the amount of air that could be introduced via a CVAD and the speed with which it could enter the pulmonary vessels. Luer locks provide a more secure connection and all equipment should have these fittings, i.e. administration sets, extension sets, injection caps. Care should be taken to clamp the catheter firmly when changing equipment. Connections must be double checked and precautions taken to prevent the introduction of air into the system when making additions to, or taking blood from, a central venous catheter.

Maintaining patency

It is important at all times for the patency of the device to be maintained. Blockage predisposes to device damage, infection, inconvenience to patients and disruption to drug delivery. Occlusion of the device is usually the result of clot formation due to:

1 An administration set or electronic infusion device being turned off accidentally and left for a prolonged period.
2 Insufficient or incorrect flushing of the device when not in use.

Precipitate formation due to inadequate flushing between incompatible medications and kinking may also impair patency of the device. Meticulous intravenous technique will prevent the majority of these problems.

Two main types of solutions are used to maintain patency in VADs: heparin is used to prevent the buildup of fibrin and sodium chloride is used to clean the internal diameter of the device of blood and drugs (ONS 1996). All devices should be flushed with 10–20 ml 0.9% sodium chloride after blood withdrawal (ONS 1996).

Maintaining patency can be achieved by either a continuous infusion to keep the vein open (KVO) or intermittent flushing (previously known as a 'heparin lock'). The advantages of intermittent flushing compared with a continuous infusion are:

1 It reduces the risk of circulatory overload.
2 It reduces the risk of vascular irritation.
3 It decreases the risk of bacterial contamination as it eliminates a continuous intravenous pathway.
4 It increases patient comfort and mobility.
5 It may reduce the cost of intravenous equipment.

One of the disadvantages is the necessity for constant vigilance and regular flushing (Weinstein 1997).

When used for intermittent therapy, the device should be flushed after each use with the appropriate flushing solution. (Guidelines for volumes, concentrations and frequency of flushing are commonly established within individual institutions.) Research has shown that flushing with 0.9% sodium chloride can also adequately maintain the patency of the cannula (Epperson 1984; Dunn & Lenihan 1987; Hamilton *et al.* 1988; Barrett & Lester 1990; Goode *et al.* 1991). Using 0.9% sodium chloride avoids side-effects such as local tissue damage, drug incompatibilities and iatrogenic haemorrhage, which can occur with heparin (Goode *et al.* 1991). Using 0.9% sodium chloride as a flushing solution could reduce the cost of maintaining peripheral devices and prevent potentially harmful side-effects. Authors are still unclear as to the volume and frequency of flushing, but it appears that daily or twice daily flushing with a volume of 2–5 ml 0.9% sodium chloride is acceptable (Goode *et al.* 1991).

However, there is a lack of consensus nationally, and even within regional health authorities, about the best practice for maintaining patency in central venous catheters, which has resulted in confusion among health care professionals and patients (Gilles & Rogers 1985; Clarke & Cox 1988; Ridley 1990; Kelly *et al.* 1992; Clemence *et al.* 1995). Heparinized saline appears to be the accepted solution for maintaining the patency of central venous catheters for intermittent use (Kelly *et al.* 1992). Use of 0.9% sodium chloride alone is not yet widespread

(except with certain types of catheters) and remains controversial. Flushing regimens ranging from once daily to once weekly have been found to be effective.

It has been suggested that one of the most important aspects of maintaining patency is the method of flushing (Baranowski 1993). It is important to use a pulsatile (push-pause) method, irrespective of the amount used and the frequency, to create turbulent flow (administer solution 1 ml at a time) and complete the procedure using a positive pressure technique. This is accomplished by clamping the catheter or extension set while flushing before the syringe completely empties. Alternatively, pressure can be maintained on the plunger of the syringe while withdrawing the syringe from the injection cap, thus preventing reflux of blood into the tip of the device and helping to prevent clotting and blockage (Baranowski 1993). Some manufacturers have produced injection caps, which create a positive pressure and thereby reduce the risk of occlusion (ICU Medical 1998).

If occlusion does occur, gentle aspiration may dislodge the clot and a flush with 0.9% sodium chloride may be all that is required to restore patency. Gentle pressure and suction may need to be repeated if the catheter has been left for a long time and a larger thrombus has formed. Silicone catheters expand on pressure and allow fluid around a clot, facilitating its dislodgment. Use of heparin solution may also be tried (Haire *et al.* 1990). However, only 10-ml syringes or larger should be used when attempting to unblock VADs. Smaller syringes appear to create a greater pressure of mmHg or pounds per square inch (psi). This may then result in rupture of the catheter and/or clots being forced into the venous system (Hadaway 1998; Macklin 1999).

Excessive force should never be used when flushing devices. However, when the catheter lumen is totally patent, internal pressure will not increase during flushing (Hadaway 1998). If resistance is felt (due to partial occlusion), and a force is applied to the plunger, this could result in a high pressure within the catheter, which may then rupture (Conn 1993; Hadaway 1998; Macklin 1999). It is, therefore, recommended that the device is checked first with a 10-ml syringe containing 0.9% sodium chloride, and if there is no pressure or occlusion, it is then safe to use a small-size syringe (Hadaway 1998; Macklin 1999). The composition of the individual device determines the maximum pressure that can be exerted.

The enzymes urokinase and streptokinase have both been used to dissolve thrombi and restore catheter patency. Although effective, these are potentially dangerous substances and their use must be approved by the medical staff and prescribed accordingly (Wachs 1990; Wickham *et al.* 1992; Richard Alexander 1994). Recently, the worldwide availability of urokinase has become a problem. An alternative fibrinolytic agent now being used is alteplase (Moureau *et al.* 1999).

When using implanted drug delivery systems, the manufacturer's literature should be consulted with reference to heparinization. The most widely stated recommendation is a flush with 500 units of heparin monthly (ONS 1996; Springhouse Corporation 1999).

Preventing damage of the VAD and performing a repair

If damage occurs to peripheral devices, they are usually removed and replaced. Most central venous catheters are made of silicone which is prone to cracking or splitting if handled incorrectly, but both temporary and permanent repairs can be performed. However, prevention of this occurrence is preferred.

Artery forceps, scissors or sharp-edged clamps should not be used on the catheter. A smooth clamp should be placed on the reinforced section of the catheter provided for this purpose. If a reinforced section is not present, placing a tape tab over part of the catheter can create one. A second alternative is to move the clamp up or down the catheter at regular intervals to reduce the risk of wear and tear at one point.

Damage can occur, however, and the nurse must be familiar with the action to be taken to minimize any risk to patient safety in this event. Immediate clamping of the catheter proximal to the fracture or split is essential to prevent blood loss or air embolism. The split area should be covered with an alcohol swab and emergency repair equipment collected, together with sterile gloves to ensure that all manipulations are aseptic. A permanent repair should be performed as soon as possible using the specific equipment provided by the manufacturer. A member of the medical staff or other designated personnel should do this.

Peripheral cannula

Definition

A cannula is a flexible tube containing a needle (stylet) which may be inserted into a blood vessel (Anderson & Anderson 1995). Cannulae are usually placed in the peripheral veins in the lower arm but may also be placed in the veins of the foot (an area used particularly in paediatric care).

Indications

1 Short-term therapy of 3–5 days.
2 Bolus injections or short infusions in the outpatient/day unit setting.

Reference material

The advantages of using a peripheral cannula are that they are usually easy to insert and have few associated complications; however, they are associated with phlebitis (either mechanical or chemical) and require constant resiting (Perdue 1995; ONS 1996; RCN 1999; Springhouse Corporation 1999).

Device information

A number of different types of peripheral cannulae are available. It has been shown that the incidence of vascular complications increases as the ratio of cannulae external diameter to vessel lumen increases. Therefore most of the literature recommends the smallest, shortest gauge cannula in any given situation (Nightingale & Bradshaw 1982; Peters et al. 1984; Lewis & Hecker 1985; Millam 1992; Perucca 1995; Weinstein 1997; Fuller & Winn 1999). The measurement used for needle and cannulae is standard wire gauge (swg), which measures the internal diameter; the smaller the gauge size, the larger the diameter. Standard wire gauge measurement is determined by how many cannulae fit into a tube with an inner diameter of 1 inch (25.4 mm) and uses consecutive numbers from 13 to 24. The diameter, e.g. 1.2 mm, may be expressed as a gauge, e.g. 18 g (BSI 1997; Nauth Misir 1998). Needles tend to be odd numbers, e.g. 19 g, 21 g, etc., while cannulae are even numbers, e.g. 18 g, 20 g, etc.

The 'over the needle' type of cannula is the most commonly used device for peripheral venous access and is available in various gauge sizes, lengths, composition and design features. The cannula is mounted on the needle (known as the stylet) and once the device is pushed off of the needle into the vein, the stylet is removed. A sharp-tipped stylet facilitates penetration into the vein and the type of graduation from the cannula to the needle can affect the degree of trauma to the vessel and the cannula tip. A thin smooth-walled cannula tapering to a scalloped end causes less damage than one that is abruptly cut off (Dougherty 1999).

The walls of the device should, therefore, be thin to provide the largest internal diameter without increasing the external diameter. This is to ensure that maximum flow rates may be achieved while reducing complications such as mechanical irritation. Flow rates vary with equipment from different manufacturers. Flow rate through a cannula is related to its internal diameter and is inversely proportional to its length. However, as the length of the cannula increases, so does the likelihood of vascular complications, for example a large-gauge device of longer length (1.6–2 cm) will fill the vessel, preventing blood flow around it, which could result in mechanical trauma to the vessel and encourage the development of phlebitis (Dougherty 1999).

The most suitable material is one that is non-irritant and does not predispose to thrombus formation (Payne-James et al. 1991). The material should also be radio-opaque or contain a stripe of radio-opaque material for radiographic visualization in the event of catheter embolus (Fuller & Winn 1999). Much controversy exists over the advantages and disadvantages of the available cannula material (Perucca 1995). Types of material include polyvinylchloride, Teflon, Vialon, and various polyurethane and elastomeric hydrogel materials. Studies have compared the different types of material available such as Teflon and Vialon, to ascertain which is most likely to be associated with the lowest potential risk of phlebitis (Gaukroger et al. 1988; McKee et al. 1989; Payne-James et al. 1991; Kerrison & Woodhull 1994; Russell et al. 1996). When considering the results of these studies, however, it must be noted that investigators often use different phlebitis scales and calculations for creating a total score for each device. Other inconsistencies relate to the differences in catheter size, skin preparation, the use of dressings and the type of solution being infused. This makes comparison between catheter materials difficult.

Other features of peripheral cannulae include winged cannulae (which help with the securing of the device to the skin in order to prevent a piston-like movement within the vein and accidental removal) and devices with small ports on the top of the device – which are favoured more in Europe that in the USA. The advantage of a ported device is the ability to administer drugs without interfering with continuous infusion. However, the caps are often not replaced correctly, which leaves the system exposed to contamination and the possible risk of air entering. It has also been found that the ports cannot be adequately sterilized with a swab, as there is no flat surface. The use of ports may encourage the practitioner to not remove the dressing and inspect the site but merely administer the drug via the port. Opinion is divided as to the risk of infection associated with ported devices (Cheeseborough & Finch 1984) and it has been recommended that if side ports are used they should be equipped with a bacterial filter (Brismar et al. 1984).

Choice of vein

The main factors to consider prior to inserting a peripheral cannula are the location for siting, condition of the vein, purpose of the infusion (that is the rate of flow required and the solution to be infused) and the duration of therapy.

The suitable vein should always be selected prior to selection of the device. The veins should feel bouncy and refill when depressed and should be straight and free of valves to ensure easy advancement of the cannula into the vein. Valves can be felt as small lumps in the vein or may be visualized at bifurcations or more commonly seen in certain vessels (see below). It is best to avoid joints as this will lead to an increased risk of mechanical phlebitis and an infusion that will infuse intermittently due to the patient's movement. It can also be very awkward for the patient and may restrict his or her ability to carry out activities.

The veins of choice are either the cephalic or basilic veins, followed by the dorsal venous network (see Fig. 45.1 in Chap. 45, Venepuncture).

The cephalic vein

The size and position of the cephalic vein make it an excellent vessel for administration of transfusions. It readily accommodates a large-gauge cannula and, by virtue of its position on the forearm, provides a natural splint (Weinstein 1997). However, its position at a joint may increase complications such as mechanical phlebitis and even general discomfort. The tendons controlling the thumb obscure the vein during insertion (Hadaway 1995), and care must be taken not to touch the radial nerve.

The basilic vein

The basilic vein is a large vessel, which is often overlooked due to its inconspicuous position on the ulnar border of the

hand and forearm. It is found on palpation when the patient's arm is placed across the chest, with the practitioner opposite the patient (Hadaway 1995). Cannulation can be awkward due to its position and its tendency to have many valves and it tends to roll easily. In addition, a haematoma may occur if the patient flexes the arm since this squeezes blood from the engorged vein into the tissues.

The dorsal venous network

Using the veins of the dorsal venous network of the hand will allow for cannulation proximally along the veins when resiting the device (Weinstein 1997; Springhouse Corporation 1999). They can usually be visualized and palpated easily.

1 The digital veins are small and may be prominent enough to accommodate a small-gauge needle as a last resort for fluid administration. With adequate taping the fingers can be immobilized, thus preventing the cannula from piercing the posterior wall of the vein, leading to bruising or infiltration.
2 The metacarpal veins are accessible, easily visualized and palpated. They are well suited for IV use, as the cannula lies flat between metacarpal bones of the hand and provides a natural splint (Weinstein 1997). The veins tend to be smaller than the forearm and therefore may prove difficult in infants due to comparatively high amounts of subcutaneous fat compared to an older child or an adult. The use of these veins is contraindicated in the elderly as there is diminished skin turgor and loss of subcutaneous tissue, making the vein difficult to stabilize and often taking longer to cannulate (Whitson 1996). Metacarpal veins are a better option for short-term or outpatient intravenous therapy.

Insertion

As the most common cause of VAD infection is the patient's own skin flora, it is important to adequately clean the skin prior to cannulation. The patient's skin should be washed with soap and water if visibly dirty (Speechley 1984); then, firm and prolonged rubbing with an antiseptic solution such as chlorhexidine in 70% alcohol or 2% aqueous solution is recommended (De Vries 1997; Maki et al. 1991). Skin cleansing is a controversial subject and it is acknowledged that a cursory wipe with an alcohol swab disturbs the skin flora and does more harm than no cleaning at all. The prepared skin area should be 4–5 cm in diameter and the solution applied with friction from the insertion site outward (Perucca 1995). It is imperative that during the skin cleansing procedure not only is the most effective antiseptic used but also the skin is cleaned for a long enough period of time: 30–60 seconds for peripheral cannulation (Millam 1992; Weinstein 1997; Dougherty 1999). In order for the antimicrobial solution to be effective and ensure coagulation of the organisms, and to prevent stinging as the needle pierces the skin, the area should be allowed to air dry for a minimum of 30 seconds. Fanning, blowing and blotting of the prepared area is contraindicated as disinfection occurs when the solution is allowed to air-dry naturally (Perucca 1995; Springhouse Corporation 1999). Once the skin has been cleaned it must not be touched or repalpated. If it is necessary to repalpate, then the cleaning regimen should be repeated.

Shaving the area prior to cannulation may cause microabrasions and result in microbial growth (Weinstein 1997; Springhouse Corporation 1999), while depilatories are not recommended because of allergic reactions which could cause skin eruptions (Perucca 1995). Weinstein (1997) suggests that antiseptics used to clean the skin also clean the hair. This is supported by Maki (1976) who could not demonstrate a relationship between the presence of hair and bacterial colonization and felt that the necessity of hair removal was doubtful. Scissors are acceptable for clipping and if hair removal is necessary, but they must be cleaned between patients to prevent cross-infection.

Skin stabilization is one of the most important elements for successful venepuncture or cannulation (Perucca 1995). Superficial veins tend to roll and to prevent this the vein must be stabilized by applying traction to the side of the insertion site or below it, using the practitioner's non-dominant hand. This also facilitates a smoother needle entry. Various methods are used:

1 The thumb can be used to stretch the skin downwards.
2 The hand of the practitioner can be placed under the patient's arm and traction applied with the thumb and forefinger on either side, creating an even traction.
3 The vein can be stretched between forefinger and thumb.

Stabilization of the vein must be maintained throughout the procedure until the needle or cannula is successfully sited. If the tension is released half way through the procedure, it can result in the needle penetrating the opposite wall of the vein, resulting in a haematoma formation.

It is important that the needle enters the skin with the bevel up, as this results in a smooth venepuncture as the sharpest part of the needle will penetrate the skin first, and this also reduces the risk of piercing the posterior wall of the vein (Weinstein 1997). The angle the needle enters the skin varies with the type of device used and the depth of the vein in the subcutaneous tissue, and ranges from 10 to 45° (Millam 1992; Perucca 1995; Weinstein 1997). Once the device is in the vein, the angle will always be reduced in order to prevent puncturing the posterior wall of the vein (Perucca 1995).

There are two main methods for approaching the vein:

1 The direct method is when the device enters the skin directly into the vein and has the advantage that the vein is entered immediately, but with small fragile veins this method may lead to puncturing of the posterior wall.
2 The indirect method is when the device is inserted through the skin, then the vein is relocated and the device advanced into the vein. This method enables a more gentle entry and may be useful in veins that are palpable and visible for only a short section.

When blood appears in the chamber of a cannula, known as 'flashback', this indicates that the initial entry into the vein has been successful. This may be accompanied by a 'giving way' sensation felt by the practitioner, which occurs due to resistance from the vein wall as the device enters the lumen of the vein (Millam 1992). If the device punctures the posterior wall, the flashback will stop. However, the flashback may be slow with small-gauge cannulae or hypotensive patients.

The cannula should be advanced gently and smoothly into the vein and a number of techniques are used by practitioners. The most common method used by nurses is the one-handed technique (see procedure for cannulation). The same hand that performs cannulation also withdraws the stylet and advances the cannula into the vein. This allows skin traction to be maintained while the device is advanced and if the patient is unable to cooperate allows the practitioner to hold onto the patient's arm (Dougherty 1999).

The one-step technique is when the cannula has entered the vein and the practitioner can slide the cannula off the stylet in one movement. The disadvantage with this method is that the stylet must remain completely still in order to prevent damage to the vein. It is best accomplished on a straight vein and when the cannula has a small fingerguard which can be used to 'push' the cannula off.

The two-handed technique is when the practitioner uses one hand to perform the cannulation and then releases skin traction to use the hand to hold and withdraw the stylet, while the dominant hand advances the cannula off the stylet. This method prevents blood spill, but as it necessitates the release of skin traction, it can often lead to the puncturing of the vein wall (Millam 1992).

Care and management in situ

Once sited, the peripheral cannula should be flushed using a heparin solution or 0.9% sodium chloride. Research has shown that the use of 0.9% sodium chloride adequately maintains patency without increasing the risk of phlebitis. Authors are still unclear as to the volume and frequency of flushing, but it appears that daily or twice daily flushing with a volume of 2–5 ml is acceptable, providing the correct technique is used, i.e. a pulsatile flush ending with positive pressure (Perucca 1995; RCN 1999; Springhouse Corporation 1999).

In order for the insertion site to be readily available for inspection, it may be necessary for the nurse to assume responsibility for taping the cannula in place as well as dressing the insertion site. Non-sterile tape should not cover the site, the equivalent of an open wound (Oldman 1991), and a method must be devised so that the site remains visible and the cannula is stable. The procedure shown in Fig. 44.1 is recommended: the site is visible during drug administration, and the tape does not cover the insertion site. Previous research has shown that dry sterile gauze and transparent dressings are associated with similar rates of skin colonization by bacteria (Maki & Ringer 1987; Hoffman et al. 1992). Low-linting gauze has been suggested as the dressing of choice for short-term peripheral sites (Madeo et al. 1997). Once the gauze is in

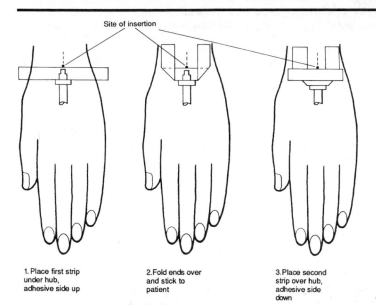

1. Place first strip under hub, adhesive side up

2. Fold ends over and stick to patient

3. Place second strip over hub, adhesive side down

Figure 44.1 Method of taping a peripheral cannula.

place a bandage is applied to aid fixation and prevent dislodgment, and is preferred by patients who may feel anxious about the necessity for resiting the device (Dougherty 1994). Transparent dressing allows the practitioner to view the site but should not be bandaged as this defeats the whole object of the transparent dressing.

Removal

It has been recommended that peripheral devices should be resited every 48–72 hours (Perucca 1995; ONS 1996; RCN 1999), although there is work that now indicates that devices may remain in up to 96 hours with no significant complications (Homer & Holmes 1998). Removal of the intravenous device or cannula should be an aseptic procedure. The device should be removed carefully using a slow, steady movement and pressure should be applied for at least a minute. This pressure should be firm and not involve any rubbing movement. A haematoma will occur if the needle is carelessly removed, causing discomfort and a focus for infection (Perucca 1995). The site should be inspected to ensure bleeding has stopped and the site should then be covered with a sterile dressing. The cannula integrity should be checked to ensure the complete device has been removed.

Midline catheter

Definition

A midline catheter is a device that provides vascular access in a larger peripheral vein without entering the central venous circulation. It is inserted into an antecubital vein and the tip is extended into the vein of the upper arm up to 20 cm, but is not extended past the axilla.

Indications

Midline catheters are used in the following circumstances:

1 When patients do not have accessible peripheral veins or have a minimal number of adequate vessels available for administration of therapy for moderate duration (less than 6 months) (ONS 1996).
2 When patients will be undergoing therapy for more than 5 days, in order to preserve the integrity of the veins and increase patient comfort by removing the need for resites, e.g. antibiotics.
3 For patient preference.

Reference material

The midline catheter offers an alternative to peripheral and central venous access. Where patients present with poor peripheral venous access and when use of a central venous catheter is contraindicated, the midline catheter provides venous accessibility along with easy, less hazardous insertion at the antecubital fossa (Goetz et al. 1998). As the catheter tip does not terminate beyond the proximal aspect of the limb being used, X-ray verification is not usually required, although the Intravenous Nursing Society (1998) supports radiological confirmation in certain clinical situations, such as if vesicant drugs are to be administered. The insertion is performed using either an over-the-needle or Seldinger technique. Benefits to the patient include less frequent resiting of the catheter and a subsequent reduction in associated venous trauma. However, mechanical phlebitis is a common side-effect and close observation and appropriate management are indicated. Once in situ, the catheter should be managed exactly as a central venous catheter, although the list of drugs that can be administered via a midline catheter does not always include vesicant or hyperosmolar solutions because of the risk of damage should the drugs extravasate (ONS 1996; Banton & Leahy Gross 1998). Therefore it is important to check the manufacturer's recommendations regarding both the device and any drugs to be administered (Rasor 1991).

Device information

Silicone or polyurethane are the most frequently used materials in the manufacture of midline catheters (Kupensky 1998) and are available as single and double lumen catheters in lengths of approximately 20 cm, which can be cut to the desired length following measurement of the arm from the selected vein.

Choice of vein

The basilic vein is the vein of choice due to its larger size, straighter course for catheter advancement and improved haemodilution capability. Data show improved catheter dwell time using the basilic compared with cephalic vein insertions.

Insertion

Adequate assessment of the patient's veins is vital and given the choice the non-dominant arm should be used. The procedure requires a sterile approach and it is recommended that sterile gloves are worn. These should be powder-free as powder on the catheter can result in mechanical phlebitis.

Care and management in situ

It is not usually appropriate to suture these devices in situ, as they can be adequately secured with Steristrips or specially designed fixing devices such as Stat Lock. The insertion site can then be covered with a moisture-permeable transparent dressing and changed according to manufacturer's recommendations, e.g. once a week. The device should be flushed with 0.9% sodium chloride after each use and then with a heparinized solution according to manufacturer's recommendations, e.g. weekly. Midline catheters can be left in situ for extended periods of time. However, it is generally recommended for a maximum of 2–4 weeks of therapy (Intravenous Nursing Society 1998). Longer dwell times should be evaluated on site assessment, length of maintaining therapy and patient condition (Kupensky 1998).

Removal

Removal requires gentle firm traction and the catheter will slide out from the insertion site. Pressure should be applied for at least 3–4 minutes and the site inspected prior to applying a dressing to ensure bleeding has stopped. The catheter integrity should be checked and its length measured to ensure that a complete device has been removed.

Table 44.2 Hazards of catheter insertion (Speer 1990)

Sepsis	Air embolism	Pneumothorax
Hydrothorax	Haemorrhage	Haemothorax
Brachial plexus injury	Thoracic duct trauma	Misdirection or kinking
Catheter embolism	Thrombosis	Cardiac tamponade Cardiac arrhythmias

Central venous access devices

Definition

A central venous access device is a device, the tip of which is placed into the superior vena cava or right atrium via direct entry site into the subclavian or jugular vein or via the antecubital veins.

Indications

1 To monitor central venous pressure in seriously ill patients.
2 For the administration of large amounts of intravenous fluid or blood, e.g. in cases of shock or major surgery.
3 To provide long-term access for:
    (a) Hydration or electrolyte maintenance.
    (b) Repeated administration of drugs, such as cytotoxic and antibiotic therapy.
    (c) Repeated transfusion of blood or blood products.
    (d) Repeated specimen collection.
4 For parenteral nutrition (Bjeletich & Hickman 1980).

Hazards of insertion

See Table 44.2.

Peripherally inserted central catheter

Definition

A peripherally inserted central catheter (PICC) is a catheter that is inserted via the antecubital veins in the arm and is advanced into the central veins, with the tip located in the superior vena cava (SVC) (Hadaway 1990; Goodwin & Carlson 1993; Gabriel 1996a). It is not to be confused with a midclavicular catheter ('long line') where the tip is located in a central vein leading to the SVC such as the subclavian, which is associated with a increased risk of thrombosis (Perdue 1995).

Indications

1 Lack of peripheral access.
2 Infusions of vesicant, irritant, parenteral nutrition or hyperosmolar solutions.
3 Long-term venous access.
4 Patient preference.

5 Patients with needle phobia to prevent repeated cannulation.

6 Clinician preference if patients are at risk of haemorrhage or pneumothorax.   (Macrae 1998)

Reference material

The PICC has many advantages over the other central
venous access devices: firstly, it eliminates the risks associated with CVC placement such as pneumothorax,
haemothorax, cardiac arrhythmia and air embolism
(Gabriel 1996b). Secondly, PICCs have been shown to be
associated with a reduction in catheter sepsis when using
these devices. [The catheter can be inserted at the bedside
under local anaesthetic (Ng et al. 1997).] Thirdly, it is easy
to use for both staff and patients and helps to preserve
peripheral veins. Finally, it has been shown to reduce patient
discomfort and provide a reliable form of access (Hadaway
1990; ONS 1996; Weinstein 1997).

Contraindications for using a PICC include the inability
to locate suitable antecubital veins; anatomical distortions
from surgery, injury or trauma, e.g. scarring from mastectomy, lymphoedema, burns, etc., which may prevent
advancement of the catheter to the desired tip location; if
a patient is unable to carry out catheter care or is confused;
if the patient is unable to lie supine for the insertion period
(Macrae 1998).

Device information

PICCs are available as single and double lumen catheters,
open-ended or valved, and may be made of silicone or
polyurethane. The majority are inserted using a 'through-
the-needle' technique, using a 'breakaway' needle or a
'peel away' introducer (ONS 1996). Catheters measure
50–65 cm long, with a diameter of 2–7 Fr. PICCs can be cut
to the required length, except for valved catheters.

Choice of vein

Adequate assessment of the patient prior to attempting
catheter placement goes a long way to ensuring success.
Examine both arms with a tourniquet in place, palpate
for the healthiest, largest vein, and preferably use the
non-dominant arm. Problems associated with vein location
have been overcome with the use of a hand-held Doppler,
which can identify forearm veins larger than 2 mm in diameter (Whitely et al. 1995). It has been found that use of this
device may aid vein location and significantly increase the
success rate of PICC insertion (Macrae 1998).

The basilic vein

The basilic vein is the vein of choice for PICC catheter
insertions due to its larger size, straighter course for
catheter advancement and improved haemodilution capability. Data show improved time in situ with the basilic
versus cephalic vein insertions (see Fig. 44.2).

The basilic vein begins in the ulnar (inner aspect) part
of the forearm, runs along the posterior, medial surface

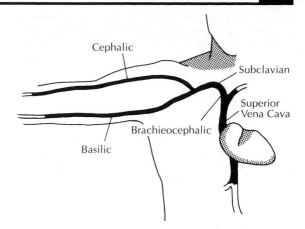

Figure 44.2   Veins of the thorax. (From BD First PICC
Clinical Education Class Manual D11 952B 5/98.)

(back of the arm) and then curves towards the antecubital
region, where it is joined by the median cubital vein. It
then progresses straight up the upper arm for approximately 5–8 cm and enters the deep tissues. It ascends medially to form the axillary vein.

The median cubital vein

The median cubital vein ascends from just below the middle
of the antecubital region and commonly divides into two
vessels, one of which joins the basilic and the other the
cephalic vein. The median cubital vein is commonly used
for blood sampling due to its size and ease of needle entry.
If a practitioner is having difficulty locating and/or cannu-
lating the basilic vein, then the median cubital vein may be
used as an alternative insertion route. The catheter will
then advance into the basilic (or cephalic) vein.

The cephalic vein

The cephalic vein begins in the radial side (thumb side) of
the hand and ascends laterally (along the outer region
of the forearm) into the antecubital region, where it forms
a junction with the axillary vein. This vein is usually
smaller and more tortuous than the basilic vein and may
make advancement of the catheter more difficult.

Insertion

Venous assessment and selection play key roles in the
successful insertion of a PICC, along with the correct
positioning of the patient and careful measurement of the
patient and the device. To obtain the correct measurement
of the length of catheter to be inserted, using a tape
measure, measure from the selected point for venepuncture along the course of the vein pathway, then across the
shoulder to the right side of the sternal notch, down to the
third intercostal space (ONS 1996; Gabriel 1999).

The use of local anaesthetic either topically or by injection should be considered to reduce the pain associated with the initial venepuncture with the introducer (ONS 1996). Topical local anaesthetic can be applied either 30 or 60 minutes prior to venepuncture, and a transparent dressing applied over the site. The cream/gel is then removed and the site is ready to be cleaned (British Medical Association and Royal Pharmaceutical Society of Great Britain 1999). Some creams may cause blanching of the skin and vasoconstriction (Bahruth 1996) or hypersensitivity and erythema of the site. Intradermal injection may also cause stinging pain and erythema at the site, but has an almost immediate action (ONS 1996).

Care and management in situ

Some practitioners prefer to suture these devices in situ, but they can be adequately secured with Steristrips or specially designed fixing devices such as Stat Lock. The insertion site is then covered with a moisture-permeable transparent dressing and changed according to manufacturer's recommendations, e.g. once a week.

Flushing solution and frequency are usually dependent on the type of catheter and so manufacturer's recommendations should be followed, e.g. valved catheters are usually flushed once a week with 0.9% sodium chloride, while open-ended catheters are flushed with a heparinized solution.

Removal

Removal requires gentle firm traction and the catheter will slide out from the insertion site. Sometimes there may be difficulty removing the device, which may be caused by venospasm, vasoconstriction or phlebitis (ONS 1996). If this occurs, then the arm should be wrapped in a warm compress and tension applied to the catheter, the dressing replaced and the removal attempted again in 24 hours. If these methods fail, then a doctor should be informed.

Following removal of the PICC, pressure should be applied for at least 3–4 minutes and the site inspected prior to applying a dressing to ensure bleeding has stopped. The catheter integrity should be checked and its length measured to ensure an intact device has been removed.

Short-term percutaneous central venous catheters (non-tunnelled)

Definition

A short-term non-tunnelled percutaneous central venous catheter is a device that enters through the skin directly into a central vein.

Indications

1 Short-term therapy of a few days up to several weeks.
2 Central venous pressure readings.

3 Emergency use, e.g. fluid replacement.
4 Absence of peripheral veins (Henderson 1997).

Reference material

Short-term use of a non-tunnelled central venous catheter such as a subclavian catheter is common practice in urgent situations and can be inserted by the doctor at the bedside, in ITU or in the emergency room (Goodman & Riley 1997). This type of catheter is easily removed and can be changed over a guidewire. It is a stiff catheter and this aids in CVP monitoring. In addition, its configuration as a multi-lumen catheter allows administration of several solutions at once. However, it is easily dislodged by patient movement and is more thrombogenic because of the catheter material, as well as being associated with a higher risk of infection (Springhouse Corporation 1999).

Device information

These catheters range from single to multi (up to five) lumen and the openings can be staggered or open ended (Fig. 44.3). Most catheters are made of polyurethane, and as the greatest hazard with these devices is risk of infection, manufacturers are now producing catheters impregnated with antibacterial, antimicrobials or silver ions which all aim to destroy bacteria and thus reduce the risk of infection (Maki et al. 1997; Raad et al. 1998).

Choice of vein

The percutaneous central venous catheter is usually placed in the subclavian or jugular veins. The subclavian vein is the entry route of choice as it requires the shortest length of catheter. As the catheter is located in the most central vein, the size of the vessel ensures a rapid blood flow around the catheter, which reduces the risk of irritation and obstruction (Weinstein 1997). Contraindications to the subclavian route are superior vena cava syndrome, irradiation to the chest, fractured clavicle or malignancy at the base of the neck (ONS 1996; Weinstein 1997).

Insertion via the internal jugular is easier than the subclavian vein and the right internal jugular provides the shortest and straightest route to the SVC, which reduces the problem of malposition. Objections to jugular insertion are catheter occlusion and irritation due to head movement, difficulty in maintaining an intact dressing and it can be disturbing for the patients and their families (Weinstein 1997).

Insertion

The hazards associated with the insertion of a central venous catheter are substantial (Table 44.2). It is recommended that the procedure should be performed in a controlled quiet environment with a minimum of activity in order to reduce the risk of contamination (Elliott et al. 1994). However, the catheter is often placed in emergency

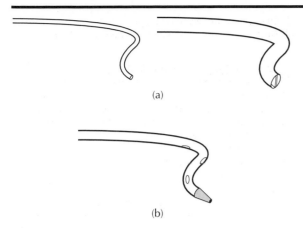

(a)

(b)

Figure 44.3 Types of catheter tips. (a) Open-ended catheter (single and double lumen). (b) Staggered exit open-ended catheter.

situations when this may not be possible. This procedure is usually performed by doctors and so the nurse's responsibilities include the following:

1 To ensure, where possible, that the patient understands and has been given a full explanation of the procedure and had the opportunity to discuss any aspects.
2 To teach the patient techniques that may be required during insertion, for example the Valsalva manoeuvre (see below).
3 To explain any specific pre- and post-procedure instructions and the appearance and function of the catheter or device.
4 To assemble the equipment requested.
5 To prepare local anaesthesia and dressing materials.
6 To ensure the correct positioning of the patient during insertion, that is, in the supine or Trendelenburg position, with the head down and a roll of towel along the spinal column. This promotes upper venous engorgement, making puncture of the chosen vessel easier and helps to prevent air embolism (ONS 1996; Henderson 1997).
7 To attend to the physical and psychological comfort of the patient during and immediately following the procedure.
8 To ensure that no fluid or medication is infused before the correct position of the catheter is confirmed on X-ray by medical staff.

The Valsalva manoeuvre

This may be performed by conscious patients to aid the insertion of the catheter. The patient is placed in the supine or Trendelenburg position which increases venous filling. He/she is asked to breathe in and then try to force the air out with the mouth and nose closed (i.e. against a closed glottis). This increases the intrathoracic pressure so that the return of blood to the heart is reduced momentar-

ily and the veins in the neck region become engorged. A distension of the vein up to 2.5 cm can be achieved in this way (Ostrow 1981).

Care and management in situ

Flushing is recommended after each use of the catheter. Since these devices are usually in constant use, 0.9% sodium chloride is the flushing solution of choice to reduce the risk of occlusion. It may be appropriate to use continuous infusions to keep the vein open. The types of dressings used at the insertion site may vary according to the type of patient and unit. Staff in some ITUs do not dress the site but clean the insertion site every 4 hours; others units may use a moisture-permeable dressing which is changed as necessary. This enables the staff to observe the site regularly for any signs of infection, as patients with these devices in situ are usually very vulnerable to infection, e.g. oncology patients, ITU, etc. (RCN 1999).

Removal

If a catheter is not tunnelled through the skin it may be removed by nursing staff. The nurse must be familiar with the procedure and confident about performing it. Aseptic technique must be adhered to and the site cleaned with chlorhexidine-soaked swabs before removal to prevent a false-positive result when the catheter tip is sent for bacteriological examination. In order to prevent air entering the vein on removal of the catheter, have the patient perform the Valsalva manoeuvre (ONS 1996). Major vessels usually heal quickly, but direct pressure must be applied to the site until cessation of bleeding confirms this. A sterile transparent or padded dressing is applied (Elliott et al. 1994; RCN 1999) and should remain in place for at least 24 hours.

Skin-tunnelled catheters

Definition

A skin-tunnelled catheter is a catheter that lies in a subcutaneous tunnel. A skin-tunnelled catheter usually exits midway from the anterior chest wall (Fig. 44.4). The tip ideally lies at the junction of the SVC and right atrium or within the SVC or upper right atrium (Davidson & Al Mufti 1997).

Indications

A skin-tunnelled catheter is used when long-term venous access is required.

Reference material

This catheter was first developed in the 1970s by Dr. Robert Hickman in the USA who wished to reduce the infections in his haematology patients. Skin tunnelling is

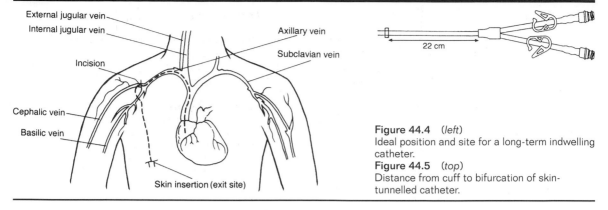

External jugular vein
Internal jugular vein
Axillary vein
Incision
Subclavian vein
Cephalic vein
Basilic vein
Skin insertion (exit site)

22 cm

Figure 44.4 (*left*)
Ideal position and site for a long-term indwelling catheter.
Figure 44.5 (*top*)
Distance from cuff to bifurcation of skin-tunnelled catheter.

usually performed if the catheter is intended to provide long-term access over a number of months or years. The purpose of the tunnel is to distance the entry site into the vein from the exit site on the skin, so providing a barrier to infection. Catheters specifically designed for skin tunnelling frequently have a cuff made of Dacron which is positioned in the subcutaneous tunnel. Tissue granulates around the cuff and reinforces the barrier to invading organisms and reduces the risk of catheter movement and possible dislodgement. However, this does not guarantee that dislodgment will not occur (ONS 1996). An example of this type of catheter is the Hickman catheter. The cuff should be sited at least 5 cm from the entry site (Stacey *et al.* 1991). The catheter currently used at The Royal Marsden Hospital has a cuff that is situated 22 cm from the top of the bifurcation (Fig. 44.5). This measurement may assist the practitioner in locating the cuff during removal of the catheter. However, the distance of the cuff from the bifurcation may vary according to the type of catheter.

Device information

Polyurethane or silicone skin-tunnelled catheters present as single, double or triple lumen catheters and may be open ended or valved. A valved catheter may have a valve located in the hub of the catheter or in the tip. Catheters such as the Groshong catheter have a round blunt tip which incorporates a two-way valve which remains closed at normal venous caval pressure. Application of a vacuum in order to withdraw blood enables the valve to open inwards; positive pressure into the catheter forces the valve to open outwards (Fig. 44.6). The advantages of valved catheters are the reduced risk of bleeding or air emboli on insertion and during subsequent care; the elimination of catheter clamping; and the elimination of the need for heparin along with a reduction in the frequency of flushing (ONS 1996; Weinstein 1997). In order for the valved catheter to function properly the tip must be situated in the midsuperior section of the vena cava and not in the right atrium, as the pressure in the atrium may force the valve permenantly open.

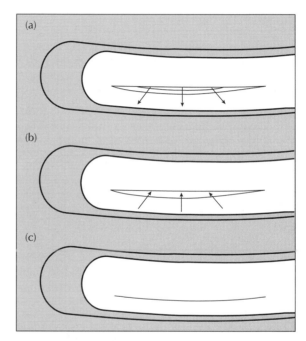

(a)

(b)

(c)

Figure 44.6 The Groshong two-way valve catheter. (a) Infusion (positive pressure). (b) Aspiration (negative pressure). (c) Closed (neutral pressure).

Choice of vein

The subclavian vein is frequently used as it is the shortest route to the SVC, and this minimizes complications. The constant anatomic location of the jugular vein makes cannulation easier than via the subclavian, and the right internal jugular is chosen as it forms the straighter and shorter route to the SVC and avoids injury to the vagus nerve, carotid artery and vein itself. The external jugular is observable and easily entered but varies in size and its junction with the subclavian is angulated, making it more difficult to cannulate (Weinstein 1997).

Insertion

Insertion of a skin-tunnelled catheter is usually performed in the operating theatre or anaesthetic room (Stacey et al. 1991). However, this procedure is now being successfully performed by clinical nurse specialists at the bedside (Hamilton et al. 1995). A general anaesthetic may be necessary for some insertions, but most procedures are performed under sedation along with the use of local anaesthesia (Stacey et al. 1991).

Access may be gained percutaneously using a needle and a guidewire or via an open surgical cutdown procedure. The percutaneous insertion involves the subclavian vein being accessed using a guidewire and Seldinger technique. After the catheter is tunnelled subcutaneously, a vein dilator is passed over the guidewire and the catheter is cut to length and introduced using a 'peel-away' sheath (Davidson & Al Mufti 1997). Reducing the likelihood of complications and preventing distress to the patient may be achieved by careful insertion techniques, strict asepsis (Elliott et al. 1994), correct positioning and radiological confirmation of the catheter placement. The catheter should be heparinized or 0.9% sodium chloride infused slowly, 10–20 ml/hour, until X-ray results confirm the correct placement of the catheter (Stacey et al. 1991; Davidson & Al Mufti 1997).

Care and management in situ

Following healing of the skin tunnel, which takes approximately 7 days, sutures at the entry site may be removed. Sutures at the exit site of a skin-tunnelled catheter should be removed after 21 days. Thereafter no dressing is usually required unless the patient requests one.

Removal

Removal techniques for skin-tunnelled catheters vary. Removal should only be performed by specially trained nurses or doctors. It is recommended that the patient is placed supine and that aseptic technique is used throughout. There are two methods for removal.

Surgical excision

This method involves locating the cuff and performing a minor surgical excision under local anaesthetic. A small incision is made over the site of the cuff and blunt dissection, i.e. using forceps, is carried out to prise apart tissues; this causes less damage to the tissues than using a scalpel. The cuff and the catheter are freed from the surrounding fibrous tissue. The catheter is then cut in order to remove the distal end via the exit site and the proximal end through the incision. Once the catheter has been removed, the wound is sutured using interrupted sutures, which can be removed after 7 days.

Traction method

With the traction method there is a greater risk of the catheter breaking, which could result in a catheter embolism. The catheter is gripped firmly and constant traction applied. It may take a few minutes for the catheter and cuff to become loose before sliding free. Constant steady pressure will remove the complete catheter; however, the catheter should be checked on removal to ensure it is complete (ONS 1996). The catheter and cuff may be pulled through, but the cuff may remain attached to tissue. This is thought to be of no significance and may be left in place. Difficulty with removal or a break in the catheter will require surgical intervention.

Since the vein closes after the catheter is removed no bleeding occurs at the exit site although there may be slight bleeding at the exit site immediately after removal of the catheter because of the passage of the cuff (Bjeletich & Hickman 1980).

Following either removal method, pressure should be applied to the site until the bleeding stops, and a dressing may be required for up to 24 hours (Weinstein 1997). The patient should be encouraged to rest for at least an hour.

If the tip is required for microbiological examination, care should be taken to clean the exit site with chlorhexidine in 70% alcohol, prior to removal, to prevent a false positive tip culture. The tip should be placed into a sterile container immediately upon removal.

Implantable ports

Definition

An implantable port is a totally implanted vascular access device which is inserted either on the chest wall or in the antecubital area. An implantable port requires access by a needle.

Indications

The portal system can be used for:

1 Bolus injections
2 Infusions of drugs
3 Blood products
4 Parenteral nutrition
5 Blood sampling

(Speechley & Davidson 1989).

Reference material

An implantable drug delivery system consists of a portal body attached to a silicone catheter (Fig. 44.7). Ports are implanted subcutaneously to provide access to the vascular system (other ports include arterial, epidural and peritoneal ports). Implanted ports require little care of the site because of the intact skin layer over the accessible port. They also require minimal flushing and permit easy access

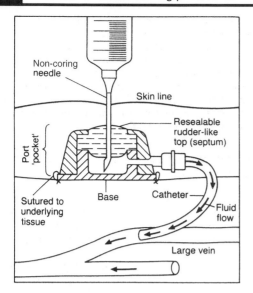

Figure 44.7 Cross-section of an implantable port, accessed with non-coring needle.

for fluids and/or medications. They are reported to offer social advantages over external central venous access such as less risk of infection. However, studies reviewed show that sample groups have not been matched and so the comparisons made should be approached with caution (Richard Alexander 1994). There is also less interference with daily activities and body image is not threatened by the presence of a catheter (Camp Sorrell 1992). The portal is accessed using a special non-coring needle (that is, one that does not damage the port by coring out the silicone on insertion) when therapy is required and the needle may remain in place for up to 1 week.

The disadvantages of a port are the discomfort associated with accessing the port (especially if placed deeply or in a difficult area to access). This can be overcome with the use of topical local anaesthetic cream. However, it still requires the insertion of a needle and for some children or adults with a fear of needles this may be unacceptable.

Device information

A variety of catheters and portals are available, the choice of which is dependent on a number of factors; for example, whether the patient is a child or an adult, amount of access necessary, etc. The majority of ports are single, although double ports are available, but require access into each septum. The portal body may be made of stainless steel, plastic or titanium and the septum is silicone along with the catheter. The self-sealing septum can withstand 1000–2000 needle punctures (Camp Sorrell 1992). Some ports need to be made up prior to insertion; others come as complete units and can weigh from 21 to 28.8 g. Non-coring needles are available and present as straight or angled in a variety of configurations, lengths and gauge sizes.

Choice of vein

The most common veins used are subclavian, internal or external jugular veins, cephalic or femoral vein (ONS 1996). Ports can also be inserted in the antecubital area of the arm.

Insertion

The port is usually inserted under general anaesthetic, either using a cut-down or a percutaneous method. The portal body is usually placed 1.25 mm under the skin over a bony area for stabilization. It is then sutured to the fascia layer (usually the pectoralis major fascia; ONS 1996). The catheter is tunnelled as previously described and the tip rests in a major vein. The septum should not be placed under the wound since access could cause stress to the suture line. The reformation of the skin barrier prevents the entry of micro-organisms, and aseptic technique during access should result in a minimal contamination rate.

Care and management in situ

The advantage of a port is that, if not required, the needle access is removed and the port only needs to be flushed once a month with a solution of heparin (100 IU per ml). If the port is accessed, a non-coring needle such as a Huber point needle should be used which should be changed every 7 days. Only practitioners specifically trained should access a port, as wrongly placed needles could lead to extravasation of drugs. The needle should be supported by gauze and covered by a transparent dressing to avoid needle dislodgment, as this has been shown to be the most frequently documented cause of extravasation (Camp Sorrell 1992).

Regular assessment of the port site is essential to check for signs of erythema, swelling or tenderness which could indicate the presence of an infection. Most manufacturers recommend the use of syringes 10 ml or larger to prevent excessive pressures which could result in separation of the catheter from the portal body.

Removal

Removal is usually performed in the theatre setting but may be undertaken in outpatients. A cut-down method is performed to remove the port from the subcutaneous pocket.

Discharging patients home with a VAD in situ

Patients may be discharged home with a VAD in situ which will allow them to receive treatment at home (e.g. continuous chemotherapy or intermittent antibiotics) or allow for easier access on each admission (e.g. via implantable ports).

Recently, patients receiving daily treatment over a 3–5 day period have maintained an indwelling peripheral cannula (Shotkin & Lombardo 1996). The degree of care is minimal compared with a central venous catheter, but patients should receive adequate information about the early signs of phlebitis, i.e. pain, redness and swelling, and what to do in the case of accidental dislodgment or removal.

Patients with long-term VADs in situ such as PICCs or skin-tunnelled catheters will require instruction and supervision to ensure adequate understanding of the care and maintenance of their devices prior to discharge. Patient education is one of the most important aspects of care, but to make teaching effective it is essential to recognize each patient's needs and limitations. It is also vital to acknowledge each patient's past experiences and use these as a resource for learning (Redman 1985); expert education of the patients by the nurse is essential to safety in the home (Dougherty et al. 1998). Educational packages should be prepared in the form of practical demonstrations and clear succinct handouts (Butler 1984). It is also important to recognize the need to prepare patients carefully to participate in their own self-care and therapy treatment (Teich & Raia 1984). Patients need an overview of what to expect from the teaching sessions and to understand the role of their own self-care and be given time to enable them to carry out the practice accurately (Howser & Meade 1987). The patient, relative and/or friends should understand the following:

1 The frequency of changing the dressing and how to care for the site.
2 How to maintain patency.
3 How to inspect for signs of infection or other complications.
4 How to problem solve and where to seek help.

Care of the site/dressing changes

The dressing of choice for PICC insertion sites is the moisture-permeable transparent dressing which usually requires changing once a week. This type of dressing and its position on the arm may make it hard for patients to perform the dressing change by themselves and requires either the help of the carer or community nurse. At the dressing change the site should be inspected for signs of infection and cleaned using an appropriate antiseptic. For patients with a skin-tunnelled catheter in situ, the sutures should only be removed once the catheter has become well established (usually 2–3 weeks after insertion) and the cuff is covered with fibrous tissue. Once the sutures are removed, there is usually no longer any need for a dressing unless the patient requests it.

Sterile, low-linting swabs and hypoallergenic tape may initially be supplied. While sutures remain in place, patients should change the dressing after their daily shower, having dried the area with clean cottonwool and wiped the exit site with a chlorhexidine-soaked swab.

When in the bath, water should not come into contact with the exit site: this should be cleaned separately using fresh water and low-linting swabs to clean and dry. The only other time that a dressing is required is when patients go swimming or take part in water sports. In this instance the whole catheter and exit site should be covered completely with an occlusive dressing before entering the water. The dressing is removed immediately afterwards to ensure no water penetrates the dressing.

Maintaining patency and handling of equipment

Before discharge the patient should observe the heparinization technique and perform it until competent to do so without supervision. Relatives and friends may be involved in this procedure. Sufficient equipment must be supplied to enable the patient to care for the catheter from the time of discharge until the next outpatient appointment or admission. A kit should be assembled containing the following:

1 Spare Luer lock caps with an injection site.
2 A spare, smooth-edged clamp.
3 A supply of heparinized saline, 50 IU in 5 ml 0.9% sodium chloride.
4 Chlorhexidine in 70% alcohol/swab saturated with isopropyl alcohol to clean the injection site on the cap.
5 A supply of sterile 5-ml syringes.
6 21-g needles to draw up the heparinized saline.
7 25-g needles to inject through the intermittent injection cap, unless using a needleless injection cap.
8 Instruction booklet to provide the patient with a point of reference.
9 A sharps container.

Early recognition of complications

Patients should be taught what early signs and symptoms to look out for and who and when to contact. The most common complications associated with VADs are infection and thrombosis. The patients should be told to report signs of redness and tracking at the exit site, along the skin tunnel or up the arm, any oozing at the exit site and fevers or rigors. Many patients are now prescribed prophylactic warfarin (either 1 mg daily or according to regular international normalized ratio screening) to prevent thrombosis (Perdue 1995). However, it should be stressed to the patient that any of the following signs or symptoms should be reported immediately: pain and/or swelling over the shoulder, across the chest and into the neck and arm. Early reporting may enable treatment and avoid removal of the device.

Problem solving and who and when to ask for help

Patients must be informed what to do if the catheter becomes occluded or splits and given a contact name and number in order to be able to seek professional advice. This will help to alleviate any anxiety (Dougherty *et al.* 1998). Most problems can be managed at home with the involvement of the community nurses and GP. This support is often crucial and should be arranged before the patient is discharged.

Quality of life issues: living with a VAD

Dániels (1995) lists the ways in which a central venous access device (CVAD) can affect body image:

1 Physical presence and alteration of body appearance and invasion of body integrity
2 It influences the type of clothes that can be worn.
3 It may interfere with bodily expressions of closeness and sexuality.

The presence of a CVAD could also have implications on how others view the role function of the individual, particularly if the patient is attached to an infusion pump (Thompson *et al.* 1989).

Patients may be well informed about access devices from the media or via the Internet. They may also have gained knowledge from friends or family experiences. While there are few physical restrictions with reference to activity, the psychological impact of an indwelling catheter on body image should not be overlooked, especially when patients are sexually active. Involving the patient in the decision-making process is vital. Patient choice about the device or even the site of insertion, e.g. use of the non-dominant arm, results in better compliance with care of the device and monitoring of problems (Hudek 1986). It also enables patients to cope better with the changes to their normal activities (Daniels 1995) and the impact on body image can be reduced by involving the individual in the choice and management of the device (Daniels 1995).

Reading central venous pressure

Central venous pressure (CVP) is the pressure within the superior vena cava or the right atrium (Woodrow 1992). Measurements of CVP reflect the relationship between the circulating blood volume (Fig. 44.8), the competence of the heart as a pump and the vascular resistance.

CVP readings are used:

1 To serve as a guide to fluid balance in critically ill patients.
2 To estimate the circulating blood volume.
3 To assist in monitoring circulatory failure.

The CVP measurement should be measured at the right atrial level as it is a measure of the pressure of the blood returning to the right atrium (Woodrow 1992). One measurement will not provide an accurate reading and several readings will be required to determine a patient's response to treatment (Henderson 1997). The most accurate method of measuring is by placing the patient in the supine

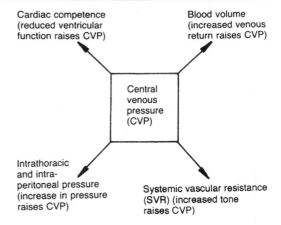

Cardiac competence (reduced ventricular function raises CVP)

Blood volume (increased venous return raises CVP)

Central venous pressure (CVP)

Intrathoracic and intra-peritoneal pressure (increase in pressure raises CVP)

Systemic vascular resistance (SVR) (increased tone raises CVP)

Figure 44.8 Determinants of central venous pressure.

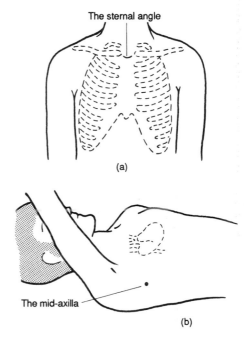

The sternal angle

(a)

The mid-axilla

(b)

Figure 44.9 Measuring central venous pressure. (a) Sternal angle. (b) Mid-axilla.

position and using either of the sites indicated in Fig. 44.9. If the patient is unable to lay flat, the mid-axilla can be used (Henderson 1997). It should be established at the outset which point is to be used, as there is a difference in pressure of about 5 cm of water between them. It is useful to mark the chosen site for future readings and note both the site and the patient's position on the CVP recording chart, the patient's care plan and even on the skin to ensure constancy of readings (Woodrow 1992). Generally, water manometers are used (Henderson 1997), but when patients are critically ill and a more accurate method is required, the CVP is transduced electronically via a central monitoring system (Woodrow 1992). Zeroing a CVP removes extraneous pressure so zero should conform to atmospheric pressure (Woodrow 1992; Henderson 1997). The normal values for CVP readings are 0–5 cm of water at the sternal angle, and 5–10 cm of water at the mid-axilla (Henderson 1997). Low readings indicate hypovolaemia, and low viscosity of fluid returning to the right atrium, right heart function and venous tone. High readings indicate hypervolaemia, high viscosity, right heart failure and user error (Woodrow 1992).

References and further reading

Anderson, K.N. & Anderson, L.E. (eds) (1995) *Mosby's Pocket Dictionary of Nursing, Medicine and Professions Allied to Medicine.* Mosby, London.

Anderson, M.A. *et al.* (1982) The double-lumen Hickman catheter. *Am J Nurs*, **82**(2), 272–7.

Bahruth, A.J. (1996) PICC insertion problems associated with topical anesthesia. *J Intraven Nurs*, **19**(1), 32–4.

Banton, J. & Leahy Gross, K. (1998) Assessing catheter performance – 4 years of tracking patient outcomes of midline, midclavicular and PICC line program. *J Vasc Access Devices*, **3**(3), 19–25.

Baranowski, L. (1993) Central venous access devices – current technologies, uses and management strategies. *J Intraven Nurs*, **16**(3), 167–94.

Barrett, P. & Lester, R. (1990) Heparin versus saline flushing solutions in a small community hospital. *Hosp Pharm*, **25**, 115–18.

Bjeletich, J. (1982) Repairing the Hickman catheter. *Am J Nurs*, **82**(2), 274.

Bjeletich, J. & Hickman, R.O. (1980) The Hickman indwelling catheter. *Am J Nurs*, **80**(1), 62–5.

Brismar, B., Malmborg, A.S., Nystrom, B. & Strandberg, A. (1984) Bacterial contamination of intravenous cannula injection ports and stopcocks. *Clin Nutr*, **3**, 23–6.

British Medical Association (1991) *A Code of Practice for the Safe Use and Disposal of Sharps*, pp. 20–21. BMA, London.

British Medical Association and Royal Pharmaceutical Society of Great Britain (1999) *British National Formulary*, no. 38, pp. 562–4. BMA and Royal Pharmaceutical Society of GB, London.

Brown, J.D. *et al.* (1997) The potential for catheter microbial contamination from a needleless connector. *J Hosp Infect*, **36**, 181–9.

BSI (1997) *Sterile Single Use Intravascular Catheters, Part 1: General Requirements*, BSEN ISO 10555-1 1997. British Standards Institution, London.

Butler, M.C. (1984) Families' response to chemotherapy by an ambulatory infusion pump. *Nurs Clin North Am*, **19**(1), 139–43.

Camp Sorrell, D. (1992) Implantable ports – everything you always wanted to know. *J Intraven Nurs*, **15**(5), 262–73.

Cella, J.H. & Watson, J. (eds) (1989) Obtaining peripheral blood specimens. In: *Nurses Manual of Laboratory Test*, pp. 481–6. F.A. Davis, Massachusetts.

Cheeseborough, J.S. & Finch, R. (1984) Side ports – an infection hazard? *Br J Parent Ther*, **5**(4), 155–7.

Clarke, J. & Cox, E. (1988) Heparinisation of Hickman catheters. *Nurs Times*, **84**(15), 51–3.

Clemence, M.A. *et al.* (1995) CVC practices: results of a survey. *J Vasc Access Devices*, **1**(1), 30–37.

Conn, C. (1993) The importance of syringe size when using an implanted vascular access device. *J Vasc Access Networks*, **3**(1), 11-18.

Daniels, L.E. (1995) The physical and psychosocial implications of central venous access devices in cancer patients: a review of the literature. *J Cancer Care*, **4**, 141–5.

Davidson, T. & Al Mufti, R. (1997) Hickman central venous catheters in cancer patients. *Cancer Topics*, **10**(8), 10–14.

Dennis, A.R., Leeson-Payne, C.G., Langham, B.T. & Aikenhead, A.R. (1995) Local anaesthesia for cannulation – has practice changed? *Anaesthesia*, **50**, 400–402.

De Vries, J.H., Van Dorp, W.T. & van Barneveld, P.W.C. (1997) A randomised trial of alcohol 70% versus alcoholic iodine 2% in skin disinfection before insertion of peripheral infusion catheters. *J Hosp Infect*, **36**, 317–20.

Dougherty, L. (1994) *A study to discover how cancer patients perceive the intravenous cannulation experience.* Unpublished MSc thesis, University of Surrey, Guildford.

Dougherty, L. (1996) Intravenous cannulation. *Nurs Stand*, **11**(2), 47–51.

Dougherty, L. (1999) Obtaining peripheral vascular access. In: *Intravenous Therapy in Nursing Practice* (eds L. Dougherty & J. Lamb). Churchill Livingstone, Edinburgh.

Dougherty, L., Viner, C. & Young, J. (1998) Establishing ambulatory chemotherapy at home. *Prof Nurse*, **13**(6), 356–60.

Dunn, D. & Lenihan, S. (1987) The case for the saline flush. *Am J Nurs*, **87**(6), 798–9.

Elliott, T.S.J., Faroqui, M.H., Armstrong, R.F. & Hanson, G.C. (1994) Guidelines for good practice in central venous catheterization. *J Hosp Inf*, **28**, 163–76.

Epperson, E.L. (1984) Efficacy of 0.9% sodium chloride injection with and without heparin for maintaining indwelling intermittent injection sites. *Clin Pharm*, **3**, 626–9.

Ford, R. (1986) History and organization of the Seattle-area Hickman catheter committee. *J Can Intraven Nurses Assoc*, **2**(2), 4–13.

Fuller, A. & Winn, C. (1999) Selecting equipment for peripheral intravenous cannulation. *Prof Nurse*, **14**(4), 233–6.

Gabriel, J. (1996a) Care and management of peripherally inserted central catheters. *Br J Nurs*, **5**(10), 594–9.

Gabriel, J. (1996b) PICC – expanding UK nurses' practice. *Surg Nurs*, **5**(2), 71–4.

Gabriel, J. (1999) Long term central venous access. In: *Intravenous Therapy in Nursing Practice* (eds L. Dougherty & J. Lamb). Churchill Livingstone, Edinburgh.

Gaukroger, P.B., Roberts, J.G. & Manners, T.A. (1988) Infusion thrombophlebitis: a prospective comparison of 645 Vialon and Teflon cannulae in anaesthetic and postoperative use. *Anaesth Intens Care*, **16**(3), 265–71.

Gilles, H. & Rogers, H.J. (1985) Is repeated flushing of Hickman catheters necessary? *Br Med J*, **290**, 1708.

Goetz, A.M., Miller, J., Wagener, M.M. & Muder, R.R. (1998) Complications related to intravenous midline catheter usage. *J Intraven Nurs*, **21**(2), 76–80.

Goode, C.J. *et al.* (1991) A meta analysis of effects of heparin flush and saline flush – quality and cost implications. *Nurs Res*, **40**(6), 324–30.

Goodman, M. & Riley, M.B. (1997) Chemotherapy administration. In: *Cancer Nursing* (eds S.L. Groenwald, M.H. Frogge, M. Goodman & C. Henke Yarbro), 4th edn., pp. 317–404. Jones & Bartlett, Boston.

Goodman, M.S. & Wickham, R. (1984) Venous access devices: an overview. *Oncol Nurses Forum*, **11**(5), 16–23.

Goodwin, M. & Carlson, I. (1993) The peripherally inserted catheter: a retrospective look at 3 years of insertions. *J Intraven Nurs*, **16**(2), 92–103.

Gyves, J. *et al.* (1982) Totally implanted system for intravenous chemotherapy in patients with cancer. *Am J Med*, **73**, 841–5.

Hadaway, L. (1995) Anatomy and physiology related to IV therapy. In: *Intravenous Therapy: Clinical Principles and Practices* (eds J. Terry, L. Baranowski, R.A. Lonsway & C. Hedrick), pp. 81–110. W.B. Saunders, Philadelphia.

Hadaway, L. (1990) An overview of vascular access devices inserted via the antecubital area. *J Intraven Nurs*, **13**(5), 297–300.

Hadaway, L. (1998) Catheter connection. *J Vasc Access Devices*, **3**(3), 40.

Haire, W.D. *et al.* (1990) Hickman catheter induced thoracic vein thrombosis. *Cancer*, **66**, 900–908.

Hamilton, H., O'Byrne, M. & Nicholai, L. (1995) Central lines inserted by clinical nurse specialists. *Nurs Times*, **91**(17), 38–9.

Hamilton, R.A. *et al.* (1988) Heparin sodium versus 0.9% sodium chloride injection for maintaining patency of indwelling intermittent infusion devices. *Clin Pharm*, **7**, 439–43.

Harrison, N., Langham, B.T. & Bogod, D.G. (1992) Appropriate use of local anaesthesia for venous cannulation. *Anaesthesia*, **47**, 210–12.

Henderson, N. (1997) Central venous lines. *Nurs Stand*, **11**(42), 49–56.

Hinds, C.T. (1988) *Intensive Care*, pp. 32–9. Baillière Tindall, Eastbourne.

Hoffman, K.K. *et al.* (1992) Transparent polyurethane film as an intravenous catheter dressing. *JAMA*, **267**(15), 2072–6.

Holmes, K. (1998) Comparison of push–pull versus discard method from central venous catheters for blood testing. *J Intraven Nurs*, **21**(5), 282–5.

Homer, L.D. & Holmes, K.R. (1998) Risks associated with 72 and 96 hour peripheral IV catheter dwell times. *J Intraven Nurs*, **21**(5), 301–305.

Howser, D.M. & Meade, C.D. (1987) Hickman catheter care – developing organised teaching strategies. *Cancer Nurs*, **10**(2), 70–76.

Hudek, K. (1986) Compliance in intravenous therapy. *J Can Intraven Assoc*, **2**(3), 3–8.

ICU Medical (1998) *Clave Connector System*. Product Information Leaflet. ICU Medical Ltd., California.

Intravenous Nursing Society (1998) Revised intravenous nursing standards of practice. *J Intraven Nurs*, **21**(15), Suppl. 1S.

Kamimoto, V. & Olson, K. (1996) Using normal saline to lock peripheral intravenous catheters in ambulatory cancer patients. *J Intraven Nurs*, **19**(2), 75–8.

Keenleyside, D. (1993) Avoiding an unnecessary outcome. A comparative trial between IV 3000 and a conventional film dressing to assess rates of catheter related sepsis. *Prof Nurse*, February, 288–91.

Keller, C.A. (1994) Method of drawing blood samples through central venous catheters in paediatric patients undergoing bone marrow transplants – results of a national survey. *Oncol Nurs Forum*, **21**(5), 879–84.

Kelly, C. *et al.* (1992) A change in flushing protocol of CVC. *Oncol Nurs Forum*, **19**(4), 599–605.

Kerrison, T. & Woodhull, J. (1994) Reducing the risk of thrombophlebitis – comparison of Teflon and Vialon cannulae. *Prof Nurse*, **9**(10), 662–6.

Kupensky, D.T. (1998) Applying current research to influence clinical practice – utilization of midline catheters. *J Intraven Nurs*, **21**(5), 271–4.

Larson, E. (1988) Guidelines for use of topical antimicrobial agents (review). *Am J Infect Contr*, **16**(6), 253–66.

Lawson, M. *et al.* (1982) The use of urokinase to restore the patency of occluded central venous catheters. *Am J IV Ther Clin Nutr*, **9**(9), 29–32.

Lewis, G.B.H. & Hecker, J.F. (1985) Infusion thrombophlebitis. *Br J Anaesth*, **57**, 220–33.

Macklin, D. (1999) A review of the physical principles of fluid administration. *J Nat Vasc Access Devices*, **4**(2), 7–11.

Macrae, K. (1998) Hand held Doppler's in central catheter insertion. *Prof Nurse*, **14**(2), 99–102.

Madeo, M. *et al.* (1997) A randomised study comparing IV 3000 (transparent polyurethane dressing) to a dry gauze dressing for peripheral intravenous catheter sites. *J Intraven Nurs*, **20**(5), 253–6.

Maki, D.G. (1976) Preventing infection in IV therapy. *Hosp Pract*, April, 95–104.

Maki, D.G. & Ringer, M. (1987) Evaluation of dressing regimes for prevention of infection with peripheral IV catheters. *J Am Med Assoc*, **258**(17), 2396–403.

Maki, D.G. *et al.* (1991) Prospective randomized trial of povidone iodine, alcohol and chlorhexidine for prevention of infection associated with CVC and arterial catheters. *Lancet*, **338**, 339–43.

Maki, D.G., Stolz, S.M., Wheeler, S. & Mermel, L.A. (1997) Prevention of central venous catheter related bloodstream infection by the use of an antiseptic impregnated catheter. *Ann Intern Med*, **127**(4), 257–66f.

Mayo, D.J. (1998) Fibrin sheath formation and chemotherapy extravasation: a case report. *Supportive Care in Cancer*, **6**, 51–6.

McKee, J.M., Shell, J.A., Warren, T.A. & Campbell, V.P. (1989) Complications of intravenous therapy: a randomised prospective study – Vialon vs Teflon. *J Intraven Nurs*, **12**(5), 288–95.

McMenamin, E.M. (1993) Catheter fracture: a complication in venous access devices. *Cancer Nurs*, **16**(6), 464–7.

Millam, D. (1992) Starting IVs – how to develop your venepuncture skills. *Nursing*, **92**, 33–46.

Millam, D. (1993) How to teach good venepuncture technique. *Am J Nurs*, **93**(7), 38–41.

Millam, D. (1995) The use of anaesthesia in IV therapy. *J Vasc Access Devices*, **1**(1), 22–9.

Moreau, N. *et al.* (1999) Multidisciplinary management of thrombotic catheter occlusions in VADs. *J Vasc Access Devices*, **4**(2), 22–9.

Nauth Misir, N. (1998) Intravascular catheters. *Prof Nurse*, **13**(7), 463–71.

Ng, P. *et al.* (1997) Peripherally inserted central catheters in general medicine. *Mayo Clin Proc*, **72**, 225–33.

Nightingale, K.W. & Bradshaw, E.G. (1982) A review of peripheral cannulae. *Br J IV Therapy*, **3**(4), 14–23.

Oldman, P. (1991) A sticky situation? *Prof Nurse*, **6**(5), 265–9.

ONS (1996) *Cancer Chemotherapy Guidelines and Recommendations for Nursing Education and Practice*. Oncology Nursing Society, Pittsburgh.

Ostrow, L.S. (1981) Air embolism and central venous lines. *Am J Nurs*, **81**(21), 40–42.

Payne-James, J.J., Rogers, J., Bray. M.J., Rana, S.K., McSwiggon, D. & Silk, D.B. (1991) Development of thrombophlebitis in peripheral veins with Vialon and PTFE-Teflon cannulas: a double blind randomised controlled trial. *Ann R Surg Engl*, **73**, 322–5.

Perdue, L. (1995) Intravenous complications. In: *Intravenous Therapy: Clinical Principles and Practices* (eds J. Terry, L. Baranowski, R.A. Lonsway & C. Hedrick), pp. 419–46. W.B. Saunders, Philadelphia.

Perucca, R. (1995) Obtaining vascular access. In: *Intravenous Therapy: Clinical Principles and Practices* (eds J. Terry, L. Baranowski, R.A. Lonsway & C. Hedrick), pp. 377–91. W.B. Saunders, Philadelphia.

Peters, J.L., Frame, J.D. & Dawson, S.M. (1984) Peripheral venous cannulation: reducing the risks. *Br J Parent Ther*, **5**, 56–8.

Petrosino, B., Becker, H. & Christian, B. (1988) Infection rates in central venous catheter dressings. *Oncol Nurs Forum*, **15**(6), 709–17.

Pinto, K.M. (1994) Accuracy of coagulation values obtained from a heparinised central venous catheter. *Oncol Nurs Forum*, **21**(3), 573–5.

Raad, I., Darouiche, R., Dupruis, J. *et al.* (1997) Central venous catheters coated with minocycline and rifampicin for the prevention of catheter related colonisation and bloodstream infections. *Ann Intern Med*, **127**, 267–74.

Rasor, J.J. (1991) Review of catheter related infection rates: comparison of conventional catheter materials with aquavene. *J Vasc Access Network*, **1**(3), 8–16.

RCN (1999) *Guidance for Nurses Giving Intravenous Therapy*. Royal College of Nursing, London.

RCN and Infection Control Nurses' Association (1992) *Intravenous Line Dressings – Principles of Infection Control*. Smith & Nephew Medical Ltd., Hull.

Redman, M. (1985) New areas of theory, development and practice in patient education. *J Adv Nurs*, **10**, 425–8.

Richard Alexander, H. (1994) Thrombotic and occlusive complications in long-term venous access. In: *Vascular Access in the Cancer Patient*, Chap. 6. J.B. Lippincott, Philadelphia.

Ridley, R.A. (1990) The use of unpreserved 0.9% sodium chloride injection for the maintenance of multilumen subclavian catheters. *Can Intraven Nurses Assoc*, **6**(1), 5–9.

Russell, W.J., Micik, S., Gourd, S., Mackay, H. & Wright, S. (1996) A prospective clinical comparison of two intravenous polyurethane cannulae. *Anaesth Intens Care*, **24**(6), 705–709.

Salzman, M.B. *et al.* (1993) Use of disinfectants to reduce microbial contamination of hubs of vascular catheters. *J Clin Microbiol*, **31**, 475–9.

Shearer, J. (1987) Normal saline flush vs dilute heparin flush. A study of peripheral intermittent IV devices. *J Intraven Nurs*, **10**, 425–7.

Shotkin, J.D. & Lombardo, F. (1996) Use of an indwelling peripheral catheter for 3–5 day chemotherapy administration in the outpatient setting. *J Intraven Nurs*, **19**(6), 315–20.

Speechley, V. (1984) The nurse's role in intravenous management. *Nurs Times*, 2 May, 31–2.

Speechley, V. & Davidson, T. (1989) Managing an implantable drug delivery system. *Prof Nurse*, **4**(6), 284–8.

Speer, E.W. (1990) CVC issues associated with the use of single and multiple lumen catheters. *J Intraven Nurs*, **13**(1), 30–39.

Springhouse Corporation (1999) *Handbook of Infusion Therapy*. Springhouse, Pennsylvania.

Stacey, R.G.W. *et al.* (1991) Percutaneous insertion of Hickman type catheters. *Br J Hosp Med*, **46**, 396–8.

Stokes, D.C. *et al.* (1989) Early detection: a simplified management of obstructed Hickman and Broviac catheters. *J Paed Surg*, **24**(3), 257–62.

Tacsak Kupensky, D. (1998) Applying current research to influence clinical practice – utilisation of midline catheters. *J Intraven Nurs*, **21**(5), 271–4.

Teich, C.J. & Raia, K. (1984) Teaching strategies for an ambulatory chemotherapy program. *Oncol Nurs Forum*, **11**(5), 24–8.

Thompson, A. *et al.* (1989) Long-term central venous access: the patient's view. *Intens Ther Clin Monit*, **10**(5), 142–5.

Treston Aurend, J., Olmsted, R.N., Allen-Bridson, K. & Craig, C.P. (1997) Impact of dressing materials on central venous catheter infection rates. *J Intraven Nurs*, **20**(4), 201–206.

Van den Berg, A.A. & Abeysekera, R.M. (1993) Rationalising venous cannulation: patient factors and lignocaine efficacy. *Anaesthesia*, **48**(1), 84.

Viall, C. (1990) Daily access of implanted venous port. *J Intraven Nurs*, **13**(5), 294–6.

Wachs, T. (1990) Urokinase administration in paediatric patients with occluded central venous catheters. *J Intraven Nurs*, **13**(2), 100–102.

Weinstein, S.M. (1997) *Plumer's Principles and Practice of Intravenous Therapy*, 6th edn. J.B. Lippincott, Philadelphia.

Whitely, M.S., Change, B.Y.P. & Marsh, H.P. (1995) Use of hand held Doppler to identify 'difficult' forearm veins for cannulation. *Ann R Coll Surg Engl*, **77**, 224–6.

Whitson, M. (1996) Intravenous therapy in the older adult: special needs and considerations. *J Intraven Nurs*, **19**(5), 251–5.

Wickham, R. *et al.* (1992) Long-term CVs: issues for care. *Semin Oncol Nurs*, **8**(2), 133–47.

Woodrow, P. (1992) Monitoring CVP. *Nurs Stand*, **6**(33), 25–9.

GUIDELINES · Reading central venous pressure

Equipment

1 Spirit level.
2 Manometer.
3 CVP monitoring intravenous administration set.

Procedure

Action	*Rationale*
1 Explain and discuss the procedure with the patient.	To ensure that the patient understands the procedure and gives his/her valid consent.
2 Ascertain the point of CVP reading, i.e. sternal angle or mid-axilla. If the patient agrees, this point should be marked on the patient and noted in the care plan chart for future reference.	CVP must always be read from the same point because the sternal angle reading is about 5 cm of water higher than the mid-axilla reading. To show an accurate trend the figure should be 0.

Guidelines • Reading central venous pressure (cont'd)

Action	Rationale
3 Assist the patient to get into a recumbent or semirecumbent position to a maximum angle of 45°.	The position of the patient must allow the baseline of the manometer to be level with the patient's right atrium. If the patient is upright or is lying on his/her side, the right atrium will not be in line with the sternal angle or the mid-axilla. However, if it is impossible for the patient to be in any other position, the CVP reading may be recorded with the patient sitting up at a 90° angle, but this must be recorded on the observation chart.
4 Position the manometer so that the baseline is level with the right atrium.	To obtain an accurate CVP reading, the baseline and the right atrium must be level.
5 Loosen the securing screw and slide the scale up or down until the baseline figure lies next to the arm of the spirit level (Fig. 44.10a). This figure should be 0 (also known as 'zeroing').	To remove effect of extraneous pressure and to ensure baseline is always the same in order to have a single point of reference.
6 Check that the baseline and right atrium are level by extending the arm of the spirit level to the sternal angle or to the mid-axilla. Move the manometer until the bubble is between the parallel lines of the spirit level (Fig. 44.10b).	
7 Care should be taken when flushing the catheter regarding the volume and type of fluid.	To ensure the patency of the catheter and to check for leaks, kinks, blockages, etc. To ensure that correct solution is used to flush, e.g. 0.9% sodium chloride or dextrose, and not a solution containing drugs.
8 Turn off the three-way tap to the patient (Fig. 44.11). Allow the manometer to fill slowly.	To allow the intravenous fluid to run into the manometer. To avoid: (a) Bubbles, which cause inaccurate readings. (b) Overfilling of, and spillage from, the manometer that would put the patient at risk from infection.

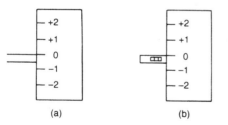

(a) (b)

Figure 44.10 (a) Setting the baseline. (b) Checking the baseline.

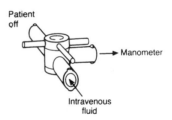

Figure 44.11 Turn off three-way tap to patient.

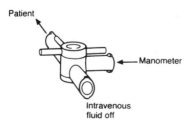

Figure 44.12 Turn off three-way tap to intravenous fluid.

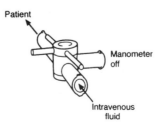

Figure 44.13 Turn off three-way tap to manometer.

9 Turn off the three-way tap to the intravenous fluid (Fig. 44.12).	To allow fluid from the manometer to enter the patient's right atrium.
10 The column of water should fall rapidly.	Indicating patency of the catheter, resulting in an accurate CVP reading.
11 When the level of fluid in the manometer ceases to drop, and oscillates with the patient's respirations, this is the CVP reading.	The pressure of the column of water in the manometer now equals the pressure in the right atrium.
12 Turn off the three-way tap to the manometer (Fig. 44.13).	To restore infusion via the intravenous catheter.
13 Readjust the infusion rate.	
14 Record the CVP measurement on the appropriate chart. Compare this measurement with the patient's acceptable CVP limits as stated by the medical team.	Acceptable CVP values vary with the patient observations and his/her overall condition. Deviations from these limits may require urgent medical intervention.

GUIDELINES • Inserting a peripheral cannula

Equipment

1 Sterile dressing pack.
2 Various gauge sizes of cannula.
3 Alcohol-based hand scrub.
4 Alcohol-based skin cleansing preparation, e.g. chlorhexidine in 70% alcohol.

5 Extension set.
6 Intermittent injection cap.
7 Hypoallergenic tape.
8 Bandage.

Procedure

Action	Rationale
1 Explain and discuss the procedure with the patient.	To ensure that the patient understands the procedure and gives his/her valid consent.
2 Assemble all the equipment necessary for cannulation.	To ensure that time is not wasted and that the procedure goes smoothly without unnecessary interruptions.
3 Check all packaging before opening and preparing the equipment to be used.	To maintain asepsis throughout and check that no equipment is damaged.
4 Carefully wash hands using bactericidal soap and water or bactericidal alcohol hand rub before commencement, and dry.	To minimize the risk of infection.
5 Check hands for any visibly broken skin, and cover with a waterproof dressing.	To minimize the risk of contamination of the nurse by the patient's blood.
6 In both an inpatient and outpatient situation, the correct lighting, ventilation, privacy and position of the patient must be ascertained.	To ensure that the operator and patient are comfortable and that adequate light is available to illuminate the procedure.
7 Support the chosen limb.	To ensure the patient's comfort and ease of access.
8 Apply the tourniquet.	To dilate the veins by obstructing the venous return. If necessary, use other methods to encourage venous access.
9 Assess and select the vein.	
10 Release the tourniquet.	To ensure that the patient does not feel discomfort while the device is selected and equipment prepared.
11 Select the device based on the vein size.	To reduce damage or trauma to the vein. To reduce the risk of phlebitis and restricted movement.

Guidelines • Inserting a peripheral cannula (cont'd)

Action	Rationale
12 Wash hands using bactericidal soap and water or bactericidal alcohol hand rub.	To minimize risk of infection.
13 Open a pack, empty all equipment onto the pack and place a sterile dressing towel under the patient's arm.	To create a sterile working area.
14 Reapply the tourniquet.	To promote venous filling.
15 Clean the patient's skin and the selected vein for at least 30 sec using an appropriate preparation and allow to dry. Do not repalpate the vein or touch the skin.	To maintain asepsis and remove skin flora.
16 Remove needle guard and inspect the device for any faults.	To detect faulty equipment, e.g. bent or barbed needles. If these are present, discard them.
17 Anchor the vein by applying manual traction on the skin a few centimeters below the proposed site of insertion.	To immobilize the vein. To provide countertension, which will facilitate a smooth needle entry.
18 Ensure the cannula is in the bevel-up position and place the device directly over the vein; insert the cannula through the skin at the selected angle according to the depth of the vein.	To ensure a successful, pain-free cannulation.
19 Wait for the first flashback of blood in the flashback chamber of the stylet.	To indicate that the needle has entered the vein.
20 Level the device by decreasing the angle between the cannula and the skin and advance the cannula slightly to ensure entry into the lumen of the vein.	To avoid advancing too far through the vein wall and causing damage to the vein wall. To stabilize the device.
21 Withdraw the stylet slightly and a second flashback of blood will be seen along the shaft of the cannula.	To ensure that the cannula is still in a patent vein. This is called the hooded technique.
22 Maintaining skin traction with the non-dominant hand, and using the dominant hand, slowly advance the cannula off the stylet and into the vein.	To ensure the vein remains immobilized and thus reducing the risk of a 'through puncture'.
23 Release the tourniquet.	To decrease the pressure within the vein.
24 Apply digital pressure to the vein above the cannula tip and remove the stylet.	To prevent blood spillage.
25 Immediately dispose of the stylet into an appropriate sharps container.	To reduce the risk of accidental needlestick injury.
26 Attach an injection cap, extension set or administration set and flush.	To ensure patency.
27 Observe the site for signs of swelling or leakage, and ask the patient if any discomfort or pain is felt.	To check that the device is positioned correctly.
28 Tape the cannula using the method illustrated in Fig. 44.1.	To ensure the device will remain stable and secure.
29 Cover with low-linting swabs and bandage firmly.	To ensure patient comfort and security of device.
30 Discard waste, making sure it is placed in appropriate containers.	To ensure safe disposal in the correct containers and avoid laceration or injury of other staff. To prevent re-use of equipment.

GUIDELINES • Inserting a midline catheter

Equipment

1 Sterile minor operation pack.
2 Sterile powder-free gloves.
3 Alcohol-based hand scrub.
4 Alcohol-based skin cleansing preparation, e.g. chlorhexidine in 70% alcohol.
5 Extension set and intermittent injection cap.
6 Sterile low-linting dressing.

7 Hypoallergenic tape.
8 Midline catheter.
9 Introducer.
10 Transparent dressing and sterile tapes.
11 10-ml syringes.
12 0.9% sodium chloride.
13 Tape measure.

Procedure

Action

1 Explain and discuss the procedure with the patient.

2 Apply tourniquet and assess venous access, assessing both limbs, and locate veins by sight and palpation.

3 Apply local anaesthetic cream/gel to chosen venepuncture site and leave for alloted time.

4 Draw screens and position patient in a comfortable position.

5 Measure using the tape measure from the selected venepuncture site up the extremity, to just below the axilla.

6 Take equipment required to patient's bedside. Open outer pack.

7 Wash hands using a bactericidal hand rub.

8 Put on powder-free sterile gloves; open sterile pack, arranging the contents as required. Prefill the syringe with 0.9% sodium chloride.

9 Remove the cap from the extension set and attach 0.9% sodium chloride; gently flush with 2 ml and leave syringe attached.

10 If the catheter tip can be trimmed, using the graduated markings along the catheter, select the marking required and pull back guidewire 1 cm from desired new tip, and using sterile scissors trim the catheter. *Never trim the guidewire!*

11 Place sterile towel under patient's arm.

12 Cleanse the skin at the selected site with an appropriate disinfectant, e.g. chlorhexidine in 70% alcohol, using concentric circles with friction and prepare an area of 15–25 cm.

13 Allow the solution to dry thoroughly.

14 Drape the patient with a fenestrated towel.

Rationale

To ensure that the patient understands the procedure and gives his/her valid consent.

To ensure the patient has adequate venous access and to select the vein for catheterization.

To minimize the pain of insertion.

To ensure privacy. To aid insertion and correct placement.

To enable selection of the most suitable catheter length and to know how far to advance the catheter in order for its tip to be located in the correct position.

To minimize the risk of infection.

To prevent contamination. Powder on gloves can increase the risk of mechanical phlebitis.

To check that the catheter is patent and to enable easy removal of guidewire.

To ensure the catheter will be the correct length for placement and to prevent damage to the vein if the guidewire is damaged.

To provide a sterile field to work on.

To ensure skin flora is destroyed and to minimize the risk of infection.

To ensure coagulation of bacteria and completion of disinfection process.

To provide a sterile field.

Guidelines • Inserting a midline catheter (cont'd)

Action	Rationale
15 Inject local anaesthetic if required using a 25-g needle to area intradermally and wait for a few minutes for it to take effect.	To enable adequate anaesthesia.
16 Reapply tourniquet.	To aid venous distension.
17 Perform venepuncture with introducer by entering the skin, 1 cm from desired point of entry, at a 15–30° angle. Advance 0.5–1 cm once flashback is seen.	To gain venous access.
18 Release tourniquet.	To prevent blood loss, 'through puncture' and enable advancement of catheter.
19 Position fingers in a V, with index finger on wings and middle finger above sheath tip, and gently remove stylet. Apply pressure.	To contain flashback, prevent contamination of the area with blood and minimize the amount of blood loss from patient.
20 Grip catheter 1 cm from the tip and thread through an introducer sheath.	To ensure tip is not contaminated.
21 Continue slow advancement of the catheter to the desired length.	To minimize damage to intima of vein.
22 Apply pressure above introducer and carefully withdraw the introducer and peel apart.	To ensure there is no movement of the catheter. To remove peel-away introducer.
23 Aspirate for blood return and flush catheter with 0.9% sodium chloride.	To check patency of device and ensure continued patency.
24 Apply gentle pressure on catheter and slowly withdraw the guidewire.	To ensure there is no withdrawal of catheter.
25 Attach an injectable cap and flush as per midline guidelines.	To ensure patency of the device.
26 Secure the catheter with sterile tape or other securing device. Apply a transparent dressing. Apply gauze and a bandage.	To ensure stability of device and protection of the site.
27 Dispose of equipment appropriately.	Dispose of sharps and clinical waste.
28 Document the procedure in the patient's notes: type, length and gauge of cannula, where it was inserted, any problem, how it was secured.	To ensure adequate records and enable continued care of device and patient.

GUIDELINES • Inserting a peripherally inserted central catheter (PICC)

Equipment

1 Sterile minor operations pack.
2 Sterile powder-free gloves.
3 Alcohol-based hand scrub.
4 Alcohol-based skin cleansing preparation, e.g. chlorhexidine in 70% alcohol.
5 Extension set and intermittent injection cap.
6 Sterile low-linting dressing.

7 Hypoallergenic tape.
8 Peripherally inserted central catheter.
9 Introducer.
10 Transparent dressing and sterile tapes.
11 10-ml syringes.
12 0.9% sodium chloride.
13 Tape measure.

Procedure

Action	Rationale
1 Gain consent from physician and assess patient's medical and IV device history.	To ensure the patient has no underlying medical problems and is suitable to undergo the procedure.

2 Explain and discuss the procedure with the patient.

To ensure that the patient understands the procedure and gives his/her valid written consent.

3 Apply tourniquet and assess venous access, assessing both extremities, and locate veins by sight and palpation.

To ensure the patient has adequate venous access and to select the vein for catheterization.

4 Apply local anaesthetic cream/gel to chosen venepuncture site and leave for alloted time.

To minimize the pain of insertion.

5 Draw screens and position patient in a supine position, with patient's arm at a 45° angle, with ability to move arm to a 90° angle.

To ensure privacy. To aid insertion of introducer and then advancement of catheter.

6 Measure using the tape measure from the selected venepuncture site up the extremity, curve at shoulder to the suprasternal notch and then down to third intercostal space (Fig. 44.14).

To enable selection of the most suitable catheter length and to establish how far to advance the catheter in order for its tip to be located in the correct position, i.e. the SVC.

7 Take equipment required to patient's bedside. Open outer pack.

To ensure appropriate equipment is available for procedure.

8 Wash hands using a bactericidal hand rub.

To minimize the risk of infection.

9 Put on sterile gown and powder-free sterile gloves; open sterile tray, arranging the contents as required. Prefill the syringe with 0.9% sodium chloride.

To prevent contamination. Powder on gloves can increase the risk of mechanical phlebitis.

10 Remove the cap from the extension set and attach 0.9% sodium chloride; gently flush with 2 ml and leave syringe attached.

To check that the catheter is patent and to enable easy removal of guidewire.

11 If the catheter tip can be trimmed, using the graduated markings along the catheter, select the marking required and pull back guidewire 1 cm from desired new tip, and using sterile scissors trim the catheter. *Never trim the guidewire!*

To ensure the catheter will be the correct length for SVC tip placement and to prevent damage to the vein if the guidewire is damaged.

12 Place sterile towel under patient's arm.

To provide a sterile field to work on.

13 Cleanse the skin at the selected site with an appropriate disinfectant, e.g. chlorhexidine in 70% alcohol, using concentric circles with friction and prepare an area of 15–25 cm.

To ensure the removal of skin flora and to minimize the risk of infection.

14 Allow the solution to dry thoroughly.

To ensure coagulation of bacteria and disinfection.

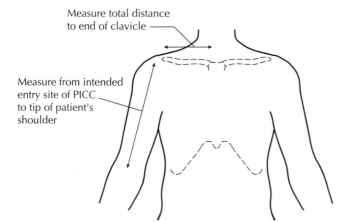

Measure total distance to end of clavicle

Measure from intended entry site of PICC to tip of patient's shoulder

Figure 44.14 Pre-insertion measurement of PICC.

Guidelines • Inserting a peripherally inserted central catheter (PICC) (cont'd)

Action	Rationale
15 Drape the patient with a fenestrated towel.	To provide a sterile field.
16 Inject local anaesthetic if required using a 25-g needle to area intradermally and wait a few minutes for it to take effect.	To enable adequate anaesthesia.
17 Reapply tourniquet.	To aid venous distension.
18 Perform venepuncture with introducer by entering the skin, 1 cm from desired point of entry, at a 15–30° angle. Advance 0.5–1 cm once flashback is seen.	To gain venous access.
19 Release tourniquet.	To prevent blood loss, 'through puncture' and enable advancement of catheter.
20 Position fingers in a V, with index finger on wings and middle finger above sheath tip, and gently remove stylet. Apply pressure.	To contain flashback, prevent contamination of the area with blood and minimize the amount of blood loss from the patient.
21 Grip catheter 1 cm from the tip and thread through introducer sheath.	
22 Ask the patient (assisted) to move the arm to a 90° angle.	To enable further advancement of catheter.
23 Turn patient's head toward the arm being cannulated and place the chin on the chest if possible.	To prevent the catheter entering the jugular veins and to ensure correct advancement of catheter downward to the SVC.
24 Continue slow advancement of the catheter to the desired length.	To minimize damage to intima of vein.
25 Apply pressure above introducer and carefully withdraw the introducer and peel apart.	To ensure there is no movement of the catheter. To remove peel-away introducer.
26 Aspirate for blood return and flush catheter with 0.9% sodium chloride.	To check patency of device and ensure continued patency.
27 Apply gentle pressure on catheter and slowly withdraw the guidewire.	To ensure there is no withdrawal of catheter.
28 Attach an injectable cap and flush as per PICC guidelines.	To ensure patency of the device.
29 Secure the catheter with sterile tape or other securing device. Apply a transparent dressing. Apply gauze and a bandage.	To ensure stability of device and protection of the site.
30 Dispose of equipment appropriately.	Dispose of sharps and clinical waste.
31 Send patient for chest X-ray. Position of catheter to be assessed by the doctor.	To allow position of tip to be assessed. To ensure correct tip location.
32 Document the procedure in the patient's notes: type, length and gauge of cannula, where it was inserted, tip confirmation, any problem, how it was secured and patient education.	To ensure adequate records and enable continued care of device and patient.

Removal

Action	Rationale
1 Wash hands using a bactericidal hand rub and gather equipment required (dressing pack, dressing, tape).	To minimize the risk of infection.
2 Remove transparent dressing and gently remove sterile tapes.	To prepare for catheter removal.

	Action	Rationale
3	Apply a pair of gloves and, using a steady and constant motion, gently pull catheter until completely removed from exit site.	To remove the catheter and prevent vein damage.
4	Apply digital pressure over exit site for about 2–3 min or until bleeding stops, and apply dressing.	To minimize blood loss and bruising. To provide protection of the entry site.
5	Check marking of length removed and check it is same as the length inserted. Document.	To ensure that complete catheter has been removed.

GUIDELINES • Changing the dressing on a central venous catheter insertion site

Before commencing the procedure it is important to check whether there is a variation to standard technique for individual patients, e.g. those receiving total parenteral nutrition, children.

Equipment

1 Sterile dressing pack.
2 Clamp for the catheter, if necessary.
3 Alcohol-based hand rub.
4 Alcohol-based skin cleansing preparation, e.g. chlorhexidine in 70% alcohol.
5 Intravenous administration set and extension set or intermittent injection cap.
6 Sterile low-linting dressing.
7 Hypoallergenic tape.
8 Bacteriological swab.

Procedure

	Action	Rationale
1	Explain and discuss the procedure with the patient.	To ensure that the patient understands the procedure and gives his/her valid consent.
2	Perform the dressing using an aseptic technique.	To prevent infection. (For further information on asepsis, see Chap. 3, Aseptic Technique.)
3	Screen the bed. Assist the patient into a supine position, if possible.	To allow dust and airborne organisms to settle before the insertion site and the sterile field are exposed. To help prevent air embolus.
4	Wash hands with bactericidal soap and water or bactericidal alcohol hand rub. Place all equipment required for the dressing on the bottom shelf of a clean dressing trolley.	To reduce the risk of cross-infection.
5	Prime the administration set, keeping the Luer lock sterile.	So that the infusion is ready for use when the current administration set is discontinued.
6	Take the trolley to the patient's bedside, disturbing the screens as little as possible.	To minimize airborne contamination.
7	Open the outer cover of the sterile dressing pack and slide the contents onto the top shelf of the trolley..	
8	Open the sterile field using the corners of the paper only. Using the forceps in the pack, arrange the sterile field with the handles of the instruments in one corner.	So that areas of potential contamination are kept to a minimum.
9	Attach a yellow clinical waste bag to the side of the trolley below the level of the top shelf.	So that contaminated material is below the level of the sterile field.
10	Open the other sterile packs, tipping their contents gently onto the centre of the sterile field. Pour lotions into gallipots or an indented plastic tray.	To reduce risk of contamination of contents.

Guidelines • Changing the dressing on a central venous catheter insertion site (cont'd)

Action	Rationale
11 Wash hands with bactericidal alcohol hand rub.	Hands may have become contaminated by handling the outer packs, etc.
12 Loosen the old dressing gently, touching only the tape, etc. securing it.	So that the dressing can be lifted off easily with the forceps.
13 Put on clean gloves.	To protect the nurse from any contact with the patient's blood.
14 Using gloved hands or forceps, remove the old dressing and discard it, together with the forceps into the yellow clinical waste bag.	
15 If the site is red or discharging, take a swab for bacteriological investigation.	For identification of pathogens. To predict colonization of the site.
16 Clean gloved hands with bactericidal alcohol hand rub.	To minimize the risk of introducing infection.
17 Clean the wound with chlorhexidine in 70% alcohol as necessary, working from the inside to the outside of the area and dealing with the cleanest parts of the wound first. Allow area to dry prior to applying the dressing.	To minimize the risk of infection spread from a 'dirty' to a 'clean' area. To enable disinfection process to be completed.
18 Apply appropriate dressing, moulding it into place so that there are no folds or creases.	To minimize skin irritation and reduce risk of dressing peeling or becoming damaged.
19 Remove gloves.	
20 Discontinue the infusion in progress. Clamp the catheter using the clamp supplied or a smooth clamp if the catheter is of silicone, or artery forceps over sterile topical swabs if it is of plastic.	To prevent entry of air or leakage of blood when the catheter is disconnected. Silicone is easily damaged so swabs prevent cracking of the catheter by artery forceps.
21 Either (a) put on gloves or (b) clean hands with bactericidal alcohol hand rub.	(a) Where potential spillage of patient's blood or certain drugs may occur, e.g. cytotoxics and (b) to minimize the risk of introducing infection into the catheter after handling unsterile parts of the system.
22 Clean connections thoroughly with chlorhexidine in 70% alcohol before disconnection. Allow to dry.	To minimize infection risk at the connection site. To enable disinfection process to be completed and to prevent skin irritation.
23 Disconnect the catheter from the old administration set and connect the prepared new set. Check that no air bubbles are present in the system. Unclamp the catheter and continue infusion. Where no clamping of the catheter is possible, the Valsalva manoeuvre should be used.	To reduce the risk of air embolism.
24 Tape the extension set into a position comfortable for the patient, and attend to his/her general comfort.	To ensure the patient's comfort and to minimize the risk of accidentally dislodging the catheter.
25 Open the roller clamp and set the rate of the infusion.	To ensure the correct rate.
26 Alternatively, attach a Luer lock intermittent injection cap and flush the catheter, and extension set, if continuous infusion is not required (see Maintaining patency, below).	To maintain a patent catheter for intermittent use.
27 Fold up the sterile field, place it in the yellow clinical waste bag and seal it before moving the trolley. Draw back the curtains. Dispose of waste in appropriate containers.	To prevent environmental contamination.

GUIDELINES • Maintaining patency of a central venous access device

This is a simple procedure which may be performed after each use or once weekly (or less frequently in some circumstances) when no therapy is necessary. For implantable ports the procedure requires accessing the port and flushing once a month (see Guidelines).

Equipment

1 Flushing solution ready prepared in a 5-ml syringe, with a 23-g needle attached, in a clinically clean container.

2 Chlorhexidine in 70% alcohol/swab saturated with 70% isopropyl alcohol.

Procedure

Action	Rationale
1 Explain and discuss the procedure with the patient.	To ensure that the patient understands the procedure and gives his/her valid consent.
2 Wash hands thoroughly or use an alcohol-based hand rub.	To reduce the risk of contamination.
3 Swab the injection cap with chlorhexidine in 70% alcohol/swab saturated with 70% isopropyl alcohol and allow to dry.	To minimize the risk of contamination at the connections.
4 Remove the needle and attach the syringe to the needleless injection cap or insert the needle into an injectable cap.	To establish connection between cap and syringe.
5 Using a push–pause method (inject 1 ml at a time), inject the contents of the syringe.	To create turbulence in order to flush the catheter thoroughly.
6 Clamp the catheter while injecting the final 0.5 ml of solution.	To maintain positive pressure and prevent back-flow of blood into the catheter, and possible clot formation.
7 Where required, remove needle from injectable cap and dispose of equipment safely.	To reduce the risk of needlestick injury to the practitioner.
8 Demonstrate the procedure clearly and methodically.	To ensure the patient is aware of each step, and the need for good hand washing/drying techniques, etc. as he/she may be performing this procedure on discharge.

GUIDELINES • Taking blood samples from a central venous catheter

Care should be taken when obtaining blood samples from a central venous catheter as inaccurate laboratory results may be reported, especially coagulation values (Pinto 1994). The proximal lumen of a multi-lumen catheter is the preferred site

1 The discard method – this is the standard accepted method (recommended by The Royal Marsden Hospital) where the first 6–10 ml of blood is withdrawn and discarded (Cella & Watson 1989). This ensures removal of any heparin or saline solution but may result in excessive blood removal in small children or those requiring multiple samples, e.g. for pharmacokinetic tests.
2 Push–pull/mixing method – a syringe is attached to the catheter and the catheter is flushed with 0.9% sodium chlo-

Whichever method is used, once the samples have been taken it is vital that the catheter is adequately flushed with sodium chloride to reduce the risk of clot formation and subsequent infection and/or occlusion.

from which to obtain the sample, and all infusions should be stopped prior to obtaining the sample. A number of methods may be used to withdraw samples:

ride and then 6 ml is withdrawn and pushed back without removing the syringe; this is repeated three times. This removes any residual solution and reduces exposure to blood and there is no blood wastage (Perucca 1995; Holmes 1998).
3 Reinfusion method – some units may take the first 6 ml of blood, cap off the syringe, take the samples and then reinfuse the blood first taken (Keller 1994).

Double- or triple-lumen catheters are now inserted routinely. Where these catheters have different-sized lumens, the largest should be reserved where possible for blood products and blood sampling only, as this will provide the easiest route for viscous solutions.

Guidelines • Taking blood samples from a central venous catheter (cont'd)

Equipment

1 Sterile dressing pack.
2 Clamp for catheter, if necessary.
3 Alcohol-based hand wash solution.
4 Extra 10-ml blood bottle without heparin or sterile 10-ml syringe.
5 Vacuum system container holder (shell).
Vacuum system adaptor.
Appropriate vacuumed blood bottles.
or
Sterile syringe of appropriate size for sample required.

6 Intermittent injection cap.
7 10-ml syringe of 0.9% sodium chloride.
8 Flushing solution, as per policy.

Procedure

Action	*Rationale*
1 Explain and discuss the procedure with the patient.	To ensure that the patient understands the procedure and gives his/her valid consent.
2 Perform procedure using an aseptic technique.	To reduce the risk of infection. (For further information on asepsis, see Chap. 3, Aseptic Technique.)
3 Wash hands with bactericidal soap and water or bactericidal alcohol hand rub.	To reduce the risk of cross-infection.
4 Prepare a tray or trolley and take it to the bedside. Cleanse hands as above. Open sterile pack and prepare equipment.	To reduce the risk of contamination of contents.
5 If intravenous fluid infusion is in progress, switch it off.	
6 Clamp the catheter with the clamp supplied or move catheter 'on/off' switch to 'off'.	To prevent entry of air or leakage of blood via the catheter.
7 Wash hands with a bactericidal alcohol hand rub. Put on non-sterile gloves. Clean hub thoroughly with chlorhexidine. Allow to dry.	To minimize the risk of introducing infection into the catheter, and prevent contamination of practitioner's hands with blood. To enable disinfection process to be completed.
8 Disconnect the administration set from the catheter and cover the end of the set with the syringe cover or remove the injection cap and discard (if a needleless injection cap is in use, it does not require removal).	To reduce the risk of contaminating the end of the administration set.
9 For vacuum sampling:	
(a) Attach vacuum container holder and adaptor and release clamp. Attach extra sample bottle: fill and discard.	To remove blood, heparin and intravenous fluids from the 'dead space' of the catheter. Samples from this 'dead space' are likely to cause inaccuracies in blood tests, because of the risk of contamination of the sample with heparin, sodium or dextrose, etc.
(b) Attach required sample bottles for requested specimens.	To obtain sample. It is not necessary to clamp the catheter when changing collection bottles, as the system is not open.
(c) Re-clamp catheter and detach vacuum container holder.	To prevent blood loss or air embolism.
10 For syringe sampling:	
(a) Attach a 10-ml syringe to the catheter. Release the clamp and withdraw 5–10 ml of blood.	To remove blood, heparin and intravenous fluids from the 'dead space' of the catheter. Samples from this 'dead space' are likely to cause inaccuracies in blood tests.
(b) Re-clamp the catheter and discard the sample and syringe.	
(c) Attach a new syringe of appropriate size. Release the clamp and withdraw the required amount of blood.	To obtain the sample.
(d) Re-clamp the catheter and detach the syringe.	To prevent blood loss or air embolism.

11 Flush with 10 ml 0.9% sodium chloride, using the push–pause method (i.e. 1 ml at a time).

To create turbulence and ensure removal of all blood in the catheter and prevent occlusion.

12 Reconnect the administration set, unclamp the catheter and recommence infusion or attach new intermittent injection cap. Release clamp and flush catheter through injection cap using the push–pause method and finishing with the positive pressure technique.

To prevent the catheter clotting in between uses.

13 Ensure that blood samples have been placed in the correct containers and agitated as necessary to prevent clotting. Label them with patient's name, number, etc. and send them to the laboratory with the appropriate forms.

To make certain that the specimens, correctly presented and identified, are delivered to the laboratory, enabling the requested tests to be performed and the results returned to the correct patient's records.

Difficulty may be encountered when taking blood samples. This is particularly true when the central catheter is made of silicone and has been in place for a period of time. The main cause is that the tip of the soft catheter lies against the wall of the vessel and the suction required to draw blood brings this into close contact, leading to temporary occlusion. There could also be a collapse of vein walls when using the vacuum system which may necessitate the use of syringes to obtain the blood.

Measures to try to dislodge the tip include asking the patient to:

1 Cough and breathe deeply.
2 Roll from side to side.

3 Raise his/her arms.
4 Perform the Valsalva manoeuvre, if possible.
5 Increase general activity, e.g. walk up and down stairs.

The tip of the catheter may be covered in a fibrin sheath. This may be resolved with rapid flushing of the catheter with 0.9% sodium chloride or a dilute solution of heparin. Occasionally this results in persistent withdrawal occlusion (PWO) and may require a fibrinolytic agent, e.g. alteplase to remove the fibrin (Richard Alexander 1994; Mayo 1998). However, it may be necessary to take blood from a peripheral vein (see Chap. 45, Venepuncture).

GUIDELINES • Unblocking an occluded catheter

Catheters may become occluded for a number of reasons, e.g. not being flushed adequately or using the incorrect technique, infusion being switched off or running too slowly, precipitation formation due to inadequate flushing between solutions/drugs. Clearance of a catheter occlusion is best performed using a negative pressure approach. The establishment of negative pressure within a catheter means creating a vacuum by aspiration of the air or dead space within a catheter (Moureau et al. 1999).

Equipment

1 Sterile dressing pack.
2 Clamp for the catheter, if necessary.
3 Bactericidal hand rub.
4 Alcohol-based skin cleansing preparation, e.g. chlorhexidine in 70% alcohol.

5 Extension set or intermittent injection cap.
6 10-ml syringes.
7 0.9% sodium chloride.
8 Three-way tap.
9 Heparin 50 IU in a saline solution.

Procedure

Action

1 Explain and discuss the procedure with the patient.

2 Perform the procedure using an aseptic technique.

3 Wash hands with bactericidal soap and water or bactericidal alcohol hand rub. Place all equipment required on bottom shelf.

Rationale

To ensure that the patient understands the procedure and gives his/her valid consent.

To minimize the risk of infection. (For further information on asepsis, see Chap. 3, Aseptic Technique.)

To minimize the risk of cross-infection.

Guidelines • *Unblocking an occluded catheter (cont'd)*

Action	Rationale
4 Open a sterile pack and empty other equipment onto it.	To create a clean working area.
5 Wash hands with bactericidal alcohol hand rub.	Hands may have become contaminated by handling the outer packs, etc.
6 Clean connections thoroughly with chlorhexidine in 70% alcohol before disconnection.	To minimize infection risk at connection site.
7 Remove any extension sets or injection caps.	Occlusion may be in extension set/cap and not in catheter.
8 Attempt to flush with 0.9% sodium chloride using a 10-ml syringe.	Smaller syringes create excessive pressure which could result in catheter rupture.
9 If there is a pressure within the catheter lumen, attempt to gently instil the 0.9% sodium chloride using a 'to and fro' motion (push–pull) over a few minutes.	To attempt to clear the catheter.
10 If nothing can be aspirated, attach a three way tap and to this add an empty 10-ml syringe and a 10-ml syringe containing heparin 50 IU in 5 ml saline.	To commence the negative pressure technique (see Fig. 44.15a).
11 Attempt to unblock catheter using the negative pressure technique (see Fig. 44.15b,c)	This enables the solution to be drawn into catheter without creating any pressure which could result in catheter rupture.

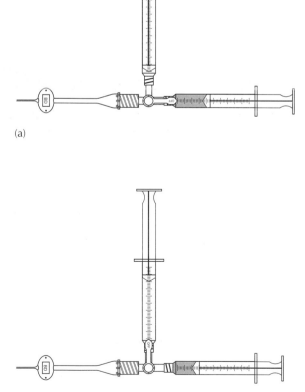

(a)

(c)

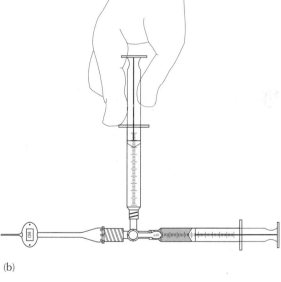

(b)

Figure 44.15 Unblocking an occluded catheter. (a) Turn tap to close off prefilled syringe and open it to empty syringe. (b) Aspirate on empty syringe, which creates a negative pressure. (c) Turn tap to close off empty syringe and open to prefilled syringe. The medication will automatically be aspirated into the catheter and repeat as necessary. (Modified from BD First PICC Clinical Education Class Manual D11952B 5/98.)

Action	Rationale
12 If still unable to aspirate, then determine the cause of the occlusion:	
(a) Blood – discuss with doctors who may prescribe alteplase.	To break down fibrin.
(b) Precipitation – discuss with pharmacy for best antidote, e.g. ethyl alcohol or hydrochloric acid.	To break down drug precipitate or fat emulsion.
13 Draw up prescribed solution.	To prepare appropriate treatment.
14 Clean gloved hands with bactericidal alcohol hand rub.	To minimize the risk of introducing infection.
15 Instil via a three way tap using negative pressure technique (see above).	To prevent catheter rupture.
16 Cap off catheter and leave for allotted time, e.g. alteplase for up to an hour or overnight.	To allow the drug to destroy fibrin.
17 Attach an empty syringe to catheter and attempt to aspirate any clots and solution.	To unblock catheter and ensure no clots are administered into the patient.
18 If blood returns, withdraw at least 10 ml and discard.	To ensure no alteplase or clots are flushed into patient.
19 Flush catheter with 10 ml 0.9% sodium chloride using a pulsatile flush and then flush with heparinized saline.	To ensure the catheter is flushed and patent.
20 Dispose of waste.	To prevent contamination of others.
21 If still unable to aspirate, discuss the use of a second instillation of alteplase. It may be necessary to remove the catheter if a single lumen or if multi-lumen, to refrain from using the occluded lumen.	To maintain some venous access for patient. If occlusion cannot be removed the catheter is no longer patent. In multi-lumen catheters there may be another patent lumen for use.

GUIDELINES • Insertion and removal of non-coring needles in implantable ports

Placement of a non-coring point needle into the implantable port should be performed by a doctor or by nurses who have been taught and assessed as being competent. The needle may be connected to an extension set and a Luer lock injection cap placed at the end of this. The needle and extension set remain in position for 7 days and will then be changed, if required, after that time.

Equipment

1 Plastic apron.
2 Sterile gloves.
3 Dressing pack.
4 10 ml Luer lock syringes containing 0.9% sodium chloride × 2.
5 21 g non-coring (Huber point) needle with extension set.
6 Chlorhexidine in 70% alcohol.
7 Heparinized saline (100 IU in 1 ml) in 10 ml Luer lock syringe.
8 Plaster.

Procedure

Action

1 Explain and discuss the procedure with the patient.

2 If required, apply topical local anaesthetic cream for 30–60 min.

3 Place the patient in a comfortable position.

Rationale

To ensure the patient understands the procedure and gives his/her valid consent.

To reduce the feeling of pain on insertion of the needle.

Guidelines • Insertion and removal of non-coring needles in implantable ports (cont'd)

Action	Rationale
4 Locate the port and identify the septum; assess the depth of the port and thickness of the skin.	In order to select correct length of needle.
5 Check length and type of therapy.	In order to select correct gauge and configuration of needle.
6 Wash hands using a bactericidal hand soap or rub.	To minimize the risk of contamination.
7 Put on sterile gloves.	To minimize the risk of contamination.
8 Flush port needle and extension set with 0.9% sodium chloride.	To check patency of needle and set.
9 Clean the skin over the port with chlorhexidine 70% alcohol in a circular pattern.	To minimize the risk of contamination and destroy skin flora.
10 Holding the needle in the dominant hand, stabilize the port between the forefinger and index finger of the non-dominant hand (see Fig. 44.16).	To ensure the port is stabilized and will not move on insertion of the needle.
11 Inform the patient you are about to insert the needle.	To prepare the patient for a pushing sensation.
12 Using a perpendicular angle, push the needle through the skin until the needle hits the back plate.	To ensure the needle is well inserted into the portal septum.
13 Draw back on the syringe and check for blood return.	To check the needle is correctly placed and the port is patent.
14 Flush with 0.9% sodium chloride and observe the site for any swelling or pain.	To check for patency and correct positioning.

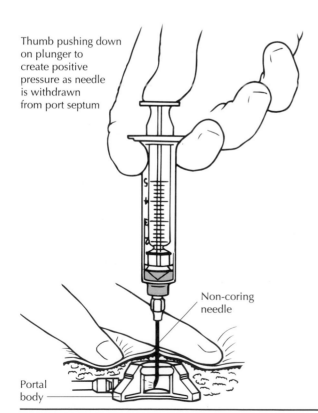

Thumb pushing down on plunger to create positive pressure as needle is withdrawn from port septum

Non-coring needle

Portal body

Figure 44.16 Flushing a port.

15 Administer the drug as required.	To carry out instructions as per prescription.
16 Flush with 10 ml 0.9% sodium chloride.	To ensure all of the drug is administered.
17 If the needle is to remain in situ, attach an injection cap and flush with heparinized saline using a pulsatile flush and ending with positive pressure.	To maintain patency.
18 Secure the needle by placing gauze under the needle if necessary and cover with transparent dressing.	To ensure the needle is well supported and will not become dislodged.
19 If needle is to be removed, then heparinize using 500 IU heparin in 5 ml 0.9% sodium chloride.	To maintain patency over a longer period of time, e.g. 1 month.
20 Clamp extension set while still maintaining positive pressure (i.e. keep thumb on syringe plunger).	To prevent back-flow of blood and possible clot formation.
21 Press down on either side of the portal of the implantable port with two fingers.	To support the port while removing the needle.
22 Withdraw the needle using steady traction (see Fig. 44.15).	To prevent trauma to the skin.
23 No dressing is usually required, but a small plaster may be applied.	To prevent oozing.

GUIDELINES • Removal of a non-skin tunnelled central venous catheter

Equipment

As for Guidelines • Changing the dressing on a central venous catheter insertion site (items 1–8; see page 641) plus:

9 Sterile scissors.
10 Small sterile specimen container.
11 Stitch cutter.

12 Additional sterile low-linting gauze swab (a new administration set, etc. is not required).

Procedure

Place patient flat in the Trendelenberg position, i.e. head slightly lower than feet (to prevent air entering vein on catheter removal) and then proceed as for a dressing procedure, steps 1–15 (pages 641–2); then continue as follows:

Action	*Rationale*
16 Clean the insertion site.	To prevent contamination of the catheter on removal, and a false-positive culture result.
17 Discontinue the infusion, if in progress. Clamp the catheter as previously described or move the catheter 'on/off' switch to 'off'.	To prevent entry of air or leakage of blood when the catheter is disconnected.
18 Clean gloved hands with a bactericidal alcohol hand rub.	To minimize the risk of infection after handling unsterile parts of the system.
19 Cut and remove any skin suture securing the catheter.	To facilitate removal.
20 Disconnect the catheter from the remainder of the infusion system.	To ease handling and removal.
21 Ask the patient to perform the Valsalva manoeuvre.	To reduce the risk of air embolus.
22 Cover the insertion site with a thick pad of several sterile topical swabs.	Swabs are used to discourage the entry of organisms into the insertion site and to absorb any leakage of blood.

Guidelines • Removal of a non-skin tunnelled central venous catheter (cont'd)

Action	Rationale
23 Hold the catheter with one hand near the point of insertion and pull firmly and gently. As the catheter begins to move, press firmly down on the site with the swabs. Maintain pressure on the swabs for about 5 min after the catheter has been removed.	Pressure is applied to prevent haemorrhage and to encourage resealing of the vein wall. It also prevents the entry of air into the vein. Continued pressure is necessary to allow time for the puncture in the vein to close.
24 When bleeding has stopped (approximately 5 min), cover site with transparent dressing.	To detect any infection at exit site. To prevent air entering the vein via the site.
25 If the catheter is removed because of infection, carefully cut off the tip (approximately 5 cm) of the catheter using sterile scissors and place it in a sterile container for microbiological investigation.	To detect any infection related to the catheter, and thus provide necessary treatment.
26 Fold up the sterile field, place it in the yellow clinical waste bag and seal it before moving the trolley. Dispose of the equipment in the appropriate containers.	To reduce the risk of environmental contamination.
27 Make the patient comfortable.	

This procedure may be adapted for removal of a skin-tunnelled catheter.

GUIDELINES • Surgical removal of a skin-tunnelled central venous catheter

Equipment

1 Plastic apron.
2 Sterile gloves.
3 Minor operations set.
4 10-ml Luer lock syringe.
5 25-g needle.
6 21-g needle.

7 10-ml plain lignocaine 1%.
8 10×10 cm low-linting gauze swabs $\times 5$.
9 3/0 Mersilk suture on a curved needle.
10 2-cm hypoallergenic tape.
11 Chlorhexidine in 70% alcohol.
12 Steristrips (to be used if necessary).

Procedure

Action

Rationale

Action	Rationale
1 Check the patient's full blood count and clotting profile for that day.	To ensure that the patient is not at risk of bleeding or infection from this invasive procedure. The platelets should be above 100×10^9/litre, the white blood count >2 and the international normalized ratio (INR) <1.3.
2 Explain and discuss the procedure with the patient.	To ensure that the patient understands the procedure and gives his/her valid consent.
3 Screen the bed and ask patient to remove clothing down to the waist.	To ensure ease of access to the patient's chest.
4 Ask patient to lie as flat as possible with his or her arms by his/her sides.	To minimize the risk of bleeding from gravitational pressure and to dissuade the patient from touching the sterile field.
5 Palpate and identify the position of the cuff in the patient.	To locate the area for the incision.
6 If the cuff cannot easily be felt, measure 22 cm up from the bifurcation at the end of the catheter distal to the patient (see Fig. 44.4), then palpate again. If it still cannot be felt ask for assistance.	To locate the probable site of the cuff. To guard against malplaced incisions.
7 Open the outer bag of the minor operation pack. Put on plastic apron and wash hands, then dry hands on sterile towel provided in the pack.	To reduce risk of infection.

8 Accept and put on sterile gloves from assistant and assemble all necessary equipment on the sterile pack.

To maintain asepsis and to prepare for the procedure and maximize efficiency.

9 Advise the patient that you will explain each step of the procedure as you go along if the patient wishes.

This should take into account the patient's individual wish for information.

10 Clean the area directly over the cuff with swabs soaked in chlorhexidine in 70% alcohol. Use a circular motion working out from the centre directly over the cuff. Allow the area to dry.

To reduce the risk of infection. To enable disinfection process to be completed. To prevent stinging on insertion of the needle.

11 Position the two sterile towels – one horizontally across the waist and the other longitudinally down the side of the patient between yourself and the patient.

To create a sterile field to operate within and therefore reduce the risk of infection.

12 Inform the patient that you are about to administer the local anaesthetic and that this will cause a stinging sensation.

To prepare the patient. The first injection can be painful and causes a stinging sensation.

13 With a 25-g needle, administer the first millilitre of local anaesthetic subcutaneously directly over the cuff site causing a raised bleb.

To commence the numbing of the area to be incised. To provide a raised area for the next injection and identification of the site.

14 Give a further 1 ml of local anaesthetic subcutaneously using the bleb as the area for the insertion of the needle, but directing the needle out and around the area of the cuff site area.

To reduce pain for the patient with repeated injections. To ensure all the incision area is numb.

15 Attach the 21-g needle and with the last remaining 4 ml of local anaesthetic give two deeper injections to either side of the cuff area.

To ensure anaesthesia at a deeper level during the blunt dissection around the cuff.

16 Test the area above the cuff for numbness and then make the incision over the cuff site. This should be about 2 cm in length. Ensure that the incision is through the . epidermis and dermis.

To ensure that the patient will not experience any pain. To facilitate identification and removal of the cuff. To allow access to the cuff which is situated below the dermis.

17 With one of the artery forceps, commence blunt dissection of tissue from around the cuff. At intervals place your finger into the site and feel the cuff.

To free the cuff from the surrounding fibrous tissue. To assess the mobility of the cuff.

18 Continue with blunt dissection around and under the cuff until it feels mobile.

To facilitate the loosening of the cuff.

19 With one artery forcep, clamp onto the cuff and lift it up out of the incision while looking down the incision to identify the catheter distal to the cuff.

To identify the catheter to allow the distal portion to be severed.

20 Once the catheter is clearly visible, maintaining your grip on the cuff with the forceps, cut through the full thickness with the blade. Then pull the portion of the catheter distal to the cuff out through the exit site.

To remove the distal half of the catheter below the cuff.

21 Still maintaining your grip on the cuff, gently dissect away the fibrous tissue from around the cuff and the first 5 mm of the catheter immediately above the catheter.

To free the cuff in readiness for removal of the proximal portion of the catheter.

22 Once the cuff is free, still maintaining your grip on the cuff gently and carefully peel away the thin straw-coloured tissue from the catheter with the blade.

To free the catheter from the anchoring fibrous bands to enable removal.

23 As the last bands are divided you should feel the catheter becoming free and you should be able to see the white of the catheter.

To ensure that you have completely freed the catheter for removal.

24 While holding a low-linting swab to the incision site, gently pull out the catheter and apply pressure.

To remove the catheter and be prepared to stop any bleeding.

Guidelines • Surgical removal of a skin-tunnelled central venous catheter (cont'd)

Action	Rationale
25 Close the incision with three or four sutures. Commence the first suture in the middle of the incision.	To close the incision efficiently. To ensure that the skin edges are brought together in alignment.
26 If there continues to be any bleeding, Steristrips can be applied across the incision over the sutures.	To minimize blood loss.
27 Apply a dressing and advise the patient that there might be some oozing and to reapply a dry dressing. Advise the patient that the sutures should be removed in 7 days.	To absorb any slight bleed and to maintain a clean site. To ensure that the incision has fully closed and healed.
28 Ask the patient to rest on the bed for the next 30–60 min, or longer if required.	To reduce the risk of bleeding as the patient sits or gets up.
29 Liaise with the nursing team and document the removal and findings in the nursing and medical notes.	To ensure there is good communication between all teams and a written record of the procedure.

Nursing care plan

Problem	Cause	Suggested action
Venous obstruction during advancement of midline or PICC.	Valves. Bifurcations. Scarring. Schlerosed veins. Venospasm. Patient position.	Midline or PICC can be flushed as it is advanced. Rotate patient's arm and move further round to a right angle. Check patient has not had any surgery/fractures, etc. which could cause scarring.
Malposition of PICC tip.	Incorrect measurement of patient. Abnormal anatomy. Incorrect positioning of patient.	With patients sitting upright, inject 20–50 ml 0.9% sodium chloride rapidly. If advanced too far, the catheter may need to be retracted several centimetres. If curled in a knot, the radiologist should attempt to straighten or remove it.
Mast cell activation syndrome: *Major* Generalized urticaria. Angioedema. Bronchospasm. Hypotension. Syncope. Upper airway obstruction. *Minor* Abdominal pain. Nausea and vomiting. Diarrhoea. Flushing. Conjunctivitis. Rhinitis.	Basophil mast cell system is activated by a non-antigen-dependent mechanism, 'trauma' of touch, vibrations, pressure, heat and cold.	Maintain airway, breathing and circulation; call for medical assistance.
Mechanical phlebitis (redness, warmth, inflammation, pain)	Traumatic insertion of catheter. Rapid advancement of catheter.	Apply heat to affected area as soon as phlebitis is observed. Rest and elevate the arm. Catheter may be used during this time, but the patient should be observed for improvement in symptoms. Continue heat until complete resolution (should be

		resolved within approximately 72 hours). If it does not resolve then catheter should be removed.
Dyspnoea, chest pain or cyanosis (may be slow in onset).	Hydrothorax, pneumothorax or haemothorax due to insertion technique.	Inform a doctor. Arrange for a chest X-ray. Assist with any immediate treatment and with chest drainage if necessary.
Change in pulse rate and rhythm after insertion of catheter.	Cardiac irritability.	Inform a doctor.
Dyspnoea, chest pain, tachypnoea, disorientation, cyanosis, raised CVP, coma, cardiac arrest.	Air embolism due to air entering circulation during the insertion procedure or via the catheter.	Monitor the patient. If signs or symptoms develop, clamp the catheter to prevent further air entry. Lay the patient on the left side in Trendelenburg position. Inform a doctor. Give oxygen or external cardiac compression in the event of cardiac arrest.
Change in pulse rate, rhythm, dyspnoea, cyanosis, cardiac arrest.	Ventricular rupture due to insertion.	Observe patient closely. Inform doctor immediately. Prepare to commence cardiac massage.
Tingling in fingers, shooting pain down arm, paralysis.	Injury to brachial plexus during insertion.	Inform a doctor. Treatment is symptomatic. Physiotherapy may be necessary.
Oedema of the arm on the side of the catheter insertion, may be associated with pain or limb discoloration.	Thoracic duct injury at insertion, resulting in alterations in lymph flow.	Inform a doctor. Removal of the catheter is usually necessary.
Oedema/pain and tenderness of arm, neck and/or chest. Engorged peripheral veins or feelings of tightness.	Thrombosis in major vessel due to irritation/damage by foreign body (catheter).	Report to doctor. Ultrasound and/or venogram may be performed and anticoagulant therapy commenced. May be prevented by use of low-dose warfarin during dwell time.
Pyrexia, tachycardia, rigors indicating systemic infection.	Infection due to poor aseptic technique. Poor technique when handling of equipment, e.g. stopcocks, overflooding of manometer.	Culture of the patient's blood is required. Take a swab of the insertion site, employing strict asepsis and minimum handling of the equipment. Administer antimicrobials as prescribed. Observe the patient closely. Removal of the catheter is sometimes indicated.
Leakage of fluid onto the dressing.	Loose connection in the system. Cracking of catheter or hub.	Check and tighten connections. Report to the relevant nursing staff and/or doctors.
Catheter required for many functions, e.g. blood sampling and extra drug administration.	Limited routes of access available to satisfy the patient's requirements.	Consider multi-lumen catheter before insertion. Use simple regimens and methods of administration. Use extension sets and administration sets available for this purpose. May require additional peripheral access.
Fluid overload resulting in dyspnoea, oedema, raised pulse rate and blood pressure.	Infusion is too fast. Inaccurate fluid monitoring.	Revise the patient's fluid intake regimen. Use flow control devices. Keep accurate records of the patient's fluid balance and weight. Inform a doctor.
Inaccurate CVP readings.	Patient in a position different from that in which the initial reading was taken.	Position should be documented in the patient's records.

Problem	Cause	Suggested action
	Reference point on the patient not observed.	Zero of the manometer must be level with the patient's right atrium at the point marked on the patient, i.e. mid-axilla or sternal angle.
	Faulty pressure reading technique.	If the CVP reading is outside the limits deemed acceptable for that patient and it is considered to be an accurate reading, recheck it after 15 or 30 min and inform a doctor if unchanged.
Elevated CVP.	Increased intrathoracic pressure caused by coughing, increased movement or pain.	Encourage coughing before taking the reading. Ensure that the patient is comfortable and pain-free.
	Lower extremities elevated.	Position the patient so that he/she is lying in a supine position.
	Patient having intermittent positive-pressure ventilation.	Read the CVP at the end expiratory level (lowest point of fluctuation). This will always be higher than the 'normal' reading.
	Anxiety and/or restlessness.	Verify the cause of the anxiety or restlessness and take action to reassure patient.
	Blood in progress via the CVP catheter.	Flush the catheter well with 0.9% sodium chloride and read again.
	Shivering and/or muscular spasm, e.g. postanaesthetic reaction (see Chap. 30, Peri-Operative Care).	Assess the patient's condition, e.g. pulse, blood pressure, temperature. Check that the patient is warm enough. Inform a doctor.
Low CVP reading.	Leak in the system or equipment adjusted inaccurately.	Check and readjust the system.
	Changing of the patient's position from recumbent to semirecumbent.	Reread with the patient in the recumbent position.
Potential pulmonary embolus due to catheter tip embolus. Symptoms include chest pain, cool clammy skin, haemoptysis, tachycardia, hypotension.	Occasionally occurs after the removal of the catheter. When using traction method, especially the skin-tunnelled type.	All skin-tunnelled catheters must be removed by competent doctors or nursing staff. Avoid using the traction method. Notify a doctor immediately if the patient develops any of the related symptoms.
Bleeding at the insertion site following removal of the catheter.	Opening in the vein wall.	Apply pressure over the site with sterile topical swabs, until bleeding has stopped. Patients prescribed warfarin or heparin will require a longer period of pressure to compensate for the prolonged clotting time. Apply sterile dressing. If bleeding persists, the doctor must be informed.
Pyrexia of unknown origin.	Could be related to CVAD.	Do not remove catheter until site of infection confirmed (unless clinical condition dictates otherwise). Inform doctors. Carry out investigations such as 'blood cultures' (from catheter and peripheral vein), swab of entry site,

full blood count, midstream urine, chest X-ray, swabs of areas that could be the source of infection, e.g. throat or wound swabs. If catheter removed, tip should be sent for bacteriological examination.

In addition, the care plan associated with intravenous management (Chap. 12, Drug Administration) may contain useful and relevant information.

Arterial cannulae

Definition

An arterial cannula is a cannula positioned in a peripheral artery (such as the radial or dorsalis pedis). If it is not possible to access a peripheral site or if the patient is critically ill and receiving high-dose inotropic drugs, the femoral artery may be used.

Reasons for arterial cannulation

1 Ease of access, thereby avoiding the discomfort of frequent punctures of the artery, e.g. tests for blood gases, serial blood lactate levels, full blood count, urea and electrolytes (Hinds 1987).
2 To gain continuous and accurate direct measurement of intra-arterial blood pressure.

Indications

1 During and following major surgery involving prolonged anaesthesia, e.g. major intracavitary surgery for longer than 1 hour.
2 Monitoring of acid–base balance and respiratory status in:
   (a) Acute respiratory failure
   (b) Mechanical ventilation
   (c) The period during and after cardiorespiratory arrest
   (d) Severe sepsis
   (e) Shock conditions
   (f) Major trauma
   (g) Acute poisoning, particularly with carbon dioxide, salicylates and paracetamol
   (h) Acute renal failure
   (i) Severe diabetic ketoacidosis.
3 Patients who require continuous arterial monitoring, e.g. those who are critically ill, or after cardiac surgery. Such patients typically receive numerous inotropic drugs, i.e. catecholamines such as dopamine or adrenalin, which have a direct effect on mean arterial pressure (MAP), making accurate measurement of MAP essential.

Reference material

Direct haemodynamic monitoring is performed more frequently because there is more awareness of the need for patient safety, and one particular method, intra-arterial pressure monitoring, is used in operating theatres, recovery rooms, intensive care units, acute general wards and during inter-hospital transfer of acutely ill patients (Allan 1984; Royal College of Anaesthetists 1990). The monitoring systems necessary and the hazard of disconnection and severe haemorrhage limit its use to intensive care units, coronary care units, theatre and recovery areas and, increasingly, high-dependency areas. Direct cannulation of the artery has been carried out safely in these settings for at least 15 years (Oh 1995).

The most convenient site for arterial cannulation is the right or left radial artery (the cannula should not be positioned close to an adjoining intravenous cannula) and vice versa. The radial artery passes down the radial or lateral side of the forearm to the wrist. Just above the wrist it lies superficially and can be felt in front of the radius, where the radial pulse is palpable. The artery then passes between the first and second metacarpal bones and enters the palm of the hand (Wilson & Waugh 1998).

Before the insertion of a radial artery cannula, circulation to the hand should be evaluated by assessing the circulation of the palmar arch using the Allen test. The Allen test consists of simultaneously compressing both the ulnar and radial arteries for approximately 1 minute. During this time, the patient rapidly opens and closes the hand to promote exsanguination.

Approximately 5 seconds after release of the artery (usually the ulnar), the extended hand should blush due to capillary refilling. This reactive hyperaemia indicates adequate circulation in the hand. If blanching occurs, palmar arch circulation is inadequate, and a radial cannula could lead to ischaemia of the hand (Hinds 1987) and an alternative route found. It should be noted that direct puncture of the artery is painful for the patient.

Complications

There are three main areas of concern:

1 Hypovolaemia. Accidental disconnection of tubing from the cannula or one of the connections can result in severe haemorrhage and hypovolaemia. Patients in shock and children are particularly vulnerable. The risk can be minimized by clearly labelling the arterial cannula (Zideman & Morgan 1981) along with the use of Luer lock sets.
2 Accidental intra-arterial injection of drugs intended for administration through a central or peripheral venous

line. This has been shown to cause distal ischaemia and necrosis, with sometimes permanent damage (Teplitz 1990; Tinker & Zapol 1991; Marieb 1998).

3 Local damage to artery. Local damage is the most common complication of arterial cannulae (Hinds 1987). Signs include change in temperature in the distal limb and mottling and blanching of the limb when the cannula is flushed. Frequent observation of the site and local digits (fingers/toes) and early removal of the cannula are necessary to minimize permanent damage.

Debate and research continue about whether the fluid used to flush the tubing and cannula should contain heparin. Some authors (e.g. Clifton *et al.* 1991; Oh 1995) claim that heparin prolongs the patency of the cannula. Others have shown that there is no statistical difference between the length of time the catheter remains patent using heparin and 0.9% sodium chloride (Kulkarni *et al.* 1994). Note: heparin-induced thrombocytopenia means that many units are moving away from use of heparin.

If the dorsalis pedis site is chosen to locate the artery, find the mid-point between the two malleoli on the dorsal surface of the foot. Then follow the midline down to the space between the first and second metatarsal. Recent work by Frezza and Mezghebe (1998) has shown there is no difference in complication rates with different positions and changes of administration sets.

In the monitoring of the critcally ill patient, especially those receiving high doses of noradrenaline, it may be necessary to move the site to the femoral artery.

References and further reading

Allan, D. (1984) Care of the patient with an arterial catheter. *Nurs Times*, **80**(46), 40–41.

Clifton, G.D. *et al.* (1991) Comparison of 0.9% sodium chloride and heparin solutions for maintenance of arterial catheter patency. *Heart Lung*, **20**(2), 115–18.

Frezza, E.E. & Mezghebe, H. (1998) Indications and complications of arterial catheter use in surgical or medical intensive care units. Analysis of 4932 patients. *Am Surg*, **64**(2), 127–31.

Hinds, C.J. (1987) *Intensive Care*. Baillière Tindall, Gillingham.

Kulkarni, M. (1994) Heparinised saline vs normal saline in maintaining patency of the radial artery catheter. *Can J Surg*, **37**(1), 37–42.

Marieb, E.N. (1998) *Human Anatomy and Physiology*. Benjamin/Cummings, California.

Morven, H. (1995) The first years of continuing arterial pressure measurement. *Br J Anaesth*, **67**, 353–9.

Oh, T.E. (1995) *Intensive Care Manual*. Butterworths, Sydney.

Royal College of Anaesthetists (1990) *The Working Party of the Commission on the Provision of Surgical Services*. Royal College of Surgeons and College of Anaesthetists, London.

Santolla, A. & Weckel, C. (1983) A new closed system for arterial lines. *Reg Nurse*, **46**(6), 49–52.

Teplitz, L. (1990) Arterial line disconnection: first aid procedure. *Nursing*, **20**(5), 33.

Tinker, J. & Zapol, W. (1991) *Care of the Critically Ill Patient*. Springer, London.

Wilson, K.J. & Waugh, A. (1998) *Ross and Wilson's Anatomy and Physiology and Illness*, 8th edn. Churchill Livingstone, Edinburgh.

Zideman, D.A. & Morgan, M. (1981) Inadvertent intra-arterial injection of flucloxacillin. *Anaesthesia*, **36**(6), 296–8.

GUIDELINES · Setting up the monitoring set and preparation for insertion of an arterial cannula

Equipment

1 500-ml pressure infuser cuff.
2 500-ml bag of 0.9% sodium chloride or prescribed solution.
3 Heparin as prescribed, plus additive label.
4 22-G cannula or other available arterial catheters.
5 Sterile intravenous pack.
6 Gloves.
7 Chlorhexidine in 70% alcohol.
8 Transparent dressing.
9 Syringes – various sizes.
10 Arterial identification label.
11 1% lignocaine injection.
12 Pressure monitoring system equipment.

Procedure

Action	Rationale
1 Explain and discuss the procedure with the patient.	To ensure that the patient understands the procedure and gives his/her valid consent.
(*Note*: most arterial cannulas are inserted when patients are anaesthetized.)	
2 Prepare infusion and additive (e.g. heparin 1 IU per ml) as prescribed. Apply additive sticker to front of bag.	To prevent duplication of treatment. To maintain accurate records. To provide a point of reference in the event of any queries.
3 Check that all Luer lock connections are secure.	To prevent disconnection.

4	Connect administration set to bag.	To prepare infusion.
5	Open roller clamp fully.	To check the flow rate.
6	Squeeze the flush device-actuator (see instructions with set).	To prime the administration set and three-way tap ports.
7	Check thoroughly for air bubbles in the circuit.	To reduce the risk of an air embolus.
8	Insert bag of heparinized saline into pressure infuser cuff. Inflate to 300 mm Hg.	This pressure is higher than arterial blood pressure, therefore an automatic flush mode is activated in the system which delivers 3 ml/hour, which maintains patency of circuit, cannula and artery (Allan 1984; Morven 1995).
9	Wash your hands with bactericidal soap and water or bactericidal alcohol hand rub before leaving clinical room.	To reduce the risk of cross-infection.
10	Prepare trolley near the patient as described in Chap. 3, Aseptic Technique.	
11	The radial site (or other site chosen by doctor) is prepared aseptically by doctor, hair is removed where necessary, the site is cleaned with chlorhexidine in 70% alcohol and a sterile towel is placed under the arm.	To maintain asepsis. To provide a clean working area.
12	Complete Allen test if radial site is used.	To assess if palmar arch circulation is adequate.
13	Local anaesthetic is administered if cannulation is performed while the patient is conscious.	To minimize pain during the procedure.
14	Nurse and doctor apply gloves. See Chap. 3, Aseptic Technique, for safe technique and practice guidelines.	To prevent contamination of hands if blood spillage occurs.
15	The nurse holds the patient's arm in order to flex the hand slightly.	To prevent movement and facilitate insertion.
16	Cannula is inserted by the doctor.	
17	Pressure is applied to artery in which cannula is inserted.	To reduce the risk of blood spillage.
18	Open roller clamp fully.	To prevent back-flow of blood.
19	Tape the tubing and cannula securely, and apply transparent dressing. Clearly label 'arterial' (Fig. 44.17).	Leaving the site visible allows the observer to recognize immediately any dislodgement or disconnection. Clear labelling prevents accidental injection of drugs.

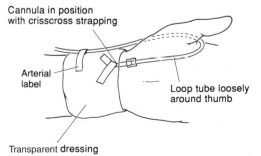

Cannula in position
with crisscross strapping

Arterial
label

Loop tube loosely
around thumb

Transparent **dressing**

Figure 44.17   Positioning, securing and labelling of cannula.

Guidelines • Setting up the monitoring set and preparation for insertion of an arterial cannula (cont'd)

Action	Rationale
20 When the patient is awake, loop the tube around the thumb.	To minimize movement of cannula and damage to vessel.
21 Inform patient of amount of movement permitted, e.g. fingers and arm may be moved gently. Discourage any stress on arm and connections.	To prevent dislodgement.

GUIDELINES • Taking a blood sample from an arterial cannula

Care must be taken not to introduce air or infection and to ensure that three-way tap is left in closed position.

Equipment

1 Intravenous sterile dressing pack.
2 Gloves.
3 Appropriate syringes and blood sample bottles, dependent on samples required.

4 Sterile Luer lock connection.
5 Chlorhexidine in 70% alcohol.
6 Bactericidal alcohol hand rub.

Procedure

Action	Rationale
1 Explain and discuss the procedure with the patient.	To ensure that the patient understands the procedure and gives his/her valid consent.
2 Prepare the trolley.	To ensure all equipment is ready.
3 Wash hands with bactericidal soap and water or bactericidal alcohol hand rub before leaving clinical room.	To minimize the risk of cross-infection.
4 Check that the three-way tap (Fig. 44.18a) is closed to air.	To prevent back-flow of blood and blood spillage.
5 Clean hands with bactericidal alcohol hand rub.	Hands have been contaminated by touching three-way tap.
6 Prepare trolley as described in Chap. 3, Guidelines: Aseptic Technique.	
7 Apply gloves. See Chap. 3 for safe technique and practice guidelines.	To prevent contamination of hand with blood.
8 Remove cap from three-way tap (Fig. 44.18a) and clean open port with a swab soaked in chlorhexidine in 70% alcohol.	To minimize the risk of infection.
9 Connect 5-ml syringe to open port.	
10 Turn three-way tap to artery and port (Fig. 44.18b).	To prevent contamination of blood sample with heparinized saline.
11 Slowly withdraw 5 ml of blood until the cannula is clear of infusion fluid.	To prevent contamination of blood with infusion fluid.
12 Turn three-way tap diagonally to close off infusion, artery and port (Fig. 44.18c).	To prevent back-flow of blood from artery, contamination with infusion fluid and blood spillage.
13 Remove syringe.	

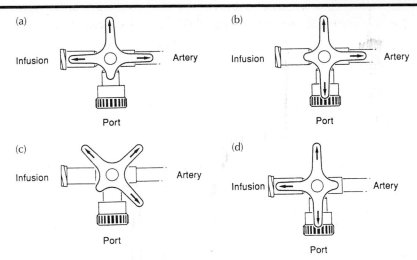

Figure 44.18 Three-way tap (a) closed to port; (b) turned to artery and port; (c) turned diagonally to close off infusion, artery and port; (d) turned to infusion and port.

14 Connect appropriately sized syringe for sample.	In order to take the required amount of blood.
15 Turn three-way tap to artery and port (Fig. 44.18b).	To prevent contamination with infusion fluid.
16 Slowly remove amount of blood required.	To prevent any spasm in vessel.
17 Turn three-way tap to infusion and artery (Fig. 44.18a).	To prevent back-flow of blood and blood spillage.
18 Remove syringe.	
19 Turn three-way tap to infusion and port (Fig. 44.18d). Flush cannula hourly by squeezing actuator (see instructions with set).	To prevent blood clotting in port.
20 Turn three-way tap to infusion and artery (Fig. 44.18a). Flush cannula gently by squeezing actuator.	To clear blood from cannula.
21 Clean port with chlorhexidine in 70% alcohol swab.	To minimize the risk of infection.
22 Apply sterile Luer lock cap and check it is secure.	To prevent haemorrhage or blood spillage.
23 Check pressure infuser cuff is inflated to 300 mm Hg.	To prevent back-flow of blood into circuit.
24 Empty blood from syringe into appropriate sample bottle, and immediately label or record blood gas.	To ensure identity of sample is correct.

GUIDELINES · Removal of an arterial cannula

Equipment

1 Intravenous sterile dressing pack.
2 Gloves.
3 Hypoallergenic tape.

4 Chlorhexidine in 70% alcohol.
5 Bactericidal skin cleanser.

Guidelines • Removal of an arterial cannula (cont'd)

Procedure

Action	*Rationale*
1 Explain and discuss the procedure with the patient.	To ensure that the patient understands the procedure and gives his/her valid consent.
2 Prepare trolley as described in Chap. 3, Guidelines: Aseptic Technique.	
3 Wash hands with bactericidal soap and water or bactericidal alcohol hand rub before leaving clinical room.	To reduce the risk of cross-infection.
4 Prepare trolley by patient as described in Chap. 3, Guidelines: Aseptic Technique.	
5 Turn three-way tap diagonally (Fig. 44.18c).	To prevent back-flow of blood into cannula.
6 Turn off intravenous set.	To prevent spillage when removing cannula.
7 Deflate pressure cuff.	Pressure no longer required.
8 Remove transparent dressing and tape from cannula site.	To enable easy removal of cannula.
9 Clean hands with a bactericidal skin cleanser solution.	
10 Apply gloves. See Chap. 3 for safe technique and practice guidelines.	To prevent contamination of hands with blood.
11 Clean cannula site area with chlorhexidine in 70% alcohol.	To reduce the risk of infection.
12 Place sterile piece of gauze over area and gently remove cannula.	To minimize bleeding.
13 Apply pressure to site for a minimum of 5 min or until bleeding stops.	To prevent a haematoma and blood loss.
14 Apply a clean, sterile, dry dressing using a non-touch technique.	To maintain asepsis.
15 Apply strapping.	To ensure pressure and prevent haematoma or blood loss.

Following this procedure, check the patient's hand hourly or as frequently as required for warmth, colour, swelling and signs of bleeding. Ask the patient to inform staff if feeling faint or if there is oozing from the dressing. The medical staff must be informed immediately if the hand or forearm becomes discoloured or swollen, or if the patient complains of pain in the limb. Then information must also be carefully documented in the patient's care plan and medical notes. Request for photograph to be taken.

Nursing care plan

Problem	*Cause*	*Suggested preventative care*
Haemorrhage. Severe haemorrhage (hypovolaemia).	Luer lock connections are loose or cracked. Blood will be lost from open connection.	Check that Luer locks are fitted securely. Do not force because the locks may crack.
	Blood may ooze around the cannula site.	Place a transparent dressing over the cannula site and observe hourly or more frequently as the situation requires.
	Accidental disconnection.	

	Cannula may have become dislodged.	Inform the patient about the danger of dislodging the cannula and amount of movement that is preferred. Take care when moving the patient. Avoid putting stress on the arm and connections. Secure the cannula well (Fig. 44.17).
Back-flow of blood into the cannula.	The pressure infusor cuff may not be inflated to the optimal pressure.	Ensure that the pressure infusor cuff is inflated to 300 mm Hg. This pressure is higher than arterial blood pressure and an automatic flush mode is activated in the system which delivers 3 ml/hour. This maintains patency of circuit, cannula and artery (Allan 1984).
Ischaemia.	A thrombosis may have formed in the circuit cannula or artery.	Ensure that heparin is added to the saline infusion (Clifton et al. 1991). Assess limb pulse, colour and temperature hourly, or more frequently as required. Absent pulses, pallor, cyanosis and coldness denote occlusion. If this occurs, medical advice must be sought and the cannula removed promptly (Hinds 1987).
Erythema or inflammation around the insertion site.	Phlebitis due to sepsis, chemical irritation or mechanical irritation.	Refer to the Nursing Care Plan in Chap. 12, Drug Administration.
Hypotension, tachycardia, cyanosis, unconsciousness.	Embolism: 　air 　particle	Refer to the procedure in Chap. 12, Drug Administration.
Arterial spasm.	Forceful flushing or forceful aspiration when withdrawing blood.	Avoid forceful flushing or aspiration and maintain a slow even pressure when withdrawing blood.
Necrosis.	Accidental injection of a drug into the artery, causing local necrosis to vessel wall.	Label the arterial cannula and circuit clearly (Fig. 44.17). In the event of accidental injection of any drug, report the error immediately to medical staff and the senior nurse and perform the following: (a) Gently withdraw blood from the three-way tap to try to withdraw the drug. (b) Stop administering the drug. (c) Assess limb pulse, colour and temperature hourly, or more frequently if required. (d) Complete an accident form and/or other relevant documentation.

Venepuncture

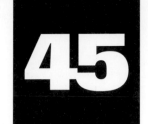

Definition

Venepuncture is the procedure of entering a vein with a needle.

Indications

Venepuncture is carried out for two reasons:

1 To obtain a blood sample for diagnostic purposes.
2 To monitor levels of blood components.

Reference material

Venepuncture is one of the most commonly performed invasive procedures (Peters *et al.* 1984; Center for Disease Control 1997). It is now becoming more routinely performed by nursing staff (Inwood 1996; Jackson 1996). In order to do this safely the nurse must have a basic knowledge of the following:

1 The relevant anatomy and physiology.
2 The criteria for choosing both the vein and device to use.
3 The potential problems which may be encountered, how to prevent them and necessary interventions.
4 The health and safety/risk management of the procedure, as well as the correct disposal of equipment.
(Intravenous Nursing Society 1998)

Certain principles, such as adherence to an aseptic technique, must be applied throughout (see Chap. 3, Aseptic Technique). The circulation is a closed sterile system and a venepuncture, however quickly completed, is a breach of this system providing a means of entry for bacteria.

The nurse must be aware of the physical and psychological comfort of the patient (Sager & Bomar 1980; Middleton 1985; Weinstein 1997). He/she must appreciate the value of adequate explanation and simple measures to prevent the complications of venepuncture, such as haematoma formation, when it is neither a natural nor acceptable consequence of the procedure.

Anatomy and physiology

The superficial veins of the upper limb are most commonly chosen for venepuncture. These veins are numerous and accessible, ensuring that the procedure can be performed safely and with minimum discomfort (Carola *et al.* 1992; Marieb 1998). Occasionally, the veins of a lower limb may be utilized. This should be avoided if possible as blood flow in this region is diminished and the risk of ensuing complications is higher (Weinstein 1997).

The veins used for venepuncture are those found in the antecubital fossa because they are sizeable veins capable of providing copious and repeated blood specimens (Weinstein 1997). However, the venous anatomy of each individual may differ. The main veins of choice are (see Fig. 45.1a):

1 The median cubital veins
2 The cephalic vein
3 The basilic vein
4 The metacarpal veins (used only when the others are not accessible) (Fig. 45.1b).

The median cubital vein may not always be visible, but its size and location make it easy to palpate. It is also well supported by subcutaneous tissue, which prevents it from rolling under the needle.

On the lateral aspect of the wrist, the cephalic vein rises from the dorsal veins and flows upwards along the radial border of the forearm, crossing the antecubital fossa as the median cephalic vein. Care must be taken to avoid accidental arterial puncture, as this vein crosses the brachial artery. It is also in close proximity to the radial nerve (Perucca 1995).

The basilic vein is often overlooked as a site for venepuncture and has its origins in the ulnar border of the hand and forearm (Wilson & Waugh 1998). It may well be prominent but is not well supported by subcutaneous tissue, making it roll easily, which can result in difficult venepuncture (Dougherty 1999). Due to its position, a haematoma may occur if the patient flexes the arm on removal of the needle, as this squeezes blood from the vein into the surrounding tissues (Weinstein 1997). Care must be taken to avoid accidental puncture of the median nerve.

The metacarpal veins are easily visualized and palpated. However, the use of these veins is contraindicated in the elderly where skin turgor and subcutaneous tissue are diminished (Dougherty 1996; Weinstein 1997).

Veins consist of three layers: the tunica intima is a smooth endothelial lining, which allows the passage of blood cells. If it becomes damaged, the lining may become roughened and there is an increased risk of thrombus formation (Hadaway 1995). Within this layer are folds of endothelium called valves, which keep blood moving

(a)

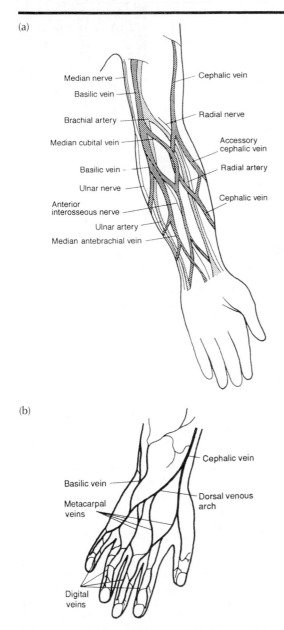

(b)

Figure 45.1 (a) Superficial veins of the forearm. (b) Superficial veins of dorsal aspect of the hand. (Reproduced by permission from Becton Dickinson and Company.)

towards the heart by preventing backflow of blood. Valves are present in larger vessels and at points of branching and are present as noticeable bulges in the veins (Hadaway 1995; Weinstein 1997; Dougherty 1999). However, when a needle touches a valve, the valve can compress and close the lumen of the vein, thus preventing the withdrawal of blood (Weinstein 1997). Therefore, if detected, venepuncture should be performed above the valve in order to facilitate collection of the sample (Weinstein 1997).

The tunica media, the middle layer of the vein wall, is composed of muscular tissue and nerve fibres, both vasoconstrictors and vasodilators, which can stimulate the vein to contract or relax. This layer is not as strong or stiff as an artery and therefore veins can distend or collapse as the pressure rises or falls (Weinstein 1997). Stimulation of this layer by a change in temperature, mechanical or chemical stimulation can produce venous spasm, which can make a venepuncture more difficult.

The tunica adventitia is the outer layer and consists of connective tissue, which surrounds and supports the vessel.

Arteries tend to be placed more deeply than veins and can be distinguished by the thicker walls, which do not collapse, the presence of a pulse and the blood is bright red. It should be noted that aberrant arteries may be present. These are arteries that are located superficially in an unusual place.

Choosing a vein

The choice of vein must be that which is best for the individual patient. The most prominent vein is not necessarily the most suitable vein for venepuncture (Weinstein 1997). There are two stages to locating a vein:

1 Visual inspection
2 Palpation

Visual inspection is the scrutiny of the veins in both arms and is essential prior to choosing a vein. Veins adjacent to foci of infection, bruising and phlebitis should not be considered, due to the risk of causing more local tissue damage or systemic infection. An oedematous limb should be avoided as there is danger of stasis of lymph, predisposing to such complications as phlebitis and cellulitis (Smith 1998). Areas of previous venepunctures should also be avoided as they can result in pain due to repeated trauma to the vein (Ahrens et al. 1991).

Palpation is an important assessment technique, as it determines the location and condition of the vein, distinguishes veins from arteries and tendons, identifies the presence of valves and detects deeper veins (Dougherty 1999). The nurse should use the same fingers for palpation as this will increase the sensitivity and ability of the nurse to know what she or he is feeling. The thumb should not be used as it is not as sensitive and has a pulse, which may lead to confusion in distinguishing veins from arteries in the patient (Weinstein 1997).

Thrombosed veins feel hard and cord-like, and should be avoided along with tortuous, sclerosed, fibrosed, inflamed or fragile veins, which may be unable to accommodate the device to be used and will result in pain and repeated venepunctures. Use of veins which cross over joints or bony prominences and those with little skin or subcutaneous cover, e.g. the inner aspect of the wrist, will also subject the patient to more discomfort. Therefore preference should be given to a vessel that is unused, easily detected by inspection and palpation, patent and healthy. These veins feel soft, bouncy and will refill when depressed (Weinstein 1997).

Influencing factors

1 Injury, disease or treatment may prevent the use of a limb for venepuncture by reducing the venous access, e.g. amputation, fracture and cerebrovascular accident. Use of a limb may be contraindicated because of an operation on one side of the body, for example mastectomy and axillary node dissection, as this can lead to impairment of lymphatic drainage, which can influence venous flow regardless of whether there is obvious lymphoedema (Rowland 1991; Smith 1998).

2 How the patient is positioned, for example having to lie on a particular side, may also dictate the site of the venepuncture (Rowland 1991; Millam 1992).

3 The age and weight of the patient will also influence choice. Young children have short fine veins, and the elderly have prominent but fragile veins. Care must be taken with fragile veins and the largest vein should be chosen along with the smallest gauge device to reduce amount of trauma to the vessel. Malnourished patients will often present with friable veins.

4 If the patient is in shock or dehydrated there will be poor superficial peripheral access. It may be necessary to take blood after the patient is rehydrated as this will promote venous filling and blood will be obtained more easily.

5 Medications can influence vein choice in that patients on anticoagulant, steroids or those who are thrombocytopenic tend to have more fragile veins and will be at greater risk of bruising both during venepuncture and on removal of the needle. Therefore choice may be limited by areas of bruising present or the inability to access the vessel without causing bruising to occur.

6 The temperature of the environment will influence venous dilation (Sager & Bomar 1980). If the patient is cold, no veins may be evident on first inspection. Application of heat, e.g. in the form of a warm compress or soaking the arm in warm water, will increase the size and visibility of the veins, thus increasing the likelihood of a successful first attempt.

7 Venepuncture itself may cause the vein to collapse or go into a spasm. This will produce discomfort and a reduction in blood flow. Careful preparation and choice of vein will reduce the likelihood of this and stroking the vein or applying heat will help resolve it.

8 Patient anxiety about the procedure may result in vasoconstriction. The nurse's manner and approach will also have a direct bearing on the patient's experience (Dougherty 1994; Weinstein 1997). Approaching the patient with a confident manner and giving an adequate explanation of the procedure may reduce anxiety. Careful preparation and an unhurried approach will help to relax the patient and this in turn will increase vasodilation (Middleton 1985; Millam 1992; Weinstein 1997; Dougherty 1999). It is important to remember that patients may dread venepuncture (Johnston-Early *et al.* 1981) and if a patient is particularly anxious, or for venepuncture in children, the use of a topical local anaesthetic cream may be appropriate (Gunawardene & Davenport 1990; Millam 1995). Involving patients in the choice of vein, even if it is simply to choose the non-dominant arm, can increase a feeling of control which in turn helps to relieve anxiety (Hudek 1986).

Improving venous access

There are a number of methods of improving venous access:

1 Application of a tourniquet – this promotes venous distension. The tourniquet should be tight enough to impede venous return but not restrict arterial flow (Hadaway 1995).

2 Opening and closing of the fist ensures the muscles will force blood into the veins and encourages distension.

3 Lowering the arm below heart level also increases blood supply to the veins.

4 Light tapping of the vein may be useful but can be painful and may result in the formation of a haematoma in patients with fragile veins, e.g. thrombocytopenic patients (Dougherty 1999).

5 The use of heat in the form of a warm pack or by immersing the arm in a bowl of warm water for 10 minutes helps to encourage venodilation and venous filling.

6 Ointment or patches containing small amounts of glyceryl trinitrate have been used to cause local vasodilatation to aid venepuncture (Hecker *et al.* 1983; Gunawardene & Davenport 1990).

Choice of device

The intravenous devices commonly used to perform a venepuncture for blood sampling are a straight steel needle and a steel winged infusion device. The optimum gauge to use is 21 swg (standard wire gauge, which measures internal diameter – the smaller the gauge size, the larger the diameter. Standard wire gauge measurement is determined by how many cannulae fit into a tube with an inner diameter of 1 inch, and uses consecutive numbers from 13 to 24). This enables blood to be withdrawn at a reasonable speed without undue discomfort to the patient or possible damage to the blood cells.

The nurse must choose the device dependent on the condition and accessibility of the individual patient's veins (Table 45.1).

Given the concern about possible contamination of the practitioner by blood, a number of new systems of collection are now available commercially. The equipment available will depend on local policy.

Skin preparation

Asepsis is vital when performing a venepuncture as the skin is breached and an alien device is introduced into a sterile circulatory system. The two major sources of microbial contamination are:

1 Cross-infection from practitioner to patient.
2 Skin flora of the patient.

Table 45.1 Choice of intravenous device

Device	swg	Advantages	Disadvantages	Use
Needle	21	Cheaper than winged infusion devices. Easy to use with large veins	Rigid. Difficult to manipulate with smaller veins in less conventional sites. May cause more discomfort	Large, accessible veins in the antecubital fossa. When small quantities of blood are to be drawn
Winged infusion device	21	Flexible due to small needle shaft. Easy to manipulate and insert at any site. Causes less discomfort	More expensive than steel needles	Veins in sites other than the antecubital fossa. When quantities of blood greater than 20 ml are required from any site
	23	Flexible due to small needle shaft. Easy to manipulate and insert at any site. Causes less discomfort. Smaller swg and therefore useful with fragile veins	More expensive than steel needles, plus there can be damage to cells which can cause inaccurate measurements in certain blood samples, e.g. sodium, potassium	Small veins in more painful sites, e.g. inner aspect of the wrist, especially if measurements are related to plasma and not cellular components

Good hand washing and drying techniques are essential on the part of the nurse; gloves should be changed between patients (see Chap. 3, Aseptic Technique).

To remove the risk presented by the patient's skin flora, firm and prolonged rubbing with an alcohol-based solution, such as chlorhexidine 70% in alcohol, is advised (Perucca 1995). This cleaning should continue for at least 30 seconds, although some authors state a minimum of 1 minute or longer (Rowland 1991; Millam 1992; Weinstein 1997). The area that has been cleaned should then be allowed to dry to (1) facilitate coagulation of the organisms, thus ensuring disinfection and (2) prevent a stinging pain on insertion of the needle due to the alcohol on the end of the needle. The skin must not be touched or the vein repalpated before puncture.

Skin cleansing is a controversial subject and it is acknowledged that a cursory wipe with an alcohol swab does more harm than no cleaning at all as it disturbs the skin flora. Good cleaning techniques in a hospital environment, where transient pathogens abound, are of value in controlling infection (Weinstein 1997).

Safety of the practitioner

Nowadays it is no longer appropriate to protect staff only when a disease is suspected or identified. Venepuncture has been associated with 13–62% of needlestick injuries reported to hospital occupational health services in the USA (Center for Disease Control 1997); therefore adherence to universal safe technique and practice is vital.

Generally, gloves should be worn when handling blood and body fluids (RCN 1995). This is to prevent contamination of the practitioner from potential blood spills. Despite this, it must always be remembered that gloves will not prevent a needlestick injury. Professional judgement

needs to be exercised as it has been shown that a loss of tactile sensation caused by wearing gloves could make a needlestick injury more likely (DoH 1990; British Medical Association 1991; RCN 1999). The Department of Health (1990) has recommended that gloves should be worn when taking blood in the following circumstances:

1 When the venepuncturist is inexperienced.
2 When the health care worker has cuts or abrasions on the hands which cannot be covered by dressings alone.
3 When the patient is restless.
4 When the patient is known to be infected with HIV or hepatitis.

There is no substitute for good technique and practitioners must always work carefully when performing this procedure.

A range of safety devices are now available for venepuncture which can reduce the risk of occupational percutaneous injuries among health care workers, in particular vacuum blood collection systems (Center for Disease Control 1997). A vacuum system consists of a plastic holder which contains or is attached to a double-ended needle or adaptor. The blood tube is vacuumed in order that the exact amount of blood required is withdrawn, when the tube is pushed into the holder. Filling ceases once the tube is full which removes the need for decanting blood and also reduces blood wastage. The system can also be attached to winged infusion devices (Perucca 1995; Dougherty 1999). It has been shown that the use of vacuum blood collection systems, particularly with winged infusion devices, is associated with a significant reduction in percutaneous injuries (Center for Disease Control 1997).

Used needles should always be discarded directly into an approved sharps container, without being resheathed. Specimens from patients with known or suspected infections such as hepatitis or HIV should be double-bagged in clear polythene bags with a biohazard label attached. The accompanying request forms should be kept separately from the specimen to avoid contamination. All other non-sharp disposables should be placed in a universal clinical waste bag.

Removal of the device

It is important to ensure that the needle is removed correctly on completion of blood sampling and that the risk of haematoma formation is minimized. Pressure should be applied as the needle is removed from the skin. If pressure is applied too early, it causes the tip of the needle to drag along the intima of the vein, resulting in sharp pain and damage to the lining of the vessel.

Digital pressure should be applied by the practitioner, as it has been shown that this results in less bruising than if the patient is left to apply the pressure (Godwin et al. 1992). The patient should also be instructed to keep his or her arm straight and not bend it as this also results in an increased risk of bruising (Dyson & Bogod 1987). A longer period of pressure may be necessary where the patients' blood may take longer to clot, for example, if the patient is receiving anticoagulants or is thrombocytopenic. The practitioner may choose to apply the tourniquet over the venepuncture site to ensure even and constant pressure on the area (Perdue 1995).

The practitioner should inspect the site carefully for bleeding or bruising before applying a dressing to the site, and the patient leaving the department. If bruising has occurred the patient should be informed of why this has happened and given instructions for what to do to reduce the bruising and any associated pain. The application of Hirudoid cream may be helpful (British Medical Association and Royal Pharmaceutical Society of Great Britain 1999).

Summary

In order to perform a safe and successful venepuncture, it is important that the practitioner

1 Considers carefully the choice of vein and device.
2 Applies the principles of asepsis.
3 Adheres to and understands safe technique and practices.

Recently there has been an increase in the number of cases of litigation involving injuries, which have occurred as a result of venepuncture (McConnell & MacKay 1996; Price & Moss 1998). It is therefore vital that nurses receive accredited and appropriate training, supervision and assessment by an experienced member of staff (Millam 1992; Dougherty 1996; Inwood 1996; RCN 1999). The nurse is then accountable and responsible for ensuring that his or her skills and competence are maintained and his or her knowledge is kept up to date, in order to fulfil the criteria set out in the Scope of Professional Practice (UKCC 1992; Dougherty 1996; Lamb 1999).

References and further reading

Ahrens, T., Wiersma, R. & Weilitz, P.B. (1991) Differences in pain perception associated with intravenous catheter insertion. *J Intraven Nurs*, **14**(2), 85–9.

British Medical Association (1991) *A Code of Practice for the Safe Use and Disposal of Sharps*, pp. 20–21. BMA, London.

British Medical Association and Royal Pharmaceutical Society of Great Britain (1999) *British National Formulary*, no. 38, p. 529. BMA and Royal Pharmaceutical Society of GB, London.

Carola, R. et al. (1992) *Human Anatomy*, p. 533. McGraw Hill, New York.

Center for Disease Control (1997) Evaluation of safety devices for preventing percutaneous injuries among health care workers during phlebotomy procedures. *JAMA*, **277**(6), 449–50.

DoH (1990) *Guidance for Clinical Health Care Workers: Protection Against Infection with HIV and Hepatitis Viruses: Recommendations of the Expert Advisory Group on AIDS*. Stationery Office, London.

Dougherty, L. (1994) *A study to Discover Cancer Patients' Perceptions of the Cannulation Experience*. MSc thesis, University of Surrey, Guildford.

Dougherty, L. (1996) Intravenous cannulation. *Nurs Stand*, **11**(2), 47–51.

Dougherty, L. (1999) Obtaining vascular access. In: *IV Therapy in Practice* (eds L. Dougherty & J. Lamb), Chap. 9. Churchill Livingstone, Edinburgh.

Dyson, A. & Bogod, D. (1987) Minimizing bruising in the antecubital fossa after venepuncture. *Br Med J*, **294**, 1659.

Godwin, P.G.R., Cuthbert, A.C. & Choyce, A. (1992) Reducing bruising after venepuncture. *Quality Health Care*, **1**, 245–6.

Gunawardene, R.D. & Davenport, H.T. (1990) Local application of EMLA and glyceryl trinitrate ointment before venepuncture. *Anaesthesia*, **45**, 52–4.

Hadaway, L. (1995) Anatomy and physiology related to IV therapy. In: *Intravenous Therapy: Clinical Principles and Practices* (eds J. Terry, L. Baranowski, R.A. Lonsway & C. Hedrick), pp. 81–110. W.B. Saunders, Philadelphia.

Hecker, J.F. et al. (1983) Nitroglycerine ointment as an aid to venepuncture. *Lancet*, 12 Feb, 332–3.

Hudek, K. (1986) Compliance in IV therapy. *J Can Intraven Nurs Assoc*, **2**(3), 3–8.

Intravenous Nursing Society (1998) Revised intravenous nursing standards of practice. *J Intraven Nurs*, **21**, Suppl. 1S.

Inwood, S. (1996) Designing a nurse training programme for venepuncture. *Nurs Stand*, **10**(21), 40–42.

Jackson, S. (1996) The case for shared training of nurses and doctors. *Nurs Times*, **92**(26), 40–41.

Johnston-Early, A. et al. (1981) Venepuncture and problem veins. *Am J Nurs*, Sept, 1636–40.

Lamb, J. (1999) Legal and professional aspects of IV therapy. In: *IV Therapy in Practice* (eds L. Dougherty & J. Lamb), Chap. 1. Churchill Livingstone, Edinburgh.

Marieb, E.N. (1998) *Essentials of Human Anatomy and Physiology*, 5th edn. Benjamin/Cummings, California.

McConnell, A.A. & MacKay, G.M. (1996) Venepuncture: the medicolegal hazards. *Postgrad Med J*, **72**, 23–4.

Michael, A. & Andrew, M. (1996) The application of EMLA and GTN ointment prior to venepuncture. *Anaesth Intens Care*, **24**(3), 360–64.

Middleton, J. (1985) Don't needle the patient. *Nurs Mirror*, **161**(4), 22–3.

Millam, D.A. (1992) Starting IVs – how to develop your venepuncture skills. *Nursing*, **92**, 33–46.

Millam, D.A. (1995) The use of anaesthesia in IV therapy. *J Vasc Access Devices*, **1**(1), 22–9.

Perdue, M. (1995) Intravenous complications. In: *Intravenous Therapy: Clinical Principles and Practices* (eds J. Terry, L. Baranowski, R.A. Lonsway & C. Hedrick), Chap. 24. W.B. Saunders, Philadelphia.

Perucca, R. (1995) Obtaining vascular access. In: *Intravenous Therapy: Clinical Principles and Practices* (eds J. Terry, L. Baranowski, R.A. Lonsway & C. Hedrick), Chap. 21. W.B. Saunders, Philadelphia.

Peters, J.L. *et al.* (1984) Peripheral venous cannulation: reducing the risks. *Br J Parent Ther*, March, 56–68.

Price, J. & Moss, J. (1998) The pitfalls of practice nursing. *Nurs Times*, **94**(30), 64–6.

RCN (1995) *Universal Precautions*. RCN, London.

RCN (1999) *Guidance for Nurses Giving Intravenous Therapy*. RCN, London.

Rowland, R. (1991) Making sense of venepuncture. *Nurs Times*, **87**(32), 41–3.

Sager, D. & Bomar, S. (1980) *Intravenous Medications – A Guide to Preparation, Administration and Nursing Management*. J.B. Lippincott, Philadelphia.

Smith, J. (1998) The practice of venepuncture in lymphoedema. *Eur J Cancer Care*, **7**, 97–8.

UKCC (1992) *Scope of Professional Practice*. United Kingdom Central Council for Nursing, Midwifery and Health Visiting, London.

Weinstein, S.M. (1997) *Plumer's Principles and Practice of Intravenous Therapy*, 6th edn. J.B. Lippincott, Philadelphia.

Wilson, K.J.W. & Waugh, A. (1998) *Anatomy and Physiology*, 8th edn. Churchill Livingstone, Edinburgh.

Yuan, R.T.W. & Cohen, M.D. (1987) Lateral antebrachial cutaneous nerve injury as a complication of phlebotomy. *J Can Intraven Nurses Assoc*, **3**(3), 16–17.

GUIDELINES • Venepuncture

Equipment

1 Clean tray or receiver.
2 Tourniquet or sphygmomanometer and cuff.
3 21 swg multiple sample needle or 21 swg winged infusion device and multiple sample luer adaptor.
4 Plastic shell holder.
5 Appropriate vacuumed specimen tubes.
6 Swab saturated with chlorohexidine in 70% alcohol, or isopropyl alcohol 70%.

7 Low-linting swabs.
8 Sterile adhesive plaster or hypoallergenic tape.
9 Specimen requisition forms.
10 Gloves, if necessary.
11 Plastic apron (optional).

A number of vacuum systems are available that can be used for taking blood samples. These are simple to use and cost effective. The manufacturer's instructions should be followed if one of these systems is used. Vacuum systems reduce the risk of health care workers being contaminated, because they offer a completely closed system during the process of blood withdrawal and there is no necessity to decant blood into bottles (Dougherty 1999). This makes them the safest method for collecting blood samples using venepuncture. If not available, the following items replace the vacuum system:

1 21 swg needle or 21 swg winged infusion device.
2 Syringe(s) of appropriate size.
3 Appropriate blood specimen bottle(s).

Procedure

Action	*Rationale*
1 Approach the patient in a confident manner and explain and discuss the procedure with the patient.	To ensure that the patient understands the procedure and gives his/her valid consent.
2 Allow the patient to ask questions and discuss any problems which have arisen previously.	Anxiety results in vasoconstriction; therefore a patient who is relaxed will have dilated veins, making access easier.
3 Consult the patient as to any preferences and problems that may have been experienced at previous venepunctures.	To involve the patient in the treatment. To acquaint the nurse fully with the patient's previous venous history and identify any changes in clinical status, e.g. mastectomy, as both may influence vein choice.
4 Check the identity of the patient matches the details on the requisition form.	To ensure the sample is taken from the correct patient.
5 Assemble the equipment necessary for venepuncture.	To ensure that time is not wasted and that the procedure goes smoothly without unnecessary interruptions.

Guidelines • Venepuncture (cont'd)

Action	Rationale
6 Carefully wash hands using bactericidal soap and water or bactericidal alcohol hand rub, and dry before commencement.	To minimize risk of infection.
7 Check hands for any visibly broken skin, and cover with a waterproof dressing.	To minimize the risk of contamination, by blood, of the practitioner.
8 Check all packaging before opening and preparing the equipment on the chosen clean receptacle.	To maintain asepsis throughout and check that no equipment is damaged.
9 Take all the requirements to the patient, exhibiting a competent manner.	To help the patient feel more at ease with the procedure.
10 In both an inpatient and an outpatient situation, lighting, ventilation, privacy and positioning must be checked.	To ensure that both patient and operator are comfortable and that adequate light is available to illuminate this procedure.
11 Support the chosen limb.	To ensure the patient's comfort and facilitate venous access.
12 (a) Apply a tourniquet to the upper arm on the chosen side, making sure it does not obstruct arterial flow. The position of the tourniquet may be varied, e.g. if a vein in the hand is to be used it may be placed on the forearm. A sphygmomanometer cuff may be used as an alternative.	To dilate the veins by obstructing the venous return.
(b) The arm may be placed in a dependent position. The patient may assist by clenching and unclenching the fist.	To increase the prominence of the veins.
(c) The veins may be tapped gently or stroked.	
(d) If all these measures are unsuccessful, remove the tourniquet and apply moist heat, e.g. a warm compress, soak limb in warm water or, with medical prescription, apply glyceryl trinitrate ointment/patch.	To promote blood flow and therefore distend the veins.
13 Select the vein using the aforementioned criteria.	
14 Select the device, based on vein size, site, etc.	To reduce damage or trauma to the vein.
15 Wash hands with bactericidal soap and water or bactericidal alcohol hand rub.	To maintain asepsis, and minimize the risk of infection.
16 Put on gloves, if appropriate.	To prevent possible contamination of practitioner.
17 Clean the patient's skin carefully for 30 sec using an appropriate preparation, e.g. chlorhexidine in 70% alcohol, and allow to dry. Do not repalpate the vein or touch the skin.	To maintain asepsis and minimize the risk of infection. To prevent pain on insertion. To minimize the risk of infection.
18 Inspect the device carefully.	To detect faulty equipment, e.g. bent or barbed needles. If these are present, discard them in a sharps bin.
19 Anchor the vein by applying manual traction on the skin a few centimetres below the proposed insertion site.	To immobilize the vein. To provide countertension to the vein which will facilitate a smoother needle entry.
20 Insert the needle smoothly at an angle of approximately 30°. The shaft of a straight needle may be bent slightly at the hub, against the inside of the lid, to enable the entry to be as flush with the skin as possible.	To facilitate a successful, pain-free venepuncture.
21 Reduce the angle of descent of the needle as soon as a flashback of blood is seen in the tubing of a winged	To prevent advancing too far through vein wall and causing damage to the vessel.

infusion device or when puncture of the vein wall is felt. If you are using a needle and syringe, pull the plunger back slightly prior to venepuncture and a flashback of blood will be seen in the barrel on vein entry.

22 Slightly advance the needle into the vein, if possible.

To stabilize the device within the vein and prevent it becoming dislodged during withdrawal of blood.

23 Do not exert any pressure on the needle.

To prevent a puncture occurring through the vein wall.

24 Withdraw the required amount of blood using a vacuumed blood collection system or syringes.

25 Release the tourniquet. In some instances this may be necessary at the beginning of sampling as inaccurate measurements may be caused by haemostasis, e.g. when taking blood to assess calcium levels.

To decrease the pressure within the vein.

26 If using a needle and syringe withdraw a small amount of blood into the syringe.

To reduce the amount of static blood in the vein and therefore the likelihood of leakage at the venepuncture site on removal of the needle.

27 Pick up a low-linting swab and place it over the puncture point.

28 Remove the needle, but do not apply pressure until the needle has been fully removed.

To prevent pain on removal and damage to the intima of the vein.

29 Discard the needle immediately in sharps bin.

To reduced the risk of accidental needlestick injury.

30 Apply digital pressure directly over the puncture site. Pressure should be applied until bleeding has ceased; approximately 1 min longer may be required if current disease or treatment interferes with clotting mechanisms.

To stop leakage and haematoma formation. To preserve vein by preventing bruising or haematoma formation.

31 The patient may apply pressure with the finger but should be discouraged from bending the arm if a vein in the antecubital fossa is used (Dyson & Bogod 1987).

To prevent leakage and haematoma formation.

32 Where a syringe has been used, transfer the blood to appropriate specimen bottles as soon as possible, making sure that the correct quantity is placed in each container.

To prevent clotting in the syringe. To ensure that an adequate amount is available for each test.

33 Mix well if the bottle contains a chemical to prevent clotting or aid accurate measurements.

To ensure that the blood is correctly presented to the laboratory and that the patient does not have to have a repeat specimen taken.

34 Label the bottles with the relevant details.

To ensure that the specimens from the right patient are delivered to the laboratory, the requested tests are performed and the results returned to the correct patient's records.

35 Inspect the puncture point before applying a dressing.

To check that the puncture point has sealed.

36 Ascertain whether the patient is allergic to adhesive plaster.

To prevent an allergic skin reaction.

37 Apply an adhesive plaster or alternative dressing.

To cover the puncture and prevent leakage or contamination.

38 Ensure that the patient is comfortable.

To ascertain whether patient wishes to rest before leaving (if an outpatient) or whether any other measures need to be taken.

39 Discard waste, making sure it is placed in the correct containers, e.g. 'sharps' into a designated receptacle.

To ensure safe disposal and avoid laceration or other injury of staff. To prevent re-use of equipment.

40 Follow hospital procedure for collection and transportation of specimens to the laboratory.

To make sure that specimens reach their intended destination.

Guidelines • Venepuncture (cont'd)

Action	Rationale
41 Remove gloves and discard in appropriate clinical waste bag.	

Nursing care plan

Problem	Cause	Prevention	Suggested action
Pain.	Puncturing an artery.	Knowledge of location of an artery. Palpate vessel for pulse.	Remove device immediately and apply pressure until bleeding stops. Explain to patient what has happened. Inform patient to contact doctor if pain continues or there is increasing swelling or bruising. Document in the patient's notes.
	Touching a nerve (sharp, shooting pain along arm and fingers).	Knowledge of location of nerves.	Remove the needle immediately and apply pressure. Explain to the patient what has happened and that the pain or numbness may last a few hours. Document in the patient's notes. Inform patient to contact doctor if pain continues or becomes worse.
	Anxiety.	(See below.)	See below.
	Use of vein in sensitive area (e.g. wrist).	Avoid using veins in sensitive areas wherever possible. Use local anaesthetic cream.	Complete procedure as quickly as possible.
Anxiety.	Previous trauma.	Minimize the risk of a traumatic venepuncture. Use all methods available to ensure successful venepuncture.	Approach patient in a calm and confident manner. Listen to the patient's fears and explain what the procedure involves. Offer patient opportunity to lie down. Suggest use of local anaesthetic cream.
	Fear of needles.		All above and perhaps referral to a psychologist if fear is of phobic proportions.
Limited venous access.	Repeated use of same veins.	Use alternate sites if possible.	Do not attempt the procedure unless experienced.
	Peripheral shutdown.	Ensure the room is not cold.	Put patient's arm in warm water. Apply glycerol trinitrate patch.

	Dehydration.		May be necessary to rehydrate patient prior to venepuncture.
	Hardened veins (due to scarring and thrombosis).		Do not use these veins as venepuncture will be unsuccessful.
Bruising and/or haematoma.	Needle has punctured the posterior wall of the vein.	Lower angle of insertion.	Remove the needle and apply pressure at the venepuncture site until bleeding stops. The following actions apply regardless of cause: (a) Elevate the limb.
	Inadequate pressure on removal of needle.	The practitioner should apply pressure.	(b) Apply ice pack if necessary. (c) Apply pressure dressing.
	Forgetting to remove the tourniquet before removing the needle.		Explain to patient what has happened. Inform patient to contact doctor if area becomes more painful as haematoma may be pressing on a nerve. Do not reapply tourniquet to affected limb.
	Poor technique/choice of vein or device.	Ensure correct device and technique are used.	
Infection at the venepuncture site.	Poor aseptic technique.	Ensure good handwashing and adequate skin cleansing.	Report to doctor as patient may require systemic or local antibiotics.
Vasovagal reaction.	Fear of needles.	Spend time listening to patient's fears. Calm, confident manner.	Place patient's head between his or her legs if patient is feeling faint. Encourage patient to lie down. Call for assistance
	Pain.		Try to secure the venepuncture device in case it is required for administration of medication.
	Hot environment.	Ensure environment is comfortable temperature.	Open a window or door.
Needle inoculation of practitioner.	Lack of safe practice.	Maintain safe practice.	Follow accident procedure for sharps injury, e.g. make site bleed and apply a waterproof dressing. Report and document. An injection of hepatitis B immunoglobulin or triple therapy may be required.
	Incorrect disposal of sharps.	Ensure sharps are disposed of immediately and safely.	
Accidental blood spillage.	Poor technique.	Use good technique.	Wear gloves if risk of spillage or if decanting into bottles.
	Damaged equipment (e.g. cracked bottles).	Use vacuumed plastic blood collection system.	Ensure blood is handled and transported correctly.
Missed vein.	Inadequate anchoring. Poor vein selection.	Ensure that only properly trained staff perform	Withdraw the needle slightly and realign it,

Problem	Cause	Prevention	Suggested action
	Wrong positioning. Lack of concentration.	venepuncture or that those who are training are supervised.	providing the patient is not feeling any discomfort. Ensure all learners are supervised. If the patient is feeling pain, then the needle should be removed immediately.
	Poor lighting.	Ensure the environment is well lit.	
	Difficult venous access.		Ask experienced colleague to perform the procedure.
Spurt of blood on entry.	Bevel tip of needle enters the vein before entire bevel is under the skin; usually occurs when the vein is very superficial.		Reassure the patient. Wipe blood away on removal of needle.
Blood stops flowing.	'Overshooting vein'.	Correct angle.	Draw back the needle, but if bruising is evident, then remove the needle immediately and apply pressure.
	Contact with valves.	Palpate to locate.	Withdraw needle slightly to move tip away from valve.
	Venous spasm.	Results from mechanical irritation and cannot be prevented.	Gently massage above the vein or apply heat.
	Vein collapse.	Use veins with large lumen.	Release tourniquet, allow veins to refill and retighten tourniquet.
	Small vein.	Avoid use of small veins wherever possible.	May require another venepuncture.
	Poor blood flow.	Use veins with large lumens.	Apply heat above vein.

Violence: Prevention and Management

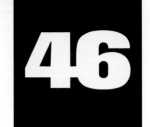

Definition

Violence is 'an act of destructive aggression which may involve injury to the self, assaulting people or objects in the environment' (Stuart & Sundeen 1991). This is a mainly physically related definition, but Robinson (1983) defines aggression as 'an assertive force which may be expressed through attitude or behaviour and is usually directed to external objects, though it may be turned inward, as reflected in self-destructive behaviour'. She states that 'aggression is a healthy force which sometimes needs to be channelled'. Thus, it can be expressed either physically or non-physically.

The Royal College of Nursing recommends the following definition of violence orientated towards staff members, which can be adapted at local level as necessary:

> Any incident in which a health professional experiences abuse, threat, fear or the application of force arising out of the course of their work, whether or not they are on duty.

(RCN 1998)

However, as violence is often directed towards other individuals and objects, the local policy should encompass these aspects.

It can therefore be concluded from the above definitions that violence is an act or type of behaviour that may take the form of aggression, abuse, threat or attack.

Indications

Management of violence is necessary:

1 When the person shows a predisposition to violence.
2 When a person makes a physical attack on another person or object.
3 When a person becomes disturbed to the extent that his/her behaviour is considered a threat to his/her own safety or the safety of others.

Reference material

Violent crime is increasing steadily (Golding 1995; Shepherd & Farrington 1995). Assaults in the UK are now the third most common type of reported accident after slips, falls and needle accidents. Nurses, ambulance and A & E staff, and those caring for psychologically disturbed patients, are particularly vulnerable (Dobson 1999). Incidents range from threats and abuse to permanently disabling injuries and, rarely, loss of life. This chapter is confined to the prevention and management of violence in the hospital setting.

Principles

The following principles underlie the management of violent persons:

1 Prevention of violent incidents is the foremost principle.
2 Restraint is always therapeutic, never punitive. As far as possible, the therapeutic regime should be maintained.
3 The risk of physical injury should be minimized. Any restraint applied must be of a degree appropriate to the actual danger or resistance shown by the person. This is particularly important with children and the elderly. Staff must receive training in the use of restraint as training can help prevent injury to staff and patients.
4 The locally agreed procedure for the nursing care of violent patients should be adhered to.

Theories of violence

Mechanisms that may combine to explain or produce a violent act are reviewed by Harrington (1972) and Gunn (1973). Generally, theories of violence may be classified as biological (Lorenz 1966; Gray 1971; Montague 1979), psychological (Freud 1955; Dollard & Miller 1961) or sociocultural (Bandura & Walters 1963; Wertham 1968; Gelles 1972). Although the latter of these cannot be completely divorced from organic or biological predisposition, certain factors may increase the risk of violent or aggressive behaviour. Early psychological traumas and cases arising from cycles of abuse are two such examples (De Zulueta 1993; Fonagy & Target 1995). Studies have shown associations between combat experience, post-traumatic stress disorder, anger and hostility, and involvement in violence (Reilly et al. 1994). In the hospital setting where reactions to stress, illness and treatment are prevalent, staff-related factors are also important in predisposing to violence by patients or visitors. Common antecedents include poor communication, negative attitudes, restrictions on patients imposed by the hospital routine or provocation by other patients or visitors (Powell et al. 1994).

Incidents of verbal or physical abuse are more likely to happen in long-term care and emergency areas and may be directed towards nurses and nursing assistants rather than doctors. Agitation and aggression preceding violent behaviour have been identified particularly among elderly confused patients, and nursing interventions such as feeding, dressing and bathing represented the most common antecedents (Campbell *et al.* 1989). Staff gender is not strongly associated with the risk of abuse (Binder & McNeil 1994; Graydon *et al.* 1994). Violence may be viewed as a behaviour influenced by various factors including personality, environment and social culture. Each perspective may add to the development of a body of knowledge about the problem of violence in the hospital setting.

Physiological considerations

Under certain circumstances patients may have little or no ability to exercise control over their aggression. In these instances aggression may be related to pathological physiology. Internal stressors may include endocrine imbalance such as hyperthyroidism, hyperglycaemia, convulsive disorders, HIV encephalopathy, dementia and brain tumours. Krakowski and Czobor (1994) confirmed an association between persistent violence and neurological impairment. The effects of alcohol and substance abuse should also be considered. Among the physiological causes given by Kerr and Taylor (1997) are pain, side-effects of medication (including neuroleptic-induced akathisia), childhood disorders such as autism and mental retardation. Preventive measures to reduce the risk of violence may not be possible and the policy for the management of violence should be adhered to.

Legislation

The law on health and safety at work applies to risks from violence, just as it does to other risks at work. Key points are summarized as follows.

1 *Health and Safety at Work etc. Act 1974*
   Employers must:
   (a) Protect the health and safety at work of their employees.
   (b) Protect the health and safety of others who might be affected, such as visitors, contractors, students and patients.
2 *Management of Health and Safety at Work Regulations 1992*
   Employers must:
   (a) Assess the risks to the health and safety of their employees.
   (b) Identify the precautions needed to reduce the risks of violence.
   (c) Make arrangements for the effective management of risks.
   (d) Appoint competent people to advise them on health and safety.
   (e) Provide information and training to employees.
3 *The Reporting of Injuries, Diseases and Dangerous Occurrences Regulations 1995*
   These Regulations state that employers must report cases in which employees have been off work for 3 days or more following an assault which has resulted in physical injury. This should be in conjunction with the local incident policy in which any psychological injury is also documented.
4 *The Safety Representatives and Safety Committees Regulations 1977* and *The Health and Safety (Consultation with Employees) Regulations 1996*
   Employers must consult with safety representatives and employees on health and safety matters (Health and Safety Commission: Health Services Advisory Committee 1997).

Policy formation

NHS trusts must establish targets for reducing violence against their staff and targets will be expected to be delivered. In addition, NHS trusts will be expected to have systems in place to monitor and record violence against staff and have published strategies in place to achieve a reduction in such incidents (Dobson 1999).

In forming a policy for managing aggression or violence, the following aspects need to be considered:

1 Environmental and organizational factors
2 Anticipation and prevention of violence
3 Action following an incident.

Environmental and organizational factors

Hospital environments can be stressful places and so certain design features can help to maximize a tranquil ambience. Calming features include creating a perception of space, ensuring there is natural daylight and fresh air and noise levels are controlled, providing smoking and non-smoking areas and ensuring privacy in toilet and bathroom areas. In creating a secure environment (in psychiatric settings) there must be a safe room for severely disturbed people, moveable objects should be of a safe weight, size and construction, and doors should be easily accessible. This list is not exhaustive and many other features are possible when considering environmental factors (Royal College of Psychiatrists 1998).

The way in which staff are deployed influences the likelihood and outcome of any violent incident. Teaching sessions on the management of violence should be held on a regular basis so that staff benefit from controlled practice of the required techniques for avoiding or containing violence. Topics may include how to help patients achieve appropriate expression of emotions, alternatives to violent behaviour or stress reduction techniques (Green 1989). Paterson *et al.* (1992) found that after a training course in the short-term management of violence, staff reported increased levels of success and confidence in their ability to manage violent incidents and reduced stress levels. It is helpful if there is an incident team in the hospital, specifically trained in violence management, that can be called if an emergency occurs (Brayley *et al.* 1984). Teamwork is essential and the leader must be seen to be confident in making the necessary decisions. It is advisable to work in teams of three wherever possible, but where a one-to-one violent confrontation arises, using a breakaway technique is usually the safest option for staff and patient (T. Swan 1995, personal communication). It is the responsibility of individual members of staff to state whether they have a physical condition, such as a back injury or pregnancy, which would render them incapable of performing such techniques. If so, then help should be summoned from other staff members at the earliest opportunity.

Anticipation and prevention of violence

The purpose of the assessment of risk of violence is to identify how and why conflict can occur and consider what measures can be taken to reduce the risks of such events within the workplace. The risk assessment process for the identification and control of violence can be separated into the following steps:

Identify hazards

It is helpful if there is an assessment form for the risks that are being assessed which can be completed in discussion with staff within the department. A review of past incidents will provide an opportunity to identify potential sources of conflict, potential aggressors and likely risk factors. For example, the assessment should consider whether any particular areas present a higher risk of violence such as:

1 Front line reception areas
2 Inpatient clinical areas
3 Outpatient clinical areas
4 Communal areas
5 Community
6 Lone working, e.g. interview rooms, isolated offices.

Identify potential aggressors

The complexities of human nature can make people unpredictable in how they will react in different situations. Illness can exacerbate the response in both patients and their relatives and health care workers need to be particularly sensitive to this. Staff will also have their own issues that may affect how they respond at different times. For example:

Patients

Patients who are at high risk of being violent should be identified. This includes those with physiological conditions as previously discussed or patients with a previous history of violent behaviour. There should be a multi-professional approach in establishing this. Patients may become violent or aggressive for a number of reasons, often these are not directly related to the environment but are as a result of a changed mental state due to treatment, e.g. drug therapy, anxiety or frustration. There may also be language or cultural differences, which can lead to confusion and aggression. Failure to recognize these issues can give the impression of indifference and further exacerbate the

situation (The Royal Marsden Hospital 1999). Violent incidents may be spontaneous, without apparent provocation. For example, a patient suffering from a psychotic illness or cerebral lesion may demonstrate these symptoms. However, there may be warning signs, such as increased agitation, which would alert staff to a potentially violent situation and therefore give nurses the opportunity to reduce the risk of violence.

Physical signs may include increased motor agitation, verbal content such as aggressive language, change in voice tone or volume, thigh tapping, fist clenching or sudden cessation of activity (Smith 1987; Benson & Den 1992). Responding to these cues to violence with an appropriate verbal interaction can prevent the escalation of an incident (Brennan & Swan 1995). Stuart and Sundeen (1991) see violence as the culmination of an escalating process, where anger and aggression are considered as precursors to violence. They suggest that preventive therapeutic interventions can be used to intercept this process, thus deferring a potentially violent situation. Three steps have been identified in calming an agitated or aroused person:

1 Diminish the anger, as the person cannot deal appropriately with the problems while remaining aroused.
2 Work at problem solving, which involves clarifying the problem, providing solutions and aiming to evaluate them with the person.
3 Carry out the actions decided upon with the person. Communication is vital and questions should be open, using 'how' and 'when' rather than 'why', which may be perceived as provocative (Brennan & Swan 1995).

Knowledge of the propensities of individual patients will enable a nurse to recognize many of the signs of impending violence, thus allowing steps to be taken to help patients find alternative outlets for their aggressive feelings.

Visitors and relatives

It is important to realize that each visitor, contractor, outpatient or patient relative visiting the hospital will have individual needs, anxieties and expectations. Tension may be released in terms of anger, and on occasions violence, towards other members of their family or staff that they encounter. Factors such as poor sign-posting, failure to find a parking space, long waiting times for an appointment, inadequate welfare facilities, perceived queue-jumping and inadequate information can all increase the risk of conflict and aggression (The Royal Marsden Hospital 1999).

Staff

The response of staff to aggressive situations may be influenced by factors such as workload, stress, illness, confidence and experience. When long hours are worked, or a heavy workload is undertaken, staff may feel under increased stress. Misunderstandings, failure to clarify task requirements or requests can lead to verbal abuse or aggression. It should not be seen as a weakness of staff if they try to avoid violence. It is important also to consider the needs of new or agency staff who may not be aware of the activities of the department. Inappropriate expectations can also lead to conflict or bullying behaviour. The level of training provided for staff (in terms of undertaking the work required, customer care skills, dealing with aggression, how to diffuse awkward situations, etc.) can also influence the degree of risk (The Royal Marsden Hospital 1999).

Agreement within the policy should be considered concerning what criteria are used before calling the police to attend an incident. This will depend on the severity of the situation and persons or property at risk (RCN 1998).

Implementing additional control measures to reduce risk

Once the hazards and risks have been identified, the next step required is a review of the procedures already in place to reduce the risks. Any additional precautions, procedures or control measures required can then be implemented. These may include providing the features previously discussed in the section on environmental and organizational factors, plus:

1 Providing comfortable seating.
2 Providing access to refreshment.
3 Providing appropriate facilities for the disabled.
4 Improving communication systems and multilingual notices and signposts.
5 Reducing waiting times.
6 Providing staff training.
7 Increasing personal security systems, such as close-circuit television.
8 Providing staff support.
9 Introducing an incident reporting system.

Action following an incident

Once violence has occurred, the following may be regarded as among the important management decisions that need to be implemented:

1 Medical personnel should be informed immediately because medication may be required as part of the management of the situation.
2 Some nurses must be delegated to attend to the needs of the remaining patients, to telephone for help and to prepare any required medication.
3 If immobilization is needed, the agreed local policy for restraining a patient must be implemented.

At all times, the *Code of Professional Conduct* must be adhered to (UKCC 1992). This is discussed in further detail in The Royal College of Nursing's guide *Dealing with Violence Against Nursing Staff* (1998). If legal advice needs to be obtained in a particular case, such as financial compensation or prosecution following personal injury or damage to property, this should be obtained from a solicitor, barrister, health and safety representative and/or trade union representative.

Following the incident, staff should be given an opportunity to discuss their feelings about the aggressor(s), other members of staff involved and the way the incident was managed. This should happen as soon as possible after the incident has resolved and with as many of the staff concerned as possible. There should be discussion on:

1 What happened
2 Any trigger factors
3 People's roles in the incident
4 How they feel now
5 How they might feel in the next few days
6 What can be done about it
7 Any measures that can be taken to avoid a repeat of the situation
(RCN 1998).

Emotional debriefing aims to recognize potential stress, acknowledge it as a normal response and provide a supportive and structured setting to allow people to cope more effectively. Discussion should not be focused on any person's performance but address the effects on them as individuals (Health and Safety Commission: Health Services Advisory Committee 1997). In addition to the debriefing procedure, the physical and psychological well-being of the staff involved and the team as a whole need to be addressed. Staff injured as a result of their involvement in the incident may be entitled to industrial injuries benefit or a payment under the criminal injuries compensation scheme and will need to be informed of their rights by the appropriate body (RCN 1998). Consideration must be given to the risk of infection in cases where injury has occurred; for example, bites or needlestick injuries. Staff must receive continued support when returning to work after a violent incident (RCN 1998). Debriefing can be supplemented by making confidential counselling available through in-house counsellors, occupational health departments or independent external bodies (Health and Safety Commission: Health Services Advisory Committee 1997).

Some staff view reporting of incidents as admission of failure, especially if violence is rare in the area in which they work (Drummond *et al.* 1989); therefore, debriefing becomes particularly relevant in order to promote reporting of incidents.

All documentation required by law (such as the reporting of staff off work for 3 days or more following an assault) or hospital policy (such as completing an incident form) should be completed and forwarded to the appropriate departments. If restraints have been used, how and by whom they were applied should be documented. Specific and accurate written records will aid recall if it is required, perhaps years later (Navis 1987).

Summary

Violent incidents often arise from a patient feeling vulnerable and attack may become the preferred means of defence. The manner in which a patient is approached may be crucial in determining whether the patient will feel secure enough to cease the behaviour or to continue to feel threatened, perhaps leading on to violent behaviour. The need for physical restraint should be seen as the application of the appropriate technique in a particular situation and not as a failure of other methods. Protection against any administrative or legal problems lies in following the appropriate guidelines and applying them in good faith and with due restraint.

References and further reading

Bandura, A. & Walters, R. (1963) *Social Learning and Personality Development*. Holt, Rinehart & Winston, New York.

Benson, S. & Den, A. (1992) Monitoring violence. *Nurs Times*, **88**(41), 46–8.

Binder, R. & McNeil, D. (1994) Staff gender and risk of assault on doctors and nurses. *Bull Am Acad Psychiatry Law*, **22**(4), 545–50.

Brayley, J. *et al.* (1994) The violence management team: an approach to aggressive behaviour in a general hospital. *Med J Aust*, **161**(4), 254–8.

Brennan, W. & Swan, T. (1995) Managing violence and aggression. In: *Royal College of General Practitioners, Members Reference Book*, pp. 443–5. Sabrecrown, London.

Campbell, B. *et al.* (1989) A high-risk occupation? *Nurs Times*, **85**(13), 37–9.

De Zulueta, F. (1993) *From Pain to Violence: The Traumatic Roots of Destructive Behaviour*. Whurr, London.

Dobson, F. (1999) *Dobson steps up major drive to protect NHS staff from assaults: violence and security*. Memorandum from NHS Executive. Press Release 15 April. Stationery Office, London.

Dollard, J. & Miller, N.E. (1961) *Frustration and Aggression*. Yale University Press, New Haven.

Drummond, D.J. *et al.* (1989) Hospital violence reduction among high-risk patients. *J Am Med Assoc*, **261**(17) 2531–4.

Fonagy, P. & Target, M. (1995) Understanding the violent patient: the use of the body and the role of the father. *Int J Psychoanalysis*, **76**, 487–501.

Freud, S. (1955) *The Complete Psychological Works of Sigmund Freud*, Vol. 18. Hogarth Press, London.

Gelles, R.J. (1972) *The Violent Home*. Sage, Beverly Hills and London.

Golding, A. (1995) Understanding and preventing violence: a review (leading article). *Public Health*, **109**(2), 91–7.

Gray, J.A. (1971) Sex differences in emotional behaviour in mammals including man: endocrine basis. *Acta Psycholog*, **35**, 29–44.

Graydon, J. *et al.* (1994) Verbal and physical abuse of nurses. *Can J Nurs Admin*, **7**(4), 70–89.

Green, E. (1989) Patient care guidelines: management of violent behavior. *J Emerg Nurs*, **15**(6), 523–8.

Gunn, J. (1973) *Violence*. David & Charles, Newton Abbot.

Harrington, J.A. (1972) Violence: a clinical viewpoint. *Br Med J*, 1, 228–31.

Health and Safety Commission: Health Services Advisory Committee (1997) *Violence and Aggression to Staff in Health Services: Guidance on Assessment and Management*, 2nd edn. HSE Books, Suffolk.

HSE (1992) *Management of Health and Safety at Work Regulations 1992*. Approved Code of Practice L21. Stationery Office, London.

HSE (1996a) *A Guide to the Reporting of Injuries, Diseases and Dangerous Occurrences Regulations 1995 (RIDDOR)*. L73. Stationery Office, London.

HSE (1996b) *A Guide to the Health and Safety (Consultation with Employees) Regulations 1996*. Guidance on Regulations L95. Stationery Office, London.

HSE (1996c) *Safety Representatives and Safety Committees*. L87. Stationery Office, London.

Kerr, I.B. & Taylor, D. (1997) Acute disturbed or violent behaviour: principles of treatment. *J Psychopharmacol*, **11**(3), 271–7.

Krakowski, M. & Czobor, P. (1994) Clinical symptoms, neurological impairment, and prediction of violence in psychiatric inpatients. *Hosp Commun Psychiatry*, **45**(7), 711–13.

Lorenz, K. (1966) *On Aggression*. Harcourt, Brace & World, New York.

Montague, M.C. (1979) Physiology of aggressive behaviour. *J Neurosurg Nurs*, **11**, 10–15.

Navis, E.S. (1987) Controlling violent patients before they control you. *Nursing*, **17**(9), 52–4.

Paterson, B. *et al.* (1992) An evaluation of a training course in the short-term management of violence. *Nurse Educ Today*, **12**, 368–75.

Powell, G., Caan, W. & Crowe, M. (1994) What events precede violent incidents in psychiatric hospitals? *Br J Psychiatry*, **165**, 107–12.

RCN (1998) *Dealing with Violence Against Nursing Staff: An RCN Guide for Nurses and Managers*. Royal College of Nursing, London.

Reilly, P. *et al.* (1994) Anger management and temper control: critical components of post traumatic stress disorder and substance abuse treatment. *J Psychoactive Drugs*, **26**(4), 401–407.

Robinson, L. (1983) *Psychiatric Nursing as a Human Experience*. W.B. Saunders, Philadelphia.

Royal College of Psychiatrists (1998) *Management of Imminent Violence – Clinical Practice Guidelines: Quick Reference Guide*. Royal College of Psychiatrists, London.

Royal Marsden Hospital (1999) *The Violence at Work Policy*. Royal Marsden Hospital, London.

Shepherd, J. & Farrington, D. (1995) Preventing crime and violence (editorial). *Br Med J*, **310**(6975), 271–2.

Smith, D. (1987) Preventing violence in nursing. *N Z Nurs J*, **80**(12), 18–19.

Stuart, G.W. & Sundeen, S.J. (1991) *Principles and Practice of Psychiatric Nursing*, 4th edn. Mosby, St Louis.

Swan, T. (1994) Definition of care and responsibility. In: *Guidance Document, Centre for Aggression Management*. Ashworth Hospital, Liverpool.

UKCC (1992) *Code of Professional Conduct*. United Kingdom Central Council for Nursing, Midwifery and Health Visiting, London.

Wertham, D.J. (1968) *A Sign For Cain*. Hale, New York.

GUIDELINES • Prevention and management of violence

Procedure

Assessment of violence

Action

1 Involve multiprofessional staff to assess if the patient is at risk of becoming violent. Some considerations are:
  (a) Endocrine imbalance, e.g. hyperthyroidism, hyperglycaemia.
  (b) Convulsive disorders.
  (c) Dementia.
  (d) Neurological impairment.
  (e) Alcohol and substance abuse.
  (f) HIV encephalopathy.
  (g) Pharmacological factors, e.g. drug toxicity.
  (h) Previous history of violence or aggressive behaviour, combat experience or post-traumatic stress disorder.
  (i) Social or psychological factors such as extreme stress.

2 Assess any nursing interventions which may be antecedents to aggression in individual patients, e.g. feeding, dressing and bathing.

3 Observe for physical signs of aggression, which may include:
  (a) Increased motor agitation.
  (b) Verbal content such as aggressive language.
  (c) Change in voice tone or volume.
  (d) Thigh tapping.
  (e) Fist clenching.
  (f) Sudden cessation of activity.

Rationale

To reduce risk of a violent situation. If the patient is at risk of becoming violent, steps should be taken to avoid violence arising.

To ascertain if aggression may be precipitated by nursing interventions and take appropriate action to reduce risk of aggression occurring.

To ascertain if the patient is at risk of becoming violent.

Prevention of violence

Action

1 Promote a safe environment and minimize risk of violence by the following:
  (a) Make other staff aware of a potentially violent situation and that they should not enter it unobserved.
  (b) Try not to encroach upon the patient's personal space. Keep at arm's length.
  (c) If possible ask other patients to leave the area.
  (d) Ensure that there is a clear exit from the situation.
  (e) Avoid cornering the patient.
  (f) Observe the area around the patient for potential weapons.
  (g) Try to appear confident, calm and relaxed. Do not fold your arms, maintain an open posture. Move slowly, showing that you have nothing in your hands.

2 Talk quietly and clearly to the patient. Do not argue or become defensive.

Rationale

To maintain a safe environment for all patients, staff and visitors present and to avoid aggravating the situation further.

The nurse may be able to ascertain the patient's reason for frustration and give an opportunity to express anger verbally by initiating conversation. Arguing or defensiveness may fuel the person's anger.

3 Ask open questions, using 'how' and 'when' to help clarify the problem.

'Why' may be perceived as provocative.

4 Work at problem solving to reduce the patient's frustration and carry out the actions decided upon with the patient.

This helps to diminish the anger as the problem is easier to deal with when the patient is less aroused.

5 Adopt an attentive expression, but do not stare.

Staring could be interpreted as an attempt at domination (Brennan & Swan 1995).

6 Address the patient by name and name yourself.

To help orientate the patient and demonstrate respect.

Management of violence

Action

Rationale

1 Nurses should consider carefully the accessories they wear. Be aware of the length of your fingernails and the way long hair is dressed. Pens, badges and other items should be removed beforehand.

To minimize the risk of physical injury to patients and others.

2 The nurse should call for assistance by shouting or using any signalling system. Ask another patient to summon help when appropriate.

It is easier to manage the situation with two or more people. It alerts others to the situation should other agencies be required.

3 Other patients should be led away from the area where the patient is to be restrained.

Violent incidents are distressing and may trigger off more violence.

4 The person in charge of the ward or unit should assess whether or not there are enough staff, and inform the senior nurse if more are needed.

To contain the violence.

5 When help arrives, the staff should be organized. A leader should be nominated (e.g. the person in charge or the patient's key worker) who should identify himself/herself to the patient as leader. He/she should give the other staff a brief history of the patient and an account of the circumstances and events leading up to the incident.

The staff will need to be informed to enable them to manage the situation.

6 A doctor, preferably the patient's own, should be called immediately. A nurse should be allocated to draw up medication and give injections if required.

Medication may be required in the management of the patient.

7 To restrain the patient, clear instructions should be given. The manager should indicate when the patient is to be restrained and coordinate staff during the procedure. Any disagreements between staff should not be voiced in front of the patient.

All staff must know the overall plan for restraint and must provide a cohesive approach.

8 Each person should know which part of the patient's body is to be held and from where to approach the patient. (The policy for immobilization may vary from area to area.)

To achieve full and safe immobilization of the patient.

9 Allocate one member of staff, preferably someone the patient knows, to talk to the patient throughout the procedure.

To inform the patient about what is happening and why.

10 Try to minimize discomfort. Restraint must be of a degree appropriate to the actual resistance given by the patient.

The procedure is not a punitive one but for safety reasons.

11 As the patient calms down, the leader should indicate when restraint can be reduced. This should be done gradually, e.g. release one wrist at a time.

The patient may still be likely to strike.

Guidelines • Prevention and management of violence (cont'd)

Action	*Rationale*
12 The leader should withdraw staff from the patient gradually. Some staff should stay with the patient.	Gradual withdrawal is safer in case of further outbursts. To observe mood and behaviour and provide reassurance to the patient.

Follow-up

Action	*Rationale*
1 Attend to any patients and staff injured during the incident. Such people should be informed of their legal rights.	To provide care and to comply with legal obligations and hospital policy.
2 Record details of any violent incidents in the appropriate documents.	To comply with legal obligations and hospital policy.
3 The entire team should discuss the incident.	To vent feelings and evaluate care provided. Violent incidents are to be regarded as learning experiences and an opportunity for reflective practice.

Wound Management

Definition of a wound

A wound can be defined as an injury to the body that involves a break in the continuity of tissues or of body structures (*Blackwell's Dictionary of Nursing* 1998). Wounds are traditionally divided into four categories:

1 Contusion (bruise)
2 Abrasion (graze)
3 Laceration (tear)
4 Incision (cut).

Puncture wounds may now also be incorporated into these groupings (*Blackwell's Dictionary of Nursing* 1998). Different causes of wounds include:

1 External, e.g. burns (chemical, electrical, fire); hypoxia; mechanical; micro-organisms; radiation; temperature extremes.
2 Internal, e.g. damage to the circulatory system (venous, arterial, lymphatic); systemic (autoimmune, endocrine, haematological, neuropathies); local (infective, neoplastic) (David 1986; Allen 1988; Lawrence & Groves 1988).

Reference material

Classification of wounds

Wounds can be classified in different ways depending on the information required and action to be taken on the data. Classifications can be utilized to assess which treatment is most appropriate. These classifications most usefully contain an appraisal of the amount of tissue loss (Westaby 1985; Flanagan 1994). The classifications of pressure ulcers are usually determined using a five point scale (James 1998); however, these can sometimes lose their reliability when transferred from one clinical area to another. As a consequence, pressure ulcers may be over- or underestimated (Reid & Morison 1994).

Further classifications that might prove valuable for assessment of treatment entail whether the wound is clean or infected or dry or wet. The following categories are described as worthwhile when considering the application of disinfectants to wounds:

1 Dry, clean surgical wounds.
2 Wet, oozing, clean surgical wounds.
3 Open, contaminated wounds or lesions (Gustafsson 1988).

A similar but more sophisticated system concerns both differing wounds and the various stages they pass through as they heal. This classification is designed for selection of a dressing:

1 Black and necrotic – covered with a hard, dry layer of skin.
2 Sloughy/necrotic – covered or filled with a soft yellow slough.
3 Clean and granulating with a significant amount of tissue loss.
4 Epithelializing.
5 Infected – redness, swelling, heat, purulent exudate and pain at wound or surrounding area.

In addition, surgical wounds can be identified as one of four types: clean, clean contaminated, contaminated or dirty. This is dependent on the infection encountered (Cruse & Foord 1980).

Some classifications consider the origin of the wound. For example: surgical trauma, accidental trauma or ulceration caused by pressure or vascular insufficiency (Turner 1983; Miller & Dyson 1996); or intentional wounds and accidental wounds (Milward 1988).

Although these classifications give an indication of the aetiology of the wound, from which some evaluation may be made of its likely nature, they are unsuitable for assessing relevant treatment. When treatment is deliberated, the most appropriate classifications will include those that consider both the degree of tissue loss and whether or not the wound is infected (Turner 1983; Westaby 1985).

Wound healing

Wound healing is the process by which tissues damaged or destroyed by injury or disease are restored to normal function (Cape & Dobson 1978; Wingate & Wingate 1988; Silver 1994; Tortora & Grabowski 1996).

> Wound healing is only one aspect of the body's response to injury and the whole person, not just the visible injury, must be treated. (Torrance 1985)

The latter statement reflects a holistic perspective and is, therefore, more appropriate as a framework for planning nursing care.

Healing may occur by first, second or third intention. Healing by first intention involves the union of the edges of a clean, incised wound under aseptic conditions without visible granulations (Cape & Dobson 1978; Dealey 1994; *Blackwell's Dictionary of Nursing* 1998).

Healing by second intention signifies the process of contraction and epithelialization. The wound edges are separated and the cavity is gradually filled with granulation tissue from the bottom and the sides (Winter 1972). Epithelial tissue grows over the granulations and forms fibrous tissue which contracts to form a scar (Cape & Dobson 1978; Westaby 1985; Thomas 1990b; Dealey 1994).

Healing by third intention occurs when the wound ulcerates and granulations are slow to form (*Blackwell's Dictionary of Nursing* 1998).

Phases of wound healing

Wound healing is a complex series of physiological events which occur in a predictable sequence (Messer 1989; Flanagan 1999). Generally, the mechanism is described in three or four stages:

1 The inflammatory phase
2 The destructive phase
3 The proliferative or reconstructive phase or fibroplasia
4 The remodelling phase or maturation phase (Torrance 1985; Westaby 1985; Jackson & Rovee 1988; Johnson 1988a; Messer 1989; Cooper 1990; Silver 1994).

These stages overlap to an extent but will be discussed individually to enhance clarity (see also Table 47.1). Contraction and epithelialization are also necessary to the wound healing process but are not usually included in the above stages. These will be considered separately.

Inflammatory stage (0–3 days)

Vasoconstriction occurs within a few seconds of tissue damage. This lasts approximately 5–10 minutes. During this time injured blood vessels bleed into the cavity and leucocytes arrive and marginate along the vessel walls.

Platelets adhere to vessel walls and edges and are stabilized by a network of fibrin to form a clot. Bleeding ceases when the blood vessels thrombose. In the absence of noradrenaline (broken down by extracellular enzymes from damaged cells), and with the release of histamine, vasodilation begins. The liberation of histamine also increases the permeability of the capillary walls, and plasma proteins, leucocytes, antibodies and electrolytes exude into the surrounding tissues. The wound becomes red, swollen and hot.

Polymorphonuclear leucocytes and macrophages are chemotactically attracted to the wound to defend against infection and begin the process of repair. The macrophage is also known as the 'director cell' of wound healing. If the number and function of macrophages is reduced, as may occur in disease, e.g. diabetes (Tooke *et al.* 1988), or due to treatment, e.g. chemotherapy in cancer patients (Souhami & Tobias 1998), healing is seriously affected.

Destructive stage (2–5 days)

Polymorphonuclear leucocytes and macrophages combine to destroy and ingest bacteria, debris and devitalized tissue. This involves a great deal of cellular activity which requires up to 20 times the normal resting rate of oxygen of phagocytic cells. Patients with hypoxic wounds are, therefore, more susceptible to wound infection.

The degradation of unwanted material causes an increased osmolarity within the area, resulting in further swelling by osmosis. This may increase pressure in restricted parts of the body, thus precipitating ischaemia.

Proliferative stage (3–24 days)

Macrophages produce factors that are chemotactic to fibroblasts and angioblasts. The macrophage secretes a fibroblast-stimulating factor which in the presence of a

Table 47.1 Factors that may delay wound healing

Disease, disorders and syndromes	Addison's disease; anaemia; arteriosclerosis; autoimmune disorders; Buerger's disease; diabetes; cardiopulmonary disease; Crohn's disease; Cushing's syndrome; hepatic failure; hypovolaemia; hypoxia; immune disorders; infection; inflammatory bowel disease; jaundice; leucopenia; malignancy; protein losing enteropathy; Raynaud's disease; renal failure; respiratory conditions; rheumatoid arthritis; thyroid deficiency; uraemia; vascular diseases; venous stasis
Drugs	Alcohol; antimicrobials; cytotoxics; immunosuppressives; nicotine; non-steroidal anti-inflammatories; penicillamine and penicillin; steroids
Poor nutritional state	Anaemia; malnutrition; mineral deficiency (particularly zinc); protein deficiency; vitamin deficiency (particularly A and C)
Micro-environment of wound	Blood supply; gas composition; humidity; infection; inflammation; high pH; low temperature; oxygen tension
Other	Aetiology of wound; age; fibrous ring round open wound; foreign body in wound; obesity; radiation; stress; suture materials; suture technique; trauma/mechanical stress; treatment (including use of antiseptics and/or linting materials)

Note: some conditions may affect the healing process via several mechanisms.
(From: Rovee *et al.* 1972; Silver 1972; Kaufman & Hirshowitz 1982; Kaufman *et al.* 1985; Westaby 1985; David 1986; Deas *et al.* 1986; Dyson *et al.* 1988; Kaufman & Alexander 1988; Kaufman & Berger 1988; Tubman Papantonio 1988a; Lycarotti & Leaper 1989; Messer 1989; Cooper 1990; Cutting 1994, Grey 1998; Donovan 1998)

growth factor released by the dead platelets causes the fibroplast to migrate into the wound soon after damage has occurred.

The fibroblasts are activated to divide and produce collagen by processes initiated by the macrophages. This develops a network of poorly organized collagen which increases the strength of the wound. Newly synthesized collagen creates a 'healing ridge' below an intact suture line, thus giving an indication of how wound healing is progressing. This mechanism is dependent on the presence of iron, vitamin C and oxygen. Therefore, appropriate levels of nutrition and oxygenation during this phase of wound healing are particularly necessary.

Angioblasts are required to form new blood vessels which grow into the wound under conditions of a hypoxic tissue gradient (Knighton *et al.* 1981; Flanagan 1996). The vessels branch and join other vessels forming loops. The fragile capillary loops are held within a framework of collagen. This complex is known as granulation tissue. Granulation tissue can grow into wound dressings such as gauze. On removal of the dressing any adhered delicate granulation tissue is also destroyed.

There is an acceleration of the inflammatory and proliferative phases in moist conditions compared to dry conditions (Dyson *et al.* 1988).

Remodelling phase (24 days onwards)

In this stage the collagen is reorganized so the fibres are enlarged and oriented along the lines of tension in the wound (at right angles to the wound margin). This occurs via a process of lysis and resynthesis. Intermolecular cross-linking aids to increase the tensile strength of the wound. Maximum strength (about 80%) is reached in approximately 3 months, although the scar never achieves the same strength as the original tissue.

(Winter 1972; Torrance 1985; Westaby 1985; David 1986; Jackson & Rovee 1988; Johnson 1988a; Pritchard & David 1988; Messer 1989; Cooper 1990; Silver 1994; Moore & Foster 1998.)

Contraction

If the wound is clean and granulating, myofibroblasts round the edge of the wound contract in unison. This can reduce significantly the size of the wound and the area that the new tissue must cover. When the edges first contract (about 4 days after injury) the wound becomes larger, but after 3 or 4 days the wound area begins to decrease, leaving a scar in approximately 3 weeks. The position of the wound is relevant to the success of healing by contracture. If the skin is attached to nearby structures this may result in its distortion and limitation of movement. However, wounds on the abdomen and breasts may close with a small amount of scarring (Torrance 1985; Westaby 1985; David 1986; Johnson 1988a; Messer 1989; Thomas 1990b; Flanagan 1996, 1999).

Oxygen-treated burns have been found to increase contraction significantly and healing of the wound in animals.

However, this was accompanied by thicker scar formation which could prove detrimental for aesthetic and rehabilitative reasons (Kaufman & Alexander 1988).

Epithelialization

Epithelial cells will migrate across healthy granulation tissue only by 'leap-frogging' over each other and will burrow under contaminated debris and unwanted material (Waldorf & Fewkes 1995). Splinters, dirt and sutures may be 'worked out' of the wound (Winter 1972; Torrance 1985; Westaby 1985; David 1986). Epidermal cells also secrete an enzyme which separates the scab from the underlying tissue. Dissolving the eschar requires nearly 50% of the cell's metabolic energy (Johnson 1988a; Messer 1989). Sources of epithelial cells include hair follicles, sweat glands and the perimeter of the wound (Torrance 1985; Johnson 1988a; Moore & Foster 1998). As the epithelial cells migrate they begin to differentiate and cannot divide (Torrance 1985). The ability of the epithelium to cover the wound surface is limited to approximately 2 cm. This means that the process of contraction is of vital importance to healing in normal wounds (Messer 1989).

Epithelialization (migration, mitosis and differentiation) is best achieved in moist conditions (Rovee *et al.* 1972; Silver 1994; Collier 1996; Moore & Foster 1998). Covering the wound in a polythene film accelerates epithelialization probably because hydration is maintained, while blowing air over wounds causes a deeper scab than normal to form and epidermal repair is delayed (Winter 1972).

Raising oxygen tension in fluid in the wound has also been found to increase epidermal migration. This suggests that in normal wound healing the availability of oxygen may be the limiting factor (Winter 1972). The epidermal migration under different types of films is perhaps directly related to their oxygen permeabilities (Winter 1972). Oxygen breathing by man was not found to increase the partial pressure of oxygen in intact skin, while vasodilation produced by warming the body or limb did raise the oxygen tension (Silver 1972). [Different results have been demonstrated in experiments involving animals (Knighton *et al.* 1981).] This suggests that warming rather than giving oxygen may be of more clinical use, although this was probably not the limiting factor in the healthy subjects studied. Another trial is necessary in hypoxic patients.

Topical acidification has also been found to increase epidermal regeneration, and may prove to be of use therapeutically (Kaufman *et al.* 1985; Glover 1992).

Growth factors

Recent research has indicated that essential cellular activity that occurs during wound healing can be attributed to specific proteins known as growth factors (Cox 1993; Garrett 1997). They are naturally occurring proteins secreted by cells in response to an injury and 'mediate, coordinate and control cellular interactions that occur during skin maintenance and wound healing' (Cox 1993). This discovery has led to advances in wound therapeutics (Devel 1987; Brown *et al.* 1991; Robson *et al.* 1992, 1993).

For example, a small study showed that a group of patients with non-healing venous ulcers showed a significantly faster healing rate following treatment with TGF-β2 growth factors (Robson *et al.* 1993). A further case study demonstrated that the addition of GM-CSF (granulocyte macrophage colony-stimulating factor) to the concurrent treatment of a patient with an ulcerative cutaneous condition (resulting from metastatic breast cancer) induced wound healing (Wandl 1997). In addition, wound healing was accelerated in postmenopausal women who had been using hormone replacement therapy (McCarthy 1997).

This is an exciting area of care which requires further research in order to ascertain its full potential. Only by understanding the different stages of wound healing will the health carer be able to provide the appropriate treatment to produce the optimum wound environment.

Factors affecting wound healing

The rate of healing of a wound varies depending on the general health of the individual, the location of the wound, the degree of the damage (David 1986) and the treatment applied.

Factors that may delay healing include systemic variables such as disease, poor nutritional state and infection. Other influences involve the local micro-environment of the wound, including temperature, pH, humidity, air gas composition (Rovee *et al.* 1972; Kaufman & Hirshowitz 1982; Dyson *et al.* 1988; Kaufman & Berger 1988; Cutting 1994), oxygen tension (Silver 1972; Kaufman & Alexander 1988), blood supply and inflammation. Whether this influence is positive or negative may depend on the stage of wound healing that has been reached. Other important considerations are external variables such as continuing trauma – possibly caused by treatment, the presence of foreign bodies, etc.

It is necessary when treating a wound to appraise all potential detrimental factors and minimize them, where possible, in order to provide the optimum systemic, local and external conditions for healing. Wound care begins with the care of the patient.

Factors known to affect wound healing are listed in Table 47.1.

Promotion of wound healing

General care of the patient

Promotion of wound healing concerns optimizing the local, internal and external environments. This includes the control of disease or underlying pathology, reduction in external risk factors such as infection and maintaining an ideal microclimate for healing in the wound (Table 47.1). Many factors need to be considered when assessing a patient with a wound.

Where possible, health care should be aimed at preventing wounding, for example, prevention of pressure ulcers by regular turning and adequate nutrition. In addition, hydrocolloid dressings have been found to be effective in preventing pressure ulcers in 'at risk' patients (Johnson 1989).

The psychological care of the patient is important to ensure acceptance of the wound and reduction in stress. It is also imperative to assess and treat pain. Apart from the obvious unpleasantness for the patient, this will also lead to stress which will then delay wound healing.

Attention must be given to adequate nutrition of the patient since this is necessary for wound healing (Roberts 1988; Lewis 1996; Casey 1998a). A dietitian's assessment is advisable. Patients are considered 'at risk' for wound healing if they have lost 20% or more of their body weight within the previous 6 months or 10% in the previous 2 months (Messer 1989).

Protein and calorie malnutrition are possible in patients with chronic or acute malabsorption. This includes diabetes, Crohn's disease, alcohol abuse, gastrointestinal surgery, liver disease and long-term steroid therapy. Malignancy, major trauma, fever, inflammatory disease, smoking, drug use, stress and iatrogenic starvation are associated with deficient intake or high energy demands (Messer 1989; Lewis 1996; Casey 1998a).

Patients at risk of inadequate vitamin A levels include those with severe diabetes and rheumatoid arthritis (Messer 1989). Vitamin A supplementation in these patients has been found to improve wound healing and should be considered as a supplement in steroid-dependent patients for at least 5 days postwounding (Messer 1989). This may be related to the fact that vitamin A is a potent immune stimulant which, when administered topically or orally, will reverse much of the steroid suppression of wound healing. However, it is not as effective in reversing the effects of non-steroidal anti-inflammatory drugs (Hunt *et al.* 1969; Cohen & Cohen 1973; Ehrlich *et al.* 1973; Hunt & Dunphy 1979).

Patients with sepsis and those having undergone major trauma are also at risk of depletion of vitamin A. Supplementation of vitamin A should be contemplated for these groups (Messer 1989). Vitamin C is necessary for collagen synthesis during the proliferative stage of the wound healing process. Deficiency of vitamin C is also associated with lowered resistance to infection (Morison 1992; Lewis 1996; Casey 1998a). Patients with poor nutritional status may benefit from zinc supplements because of the role of zinc in DNA synthesis and the immune response (Wells 1994; Lewis 1996).

A thorough nutritional assessment is essential to identify actual or potential problems and to guide treatment. Nutritional risk assessment tools are available and the dietetic support staff are a useful resource to discuss patients who may be considered to be at risk (Casey 1998a).

The majority of chronic non-malignant wounds are hypoxic wounds (Messer 1989). The major conditions that predispose to this are diabetes, venous stasis, vascular insufficiency, cardiopulmonary disease, irradiation, oedema, hypovolaemia and smoking (Messer 1989). It is possible that hyperbaric oxygen therapy may be helpful for healing wounds in these patients. This involves the patient breathing 100% oxygen while in a chamber where the pressure is elevated above atmospheric pressure, and enables the amount of oxygen in solution to be increased. This has been used to successfully treat chronic unhealed wounds (Barr *et al.* 1990).

However, it is not always possible to overcome the deleterious effects of smoking with hyperbaric oxygen therapy while the patient continues to smoke (Messer 1989). It is, therefore, important to educate patients and assist them in this aspect of their care by helping them to reduce or stop smoking.

Drugs that may delay wound healing should be reduced or withdrawn where therapeutically possible. This includes penicillamine which prevents collagen cross-linking (Messer 1989).

Other factors that require consideration are: the necessity to maintain adequate fluid replacement postoperatively or post-trauma to prevent hypovolaemia (Messer 1989); containing and removing infection (both local and systemic) (Donovan 1998); use of measures to assist healing, for example, using mattresses which can reduce the healing time of sores (Andrews & Balai 1989), etc.

Physical and psychological rehabilitation may be necessary if the results of wounding and wound healing are debilitating and disfiguring and adjustment to changes in body image are necessary. This includes physiotherapy, counselling and occupational therapy.

Infection

All wounds are prone to colonization which is a precursor to infection. Careful wound assessment is essential to identify potential sites for infection to occur, although routine swabbing of the area is not considered to be beneficial (Donovan 1998). Appropriate treatment of the infection should be determined from a positive wound swab(s).

Care of the microscopic wound environment

A considerable percentage of nurses' time is spent carrying out dressing procedures. Although research has examined wound physiology (Winter 1971; Johnson 1984; Ayton 1985; Torrance 1985; Westaby 1985; Leaper 1986; Turner *et al.* 1986; Garrett 1997; Miller 1998) and wound dressings (Johnson 1984; Ayton 1985; Draper 1985; Harkiss 1985a,b; Silver 1994; Thomas 1996, 1997; Grocott 1999; Williams 1999) there is little that appraises different dressing packs and procedures.

Packs and procedures should be designed for safety, comfort and ease and speed of use. Opinion and research indicate that forceps (especially those made of plastic) are clumsy, can cause pain and damage and are difficult to use (Wells 1984; Mallett 1988). Gloves are a more suitable alternative and, in addition, should assist in reducing the risk of cross-infection.

Cotton wool or gauze used in cleaning can leave fibres in the wound. This may stimulate foreign body reaction and lengthen the inflammatory phase. Not only will this act as a focus for infection and damage new epidermis, but also it will retard wound healing (Winter 1971, 1972; Turner 1979; Johnson 1984). Medical foam or low-linting material

may be used instead. Appropriate use of hydrotherapy via a bath, shower or 0.9% sodium chloride stream can be utilized to remove debris or for debridement (Zederfeldt *et al.* 1980; Gogia *et al.* 1988; Jeter & Tintle 1988; Trelstad & Osmundson 1989). It is important to consider the appropriate cleaning mechanism of these baths to minimize the risk of cross infection; guidelines can be obtained from the relevant manufacturers.

Introduction of a less complicated wound dressing procedure and new pack containing medical foam and gloves instead of cotton wool and forceps was evaluated in one London hospital. This demonstrated that not only was it quicker to use but also nurses preferred the new pack to the original pack (Mallett 1988).

The implications of research suggest that traditional packs are likely to be detrimental to the patient and are also more difficult to use by the health care professional. Studies of packs and procedures indicate that foam and gloves may be suitable subsitutes. Further research in this area is necessary.

Evaluation of the wound

The wound should be evaluated each time a dressing is applied or if it gives rise for concern. The aim of evaluating the wound is to assess healing and to establish which treatment will best provide the ideal environment for healing. The different classifications of wounds that relate to tissue loss and regeneration and absence or presence of infection may be of assistance in this process.

Factors that should be appraised include the underlying pathology of the wound. For example, if an ulcer is present on the leg, is it venous, arterial, lymphatic, malignant, etc? In addition, the surface area or volume of the wound should be measured. This can be carried out using a number of methods (Fincham Gee 1990; McTaggart 1994), and is necessary to ascertain the rate of healing. The amount and type of drainage is also important, both in traumatic and surgical wounds.

A list of variables that require regular assessment is shown in Table 47.2.

Principles of cleaning the wound

The aim of wound cleansing is to help create the optimum local condition for wound healing by removal of excess debris, exudate, foreign and necrotic material, toxic components, the food source of potential infecting microorganisms, bacteria and other micro-organisms (Wells 1984; Turner *et al.* 1986; Gustafsson 1988; Jeter & Tintle 1988; Morison 1989). Debridement is necessary to remove necrotic tissue which provides the ideal environment for bacterial growth and can hinder the healing process (Jackson & Rovee 1988).

If the wound is clean and little exudate is present, repeated cleansing is contraindicated since it may damage new tissue, decrease the temperature of the wound unnecessarily and remove exudate (Morison 1989). A fall in the temperature of the wound of 12°C is possible if the procedure is prolonged or the lotions are cold. This can take 3 hours or longer to return to normal warmth, during which

Table 47.2 Assessment of wounds

Factor	Variables
General	Aetiology; location; presence of haematoma, seroma, oedema; amount of necrosis; open/closed; number of times requires dressing per unit time
Pain	Amount; at change of dressing; only when traumatized; intermittent; continuous; time of day; type of pain (e.g. sharp, stabbing, dull, etc.)
Stage of healing	Original tissue loss; amount of granulation and epithelial tissue; area/volume/depth of wound; temperature; sensation; inflammation
Drainage	Colour; consistency; nature/type; volume over time; odour
Area surrounding wound	Colour; oedema; erythema; sensation; turgor; other skin conditions
Infection	Amount of pus and exudate; pain; temperature; positive swab culture; inflammation; friable granulation tissue; odour

time the cellular activity is reduced and therefore the healing process slowed (Stronge 1984).

Sodium chloride (0.9%) is a physiological balanced solution that has a similar osmotic pressure to that already present in living cells and is therefore compatible with human tissue (Lawrence 1997). Used at body temperature, it is the safest and best cleansing solution for non-contaminated wounds (Ferguson 1988; Jeter & Tintle 1988; Tubman Papantonio 1988b; Morgan 1990). Although sodium chloride has no antiseptic properties it dilutes bacteria and is non-toxic to tissue (Morgan 1990). Tap water is also advocated for cleansing wounds (Riyat & Quinton 1997). A study demonstrated that, in comparison to sterile 0.9% sodium chloride, lower rates of infection were found in the group where tap water was used (Angeras et al. 1992). However, caution should be exercised when using tap water because it can cause pain if applied to raw tissue and lead to further tissue damage if the force of flow is too strong (Clide 1992).

A number of other solutions have been used traditionally to clean wounds, some of which need to be used with caution (Table 47.3). An example of this is povidone-iodine. This is sometimes used in a weak aqueous solution (1%) as an antiseptic. However, solutions of 5% povidone-iodine have been found to reduce blood flow in granulation tissue (Brennan & Leaper 1985). A recent consensus meeting discussed the use of iodine in wound management. Although there is insufficient research to evaluate its effectiveness, it was demonstrated that the newer preparations of iodine now available appear to be effective and non-toxic due to their lower concentrations of iodine at the wound surface (Gilchrist 1997).

Some compounds used to clean wounds have documented deleterious effects on tissue or have been found to have detrimental effects in mammals. These include the much discussed sodium hypochlorite which is found in several wound cleansing solutions (Table 47.3). Eusol is a particularly well-known solution containing sodium hypochlorite. Debate about its use has continued for a number of years. Many clinicians and researchers have recommended that it should not be used (Ferguson 1988;

Johnson 1988b; Morgan 1990; Spanswick et al. 1990) or should not be used routinely (Morison 1989). In view of the mounting evidence against sodium hypochlorite (Bloomfield & Sizer 1985; Brennan & Leaper 1985; Deas et al. 1986; Thorp et al. 1987) and the availability of a range of alternatives, the use of sodium hypochlorite is not recommended in this manual except for short-term use in exceptional circumstances, such as in recent war wounds, chronic sloughy wounds where other recognized measures have failed, and some patients' wounds in accident and emergency departments. Its use should be defined only by the clinical specialist.

Principles of dressing the wound

With the exception of wounds where the main aim is to ameliorate symptoms such as malignant wounds, an ideal wound dressing may be described in general terms as follows:

> A material which, when applied to the surface of a wound, provides and maintains an environment in which healing can take place at the maximum rate. (Turner *et al.* 1986)

More specifically, to provide such an environment the dressing must be capable of fulfilling the following functions:

1 To remove excess exudate and toxic components.
2 To maintain a high humidity at the wound–dressing interface (Field & Kerstein 1994).
3 To allow gaseous exchange.
4 To provide thermal insulation.
5 To be impermeable to bacteria.
6 To be free from particulate or toxic components.
7 To allow change without trauma (Turner 1985).

In addition, the dressing should minimize pain, odour and bleeding and be comfortable and acceptable to the patient.

Occlusive dressings achieve many of these criteria. They affect the wound and healing in several ways. Occlusive dressings have the ability to maintain hydration and prevent the formation of an eschar. This leads to a more

Table 47.3 Suitability of products used on wounds

Suitable	Sodium chloride (0.9%) (safe, non-irritant and non-toxic) Tap water (used more frequently, especially on areas already colonized. Some patients prefer to shower prior to dressing changes)
Not ideal, use with caution	Chlorhexidine – antiseptic (can cause sensitization and irritation; do not use alcoholic solutions) Hydrogen peroxide – antiseptic (use on dirty, infected, necrotic wounds only; do not use on large or deep wounds as may cause air embolism; may be caustic to skin and wound) Metronidazole – antibacterial (anaerobes only) (can cause nausea, neuropathy if used systemically) Potassium permanganate (0.01%) – mild antiseptic properties (causes staining of skin) Povidone-iodine – antiseptic (do not use alcoholic solution; rarely causes skin reactions; some sources suggest that it should not be used on severe or extensive burns, if non-toxic goitre is present, in pregnancy or on lactating women)
Not suitable	Cetrimide – antibacterial and antifungal (toxic to wound tissue and causes skin hypersensitivity) Gentian violet – astringent, antiseptic (carcinogenic; is sometimes used on excoriating radiotherapy burns) Mercurochrome – weak bacteriostatic agent (toxic to tissue) Sodium hypochlorite – antiseptic (powerful oxidizing agent which is toxic to tissue)

From: Valdes-Dapena & Arey 1962; Bloomfield & Sizer 1985; Brennan & Leaper 1985; Deas *et al.* 1986; *Nurses' Drug Alert* 1987; Thorp *et al.* 1987; Johnson 1988a; Morison 1989; Morgan 1990; Farrow & Toth 1991; Lawrence 1997.

rapid epithelial migration. The lag phase before epithelial cell proliferation and the time for epidermal differentiation is reduced. Wound contraction occurs more quickly and there is a decrease in some signs of inflammation (redness, oedema) as well as pain. Dermal repair is also accelerated (Rovee *et al.* 1972; Dyson *et al.* 1988; Jackson & Rovee 1988; Winter & Hewitt 1990).

Protocols have been developed which suggest different types of treatment depending on whether the wound is clean, infected or necrotic or shallow or deep (Johnson 1988d). Dry dressings do not afford most of the criteria for an ideal dressing and should not be used as a primary contact layer (Dealey 1991). Care should be taken with wounds that are difficult shapes to treat. These include long, narrow cavities which require a dressing that can be comfortably inserted into the space but removed easily without leaving any fibres behind (Bale 1991) and without trauma. (See Table 47.4 for details of groups of dressings.)

Other treatments

Other treatments for wounds include the possibility of topical acidification (Kaufman *et al.* 1985) and active treatment using growth factors or autologous platelet-derived factors (Jackson & Rovee 1988).

Small, full-thickness skin loss can be repaired easily using skin grafts (Westaby 1985). Where possible, it is preferable to use autografts. However, if donor sites are limited, homografts can be utilized. Muscle, tendon and bone may also be used to replace lost tissue (Pritchard & David 1988).

Recently, the use of complementary therapies in wound management has gained more attention. Much of the evidence is anecdotal, but there have been trials using essential oils in relation to the reduction in the symptoms of pain and odour, the promotion of granulation tissue and managing wound cleansing (Price & Price 1995; Baker 1998). Therapeutic touch has also been evaluated (Finch 1997). It was shown to be of benefit in symptom management, e.g. reducing pain (Meehan 1993) and reducing levels of anxiety (Heidt 1981).

These are areas that require further research before they gain more approval and acceptance. Nurses should exercise caution when considering the use of these products when there is clearly insufficient research and knowledge to support these interventions.

Conclusions

Taking into consideration all of the factors regarding wound pressure, prevention and management, it may be useful for nurses to collect and collate statistics and build up an accurate profile of patients and the nature of their problems. In this way it would be possible to evaluate the care given and provide information on potential areas of concern that further research could be based upon. This could result in an increase in the efficiency and cost effectiveness of wound and pressure sore management within a hospital or in the community.

Particular wounds: leg ulceration

Reference material

Ulceration of the skin of the lower limb has been an affliction of the human race since the time of Hippocrates. It is almost certainly the price we pay for having emerged from the ocean and learnt to stand erect.   (Burnand 1990)

Table 47.4 Dressing groups

Dressing	Advantages	Disadvantages
Polymeric films	Only suitable for shallow wounds; prophylactic use against pressure sores; retention dressings; cool the surface of the wound; allow passage of water vapour; allow monitoring of wound	Possibility of adhesive trauma on removal; cool the surface of the wound
Dextranomers	Form stiff hydrophilic paste; useful in the treatment of infected wound cavities	Require retaining dressing
Hydrogels	Suitable for light to medium exuding wounds; reduce pain; cool the wound surface; desloughing abilities allow monitoring of wound; carrier for medications; good permeability gas profile; low trauma at change; non-allergenic; non-sensitizing; easy to use	Cool the surface of the wound; some hydrogels cannot be used on infected wounds. Please refer to manufacturers' recommendations with regard to particular products
Hydrocolloid gel	Suitable for light to medium exuding wounds; has the same benefits as hydrogels but due to its hydrocolloid content it accelerates wound healing	Do not apply too much to wound bed – can cause skin maceration
Hydrocolloids	Provide a moist wound environment suitable for assisting debridement of wound; swelling of hydrocolloid increases pressure on the base of the wound, and *may* aid healthy granulation; pain relief; waterproof; provide thermal insulation; most provide a barrier to micro-organisms; low trauma at change; non-allergenic; non-sensitizing; easy to use	May release degradation products into the wound; strong odour produced as dressing interacts with exudate; some hydrocolloids cannot be used on infected wounds. Please refer to manufacturers' recommendations with regard to particular products
Alginates	Suitable for heavily exuding wounds; highly absorbent; can be used on infected wounds; useful for sinus and fissure drainage; hydrophilic gel formed in the presence of sodium ions provides a moist wound environment; sodium chloride (0.9%) can be used to flush away some alginates; fibres trapped in the wound are biodegradable; some alginates are haemostatic in action; odour remission	Cannot be used on wounds that are not exuding or exuding lightly; cannot be used on wounds with hard necrotic tissue; sometimes a mild burning sensation occurs on application
Hydrofibre dressings	Suitable for highly exuding wounds; soft to touch but hold fluid directly into their fibre structure and holds it away from the surrounding skin; very easy to remove	Require a retaining dressing
Polyurethane foams	Suitable for use with open, exuding wounds; provide high thermal insulation; left in situ for long time	May be difficult to use in wounds with deep tracks

From: Fraser & Gilchrist 1983; Gilchrist & Martin 1983; Lawrence 1985; Mertz *et al*. 1985; Pottle 1987; Johnson 1988c; Dealey 1989; Goren 1989; Piper 1989; Margolin *et al*. 1990; Thomas & Loveless 1992; Benbow 1994; Grocott 1999; Williams 1999.

Prevalence and cost

Approximately 1.5–3 people per 1000 head of population are affected by leg ulceration during their lifetime and prevalence increases with age (20 in 1000 people over the age of 80 years; Lees & Lambert 1992). Ulceration is often recurrent (Callam *et al.* 1987b), persistent (Dale & Gibson 1986a; Franks *et al.* 1995), and affects more women than men (Anning 1954; Dale & Gibson 1986a; Callam *et al.* 1987b; Ryan 1987).

The annual cost of treatment to the National Health Service of leg ulceration is between £300 million and £600 million (Thomas 1990a; West & Priestly 1994). Leg ulceration treated by community nurses was estimated to use over £400 000 of resources in Paddington and North Kensington Health District in 1988 (Mallett & Charles

1989); much of this is borne by the cost of the district nursing service (Callam *et al*. 1987b).

Aetiology

The most common predisposing factor to leg ulceration is hypoxia due to obstruction and/or disease (Casey 1998a).

Venous disease

Venous disease has been found to be prevalent in 70–95% of cases (Fangrell 1979; Callam *et al*. 1987b; Williamson 1988; Perkins 1989). Venous hypertension precipitating micro-oedema is probably the main cause of venous leg ulcers (Fangrell 1979; Ryan 1985b; Hollinworth 1998). This, in turn, can lead to lymphatic damage with resulting lymphoedema, fibrosis or liposclerosis (Robinson 1988; Ryan 1988a).

The reason that more women than men are prone to leg ulceration is due to the presence of varicose veins and episodes of deep vein thrombosis associated with pregnancy, which can lead to venous damage and ulceration in the affected leg (Dale & Gibson 1986a; Ryan 1987; Knight 1990). In one study, only 12% of women with varicose veins had never been pregnant, compared with 57% who had four or more pregnancies (Henry & Corless 1989). In addition, further research indicates that multiple pregnancies enlarge the gonadal veins, leading to vulvar, inner and posterior thigh and leg varicosities which do not follow the saphenous system. Symptoms are pain and heaviness in the thigh and legs and lateral aspects of the leg and foot (Lechter *et al*. 1987). Venous pathology is also related to the menstrual cycle, when the level of circulating oestrogens is at its lowest (Marcelon *et al*. 1988).

Warming can induce venous dilation resulting in decreased venous return and 'heavy legs' (Marcelon & Vanhoutte 1988; Morison & Moffatt 1994), and disorders relating to chronic venous insufficiency appear especially when the ambient temperature is high (Boccalon & Ginestet 1988).

Venous ulcers are often described as occurring in the area around or on the medial malleolus, shallow and extensive and on the left leg (Falanga & Eaglstein 1986; Matthews 1986; Callam *et al*. 1987b; Ryan 1987; Swanwick & MacLellan 1988; Thomas 1988a; Williamson 1988). This may be associated with iliocaval syndrome which occurs when the left common iliac vein is compressed by the common iliac artery (Ryan 1987; Taheri *et al*. 1987). These findings were not supported by the Paddington and North Kensington Health District survey, which suggested that significantly more ulcers were found on the anterolateral aspect of the lower leg. Ulceration was also statistically more likely to be on the right leg (Mallett & Charles 1990). A larger, more recent survey has not strengthened either claim (Mallett and Charles, unpublished data).

Venous ulcers develop gradually and produce intermittent pain (Dale & Gibson 1986a; Thomas 1988a). Data from a survey in Parkside Health District do not support this.

Arterial disease

Between 4 and 30% of patients with leg ulceration have been reported to have arterial insufficiency. This proportion increases with age to 50% in the very elderly (Matthews 1986; Callam *et al*. 1987a,b; Williamson 1988; Perkins 1989). Women are also more prone to arterial ulceration than men (Knight 1990), although some research contradicts this (Callam *et al*. 1987a).

Arterial ulcers are deep and 'punched out' (Dale & Gibson 1986b; Mani *et al*. 1988; Williamson 1988; Perkins 1989), and found on the feet or the anterior or lateral aspect of the ankle (Thomas 1988a). These ulcers develop rapidly and give continuous or persistent pain, especially at night (Dale & Gibson 1986c; Thomas 1988a; Perkins 1989; RCN 1998).

Other predisposing and aggravating factors

Rheumatoid arthritis causes vasculitis which can lead to small, painful, 'punched out' ulcers (Williamson 1988; Baker *et al*. 1991). In addition, treatment with steroids leads to thinning of the skin and susceptibility to trauma.

Diabetes is also associated with vasculitis and neuropathy, and has been found to be five times more common in patients with leg ulceration (Callam *et al*. 1987b; Rosenberg 1990).

Vowden (1998) showed that venous ulceration was more common in Caucasians than ethnic minorities. However, this may be due to fewer ethnic patients presenting for treatment.

Diastolic hypertension can lead to (usually) painful bilateral ischaemic ulceration, known as 'Martorell's ulcer' (Alberdi 1988).

Blood disease, such as sickle cell anaemia or thalassaemia, can cause haematological ulcers (Hallows 1987; Williamson 1988).

Obesity, immobilization and dependency of the lower limb, limitation of ankle joint and poor gait due to ulceration (the last two both leading to an inadequately functioning calf muscle pump) can aggravate ulceration and contribute to its persistence (Callam *et al*. 1987b; Autar 1998).

Poor nutrition, especially relating to older patients with multiple pathologies, may hinder healing (Casey 1998a).

Treatment

It is imperative to distinguish between ulcers of varying pathologies as the management and treatment are very different. Assessment must be carried out to elicit which of the three vascular systems (arterial, venous and/or lymphatic) are diseased to provide the most appropriate care (Ryan 1988a; Vowden 1998). Understanding and systematic management of the underlying disease, as well as topical wound care are necessary for a therapeutic approach (Falanga & Eaglstein 1986).

Recently, the management of oedema has been established as the mainstay of treatment. The presence of oedema inhibits the microcirculation, thus preventing the perfusion exchange of nutrients (Hofman 1998).

It is important to note that often these wounds can be of a chronic nature. In this situation, emphasis should be placed on symptom management and quality of life issues (Armstrong et al. 1998; Nelson 1998). The original terms of describing leg ulcers (e.g. shallow, punched out) are difficult to measure but are still used as a means of defining underlying technology (RCN 1998).

Venous and lymphatic disease can be treated by improving the function of the calf muscle pump by graduated compression (Callam et al. 1987b; Dale & Gibson 1987, 1990; Blair et al. 1988b; Evans 1988; Smith 1988; Thompson 1990; McCulloch 1998). This has been found to be more important than certain types of dressing (Blair et al. 1988a). High compression, e.g. multiple-layer bandaging and the use of elastic layered compression, have been shown to be cost effective in the treatment of venous ulceration (Dale 1998; Nelson 1998). However, the practical problems of applying compression stockings have been shown to adversely affect compliance with this treatment (Moffat & Dorman 1995). Compression bandaging is detrimental to those with arterial insufficiency.

The physiotherapist can play a major role in improving the calf muscle pump function and intermittent compression therapy (McCulloch 1998). If compression therapy is the treatment of choice, careful consideration must be given to the selection of hosiery so that an informed decision can be made regarding the layer of hosiery required (Jones & Nelson 1998). Surgery may be necessary in cases to increase the perfusion of the tissues, although it should be noted that arterial surgery can also lead to a decrease in the venous return time (Struckmann 1988).

Many additional therapies have been successfully tried in the management of leg ulcers. Advanced technology applied to the theory of ulceration means that techniques such as laser, hyperbaric oxygen, growth factors and gene therapies have received additional attention (Gilchrist 1997). Complementary therapists are also endeavouring to adopt a more scientific evaluative approach in order to promote the possibility of using alternative therapies (Gilchrist 1997).

As with all wound care, careful consideration must be given to the choice of dressing, which should be dictated by the nature of the wound and the symptoms present (Armstrong et al. 1998).

Pressure ulcers or decubitus ulcers

Definition

The terms 'decubitus ulcer' or 'pressure ulcer or sore' are used to describe any area of damage to the skin or underlying tissues caused by direct pressure or shearing forces. The extent of this damage can range from persistent erythema to necrotic ulceration involving muscle, tendon and bone.

Reference material

Cost

The cost of prevention and management of pressure sores has been a key issue in some reports (e.g. DoH 1994). It is estimated that the cost to the NHS may be as high as £400 million per year (McSweeney 1994). There are no established criteria for assessing the cost of pressure ulcers, and while the cost of bed hire and wound care products can be calculated, it is difficult to estimate the cost of nursing care (West & Priestley 1994), or the cost to the patient.

A pressure ulcer prevention programme may be beneficial but if comprehensive could also be costly. West and Priestly (1994) argue that although a prevention programme would involve costs in the short term, benefits would occur in the medium and long term (see also Taylor & Clark 1994).

Prevalence

The prevalance of pressure ulcers in hospital was shown to be 6.65% of total in-patients (DoH 1993). In the community setting it is often more difficult to determine, although one study in Preston (1991) showed a prevalence of 6.7%.

The Health of the Nation document (DoH 1992) highlighted a recommendation to reduce the annual incidence by 5–10%, although since the *Community Care Act (1993)* and the recommendations that more patients were cared for in their own homes, limited manpower and financial resources in the community are being stretched (Inman & Firth 1998).

Aetiology

Three major factors have been identified as being significant contributory factors in the development of pressure ulcers:

1 Pressure. The blood pressure at the arterial end of the capillaries is approximately 30 mm Hg, while at the venous end this drops to 10 mm Hg (the average mean capillary pressure equals about 17 mm Hg; Guyton 1984). Any external pressures exceeding this will cause capillary obstruction. Tissues that are dependant on these capillaries are deprived of their blood supply. Eventually, the ischaemic tissues will die (David 1986; Waterlow 1988; Wyngaarden & Smith 1988; Department of Infection Control, Memorial Hospital 1989; Johnson 1989). However, research has demonstrated that with constant pressure, even in denigrated tissues, a critical period of 1–2 hours exists before pathological changes occur (Kosiak 1958, 1976).

2 Shearing. This may occur when the patient slips down the bed or is dragged up the bed. As the skeleton moves over the underlying tissue the microcirculation is destroyed and the tissue dies of anoxia. In more serious cases, lymphatic vessels and muscle fibres may also become torn, resulting in a deep pressure ulcer (Pritchard & David 1988; Waterlow 1988; Wyngaarden

& Smith 1988; Department of Infection Control, Memorial Hospital 1989; Johnson 1989).

3 Friction. This is a component of shearing, which causes stripping of the stratum corneum, leading to superficial ulceration (Waterlow 1988; Wyngaarden & Smith 1988; Johnson 1989).

The most likely sites for pressure ulcer development are:

1 Sacral area
2 Coccygeal area
3 Ischial tuberosities
4 Greater trochanters (Wyngaarden & Smith 1988).

Identification of at-risk patients

Many predisposing factors are involved in the development of pressure ulcers:

1 Immunosuppression (Waterlow 1987)
2 Immobility (Waterlow 1988; European Pressure Ulcer Advisory Panel 1998)
3 Moisture (Wyngaarden & Smith 1988)
4 Inactivity (European Pressure Ulcer Advisory Panel 1998)
5 Faecal and urinary incontinence (Waterlow 1988; Department of Infection Control, Memorial Hospital 1989; European Pressure Ulcer Advisory Panel 1998)
6 Decreased level of consciousness (Department of Infection Control, Memorial Hospital 1989; European Pressure Ulcer Advisory Panel 1998)
7 Infection (Waterlow 1988)
8 Circulatory diseases, for example, peripheral vascular disease, cardiac disease (Barton 1988; Department of Infection Control, Memorial Hospital 1989)
9 Personal hygiene (Waterlow 1988)
10 Neurological diseases, for example, multiple sclerosis (Waterlow 1988; Department of Infection Control, Memorial Hospital 1989)
11 Weight distribution (Waterlow 1988)
12 Treatment regimes (Waterlow 1988)
13 Malnutrition/nutritional status (Waterlow 1988; Department of Infection Control, Memorial Hospital 1989)
14 Drugs that affect mobility, for example, sedatives (Waterlow 1988; Department of Infection Control, Memorial Hospital 1989)
15 Anaemia (Waterlow 1988)
16 Malignancy (Waterlow 1988)
17 Patient-handling methods (Waterlow 1988; Department of Infection Control, Memorial Hospital 1989)
18 Shortage of nursing staff where patients require regular positioning (Department of Infection Control, Memorial Hospital 1989; Clark 1998)
19 Design of beds, mattresses, chairs and wheelchairs (Department of Infection Control, Memorial Hospital 1989)
20 Advanced age (European Pressure Ulcer Advisory Panel 1998)
21 Fracture (European Pressure Ulcer Advisory Panel 1998)
22 Chronic systemic illness (European Pressure Ulcer Advisory Panel 1998)

A patient's risk of developing a pressure ulcer should be assessed either on admission to hospital or in the community when the patient first comes into contact with health services. The UKCC Code of Professional Conduct states that nurses have a responsibility to identify patients at risk (UKCC 1993). Norton et al. (1985) and Waterlow (1991) developed 'at risk' scales, which are shown in Table 47.5 and Fig. 47.1. In Norton's scale, patients with scores of 14 or below are considered to run the greatest risk of developing pressure ulcers. Patients with scores of 14–18 are not considered to be at risk, but they will require reassessment immediately any change in their condition is observed. Scores of 18–20 indicate patients at minimal risk. Waterlow's scale defines patients with a score of 11–15 as being 'at risk', 16–20 as 'high risk' and over 20 as 'very high risk' (Fig. 47.1; Waterlow 1991, 1998). In one study (Smith 1989), 22 (75.7%) of patients identified as being 'at risk' (scores of 10 and over) on admission using an earlier Waterlow scale developed pressure ulcers. In the same study, 18 (62%) of patients with scores of 16 or less on the Norton scale developed ulcers. The author concludes that the Waterlow scale is more accurate at predicting formation of pressure ulcers.

Another study (Edwards 1994) analysed the use of the Waterlow scale with elderly people in the community. The criteria for allocating scores do not have clear operational definitions and can be ambiguous. The risk factor was found to be overestimated in some cases, and therefore not an accurate guide to allocating resources. The author concludes that the Waterlow scale on its own is not a sufficient means of deciding how preventive resources are to be allocated to patients in the community. However, Waterlow has also produced a Pressure Sore Prevention Manual (Waterlow 1995).

Table 47.5 The Norton scale (Norton et al. 1985)

Physical condition	Score	Mental condition	Score	Activity	Score	Mobility	Score	Incontinent	Score
Good	4	Alert	4	Ambulant	4	Full	4	Not	4
Fair	3	Apathetic	3	Walk/help	3	Slightly limited	3	Occasionally	3
Poor	2	Confused	2	Chairbound	2	Very limited	2	Usually/urine	2
Very bad	1	Stuporous	1	Bedfast	1	Immobile	1	Doubly	1

WATERLOW PRESSURE SORE PREVENTION/TREATMENT POLICY

RING SCORES IN TABLE, ADD TOTAL. SEVERAL SCORES PER CATEGORY CAN BE USED

BUILD/WEIGHT FOR HEIGHT	★	SKIN TYPE VISUAL RISK AREAS	★	SEX AGE	★	SPECIAL RISKS	★
AVERAGE	0	HEALTHY	0	MALE	1	**TISSUE MALNUTRITION**	★
ABOVE AVERAGE	1	TISSUE PAPER	1	FEMALE	2		
OBESE	2	DRY	1	14 - 49	1	e.g.: TERMINAL CACHEXIA	8
BELOW AVERAGE	3	OEDEMATOUS	1	50 - 64	2	CARDIAC FAILURE	5
		CLAMMY (TEMP↑)	1	65 - 74	3	PERIPHERAL VASCULAR	
CONTINENCE	★	DISCOLOURED	2	75 - 80	4	DISEASE	5
		BROKEN/SPOT	3	81+	5	ANAEMIA	2
COMPLETE/						SMOKING	1
CATHETERISED	0	**MOBILITY**	★	**APPETITE**	★	**NEUROLOGICAL DEFICIT**	★
OCCASION INCONT	1						
CATH/INCONTINENT							
OF FAECES	2	FULLY	0	AVERAGE	0	eg: DIABETES, M.S, CVA,	
DOUBLY INCONT	3	RESTLESS/FIDGETY	1	POOR	1	MOTOR/SENSORY	
		APATHETIC	2	N.G. TUBE/		PARAPLEGIA	4 - 6
		RESTRICTED	3	FLUIDS ONLY	2	**MAJOR SURGERY/TRAUMA**	★
		INERT/TRACTION	4	NBM/ANOREXIC	3		
		CHAIRBOUND	5			ORTHOPAEDIC -	
						BELOW WAIST,SPINAL	5
						ON TABLE > 2 HOURS	5

SCORE	10+ AT RISK	15+ HIGH RISK	20+ VERY HIGH RISK

MEDICATION	★
CYTOTOXICS, HIGH DOSE STEROIDS ANTI-INFLAMMATORY	4

REMEMBER   TISSUE DAMAGE OFTEN STARTS PRIOR TO ADMISSION, IN CASUALTY. A SEATED PATIENT IS ALSO AT RISK

ASSESSMENT: (See Over) **IF THE PATIENT FALLS INTO ANY OF THE RISK CATEGORIES THEN PREVENTATIVE NURSING IS REQUIRED. A COMBINATION OF GOOD NURSING TECHNIQUES AND PREVENTATIVE AIDS WILL DEFINITELY BE NECESSARY.**

PREVENTION:
PREVENTATIVE AIDS:

Special Mattress/ Bed:
10+Overlays or specialist foam mattresses
15+Alternating pressure overlays, mattresses and bed systems.
20+Bed Systems: Fluidised, bead, low air loss and alternating pressure mattresses.
Note: Preventative aids cover a wide spectrum of specialist features. Efficacy should be judged, if possible, on the basis of independent evidence.

Cushions:
No patient should sit in a wheelchair without some form of cushioning. If nothing else is available - use the patient's own pillow.
10+ 4" Foam cushion.
15+ Specialist Gell and/or foam cushion
20+ Cushion capable of adjustment to suit individual patient.

Bed Clothing:
Avoid plastic draw sheets, inco pads and tightly tucked in sheets/sheet covers, especially when using Specialist bed and mattress overlay systems.
Use Duvet - plus vapour permeable cover

NURSING CARE
General: Frequent changes of position,lying/sitting. Use of pillows.
Pain: Appropriate pain control.
Nutrition: High protein, vitamins, minerals
Patient Handling: Correct lifting technique - Hoists - Monkey Pole - Transfer Devices
Patient Comfort Aids: Real sheepskins - Bed Cradle.
Operating Table: 4' cover plus adequate protection.
Theatre/A&E Trolley
Skin Care: General Hygiene, NO rubbing, cover with an appropriate dressing.

IF TREATMENT IS REQUIRED, FIRST REMOVE PRESSURE

WOUND CLASSIFICATION

Stirling Pressure Sore Severity Scale (SPSSS)
Stage 0 - No clinical evidence of a pressure sore.
0.1 - Healed with scarring.
0.2 - Tissue damage not assessed as a pressure sore. (a) see below

Stage 1 - Discolouration of intact skin.
1.1 - Non blanchable erythema with increased local heat.
1.2 - Blue/purple/black discolouration - The sore is at least **Stage 1** (a or b).

Stage 2 - Partial-thickness skin loss or damage.
2.1 Blister   **2.2** Abrasion
2.3 Shallow ulcer, no underming of adjacent tissue.
2.4 Any of these with underlying blue/purple/black discolouration or induration. The sore is at least **Stage 2** (a,b or c+d for **2.3**, + e for **2.4**)

Stage 3 - Full thickness skin loss involving damage/necrosis of subcutaneous tissue, not extending to underlying bone, tendon or joint capsule.
3.1 - Crater, without undermining adjacent tissue.
3.2 - Crater, with undermining of adjacent tissue.
3.3 - Sinus, the full extent of which is uncertain.
3.4 - Necrotic tissue masking full extent of damage.
The sore is at least **Stage 3** (b, +/- e, f, g, +h for **3.4**)

Stage 4 - Full thickness loss with extensive destruction and tissue necrosis extending to underlying bone, tendon or capsule.
4.1 Visible exposure of bone tendon or capsule.
4.2 Sinus assessed as extending to same. (b+/-e, f,g,h,i)

Guide to types of Dressings/Treatment
a. Semi-permeable membrane   f. Alginate rope/ribbon
b. Hydrocolloid   g. Foam cavity filler
c. Foam dressing   h. Enzymatic debridement
d. Alginate   i. Surgical debridement
e. Hydrogel

Figure 47.1   The Waterlow Pressure Sore Prevention/Treatment Policy. (With permission of copyright holder J. Waterlow 1991, revised 1995 and 1998. Copies obtainable from Newtons, Curland, Taunton, TA3 5SG.)

Some departments have successfully devised their own risk assessment tools in response to local conditions (Birtwistle 1994). While assessment of risk is essential, the validity and reliability of tools should not be taken for granted (Nuffield Institute of Health 1995).

Grades of pressure ulcers

If a pressure ulcer develops then classification of the wound will assist in determining the most appropriate treatment (see 'Reference material', above). However, grading systems have been produced specifically for use with pressure ulcers, such as that by David *et al.* (1983) (Table 47.6), or the National Pressure Ulcer Advisory Panel (1989). These are valuable in describing the state of the ulcer and the most pertinent care required by the patient.

A recent report suggested a new four stage classification scale. The scoring is dependent on observation alone and consists of four stages which relate to discoloration of skin, degree of tissue involvement, nature of the wound bed and infective complications. The user can choose the level of detail required, but it is recommended that at least two of the categories are used. The scale can be adapted for local conditions (Reid & Morison 1994).

Treatment

Treatment of pressure ulcers is the same as for any other wound. The aetiology and underlying or related pathology, as well as the wound itself, must be assessed in order to provide the most appropriate treatment. Care should be aimed at relief of pressure, the minimization of symptoms from predisposing factors and the provision of the ideal micro-environment for wound healing.

The most effective treatment for and prevention of pressure ulcers includes frequent turning or moving the patient (for example, at least every 2 hours), keeping the skin clean and using an air or foam mattress (David 1986; Wyngaarden & Smith 1988; Andrews & Balai 1989). Of prime consideration in nursing care is the positioning and regular repositioning of the patient (Barbenel 1990) and an awareness of interface pressures, e.g. creased bed linen and night clothing that can create friction and lead to further skin breakdown.

There has been no evidence that regular turning and repositioning stops pressure sores occurring, but this could

Table 47.6   Pressure sore grades (David *et al.* 1983)

Grade	Description
1	(a) Where the skin is likely to break down (red, black and blistered areas)
	(b) Healed areas still covered by a scab
2	Superficial break in the skin
3	Destruction of the skin without cavity (full skin thickness)
4	Destruction of the skin with cavity (involving underlying tissues)

be because there are no firm guidelines on the ideal timing of this procedure (Clark 1998).

The affected area should not be rubbed as this causes maceration and degeneration of the subcutaneous tissues, especially in elderly patients (Dyson 1978).

Devices used for relief of pressure

The most effective way of preventing pressure ulcers or facilitating healing is to minimize the pressure in the affected area(s). Usually it is sufficient for the patient to be nursed on alternating aspects of the body surface, provided the patient is repositioned regularly. Sometimes this is inappropriate or impossible due to individual patients' circumstances, for example, surgical intervention, body deformities, etc. (Barton & Barton 1981).

A wide variety of devices are available to help relieve pressure over susceptible areas, e.g. cushions, overlays, static/dynamic mattresses and replacement beds. These devices differ in function and complexity, and choice must be based on meeting the patient's individual need, sound criteria for decision-making, and effective use of available resources (Table 47.7) (Pritchard & David 1988; Lockyer-Stevens 1994). Research on the effectiveness of pressure-relieving devices is largely insufficient and inconclusive and does not provide clear guidelines on which equipment is cost effective (Nuffield Institute for Health 1995).

Fungating wounds

Definition

A fungating wound is the result of a cancerous mass that infiltrates the epithelium and surrounding lymph and blood vessels. It can present as an ulcerating crater with a distinct margin or a raised fungating nodule (Moody & Grocott 1993).

Reference material

Aetiology

Fungating wounds can occur almost anywhere on the body. They arise most commonly from cancer of the breast or head and neck, melanoma, soft tissue sarcoma and some cancers of the genito-urinary system (Thomas 1992). No two fungating wounds are completely alike. Each patient responds individually to having such a wound, the consequences of which impinge on physical, psychological, social, sexual as well as spiritual wellbeing. The highest level of nursing expertise is required.

The incidence of fungating lesions is difficult to establish precisely. Thomas (1992), who conducted a survey of radiotherapy centres across the UK and received 114 completed questionnaires, reported that 295 patients with fungating wounds were seen in 1 month, and 2417 in 1 year; 62% of the wounds were breast lesions. He concludes that 'fungating wounds occur in sufficient numbers to represent a significant problem'.

Table 47.7 A selection of mechanical methods for relieving pressure

Aid	Use	Advantages	Disadvantages
Sheepskin	Low risk patients, Waterlow < 10. Good for under heels	Warm and comfortable. Decreases friction	Does *not* relieve pressure. Hardens and matts with washing. Needs to be changed frequently. *Not recommended* for regularly incontinent patients
Heel and elbow pads: sheepskin, foam, silicone	Waterlow 10+ or patients on prolonged bedrest	Reduce friction and shearing over the elbow and heel	Often have inadequate methods of keeping them on. Become hardened by washing
Silicone-filled mattress pad/cushion (e.g. Transoft)	Waterlow 10+ or patients on prolonged bedrest, able to move spontaneously	Relieves pressure by distributing it over a greater area. Comfortable. Machine (industrial) washable. Acceptable in community settings as well as in hospital. Can be used for incontinent patients. Relatively cheap purchase price. Plastic protective covers available	If the patient is very incontinent of urine, even if the plastic side is uppermost, there is seepage into the core material. Stitching comes undone after several launderings
Roho air-filled mattress/cushions	High–medium risk patients, Waterlow 10–15. To wear off pressure equalizing beds	Interlinked air cells transfer air with movement. Patient can be nursed sitting or recumbent. Non-mechanical. Washable	Can be punctured and is expensive to repair. Often incorrectly inflated due to lack of understanding and education. Can be mechanically cleaned in Sterile Supply Department
Alternating pressure beds (Pegasus, ripple, Nimbus)	High–medium risk patients, Waterlow 15+	Mechanical alteration of pressure. Reduce the frequency of (but not need for) repositioning. Available on hire at short notice	Must be checked and maintained. May increase pressures in very thin patients. Punctures possible
Mechanaid netbed	Moderate risk patients, Waterlow 15	Fits any bed. Easy to assemble and dismantle. Easy to store. No servicing, maintenance or laundry difficulties. Patients can be repositioned by one nurse. Appears to encourage relaxation and sleep. Can be lowered onto the bed surface when a firm base is required	Patients do not always like it. Wedge of pillows needed to sit patient up. Patients may lose heat. Not always easy for patients to communicate with people sitting by bed
Water bed	Moderate risk patients, Waterlow 15+	Spreads pressure. Is warm and comfortable. Available on hire at short notice	Patient is supported on the skin of the water sac thus reducing the pressure-relieving properties. Difficult to get the patient in and out
Water flotation bed	Moderate–high risk patients, Waterlow 15+	Equalizes pressure and weight. Heated	Expensive to buy, run and maintain. Makes some patients feel 'sea-sick'. Reduces self-motivated movement. Heavy to move. If not filled correctly can create more pressure than conventional bed. Not to be confused with water bed above
Fluidized air bed	High risk patients, Waterlow 20+, or indicated because of medical condition	As near to levitation as possible. Warm, sterile air produces a beneficial environment for healing wounds. One nurse can manage even a very heavy or debilitated patient on his/her own. Can be used for incontinent patients or those with heavy wound exudate. May help to alleviate severe pain	Expensive to hire. Need to reinforce floors before it can be installed. Minimizes self-motivation. Can be difficult for the patient to get in and out of bed even with help. Available on hire basis only
Low air loss bed	High risk patients, Waterlow 20+. Orientated and immobile patients	Pressure-equalizing properties equal to the fluidized air bed. Patient can be nursed in any position including prone. (Patient can control position.) Mobilization easy	Expensive to buy but can be hired. Nurses need education in the use of the equipment. Noise can be disturbing

Adapted from Pritchard & David (1988).
It is important to remember the risk of cross-infection with the use of special beds. Most companies provide adequate cleaning/sterilizing of their equipment (Pegasus 1998).

Assessment

Assessment and evaluation of a wound are discussed earlier in the chapter, but it is important to emphasize that an accurate history of a malignant lesion should be taken, and that the management of the wound should be documented clearly from the beginning. A wound assessment tool to record the amount and type of odour/exudate/pain, and the dressings used, is a helpful means of evaluating care strategies.

Grocott (1997) evaluated a tool that measured outcomes using the TELER system (Le Roux 1995) for the key variables of symptom management, dressing performance and the impact that the wound had on the patient's life. This showed that further work was required to address the wound products in order to answer patients' needs.

Problems associated with fungating wounds

Physical

1 Wound is conspicuous
2 Pain/discomfort
3 Irritation/itching
4 Exudate
5 Odour
6 Bleeding/haemorrhage
7 Infection
8 Side-effects of treatment, e.g. radiotherapy.

Psychological/social/sexual

1 Altered body image/relationship with partner
2 Embarrassment
3 Social isolation
4 Chronic nature of condition: situation may deteriorate
5 Impact on life: frequent dressing changes; hospital admissions/visits; treatment.

Aims of treatment

Malignant fungating lesions are an immense challenge. The aim of treatment is rarely to heal: care is focused on reducing the impact of symptoms and maximizing comfort (Saunders & Regnard 1989; Fairburn 1994; Laverty *et al.* 1997). Quality of life is the guiding principle of care planning, which should be undertaken in partnership with the patient.

Nurses must ensure that patients are aware that comfort, not cure, is the aim, and respond to patients' needs sensitively. The chronic nature of malignant wounds means that patients are involved in an ongoing process of adjustment. Wounds are also a constant reminder to patients of advanced disease (Laverty *et al.* 1997).

Management of symptoms

1 *Pain.* Localized pain is sometimes experienced with wounds in addition to generalized pain which is addressed separately (see Chap. 29, Pain Assessment and Management). A short-acting analgesic such as dextromoramide (e.g. Palfium) or nitrous oxide (e.g. Entonox) may be required to supplement the regular analgesic, for instance when dressings are changed. A recent small-scale study looked at the use of a mix of diamorphine and a hydrogel which was applied onto the wound site. This was based on the presumption that peripheral opioid receptors are present. The results (although on a small group of patients) suggest that the use of topically based analgesia may have a clinically useful analgesic effect (Back & Finlay 1995).

2 *Itching.* Irritation may occur around the margin of the wound (Fairburn 1993). A gentle moisturising cream (e.g. Diprobase) or a barrier cream (e.g. Metanium) may provide relief. The use of a hydrogel sheet can also reduce itching and promote comfort. Irritation caused by radiotherapy may respond to topical hydrocortisone.

3 *Exudate.* Exudate from a fungating lesion can act as a reservoir for infection (especially bacterial infection) (Collinson 1992). Surgical debridement of necrotic and sloughy areas can control the production of exudate, but may be too extensive a procedure for some patients with advanced disease (Collinson 1992; Fairburn 1993). Plastic surgical procedures are often not feasible because of local invasion by the tumour (Moss 1989). Less invasive measures (e.g. radiotherapy) may be beneficial in the short term (Thomas 1992; Fairburn 1993). Wound dressings should be absorbent and non-adhesive (Fairburn 1994), but can be bulky. The social and psychological effects of large, conspicuous dressings must be taken into account when selecting a suitable dressing (Thomas 1992).

4 *Malodour/infection.* Malodour is often an indication that a wound is infected (Dealey 1994). Swabs should be taken to identify the causative organism before systemic measures are adopted. Metronidazole as a gel has proved an effective agent for deodorization of fungating lesions (Newman *et al.* 1989; Thomas & Hay 1991; Bower *et al.* 1992; Finlay *et al.* 1996). It can be combined with a hydrogel for debridement of sloughy areas (Thomas & Hay 1991). Charcoal dressings are also effective at controlling odour in less heavily exuding and less extensively infected wounds (Thomas 1992; Fairburn 1994). Small studies have been conducted on some other topical applications, but there is little substantial research evidence available:

(a) *Natural live yoghurt.* The wound is cleaned with 0.9% sodium chloride and the yoghurt applied for 10 minutes. The yoghurt is then rinsed away thoroughly, again with 0.9% sodium chloride. The wound is dressed according to the plan of care. The process may be repeated three to four times daily (Welch 1981; Schulte 1993).

(b) *Sugar paste.* Useful for debridement and to aid regranulation of tissue. Twice daily application has been recommended for 'optimum antibacterial effect' (Middleton 1990; Topham 1996).

(c) *Icing sugar.* May be effective for deodorizing lesions. The powder is sprinkled over the affected area, washed off and then reapplied as a viscid liquid (Thomlinson 1980).

5 *Bleeding/haemorrhage.* As the lesion increases in depth and extends at the margins, capillary bleeding may occur (Fairburn 1994). Dressings should be loosened off by showering or soaking to prevent trauma. Alginate dressings may be useful for controlling capillary bleeding (Thomas 1992). If bleeding is profuse, measures with an immediate effect may be taken:

(a) *Adrenaline 1:1000.* Acts as a vasoconstrictor when applied topically, but must be applied with caution because it is absorbed systemically (Dealey 1994; British Medical Association and Royal Pharmaceutical Society of Great Britain 1999).

(b) *Transexamic acid.* Applied topically it stems bleeding by inhibiting fibrinolysis (removal of clots from a wound). The literature on its mode of action refers only to cases of epistaxis (Jash 1973).

(c) *Haemostatic swabs.* Stimulate rapid capillary coagulation. They are most commonly applied in surgical procedures, but are becoming established in primary care to control bleeding in urgent cases (Twycross & Lack 1990).

(d) *Sucralfate.* A letter in the *Wound Care Journal* purports to its use, in paste form, in controlling bleeding (Emflorgo 1998).

6 *Radiotherapy.* This can reduce the amount of exudate and control bleeding in malignant wounds. It is given either as a single fraction to avoid frequent hospital visits, or in divided doses over 2–3 weeks, in which case patients are admitted for the full course of treatment (Ashby 1991). Occasionally, radiotherapy is used prophylactically to prevent fungation if the skin is intact. If fungation has already occurred, radiotherapy may still be of value in reducing tumour bulk and enabling a degree of healing. Palliative radiotherapy of this kind is designed to spare healthy skin cells surrounding the wound and to avoid damage to the bed and margins of the wound (Horwich 1992).

7 *Hormone therapy.* Hormone therapy can reduce the rate at which a fungating wound progresses and deteriorates (Fairburn 1993). Chemotherapy is occasionally used for this purpose, but hormone therapy has fewer side-effects and can enhance the patient's sense of wellbeing.

Dressings

Numerous dressings are available to help overcome the problems associated with malignant wounds. Table 47.8 lists types of wound and recommended dressings. The FP10 index is the drug tariff that general practitioners use to prescribe wound dressings for patients in the community. There are several limitations to this guide and it is important that hospital nurses are aware of dressing availability before they do their selection process (Dale 1995).

Table 47.8 Dressings for managment of fungating wounds

Wound type	Aim	Suggested intervention
Necrotic	Debridement of eschar	Enzymes Hydrogel (Surgical intervention if appropriate)
Sloughy	Debride slough. Prevent infection	Hydrogel Alginate/hydrofibre (if high exudate is present) Enzymes (rarely)
Infected	Treat infection. Prevent associated symptoms (odour, exudate)	Metronidazole gel (topical) (can be mixed with hydrogel or hydrocolloid gel to manage associated symptoms)
Malodorous	Remove odour	Metronidazole gel (topical) Charcoal sheet Sugar paste prepared under sterile conditions Icing sugar Honey
Highly exuding (cavity)	Contain exudate	Alginate (sheet/ribbon) Hydrofibre (sheet/ribbon) Foam sheet Foam cavity dressings
Lightly exuding	Contain exudate. Prevent increase	Hydrocolloid Hydrogel/hydrocolloid gel Semipermeable film
Bleeding	Control bleeding	Alginate Surgical haemostatic sponges
Itching	Control itching	Hydrogel sheets

A mixture of these products can be used, depending on the current status of the wound and the number of presenting problems (Mallett *et al.* 1999).

District nurses and health visitors are preparing themselves to be able to prescribe. A limited amount of drugs and wound management products will be available in a formulary from the end of 1999 (Gooch 1999).

Some centres are also exploring the concept of using protocolized prescribing (Laverty *et al.* 1997) to ensure that those professionals with appropriate experience can advise the medical staff.

Securing dressings

Tapes should only be applied to healthy skin in order to avoid further tissue damage. Care should be taken to leave a large margin around the wound including any existing cutaneous nodules.

Plain bandaging or the use of Netelast/Tubifast is helpful where a wound is positioned in a difficult area. Tapeless retention dressings are ideal to use in difficult-to-dress areas and for delicate skin. They are also reusable and can be adapted to suit the individual patient (McGregor 1998; McGregor & Baxter 1999).

Conclusions

Fungating wounds pose a challenge in primary care, where district and Macmillan nurses are an invaluable resource in the important work of assessing wounds and liaising with hospitals and hospices about individual care plans. Clear, rational decision-making is vital to establishing trust with the patient and achieving maximum levels of comfort and quality of life.

Skilful communication is needed to help patients to adjust to the dependence that serious wounds may cause. Frequent hospital admissions and dressing changes, and deteriorating health, may leave patients and family feeling that their lives are being taken over by the illness. Psychological wounds, caused by embarrassment, changes in body image and, sometimes, social isolation, may never heal completely, but patients can be greatly helped by tact, understanding and supportive care.

Radiotherapy skin damage

Definition

Skin damage from radiotherapy can be defined as a local irritation/erythema or a loss in integrity of the skin, on or in the immediate surrounding area where the treatment is directed.

Reference material

Aetiology

Skin damage from radiotherapy results from prolonged treatment periods, existing friable/broken skin integrity, poor general health (due to disease or concurrent treatment, e.g. surgery, chemotherapy) and treatment directed at particular body areas (e.g. inframammary folds).

The degree of damage depends on the amount of treatment (often reliant on curative versus palliative), the patient's performance status and the body area that is being irradiated (e.g. skin folds, groins, natal cleft). Extensive experience has indicated that the patient can experience a range of symptoms, from areas of dry desquamation and associated erythema to areas of moist desquamation that can lead to sloughy and/or necrotic wounds that can take a long time to heal.

Healing will be delayed while the patient is still undergoing treatment and for 2–4 weeks after treatment has finished due to the cell damage caused as a result of radiation.

Emphasis of care is on prevention initially, and then focuses on comfort if skin breakdown occurs.

Assessment

Assessment of the treatment area is imperative and should be ongoing. Constant checking of the site of irradiation at each treatment is important in order to monitor the skin and observe for any signs of breakdown. Measures to promote comfort and ease any 'burning' sensation should be initiated early on in the treatment plan.

Symptom management

A dearth of research is available relating to the treatment of radiotherapy skin reactions (Campbell & Lane 1996). Much of the treatment relies on anecdotal evidence and specialist practitioners' experiences (Table 47.9).

Conclusions

It is important to remember that most dressings will have to be removed before the patient receives his or her radiotherapy because the dressing bulk can affect the dosage of radiotherapy that the patient receives (Lochhead 1983).

Table 47.9 Management of radiotherapy reactions

Problem	Suggested treatment
Erythema	Hydrogel sheets
	Aqueous cream (with menthol)
	Hydrocortisone cream
	Johnson's baby talc
	Aloe vera cream
Dry desquamation	Aqueous cream (with menthol)
	Hydrogel sheets
	Hydroocolloid sheets
Moist desquamation (low exudate)	Hydrogel/hydrocolloid gel
	Hydrocolloid sheet
	Secondary dressing
Moist desquamation (high exudate)	Alginate/hydrofibre
	Secondary dressing (foam sheet)
Necrosis/sloughy	Debride eschar/slough

Sometimes this can be of benefit, especially if an increased dose is required at the skin surface.

Particular areas of the body may require specialist attention and the location of these wounds frequently provides a challenge for the practitioner in relation to securing wound care products and being innovative to promote a positive body image.

Plastic surgery wounds

Definition

Plastic surgery wounds is the collective term that refers to surgical procedures that are performed to restore function and cosmesis. This is achieved by using flaps and skin grafts for reconstruction purposes, in addition to using the natural elasticity and mobility of the skin. A surgical flap is a strip of tissue, usually consisting of skin, underlying fat, fascia, muscle or bone, which is transferred from one part of the body (known as the donor site) to another (known as the recipient site) (Coull 1992), for example, a free radial forearm flap repair to reconstruct the anterior part of the tongue.

A skin graft is living tissue which is removed from one person and then applied to another area of the body or to another person (Coull 1991), for example, a skin graft taken from the upper arm to cover the radial forearm defect. There are two types of skin grafts: full thickness and split thickness. In full thickness the entire epidermis and dermis are removed (Rodzwic & Donnard 1986), whereas in split thickness (also known as split skin) the graft consists of the epidermis and upper layers of the dermis only (Coull 1991).

Reference material

Aetiology

Plastic surgery is performed following trauma, e.g. burns, or surgery, e.g. excision of a carinoma, or congenital defects, e.g. cleft palate. Surgical reconstruction is often required, particularly following extensive surgery for cancer of the breast, head and neck, melanoma, soft tissue sarcomas, gynaecological and genito-urinary systems. The aim is to perform the simplest procedure that will provide the desired aesthetic and functional outcome (Clamon & Netscher 1994). Each patient is therefore entirely unique in undergoing such surgery, which can result in altered anatomy. Consequently, each can be affected differently by the psychological and physical impact such trauma or disease has on them as individuals.

Assessment

The pre-operative patient history must be as detailed as possible, including information on past and present medical conditions, e.g. diabetes and radiotherapy, both of which can delay the wound healing process. Other factors

to take into consideration are medication, e.g. aspirin which will affect clotting ability, impaired nutritional status which can delay wound healing, and a history of smoking which can impair circulation (see Chap. 30, Peri-Operative Care). For certain patient groups, e.g. those with recurrence of head and neck cancer, anatomy may already have been altered, through previous surgery, thereby narrowing down the possible options for reconstruction.

Postoperative observation of the wound sites, dressings and drains is crucial as deterioration of a wound can occur suddenly, e.g. fluid-filled seromas, necessitating the need for prompt nursing action (see below).

Associated problems

Split skin graft donor site

The two most common problems associated with a split skin graft donor site are slipping of dressing and infection.

Slipping of dressing, resulting in pain and discomfort

The donor sites chosen for this procedure are usually the upper thigh, upper arm and upper buttock. Less conspicuous areas of the body are chosen wherever possible. Due to gravity, the dressing has a tendency to slip, resulting in the exposure of raw skin. The excision of the thin layer of skin leaves nerve endings exposed, resulting in pain at the donor site (Wilkinson 1997). Analgesia should therefore be given prior to performing or renewing a dressing. A non-steroidal anti-inflammatory, e.g. diclofenac, used in conjunction with a compound analgesic, e.g. codydramol or co-codamol, is suitable unless contraindicated. Exposed areas of raw skin should be dressed with an alginate and covered with low-linting gauze. The combination of these two dressings will assist in absorbing exudate. A bandage and tape, with a few pieces of tape placed vertically at the top of the dressing to prevent slipping, are then used to secure the dressings. Alternatively, a tapeless dressing can be used instead of a bandage and tape. This is a hypoallergenic, non-latex stretchy material which does not require tape to secure it to the primary dressing or to the patient (McGregor & Baxter 1999).

Infection

A high amount of exudate on the dressing, evident by new and excessive strikethrough, can indicate the presence of infection. For example, *Pseudomonas aeruginosa* is characterized by a strong, musty smell and a bright blue–green discharge (Wilkinson 1997). The entire dressing should be soaked off in order to assess the wound site, and the site should be swabbed for microbial culture and sensitivity. While infected, the wound site should be dressed daily. *Pseudomonas aeruginosa* is known to be sensitive to flamazine (Hamilton-Miller *et al.* 1993). This is an antibacterial cream containing silver sulphadiazine 1% w/w, and is applied topically to the wound site, then covered with a non-adherent dressing. If the patient experiences a raised temperature, increased pain or appears unwell, this may indicate the presence of a systemic infection and will require a course of antibiotics (Wilkinson 1997).

Split skin recipient site (flap donor site)

When a flap is transferred from its original site it leaves a deficit of tissue. Split skin is applied to this site as primary closure is not possible. The most common problem with flap donor sites is fluid-filled seromas.

Fluid-filled seromas

On removing the dressing after 5 days, the split skin should be smooth and pink or red in colour. Any seromas, characterized by blisters containing air and haemoserous fluid, must be expelled. Without performing this the graft will not take. A sterile needle is used to evacuate the fluid, enabling the graft to be carefully rolled from the centre outwards (Coull 1991). This can be performed by using a cotton bud and enables the graft to adhere to the underlying tissue. A tulle dressing, low-linting gauze and a bandage, or a tapeless dressing are then applied. The pressure from the dressing assists in expelling the blisters (Coull 1991).

Scarring

Definition

A scar is defined as the mark left after a wound has healed with the formation of connective tissue (Davis et al. 1993). Initially the scar is red and raised; then over a period of 6–12 months this matures to produce a hypopigmented, flat scar (Davies 1985a). With regular massage, using an unperfumed moisturising cream, the condition of the scar can improve (Allsworth 1985).

Hypertrophic and keloid scars

Occasionally the scar continues to become increasingly red, raised and itchy, defined as hypertrophic. If these symptoms continue, with the scar tissue invading surrounding unaffected tissue as well as increasing in height, a keloid scar is formed (Davies 1985a). The areas that are most susceptible are the upper back, shoulders, anterior chest, presternal area and the upper arms (Munro 1995a). Dark-skinned people have a greater susceptibility to developing keloid scars than those who are lighter skinned (Davies 1985a).

Reference material

Aetiology

There are a number of possible predisposing factors, as stated by Munro (1995a):

1 Increased skin tension can contribute to the formation of keloid and hypertrophic scars; however, earlobes, which are free of tension, can also develop keloid scars.

2 These scars appear to have a genetic basis. In addition to this, keloid formation has been associated with some dermatological conditions and inherited connective tissue disorders.

3 There is thought to be a relationship between endocrine changes and keloid formation, e.g. keloids have been known to occur after a thyroidectomy.

4 The production of hypertrophic and keloid scars may have an immunological basis.

5 Biochemical differences between healthy scars, keloid and hypertrophic scars have been found, indicating that collagen synthesis is altered.

6 Hypoxia may contribute to the formation of abnormal scars. Kischer et al. (1982) found that microvessels in these scars are partially or completely occluded, causing excessive fibroblast activity in the scar.

7 Several studies have suggested that growth factors may have a role in keloid formation. Russell et al. (1988) found that cultured keloid fibroblasts grew more readily in a medium with reduced growth factors than normal fibroblasts.

Further studies are needed to provide confirmation.

Assessment

The disfigurement and dysfunction that can result from hypertrophic and keloid scarring will have a differing impact on the individual concerned. From the initial assessment, it may be possible to perform further minor surgery, e.g. Z or Y plasty, where the scar is eased by cutting it in the line of relaxed skin tension (Allsworth 1985) or to use intralesional steroid injections. Pressure garments are also used to flatten the scars. Surgery is often used to debulk larger lesions, while smaller lesions are treated with other therapies (Munro 1995b).

Various non-surgical techniques can be implemented. The use of a silicone gel sheet, e.g. Cica-care (Williams 1996) or a glycerine gel sheet, e.g. Novogel (Baum & Busuito 1998) appears to soften, flatten and blanch scars, preventing their development.

Cosmetic camouflage can cleverly assist in concealing some scarring. This service is provided by skilled professionals, enabling the clients to develop their own techniques with guidance. Education and support are crucial in assisting the patient to reintegrate into society. Advice may be required regarding specific problems, e.g. patients with a known history of keloid formation should avoid elective surgery and trauma such as ear piercing (Munro 1995b).

Disfigurement should be approached as a total problem, skin deep, mind deep and societal, as stated by Doreen Trust, founder and director of the Disfigurement Guidance Centre in Cupar, Fife, cited in Trevelyan (1996).

References and further reading

Alberdi, J.M.Z. (1988) Hypertensive ulcer: Martorell's ulcer. *Phlebology*, 3, 139–42.

Allen, S. (1988) Ulcers: treating the cause. *Nurs Times*, **84**(51), 62–3.

Allsworth, J. (1985) *Skin Camouflage. A Guide To Remedial Techniques.* Arnould–Taylor, Cheltenham.

Andrews, J. & Balai, R. (1989) The prevention and treatment of pressure sores by use of pressure distributing mattresses. *Care Sci Pract*, **7**(3), 72–6.

Angeras, M.H., Brandberg, A., Falk, A. & Seeman, T. (1992) Comparison between sterile saline and tap water for the cleaning of acute traumatic soft tissue wounds. *Eur J Surg*, **58**, 347–50.

Anning, S.T. (1954) Leg ulcers, their cause and treatment. Churchill, London. In: *The Management of Leg Ulcers* (1987), 2nd edn. (ed. T.J. Ryan). Oxford University Press, Oxford.

Armstrong, S., Duncan, V. & Gibson B. (1998) Venous leg ulcers, Part 4. Wound care. *Prof Nurse*, **13**(11), 798–802.

Ashby, M. (1991) The role of radiotherapy in palliative care. *J Pain Symp Manage*, **6**(6), 380–88.

Autar, R. (1998) Calculating patients' risk of deep vein thrombosis. *Br J Nurs*, **7**(1), 7–12.

Ayton, A. (1985) Wounds that won't heal: wound care. *Commun Outlook*, November, 16–19.

Back, I. & Finlay, I. (1995) Analgesic effect of topical opioids on painful skin ulcers. (Letter.) *J Pain Sympt Manage*, **10**(7), 493.

Baker, J. (1998) Essential oils: a complementary therapy in wound management. *J Wound Care*, **7**(7), 355–7.

Baker, S.R., Stacey, M.C., Jopp-McKay, A.G. et al. (1991) Epidemiology of chronic venous ulcers. *Br J Surg*, **78**, 864–7.

Balakrishnan, C. (1994) Simple method of applying pressure to skin grafts of neck with foam dressing and staples. *J Burn Care Rehab*, Sept/Oct, 432–3.

Bale, S. (1991) A holistic approach and the ideal dressing. *Prof Nurse*, **6**(6), 316–23.

Bale, S. & Jones, V. (1997) *Wound Care Nursing: A Patient Centred Approach.* Baillière Tindall, London.

Barbenel, J.C. (1990) Movement studies during sleep. In: *Pressure Sores – Clinical Practice and Scientific Approach* (ed. D. L. Bader), pp. 249–60. Macmillan, London.

Barr, P.O. et al. (1990) Hyperbaric oxygen and problem wounds. *Care Sci Pract*, **8**(1), 3–6.

Barton, A.A. (1988) Prevention of pressure sores. *Nurs Times*, **73**, 1593–5.

Barton, A. & Barton, M. (1981) *The Management and Prevention of Pressure Sores.* Faber & Faber, London.

Baum, T.M. & Busuito, M.J. (1998) Use of a glycerin-based gel sheeting in scar management. *Adv Wound Care*, **11**(1), 40–43.

Benbow, M. (1994) The benefits of hydrogel dressings. *Commun Outlook*, October, 29–34.

Birtwistle, J. (1994) Pressure sore formation and risk assessment in intensive care. *Care Crit Ill*, **10**(4), 154–5; 157–9.

Blackwell's Dictionary of Nursing (1998). Blackwell Science, Oxford.

Blair, S.D. et al. (1988a) Do dressings influence the healing of chronic venous ulcers? *Phlebology*, **3**, 129–34.

Blair, S.D. et al. (1988b) Sustained compression and healing of chronic leg ulcers. *Br Med J*, **297**(6657), 1159–61.

Bloomfield, S.F. & Sizer, T.J. (1985) Eusol BPC and other hypochlorite formulations used in hospitals. *Pharm J*, 3 August, 153–7.

Boccalon, H. & Ginestet, M.C. (1988) Influence of temperature variations on venous return: clinical observations. *Phlebology*, **3**, Suppl. 1, 47–9.

Bower, M., Stein, R., Evans, T., Hedley, A., Pert, P. & Coombes, R. (1992) A double-blind study of the efficacy of metronidazole gel in the treatment of malodorous fungating tumours. *Eur J Cancer*, **28**(4/5), 888–9.

Brennan, S.S. & Leaper, D.J. (1985) The effect of antiseptics on the healing wound: a study using the rabbit ear chamber. *Br J Surg*, **72**, 780–782.

British Medical Association and Royal Pharmaceutical Society of Great Britain (1999) *British National Formulary.* Pharmaceutical Press, Oxford.

Brown, G.L. et al. (1989) Enhancement of wound healing by topical treatment with epidermal growth factor. *New Engl J Med*, **321**(2), 76–9.

Brown, G.L. et al. (1991) Stimulation of healing of chronic wounds by epidermal growth factor. *Plastic Reconstr Surg*, **88**, 189–94.

Burnand, K.G. (1990) Aetiology of venous ulceration. *Br J Surg*, **77**, 483–4.

Callam, M.J. et al. (1985) Chronic ulceration of the leg: extent of the problem and provision of care. *Br Med J*, **290**, 1855–6.

Callam, M.J. et al. (1987a) Arterial disease in chronic leg ulceration: an underestimated hazard? Lothian and Forth Valley Leg Ulcer Study. *Br Med J*, **294**, 929–31.

Callam, M.J. et al. (1987b) *Lothian and Forth Valley Leg Ulcer Study.* Buccleuch, Hawick.

Campbell, J. & Lane, C. (1996) Developing a skin-care protocol in radiotherapy. *Prof Nurse*, **12**(2), 105–108.

Casey, G. (1998) Three steps to effective wound care. *Nurs Stand*, **12**(49), 43–4.

Casey, G. (1998a) The importance of nutrition in wound healing. *Nurs Stand*, **13**(3), 51–6.

Casey, G. (1998b) The management of pain in wound care. *Nurs Stand*, **13**(12), 49–54.

Cherry, G.W. & Ryan, T.J. (1987) *Blueprint for the Treatment of Leg Ulcers and the Prevention of Recurrence.* Squibb Surgicare, Hounslow.

Clamon, J. & Netscher, D.T. (1994) General principles of flap reconstruction: goals for aesthetic and functional outcome. *Plastic Surg Nurs*, **14**(1), 9–14.

Clark, M. (1998) Repositioning to prevent pressure sores – what is the evidence? *Nurs Stand*, **13**(3), 58–64.

Clarke, R. & Stewart–Smith, J. (1993) Speedy recovery. *Nurs Times*, **89**(25), 72 & 75.

Clide, S. (1992) Cleaning choices. *Nurs Times*, **88**(19), 74–8.

Cohen, B.E. & Cohen, I.K. (1973) Vitamin A: adjuvant and steroid antagonist in the immune response. *J Immunol*, **3**(5), 1376–1380. In: Wound care (1989). (M.S. Messer). *Crit Care Nurs Q*, **11**(4), 17–27.

Collier, M. (1996) The principles of optimum wound management. *Nurs Stand*, **10**(43), 47–52.

Collinson, G. (1992) Improving quality of life in patients with malignant fungating wounds. *Proc 2nd Eur Conf on Wound Management.* Macmillan, London.

Cooper, D.M. (1990) Optimizing wound healing. *Nurs Clin North Am*, **25**(1), 165–80.

Cooper, J. (1997) *Occupational Therapy in Oncology and Palliative Care.* Whurr, London.

Coull, A. (1991) Making sense of split skin grafts. *Nurs Times*, **87**(27), 54–5.

Coull, A. (1992) Making sense of surgical flaps. *Nurs Times*, **88**(1) 32–4.

Cox, B.D. et al. (1987) *The Health and Lifestyle Survey.* Health Promotion Trust, London.

Cox, D.A. (1993) Growth factors in wound healing. *J Wound Care*, **12**(6), 339–42.

Cruse, P.J.E. & Foord, R. (1980) The epidemiology of wound infection. *Surg Clin North Am*, **60**(1), 27–40. In: *The Royal Marsden Hospital Manual of Clinical Nursing Procedures* (1988) 2nd edn. (eds A.P. Pritchard & J.A. David). Harper & Row, London.

Cunliffe, W.J. (1990) Eusol – to use or not to use? *Dermatol Pract*, **8**(2), 5–7.

Cutting, K. (1994) Factors influencing wound healing. *Nurs Stand*, **8**(50), 33–7.

Dale, J. (1995) Wound dressings on the Drug Tariff. *Prof Nurse*, **10**(7), 461–5.

Dale, J.J. & Gibson, B. (1986a) Leg ulcers: a disease affecting all ages. *Prof Nurse*, **1**(8), 213–16.

Dale, J.J. & Gibson, B. (1986b) Leg ulcers: the nursing assessment. *Prof Nurse*, **1**(9), 236–8.

Dale, J.J. & Gibson, B. (1986c) The treatment of leg ulcers. *Prof Nurse*, **1**(12), 321–4.

Dale, J.J. & Gibson, B. (1987) Compression bandaging for venous ulcers. *Prof Nurse*, **2**(7), 211–14.

Dale, J.J. & Gibson, B. (1990) Back-up for the venous pump. *Prof Nurse*, **5**(9), 481–6.

Dale, J. (1998) Venous leg ulcers. Part 3: compression. *Prof Nurse*, **13**(10), 715–19.

David, J.A. (1983) Normal physiology from injury to repair. *Nursing*, **2**(11), 296–7.

David, J.A. (1986) *Wound Management: A Comprehensive Guide to Dressing and Healing*. Martin Dunitz, London.

David, J.A. (1987) Beds. *Nursing*, **3**(13), 503–505.

David, J.A. (1990) Recent venous ulcer treatments. *Nurs Stand*, **4**(23), 24–6.

David, J.A. *et al.* (1983) *An Investigation of the Current Methods Used in Nursing for the Care of Patients with Established Pressure Sores*. Nursing Practice Research Unit, University of Surrey.

Davies, D.M. (1985a) Plastic and reconstructive surgery. *Br Med J*, **290**, 1056–8.

Davies, D.M. (1985b) *ABC of plastic and reconstructive surgery*. British Medical Journal, London.

Davis, M.H., Dunkley, P., Harden, R., *et al.* (1993) *The Wound Handbook*. Centre for Medical Education, Dundee, and Perspective, London.

Dealey, C. (1988) The role of the tissue viability nurse. *Nurs Stand*, **2**(51), Suppl., 4–5.

Dealey, C. (1989) Management of cavity wounds. *Nursing*, **3**(39), 25–7.

Dealey, C. (1991) Criteria for wound healing. *Nursing*, **4**(29), 20–21.

Dealey, C. (1994) *The Care of Wounds*. Blackwell Science, Oxford.

Deas, J. *et al.* (1986) The toxicity of commonly used antiseptics on fibroblasts in tissue culture. *Phlebology*, **1**, 205–209.

Department of Infection Control, Memorial Hospital (1989) *Blueprint for the Prevention and Management of Pressure Sores*. Convatec Ltd., Ickenham, Uxbridge.

Devel, T.F. (1987) Polypeptide growth factors: roles in normal and abnormal cell growth. *Annu Rev Cell Biol*, **3**, 443–64.

DoH (1992) *The Health of the Nation: A Strategy for Health in England*. Stationery Office, London.

DoH (1993) *The Health of the Nation: Pressure Sores – A Key Quality Indicator*. Stationery Office, London.

DoH (1994) *Pressure Sores: A Key Quality Indicator*. Department of Health, Leeds.

Donovan, S. (1998) Wound infection and wound swabbing. *Prof Nurse*, **13**(11), 757–9.

Draper, J. (1985) Make the dressing fit the wound. *Nurs Times*, **81**(41), 32–5.

Dyson, M. *et al.* (1988) Comparison of the effects of moist and dry conditions on dermal repair. *J Invest Dermatol*, **91**(5), 434–9.

Dyson, R. (1978) Bed sores – the injuries hospital staff inflict on patients. *Nurs Mirror*, **146**(24), 30–32.

Edwards, M. (1994) *The reliability and validity of the Waterlow pressure sore risk scale when used within district nursing to assess elders nursed in a domiciliary setting*. MSc dissertation, University of London.

Ehrlich, H.P. *et al.* (1973) The effects of vitamin A and glucocorticoids upon inflammation and collagen synthesis. *Ann Surg*, **2**, 222–7. In: Wound care (1989) (M.S. Messer). *Crit Care Nurs Q*, **11**(4), 17–27.

Emflorgo, C. (1998) Controlling bleeding in fungating wounds. (Letter.) *J Wound Care*, **7**(5), 235.

European Pressure Ulcer Advisory Panel (1998) A policy statement on the prevention of pressure ulcers. *Br J Nurs*, **7**(15), 888–90.

Evans, P. (1988) Venous disorders of the leg. *Nurs Times*, **84**(49), 46–7.

Fader, R.C. *et al.* (1983) Sodium hypochlorite decontamination of split-thickness cadaveric skin infected with bacteria and yeast with subsequent isolation and growth of basal cells to confluency in tissue culture. *Antimicrob Agents Chemother*, **24**(2), 181–5.

Fairburn, K. (1993) Towards better care for women. *Prof Nurse*, **9**(30), 204–12.

Fairburn, K. (1994) A challenge that requires further research. *Prof Nurse*, **9**(4), 272–7.

Falanga, V. & Eaglstein, W. (1986) A therapeutic approach to venous ulcers. *J Am Acad Dermatol*, **14**(5), 777–84.

Fangrell, B. (1979) Local microcirculaton in chronic venous incompetence and leg ulcers. *Vasc Surg*, **13**(4), 217–25.

Farrow, S. & Toth, B. (1991) The place of Eusol in wound management. *Nurs Stand*, **5**(22), 25–7.

Ferguson, A. (1988) Best performer. *Nurs Times*, **84**(14), 52–5.

Field, C.K. & Kerstein, M.D. (1994) Overview of wound healing in a moist environment. *Am J Surg*, **167**, Suppl. 1a, 2s–6s.

Finch, A. (1997) Therapeutic touch and wound healing. *J Wound Care*, **6**(10), 501–504.

Fincham Gee, C. (1990) Measuring the wound size. *Nursing*, **4**(2), 34–5.

Finlay, I., Bowszyc, J. & Ramlav, C. (1996) The effect of topical 0.75% metronidazole gel on malodorous cutaneous ulcers. *J Pain Sympt Manage*, **11**(3), 158–62.

Flanagan, M. (1994) Wound care: assessment criteria. *Nurs Times*, **90**(35), 76–88.

Flanagan, M. (1995) Who is at risk of a pressure sore? *Prof Nurse*, **10**(5), 305–308.

Flanagan, M. (1996) A practical framework for wound assessment 1: physiology. *Br J Nurs*, **5**(22), 1391–7.

Flanagan, M. (1999) The physiology of wound healing. In: *Wound Management: Theory and Practice* (eds M. Miller & D. Glover). Nursing Times Books, London.

Florey, C. du V. (1982) Diabetes mellitus (Chap. 25). In: *Epidemiology of Diseases* (eds D.L. Miller & R.D.T. Farmer). Blackwell Scientific Publications, Oxford.

Forrest, R.D. (1980) The treatment of pressure sores. *J Int Med Res*, **8**, 430–35.

Fowler, A. & Dempsey, A. (1998) Split-thickness skin graft donor sites. *J Wound Care*, **7**(8), 399–402.

Francis, A. (1998) Nursing management of skin graft sites. *Nurs Stand*, **12**(33), 41–4.

Franks, P., Oldroyd, M. & Dickson, D. (1995) Risk factors for leg ulceration recurrence: a randomised trial of two types of compression stocking. *Age Ageing*, **24**, 490–94.

Fraser, R. & Gilchrist, T. (1983) Sorbsan calcium alginate fibre dressings in footcare. *Biomaterials*, **4**, 222–4.

Garrett, B. (1997) The proliferation and movement of cells during re-epithelialisation. *J Wound Care*, **6**(4), 174–7.

Garrett, B. (1998) Re-epithelialisation. *J Wound Care*, **7**(7), 358–9.

General Household Survey, 1986 (1989) pp. 290–93. Stationery Office, London.

Gilchrist, B. (1989) The treatment of leg ulcers with occlusive hydrocolloid dressings: a microbiological study. In: *Directions in Nursing Research* (eds J. Wilson-Barnett & S. Robinson), pp. 51–8. Scutari Press, London.

Gilchrist, B. (1997) Should iodine be considered in wound management? *J Wound Care*, **6**(3), 148–50.

Gilchrist, B. (1998) Innovations in leg ulcer care. *J Wound Care*, **7**(3), 151–2.

Gilchrist, T. & Martin, A.M. (1983) Wound treatment with Sorbsan – an alginate fibre dressing. *Biomaterials*, **4**, 317–20.

Glover, M. (1992) Growth factors and wound healing. *Wound Manag*, **2**(1), 9–11.

Gogia, P.P. *et al.* (1988) Wound management with whirlpool and infrared cold laser treatment. *Phys Ther*, **68**(8), 1239–42.

Gooch, S. (1999) Nurse prescribing and the Crown Report. *Prof Nurse*, **14**(10), 678–80.

Goren, D. (1989) Use of Omniderm in treatment of low-degree pressure sores in terminally ill cancer patients. *Cancer Nurs* **12**(3), 165–9.

Gould, D. (1984) Clinical forum. *Nurs Mirror*, **159**(16), iii–vi.

Grey, J.E. (1998) Cellulitis associated with wounds. *J Wound Care*, **7**(70), 338–9.

Griffin, T. (ed.) (1989) *Social Trends 19. Central Statistical Office.* Stationery Office, London.

Grocott, P. (1997) Evaluation of a tool used to assess the management of fungating wounds. *J Wound Care*, **6**(9), 421–4.

Grocott, P. (1999) The management of fungating wounds. *J Wound Care*, **8**(5), 232–4.

Gustafsson, G. (1988) Guidelines for the application of disinfectants in wound care. *Nurs RSA Verpleging*, **3**(11/12), 8–9.

Guttman, L. (1976) The prevention and treatment of pressure sores. In: *Bed Sore Biomechanics* (eds R.M. Kenedi *et al.*). Macmillan, London.

Guyton, A.C. (1984) *Physiology of the Human Body*, 6th edn. CBS College Publishing, Philadelphia.

Hallows, L. (1987) Leg ulcers. An underlying problem. *Commun Outlook*, September, 6–14.

Hamilton-Miller, J.M.T., Shah, S. & Smith, C. (1993) Silver sulphadiazine: a comprehensive in vitro reassessment. *Chemotherapy*, **39**, 405–409.

Hansbrough, W. (1995) Management of skin-grafted burn wounds with xeroform and layers of dry coarse-mesh gauze dressing results in excellent graft take and minimal nursing time. *J Burn Care Rehab*, **16**(5), 531–4.

Harkiss, K.J. (ed.) (1971) *Surgical Dressings and Wound Healing.* Bradford University Press, Bradford.

Harkiss, K.J. (1985a) Leg ulcers: cheaper in the long run. *Commun Outlook*, August, 19–28.

Harkiss, K.J. (1985b) Wound management: cost analysis of dressing materials used in venous leg ulcers. *Pharm J*, 31 August, 268–9.

Heidt, P. (1981) Effect of therapeutic touch on anxiety levels of hospitalised patients. *Nurs Res*, **30**(1), 32–7.

Henry, M. & Corless, C. (1989) The incidence of varicose veins in Ireland. *Phlebology*, **41**, 133–7.

Hofman, D. (1998) Oedema and the management of leg ulcers. *J Wound Care*, **7**(7), 345–8.

Hollinworth, H. (1998) Venous leg ulcers. Part 1: aetiology. *Prof Nurse*, **13**(8), 553–8.

Holmes, S. (1990) Good food for long life. *Prof Nurse*, **6**(1), 43–6.

Horwich, A. (1992) Radiotherapy update. *Br Med J*, **304**, 1554–7.

Hunt, T.K. & Dunphy, J.E. (1979) *Fundamentals of Wound Management.* Appleton-Century-Crofts, New York. In: Wound care (1989) (M.S. Messer). *Crit Care Nurs Q*, **11**(4), 17–27.

Hunt, T.K. *et al.* (1969) Effect of vitamin A on reversing the inhibitory effect of cortisone on healing of open wounds in animals and man. *Ann Surg*, **170**, 633–41. In: Wound care (1989) (M.S. Messer). *Crit Care Nurs Q*, **11**(4), 17–27.

Husian, T. (1953) An experimental study of some pressure effects on tissues, with reference to the bed-sore problems. *J Pathol Bacteriol*, **66**, 347–58.

Inman, C. & Firth, J. (1998) Pressure sore prevention in the community. *Prof Nurse*, **13**(7), 515–20.

Ivetic, O. & Lyne, P.A. (1990) Fungating and ulcerating malignant lesions: a review of the literature. *J Adv Nurs*, **15**, 83–8.

Jackson, D.S. & Rovee, D.T. (1988) Current concepts in wound healing: research and theory. *J Enterostomal Ther*, **15**(3), 133–7.

James, H. (1998) Classification and grading of pressure sores. *Prof Nurse*, **13**(10), 669–72.

Jash, D.K. (1973) Epistaxis: topical use of aminocapoic acid in its management. *J Laryngol Otol*, **87**, 895–8.

Jeter, K.F. & Tintle, T. (1988) Principles of wound cleaning and wound care. *J Home Health Care Pract*, **1**, 43–7.

Johnson, A. (1984) Towards rapid tissue healing. *Nurs Times*, **80**(48), 39–43.

Johnson, A. (1988a) Natural healing processes: an essential update. *Prof Nurse*, **3**, 149–52.

Johnson, A. (1988b) The case against the use of hypochlorites in the treatment of open wounds. *Care Sci Pract*, **6**(3), 86–8.

Johnson, A. (1988c) Modern wound care products. *Prof Nurse*, **3**, 392–8.

Johnson, A. (1988d) Standard protocols for treating open wounds. *Prof Nurse*, **3**(12), 498–501.

Johnson, A. (1989) Granuflex wafers as a prophylactic pressure sore dressing. *Care Sci Pract*, **7**(2), 55–8.

Jones, J.E. & Nelson, E.A. (1998) Compression hosiery in the management of venous leg ulcers. *J Wound Care*, **7**(6), 293–6.

Kaufman, T. & Alexander, J.W. (1988) Topical oxygen treatment promoted healing and enhanced scar formation of experimental full-thickness burns. In: *Beyond Occlusion: Wound Care Proceedings. Royal Society of Medicine International Congress and Symposium Series* (ed. T.J. Ryan), pp. 61–6. Royal Society of Medicine, London.

Kaufman, T. & Berger (1988) Topical pH and burn wound healing: a review. In: *Beyond Occlusion: Wound Care Proceedings. Royal Society of Medicine International Congress and Symposium Series* (ed. T.J. Ryan), pp. 55–60. Royal Society of Medicine, London.

Kaufman, T. & Hirshowitz, B. (1982) The influence of various microclimate conditions on the burn wound: a review. *Burns*, **9**, 84–90.

Kaufman, T. *et al.* (1985) Topical acidification promotes healing of experimental deep partial thickness skin burns: a randomized double-blind preliminary study. *Burns*, **12**, 84–90.

Kischer, C.W., Shetlar, M.R. & Chvapil, M. (1982) Hypertrophic scars and keloids: a review and new concept concerning their origin. *Scan Microsc*, **4**, 1699–713.

Knight, A. (1990) The skin clinic. *Mod Med*, **35**(8), 608.

Knighton, D.R. *et al.* (1981) Regulation of wound healing angiogenesis. Effect of oxygen gradients and inspired oxygen concentration. *Surgery*, **90**(2), 262–70.

Kosiak, M. (1958) Evaluation of pressure as a factor in the production of ischial ulcers. *Arch Phys Med Rehab*, **40**, 62–9.

Kosiak, M. (1976) A mechanical resting surface: its effect on pressure distribution. *Arch Phys Med Rehab*, **57**, 481–3.

Lait, M.E. & Smith, L.N. (1998) Wound management: a literature review. *J Clin Nurs*, **7**, 11–17.

Laverty, D., Mallett, J. & Mulholland, J. (1997) Protocols and guidelines for managing wounds. *Prof Nurse*, **13**(2), 79–81.

Lawrence, J.C. (1997) Wound irrigation. *J Wound Care*, **6**(1), 23–6.

Lawrence, J.D. (1985) The physical properties of a new hydrocolloid dressing. In: *An Environment for Healing: The Role of Occlusion. Royal Society of Medicine International Congress and Symposium Series* (ed. T.J. Ryan), pp. 69–76. Royal Society of Medicine, London.

Lawrence, J.D. & Groves, A.R. (1988) *Blueprint for the Management of Minor Burns*. Squibb Surgicare, Hounslow.

Leaper, D. (1986) Antiseptics and their effects on healing tissue. *Nurs Times*, **82**(22), 45–6.

Lechter, A. *et al.* (1987) Pelvic varices and gonadal veins. *Phlebology*, **2**, 181–8.

Lees, T.A. & Lambert, D. (1992) Prevalence of lower limb ulceration in an urban health district. *Br J Surg*, **79**, 1032–4.

Le Roux, A.A. (1995) TELER: the concept. *Physiotherapy*, **79**(11), 755–8.

Lewis, B. (1996) Zinc and vitamin C in the aetiology of pressure sores. *J Wound Care*, **5**(10), 483–4.

Lochhead, J.N. (1983) *Care of the Patient in Radiotherapy*, p. 113. Blackwell Science, Oxford.

Lockyer-Stevens, N. (1994) A developing information base for purchasing decisions. *Prof Nurse*, **9**(8), 534–42.

Lycarotti, M.E. & Leaper, D.J. (1989) Measurement in wound healing. *Care Sci Pract*, **7**(3), 68–71.

McCain, D. & Sutherland, S. (1998) Nursing essentials: skin grafts for patients with burns. *Am J Nurs*, **98**(7), 34–8.

McCarthy, M. (1997) Oestrogen accelerates wound healing in post menopausal women. *Lancet*, **350**(9087), 1301.

McCulloch, J.M. (1998) The role of physiotherapy in managing patients with wounds. *J Wound Care*, **7**(5), 241–4.

McGregor, F. (1998) *Reusable Non-Adhesive Secondary Dressing System for Difficult to Dress Areas and Delicate Skin*. Guy's and St Thomas' Hospital Trust, London.

McGregor, F. & Baxter, H. (1999) Staying power. *Nurs Times*, **95**(19), 66, 68 & 71.

McSweeney, P. (1994) Assessing the cost of pressure sores. *Nurs Stand*, **8**(52), 25–6.

McTaggart, J.H. (1994) An area of clinical neglect. *Prof Nurse*, **9**(9), 600–606.

Mahon, S.M. (1987) Nursing interventions for the patient with a myocutaneous flap. *Cancer Nurs*, **10**(1), 21–31.

Maibach, H.I. & Rovee, D.T. (1972) *Epidermal Wound Healing*. Year Book Medical Publishers, Chicago.

Mallett, J. (1988) Wound dressing made easier. *Senior Nurse*, **8**(5), 31–3.

Mallett, J. & Charles, H. (1989) *Survey of Clients with Leg Ulceration Treated by District Nurses in Paddington and North Kensington*. Report produced for Paddington and North Kensington Health Authority.

Mallett, J. & Charles, H. (1990) Defining the leg ulcer problem. *J Distr Nurs*, **9**(1), 5–10.

Mallett, J., Mulholland, J., Laverty, D., *et al.* (1999) An integrated approach to wound management. *Int J Palliat Nurs*, **5**(3), 124–32.

Mani, R. *et al.* (1988) Non-invasive oxygen measurements: have they a role in ulcer investigations? In: *Beyond Occlusion: Wound Care Proceedings. Royal Society of Medicine International Congress and Symposium Series* (ed. T.J. Ryan). Royal Society of Medicine, London.

Marcelon, G. & Vanhoutte, P.M. (1988) Venotonic effect of ruscus under variable temperature conditions in vitro. *Phlebology*, **3**, Suppl. 1, 51–4.

Marcelon, G. *et al.* (1988) Oestrogens impregnation and ruscus action on the human vein in vitro, depending on preliminary results. *Phlebology*, **3**, Suppl. 1, 83–5.

Margolin *et al.* (1990) Management of radiation-induced moist skin desquamation using hydrocolloid dressing. *Cancer Nurs*, **13**(2), 71–80.

Martindale, W. (1982) *The Extra Pharmacopoeia*, 28th edn. Pharmaceutical Press, London.

Masi, A.T. & Medsger, T.A. (1979) Epidemiology of the rheumatic diseases. In: *Arthritis and Allied Conditions* (ed. D.J. McCarty), pp. 11–35. Lea & Febiger, Philadelphia. In: The nursing management of pain in the community: a theoretical framework (1989) (J.M. Walker). *J Adv Nurs*, **14**, 240–47.

Matthews, R.N. (1986) Leg ulcers. *Surgery*, **1**(33), 790–95.

Meehan, T.C. (1993) Therapeutic touch – post-operative pain: a rogerian research study. *Nurs Sci*, **6**(2), 69–79.

Mertz, P.M. *et al.* (1985) Occlusive wound dressings to prevent bacterial invasion and wound infection. *J Am Acad Dermatol*, **12**(4), 662–8.

Messer, M.S. (1989) Wound care. *Crit Care Nurs Q*, **11**(4), 17–27.

Middleton, K. (1990) Sugar pastes in wound management. *Dressing Times*, **3**(2). Surgical Materials Testing Laboratory, Bridgend.

Miller, D.L. & Farmer, R.D.T. (eds) (1982) *Epidemiology of Diseases*. Blackwell Scientific Publications, Oxford.

Miller, M. (1998) Moist wound healing: the evidence. *Nurs Times*, **94**(45), 74–6.

Miller, M. & Dyson, M. (1996) *Principles of Wound Care. A Professional Nurse Publication*. Macmillan Magazines, London.

Milward, P. (1988) The healing process. *Care Sci Pract*, **6**(3), Educ Leaflet Suppl.

Moffat, C.J. & Dorman, M.C.R. (1995) Recurrence of leg ulcers within a community ulcer service. *J Wound Care*, **4**(2), 57–61.

Moody, M. & Grocott, P. (1993) Let us extend our knowledge base. *Prof Nurse*, **8**(9), 586–90.

Moore, P. & Foster, L. (1998) Acute surgical wound care 2: the wound healing process. *Br J Nurs*, **7**(19), 1183–7.

Morgan, D.A. (1990) *Formulary of Wound Management Products. A Guide for Health Care Staff*, 6th edn. Convatec Ltd, Ickenham, Uxbridge.

Morison, M.J. (1989) Wound cleansing – which solution? *Prof Nurse*, **4**, 220–25.

Morison, M.J. (1992) *A Colour Guide to the Nursing Management of Wounds*. Wolfe, London.

Morison, M.J. & Moffatt, C.J. (1994) *A Colour Guide to the Assessment and Management of Leg Ulcers*, 2nd edn. Times Mirror, London.

Moss, A. (1989) Treatment of terminal breast cancer. *Br Med J*, **298**, 10.

Munro, K.J.G. (1995a) Hypertrophic and keloid scars. *J Wound Care*, **4**(3), 143–8.

Munro, K.J.G. (1995b) Treatment of hypertrophic and keloid scars. *J Wound Care*, **4**(5), 243–5.

Nelson, E.A. (1998) The evidence in support of compression bandaging. *J Wound Care*, **7**(3), 148–50.

Negus, D. (1992) *Leg Ulcers. A Pratical Approach to Management*. Butterworth–Heinemann, Oxford.

Newman, V. *et al.* (1989) The use of metronidazole gel to control the smell of malodorous lesions. *Palliat Med*, **3**, 303–305.

Nicholls, R. (1989) Leg ulcers: collecting the facts. *Nurs Stand*, Spec Suppl, **6**, 12–13.

Nicholls, R. (1990) Leg ulcers: a study in the community. *Nurs Stand*, Spec Suppl, **7**, 4–6.

Norton, D. *et al.* (1985) *An Investigation of Geriatric Nursing Problems in Hospital*. Churchill Livingstone, Edinburgh.

Nuffield Institute for Health (1995) *Effective health care: the prevention and treatment of pressure sores*, October, **2**(1). NHS Centre for Reviews and Dissemination, University of York.

Nurses' Drug Alert (1987) *Avoid Use of Hydrogen Peroxide and Povidone-Iodine in Open Wounds*. M.J. Powers, New Jersey.

Official Population Census Statistics (1983) *Midyear Population Estimates for Parkside Health District*. Stationery Office, London.

Pattie, A.H. & Gilleard, C.J. (1979) *Manual of the Clifton Assessment Procedures of the Elderly* (CAPE). Hodder & Stoughton, London.

Pegasus Airwave Ltd (1998) *Infection Control Policy*. Pegasus, Waterlooville.

Perkins, P. (1989) A clinic to cope with leg ulcers. *Mims Mag*, April, 73–4.

Piper, S.M. (1989) Effective use of occlusive dressings. *Prof Nurse*, **4**(8), 402–404.

Pottle, B. (1987) Trial of a dressing for non-healing ulcers. *Nurs Times*, **83**(12), 54–8.

Price, S. & Price, L. (1995) *Aromatherapy for Health Professionals*. Churchill Livingstone, New York.

Pritchard, A.P. & David, J.A. (eds) (1988) *The Royal Marsden Manual of Clinical Nursing Procedures*, 2nd edn. Harper & Row, London.

Raiman, J. (1986) Pain relief – a two-way process. *Nurs Times*, **82**(15), 24–8.

RCN (1998) *The Management of Patients with Venous Leg Ulcers*. (Recommendations.) RCN Institute, York.

Reid, J. & Morison, M. (1994) Towards a consensus classification of pressure sores. *J Wound Care*, **3**(3), 157–9.

Riyat, M.S. & Quinton, D.N. (1997) Tap water as a wound cleansing agent in accident and emergency. *J Accid Emerg*, **14**, 165–6.

Roberts, G. (1988) Nutrition and wound healing. *Nurs Stand*, **2**(51), Suppl., 8–12.

Robinson, B. (1988) Aetiology and treatment of leg ulcers. Focus on wound healing. *Mims Mag*, July, Suppl., 23.

Robson, M.C. *et al.* (1992) Platelet derived growth factor BB for the treatment of chronic pressure ulcers. *Lancet*, **339**(8784), 23–5.

Robson, M.C. *et al.* (1993) Transforming growth factor beta-2 accelerates healing of venous stasis ulcers in an open-label, placebo-controlled clinical study. *Wound Repair Regen*, **1**, 91.

Rodzwic, D. & Donnard, J. (1986) The use of myocutaneous flaps in reconstructive surgery for head and neck cancer: guidelines for nursing care. *Oncol Nurs Forum*, **13**(3), 29–34.

Rosenberg, C.S. (1990) Wound healing in the patient with diabetes mellitus. *Nurs Clin North Am*, **25**(1), 247–61.

Rovee, D.T. *et al.* (1972) Effect of local wound environment on epidermal healing. In: *Epidermal Wound Healing* (eds H.I. Maibach & D.T. Rovee), pp. 159–81. Year Book Medical Publishers, Chicago.

Royal College of General Practitioners (1986) *Alcohol: A Balanced View* (Report from General Practice, 24). Royal College of General Practitioners, Exeter.

Russell, S.B., Trupin, K.M., Rodriguez-Eaton, S., Russell, J.D. & Trupin, J.S. (1988) Reduced growth-factor requirement of keloid-derived fibroblasts may account for tumor growth. *Proc Natl Sci USA*, **85**, January, 587–91.

Ryan, T.J. (ed) (1985a) *An Environment for Healing: The Role of Occlusion*. Royal Society of Medicine, International Congress and Symposium Series, pp. 5–14. Royal Society of Medicine, London.

Ryan, T.J. (1985b) Current management of leg ulcers. *Drugs*, **30**(5), 461–8.

Ryan, T.J. (1987) *The Management of Leg Ulcers*, 2nd edn. Oxford University Press, Oxford.

Ryan, T.J. (1988a) Management of leg ulcers. *The Practitioner*, **232**, 1014–21.

Ryan, T.J. (ed) (1988b) *Beyond Occlusion: Wound Care Proceedings*. Royal Society of Medicine, International Congress and Symposium Series. Royal Society of Medicine, London.

Saunders, C.M. (1978) *The Management of Terminal Disease*. Edward Arnold, Sevenoaks.

Saunders, J. (1989) Toilet cleaner for wound care? *Commun Outlook*, pp. 11–13. *Nurs Times*, **85**(10).

Saunders, Y. & Regnard, C. (1989) Management of malignant ulcers: a flow diagram. *Palliat Med*, **3**, 153–5.

Schulte, M. (1993) Yoghurt helps to control wound odour. *Oncol Nurs Forum*, **20**(8), 1262.

Silver, I.A. (1972) Oxygen tension and epithelialization (Chap. 17). In: *Epidermal Wound Healing* (eds H.I. Maibach & D.T. Rovee), pp. 291–305. Year Book Medical Publishers, Chicago.

Silver, I.A. (1994) The physiology of wound healing. *J Wound Care*, **3**(2), 100–109.

Smith, I. (1989) Waterlow/Norton scoring system – a ward view. *Care Sci Pract*, **7**(4), 93–5.

Smith, S. (1988) Doing the leg work. *Commun Outlook*, pp. 17–18. *Nurs Times*, **84**(33).

Souhami, R. & Tobias, J. (1998) *Cancer and Its Management*, 3rd edn., p. 74. Blackwell Science, Oxford.

Spanswick, A. *et al.* (1990) Eusol – the final word. *Prof Nurse*, **5**(4), 211–14.

Stronge, J.L. (1984) Principles of wound care. *Nursing*, **2**(26), Suppl., 7–10.

Struckmann, J.R. (1988) Venous muscle pump function following reconstructive arterial surgery. *Phlebology*, **3**, 169–73.

Swanwick, T. & MacLellan, D. (1988) The treatment of venous ulceration. *Nursing*, **3**(32), 40–43.

Taheri, S.A. *et al.* (1987) Iliocaval compression syndrome. *Phlebology*, **2**, 173–9.

Taylor, A. & Clark, M. (1994) Management of pressure sore prevention: recent initiatives. *Nurs Stand*, **8**(48), 54–5.

The Dressing Times (1988) 1(2). Welsh Centre for the Quality Control of Surgical Dressings, East Glamorgan Hospital, Glamorgan.

The Dressing Times (1989) 2(1). Welsh Centre for the Quality Control of Surgical Dressings, East Glamorgan Hospital, Glamorgan.

Thomas, L. (1988a) Treating leg ulcers. *Nurs Stand*, **2**(18), 22–3.

Thomas, L. (1988b) Treating leg ulcers. *Nurs Stand*, **2**(19), 28.

Thomas, S. (1990a) Cost-effective management of leg ulcers. *Commun Outlook*, pp. 21–2. *Nurs Times*, **86**(11).

Thomas, S. (1990b) *Wound Management and Dressings*. Pharmaceutical Press, London.

Thomas, S. (1992) *Current Practices in the Management of Fungating Lesions and Radiation Damaged Skin*. Surgical Materials Testing Laboratory, Bridgend.

Thomas, S. (1997) A structured approach to the selection of dressings. URL: http://www.smtl.co.uk/world-wide-wounds/1997/july/thomas-guide/dress-select.html.

Thomas, S. & Hay, N. (1991) The antimicrobial properties of 2 metronidazole-mediated dressings used to treat malodorous wounds. *Pharm J*, 2 March, 264–6.

Thomas, S. & Hay, N.P. (1996) In vitro investigations of a new hydrogel dressing. *J Wound Care*, **5**(3), 130–31.

Thomas, S. & Loveless, P. (1992) Observations on the fluid handling properties of alginate dressings. *Pharm J*, **248**, 850–51.

Thomlinson, R. (1980) Kitchen remedy for necrotic malignant breast ulcers (letter). *Lancet*, 27 September, 707.

Thompson, J. (1990) Foot and leg care. *Community Outlook*, pp. 14–17. *Nurs Times*, **86**(8).

Thorp, J.M. *et al.* (1987) Gross hypernatraemia associated with the use of antiseptic surgical packs. *Anaesthesia*, **42**, 750–53.

Tomlinson, D. (1987) To clean or not to clean? *J Infect Control/Nurs Times*, **83**(9), 71–5.

Tooke, J.E. *et al.* (1988) Diabetes and wound healing: the skin response to injury, and white cell behaviour in vivo in diabetic patients. In: *Beyond Occlusion: Wound Care Proceedings. Royal Society of Medicine International Congress and Symposium Series* (ed. T.J. Ryan), pp. 71–4. Royal Society Medicine, London.

Topham, J. (1996) Sugar paste and povidone-iodine in the treatment of wounds. *J Wound Care*, **5**(8), 364–5.

Torrance, C. (1985) Wound care in accident and emergency. *Nursing*, **2**(42), Suppl., 1–3.

Tortora, G.J. & Grabowski, S.R. (1996) *Principles of Anatomy and Physiology*, 8th edn. Harper Collins, Menlo Park, California.

Trelstad, A. & Osmundson, D. (1989) Water piks: wound cleansing alternative. *Plastic Surg Nurs*, **9**(3), 117–19.

Trevelyan, J. (1996) Looking good. Wigs and camouflage. *Nurs Times*, **92**(39), 44–5.

Tubman Papantonio, C. (1988a) Holistic approach to healing: part I. *Home Healthcare Nurse*, **6**(5), 31–4.

Tubman Papantonio, C. (1988b) Holistic approach to healing: part II. *Home Healthcare Nurse*, **6**, 31–5.

Turner, T.D. (1979) Hospital usage of absorbent dressings. *Pharm J*, May, 421–2.

Turner, T.D. (1983) A practical guide to absorbent dressings. *Nursing*, **12**, Suppl.

Turner, T.D. (1985) Semiocclusive and occlusive dressings. In: *An Environment for Healing: The Role of Occlusion. Royal Society of Medicine International Congress and Symposium Series* (ed. T.J. Ryan). Royal Society of Medicine, London.

Turner, T.D. *et al.* (1986) Advances in wound management symposium proceedings. John Wiley, Cardiff. In: *Blueprint for the Treatment of Leg Ulcers and the Prevention of Recurrence* (1987) (eds G.W. Cherry & T.J. Ryan). Squibb Surgicare, Hounslow.

Twycross, R.G. & Lack, S.A. (1990) *Therapeutics in Terminal Cancer*, 2nd edn. Churchill Livingstone, Edinburgh.

United Kingdom Central Council for Nursing, Midwifery and Health Visiting (1993) *UKCC Code of Professional Conduct*. UKCC, London.

Valdes-Dapena, M.A. & Arey, J.B. (1962) Boric acid poisoning. *J Pediatr*, **61**(4), 531–46.

Vowden, K. (1997) Ethnic origin and venous leg ulceration. *Wound Care Soc Newsl No. 28*. Wound Care Society, Huntingdon.

Vowden, K. (1998) Venous leg ulcers, Part 2: assessment. *Prof Nurse*, **13**(9), 633–8.

Waldorf, H. & Fewkes, J. (1995) Advances in dermatology. *J Wound Heal*, **10**, 77–97.

Walker, J.M. *et al.* (1989) The nursing management of pain in the community: a theoretical framework. *J Adv Nurs*, **14**, 240–47.

Wandl, U.B. (1997) GM-CSF in the treatment of skin ulceration in breast cancer. *J Wound Care*, **6**(4), 165–6.

Waterlow, J. (1987) Calculating the risk. *Nurs Times*, **83**(39), 58–60.

Waterlow, J. (1988) Prevention is cheaper than cure. *Nurs Times*, **84**(25), 69–70.

Waterlow, J. (1991) A policy that protects. *Prof Nurse*, **6**(5), 258–64.

Waterlow, J. (1995) *Pressure Sore Prevention Manual*. Newtons, Curland, Taunton.

Waterlow, J. (1998) The treatment and use of the Waterlow card. *Nurs Times*, **94**(7), 63–7.

Welch, L. (1981) Simple new remedy for the odour of open lesion. *Reg Nurse*, February, 42–3.

Wells, L. (1994) At the front line of care. *Prof Nurse*, **9**(8), 525–30.

Wells, R.J. (1984) Controversial issues in wound care. *J Clin Nurs*, Suppl., June, 10–11.

West, P. & Priestly, J. (1994) Money under the mattress. *Health Serv J*, **104**(5398), 20–22.

Westaby, S. (1985) *Wound Care*. Heinemann, London.

Wilkinson, B. (1997) Hard graft. *Nurs Times*, **93**(16), 63–4, 66 & 68.

Williams, C. (1994) Kaltostat. *Br J Nurs*, **3**(18), 965–7.

Williams, C. (1996) Cica-care: adhesive gel sheet. *Br J Nurs*, **5**(14), 875–6.

Williams, C. (1999) An investigation of the benefits of Aquacel Hydrofibre wound dressing. *Br J Nurs*, **8**(10), 676–80.

Williams, I. (1989) A company wraps up the bandage market with new deal for wounded. *The Guardian*, 13 March.

Williamson, D. (1988) Leg ulcers. Taking your time with leg ulcers. *Mims Mag*, 1 May, 105–108.

Willington, F.L. (1977) The use of non-ionic detergents in sanitary cleansing: a report of a preliminary trial. *J Adv Nurs*, **3**, 373–82.

Wilson-Barnett, J. & Robinson, S. (eds) (1989) *Directions in Nursing Research*. Scutari Press, London.

Wingate, P. & Wingate, R. (1988) *The Penguin Medical Enclyopedia*, 3rd edn. Penguin, West Drayton.

Winter, A. & Hewitt, H. (1990) Testing a hydrocolloid. *Nurs Times*, **86**(50), 59–62.

Winter, G.D. (1971) Healing of skin wounds and the influence of dressings on the repair process. In: *Surgical Dressings and Wound Healing* (ed. K.J. Harkiss), pp. 46–50. Bradford University Press, Bradford.

Winter, G.D. (1972) Epidermal regeneration studied in the domestic pig. In: *Epidermal Wound Healing* (eds H.I. Maibach & D.T. Rovee), pp. 71–112. Year Book Medical Publishers, Chicago.

Wood, P.H.N. (1977) In: *Epidemiology of Diseases* (1982) (eds D.L. Miller & R.D.T. Farmer). Blackwell Scientific Publications, Oxford.

Wyngaarden, J.B. & Smith, L.H. (1988) *Cecil Textbook of Medicine*, 18th edn. W.B. Saunders, Philadelphia.

Young, T. & Fowler, A. (1998) Nursing management of skin grafts and donor sites. *Br J Nurs*, **7**(6), 324, 326, 328, 330, 332–4.

Zederfeldt, B. *et al.* (1980) *Wounds and Wound Healing*. Wolfe, New York.

GUIDELINES • Changing wound dressings

Equipment

1 As for 'Guidelines • Aseptic technique' (Chap. 3, page 44).
2 Cleansing fluid for irrigation (see Table 47.3).
3 Appropriate dressing (see Table 47.4).

Procedure

See procedure for 'Aseptic technique' (Chap. 3, page 45) up to and including step 11, then loosen the dressing.

Guidelines • Changing wound dressings (cont'd)

Action	Rationale
12 Where appropriate, loosen the old dressing.	The dressing can then be lifted off without causing trauma.
13 Clean hands with a bactericidal alcohol hand rub.	Hands may become contaminated by handling outer packets, dressing, etc.
14 Using the plastic bag in the pack, arrange the sterile field. Tear open sachet and pour lotion into gallipots or an indented plastic tray (Table 47.3).	The time the wound is exposed should be kept to a minimum to reduce the risk of contamination. To prevent contamination of the environment. To minimize risk of contamination of lotion.
15 Remove dressing by placing a hand in the plastic bag, lifting the dressing off and inverting the plastic bag so that the dressing is now inside the bag. Thereafter use this as the 'dirty' bag.	To reduce the risk of cross-infection. To prevent contamination of the environment.
16 Attach the bag with the dressing to the side of the trolley below the top shelf.	Contaminated material should be below the level of the sterile field.
17 Assess the wound healing with reference to volume, amount of granulation tissue and epithelialization, signs of infection, underlying pathology, etc. (Table 47.2). (Record assessment in relevant documentation at the end of the procedure.)	To evaluate wound care.
18 Put on gloves, touching only the inside wrist end.	To reduce the risk of infection to the wound and contamination of the nurse. Gloves provide greater sensitivity than forceps and are less likely to traumatize the wound or the patient's skin.
19 If necessary, gently clean the wound with a gloved hand using 0.9% sodium chloride, unless another solution is indicated (Table 47.3). If appropriate, irrigate by flushing with water or 0.9% sodium chloride.	To reduce the possibility of physical and chemical trauma to granulation and epithelial tissue.
20 Apply the dressing that is most suitable for the wound using the criteria for dressings (Table 47.4).	To promote healing and/or reduce symptoms.
21 Remove gloves; fasten dressing with hypoallergenic tape/Netelast/bandaging/tapeless retention dressings.	To prevent irritation of skin and to avoid trauma to wound.
22 Make sure the patient is comfortable and the dressing is secure.	A dressing may slip or feel uncomfortable as the patient changes position.

Continue with steps 18–21 from the procedure for Aseptic technique.

GUIDELINES • Removal of sutures, clips or staples

Equipment

1 As for 'Guidelines • Aseptic technique' (Chap. 3, page 44).
2 Sterile scissors, stitch cutter, staple remover.
3 Sterile adhesive sutures.

Procedure

Action	Rationale
1 Explain and discuss the procedure with the patient.	To ensure that the patient understands the procedure and gives his/her valid consent.

2 Perform procedure using aseptic technique.

To prevent infection (for further information see procedure on aseptic technique, Chap. 3).

3 Clean the wound with an appropriate sterile solution such as 0.9% sodium chloride (Table 47.3).

To prevent infection.

For removal of sutures

4 Lift knot of suture with metal forceps. Snip stitch close to the skin. Pull suture out gently.

Plastic forceps tend to slip against nylon sutures. To prevent infection by drawing exposed suture through the tissue.

5 Use tips of scissors slightly open or the side of the stitch cutter to gently press the skin when the suture is being drawn out.

To minimize pain by counteracting the adhesion between the suture and surrounding tissue.

For removal of clips

6 Squeeze wings of Royal clips together with forceps to release from skin.

To release clips atraumatically from the wound.

7 If the wound gapes use adhesive sutures to oppose the wound edges.

To improve the cosmetic effect.

8 When necessary, cover the wound with an appropriate dressing (Tables 47.4 and 47.8).

To provide the best possible environmemt for wound healing to take place. To reduce the risk of infection. To prevent the suture line from rubbing against clothing.

For removal of staples

9 Slide the lower bar of the staple remover with the V-shaped groove under the staple at an angle of 90°. Squeeze the handles of the staple removers together to open the staple.

To release the staple atraumatically from the wound. If the angle of the staple remover is not correct, the staple will not come out freely.

If the suture line is under tension, use free hand to gently squeeze the skin either side of the suture line.

To reduce tension of skin around suture line and lessen pain on removal of staple.

10 If the wound gapes use adhesive sutures to oppose the wound edges.

To improve the cosmetic effect.

For all suture lines

11 Record condition of suture line and surrounding skin (for example, amount of exudate, pus, inflammation, pain, etc.; see Table 47.2).

To document care and enable evaluation of the wound.

GUIDELINES • Drain dressing (Redivac – closed drainage systems)

Equipment

1 As for Guidelines • Aseptic technique (Chap. 3, page 44).
2 Non-adherent, absorbent dressing.

Procedure

Action

1 Explain and discuss the procedure with the patient.

Rationale

To ensure that the patient understands the procedure and gives his/her valid consent.

2 Perform procedure using aseptic technique.

To prevent infection (for further information on asepsis, see procedure on aseptic technique, Chap. 3).

Guidelines • Drain dressing (Redivac – closed drainage systems) (cont'd)

Action	Rationale
3 Clean the surrounding skin with an appropriate sterile solution such as 0.9% sodium chloride (Table 47.3).	To prevent infection and remove excess debris.
4 Ensure that the skin suture holding the drain site in position is intact.	To prevent the drain from leaving the wound.
5 Cover the drain site with a non-adherent, absorbent dressing.	To protect the drain site, prevent infection entering the wound and absorb exudate.
6 Tape securely.	To prevent drain coming loose.
7 Ensure that the drain is primed or that the suction pump is in working order.	To ensure continuity of drainage.

GUIDELINES • Change of vacuum drainage system

(See Chap. 21, Intrapleural Drainage.)

Equipment

1 Sterile topical swab.
2 Artery forceps.
3 Dressing pack.

Procedure

Action	Rationale
1 Explain and discuss the procedure with the patient.	To ensure that the patient understands the procedure and gives his/her valid consent.
2 Perform procedure using aseptic technique.	To prevent infection (see procedure on aseptic technique, Chap. 3).
3 Wash hands using bactericidal soap and water or bactericidal alcohol hand rub.	To minimize the risk of infection.
4 Ensure sterile drainage system is readily available.	To ensure sterility during change of system.
5 Measure the contents of the bottle to be changed and record this in the appropriate documents.	To maintain an accurate record of drainage from the wound and enable evaluation of state of wound.
6 Clamp the tube with artery forceps and remove the bottle.	To prevent air and contamination entering the wound via the drain.
7 Clean the end of the tube and attach it to the sterile bottle.	To maintain sterility.
8 Remove the artery forceps.	To re-establish the drainage system.
9 Place used vacuum drainage system into the clinical waste bag.	To safely dispose of used system.

GUIDELINES • Removal of drain (Yeates vacuum drainage system)

Equipment

1 As for Guidelines • Aseptic technique (Chap. 3, page 44).
2 Sterile scissors or suture cutter.

Procedure

Action	*Rationale*
1 Check the patient's operation notes.	To establish the number and site(s) of internal and external sutures.
2 Explain and discuss the procedure with the patient.	To ensure that the patient understands the procedure and gives his/her valid consent.
3 If appropriate (in closed drainage systems) release vacuum.	To prevent pulling at wound tissue, causing pain and tissue damage.
4 Perform the procedure using aseptic technique.	To minimize the risk of infection. (For further information on asepsis, see Chap. 3.)
5 Where the wound is covered with an occlusive dressing (e.g. following lumpectomy in the breast), lift and snip the dressing from around the drain. Do not remove it from the entire wound.	To prevent disturbing the incision or contaminating the wound.
6 Only clean the wound if necessary, using an appropriate sterile solution, such as 0.9% sodium chloride (Table 47.3).	To reduce risk of infection.
7 Hold the knot of the suture with metal forceps and gently lift upwards.	Plastic forceps tend to slip against nylon sutures. To allow space for the scissors or stitch cutter to be placed underneath.
8 Cut the shortest end of the suture as close to the skin as possible.	To prevent infection by allowing the suture to be liberated from the drain without drawing the exposed part through tissue.
9 Remove drain gently. If there is resistance, place free gloved hand against the tissue to oppose the tugging of the drain being removed. If the resistance is felt to be excessive, nitrous oxide (e.g. Entonox) may be required.	To minimize pain and reduce trauma.
10 Cover the drain site with a sterile dressing and tape securely.	To prevent infection entering the drain site.
11 Measure and record the contents of the drainage bottle in the appropriate documents.	To maintain an accurate record of drainage from the wound and enable evaluation of state of wound.
12 Dispose of used drainage system in clinical waste bag.	To ensure safe disposal.

GUIDELINES • Shortening of drain (Penrose, etc. open drainage systems)

Procedure

Action	*Rationale*
1 Follow steps 1–8 above (removal of drain), i.e. to the stage where the suture has been cut.	
2 Using gloved hand, gently ease the drain out of wound to the length requested by surgeons (usually 3–5 cm).	To allow healing to take place from base of wound.
3 Using gloved hand, place a sterile safety pin through the drain as close to the skin as possible, taking great care not to stab either the nurse or patient.	To prevent retraction into the wound and minimize the risk of cross-infection.
4 Cut same amount of tubing from distal end of drain as withdrawn from wound.	So there is a convenient length of tubing to drain into the bag. To ensure patient comfort.
5 Place a sterile, suitably sized drainage bag over the drain site.	To allow effluent to drain into the bag. To prevent excoriation of the skin. To contain any odour.

Guidelines • Shortening of drain (Penrose, etc. open drainage systems) (cont'd)

Action	Rationale
6 Check bag is secure and comfortable for the patient.	For patient comfort.
7 Record by how much the drainage tube was shortened.	To ensure the length remaining in the wound is known.

GUIDELINES • Prevention of pressure ulcers

Procedure

Action	Rationale
1 Assess every patient on admission using a recognized scale, such as the Norton (Table 47.5) or Waterlow (Fig. 47.1) scale.	To identify the patient at risk of developing decubitus ulcers.
2 Reassess every patient on a regular basis and/or if there has been any deterioration or change in condition.	To provide appropriate data on which to base treatment.
3 Do not rub any area at risk.	Rubbing causes maceration and degeneration of subcutaneous tissues, especially in the elderly.
4 Wash areas at risk only if the patient is incontinent or sweating profusely. Use mild soap or a liquid detergent. Ensure that all detergent or soap is rinsed off and that the area is patted dry. Use moisturizer if the skin is very dry. Ask the patient what suits his/her skin.	To maintain skin integrity and prevent the formation of sores. Excessive use of soap can be harmful to the skin. Thorough gentle drying of the skin promotes comfort and discourages the growth of micro-organisms. Dry skin cracks allow entry of micro-organisms (Morison 1992).
5 Use barrier creams only when indicated.	Barrier creams prevent damage to the epidermis. They are, however, occlusive and prevent moisture exchange from the skin (Pritchard & David 1988).
6 Educate the patient to shift position, to pull or push up regularly and to examine the vulnerable areas.	After discharge the patient may be self-caring and possibly still vulnerable to pressure ulcers/tissue damage. To encourage the patient to participate in own care.
7 Initiate a mobility programme for the patient. Call on the physiotherapist, occupational therapist or dietician as appropriate.	To reduce further tissue damage and improve the circulation.
8 Where possible, relieve the pressure over areas vulnerable to tissue breakdown. Use appropriate pressure relief devices (Table 47.7). If necessary, turn the patient at least 2-hourly and record the position on the relevant charts (Clark 1998).	To reduce pressure where possible. Use of inappropriate aids may increase pressure to vulnerable areas.
9 Have the patient recumbent whenever possible. Support with bead bags or pillows in bed. Reduce period spent sitting in chair if pelvic sores develop.	Avoid the use of bedrests as these increase shearing by allowing the patient to slide down the bed.

Index